ALREADY REGISTERED?

1. Log in at expertconsult.com
2. Scratch off your Activation Code below
3. Enter it into the "Add a Title" box
4. Click "Activate Now"
5. Click the title under "My Titles"

FIRST-TIME USER?

1. *REGISTER*
   - Click "Register Now" at expertconsult.com
   - Fill in your user information and click "Continue"
2. *ACTIVATE YOUR BOOK*
   - Scratch off your Activation Code below
   - Enter it into the "Enter Activation Code" box
   - Click "Activate Now"
   - Click the title under "My Titles"

Plastic Surgery

THIRD EDITION

Volume Two

Aesthetic

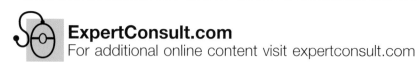

ExpertConsult.com

For additional online content visit expertconsult.com

Content Strategists: Sue Hodgson, Belinda Kuhn
Content Development Specialists: Alexandra Mortimer, Louise Cook, Poppy Garraway
Content Coordinators: Emma Cole, Trinity Hutton, Sam Crowe
Project Managers: Caroline Jones, Cheryl Brant
Design: Stewart Larking, Miles Hitchen
Illustration Manager: Jennifer Rose
Illustrator: Antbits
Marketing Manager: Helena Mutak
Technical Copyeditors: Darren Smith, Colin Woon
Video Reviewers: Leigh Jansen, James Saunders
Artwork Reviewer: Priya Chadha

Plastic Surgery

THIRD EDITION

Volume Two

Aesthetic

Editor in Chief:

Peter C. Neligan
MB, FRCS(I), FRCSC, FACS
Professor of Surgery
Department of Surgery, Division of Plastic Surgery
University of Washington
Seattle, WA, USA

Volume Editor:

Richard J. Warren
MD, FRCSC
Clinical Professor
Division of Plastic Surgery
University of British Columbia
Vancouver, BC, Canada

Video Editor:

Allen L. Van Beek
MD, FACS
Adjunct Professor
University Minnesota School of Medicine
Division Plastic Surgery
Minneapolis, MN, USA

ELSEVIER
SAUNDERS

London, New York, Oxford, St Louis, Sydney, Toronto

ELSEVIER
SAUNDERS

SAUNDERS an imprint of Elsevier Inc

First edition 1990
Second edition 2006
Third edition 2013

Notices
Knowledge and best practice in this field are constantly changing. As new research and experience broaden our understanding, changes in research methods, professional practices, or medical treatment may become necessary.

Practitioners and researchers must always rely on their own experience and knowledge in evaluating and using any information, methods, compounds, or experiments described herein. In using such information or methods they should be mindful of their own safety and the safety of others, including parties for whom they have a professional responsibility.

With respect to any drug or pharmaceutical products identified, readers are advised to check the most current information provided (i) on procedures featured or (ii) by the manufacturer of each product to be administered, to verify the recommended dose or formula, the method and duration of administration, and contraindications. It is the responsibility of practitioners, relying on their own experience and knowledge of their patients, to make diagnoses, to determine dosages and the best treatment for each individual patient, and to take all appropriate safety precautions.

To the fullest extent of the law, neither the Publisher nor the authors, contributors, or editors, assume any liability for any injury and/or damage to persons or property as a matter of products liability, negligence or otherwise, or from any use or operation of any methods, products, instructions, or ideas contained in the material herein.

Volume 2 ISBN: 978-1-4557-1053-9
Volume 2 Ebook ISBN: 978-1-4557-4049-9
Volume set ISBN: 978-1-4377-1733-4

ELSEVIER your source for books, journals and multimedia in the health sciences
www.elsevierhealth.com

Working together to grow
libraries in developing countries

www.elsevier.com | www.bookaid.org | www.sabre.org

ELSEVIER   **BOOK AID International**   **Sabre Foundation**

The publisher's policy is to use **paper manufactured from sustainable forests**

Printed in China
Last digit is the print number: 9   8   7   6   5   4   3   2   1

Contents

Volume Six: Hand and Upper Extremity
James Chang

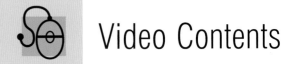

Video Contents

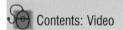

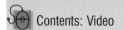

Foreword

In many ways, a textbook defines a particular discipline, and this is especially true in the evolution of modern plastic surgery. The publication of Zeis's *Handbuch der Plastischen Chirurgie* in 1838 popularized the name of the specialty but von Graefe in his monograph *Rhinoplastik*, published in 1818, had first used the title "plastic". At the turn of the last century, Nélaton and Ombredanne compiled what was available in the nineteenth century literature and published in Paris a two volume text in 1904 and 1907. A pivotal book, published across the Atlantic, was that of Vilray Blair, entitled *Surgery and Diseases of the Jaws* (1912). It was, however, limited to a specific anatomic region of the human body, but it became an important handbook for the military surgeons of World War I. Gillies' classic *Plastic Surgery of the Face* (1920) was also limited to a single anatomic region and recapitulated his remarkable and pioneering World War I experience with reconstructive plastic surgery of the face. Davis' textbook, *Plastic Surgery: Its Principles and Practice* (1919), was probably the first comprehensive definition of this young specialty with its emphasis on plastic surgery as ranging from the "top of the head to the soles of the feet." Fomon's *The Surgery of Injury and Plastic Repair* (1939) reviewed all of the plastic surgery techniques available at that time, and it also served as a handbook for the military surgeons of World War II. Kazanjian and Converse's *The Surgical Treatment of Facial Injuries* (1949) was a review of the former's lifetime experience as a plastic surgeon, and the junior author's World War II experience. The comprehensive plastic surgery text entitled *Plastic and Reconstructive Surgery,* published in 1948 by Padgett and Stephenson, was modeled more on the 1919 Davis text.

The lineage of the Neligan text began with the publication of Converse's five volume *Reconstructive Plastic Surgery* in 1964. Unlike his co-authored book with Kazanjian 15 years earlier, Converse undertook a comprehensive view of plastic surgery as the specialty existed in mid-20th century. Chapters were also devoted to pertinent anatomy, research and the role of relevant specialties like anesthesiology and radiology. It immediately became the bible of the specialty. He followed up with a second edition published in 1977, and I was the Assistant Editor. The second edition had grown from five to seven volumes (3970 pages) because the specialty had also grown. I edited the 1990 edition which had grown to eight volumes and 5556 pages; the hand section was edited by J. William Littler and James W. May. I changed the name of the text from *Reconstructive Plastic Surgery* to *Plastic Surgery* because in my mind I could not fathom the distinction between both titles. To the mother of a child with cleft lip, the surgery is "cosmetic," and many of the facelift procedures at that time were truly reconstructive because of the multiple layers at which the facial soft tissues were being readjusted. The late Steve Mathes edited the 2006 edition in eight volumes. He changed the format somewhat and V.R. Hentz was the hand editor. At that time, the text had grown to more than 7000 pages.

The education of the plastic surgeon and the reference material that is critically needed are no longer limited to the printed page or what is described in modern parlance as "hard copy". Certainly, Gutenberg's invention of movable type printing around 1439 allowed publication and distribution of the classic texts of Vesalius (*Fabrica*, 1543) and Tagliacozzi (*De Curtorum Chirurgia Per Insitionem* (1597) and for many years, this was the only medium in which surgeons could be educated. However, by the nineteenth century, travel had become easier with the development of reliable railroads and oceangoing ships, and surgeons conscientiously visited different surgical centers and attended organized meetings. The American College of Surgeons after World War II pioneered the use of operating room movies, and this was followed by videos. The development of the internet has, however, placed almost all information at the fingertips of surgeons around the world with computer access. In turn, we now have virtual surgery education in which the student or surgeon sitting at a computer is interactive with a software program containing animations, intraoperative videos with sound overlay, and access to the world literature on a particular subject. We are rapidly progressing from the bound book of the Gutenberg era to the currently ubiquitous hand held device or tablet for the mastery of surgical/knowledge.

The Neligan text continues this grand tradition of surgical education by bringing the reader into the modern communications world. In line with advances of the electronic era, there is extra online content such as relevant history, complete reference lists and videos. The book is also available as an e-book. It has been a monumental task, consuming hours of work by the editor and all of its participants. The "text" still defines the specialty of plastic surgery. Moreover, it ensures that a new generation of plastic surgeons will have access to all that is known. They, in turn, will not only carry this information into the future but will also build on it. Kudos to Peter Neligan and his colleagues for continuing the chronicle of the plastic surgery saga that has been evolving over two millennia.

Joseph G. McCarthy, MD
2012

Preface

I have always loved textbooks. When I first started my training I was introduced to Converse's *Reconstructive Plastic Surgery*, then in its second edition. I was over-awed by the breadth of the specialty and the expertise contained within its pages. As a young plastic surgeon in practice I bought the first edition of this book, *Plastic Surgery*, edited by Dr. Joseph McCarthy and found it an invaluable resource to which I constantly referred. I was proud to be asked to contribute a chapter to the second edition, edited by Dr. Stephen Mathes and never thought that I would one day be given the responsibility for editing the next edition of the book. I consider this to be the definitive text on our specialty so I took that responsibility very seriously. The result is a very changed book from the previous edition, reflecting changes in the specialty, changes in presentation styles and changes in how textbooks are used.

In preparation for the task, I read the previous edition from cover to cover and tried to identify where major changes could occur. Inevitably in a text this size, there is some repetition and overlap. So the first job was to identify where the repetition and overlap occurred and try to eliminate it. This allowed me to condense some of the material and, along with some other changes, enabled me to reduce the number of volumes from 8 to 6. Reading the text led me to another realization. That is that the breadth of the specialty, impressive when I was first introduced to it, is even more impressive now, 30 years later and it continues to evolve. For this reason I quickly realized that in order to do this project justice, I could not do it on my own. My solution was to recruit volume editors for each of the major areas of practice as well as a video editor for the procedural videos. Drs. Gurtner, Warren, Rodriguez, Losee, Song, Grotting, Chang and Van Beek have done an outstanding job and this book truly represents a team effort.

Publishing is at a crossroads. The digital age has made information much more immediate, much more easy to access and much more flexible in how it is presented. We have tried to reflect that in this edition. The first big change is that everything is in color. All the illustrations have been re-drawn and the vast majority of patient photographs are in color. Chapters on anatomy have been highlighted with a red tone to make them easier to find as have pediatric chapters which have been highlighted in green. Reflecting on the way I personally use textbooks, I realized that while I like access to references, I rarely read the list of references at the end of a chapter. When I do though, I frequently pull some papers to read. So you will notice that we have kept the most important references in the printed text but we have moved the rest to the web. However, this has allowed us to greatly enhance the usefulness of the references. All the references are hyperlinked to PubMed and expertconsult facilitates a search across all volumes. Furthermore, while every chapter has a section devoted to the history of the topic, this is again something I like to be able to access but rarely have the leisure to read. That section in each of the chapters has also been moved to the web. This not only relieved the pressure on space in the printed text but also allowed us to give the authors more freedom in presenting the history of the topic. As well, there are extra illustrations in the web version that we simply could not accommodate in the printed version. The web edition of the book is therefore more complete than the printed version and owning the book, automatically gets one access to the web. A mouse icon has been added to the text to mark where further content is available online. In this digital age, video has become a very important way to impart knowledge. More than 160 procedural videos contributed by leading experts around the world accompany these volumes. These videos cover the full scope of our specialty. This text is also available as an e-Book.

This book then is very different from its predecessors. It is a reflection of a changing age in communication. However I will be extremely pleased if it fulfils its task of defining the current state of knowledge of the specialty as its predecessors did.

Peter C. Neligan, MB, FRCS(I), FRCSC, FACS
2012

List of Contributors

Neta Adler, MD
Senior Surgeon
Department of Plastic and Reconstructive
Surgery
Hadassah University Hospital
Jerusalem, Israel
*Volume 3, Chapter 40 Congenital melanocytic
nevi*

Ahmed M. Afifi, MD
Assistant Professor of Plastic Surgery
University of Winsconsin
Madison, WI, USA
Associate Professor of Plastic Surgery
Cairo University
Cairo, Egypt
*Volume 3, Chapter 1 Anatomy of the head and
neck*

Maryam Afshar, MD
Post Doctoral Fellow
Department of Surgery (Plastic and
Reconstructive Surgery)
Stanford University School of Medicine
Stanford, CA, USA
*Volume 3, Chapter 22 Embryology of the
craniofacial complex*

Jamil Ahmad, MD, FRCSC
Staff Plastic Surgeon
The Plastic Surgery Clinic
Mississauga, ON, Canada
*Volume 2, Chapter 18 Open technique
rhinoplasty*
*Volume 5, Chapter 8.3 Superior or medial
pedicle*

Hee Chang Ahn, MD, PhD
Professor
Department of Plastic and Reconstructive
Surgery
Hanyang University Hospital, School of
Medicine
Seoul, South Korea
Volume 6, Chapter 22 Ischemia of the hand
*Volume 6, Video 22.01 Radial artery periarterial
sympathectomy*
*Volume 6, Video 22.02 Ulnar artery periarterial
sympathectomy*
*Volume 6, Video 22.03 Digital artery periarterial
sympathectomy*

Tae-Joo Ahn, MD
Jeong-Won Aesthetic Plastic Surgical Clinic
Seoul, South Korea
*Volume 2, Video 10.01 Eyelidplasty non-
incisional method*
Volume 2, Video 10.02 Incisional method

Lisa E. Airan, MD
Assistant Clinical Professor
Department of Dermatology
Mount Sinai Hospital
Aesthetic Dermatologist
Private Practice
New York, NY, USA
Volume 2, Chapter 4 Soft-tissue fillers

Sammy Al-Benna, MD, PhD
Specialist in Plastic and Aesthetic Surgery
Department of Plastic Surgery
Burn Centre, Hand Centre, Operative
Reference Centre for Soft Tissue Sarcoma
BG University Hospital Bergmannsheil, Ruhr
University Bochum
Bochum, North Rhine-Westphalia, Germany
*Volume 4, Chapter 18 Acute management of
burn/electrical injuries*

Amy K. Alderman, MD, MPH
Private Practice
Atlanta, GA, USA
*Volume 1, Chapter 10 Evidence-based medicine
and health services research in plastic surgery*

Robert J. Allen, MD
Clinical Professor of Plastic Surgery
Department of Plastic Surgery
New York University Medical Centre
Charleston, SC, USA
*Volume 5, Chapter 18 The deep inferior
epigastric artery perforator (DIEAP) flap*
*Volume 5, Chapter 19 Alternative flaps for breast
reconstruction*
*Volume 5, Video 18.02 DIEP flap breast
reconstruction*

Mohammed M. Al Kahtani, MD, FRCSC
Clinical Fellow
Division of Plastic Surgery
Department of Surgery
University of Alberta
Edmonton, AB, Canada
*Volume 1, Chapter 33 Facial prosthetics in
plastic surgery*

Faisal Al-Mufarrej, MB, BCh
Chief Resident in Plastic Surgery
Division of Plastic Surgery
Department of Surgery
Mayo Clinic
Rochester, MN, USA
*Volume 6, Chapter 20 Osteoarthritis in the hand
and wrist*

Gary J. Alter, MD
Assistant Clinical Professor
Division of Plastic Surgery
University of Califronia at Los Angeles School
of Medicine
Los Angeles, CA, USA
Volume 2, Chapter 31 Aesthetic genital surgery

Al Aly, MD, FACS
Director of Aesthetic Surgery
Professor of Plastic Surgery
Aesthetic and Plastic Surgery Institute
University of California
Irvine, CA, USA
Volume 2, Chapter 27 Lower bodylifts

Khalid Al-Zahrani, MD, SSC-PLAST
Assistant Professor
Consultant Plastic Surgeon
King Khalid University Hospital
King Saud University
Riyadh, Saudi Arabia
Volume 2, Chapter 27 Lower bodylifts

Kenneth W. Anderson, MD
Marietta Facial Plastic Surgery & Aesthetics
Center
Mareitta, GA, USA
Volume 2, Video 23.04 FUE FOX procedure

Alice Andrews, PhD
Instructor
The Dartmouth Institute for Health Policy and
Clinical Practice
Lebanon, NH, USA
*Volume 5, Chapter 12 Patient-centered health
communication*

Louis C. Argenta, MD
Professor of Plastic and Reconstructive Surgery
Department of Plastic Surgery
Wake Forest Medical Center
Winston Salem, NC, USA
*Volume 1, Chapter 27 Principles and applications
of tissue expansion*

Charlotte E. Ariyan, MD, PhD
Surgical Oncologist
Gastric and Mixed Tumor Service
Memorial Sloan-Kettering Cancer Center
New York, NY, USA
Volume 3, Chapter 14 Salivary gland tumors

Stephan Ariyan, MD, MBA
Clinical Professor of Surgery
Plastic Surgery
Otolaryngology Yale University School of
Medicine Associate Chief
Department of Surgery
Yale New Haven Hospital Director
Yale Cancer Center Melanoma Program
New Haven, CT, USA
Volume 1, Chapter 31 Melanoma
Volume 3, Chapter 14 Salivary gland tumors

Bryan S. Armijo, MD
Plastic Surgery Chief Resident
Department of Plastic and Reconstructive
Surgery
Case Western Reserve/University Hospitals
Cleveland, OH, USA
*Volume 2, Chapter 20 Airway issues and the
deviated nose*

Eric Arnaud, MD
Chirurgie Plastique et Esthétique
Chirurgie Plastique Crânio-faciale
Unité de chirurgie crânio-faciale du
departement de neurochirurgie
Hôpital Necker Enfants Malades
Paris, France
Volume 3, Chapter 32 Orbital hypertelorism

Christopher E. Attinger, MD
Chief, Division of Wound Healing
Department of Plastic Surgery
Georgetown University Hospital
Georgetown, WA, USA
Volume 4, Chapter 8 Foot reconstruction

Tomer Avraham, MD
Resident, Plastic Surgery
Institute of Reconstructive Plastic Surgery
NYU Medical Center
New York, NY, USA
*Volume 1, Chapter 12 Principles of cancer
management*

Kodi K. Azari, MD, FACS
Associate Professor of Orthopaedic Surgery
Plastic Surgery Chief
Section of Reconstructive Transplantation
Department of Orthopaedic Surgery and
Surgery
David Geffen School of Medicine at UCLA
Los Angeles, CA, USA
*Volume 6, Chapter 15 Benign and malignant
tumors of the hand*

Sérgio Fernando Dantas de Azevedo, MD
Member
Brazilian Society of Plastic Surgery
Volunteer Professor of Plastic Surgery
Department of Plastic Surgery
Federal University of Pernambuco
Permambuco, Brazil
Volume 2, Chapter 26 Lipoabdominoplasty
*Volume 2, Video 26.01 Lipobdominoplasty
(including secondary lipo)*

Daniel C. Baker, MD
Professor of Surgery
Insitiute of Reconstructive Plastic Surgery
New York University Medical Center
Department of Plastic Surgery
New York, NY, USA
*Volume 2, Chapter 11.5 Facelift: Lateral
SMASectomy*

Steven B. Baker, MD, DDS, FACS
Associate Professor and Program Director
Co-director Inova Hospital for Children
Craniofacial Clinic
Department of Plastic Surgery
Georgetown University Hospital
Georgetown, WA, USA
*Volume 3, Chapter 30 Cleft and craniofacial
orthognathic surgery*

Karim Bakri, MD, MRCS
Chief Resident
Division of Plastic Surgery
Mayo Clinic
Rochester, MN, USA
*Volume 6, Chapter 20 Osteoarthritis in the hand
and wrist*

Carla Baldrighi, MD
Staff Surgeon
Reconstructive Microsurgery Unit
Azienda Ospedaliera Universitaria Careggi
Florence, Italy
*Volume 6, Chapter 30 Growth considerations in
pediatric upper extremity trauma and
reconstruction*
*Volume 6, Video 30.01 Epiphyseal transplant
harvesting technique*

Jonathan Bank, MD
Resident, Section of Plastic and Reconstructive
Surgery
Department of Surgery
Pritzker School of Medicine
University of Chicago Medical Center
Chicago, IL, USA
*Volume 4, Chapter 12 Abdominal wall
reconstruction*

A. Sina Bari, MD
Chief Resident
Division of Plastic and Reconstructive Surgery
Stanford University Hospital and Clinics
Stanford, CA, USA
*Volume 1, Chapter 16 Scar prevention,
treatment, and revision*

Scott P. Bartlett, MD
Professor of Surgery
Peter Randall Endowed Chair in Pediatric
Plastic Surgery
Childrens Hospital of Philadelphia, University of
Philadelphia
Philadelphia, PA, USA
*Volume 3, Chapter 34 Nonsyndromic
craniosynostosis*

Fritz E. Barton, Jr., MD
Clinical Professor
Department of Plastic Surgery
University of Texas Southwestern Medical
Center
Dallas, TX, USA
*Volume 2, Chapter 11.7 Facelift: SMAS with skin
attached – the "high SMAS" technique*
*Volume 2, Video 11.07.01 The High SMAS
technique with septal reset*

Bruce S. Bauer, MD, FACS, FAAP
Director of Pediatric Plastic Surgery, Clinical
Professor of Surgery
Northshore University Healthsystem
University of Chicago, Pritzker School of
Medicine, Highland Park Hospital
Chicago, IL, USA
*Volume 3, Chapter 40 Congenital melanocytic
nevi*

Ruediger G.H. Baumeister, MD, PhD
Professor of Surgery Emeritus
Consultant in Lymphology
Ludwig Maximilians University
Munich, Germany
*Volume 4, Chapter 3 Lymphatic reconstruction of
the extremities*

Leslie Baumann, MD
CEO
Baumann Cosmetic and Research Institute
Miami, FL, USA
*Volume 2, Chapter 2 Non surgical skin care and
rejuvenation*

Adriane L. Baylis, PhD
Speech Scientist
Section of Plastic and Reconstructive Surgery
Nationwide Children's Hospital
Columbus, OH, USA
*Volume 3, Chapter 28 Velopharyngeal
dysfunction*
*Volume 3, Video 28 Velopharyngeal
incompetence (1-3)*

Elisabeth Beahm, MD, FACS
Professor
Department of Plastic Surgery
University of Texas MD Anderson Cancer
Center
Houston, TX, USA
*Volume 5, Chapter 10 Breast cancer: Diagnosis
therapy and oncoplastic techniques*
*Volume 5, Video 10.01 Breast cancer: diagnosis
and therapy*

Michael L. Bentz, MD, FAAP, FACS
Professor of Surgery Pediatrics and
Neurosurgery Chairman
Chairman of Clinical Affairs
Department of Surgery
Division of Plastic Surgery Vice
University of Winconsin School of Medicine and
Public Health
Madison, WI, USA
Volume 3, Chapter 42 Pediatric tumors

Aaron Berger, MD, PhD
Resident
Division of Plastic Surgery, Department of Surgery
Stanford University Medical Center
Palo Alto, CA, USA
Volume 1, Chapter 31 Melanoma

Pietro Berrino, MD
Teaching Professor
University of Milan
Director
Chirurgia Plastica Genova SRL
Genoa, Italy
Volume 5, Chapter 23 Poland's syndrome

Valeria Berrino, MS
In Training
Chirurgia Plastica Genova SRL
Genoa, Italy
Volume 5, Chapter 23 Poland's syndrome

Miles G. Berry, MS, FRCS(Plast)
Consultant Plastic and Aesthetic Surgeon
Institute of Cosmetic and Reconstructive Surgery
London, UK
Volume 2, Chapter 11.3 Facelift: Platysma-SMAS plication
Volume 2, Video 11.03.01 Facelift – Platysma SMAS plication

Robert M. Bernstein, MD, FAAD
Associate Clinical Professor
Department of Dermatology
College of Physicians and Surgeons
Columbia University
Director
Private Practice
Bernstein Medical Center for Hair Restoration
New York, NY, USA
Volume 2, Video 23.04 FUE FOX procedure
Volume 2, Video 23.02 Follicular unit hair transplantation

Michael Bezuhly, MD, MSc, SM, FRCSC
Assistant Professor
Department of Surgery, Division of Plastic and Reconstructive Surgery
IWK Health Centre, Dalhousie University
Halifax, NS, Canada
Volume 6, Chapter 23 Nerve entrapment syndromes
Volume 6, Video 23.01-04 Carpal tunnel and cubital tunnel releases in the same patient in one procedure with field sterility – local anaesthetic and surgery

Sean M. Bidic, MD, MFA, FAAP, FACS
Private Practice
American Surgical Arts
Vineland, NJ, USA
Volume 6, Chapter 16 Infections of the hand

Phillip N. Blondeel, MD, PhD, FCCP
Professor of Plastic Surgery
Department of Plastic and Reconstructive Surgery
University Hospital Gent
Gent, Belgium
Volume 5, Chapter 18 The deep inferior epigastric artery perforator (DIEAP) Flap
Volume 5, Chapter 19 Alternative flaps for breast reconstruction
Volume 5, Video 18.02 DIEP flap breast reconstruction

Sean G. Boutros, MD
Assistant Professor of Surgery
Weill Cornell Medical College (Houston)
Clinical Instructor
University of Texas School of Medicine (Houston)
Houston Plastic and Craniofacial Surgery
Houston, TX, USA
Volume 3, Video 7.02 Reconstruction of acquired ear deformities

Lorenzo Borghese, MD
Plastic Surgeon
General Surgeon
Department of Plastic and Maxillo Facial Surgery
Director of International Cooperation South East Asia
Pediatric Hospital "Bambino Gesu'"
Rome, Italy
Volume 4, Chapter 19 Extremity burn reconstruction
Volume 4, Video 19.01 Extremity burn reconstruction

Trevor M. Born, MD, FRCSC
Lecturer
Division of Plastic and Reconstructive Surgery
The University of Toronto
Toronto, Ontario, Canada
Attending Physician
Lenox Hill Hospital
New York, NY, USA
Volume 2, Chapter 4 Soft-tissue fillers

Gregory H. Borschel, MD, FAAP, FACS
Assistant Professor
University of Toronto Division of Plastic and Reconstructive Surgery
Assistant Professor
Institute of Biomaterials and Biomedical Engineering
Associate Scientist
The SickKids Research Institute
The Hospital for Sick Children
Toronto, ON, Canada
Volume 6, Chapter 35 Free functioning muscle transfer in the upper extremity

Kirsty U. Boyd, MD, FRCSC
Clinical Fellow – Hand Surgery
Department of Surgery – Division of Plastic Surgery
Washington University School of Medicine
St. Louis, MO, USA
Volume 1, Chapter 22 Repair and grafting of peripheral nerve
Volume 6, Chapter 33 Nerve transfers

James P. Bradley, MD
Professor of Plastic and Reconstructive Surgery
Department of Surgery
University of California, Los Angeles David Geffen School of Medicine
Los Angeles, CA, USA
Volume 3, Chapter 33 Craniofacial clefts

Burton D. Brent, MD
Private Practice
Woodside, CA, USA
Volume 3, Chapter 7 Reconstruction of the ear

Mitchell H. Brown, MD, Med, FRCSC
Associate Professor of Plastic Surgery
Department of Surgery
University of Toronto
Toronto, ON, Canada
Volume 5, Chapter 3 Secondary breast augmentation

Samantha A. Brugmann, PHD
Postdoctoral Fellow
Department of Surgery
Stanford University
Stanford, CA, USA
Volume 3, Chapter 22 Embryology of the craniofacial complex

Terrence W. Bruner, MD, MBA
Private Practice
Greenville, SC, USA
Volume 2, Chapter 28 Buttock augmentation
Volume 2, Video 28.01 Buttock augmentation

Todd E. Burdette, MD
Staff Plastic Surgeon
Concord Plastic Surgery
Concord Hospital Medical Group
Concord, NH, USA
Volume 1, Chapter 36 Robotics, simulation, and telemedicine in plastic surgery

Renee M. Burke, MD
Attending Plastic Surgeon
Department of Plastic Surgery
St. Alexius Medical Center
Hoffman Estates, IL, USA
Volume 3, Chapter 8 Acquired cranial and facial bone deformities
Volume 3, Video 8.01 Removal of venous malformation enveloping intraconal optic nerve

Charles E. Butler, MD, FACS
Professor, Department of Plastic Surgery
The University of Texas MD Anderson Cancer
Center
Houston, TX, USA
Volume 1, Chapter 32 Implants and biomaterials

**Peter E. M. Butler, MD, FRCSI, FRCS,
FRCS(Plast)**
Consultant Plastic Surgeon
Honorary Senior Lecturer
Royal Free Hospital
London, UK
*Volume 1, Chapter 34 Transplantation in plastic
surgery*

Yilin Cao, MD
Director, Department of Plastic and
Reconstructive Surgery
Shanghai 9th People's Hospital
Vice-Dean
Shanghai Jiao Tong University Medical School
Shanghai, The People's Republic of China
*Volume 1, Chapter 18 Tissue graft, tissue repair,
and regeneration*
*Volume 1, Chapter 20 Repair, grafting, and
engineering of cartilage*

Joseph F. Capella, MD, FACS
Chief, Post-Bariatric Body Contouring
Division of Plastic Surgery
Hackensack University Medical Center
Hackensack, NJ, USA
Volume 2, Chapter 29 Upper limb contouring
Volume 2, Video 29.01 Upper limb contouring

Brian T. Carlsen, MD
Assistant Professor of Plastic Surgery
Department of Surgery
Mayo Clinic
Rochester, MN, USA
*Volume 6, Chapter 20 Osteoarthritis in the hand
and wrist*

Robert C. Cartotto, MD, FRCS(C)
Attending Surgeon
Ross Tilley Burn Centre
Health Sciences Centre
Toronto, ON, Canada
*Volume 4, Chapter 23 Management of patients
with exfoliative disorders, epidermolysis bullosa,
and TEN*

Giuseppe Catanuto, MD, PhD
Research Fellow
The School of Oncological Reconstructive
Surgery
Milan, Italy
*Volume 5, Chapter 14 Expander/implant breast
reconstructions*
*Volume 5, Video 14.01 Mastectomy and
expander insertion: first stage*
*Volume 5, Video 14.02 Mastectomy and
expander insertion: second stage*

Peter Ceulemans, MD
Assistant Professor
Department of Plastic Surgery
Ghent University Hospital
Ghent, Belgium
*Volume 4, Chapter 13 Reconstruction of male
genital defects*

Rodney K. Chan, MD
Staff Plastic and Reconstructive Surgeon
Burn Center
United States Army Institute of Surgical
Research
Fort Sam
Houston, TX, USA
*Volume 3, Chapter 19 Secondary facial
reconstruction*

David W. Chang, MD, FACS
Professor
Department of Plastic Surgery
MD. Anderson Centre
Houston, TX, USA
*Volume 4, Chapter 3 Lymphatic reconstruction of
the extremities*
*Volume 4, Video 3.01 Lymphatico-venous
anastomosis*
*Volume 6, Chapter 15 Benign and malignant
tumors of the hand*

Edward I. Chang, MD
Assistant Professor
Department of Plastic Surgery
The University of Texas M.D. Anderson Cancer
Center
Houston, TX, USA
*Volume 3, Chapter 17 Carcinoma of the upper
aerodigestive tract*

James Chang, MD
Professor and Chief
Division of Plastic and Reconstructive Surgery
Stanford University Medical Center
Stanford, CA, USA
*Volume 6, Introduction: Plastic surgery
contributions to hand surgery*
*Volume 6, Chapter 1 Anatomy and biomechanics
of the hand*
Volume 6, Video 11.01 Hand replantation
Volume 6, Video 12.01 Debridement technique
*Volume 6, Video 19.01 Extensor tendon rupture
and end-side tendon transfer*
*Volume 6, Video 29.01 Addendum pediatric
trigger thumb release*

Robert A. Chase, MD
Holman Professor of Surgery – Emeritus
Stanford University Medical Center
Stanford, CA, USA
*Volume 6, Chapter 1 Anatomy and biomechanics
of the hand*

Constance M. Chen, MD, MPH
Plastic and Reconstructive Surgeon
Division of Plastic and Reconstructive Surgery
Lenox Hill Hospital
New York, NY, USA
Volume 3, Chapter 9 Midface reconstruction

Philip Kuo-Ting Chen, MD
Director
Department of Plastic and Reconstructive
Surgery
Chang Gung Memorial Hospital and Chang
Gung University
Taipei, Taiwan, The People's Republic of China
Volume 3, Chapter 23 Repair of unilateral cleft lip

Yu-Ray Chen, MD
Professor of Surgery
Department of Plastic and Reconstructive
Surgery
Chang Gung Memorial Hospital
Chang Gung University
Tao-Yuan, Taiwan, The People's Republic of
China
*Volume 3, Chapter 15 Tumors of the facial
skeleton: Fibrous dysplasia*

Ming-Huei Cheng, MD, MBA, FACS
Professor and Chief, Division of Reconstructive
Microsurgery
Department of Plastic and Reconstructive
Surgery
Chang Gung Memorial Hospital
Chang Gung Medical College
Chang Gung University
Taoyuan, Taiwan, The People's Republic of
China
*Volume 3, Chapter 12 Oral cavity, tongue, and
mandibular reconstructions*
*Volume 3, Video 12.02 Ulnar forearm flap for
buccal reconstruction*

You-Wei Cheong, MBBS, MS
Consultant Plastic Surgeon
Department of Surgery
Faculty of Medicine and Health Sciences,
University of Putra Malaysia
Selangor, Malaysia
*Volume 3, Chapter 15 Tumors of the facial
skeleton: Fibrous dysplasia*

Armando Chiari Jr., MD, PhD
Adjunct Professor
Department of Surgery
School of Medicine of the Federal University of
Minas Gerais
Belo Horzonti, Minas Gerais, Brazil
*Volume 5, Chapter 8.5 The L short scar
mammaplasty*

Ernest S. Chiu, MD, FACS
Associate Professor of Plastic Surgery
Department of Plastic Surgery
New York University
New York
USA
*Volume 2, Chapter 9 Secondary blepharoplasty:
Techniques*

Hong-Lim Choi, MD, PhD
Jeong-Won Aesthetic Plastic Surgical Clinic
Seoul, South Korea
Volume 2, Video 10.01 Eyelidplasty non-incisional method
Volume 2, Video 10.02 Incisional method

Jong Woo Choi, MD, PhD
Associate Professor
Department of Plastic and Reconstructive
Surgery
Asan Medical Center
Ulsan University
College of Medicine
Seoul, South Korea
Volume 2, Chapter 10 Asian facial cosmetic surgery

**Alphonsus K. Chong, MBBS, MRCS,
MMed(Orth), FAMS(Hand Surgery)**
Consultant Hand Surgeon
Department of Hand and Reconstructive
Microsurgery
National University Hospital
Assistant Professor
Department of Orthopaedic Surgery
Yong Loo Lin School of Medicine
National University of Singapore
Singapore
Volume 6, Chapter 3 Diagnostic imaging of the hand and wrist
Volume 6, Video 3.01 Diagnostic imaging of the hand and wrist – Scaphoid lunate dislocation

David Chwei-Chin Chuang, MD
Senior Consultant, Ex-President, Professor
Department of Plastic Surgery
Chang Gung University Hospital
Tao-Yuan, Taiwan, The People's Republic of
China
Volume 6, Chapter 36 Brachial plexus injuries-adult and pediatric
Volume 6, Video 36.01-02 Brachial plexus injuries

Kevin C. Chung, MD, MS
Charles B. G. de Nancrede, MD Professor
Section of Plastic Surgery, Department of
Surgery
Assistant Dean for Faculty Affairs
University of Michigan Medical School
Ann Arbor, MI, USA
Volume 6, Chapter 8 Fractures and dislocations of the carpus and distal radius
Volume 6, Chapter 19 Rheumatologic conditions of the hand and wrist
Volume 6, Video 8.01 Scaphoid fixation
Volume 6, Video 19.01 Silicone MCP arthroplasty

Juan A. Clavero, MD, PhD
Radiologist Consultant
Radiology Department
Clínica Creu Blanca
Barcelona, Spain
Volume 5, Chapter 13 Imaging in reconstructive breast surgery

Mark W. Clemens, MD
Assistant Professor
Department of Plastic Surgery
Anderson Cancer Center University of Texas
Houston, TX, USA
Volume 4, Chapter 8 Foot reconstruction
Volume 5, Chapter 15 Latissimus dorsi flap breast reconstruction
Volume 5, Video 15.01 Latissimus dorsi flap technique

Steven R. Cohen, MD
Senior Clinical Research Fellow, Clinical
Professor
Plastic Surgery
University of California
San Diego, CA
Director
Craniofacial Surgery
Rady Children's Hospital, Private Practice,
FACES+ Plastic Surgery, Skin and Laser Center
La Jolla, CA, USA
Volume 2, Chapter 5 Facial skin resurfacing

Sydney R. Coleman, MD
Clinical Assistant Professor
Department of Plastic Surgery
New York University Medical Center
New York, NY, USA
Volume 2, Chapter 14 Structural fat grafting
Volume 2, Video 14.01 Structural fat grafting of the face

John Joseph Coleman III, MD
James E. Bennett Professor of Surgery,
Department of Dermatology and Cutaneuous
Surgery
University of Miami Miller School of Medicine
Miami, FA
Chief of Plastic Surgery
Department of Surgery
Indiana University School of Medicine
Indianapolis, IN, USA
Volume 3, Chapter 16 Tumors of the lips, oral cavity, oropharynx, and mandible

Lawrence B. Colen, MD
Associate Professor of Surgery
Eastern Virginia Medical School
Norfolk, VA, USA
Volume 4, Chapter 8 Foot reconstruction

E. Dale Collins Vidal, MD, MS
Chief
Section of Plastic Surgery
Dartmouth-Hitchcock Medical Center
Professor of Surgery
Dartmouth Medical School
Director of the Center for Informed Choice
The Dartmouth Institute (TDI) for Health Policy
and Clinical Practice
Hanover, NH, USA
Volume 1, Chapter 10 Evidence-based medicine and health services research in plastic surgery
Volume 5, Chapter 12 Patient-centered health communication

Shannon Colohan, MD, FRCSC
Clinical Instructor, Plastic Surgery
Department of Plastic Surgery
University of Texas Southwestern Medical
Center
Dallas, TX, USA
Volume 4, Chapter 2 Management of lower extremity trauma

Mark B. Constantian, MD, FACS
Active Staff
Saint Joseph Hospital
Nashua, NH (private practice)
Assistant Clinical Professor of Plastic Surgery
Division of Plastic Surgery
Department of Surgery
University of Wisconsin
Madison, WI, USA
Volume 2, Chapter 19 Closed technique rhinoplasty

Peter G. Cordeiro, MD, FACS
Chief
Plastic and Reconstructive Surgery
Memorial Sloan-Kettering Cancer Center
Professor of Surgery
Weill Cornell Medical College
New York, NY, USA
Volume 3, Chapter 9 Midface reconstruction
Volume 4, Chapter 14 Reconstruction of acquired vaginal defects

Christopher Cox, MD
Chief Resident
Department of Orthopaedic Surgery
Stanford University Medical School
Stanford, CA, USA
Volume 6, Chapter 5 Principles of internal fixation as applied to the hand and wrist
Volume 6, Video 5.01 Dynamic compression plating and lag screw technique

Albert Cram, MD
Professor Emeritus
University of Iowa
Iowa City Plastic Surgery
Coralville, IO, USA
Volume 2, Chapter 27 Lower bodylifts

Catherine Curtin, MD
Assistant Professor
Department of Surgery Division of Plastic
Stanford University
Stanford, CA, USA
*Volume 6, Chapter 37 Restoration of upper
extremity function*
*Volume 6, Video 37.01 1 Stage grasp IC 6 short
term*
*Volume 6, Video 37.02 2 Stage grasp release
outcome*

Lars B. Dahlin, MD, PhD
Professor and Consultant
Department of Clinical Sciences, Malmö-Hand
Surgery
University of Lund
Malmö, Sweden
*Volume 6, Chapter 32 Peripheral nerve injuries of
the upper extremity*
Volume 6, Video 32.01 Digital Nerve Suture
Volume 6, Video 32.02 Median Nerve Suture

Dai M. Davies, FRCS
Consultant and Institute Director
Institute of Cosmetic and Reconstructive
Surgery
London, UK
*Volume 2, Chapter 11.3 Facelift: Platysma-SMAS
plication*
*Volume 2, Video 11.03.01 Platysma SMAS
plication*

**Michael R. Davis, MD, FACS, LtCol,
USAF, MC**
Chief
Reconstructive Surgery and Regenerative
Medicine
Plastic and Reconstructive Surgeon
San Antonio Military Medical Center
Houston, TX, USA
*Volume 5, Chapter 1 Anatomy for plastic surgery
of the breast*

Jorge I. De La Torre, MD
Professor and Chief
Division of Plastic Surgery
University of Alabama at Birmingham
Birmingham, AL, USA
*Volume 5, Chapter 1 Anatomy for plastic surgery
of the breast*

A. Lee Dellon, MD, PhD
Professor of Plastic Surgery
Professor of Neurosurgery
Johns Hopkins University
Baltimore, MD, USA
*Volume 4, Chapter 6 Diagnosis and treatment of
painful neuroma and of nerve compression in the
lower extremity*
*Volume 4, Video 6.01 Diagnosis and treatment
of painful neuroma and of nerve compression in
the lower extremity*

Sara R. Dickie, MD
Resident, Section of Plastic and Reconstructive
Surgery
Department of Surgery
University of Chicago Medical Center
Chicago, IL, USA
*Volume 4, Chapter 9 Comprehensive trunk
anatomy*

Joseph J. Disa, MD, FACS
Attending Surgeon
Plastic and Reconstructive Surgery in the
Department of Surgery
Memorial Sloan Kettering Cancer Center
New York, NY, USA
Volume 3, Chapter 9 Midface reconstruction
*Volume 4, Chapter 14 Reconstruction of
acquired vaginal defects*

Risal Djohan, MD
Head of Regional Medical Practice
Department of Plastic Surgery
Cleveland Clinic
Cleveland, OH, USA
*Volume 3, Chapter 1 Anatomy of the head and
neck*

Erin Donaldson, MS
Instructor
Department of Otolaryngology
New York Medical College
Valhalla, NY, USA
*Volume 1, Chapter 36 Robotics, simulation, and
telemedicine in plastic surgery*

Amir H. Dorafshar, MBChB
Assistant Professor
Department of Plastic and Reconstructive
surgery
John Hopkins Medical Institute
John Hopkins Outpatient Center
Baltimore, MD, USA
Volume 3, Chapter 3 Facial fractures

Ivica Ducic, MD, PhD
Professor – Plastic Surgery
Director – Peripheral Nerve Surgery Institute
Department of Plastic Surgery
Georgetown University Hospital
Washington, DC, USA
*Volume 6, Chapter 23 Complex regional pain
syndrome in the upper extremity*

Gregory A. Dumanian, MD, FACS
Chief of Plastic Surgery
Division of Plastic Surgery, Department of
Surgery
Northwestern Feinberg School of Medicine
Chicago, IL, USA
*Volume 4, Chapter 11 Reconstruction of the soft
tissues of the back*
*Volume 6, Chapter 40 Treatment of the upper
extremity amputee*
*Volume 6, Video 40.01 Targeted muscle
reinnervation in the transhumeral amputee –
Surgical technique and guidelines for restoring
intuitive neural control*

William W. Dzwierzynski, MD
Professor and Program Director
Department of Plastic Surgery
Medical College of Wisconsin
Milwaukee, WI, USA
*Volume 6, Chapter 11 Replantation and
revascularization*

L. Franklyn Elliott, MD
Assistant Clinical Professor
Emory Section of Plastic Surgery
Emory University
Atlanta, GA, USA
*Volume 5, Chapter 16 The bilateral pedicled
TRAM flap*
*Volume 5, Video 16.01 Pedicle TRAM breast
reconstruction*

Marco Ellis, MD
Chief Resident
Division of Plastic Surgery
Northwestern Memorial Hospital
Northwestern University, Feinberg School of
Medicine
Chicago, IL, USA
Volume 2, Chapter 8 Blepharoplasty
Volume 2, Video 8.01 Periorbital rejuvenation

Dino Elyassnia, MD
Associate Plastic Surgeon
Marten Clinic of Plastic Surgery
San Francisco, CA, USA
*Volume 2, Chapter 12 Secondary deformities
and the secondary facelift*

Surak Eo, MD, PhD
Chief, Associate Professor
Plastic and Reconstructive Surgery
DongGuk University Medical Center
DongGuk University Graduate School of
Medicine
Gyeonggi-do, South Korea
*Volume 6, Video 34.01 EIP to EPL tendon
transfer*

Elof Eriksson, MD, PhD
Chief
Department of Plastic Surgery
Joseph E. Murray Professor of Plastic and
Reconstructive Surgery
Brigham and Women's Hospital
Boston, MA, USA
*Volume 1, Chapter 11 Genetics and prenatal
diagnosis*

Simon Farnebo, MD, PhD
Consultant Hand Surgeon
Department of Plastic Surgery, Hand Surgery
and Burns
Institution of Clinical and Experimental
Medicine, University of Linköping
Linköping, Sweden
*Volume 6, Chapter 32 Peripheral nerve injuries of
the upper extremity*
Volume 6, Video 32.01 Digital Nerve Suture
Volume 6, Video 32.02 Median Nerve Suture

Jeffrey A. Fearon, MD
Director
The Craniofacial Center
Medical City Children's Hospital
Dallas, TX, USA
*Volume 3, Chapter 35 Syndromic
craniosynostosis*

John M. Felder III, MD
Resident Physician
Department of Plastic Surgery
Georgetown University Hospital
Washington, DC, USA
*Volume 6, Chapter 23 Complex regional pain
syndrome in the upper extremity*

Evan M. Feldman, MD
Chief Resident
Division of Plastic Surgery
Baylor College of Medicine
Houston, TX, USA
*Volume 3, Chapter 29 Secondary deformities of
the cleft lip, nose, and palate*
Volume 3, Video 29.01 Complete takedown
Volume 3, Video 29.02 Abbé flap
*Volume 3, Video 29.03 Thick lip and buccal
sulcus deformities*
Volume 3, Video 29.04 Alveolar bone grafting
Volume 3, Video 29.05 Definitive rhinoplasty

Julius Few Jr., MD
Director
The Few Institute for Aesthetic Plastic Surgery
Clinical Associate
Division of Plastic Surgery
University of Chicago
Chicago, IL, USA
Volume 2, Chapter 8 Blepharoplasty
Volume 2, Video 8.01 Periorbital rejuvenation

Alvaro A. Figueroa, DDS, MS
Director
Rush Craniofacial Center
Rush University Medical Center
Chicago, IL, USA
*Volume 3, Chapter 27 Orthodontics in cleft lip
and palate management*

Neil A. Fine, MD
Associate Professor of Clinical Surgery
Department of Surgery
Northwestern University
Chicago, IL, USA
*Volume 5, Chapter 5 Endoscopic approaches to
the breast*
*Volume 5, Video 5.01 Endoscopic transaxillary
breast augmentation*
*Volume 5, Video 5.02 Endoscopic approaches
to the breast*
*Volume 5, Video 11.02 Partial breast
reconstruction with a latissimus D*

Joel S. Fish, MD, MSc, FRCSC
Medical Director Burn Program
Department of Surgery, University of Toronto,
Division of Plastic and Reconstructive Surgery
Hospital for Sick Children
Toronto, ON, Canada
*Volume 4, Chapter 23 Management of patients
with exfoliative disorders, epidermolysis bullosa,
and TEN*

David M. Fisher, MB, BCh, FRCSC, FACS
Medical Director, Cleft Lip and Palate Program
Division of Plastic and Reconstructive Surgery
The Hospital for Sick Children
Toronto, ON, Canada
*Volume 3, Video 23.02 Unilateral cleft lip repair
– anatomic subunit approximation technique*

Jack Fisher, MD
Department of Plastic Surgery
Vanderbilt University
Nashville, TN, USA
Volume 2, Chapter 23 Hair restoration
Volume 5, Chapter 8.1 Reduction mammaplasty
*Volume 5, Chapter 8.2 Inferior pedicle breast
reduction*

James W. Fletcher, MD, FACS
Chief Hand Surgery
Department Plastic and Hand Surgery
Regions Hospital
Assistant Prof. U MN Dept of Surgery and Dept
Orthopedics
St. Paul, MN, USA
*Volume 6, Video 20.01 Ligament reconstruction
tendon interposition arthroplasty of the thumb
CMC joint*

Joshua Fosnot, MD
Resident
Division of Plastic Surgery
The University of Pennsylvania Health System
Philadelphia, PA, USA
*Volume 5, Chapter 17 Free TRAM breast
reconstruction*
*Volume 5, Video 17.01 The muscle sparing free
TRAM flap*

Ida K. Fox, MD
Assistant Professor of Plastic Surgery
Department of Surgery
Washington University School of Medicine
Saint Louis, MO, USA
Volume 6, Chapter 33 Nerve transfers
Volume 6, Video 33.01 Nerve transfers

Ryan C. Frank, MD, FRCSC
Attending Surgeon
Plastic and Craniofacial Surgery
Alberta Children's Hospital
University of Calgary
Calgary, AB, Canada
Volume 2, Chapter 5 Facial skin resurfacing

Gary L. Freed, MD
Assistant Professor Plastic Surgery
Dartmouth-Hitchcock Medical Center
Lebanon, NH, USA
*Volume 5, Chapter 12 Patient-centered health
communication*

Jeffrey B. Friedrich, MD
Assistant Professor of Surgery, Orthopedics
and Urology (Adjunct)
Department of Surgery, Division of Plastic
Surgery
University of Washington
Seattle, WA, USA
*Volume 6, Chapter 13 Thumb reconstruction
(non microsurgical)*

Allen Gabriel, MD
Assitant Professor
Department of Plastic Surgery
Loma Linda University Medical Center
Chief of Plastic Surgery
Southwest Washington Medical Center
Vancouver, WA, USA
Volume 5, Chapter 2 Breast augmentation
*Volume 5, Chapter 4 Current concepts in
revisionary breast surgery*
*Volume 5, Video 4.01 Current concepts in
revisionary breast surgery*

Günter Germann, MD, PhD
Professor of Plastic Surgery
Clinic for Plastic and Reconstructive Surgery
Heidelberg University Hospital
Heidelberg, Germany
*Volume 6, Chapter 10 Extensor tendon injuries
and reconstruction*

Goetz A. Giessler, MD, PhD
Plastic Surgeon, Hand Surgeon, Associate
Professor of Plastic Surgery, Fellow of the
European Board of Plastic Reconstructive and
Aesthetic Surgery
BG Trauma Center Murnau
Murnau am Staffelsee, Germany
*Volume 4, Chapter 4 Lower extremity sarcoma
reconstruction*
*Volume 4, Video 4.01 Management of lower
extremity sarcoma reconstruction*

Jesse A. Goldstein, MD
Chief Resident
Department of Plastic Surgery
Georgetown University Hospital
Washington, DC, USA
*Volume 3, Chapter 30 Cleft and craniofacial
orthognathic surgery*

Vijay S. Gorantla, MD, PhD
Associate Professor of Surgery
Department of Surgery, Division of Plastic and
Reconstructive Surgery
University of Pittsburgh Medical Center
Administrative Medical Director
Pittsburgh Reconstructive Transplantation
Program
Pittsburgh, PA, USA
*Volume 6, Chapter 38 Upper extremity
composite allotransplantation*
*Volume 6, Video 38.01 Upper extremity
composite allotransplantation*

Arun K. Gosain, MD
DeWayne Richey Professor and Vice Chair
Department of Plastic Surgery
University Hospitals Case Medical Center
Chief, Pediatric Plastic Surgery
Rainbow Babies and Children's Hospital
Cleveland, OH, USA
Volume 3, Chapter 38 Pierre Robin sequence

Lawrence J. Gottlieb, MD, FACS
Professor of Surgery
Director of Burn and Complex Wound Center
Director of Reconstructive Microsurgery
Fellowship
Section of Plastic and Reconstructive Surgery
Department of Surgery
University of Chicago
Chicago, IL, USA
*Volume 3, Chapter 41 Pediatric chest and trunk
defects*

Barry H. Grayson, DDS
Associate Professor of Surgery (Craniofacial
Orthodontics)
New York University Langone Medical Centre
Institute of Reconstructive Plastic Surgery
New York, NY, USA
Volume 3, Chapter 36 Craniofacial microsomia
Volume 3, Video 24.01 Repair of bilateral cleft lip

Arin K. Greene, MD, MMSc
Associate Professor of Surgery
Department of Plastic and Oral Surgery
Children's Hospital Boston
Harvard Medical School
Boston, MA, USA
Volume 1, Chapter 29 Vascular anomalies

James C. Grotting, MD, FACS
Clinical Professor of Plastic Surgery
University of Alabama at Birmingham;
The University of Wisconsin, Madison, WI;
Grotting and Cohn Plastic Surgery
Birmingham, AL, USA
Volume 5, Chapter 7 Mastopexy
Volume 5, Chapter 8.7 Sculpted pillar vertical
*Volume 5, Video 8.7.01 Marking the sculpted
pillar breast reduction*
Volume 5, Video 8.7.02 Breast reduction surgery

Ronald P. Gruber, MD
Associate Adjunct Clinical Professor
Division of Plastic and Reconstructive Surgery
Stanford University
Associate Clinical Professor
Division of Plastic and Reconstructive Surgery
University of California, San Francisco
San Francisco, CA, USA
Volume 2, Chapter 21 Secondary rhinoplasty

**Mohan S. Gundeti, MB, MCh, FEBU,
FRCS, FEAPU**
Associate Professor of Urology in Surgery and
Pediatrics, Director Pediatric Urology, Director
Centre for Pediatric Robotics and Minimal
Invasive Surgery
University of Chicago and Pritzker Medical
School Comer Children's Hospital
Chicago, IL, USA
*Volume 3, Chapter 44 Reconstruction of
urogenital defects: Congenital*
*Volume 3, Video 44.01 First stage hypospadias
repair with free inner preputial graft*
*Volume 3, Video 44.02 Second stage
hypospadias repair with tunica vaginalis flap*

Eyal Gur, MD
Head
Department of Plastic and Reconstructive
Surgery
The Tel Aviv Sourasky Medical Center
The Tel Aviv University School of Medicine
Tel Aviv, Israel
Volume 3, Chapter 11 Facial paralysis
Volume 3, Video 11.01 Facial paralysis

Geoffrey C. Gurtner, MD, FACS
Professor and Associate Chairman
Stanford University Department of Surgery
Stanford, CA, USA
*Volume 1, Chapter 13 Stem cells and
regenerative medecine*
*Volume 1, Chapter 35 Technology innovation in
plastic surgery*

Bahman Guyuron, MD
Kiehn-DesPrez Professor and Chairman
Department of Plastic Surgery
Case Western Reserve University School of
Medicine
Cleveland, OH, USA
*Volume 2, Chapter 20 Airway issues and the
deviated nose*
*Volume 3, Chapter 21 Surgical management of
migraine headaches*
Volume 2, Video 3.02 Botulinum toxin

Steven C. Haase, MD
Clinical Associate Professor
Department of Surgery, Section of Plastic
Surgery
University of Michigan Health
Ann Arbor, MI, USA
*Volume 6, Chapter 8 Fractures and dislocations
of the carpus and distal radius*

Robert S. Haber, MD, FAAD, FAAP
Assistant Professor, Dermatology and
Pediatrics
Case Western Reserve University School of
Medicine
Director
University Hair Transplant Center
Cleveland, OH, USA
*Volume 2, Video 23.08 Strip harvesting the
haber spreader*

Florian Hackl, MD
Research Fellow
Division of Plastic Surgery
Brigham and Women's Hospital
Harvard Medical School
Boston, MA, USA
*Volume 1, Chapter 11 Genetics and prenatal
diagnosis*

Phillip C. Haeck, MD
Private Practice
Seattle, WA, USA
*Volume 1, Chapter 4 The role of ethics in plastic
surgery*

Bruce Halperin, MD
Adjunct Associate Clinical Professor of
Anesthesia
Department of Anesthesia
Stanford University School of Medicine
Palo Alto, CA, USA
*Volume 1, Chapter 8 Patient safety in plastic
surgery*

Moustapha Hamdi, MD, PhD
Professor and Chairman of Plastic and
Reconstructive Surgery
Department of Plastic Surgery
Brussels University Hospital
Brussels, Belgium
*Volume 5, Chapter 21 Local flaps in partial
breast reconstruction*

Warren C. Hammert, MD
Associate Professor of Orthopaedic and
Plastic Surgery
Department of Orthopaedic Surgery
University of Rochester Medical Center
Rochester, NY, USA
*Volume 6, Chapter 7 Hand fractures and joint
injuries*

Dennis C. Hammond, MD
Clinical Assistant Professor
Department of Surgery
Michigan State University College of Human
Medicine
East Lansing
Associate Program Director
Plastic and Reconstructive Surgery
Grand Rapids Medical Education and Research
Center for Health Professions
Grand Rapids, MI, USA
*Volume 5, Chapter 8.4 Short scar periareolar
inferior pedicle reduction (SPAIR) mammaplasty*
Volume 5, Video 8.4.01 Spair technique

Scott L. Hansen, MD, FACS
Assistant Professor of Plastic and
Reconstructive Surgery
Chief, Hand and Microvascular Surgery
University of California, San Francisco
Chief, Plastic and Reconstructive Surgery
San Francisco General Hospital
San Francisco, CA, USA
*Volume 1, Chapter 24 Flap classification and
applications*

James A. Harris, MD
Cosmetic Surgeon
Private Practice
Hasson & Wong Aesthetic Surgery
Vancouver, BC, Canada
Volume 2, Video 23.05 FUE Harris safe system

Isaac Harvey, MD
Clinical Fellow
Department of Paediatric Plastic and
Reconstructive Surgery
Hospital for Sick Kids
Toronto, ON, Canada
*Volume 6, Chapter 35 Free functional muscle
transfers in the upper extremity*

Victor Hasson, MD
Cosmetic Surgeon
Private Practice
Hasson & Wong Aesthetic Surgery
Vancouver, BC, Canada
*Volume 2, Video 23.07 Perpendicular angle
grafting technique*

Theresa A Hegge, MD, MPH
Resident of Plastic Surgery
Division of Plastic Surgery
Southern Illinois University
Springfield, IL, USA
*Volume 6, Chapter 6 Nail and fingertip
reconstruction*

Jill A. Helms, DDS, PhD
Division of Plastic and Reconstructive Surgery
Department of Surgery
School of Medicine
Stanford University
Stanford, CA, USA
*Volume 3, Chapter 22 Embryology of the
craniofacial complex*

Ginard I. Henry, MD
Assistant Professor of Surgery
Section of Plastic Surgery
University of Chicago Medical Center
Chicago, IL, USA
*Volume 4, Chapter 1 Comprehensive lower
extremity anatomy, embryology, surgical exposure*

Vincent R. Hentz, MD
Emeritus Professor of Surgery and Orthopedic
Surgery (by courtesy)
Stanford University
Stanford, CA, USA
*Volume 6, Chapter 1 Anatomy and biomechanics
of the hand*
*Volume 6, Chapter 37 Restoration of upper
extremity function in tetraplegia*
*Volume 6, Video 37.01 1 Stage grasp IC 6 short
term*
*Volume 6, Video 37.02 2 Stage grasp release
outcome*

**Rebecca L. von der Heyde, PhD,
OTR/L, CHT**
Associate Professor
Program in Occupational Therapy
Maryville University
St. Louis, MO, USA
Volume 6, Chapter 39 Hand therapy
*Volume 6, Video 39.01 Hand therapy
Goniometric measurement*
Volume 6, Video 39.02 Threshold testing
*Volume 6, Video 39.03 Fabrication of a
synergistic splint*

Kent K. Higdon, MD
Former Aesthetic Fellow
Grotting and Cohn Plastic Surgery;
Current Assistant Professor
Vanderbilt University
Nashville, TN, USA
Volume 5, Chapter 7 Mastopexy
Volume 5, Chapter 8.1 Reduction mammaplasty
*Volume 5, Chapter 8.7 Sculpted pillar vertical
mammaplasty*

John Hijjawi, MD, FACS
Assistant Professor
Department of Plastic Surgery, Department of
General Surgery
Medical College of Wisconsin
Milwaukee, WI, USA
*Volume 4, Chapter 20 Cold and chemical injury
to the upper extremity*

Jonay Hill, MD
Clinical Assistant Professor
Anesthesiology Department
Anesthesia and Critical Care
Stanford University School of Medicine
Stanford, CA, USA
*Volume 6, Chapter 4 Anesthesia for upper
extremity surgery*

Piet Hoebeke, MD, PhD
Full Senior Professor of Paediatric Urology
Department of Urology
Ghent University Hospital
Ghent, Belgium
*Volume 4, Chapter 13 Reconstruction of male
genital defects*
*Volume 4, Video 13.01 Complete and partial
penile reconstruction*

William Y. Hoffman, MD
Professor and Chief
Division of Plastic and Reconstructive Surgery
University of California, San Francisco
San Francisco, CA, USA
Volume 3, Chapter 25 Cleft palate

Larry H. Hollier Jr., MD, FACS
Professor and Program Director
Division of Plastic Surgery
Baylor College of Medicine and Texas
Children's Hospital
Houston, TX, USA
*Volume 3, Chapter 29 Secondary deformities of
the cleft lip, nose, and palate*
Volume 3, Video 29.01 Complete takedown
Volume 3, Video 29.02 Abbé flap
*Volume 3, Video 29.03 Thick lip and buccal
sulcus deformities*
Volume 3, Video 29.04 Alveolar bone grafting
Volume 3, Video 29.05 Definitive rhinoplasty

Joon Pio Hong, MD, PhD, MMM
Chief and Associate Professor
Department of Plastic Surgery
Asian Medical Center University of Ulsan
School of Medicine
Seoul, Korea
*Volume 4, Chapter 5 Reconstructive surgery:
Lower extremity coverage*

Richard A. Hopper, MD, MS
Chief
Division of Pediatric Plastic Surgery
University of Washington
Surgical Director
Craniofacial Center
Seattle Childrens Hospital
Associate Professor
Division of Plastic Surgery
Seattle, WA, USA
Volume 3, Chapter 26 Alveolar clefts
Volume 3, Chapter 36 Craniofacial microsomia

Philippe Houtmeyers, MD
Resident
Plastic Surgery
Ghent University Hospital
Ghent, Belgium
*Volume 4, Chapter 13 Reconstruction of male
genital defects*
*Volume 4, Video 13.01 Complete and partial
penile reconstruction*

Steven E.R. Hovius, MD, PhD
Head
Department of Plastic, Reconstructive and
Hand Surgery
ErasmusmMC
University Medical Center
Rotterdam, The Netherlands
*Volume 6, Chapter 28 Congenital hand IV
disorders of differentiation and duplication*

Michael A. Howard, MD
Clinical Assistant Professor of Surgery
Division of Plastic Surgery
University of Chicago, Pritzker School of
Medicine
Northbrook, IL, USA
*Volume 4, Chapter 9 Comprehensive trunk
anatomy*

Jung-Ju Huang, MD
Assistant Professor
Division of Microsurgery
Plastic and Reconstructive Surgery
Chang Gung Memorial Hospital
Taoyuan, Taiwan, The People's Republic of
China
*Volume 3, Chapter 12 Oral cavity, tongue, and
mandibular reconstructions*
*Volume 3, Video 12.01 Fibula
osteoseptocutaneous flap for composite
mandibular reconstruction*
*Volume 3, Video 12.02 Ulnar forearm flap for
buccal reconstruction*

C. Scott Hultman, MD, MBA, FACS
Ethel and James Valone Distinguished
Professor of Surgery
Division of Plastic Surgery
University of North Carolina
Chapel Hill, NC, USA
*Volume 1, Chapter 5 Business principles for
plastic surgeons*

Leung-Kim Hung, MChOrtho (Liv)
Professor
Department of Orthopaedics and Traumatology
Faculty of Medicine
The Chinese University of Hong Kong
Hong Kong, The People's Republic of China
*Volume 6, Chapter 29 Congenital hand V
disorders of overgrowth, undergrowth, and
generalized skeletal deformities*

Gazi Hussain, MBBS, FRACS
Clinical Senior Lecturer
Macquarie Cosmetic and Plastic Surgery
Macquarie University
Sydney, Australia
Volume 3, Chapter 11 Facial paralysis

Marco Innocenti, MD
Director Reconstructive Microsurgery
Department of Oncology
Careggi University Hospital
Florence, Italy
*Volume 6, Chapter 30 Growth considerations in
pediatric upper extremity trauma and
reconstruction*
*Volume 6, Video 30.01 Epiphyseal transplant
harvesting technique*

Clyde H. Ishii, MD, FACS
Assistant Clinical Professor of Surgery
John A. Burns School of Medicine
Chief, Department of Plastic Surgery
Shriners Hospital
Honolulu Unit
Honolulu, HI, USA
*Volume 2, Chapter 10 Asian facial cosmetic
surgery*

Jonathan S. Jacobs, DMD, MD
Associate Professor of Clinical Plastic Surgery
Eastern Virginia Medical School
Norfolk, VA, USA
*Volume 2, Chapter 16 Anthropometry,
cephalometry, and orthognathic surgery*
*Volume 2, Video 16.01 Anthropometry,
cephalometry, and orthognathic surgery*

Jordan M.S. Jacobs, MD
Craniofacial Fellow
Department of Plastic Surgery
New York University Langone Medical Center
New York, NY, USA
*Volume 2, Chapter 16 Anthropometry,
cephalometry, and orthognathic surgery*
*Volume 2, Video 16.01 Anthropometry,
cephalometry, and orthognathic surgery*

**Ian T. Jackson, MD, DSc(Hon), FRCS,
FACS, FRACS (Hon)**
Emeritus Surgeon
Surgical Services Administration
William Beaumont Hospitals
Royal Oak, MI, USA
*Volume 3, Chapter 18 Local flaps for facial
coverage*

Oksana Jackson, MD
Assistant Professor of Surgery
Division of Plastic Surgery
University of Pennsylvania School of Medicine
Clinical Associate
The Children's Hospital of Philadelphia
Philadelphia, PA, USA
Volume 3, Chapter 43 Conjoined twins

Jeffrey E. Janis, MD, FACS
Associate Professor
Program Director
Department of Plastic Surgery
University of Texas Southwestern Medical
Center
Chief of Plastic Surgery
Chief of Wound Care
President-Elect
Medical Staff
Parkland Health and Hospital System
Dallas, TX, USA
Volume 4, Chapter 16 Pressure sores

Leila Jazayeri, MD
Resident
Stanford University Plastic and Reconstructive
Surgery
Stanford, CA, USA
*Volume 1, Chapter 35 Technology innovation in
plastic surgery*

Elizabeth B. Jelks, MD
Private Practice
Jelks Medical
New York, NY, USA
*Volume 2, Chapter 9 Secondary blepharoplasty:
Techniques*

Glenn W. Jelks, MD
Associate Professor
Department of Ophthalmology
Department of Plastic Surgery
New York University School of Medicine
New York, NY, USA
*Volume 2, Chapter 9 Secondary blepharoplasty:
Techniques*

Mark Laurence Jewell, MD
Assistant Clinical Professor of Plastic Surgery
Oregon Health Science University
Jewell Plastic Surgery Center
Eugene, OR, USA
*Volume 2, Chapter 11.4 Facelift: Facial
rejuvenation with loop sutures, the MACS lift and
its derivatives*

Andreas Jokuszies, MD
Consultant Plastic, Aesthetic and Hand
Surgeon
Department of Plastic, Hand and
Reconstructive Surgery
Hanover Medical School
Hanover, Germany
*Volume 1, Chapter 15 Skin wound healing:
Repair biology, wound, and scar treatment*

Neil F. Jones, MD, FRCS
Chief of Hand Surgery
University of California Medical Center
Professor of Orthopedic Surgery
Professor of Plastic and Reconstructive Surgery
University of California Irvine
Irvine, CA, USA
Volume 6, Chapter 22 Ischemia of the hand
*Volume 6, Chapter 34 Tendon transfers in the
upper extremity*
*Volume 6, Video 34.01 EIP to EPL tendon
transfer*

David M. Kahn, MD
Clinical Associate Professor of Plastic Surgery
Department of Surgery
Stanford University School of Medicine
Stanford, CA, USA
Volume 2, Chapter 21 Secondary rhinoplasty

Ryosuke Kakinoki, MD, PhD
Associate Professor
Chief of the Hand Surgery and Microsurgery
Unit
Department of Orthopedic Surgery and
Rehabilitation Medicine
Graduate School of Medicine
Kyoto University
Kyoto, Japan
*Volume 6, Chapter 2 Examination of the upper
extremity*
*Volume 2, Video 2.01-2.17 Examination of the
upper extremity*

Alex Kane, MD
Associate Professor of Surgery
Washington University School of Medicine
St. Louis, WO, USA
Volume 3, Chapter 23 Repair of unilateral cleft lip

Gabrielle M. Kane, MBBCh, EdD, FRCPC
Medical Director, Associate Professor
Department of Radiation Oncology
Associate Professor
Department of Medical Education and
Biomedical Informatics
University of Washington School of Medicine
Seattle, WA, USA
*Volume 1, Chapter 28 Therapeutic radiation:
Principles, effects, and complications*

Michael A. C. Kane, MD
Attending Surgeon Manhattan Eye, Ear and
Throat Institute
Department of Plastic Surgery
New York, NY, USA
Volume 2, Chapter 3 Botulinum toxin (BoNT-A)

Dennis S. Kao, MD
Hand Fellow
Department of Plastic Surgery
Medical College of Wisconsin
Milwaukee, WI, USA
*Volume 4, Chapter 20 Cold and chemical injury
to the upper extremity*

Sahil Kapur, MD
Resident, Plastic and Reconstructive Surgery
Department of Surgery, Division of Plastic and
Reconstructive Surgery
University of Wisconsin
Madison, WI, USA
Volume 3, Chapter 42 Pediatric tumors

Leila Kasrai, MD, MPH, FRCSC
Head, Division of Plastic Surgery
St Joseph's Hospital
Toronto, ON, Canada
Volume 2, Video 22.01 Setback otoplasty

Abdullah E. Kattan, MBBS, FRCS(C)
Clinical Fellow
Division of Plastic Surgery
Department of Surgery
University of Toronto
Toronto, ON, Canada
*Volume 4, Chapter 23 Management of patients
with exfoliative disorders, epidermolysis bullosa,
and TEN*

David L. Kaufman, MD, FACS
Private Practice Plastic Surgery
Aesthetic Artistry Surgical and Medical Center
Folsom, CA, USA
Volume 2, Chapter 21 Secondary rhinoplasty

Lindsay B. Katona, BA
Research Associate
Thayer School of Engineering
Dartmouth College
Hanover, NH, USA
*Volume 1, Chapter 36 Robotics, simulation, and
telemedicine in plastic surgery*

Henry K. Kawamoto, Jr., MD, DDS
Clinical Professor
Division of Plastic Surgery
University of California at Los Angeles
Los Angeles, CA, USA
Volume 3, Chapter 33 Craniofacial clefts

Jeffrey M. Kenkel, MD, FACS
Professor and Vice-Chairman
Rod J Rohrich MD Distinguished Professorship
in Wound Healing and Plastic Surgery
Department of Plastic Surgery
Southwestern Medical School
Director
Clinical Center for Cosmetic Laser Treatment
Dallas, TX, USA
*Volume 2, Chapter 24 Liposuction: A
comprehensive review of techniques and safety*

Carolyn L. Kerrigan, MD, MSc
Professor of Surgery
Section of Plastic Surgery
Dartmouth Hitchcock Medical Center
Lebanon, NH, USA
*Volume 1, Chapter 10 Evidence-based medicine
and health services research in plastic surgery*

Marwan R. Khalifeh, MD
Instructor of Plastic Surgery
Department of Plastic Surgery
Johns Hopkins University School of Medicine
Washington, DC, USA
*Volume 4, Chapter 12 Abdominal wall
reconstruction*

Jae-Hoon Kim, MD
April 31 Aesthetic Plastic Surgical Clinic
Seoul, South Korea
*Volume 2, Video 10.03 Secondary rhinoplasty:
septal extension graft and costal cartilage strut
fixed with K-wire*

**Timothy W. King, MD, PhD, MSBE,
FACS, FAAP**
Assistant Professor of Surgery and Pediatrics
Director of Research
Division of Plastic Surgery, Department of
Surgery
University of Wisconsin School of Medicine and
Public Health
Madison, WI, USA
Volume 1, Chapter 32 Implants and biomaterials

Brian M. Kinney, MD, FACS, MSME
Clinical Assistant Professor of Plastic Surgery
University of Southern California School of
Medicine
Los Angeles, CA, USA
*Volume 1, Chapter 7 Photography in plastic
surgery*

Richard E. Kirschner, MD
Chief, Section of Plastic and Reconstructive
Surgery
Director, Ambulatory Surgical Services
Director, Cleft Lip and Palate Center
Co-Director Nationwide Children's Hospital
Professor of Surgery and Pediatrics
Senior Vice Chair, Department of Plastic Surgery
The Ohio State University College of Medicine
Columbus, OH, USA
Volume 3, Chapter 28 Velopharyngeal dysfunction
*Volume 3, Video 28.01-28.03 Velopharyngeal
incompetence*

Elizabeth Kiwanuka, MD
Division of Plastic Surgery
Brigham and Women's Hospital
Harvard Medical School
Boston, MA, USA
*Volume 1, Chapter 11 Genetics and prenatal
diagnosis*

Grant M. Kleiber, MD
Plastic Surgery Resident
Section of Plastic and Reconstructive Surgery
University of Chicago Medical Center
Chicago, IL, USA
*Volume 4, Chapter 1 Comprehensive lower
extremity anatomy, embryology, surgical exposure*

Mathew B. Klein, MD, MS
David and Nancy Auth-Washington Research
Foundation Endowed Chair for Restorative
Burn Surgery
Division of Plastic Surgery
University of Washington
Program Director and Associate Professor
Division of Plastic Surgery
Harborview Medical Center
Seattle, WA, USA
Volume 4, Chapter 22 Reconstructive burn surgery

Kyung S Koh, MD, PhD
Professor of Plastic Surgery
Asan Medical Center, University of Ulsan
School of Medicine
Seoul, Korea
*Volume 2, Chapter 10 Asian facial cosmetic
surgery*

John C. Koshy, MD
Postdoctoral Research Fellow
Division of Plastic Surgery
Baylor College of Medicine
Houston, TX, USA
*Volume 3, Chapter 29 Secondary deformities of
the cleft lip, nose, and palate*
Volume 3, Video 29.01 Complete takedown
Volume 3, Video 29.02 Abbé flap
*Volume 3, Video 29.03 Thick lip and buccal
sulcus deformities*
Volume 3, Video 29.04 Alveolar bone grafting
Volume 3, Video 29.05 Definitive rhinoplasty

Evan Kowalski, BS
Section of Plastic Surgery
University of Michigan Health System
Ann Arbor, MI, USA
Volume 6, Video 19.02 Silicone MCP arthroplasty

Stephen J. Kovach, MD
Assistant Professor of Surgery
Division of Plastic and Reconstructive Surgery
University of Pennsylvannia Health System
Assistant Professor of Surgery
Department of Orthopaedic Surgery
University of Pennsylvannia Health System
Philadelphia, PA, USA
Volume 4, Chapter 7 Skeletal reconstruction

Steven J. Kronowitz, MD, FACS
Professor, Department of Plastic Surgery
MD Anderson Cancer Center
The University of Texas
Houston, TX, USA
Volume 1, Chapter 28 Therapeutic radiation principles, effects, and complications

Todd A. Kuiken, MD, PhD
Director
Center for Bionic Medicine
Rehabilitation Institute of Chicago
Professor
Department of PMandR
Fienberg School of Medicine
Northwestern University
Chicago, IL, USA
Volume 6, Chapter 40 Treatment of the upper extremity amputee
Volume 6, Video 40.01 Targeted muscle reinnervation in the transhumeral amputee

Michael E. Kupferman, MD
Assistant Professor
Department of Head and Neck Surgery
Division of Surgery
The University of Texas MD Anderson Cancer Center
Houston, TX, USA
Volume 3, Chapter 17 Carcinoma of the upper aerodigestive tract

Robert Kwon, MD
Plastic Surgeon
Regional Plastic Surgery Center
Richardson, TX, USA
Volume 4, Chapter 16 Pressure sores

Eugenia J. Kyriopoulos, MD, MSc, PhD, FEBOPRAS
Attending Plastic Surgeon
Department of Plastic Surgery and Burn Center
Athens General Hospital "G. Gennimatas"
Athens, Greece
Volume 5, Chapter 21 Local flaps in partial breast reconstruction

Donald Lalonde, BSC, MD, MSc, FRCSC
Professor Surgery
Division of Plastic Surgery
Saint John Campus of Dalhousie University
Saint John, NB, Canada
Volume 6, Chapter 24 Nerve entrapment syndromes
Volume 6, Video 24.01 Carpal tunnel and cubital tunnel releases

Wee Leon Lam, MB, ChB, M Phil, FRCS
Microsurgery Fellow
Department of Plastic and Reconstructive Surgery
Chang Gung Memorial Hospital
Taipei, Taiwan, The People's Republic of China
Volume 6, Chapter 14 Thumb and finger reconstruction – microsurgical techniques
Volume 6, Video 14.01 Trimmed great toe
Volume 6, Video 14.02 Second toe for index
Volume 6, Video 14.03 Combined second and third toe for metacarpal hand

Julie E. Lang, MD, FACS
Assistant Professor of Surgery
Department of surgery
Director of Breast Surgical Oncology
University of Arizona
Tucson, AZ, USA
Volume 5, Chapter 10 Breast cancer: Diagnosis therapy and oncoplastic techniques
Volume 5, Video 10.01 Breast cancer: diagnosis and therapy

Patrick Lang, MD
Plastic Surgery Resident
University of California
San Francisco, CA, USA
Volume 1, Chapter 24 Flap classification and applications

Claude-Jean Langevin, MD, DMD
Assistant Professor University of Central Florida
Department of Surgery MD Anderson Cancer Center
Plastic and Reconstructive Surgeon
University of Central Florida
Orlando, FL, USA
Volume 2, Chapter 13 Neck rejuvenation

Laurent Lantieri, MD
Department of Plastic Surgery
Hôpital Européen Georges Pompidou
Assistance Publique Hôpitaux de Paris
Paris Descartes University
Paris, France
Volume 3, Chapter 20 Facial transplant
Volume 3, Video 20.1 and 20.2 Facial transplant

Michael C. Large, MD
Urology Resident
Department of Surgery, Division of Urology
University of Chicago Hospitals
Chicago, IL, USA
Volume 3, Chapter 44 Reconstruction of urogenital defects: Congenital
Volume 3, Video 44.01 First stage hypospadias repair with free inner preputial graft
Volume 3, Video 44.02 Second stage hypospadias repair with tunica vaginalis flap

Don LaRossa, MD
Emeritus Professor of Surgery
Division of Plastic and Reconstructive Surgery
Perelman School of Medicine
University of Pennsylvania
Philadelphia, PA, USA
Volume 3, Chapter 43 Conjoined twins

Caroline Leclercq, MD
Consultant Hand Surgeon
Institut de la Main
Paris, France
Volume 6, Chapter 17 Management of Dupuytren's disease

Justine C. Lee, MD, PhD
Chief Resident
Section of Plastic and Reconstructive Surgery Department
University of Chicago Medical Center
Chicago, IL, USA
Volume 3, Chapter 41 Pediatric chest and trunk defects

W. P. Andrew Lee, MD
The Milton T. Edgerton, MD, Professor and Chairman
Department of Plastic and Reconstructive Surgery
Johns Hopkins University School of Medicine
Baltimore, MD, USA
Volume 1, Chapter 34 Transplantation in plastic surgery
Volume 6, Chapter 38 Upper extremity composite allotransplantation
Volume 6, Video 38.01 Upper extremity composite tissue allotransplantation

Valerie Lemaine, MD, MPH, FRCSC
Assistant Professor of Plastic Surgery
Department of Surgery
Division of Plastic Surgery
Mayo Clinic
Rochester, MN, USA
Volume 1, Chapter 10 Evidence-based medicine and health services research in plastic surgery

Ping-Chung Leung, SBS, OBE, JP, MBBS, MS, DSc, Hon DSocSc, FRACS, FRCS, FHKCOS, FHKAM (ORTH)
Professor Emeritus
Orthopaedics and Traumatology
The Chinese University of Hong Kong
Hong Kong, The People's Republic of China
Volume 6, Chapter 29 Congenital hand V disorders of overgrowth, undergrowth, and generalized skeletal deformities

Benjamin Levi, MD
Post Doctoral Research Fellow
Division of Plastic and Reconstructive Surgery
Stanford University
Stanford, CA
House Officer
Division of Plastic and Reconstructive Surgery
University of Michigan
Ann Arbor, MI, USA
Volume 1, Chapter 13 Stem cells and regenerative medicine

L. Scott Levin, MD, FACS
Chairman of Orthopedic Surgery
Department of Orthopaedic Surgery
University of Pennsylvania School of Medicine
Philadelphia, PA, USA
Volume 4, Chapter 7 Skeletal reconstruction

Bradley Limmer, MD
Assistant Clinical Professor
Department of Internal Medicine
Division of Dermatology
Associate Clinical Professor
Department of Plastic and Reconstructive
Surgery
Surgeon, Private Practice
Limmer Clinic
San Antonio, TX, USA
*Volume 2, Video 23.02 Follicular unit hair
transplantation*

Bobby L. Limmer, MD
Professor of Dermatology
University of Texas
Surgeon, Private Practice
Limmer Clinic
San Antonio, TX, USA
*Volume 2, Video 23.02 Follicular unit hair
transplantation*

Frank Lista, MD, FRCSC
Medical Director
Burn Program
The Plastic Surgery Clinic
Mississauga, ON, Canada
*Volume 5, Chapter 8.3 Superior or medial
pedicle*

Wei Liu, MD, PhD
Professor of Plastic Surgery
Associate Director of National Tissue
Engineering Research Center
Department of Plastic and Reconstructive
Surgery
Shanghai 9th People's Hospital
Shanghai Jiao Tong University School of
Medcine
Shanghai, The People's Republic of China
*Volume 1, Chapter 18 Tissue graft, tissue repair,
and regeneration*
*Volume 1, Chapter 20 Repair, grafting, and
engineering of cartilage*

Michelle B. Locke, MBChB, MD
Honourary Lecturer
University of Auckland Department of Surgery
Auckland City Hospital Support Building
Grafton, Auckland, New Zealand
*Volume 2, Chapter 1 Managing the cosmetic
patient*

Sarah A. Long, BA
Research Associate
Thayer School of Engineering
Dartmouth College
San Mateo, CA, USA
*Volume 1, Chapter 36 Robotics, simulation, and
telemedicine in plastic surgery*

Michael T. Longaker, MD, MBA, FACS
Deane P. and Louise Mitchell Professor and
Vice Chair
Department of Surgery
Stanford University
Stanford, CA, USA
*Volume 1, Chapter 13 Stem cells and
regenerative medicine*

Peter Lorenz, MD
Chief of Pediatric Plastic Surgery, Director
Craniofacial Surgery Fellowship
Department of Surgery, Division of Plastic
Surgery
Stanford University School of Medicine
Stanford, CA, USA
*Volume 1, Chapter 16 Scar prevention,
treatment, and revision*

Joseph E. Losee, MD, FACS, FAAP
Professor of Surgery and Pediatrics
Chief, Division Pediatric Plastic Surgery
Children's Hospital of Pittsburgh
University of Pittsburgh Medical Center
Pittsburgh, PA, USA
Volume 3, Chapter 31 Pediatric facial fractures

Albert Losken, MD, FACS
Associate Professor Program Director
Emory Division of Plastic and Reconstructive
Surgery
Emory University School of Medicine
Atlanta, GA, USA
*Volume 5, Chapter 11 The oncoplastic approach
to partial breast reconstruction*

Maria M. LoTempio, MD
Assistant Professor in Plastic Surgery
Medical University of South Carolina
Charleston, SC
Adjunct Assistant Professor in Plastic Surgery
New York Eye and Ear Infirmary
New York, NY, USA
*Volume 5, Chapter 19 Alternative flaps for breast
reconstruction*

Otway Louie, MD
Assistant Professor
Division of Plastic and Reconstructive Surgery
Department of Surgery
University of Washington Medical Center
Seattle, WA, USA
Volume 4, Chapter 17 Perineal reconstruction

David W. Low, MD
Professor of Surgery
Division of Plastic Surgery
University of Pennsylvania School of Medicine
Clinical Associate
The Children's Hospital of Philadelphia
Philadelphia, PA, USA
Volume 3, Chapter 43 Conjoined twins

Nicholas Lumen, MD, PhD
Assistant Professor of Urology
Urology
Ghent University Hospital
Ghent, Belgium
*Volume 4, Chapter 13 Reconstruction of male
genital defects*
*Volume 4, Video 13.01 Complete and partial
penile reconstruction*

Antonio Luiz de Vasconcellos Macedo, MD
General Surgery
Director of Robotic Surgery
President of Oncology
Board of Albert Einstein Hospital
Sao Paulo, Brazil
*Volume 5, Chapter 20 Omentum reconstruction
of the breast*

Gustavo R. Machado, MD
University of California Irvine Medical Center
Department of Orthopaedic Surgery, Orange,
CA, USA
*Volume 6, Video 34.01 EIP to EPL tendon
transfer*

Susan E. Mackinnon, MD
Sydney M. Shoenberg, Jr. and Robert H.
Shoenberg Professor
Department of Surgery, Division of Plastic and
Reconstructive Surgery
Washington University School of Medicine
St. Louis, MO, USA
*Volume 1, Chapter 22 Repair and grafting of
peripheral nerve*
Volume 6, Chapter 33 Nerve transfers
Volume 6, Video 33.01 Nerve transfers

Ralph T. Manktelow, BA, MD, FRCS(C)
Professor
Department of Surgery
University of Toronto
Toronto, ON, Canada
Volume 3, Chapter 11 Facial paralysis

Paul N. Manson, MD
Professor of Plastic Surgery
University of Maryland Shock Trauma Unit
University of Maryland and Johns Hopkins
Schools of Medicine
Baltimore, MD, USA
Volume 3, Chapter 3 Facial fractures

Daniel Marchac, MD
Professor
Plastic, Reconstructive and Aesthetic
College of Medicine of Paris Hospitals
Paris, France
Volume 3, Chapter 32 Orbital hypertelorism

Malcom W. Marks, MD
Professor and Chairman
Department of Plastic Surgery
Wake Forest University School of Medicine
Winston-Salem, NC, USA
*Volume 1, Chapter 27 Principles and applications
of tissue expansion*

Timothy J. Marten, MD, FACS
Founder and Director
Marten Clinic of Plastic Surgery
Medical Director
San Francisco Center for the Surgical Arts
San Francisco, CA, USA
*Volume 2, Chapter 12 Secondary deformities
and the secondary facelift*

Mario Marzola, MBBS
Private Practice
Norwood, SA, Australia
Volume 2, Video 23.01 Donor closure tricophytic technique

Alessandro Masellis, MD
Plastic Surgeon
Department of Plastic Surgery and Burn Therapy
Ospedale Civico ARNAS Palermo
Palermo, Italy
Volume 4, Chapter 19 Extremity burn reconstruction

Michele Masellis, MD, PhD
Plastic Surgeon
Former Chief
Professor Emeritus
Department of Plastic Surgery and Burn Unit
ARNAS Civico Hospital
Palermo, Italy
Volume 4, Chapter 19 Extremity burn reconstruction

Jaume Masia, MD, PhD
Professor and Chief
Plastic Surgery Department
Hospital de la Santa Creu i Sant Pau
Universidad Autónoma de Barcelona
Barcelona, Spain
Volume 5, Chapter 13 Imaging in reconstructive breast surgery

David W. Mathes, MD
Associate Professor of Surgery
Department of Surgery, Division of Plastic and Reconstructive Surgery
University of Washington School of Medicine
Chief of Plastic Surgery
Puget Sound Veterans Affairs Hospital
Seattle, WA, USA
Volume 1, Chapter 34 Transplantation in plastic surgery

Evan Matros, MD
Assistant Attending Surgeon
Department of Surgery
Memorial Sloan-Kettering Cancer Center
Assistant Professor of Surgery (Plastic)
Weill Cornell University Medical Center
New York, NY, USA
Volume 1, Chapter 12 Principles of cancer management

G. Patrick Maxwell, MD, FACS
Clinical Professor of Surgery
Department of Plastic Surgery
Loma Linda University Medical Center
Loma Linda, CA, USA
Volume 5, Chapter 2 Breast augmentation
Volume 5, Chapter 4 Current concepts in revisionary breast surgery

Isabella C. Mazzola
Milan, Italy
Volume 1, Chapter 2 History of reconstructive and aesthetic surgery

Riccardo F. Mazzola, MD
Professor of Plastic Surgery
Postgraduate School Plastic Surgery
Maxillo-Facial and Otolaryngolog
Department of Specialistic Surgical Science
School of Medicine
University of Milan
Milan, Italy
Volume 1, Chapter 2 History of reconstructive and aesthetic surgery

Steven J. McCabe, MD, MSc
Assistant Professor
Department of Bioinformatics and Biostatistics
University of Louisville School of Public Health and Information Sciences
Louisville, KY, USA
Volume 6, Chapter 18 Occupational hand disorders

Joseph G. McCarthy, MD
Lawrence D. Bell Professor of Plastic Surgery,
Director Institute of Reconstructive Plastic Surgery and Chair
Department of Plastic Surgery
New York University Langone Medical Center
New York, NY, USA
Volume 3, Chapter 36 Craniofacial microsomia

Mary H. McGrath, MD, MPH
Plastic Surgeon
Division of Plastic Surgery
University of California San Francisco
San Francisco, CA, USA
Volume 1, Chapter 3 Psychological aspects of plastic surgery

Kai Megerle, MD
Research Fellow
Division of Plastic and Reconstructive Surgery
Stanford Medical Center
Stanford, CA, USA
Volume 6, Chapter 10 Extensor tendon injuries

Babak J. Mehrara, MD, FACS
Associate Member, Associate Professor of Surgery (Plastic)
Memorial Sloan-Kettering Cancer Center
Weil Cornell University Medical Center
New York, NY, USA
Volume 1, Chapter 12 Principles of cancer management

Bryan Mendelson, FRCSE, FRACS, FACS
Private Plastic Surgeon
The Centre for Facial Plastic Surgery
Melbourne, Australia
Volume 2, Chapter 6 Anatomy of the aging face

Constantino G. Mendieta, MD, FACS
Private Practice
Miami, FL, USA
Volume 2, Chapter 28 Buttock augmentation
Volume 2, Video 28.01 Buttock augmentation

Frederick J. Menick, MD
Private Practitioner
Tucson, AZ, USA
Volume 3, Chapter 6 Aesthetic nasal reconstruction
Volume 3, Video 6.01 Aesthetic reconstruction of the nose – The 3-stage folded forehead flap for cover and lining,
Volume 3, Video 6.02 Aesthetic reconstruction of the nose-First stage transfer and intermediate operation

Ursula Mirastschijski, MD, PhD
Assistant Professor
Department of Plastic, Hand and Reconstructive Surgery, Burn Center Lower Saxony, Replantation Center
Hannover Medical School
Hannover, Germany
Volume 1, Chapter 15 Skin wound healing: Repair biology, wound, and scar treatment

Takayuki Miura, MD
Emeritus Professor of Orthopedic Surgery
Department of Orthopedic Surgery
Nagoya University School of Medicine
Nagoya, Japan
Volume 6, Chapter 29 Congenital hand V: Disorders of overgrowth, undergrowth, and generalized skeletal deformities

Fernando Molina, MD
Professor of Plastic, Aesthetic and Reconstructive Surgery
Reconstructive and Plastic Surgery
Hospital General "Dr. Manuel Gea Gonzalez"
Universidad Nacional Autonoma de Mexico
Mexico City, Mexico
Volume 3, Chapter 39 Treacher-Collins syndrome

Stan Monstrey, MD, PhD
Professor in Plastic Surgery
Department of Plastic Surgery
Ghent University Hospital
Ghent, Belgium
Volume 4, Chapter 13 Reconstruction of male genital defects
Volume 4, Video 13.01 Complete and partial penile reconstruction

Steven L. Moran, MD
Professor and Chair of Plastic Surgery
Division of Plastic Surgery, Division of Hand and Microsurgery
Professor of Orthopedics
Rochester, MN, USA
Volume 6, Chapter 20 Management of osteoarthritis of the hand and wrist

Luis Humberto Uribe Morelli, MD
Resident of Plastic Surgery
Unisanta Plastic Surgery Department
Sao Paulo, Brazil
Volume 2, Chapter 26 Lipoabdominoplasty
Volume 2, Video 26.01 Lipobdominoplasty
(including secondary lipo)

Robert J. Morin, MD
Plastic Surgeon and Craniofacial Surgeon
Department of Plastic Surgery
Hackensack University Medical Center
Hackensack, NJ
New York Eye and Ear Infirmary
New York, NY, USA
Volume 3, Chapter 8 Acquired cranial and facial
bone deformities

Steven F. Morris, MD, MSc, FRCS(C)
Professor of Surgery
Professor of Anatomy and Neurobiology
Dalhousie University
Halifax, NS, Canada
Volume 1, Chapter 23 Vascular territories

Colin Myles Morrison, MSc (Hons),
FRCSI (Plast)
Consultant Plastic Surgeon
Department of Plastic and Reconstructive
Surgery
St. Vincent's University Hospital
Dublin, Ireland
Volume 2, Chapter 13 Neck rejuvenation
Volume 5, Chapter 18 The deep inferior
epigastric artery perforator (DIEAP) flap

Wayne A. Morrison, MBBS, MD, FRACS
Director
O'Brien Institute
Professorial Fellow
Department of Surgery
St Vincent's Hospital
University of Melbourne
Plastic Surgeon
St Vincent's Hospital
Melbourne, Australia
Volume 1, Chapter 19 Tissue engineering

Robyn Mosher, MS
Medical Editor/Project Manager
Thayer School of Engineering (contract)
Dartmouth College
Norwich, VT, USA
Volume 1, Chapter 36 Robotics, simulation, and
telemedicine in plastic surgery

Dimitrios Motakis, MD, PhD, FRCSC
Plastic and Reconstructive Surgeon
Private Practice
University Lecturer
Department of Surgery
University of Toronto
Toronto, ON, Canada
Volume 2, Chapter 4 Soft-tissue fillers

A. Aldo Mottura, MD, PhD
Associate Professor of Surgery
School of Medicine
National University of Córdoba
Cordoba, Argentina
Volume 1, Chapter 9 Local anesthetics in plastic
surgery

Hunter R. Moyer, MD
Fellow
Department of Plastic and Reconstructive
Surgery
Emory University, Atlanta, GA, USA
Volume 5, Chapter 16 The bilateral Pedicled
TRAM flap

Gustavo Muchado, MD
Plastic surgeon
Division of Plastic and Reconstructive Surgery
and Department of Orthopaedic Surgery
University of California Irvine Medical Center
Orange, CA, USA
Volume 6, Video 34.01 EIP to EPL tendon
transfer

Reid V. Mueller, MD
Associate Professor
Division of Plastic and Reconstructive Surgery
Oregon Health and Science University
Portland, OR, USA
Volume 3, Chapter 2 Facial trauma: soft tissue
injuries

John B. Mulliken, MD
Director, Craniofacial Centre
Department of Plastic and Oral Surgery
Children's Hospital
Boston, MA, USA
Volume 1, Chapter 29 Vascular anomalies
Volume 3, Chapter 24 Repair of bilateral cleft lip

Egle Muti, MD
Associate Professor of Plastic Reconstructive
and Aesthetic Surgery
Department of Plastic Surgery
University of Turin School of Medicine
Turin, Italy
Volume 5, Chapter 23.1 Congenital anomalies of
the breast
Volume 5, Video 23.01.01 Congenital anomalies
of the breast: An example of tuberous breast
type 1 corrected with glandular flap type 1

Maurice Y. Nahabedian, MD
Associate Professor Plastic Surgery
Department of Plastic Surgery
Georgetown University and Johns Hopkins
University
Northwest, WA, USA
Volume 5, Chapter 22 Reconstruction of the
nipple-areola complex
Volume 5, Video 11.01 Partial breast
reconstruction using reduction mammaplasty
Volume 5, Video 11.03 Partial breast
reconstruction with a pedicle TRAM

Foad Nahai, MD, FACS
Clinical Professor of Plastic Surgery
Department of Surgery
Emory University School of Medicine
Atlanta, GA, USA
Volume 2, Chapter 1 Managing the cosmetic
patient

Fabio X. Nahas, MD, PhD
Associate Professor
Division of Plastic Surgery
Federal University of São Paulo
São Paulo, Brazil
Volume 2, Video 24.01 Liposculpture

Deepak Narayan, MS, FRCS (Eng),
FRCS (Edin)
Associate Professor of Surgery
Yale University School of Medicine
Chief
Plastic Surgery
VA Medical Center
West Haven, CT, USA
Volume 3, Chapter 14 Salivary gland tumors

Maurizio B. Nava, MD
Chief of Plastic Surgery Unit
Istituto Nazionale dei Tumori
Milano, Italy
Volume 5, Chapter 14 Expander/implant
reconstruction of the breast
Volume 5, Video 14.01 Mastectomy and
expander insertion: first stage
Volume 5, Video 14.02 Mastectomy and
expander insertion: second stage

Carmen Navarro, MD
Plastic Surgery Consultant
Plastic Surgery Department
Hospital de la Santa Creu i Sant Pau
Universidad Autónoma de Barcelona
Barcelona, Spain
Volume 5, Chapter 13 Imaging in reconstructive
breast surgery

Peter C. Neligan, MB, FRCS(I), FRCSC,
FACS
Professor of Surgery
Department of Surgery, Division of Plastic
Surgery
University of Washington
Seattle, WA, USA
Volume 1, Chapter 1 Plastic surgery and
innovation in medicine
Volume 1, Chapter 25 Flap pathophysiology and
pharmacology
Volume 3, Chapter 10 Cheek and lip
reconstruction
Volume 4, Chapter 3 Lymphatic reconstruction of
the extremities
Volume 3, Video 11.01-03 (1) Facial paralysis (2)
cross fact graft, (3) gracilis harvest
Volume 3, Video 18.01 Facial artery perforator
flap
Volume 4, Video 3.02 Charles Procedure
Volume 5, Video 18.01 SIEA
Volume 5, Video 19.01-19.03 Alternative free
flaps

Jonas A Nelson, MD
Integrated General/Plastic Surgery Resident
Department of Surgery
Division of Plastic Surgery
Perelman School of Medicine
University of Pennsylvania
Philadelphia, PA, USA
*Volume 5, Video 17.01 The muscle sparing free
TRAM flap*

David T. Netscher, MD
Clinical Professor
Division of Plastic Surgery
Baylor College of Medicine
Houston, TX, USA
*Volume 6, Chapter 21 The stiff hand and the
spastic hand*

Michael W. Neumeister, MD
Professor and Chairman
Division of Plastic Surgery
SIU School of Medicine
Springfield, IL, USA
*Volume 6, Chapter 6 Nail and fingertip
reconstruction*

M. Samuel Noordhoff, MD, FACS
Emeritus Superintendent
Chang Gung Memorial Hospitals
Taipei, Taiwan, The People's Republic of China
Volume 3, Chapter 23 Repair of unilateral cleft lip

Christine B. Novak, PT, PhD
Research Associate
Hand Program, Division of Plastic and
Reconstructive Surgery
University Health Network, University of Toronto
Toronto, ON, Canada
Volume 6, Chapter 39 Hand therapy

Daniel Nowinski, MD, PhD
Director
Department of Plastic and Maxillofacial Surgery
Uppsala Craniofacial Center
Uppsala University Hospital
Uppsala, Sweden
*Volume 1, Chapter 11 Genetics and prenatal
diagnosis*

Scott Oates, MD
Professor
Department of Plastic Surgery
The University of Texas MD Anderson Cancer
Center
Houston, TX, USA
*Volume 6, Chapter 15 Benign and malignant
tumors of the hand*

Kerby Oberg, MD, PhD
Associate Professor
Department of Pathology and Human Anatomy
Loma Linda University School of Medicine
Loma Linda, CA, USA
*Volume 6, Chapter 25 Congenital hand 1:
embryology, classification, and principles*

James P. O'Brien, MD, FRCSC
Associate Professor of Surgery
Dalhousie University
Halifax Nova Scotia
Clinical Associate Professor of Surgery
Memorial University
St. John's Newfoundland
Vice President Research
Innovation and Development
Horizon Health Network
New Brunswick, NB, Canada
*Volume 6, Chapter 24 Nerve entrapment
syndromes*

Andrea J. O'Connor, BE(Hons), PhD
Associate Professor of Chemical and
Biomolecular Engineering
Department of Chemical and Biomolecular
Engineering
University of Melbourne
Melbourne, VIC, Australia
Volume 1, Chapter 19 Tissue engineering

Rei Ogawa, MD, PhD
Associate Professor
Department of Plastic
Reconstructive and Aesthetic Surgery Nippon
Medical School
Tokyo, Japan
*Volume 1, Chapter 30 Benign and malignant
nonmelanocytic tumors of the skin and soft
tissue*

Dennis P. Orgill, MD, PhD
Professor of Surgery
Division of Plastic Surgery, Brigham and
Women's Hospital
Harvard Medical School
Boston, MA, USA
Volume 1, Chapter 17 Skin graft

Cho Y. Pang, PhD
Senior Scientist
Research Institute
The Hospital for Sick Children
Professor
Departments of Surgery/Physiology
University of Toronto
Toronto, ON, Canada
*Volume 1, Chapter 25 Flap pathophysiology and
pharmacology*

Ketan M. Patel, MD
Resident Physician
Department of Plastic Surgery
Georgetown University Hospital
Washington DC, USA
*Volume 5, Chapter 22 Reconstruction of the
nipple-areola complex*

William C. Pederson, MD, FACS
President and Fellowship Director
The Hand Center of San Antonio
Adjunct Professor of Surgery
The University of Texas Health Science Center
at San Antonio
San Antonio, TX, USA
*Volume 6, Chapter 12 Reconstructive surgery of
the mutilated hand*

José Abel de la Peña Salcedo, MD
Secretario Nacional
Federación Iberolatinoamericana de Cirugía
Plástica, Estética y Reconstructiva
Director del Instituto de Cirugia Plastica, S.C.
Hospital Angeles de las Lomas
Col.Valle de las Palmas
Huixquilucan, Edo de Mexico, Mexico
Volume 2, Chapter 28 Buttock augmentation
Volume 2, Video 28.01 Buttock augmentation

Angela Pennati, MD
Assistant Plastic Surgeon
Unit of Plastic Surgery
Istituto Nazionale dei Tumori
Milano, Italy
*Volume 5, Chapter 14 Expander/implant breast
reconstructions*
*Volume 5, Video 14.01 Mastectomy and
expander insertion: first stage*
*Volume 5, Video 14.02 Mastectomy and
expander insertion: second stage*

Joel E. Pessa, MD
Clinical Associate Professor of Plastic Surgery
UTSW Medical School
Dallas, TX
Hand and Microsurgery Fellow
Christine M. Kleinert Hand and Microsurgery
Louisville, KY, USA
*Volume 2, Chapter 17 Nasal analysis and
anatomy*

Walter Peters, MD, PhD, FRCSC
Professor of Surgery
Department of Plastic Surgery
University of Toronto
Toronto, ON, Canada
*Volume 5, Chapter 6 Iatrogenic disorders
following breast surgery*

Giorgio Pietramaggiori, MD, PhD
Plastic Surgery Resident
Department of Plastic and Reconstructive
Surgery
University Hospital of Lausanne
Lausanne, Switzerland
Volume 1, Chapter 17 Skin graft

John W. Polley, MD
Professor and Chairman
Rush University Medical Center
Department of Plastic and Reconstructive
Surgery
John W. Curtin – Chair
Co-Director, Rush Craniofacial Center
Chicago, IL, USA
*Volume 3, Chapter 27 Orthodontics in cleft lip
and palate management*

Bohdan Pomahac, MD
Assistant Professor
Harvard Medical School
Director
Plastic Surgery Transplantation
Medical Director
Burn Center
Division of Plastic Surgery
Brigham and Women's Hospital
Boston, MA, USA
Volume 1, Chapter 11 Genetics and prenatal diagnosis

Julian J. Pribaz, MD
Professor of Surgery Harvard Medical School
Division of Plastic Surgery
Brigham and Women's Hospital
Boston, MA, USA
Volume 3, Chapter 19 Secondary facial reconstruction

Andrea L. Pusic, MD, MHS, FRCSC
Associate Attending Surgeon
Department of Plastic and Reconstructive
Memorial Sloan-Kettering Cancer Center
New York, NY, USA
Volume 1, Chapter 10 Evidence-based medicine and health services research in plastic surgery
Volume 4, Chapter 14 Reconstruction of acquired vaginal defects

Oscar M. Ramirez, MD, FACS
Adjunct Clinical Faculty
Plastic Surgery Division
Cleveland Clinic Florida
Boca Raton, FL, USA
Volume 2, Chapter 11.8 Facelift: Subperiosteal facelift
Volume 2, Video 11.08.01 Facelift: Subperiosteal mid facelift endoscopic temporo-midface

William R. Rassman, MD
Director
Private Practice
New Hair Institution
Los Angeles, CA, USA
Volume 2, Video 23.04 FUE FOX procedure

Russell R. Reid, MD, PhD
Assistant Professor of Surgery, Bernard Sarnat Scholar
Section of Plastic and Reconstructive Surgery
University of Chicago
Chicago, IL, USA
Volume 1, Chapter 21 Repair and grafting of bone
Volume 3, Chapter 41 Pediatric chest and trunk defects

Neal R. Reisman, MD, JD
Chief of Plastic Surgery, Clinical Professor
Plastic Surgery
St. Luke's Episcopal Hospital
Baylor College of Medicine
Houston, TX, USA
Volume 1, Chapter 6 Medico-legal issues in plastic surgery

Dominique Renier, MD, PhD
Pediatric Neurosurgeon
Service de Neurochirurgie Pédiatrique
Hôpital Necker-Enfants Malades
Paris, France
Volume 3, Chapter 32 Orbital hypertelorism

Dirk F. Richter, MD, PhD
Clinical Director
Department of Plastic Surgery
Dreifaltigkeits-Hospital Wesseling
Wesseling, Germany
Volume 2, Chapter 25 Abdominoplasty procedures
Volume 2, Video 25.01 Abdominoplasty

Thomas L. Roberts III, FACS
Plastic Surgery Center of the Carolinas
Spartanburg, SC, USA
Volume 2, Chapter 28 Buttock augmentation
Volume 2, Video 28.01 Buttock augmentation

Federico Di Rocco, MD, PhD
Pediatric Neurosurgery
Hôpital Necker Enfants Malades
Paris, France
Volume 3, Chapter 32 Orbital hypertelorism

Natalie Roche, MD
Associate Professor
Department of Plastic Surgery
Ghent University Hospital
Ghent, Belgium
Volume 4, Chapter 13 Reconstruction of male genital defects
Volume 4, Video 13.01 Complete and partial penile reconstruction

Eduardo D. Rodriguez, MD, DDS
Chief, Plastic Reconstructive and Maxillofacial Surgery, R Adams Cowley Shock Trauma Center
Professor of Surgery
University of Maryland School of Medicine
Baltimore, MD, USA
Volume 3, Chapter 3 Facial fractures

Thomas E. Rohrer, MD
Director, Mohs Surgery
SkinCare Physicians of Chestnut Hill
Clinical Associate Professor
Department of Dermatology
Boston University
Boston, MA, USA
Volume 2, Video 5.02 Facial resurfacing

Rod J. Rohrich, MD, FACS
Professor and Chairman Crystal Charity Ball
Distinguished Chair in Plastic Surgery
Department of Plastic Surgery
Professor and Chairman Betty and Warren
Woodward Chair in Plastic and Reconstructive Surgery
University of Texas Southwestern Medical Center at Dallas
Dallas, TX, USA
Volume 2, Chapter 17 Nasal analysis and anatomy
Volume 2, Chapter 18 Open technique rhinoplasty

Joseph M. Rosen, MD
Professor of Surgery
Division of Plastic Surgery, Department of Surgery
Dartmouth-Hitchcock Medical Center
Lyme, NH, USA
Volume 1, Chapter 36 Robotics, simulation, and telemedicine in plastic surgery

E. Victor Ross, MD
Director of Laser and Cosmetic Dermatology
Scripps Clinic
San Diego, CA, USA
Volume 2, Chapter 5 Facial skin resurfacing

Michelle C. Roughton, MD
Chief Resident
Section of Plastic and Reconstructive Surgery
University of Chicago Medical Center
Chicago, IL, USA
Volume 4, Chapter 10 Reconstruction of the chest

Sashwati Roy, PhD
Associate Professor of Surgery
Department of Surgery
The Ohio State University Medical Center
Columbus, OH, USA
Volume 1, Chapter 14 Wound healing

J. Peter Rubin, MD, FACS
Chief of Plastic Surgery
Director, Life After Weight Loss Body Contouring Program
University of Pittsburgh
Pittsburgh, PA, USA
Volume 2, Chapter 30 Post-bariatric reconstruction
Volume 2, Video 30.01 Post bariatric reconstruction – bodylift procedure
Volume 5, Chapter 25 Contouring of the arms, breast, upper trunk, and male chest in the massive weight loss patient
Volume 5, Video 25.01 Brachioplasty part 1: contouring of the arms
Volume 5, Video 25.02 Bracioplasty part 2: contouring of the arms

Alesia P. Saboeiro, MD
Attending Physician
Private Practice
New York, NY, USA
Volume 2, Chapter 14 Structural fat grafting
Volume 2, Video 14.01 Structural fat grafting of
the face

Justin M. Sacks, MD
Assistant Professor
Department of Plastic and Reconstructive
Surgery
The Johns Hopkins University School of
Medicine
Baltimore, MD, USA
Volume 3, Chapter 17 Carcinoma of the upper
aerodigestive tract
Volume 6, Chapter 15 Benign and malignant
tumors of the hand

Hakim K. Said, MD
Assistant Professor of Surgery
Division of Plastic Surgery
University of Washington
Seattle, WA, USA
Volume 4, Chapter 17 Perineal reconstruction

Michel Saint-Cyr, MD, FRCSC
Associate Professor Plastic Surgery
Department of Plastic Surgery
University of Texas Southwestern Medical
Center
Dallas, TX, USA
Volume 4, Chapter 2 Management of lower
extremity trauma
Volume 4, Video 2.01 Alternative flap harvest

Cristianna Bonneto Saldanha, MD
Resident
General Surgery Department
Santa Casa of Santos Hospital
São Paulo, Brazil
Volume 2, Chapter 26 Lipoabdominoplasty
Volume 2, Video 26.01 Lipobdominoplasty
(including secondary lipo)

Osvaldo Ribeiro Saldanha, MD
Chairman of Plastic Surgery
Unisanta
Santos
Past President of the Brazilian Society of
Plastic Surgery (SBCP)
International Associate Editor of Plastic and
Reconstructive Surgery
São Paulo, Brazil
Volume 2, Chapter 26 Lipoabdominoplasty
Volume 2, Video 26.01 Lipobdominoplasty
(including secondary lipo)

Osvaldo Ribeiro Saldanha Filho, MD
São Paulo, Brazil
Volume 2, Chapter 26 Lipoabdominoplasty
Volume 2, Video 26.01 Lipobdominoplasty
(including secondary lipo)

Douglas M. Sammer, MD
Assistant Professor of Plastic Surgery
Department of Plastic Surgery
University of Texas Southwestern Medical
Center
Dallas, TX, USA
Volume 6, Chapter 19 Rheumatologic conditions
of the hand and wrist

Joao Carlos Sampaio Goes, MD, PhD
Director Instituto Brasileiro Controle Cancer
Chairman
Department Plastic Surgery and Mastology of
IBCC
Sao Paulo, Brazil
Volume 5, Chapter 8.6 Periareolar technique with
mesh support
Volume 5, Chapter 20 Omentum reconstruction
of the breast

Michael Sauerbier, MD, PhD
Chairman and Professor
Department for Plastic, Hand and
Reconstructive Surgery
Cooperation Hospital for Plastic Surgery of the
University Hospital Frankfurt
Academic Hospital University of Frankfurt a.
Main
Frankfurt, Germany
Volume 4, Chapter 4 Lower extremity sarcoma
reconstruction
Volume 4, Video 4.01 Management of lower
extremity sarcoma reconstruction

Hani Sbitany, MD
Plastic and Reconstructive Surgery
Assistant Professor of Surgery
University of California
San Francisco, CA, USA
Volume 1, Chapter 24 Flap classification and
applications

Tim Schaub, MD
Private Practice
Arizona Center for Hand Surgery, PC
Phoenix, AZ, USA
Volume 6, Chapter 16 Infections of the hand

Loren S. Schechter, MD, FACS
Assistant Professor of Surgery
Chief, Division of Plastic Surgery
Chicago Medical School
Chicago, IL, USA
Volume 4, Chapter 15 Surgery for gender identity
disorder

Stephen A. Schendel, MD
Professor Emeritus of Surgery and Clinical
Adjunct Professor of Neurosurgery
Department of Surgery and Neurosurgery
Stanford University Medical Center
Stanford, CA, USA
Volume 3, Chapter 4 TMJ dysfunction and
obstructive sleep apnea

Saja S. Scherer-Pietramaggiori, MD
Plastic Surgery Resident
Department of Plastic and Reconstructive
Surgery
University Hospital of Lausanne
Lausanne, Switzerland
Volume 1, Chapter 17 Skin graft

Clark F. Schierle, MD, PhD
Vice President
Aesthetic and Reconstructive Plastic Surgery
Northwestern Plastic Surgery Associates
Chicaho, IL, USA
Volume 5, Chapter 5 Endoscopic approaches to
the breast

Stefan S. Schneeberger, MD
Visiting Associate Professor of Surgery
Department of Plastic Surgery
Johns Hopkins Medical University
Baltimore, MD, USA
Associate Professor of Surgery
Center for Operative Medicine
Department for Viszeral
Transplant and Thoracic Surgery
Innsbruck Medical University
Innsbruck, Austria
Volume 6, Chapter 38 Upper extremity
composite allotransplantation

Iris A. Seitz, MD, PhD
Director of Research and International
Collaboration
University Plastic Surgery
Rosalind Franklin University
Clinical Instructor of Surgery
Chicago Medical School
University Plastic Surgery, affiliated with
Chicago Medical School, Rosalind Franklin
University
Morton Grove, IL, USA
Volume 1, Chapter 21 Repair and grafting of
bone

Chandan K. Sen, PhD, FACSM, FACN
Professor and Vice Chairman (Research) of
Surgery
Department of Surgery
The Ohio State University Medical Center
Associate Dean
Translational and Applied Research
College of Medicine
Executive Director
OSU Comprehensive Wound Center
Columbus, OH, USA
Volume 1, Chapter 14 Wound healing

Subhro K. Sen, MD
Clinical Assistant Professor
Division of Plastic and Reconstructive Surgery
Robert A. Chase Hand and Upper Limb
Center, Stanford University Medical Center
Palo Alto, CA, USA
Volume 1, Chapter 14 Wound healing
Volume 6, Chapter 4 Anesthesia for upper
extremity surgery
Volume 6, Video 4.01 Anesthesia for upper
extremity surgery

Joseph M. Serletti, MD, FACS
Henry Royster – William Maul Measey
Professor of Surgery and Chief
Division of Plastic Surgery
Vice Chair (Finance)
Department of Surgery
University of Pennsylvania
Philadelphia, PA, USA
Volume 5, Chapter 17 Free TRAM breast
reconstruction
Volume 5, Video 17.01 The muscle sparing free
TRAM flap

Randolph Sherman, MD
Vice Chair
Department of Surgery
Cedars-Sinai Medical Center
Los Angeles, CA, USA
Volume 6, Chapter 12 Reconstructive surgery of
the mutilated hand

Kenneth C. Shestak, MD
Professor of Plastic Surgery
Division of Plastic Surgery
University of Pittsburgh
Pittsburgh, PA, USA
Volume 5, Chapter 9 Revision surgery following
breast reduction and mastopexy
Volume 5, Video 7.01 Circum areola mastopexy

Lester Silver, MD, MS
Professor of Surgery
Department of Surgery/Division of Plastic
Surgery
Mount Sinai School of Medicine
New York, NY, USA
Volume 3, Chapter 37 Hemifacial atrophy

Navin K. Singh, MD, MSc
Assistant Professor of Plastic Surgery
Department of Plastic Surgery
Johns Hopkins University School of Medicine
Washington, DC, USA
Volume 4, Chapter 12 Abdominal wall
reconstruction

Vanila M. Singh, MD
Clinical Associate Professor
Stanford University Medical Center
Department of Anesthesiology and Pain
Management
Stanford, CA, USA
Volume 6, Chapter 4 Anesthesia for upper
extremity surgery

Carla Skytta, DO
Resident
Department of Surgery
Doctors Hospital
Columbus, OH, USA
Volume 3, Chapter 5 Scalp and forehead
reconstruction

Darren M. Smith, MD
Resident
Division of Plastic Surgery
University of Pittsburgh Medical Center
Pittsburgh, PA, USA
Volume 3, Chapter 31 Pediatric facial fractures

**Gill Smith, MB, BCh, FRCS(Ed),
FRCS(Plast)**
Consultant Hand, Plastic and Reconstructive
Surgeon
Great Ormond Street Hospital
London, UK
Volume 6, Chapter 26 Congenital hand II Failure
of formation (transverse and longitudinal arrest)

Paul Smith, MBBS, FRCS
Honorary Consultant Plastic Surgeon
Great Ormond Street Hospital London, UK
Volume 6, Chapter 26 Congenital hand II Failure
of formation (transverse and longitudinal arrest)

Laura Snell, MSc, MD, FRCSC
Assistant Professor
Division of Plastic Surgery
University of Toronto
Toronto, ON, Canada
Volume 4, Chapter 14 Reconstruction of
acquired vaginal defects

Nicole Z. Sommer, MD
Assistant Professor of Plastic Surgery
Southern Illinois University School of Medicine
Springfield, IL, USA
Volume 6, Chapter 6 Nail and fingertip
reconstruction

David H. Song, MD, MBA, FACS
Cynthia Chow Professor of Surgery
Chief, Section of Plastic and Reconstructive
Surgery
Vice-Chairman, Department of Surgery
The University of Chicago Medicine & Biological
Sciences
Chicago, IL, USA
Volume 4, Chapter 10 Reconstruction of the
chest

Andrea Spano, MD
Senior Assistant Plastic Surgeon
Unit of Plastic Surgery
Istituto Nazionale dei Tumori
Milano, Italy
Volume 5, Chapter 14 Expander/implant breast
reconstructions
Volume 5, Video 14.01 Mastectomy and
expander insertion: first stage
Volume 5, Video 14.02 Mastectomy and
expander insertion: second stage

Scott L. Spear, MD, FACS
Professor and Chairman
Department of Plastic Surgery
Georgetown University Hospital
Georgetown, WA, USA
Volume 5, Chapter 15 Latissimus dorsi flap
breast reconstruction
Volume 5, Chapter 26 Fat grafting to the breast
Volume 5, Video 15.01 Latissimus dorsi flap
technique

Robert J. Spence, MD
Director
National Burn Reconstruction Center
Good Samaritan Hospital
Baltimore, MD, USA
Volume 4, Chapter 21 Management of facial
burns
Volume 4, Video 21.01 Management of the
burned face intra-dermal skin closure
Volume 4, Video 21.02 Management of the
burned face full-thickness skin graft defatting
technique

Samuel Stal, MD, FACS
Professor and Chief
Division of Plastic Surgery, Baylor College of
Medicine and Texas Children's Hospital
Houston, TX, USA
Volume 3, Chapter 29 Secondary deformities of
the cleft lip, nose, and palate
Volume 3, Video 29.01 Complete takedown
Volume 3, Video 29.02 Abbé flap
Volume 3, Video 29.03 Thick lip and buccal
sulcus deformities
Volume 3, Video 29.04 Alveolar bone grafting
Volume 3, Video 29.05 Definitive rhinoplasty

Derek M. Steinbacher, MD, DMD
Assistant Professor
Plastic and Carniomaxillofacial Surgery
Yale University, School of Medicine
New Haven, CT, USA
Volume 3, Chapter 34 Nonsyndromic
craniosynostosis

Douglas S. Steinbrech, MD, FACS
Gotham Plastic Surgery
New York, NY, USA
Volume 2, Chapter 9 Secondary blepharoplasty:
Techniques

Lars Steinstraesser, MD
Heisenberg-Professor for Molecular Oncology
and Wound Healing
Department of Plastic and Reconstructive
Surgery, Burn Center
BG University Hospital Bergmannsheil, Ruhr
University
Bochum, North Rhine-Westphalia, Germany
Volume 4, Chapter 18 Acute management of
burn/electrical injuries

Phillip J. Stephan, MD
Clinical Instructor
Department of Plastic Surgery
University of Texas Southwestern
Wichita Falls, TX, USA
*Volume 2, Chapter 24 Liposuction: A
comprehensive review of techniques and safety*

Laurie A. Stevens, MD
Associate Clinical Professor of Psychiatry
Columbia University College of Physicians and
Surgeons
New York, NY, USA
*Volume 1, Chapter 3 Psychological aspects of
plastic surgery*

Alexander Stoff, MD, PhD
Senior Fellow
Department of Plastic Surgery
Dreifaltigkeits-Hospital Wesseling
Wesseling, Germany
*Volume 2, Chapter 25 Abdominoplasty
procedures*
Volume 2, Video 25.01 Abdominoplasty

Dowling B. Stough, MD
Medical Director
The Dermatology Clinic
Clinical Assistant Professor
Department of Dermatology
University of Arkansas for Medical Sciences
Little Rock, AR, USA
Volume 2, Video 23.09 Tension donor dissection

James M. Stuzin, MD
Associate Professor of Surgery (Plastic)
Voluntary
University of Miami Leonard M. Miller School of
Medicine
Miami, FL, USA
*Volume 2, Chapter 11.6 Facelift: The extended
SMAS technique in facial rejuvenation*
*Volume 2, Video 11.06.01 Facelift – Extended
SMAS technique in facial shaping*

John D. Symbas, MD
Plastic and Reconstructive Surgeon
Private Practice
Marietta Plastic Surgery
Marietta, GA, USA
*Volume 5, Chapter 16 The bilateral pedicled
TRAM flap*
*Volume 5, Video 16.01 Pedicle TRAM breast
reconstruction*

Amir Taghinia, MD
Instructor in Surgery
Harvard Medical School
Staff Surgeon
Department of Plastic and Oral Surgery
Children's Hospital
Boston, MA, USA
*Volume 6, Chapter 27 Congenital hand III
disorders of formation – thumb hypoplasia*
*Volume 6, Video 27.01 Congenital hand III
disorders of formation – thumb hypoplasia*
*Volume 6, Video 31.01 Vascular anomalies of
the upper extremity*

David M.K. Tan, MBBS
Consultant
Department of Hand and Reconstructive
Microsurgery
National University Hospital
Yong Loo Lin School of Medicine
National University Singapore
Kent Ridge, Singapore
*Volume 6, Chapter 3 Diagnostic imaging of the
hand and wrist*
*Volume 6, Video 3.01 Diagnostic imaging of the
hand and wrist – Scaphoid lunate dislocation*

Jin Bo Tang, MD
Professor and Chair
Department of Hand Surgery
Chair
The Hand Surgery Research Center
Affiliated Hospital of Nantong University
Nantong, The People's Republic of China
*Volume 6, Chapter 9 Flexor tendon injuries and
reconstruction*
*Volume 6, Video 9.01 Flexor tendon injuries and
reconstruction – Partial venting of the A2 pulley*
*Volume 6, Video 9.02 Flexor tendon injuries and
reconstruction – Making a 6-strand repair*
*Volume 6, Video 9.03 Complete flexor-extension
without bowstringing*

Daniel I. Taub, DDS, MD
Assistant Professor
Oral and Maxillofacial Surgery
Thomas Jefferson University Hospital
Philadelphia, PA, USA
*Volume 2, Chapter 16 Anthropometry,
cephalometry, and orthognathic surgery*
*Volume 2, Video 16.01 Anthropometry,
cephalometry, and orthognathic surgery*

Peter J. Taub, MD, FACS, FAAP
Associate Professor, Surgery and Pediatrics
Division of Plastic and Reconstructive Surgery
Mount Sinai School of Medicine
New York, NY, USA
Volume 3, Chapter 37 Hemifacial atrophy

**Sherilyn Keng Lin Tay, MBChB,
MRCS, MSc**
Microsurgical Fellow
Department of Plastic Surgery
Chang Gung Memorial Hospital
Taoyuan, Taiwan, The People's Republic of
China
Specialist Registrar
Department of Reconstructive and Plastic
Surgery
St George's Hospital
London, UK
*Volume 1, Chapter 26 Principles and techniques
of microvascular surgery*

**G. Ian Taylor, AO, MBBS, MD, MD
(HonBrodeaux), FRACS, FRCS (Eng),
FRCS (Hon Edinburgh), FRCSI (Hon),
FRSC (Hon Canada), FACS (Hon)**
Professor
Deparment of Plastic Surgery
Royal Melbourne Hospital
Professor
Department of Anatomy
University of Melbourne
Melbourne, Australia
Volume 1, Chapter 23 Vascular territories

Oren M. Tepper, MD
Assistant Professor
Plastic and Reconstructive Surgery
Montefiore Medical Center
Albert Einstein College of Medicine
New York, NY, USA
Volume 3, Chapter 36 Craniofacial microsomia

Chad M. Teven, BS
Research Associate
Section of Plastic and Reconstructive Surgery
University of Chicago
Chicago, IL, USA
*Volume 1, Chapter 21 Repair and grafting of
bone*

Brinda Thimmappa, MD
Adjunct Assistant Professor
Department of Plastic and Reconstructive
Surgery
Loma Linda Medical Center
Loma Linda, CA
Plastic Surgeon
Division of Plastic and Maxillofacial Surgery
Southwest Washington Medical Center
Vancouver, WA, USA
*Volume 3, Chapter 4 TMJ dysfunction and
obstructive sleep apnea*

Johan Thorfinn, MD, PhD
Senior Consultant of Plastic Surgery, Burn Unit
Co-Director
Department of Plastic Surgery, Hand Surgery,
and Burns
Linköping University Hospital
Linköping, Sweden
*Volume 6, Chapter 32 Peripheral nerve injuries of
the upper extremity*
*Volume 6, Video 32.01-02 Peripheral nerve
injuries (1) Digital Nerve Suture (2) Median Nerve
Suture*

Charles H. Thorne, MD
Associate Professor of Plastic Surgery
Department of Plastic Surgery
NYU School of Medicine
New York, NY, USA
Volume 2, Chapter 22 Otoplasty

Michael Tonkin, MBBS, MD, FRACS (Orth), FRCS Ed Orth
Professor of Hand Surgery
Department of Hand Surgery and Peripheral Nerve Surgery
Royal North Shore Hospital
The Childrens Hospital at Westmead
University of Sydney Medical School
Sydney, Australia
Volume 6, Chapter 25 Congenital hand 1 Principles, embryology, and classification
Volume 6, Chapter 29 Congenital hand V Disorders of Overgrowth, Undergrowth, and Generalized Skeletal Deformities (addendum)

Patrick L Tonnard, MD
Coupure Centrum Voor Plastische Chirurgie
Ghent, Belgium
Volume 2, Video 11.04.01 Loop sutures MACS facelift

Kathryn S. Torok, MD
Assistant Professor
Division of Pediatric Rheumatology
Department of Pediatrics
Univeristy of Pittsburgh School of Medicine
Childrens Hospital of Pittsburgh
Pittsburgh, PA, USA
Volume 3, Chapter 37 Hemifacial atrophy

Ali Totonchi, MD
Assistant Professor of Surgery
Division of Plastic Surgery
MetroHealth Medical Center
Case Western Reserve University
Cleveland, OH, USA
Volume 3, Chapter 21 Surgical management of migraine headaches

Jonathan W. Toy, MD
Body Contouring Fellow
Division of Plastic and Reconstructive Surgery
University of Pittsburgh
University of Pittsburgh Medical Center Suite
Pittsburg, PA, USA
Volume 2, Chapter 30 Post-bariatric reconstruction
Volume 5, Chapter 25 Contouring of the arms, breast, upper trunk, and male chest in the massive weight loss patient

Matthew J. Trovato, MD
Dallas Plastic Surgery Institute
Dallas, TX, USA
Volume 2, Chapter 29 Upper limb contouring
Volume 2, Video 29.01 Upper limb contouring

Anthony P. Tufaro, DDS, MD, FACS
Associate Professor of Surgery and Oncology
Departments of Plastic Surgery and Oncology
Johns Hopkins University
Baltimore, MD, USA
Volume 3, Chapter 16 Tumors of the lips, oral cavity, oropharynx, and mandible

Joseph Upton III, MD
Clinical Professor of Surgery
Department of Plastic Surgery
Children's Hospital Boston
Shriner's Burn Hospital Boston
Beth Israel Deaconess Hospital
Harvard Medical School
Boston, MA, USA
Volume 6, Chapter 27 Congenital hand III disorders of formation – thumb hypoplasia
Volume 6, Chapter 31 Vascular anomalies of the upper extremity
Volume 6, Video 27.01 Congenital hand III disorders of formation – thumb hypoplasia
Volume 6, Video 31.01 Vascular anomalies of the upper extremity

Walter Unger, MD
Clinical Professor
Department of Dermatology
Mount Sinai School of Medicine
New York, NY
Associate Professor (Dermatology)
University of Toronto
Private Practice
New York, NY, USA
Toronto, ON, Canada
Volume 2, Video 23.06 Hair transplantation

Francisco Valero-Cuevas, PhD
Director
Brain-Body Dynamics Laboratory
Professor of Biomedical Engineering
Professor of Biokinesiology and Physical Therapy
By courtesy Professor of Computer Science and Aerospace and Mechanical Engineering
The University of Southern California
Los Angeles, CA, USA
Volume 6, Chapter 1 Anatomy and biomechanics of the hand

Allen L. Van Beek, MD, FACS
Adjunct Professor
University Minnesota School of Medicine
Division Plastic Surgery
Minneapolis, MN, USA
Volume 2, Video 3.01 Botulinum toxin
Volume 2, Video 4.01 Soft tissue fillers
Volume 2, Video 5.01 Chemical peel
Volume 2, Video 18.01 Open technique rhinoplasty

Nicholas B. Vedder
Professor of Surgery and Orthopaedics
Chief of Plastic Surgery Vice Chair, Department of Surgery
University of Washington
Seattle, WA, USA
Volume 6, Chapter 13 Thumb reconstruction: non microsurgical techniques

Valentina Visintini Cividin, MD
Assistant Plastic Surgeon
Unit of Plastic Surgery
Istituto Nazionale dei Tumori
Milano, Italy
Volume 5, Chapter 14 Expander/implant reconstruction of the breast
Volume 5, Video 14.01 Mastectomy and expander insertion: first stage
Volume 5, Video 14.02 Mastectomy and expander insertion: second stage

Peter M. Vogt, MD, PhD
Professor and Chairman
Department of Plastic Hand and Reconstructive Surgery
Hannover Medical School
Hannover, Germany
Volume 1, Chapter 15 Skin wound healing: Repair biology, wound, and scar treatment

Richard J. Warren, MD, FRCSC
Clinical Professor
Division of Plastic Surgery
University of British Columbia
Vancouver, BC, Canada
Volume 2, Chapter 7 Forehead rejuvenation
Volume 2, Chapter 11.1 Facelift: Principles
Volume 2, Chapter 11.2 Facelift: Introduction to deep tissue techniques
Volume 2, Video 7.01 Modified Lateral Brow Lift
Volume 2, Video 11.1.01 Parotid masseteric fascia
Volume 2, Video 11.1.02 Anterior incision
Volume 2, Video 11.1.03 Posterior Incision
Volume 2, Video 11.1.04 Facelift skin flap
Volume 2, Video 11.1.05 Facial fat injection

Andrew J. Watt, MD
Plastic Surgeon
Department of Surgery
Division of Plastic and Reconstructive Surgery
Stanford University Medical Center
Stanford University Hospital and Clinics
Palo Alto, CA, USA
Volume 6, Chapter 17 Management of Dupuytren's disease
Volume 6, Video 17.01 Management of Dupuytren's disease

Simeon H. Wall, Jr., MD, FACS
Private Practice
The Wall Center for Plastic Surgery
Gratis Faculty
Division of Plastic Surgery
Department of Surgery
LSU Health Sciences Center at Shreveport
Shreveport, LA, USA
Volume 2, Chapter 21 Secondary rhinoplasty

Derrick C. Wan, MD
Assistant Professor
Department of Surgery
Stanford University School of Medicine
Stanford, CA, USA
Volume 1, Chapter 13 Stem cells and regenerative medicine

Renata V. Weber, MD
Assistant Professor Surgery (Plastics)
Division of Plastic and Reconstructive Surgery
Albert Einstein College of Medicine
Bronx, NY, USA
Volume 1, Chapter 22 Repair and grafting of peripheral nerve

Fu Chan Wei, MD
Professor
Department of Plastic Surgery
Chang Gung Memorial Hospital
Taoyuan, Taiwan, The People's Republic of China
Volume 1, Chapter 26 Principles and techniques of microvascular surgery
Volume 6, Chapter 14 Thumb and finger reconstruction – microsurgical techniques
Volume 6, Video 14.01 Trimmed great toe
Volume 6, Video 14.02 Second toe for index
Volume 6, Video 14.03 Combined second and third toe for metacarpal hand

Mark D. Wells, MD, FRCS, FACS
Clinical Assistant Professor of Surgery
The Ohio State University
Columbus, OH, USA
Volume 3, Chapter 5 Scalp and forehead reconstruction

Gordon H. Wilkes, MD
Clinical Professor and Divisional Director
Division of Plastic Surgery
University of Alberta Faculty of Medicine
Alberta, AB, Canada
Volume 1, Chapter 33 Facial prosthetics in plastic surgery

Henry Wilson, MD, FACS
Attending Plastic Surgeon
Private Practice
Plastic Surgery Associates
Lynchburg, VA, USA
Volume 5, Chapter 26 Fat grafting to the breast

Scott Woehrle, MS, BS
Physician Assistant
Department of Plastic Surgery
Jospeh Capella Plastic Surgery
Ramsey, NJ, USA
Volume 2, Chapter 29 Upper limb contouring
Volume 2, Video 29.01 Upper limb contouring

Johan F. Wolfaardt, BDS, MDent (Prosthodontics), PhD
Professor
Division of Otolaryngology-Head and Neck Surgery
Department of Surgery
Faculty of Medicine and Dentistry
Director of Clinics and International Relations
Institute for Reconstructive Sciences in Medicine
University of Alberta
Covenant Health Group
Alberta Health Services
Alberta, AB, Canada
Volume 1, Chapter 33 Facial prosthetics in plastic surgery

S. Anthony Wolfe, MD
Chief
Division of Plastic Surgery
Miami Children's Hospital
Miami, FL, USA
Volume 3, Chapter 8 Acquired cranial and facial bone deformities
Volume 3, Video 8.01 Removal of venous malformation enveloping intraconal optic nerve

Chin-Ho Wong, MBBS, MRCS, MMed (Surg), FAMS (Plast. Surg)
Consultant
Department of Plastic Reconstructive and Aesthetic Surgery
Singapore General Hospital
Singapore
Volume 2, Chapter 6 Anatomy of the aging face

Victor W. Wong, MD
Postdoctoral Research Fellow
Department of Surgery
Stanford University
Stanford, CA, USA
Volume 1, Chapter 13 Stem cells and regenerative medecine

Jeffrey Yao, MD
Assistant Professor
Department of Orthopaedic Surgery
Stanford University Medical Center
Palo Alto, CA, USA
Volume 6, Chapter 5 Principles of internal fixation as applied to the hand and wrist

Akira Yamada, MD
Assistant Professor
Department of Plastic and Reconstructive Surgery
Osaka Medical College
Osaka, Japan
Volume 3, Video 7.01 Microtia: auricular reconstruction

Michael J. Yaremchuk, MD, FACS
Chief of Craniofacial Surgery-Massachusetts General Hospital
Program Director-Plastic Surgery Training Program
Massachusetts General Hospital
Professor of Surgery
Harvard Medical School
Boston, MA, USA
Volume 2, Chapter 15 Skeletal augmentation
Volume 2, Video 15.01 Midface skeletal augmentation and rejuvenation

David M. Young, MD
Professor of Plastic Surgery
Department of Surgery
University of California
San Francisco, CA, USA
Volume 1, Chapter 24 Flap classification and applications

Peirong Yu, MD
Professor
Department of Plastic Surgery
The University of Texas M.D. Anderson Cancer Center
Houston, TX, USA
Volume 3, Chapter 13 Hypopharyngeal, esophageal, and neck reconstruction
Volume 3, Video 13.01 Reconstruction of pharyngoesophageal defects with the anterolateral thigh flap

James E. Zins, MD
Chairman
Department of Plastic Surgery
Dermatology and Plastic Surgery Institute
Cleveland Clinic
Cleveland, OH, USA
Volume 2, Chapter 13 Neck rejuvenation

Christopher G. Zochowski, MD
Chief Resident
Department of Plastic and Reconstructive Surgery
Case Western Reserve University
Cleveland, OH, USA
Volume 3, Chapter 38 Pierre Robin sequence

Elvin G. Zook, MD
Professor Emeritus
Division of Plastic Surgery
Southern Illinois University School of Medicine
Springfield, IL, USA
Volume 6, Chapter 6 Nail and fingertip reconstruction

Ronald M. Zuker, MD, FRCSC, FACS, FRCSEd(Hon)
Staff Plastic Surgeon
The Hospital for Sick Children
Professor of Surgery
Department of Surgery
The University of Toronto
Toronto, ON, Canada
Volume 3, Chapter 11 Facial paralysis

Acknowledgments

Editing a textbook such as this is an exciting, if daunting job. Only at the end of the project, over 4 years later, does one realize how much work it entailed and how many people helped make it happen. Sue Hodgson was the Commissioning Editor who trusted me to undertake this. Together, over several weekends in Seattle and countless e-mails and phone calls, we planned the format of this edition and laid the groundwork for a planning meeting in Chicago that included the volume editors and the Elsevier team with whom we have worked. I thank Drs. Gurtner, Warren, Rodriguez, Losee, Song, Grotting, Chang and Van Beek for tirelessly ensuring that each volume was as good as it could possibly be.

I had a weekly call with the Elsevier team as well as several visits to the offices in London. I will miss working with them. Louise Cook, Alexandra Mortimer and Poppy Garraway have been professional, thorough, and most of all, fun to work with. Emma Cole and Sam Crowe helped enormously with video content. Sadly, Sue Hodgson has left Elsevier, however Belinda Kuhn ably filled her shoes and ensured that we kept to our timeline, didn't lose momentum, and that the final product was something we would all be proud of.

Several residents helped, in focus groups to define format and style as well as specifically engaging in the editing process. I thank Darren Smith and Colin Woon for their help as technical copyeditors. Thanks to James Saunders and Leigh Jansen for reviewing video content and thanks also to Donnie Buck for all of his help with the electronic content. Of course we edited the book, we didn't write it. The writers were our contributing authors, all of whom engaged with enthusiasm. I thank them for defining Plastic Surgery, the book and the specialty.

Finally, I would like to thank my residents and fellows, who challenge me and make work fun. My partners in the Division of Plastic Surgery at the University of Washington, under the leadership of Nick Vedder, are a constant source of support and encouragement and I thank them. Finally, my family, Kate and David and most of all, my wife Gabrielle are unwavering in their love and support and I will never be able to thank them enough.

Peter C. Neligan, MB, FRCS(I), FRCSC, FACS
2012

It has been an honor to be involved with the Elsevier publishing team, Peter Neligan and all the contributing authors to the Aesthetic volume – outstanding leaders in plastic surgery who have invested precious time in the creation of this text.

I would like to personally thank A.D. Courtemanche, a wise, talented man who taught me plastic surgery and offered me an appointment at the University of British Columbia. Later, Foad Nahai, a man of tremendous energy, gave me a chance on the international stage.

I am grateful to my late parents, Harold and Dolly Warren, who provided a lifetime of encouragement and to my children, Dallas and Alex who saw their dad a lot less than they should. Lastly, my wife and lifelong partner, Betty, has been an unstoppable force which has kept me going throughout this fantastic project.

Richard J. Warren, MD, FRCSC
2012

Dedicated to the memory of Stephen J. Mathes

1

Managing the cosmetic patient

Michelle B. Locke and Foad Nahai

Understanding the motives, expectations, and desires of a patient seeking cosmetic surgery is at least as important as manual dexterity for achieving consistently satisfactory results.[1]

SYNOPSIS

- Societal interest in plastic surgery is increasing:
  - The number of plastic surgery procedures performed by ASAPS members has increased 72.5% since 1997
  - Women between the ages of 35 and 50 comprise the largest group of patients for both surgical and nonsurgical procedures.
- Understanding the patients motivations for surgery and their expectations of the outcomes are the keys to achieving satisfied patients postoperatively:
  - Managing the patients expectations requires full patient education
  - Second consultations are almost always necessary preoperatively
  - Be sure to discuss your policy for revisional surgery during the preoperative period.
- Postoperative follow up should include detailed written instructions and the surgeon's contact details:
  - Regular follow up visits are needed during the early post-operative period to assist the patient through the recovery
  - Unhappy patients or those with unsatisfactory outcomes should be seen more often to improve communication.
- Societal interest in plastic surgery is increasing:
  - The number of plastic surgery procedures performed by ASAPS members has increased 72.5% since 1997
  - Women between the ages of 35 and 50 comprise the largest group of patients for both surgical and nonsurgical procedures.

Societal interest in cosmetic surgery

The concept of beauty

What is beauty? The concept of attractiveness seems to be innate and is similar across cultures and religions. While it can be influenced somewhat by social trends and advertising, research shows that subjective attractiveness is largely biological, overlaid with only a small amount of personal preference. Studies looking at the consistency of physical attractiveness ratings across cultural groups agree that facial attractiveness is species-specific, not race-specific.[2,3] Research in the US has shown that the ratings provided by Asians, Hispanics, Caucasians, and African Americans correlate well for facial attractiveness overall, although features such as expression and sexual maturity influenced some cultural groups more than others.[3] Also, Caucasians and African Americans differed on their judgment of bodies. Judgments can potentially be influenced by cultural norms, for example, the classical Roman nose is very different in size and shape than the African American nose, so what may be considered a deformity in one person may be attractive on another. There is no simple answer to the question of what constitutes beauty, or even an attractive face.

In order to ascertain what makes an attractive face, some researchers have assessed facial features by judging individual faces, then comparing the results with computer-generated composite faces, averaging the individuals.[4,5] This research showed there was a trend towards the composite face being more attractive than the faces individually, producing a claim that "attractive faces are only average." Others have disputed this claim, saying that a mathematically averaged face is not the same as an average face.[6,7] Interestingly, functional magnetic resonance imaging scanning of subjects during judgment on the facial attractiveness of strangers has shown that perceived facial attractiveness increases with eye contact rather than with increased physical attractiveness *per se*.[8,9] These studies have also shown that facial attractiveness is a fundamental condition which a stranger can read rapidly. In fact, it takes only 150 ms and no eye movement to judge a stranger's attractiveness.

Over 2000 articles on the study of facial attractiveness have been published in the past 30 years. Social and psychological literature from the 1970s and 1980s extensively studied the response to physical attractiveness and showed that physical attractiveness has a statistically significant effect on the person's self-esteem and well-being.[2] This implies that beauty has influence which is more than "just skin deep."[10] Pediatric studies have revealed that parents provide better parenting to attractive children and have higher expectations of success for them. Conversely, children with craniofacial deformities have behavioral and anxiety problems.[11] Studies have also shown that attractive women receive more dates and are perceived to have more positive social attributes. Housman suggested that physically attractive people are offered greater opportunities for success and happiness throughout their life.[10] Attractive individuals are more likely to be hired, promoted, and earn higher salaries than their less attractive counterparts. As the potential benefits go far beyond improved self-esteem, it is perhaps not surprising that individuals are attending their plastic surgeons with requests for surgical and non-surgical options in an attempt to increase their perceived attractiveness or correct a deformity.

Increasing societal acceptance of cosmetic surgery

The specialty of plastic surgery is rooted in reconstructive surgery for congenital abnormalities and acquired injuries. Surgery for purely aesthetic reasons was incorporated into the field somewhat later. Research from the American Society for Aesthetic Plastic Surgery (ASAPS) has shown that societal acceptance of plastic surgery is increasing. The ASAPS Quick Facts consumer attitudes survey of 2010 found that 53% of women and 49% of men approve of cosmetic surgery, while 27% of married Americans and 33% of unmarried Americans would consider cosmetic surgery for themselves in the future.[11] If you compare these attitudes with previous results, 20% of Americans are more favorably disposed towards cosmetic surgery now than they were 5 years ago. This increased acceptance may be related to the extensive media coverage which essentially normalizes plastic surgery. This includes

celebrities openly discussing their plastic surgical procedures, as well as popular television programs such as Dr 90210 and Extreme Makeover. Unfortunately, the downside of making plastic surgery a form of mainstream entertainment is the misrepresentation of the significance, complexity, downtime, and potential complications of undergoing surgery. These issues increase the chance that the patient will present with unrealistic expectations which must be clearly addressed by the plastic surgeon at preoperative consultations.

ASAPS statistics for surgical procedures performed by its members in 2011 show that the most commonly performed plastic surgery operations are breast augmentation and liposuction *(Fig. 1.1)*.[11] Compared with the surgical statistics from 1997, there has been a significant increase in these procedures *(Fig. 1.2)*. This is in line with the overall 72.5% increase in plastic surgical operations performed over this period. Over this same time period there has also been a significant rise in nonsurgical cosmetic procedures, such as injectables (botulinum toxin, hyaluronic acid, and so forth), laser hair removal, and skin-resurfacing techniques, which have outpaced the growth in surgical procedures, growing 355.6% since 1997. This trend also highlights the public's acceptance of cosmetic

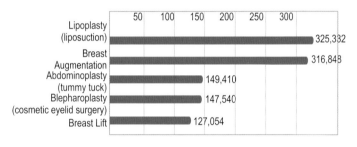

Fig. 1.1 Top five surgical procedures in 2011 (American Society for Aesthetic Plastic Surgery 2011 data.)

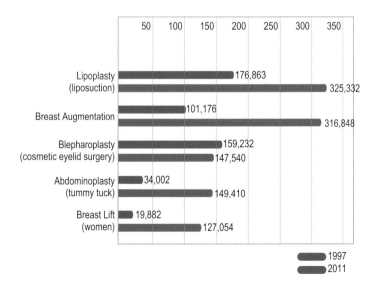

Fig. 1.2 Change in procedure numbers 1997–2011 (American Society for Aesthetic Plastic Surgery 2011 data.)

Table 1.1 Age distribution of plastic surgery patients (American Society for Aesthetic Plastic Surgery 2011 data)

	<18 years	19–34 years	35–50 years	51–64 years	65+ years
Surgical procedures	2.1%	27.9%	40.6%	23.3%	6.1%
Nonsurgical procedures	1.3%	17.7%	43.4%	28.8%	8.8%
Total for all procedures	1.4%	19.5%	42.9%	27.8%	8.3%

Table 1.2 Sex distribution of plastic surgical patients (American Society for Aesthetic Plastic Surgery 2011 data)

	Female		Male	
	Number	Percentage	Number	Percentage
Surgical procedures	1 493 615	91.2%	144 909	8.8%
Nonsurgical procedures	6 904 810	91.4%	651 176	8.6%
Overall	8 398 424	91.3%	796 086	8.7%

procedures overall, and the popularity of nonsurgical procedures may indicate a pool of potential patients who will consider operative procedures in the future.

The largest age group of patients undergoing surgical and nonsurgical procedures is between 35 and 50 years of age. Interestingly, statistics show that patients in the younger age group than this (19–34 years) represent a greater proportion of patients who undergo surgical procedures (27.9%) than patients in the older group (51–64 years: 23.3%), while the older group more commonly underwent more nonsurgical procedures than the younger (*Table 1.1*). This may be related to the increasing societal acceptance of plastic surgery, as younger people tend to be quicker adopters of a new trend than older persons. Not surprisingly, the majority of plastic surgical and nonsurgical patients are female (*Table 1.2*).

Surgeon advertising

When aesthetic plastic surgery first developed, advertising the surgeon's services was considered distasteful and was frowned upon by most practitioners. However, as times have changed, advertising of services has become commonplace. In these authors' opinion, advertising should be discreet, professional, and truthful. A professional, thorough website, which can be accessed by public search engines and via links from the websites of professional bodies with whom the surgeon is affiliated, is essentially a common form of advertising. Many patients say they wish to see before-and-after photos if possible, while the surgeon must of course be

cognizant of maintaining patient privacy. As a minimum, the website should cover the surgeon's personal philosophy and procedures offered, and provide contact details and a location map. Additionally, advertising in local magazines or newspapers may be appropriate. However, it is important that plastic surgery is not seen to be trying to sell a service to the patient, but instead is advertised as available and able to meet the patient's needs and requirements with competence and care. The American Board of Plastic Surgery, the American Society of Plastic Surgeons (ASPS), and ASAPS all have ethical codes and guidelines governing advertising to which diplomats and members must adhere.

Patient motivation for cosmetic surgery

As Greer stated in 1984, "Understanding the motives, expectations, and desires of a patient seeking cosmetic surgery is at least as important as manual dexterity for achieving consistently satisfactory results."[1] The patient may seek cosmetic surgery for any number of reasons. Elucidating the patient's motivation is a goal of your first patient encounter. The best reason for wanting plastic surgery is for self-improvement. However, there are many other potential reasons. Patients may feel that surgery will alter their life in some way, perhaps make them more outgoing, help them secure a partner, or save their marriage. The surgeon must be wary of patients with hidden agendas, as an excellent surgical outcome may still not result in a happy patient postoperatively.

During the initial consultation, the surgeon must attempt to ascertain what the patient actually wants. This may be different from what the spouse or partner or parents want. If the patient is not initiating the surgery, then beware operating on the patient. If the patient has attended the first appointment with his or her partner and the surgeon feels the partner is the driving force behind the consultation, a second appointment should be scheduled with the patient alone. It is important to ensure that it is the patient who wants the surgery and that s/he fully understands the ramifications of surgery before going ahead with any procedures.

Another potential warning sign regarding patient motivation is "doctor shopping." While we encourage any patient to seek a second, or even third, opinion if they wish, if the surgeon is aware that the patient has seen several doctors already, this should strike a warning bell. The surgeon should inquire as to the reason for this. Perhaps the patient's request for surgery has been declined by other surgeons with good reason. The patient's expectations may be excessively high and unrealistic. The patient may simply be indecisive. The surgeon should be cautious about offering surgery to these patients unless there is a thorough understanding about the reasons for that patient shopping around.

The ideal patient

The ideal patient for cosmetic plastic surgery is one with whom the surgeon can develop rapport and understanding. The patient should be pleasant to the surgeon and the

Top 5 Cosmetic Surgeries for Men in 2011

Lipoplasty (liposuction)	41,663
Rhinoplasty	24,533
Blepharoplasty (cosmetic eyelid surgery)	22,905
Gynecomastia	17,645
Facelift	10,400

Fig. 1.3 Top five cosmetic surgeries for men. (American Society for Aesthetic Plastic Surgery 2011 data.)

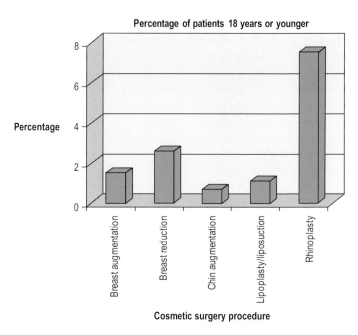

Fig. 1.4 Percentage of patients for cosmetic surgery procedures who are 18 years and younger. (American Society for Aesthetic Plastic Surgery 2011 data.)

office staff, have effective communication skills, and be intelligent, well educated, and well informed regarding their potential treatment. They must have an identifiable deformity for correction, with realistic expectations of the outcome and a full understanding of potential complications. They should be sensible and compliant with pre- and postoperative instructions. Unfortunately, not all of our patients fit this profile!

Special patient groups

The male cosmetic surgery patient

Male patients account for nearly 9% of all cosmetic surgery in the US and men underwent nearly 145 000 cosmetic surgery operations in 2011.[11] While the most common operations include lipoplasty and rhinoplasty (**Fig. 1.3**), men also represented 9% of all facelift (rhytidectomy) procedures in 2011.

Importantly, men are often overrepresented in the complication data for their procedures, particularly hematoma rates. This should be thoroughly discussed with patients before surgery. The reported incidence of hematoma following male rhytidectomy ranges from 8 to 13% in most series, twice as high as for females. This may be related to the greater vascularity of the male facial skin, with a higher number of microvessels to supply the hair follicles.[12] Strict perioperative blood pressure control may be the most important aspect of care to reduce this rate. To this end, we routinely give males clonidine (a centrally acting, alpha$_2$ adrenergic receptor agonist) 0.1 mg postoperatively. This helps stabilize their blood pressure and is long-acting, with a half-life of about 12 hours.

The young cosmetic surgery patient

How young is too young for plastic surgery? This is not a straightforward question and the answer usually depends on the reason for the surgery and the degree of patient deformity and concern. The number of teenage patients is small – only 2.1% of all patients undergoing plastic surgery in 2011.[11] Data

from the last 12 years of reporting from both the ASAPS and the ASPS show similar rates every year over the time period, ranging between 1 and 3%. Excluding otoplasty (cosmetic ear surgery), rhinoplasty is the most common surgery for teenagers overall (**Fig. 1.4**). While ASAPS 2011 data show that only 1.5% of all breast augmentations were performed on women 18 years of age and under, over 44% of these were performed for purely cosmetic purposes (**Fig. 1.5**). This is despite the fact that the US Food and Drug Administration (FDA) only approves saline-filled breast implants for cosmetic augmentation in women age 18 years and over, and silicone-filled implants for women 22 years and older. The FDA states that this restriction is placed because "breasts continue to develop through late teens and early 20s and because there is a concern that a young woman may not be mature enough to make an informed decision about the potential risks."

As the FDA implies, the greatest concern when operating on a young patient is that the teen will have unrealistic expectations from the surgery. Clearly, plastic surgeons need to assess the mental as well as the physical maturity of younger patients before undertaking any surgical procedures. The young patient must understand that the surgery itself results in a permanent change. In particular, patients must understand that there will be permanent scars and there are potential complications which will be with them for life. A thorough preoperative assessment of why the young patient wishes to have the surgery, and what difference the patient thinks it will make to her life should be undertaken. Any unrealistic expectations of the changes that the surgery may make should warn the surgeon against operating until the patient is more emotionally mature and may prompt a psychological referral instead.

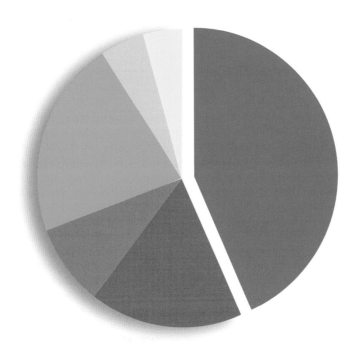

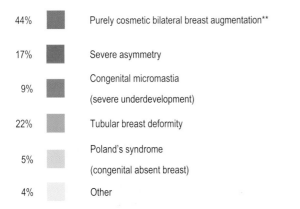

44% Purely cosmetic bilateral breast augmentation**

17% Severe asymmetry

9% Congenital micromastia
(severe underdevelopment)

22% Tubular breast deformity

5% Poland's syndrome
(congenital absent breast)

4% Other

Fig. 1.5 Breast augmentation in women 18 years and under. *In 2011, 4830 procedures were performed on women 18 and under, less than 2% of the total number of breast augmentations. **The Food and Drug Administration recommends that cosmetic breast augmentation be restricted to women age 18 and above. (American Society for Aesthetic Plastic Surgery 2011 data.)

Younger patients need support people during and after surgery as much, or even more, than older adults. During the preoperative assessments, make note of who attends with the patient. Is it a parent or caregiver? Or is it a boyfriend or girlfriend? While patients over 18 are not required to inform their parents of their request for surgery, it can show a level of maturity if the patient has discussed the surgery with parents and have family support before going ahead. Contrast this with young patients who do not want to tell anyone they are undergoing surgery. Who will look after them during their postoperative recovery period? Who will bring them to their follow-up visits? Who will support them if there are complications? Also, plastic surgery for cosmetic purposes is not normally covered by insurance, raising the question of how patients will pay for the primary surgery and what arrangements they can make to pay for revisions and complications. Parental and family support assists both emotionally and physically, and the plastic surgeon should be wary of operating on a young patient without an obvious support network.

Friends or family as your cosmetic surgery patient

It is a strong endorsement of your skills and reputation as a plastic surgeon when friends or family consult you and desire your surgical expertise. However, this flattery can be expensive, as family and friends often have an expectation of free or heavily discounted procedures. Not only does such discounting generate little revenue to help meet the overheads of the practice, it also takes up time in your surgical schedule that could have been spent operating profitably on another patient. It is important to have a clear policy to manage these expectations ahead of time.

If you don't wish (or cannot afford) to discount your surgery, one strategy is to explain to the patient that you provide a professional service and therefore there will be a bill for your services. However, as the individual is an important person to you, you will endeavour to provide added value in different ways. For example, increasing your availability to see the patient outside your regular office hours, such as evenings or weekend, may be very valuable to a friend or medical colleague who works full-time. The cost of this, even if you pay a practice nurse overtime to see the patient with you, can be significantly less than discounting the surgery.

It is the practice of the senior author to discount my surgical fee for family, friends, other healthcare professionals, and office staff. However, the amount of discount that is offered will vary with the relationship. It can be embarrassing and challenging to discuss this face to face with the patient. To avoid this, I provide a letter to the patient explaining my position on this matter, which is a modified version of one which Dr. Tom Rees shared with me years ago *(Fig. 1.6)*.

FIG 1.6 APPEARS ONLINE ONLY

Of course, these comments ignore the ethical issue of whether one should operate on one's family and friends. The Code of Ethics states that physicians should not, except in

In almost all of the US, individuals are considered minors and therefore unable to consent to surgery until they reach the age of 18. State legislation requires parental consent for surgery on any patient under 18 years. However, the state recognizes that the legal age of majority is arbitrary and that there are minors who are competent and others, of legal age, who are not. While this can be confusing, the fundamental basis of the legislation is to protect minors from the consequences of poor decisions. A responsible plastic surgeon also has a role to play in protecting young patients from the consequences of unnecessary surgery, even if the patient is over the age of majority. First and foremost, it is the surgeon's job to care about the patient's overall well-being.

emergencies or when the illness is minor, treat themselves or anyone with whom they have a relationship, such as their spouse or child. This is due to the fact that your emotional bond with the patient could compromise the quality of your care and impair your judgment. Despite this, operating on family seems to be common in our profession. If you do undertake this surgery, ensure that you can do so safely and to a high standard. If you feel that your judgment may be impaired by the relationship, do not hesitate to refer the patient to a colleague.

The initial consultation

First contact with the office

Although your website may well be the patient's first contact with, and first impression of, your practice and you, the receptionist is usually the first person the patient will have contact with in the office. It is important that the reception staff leave a favorable first impression on the patient. Make sure that the person answering your phone calls provides friendly, efficient, personal service. The receptionist should be able to answer questions about you and your facility, as well as provide information about the services you offer. This could include approximate cost information, as many patients wish to know this before they make an appointment. If the reception staff do not know the answers to the questions asked, they should be able to put potential patients through to someone who can answer them, possibly your patient coordinator, administrative assistant, or nurse.

It is useful to have the reception staff inquire how the patient found out about you. They may have been referred from friends or family, have found you on an internet search, or seen your advertising. This information should be recorded and you should assess it regularly, to see whether your advertising dollar has been usefully spent.

When making the patient an appointment to see you, ensure that the receptionist checks how the patient prefers to be contacted. Some patients may not be happy to receive calls at their place of work, or at home, or they may not want you to leave messages for them if they do not have a private voice mailbox. This information is especially important as new patient management systems are integrated into more and more practices. These can automatically contact the patient for you, to remind them of their appointment times or request feedback on their visit. If the preferred method of contact is not clearly indicated in the patient's paper or electronic record, breaches of the patient's privacy can occur.

Once an appointment time has been made for the patient, an information pack is sent out from the office, although all the information may alternatively be available on a practice website. This includes information regarding the surgeon and the practice, including its location, a map, and parking instructions. A health questionnaire is included, which the patient is requested to complete and bring along to the appointment (*Fig. 1.7*). The pack can also be personalized to include a brochure on the procedure that the patient is considering. While all of this information is likely to be on your website, not all patients are computer-literate and printed material can be brought along at the time of the appointment to assist with directions. FIG **1.7** APPEARS ONLINE ONLY

Nurse assessment

In the senior author's practice, the first person to see and assess the patient is my nurse. The patient is brought into a private consultation room and the nurse goes over the preassessment forms with the patient. This includes checking that the health questionnaire forms are accurately completed and that any allergies are correctly recorded, and confirming the reason for today's appointment. Depending on the patient and the likely surgery, sometimes the nurse will spend time looking through pre- and postoperative photographs with the patient. At the end of this time, the nurse leaves the information for me to read over before I see the patient. The nurse can also provide valuable feedback on the patient. It is helpful to be warned about any potential issues with the patient before entering the room yourself. Also, some patients can be polite and sociable to the surgeon but rude to the other staff members, so it is always useful to be aware of the nurse's first impression of the patient, along with your own.

Surgeon's assessment

After reviewing the information, I then introduce myself and ask the patient what I can do for the patient. I spend between 15 and 30 minutes with the patient. Initially we will discuss the patient's goals and aims from surgery. This time helps me assess the patient and whether his or her expectations are reasonable, and whether I can meet them. It also develops rapport with the patient much more effectively than beginning the consultation with closed questions. Then I will review all the health information with the patient, including personal history of smoking and deep-vein thrombosis, as well as adding any pertinent procedure-specific questions. After reviewing the history, we return to the reason for the consultation.

Throughout the appointment, I am assessing the patient by appearance, grooming, manner, body language, and enthusiasm for any surgery. I want to know whether the patient is a realistic person with reasonable expectations. Do I think that I can achieve these goals? Do I like the patient? If we have a complication, will I be happy to see the patient regularly in my clinic and will I be able to support him or her throughout the issue? I am sure that the patient will be making similar judgments about me, so I strive to be attentive, to maintain eye contact rather than looking at the notes, and to be friendly and caring in my demeanor. I always provide feedback at the end of the consultation regarding whether I think the patient is a suitable candidate for the procedure or not.

Photography

Formal, standardized photographs are taken of the patient at the first appointment. These must be suitably consented and the intended use of the images should be clear to the patient on a signed consent form (*Fig. 1.8*). The consent could allow display of the images for the patient's record only, for teaching purposes, for publications, website use, or to show other patients. I have a separate consent form for any patient who consents to the use of photographs on the website, to ensure complete understanding of this process and avoid any unwanted legal issues. 😻 FIG **1.8** APPEARS ONLINE ONLY

My practice has a professional photographer who takes images and also provides digitally altered images to predict the postoperative appearance. This is particularly helpful for rhytidectomy and rhinoplasty procedures. Often rhinoplasty patients will be offered more than one postoperative option, so that they can see how their nose might look if set further back, or with more hump reduction. This is helpful to ensure that both you and the patient have similar goals in mind for the surgery. However, it is important to make it clear to the patient that these photographs do not guarantee the outcome.

Patient coordinator

After seeing me and having photographs taken, the patient then sees my patient coordinator. While I do not pressure the patient to make any decisions at the first appointment, the issue of fees and the waiting time for scheduling are covered. If an overnight stay is being considered, the patient is shown photographs of the overnight suites, or tours the facilities if there are empty rooms available for viewing. The coordinator will also go over the surgery, complications, and recovery time with the patient again. The coordinator then becomes the liaison person for the patient, to answer questions and schedule surgery or further appointments.

After the appointment

The patient is always given written material to take home regarding the procedure and the facility. Once the patient has left, I dictate a letter to the patient at the same time as my clinical note. This letter reiterates our discussions and the potential surgical plan *(Fig. 1.9)*. I routinely request that the patient comes back for a second appointment at no charge, prior to scheduling surgery. 😻 FIG **1.9** APPEARS ONLINE ONLY

Second and subsequent consultations

A second appointment allows me the opportunity of answering any further questions and reviewing my surgical plan with the patient. It also provides another chance to go over the limitations of each procedure, the scars, and potential complications for a second time. We also discuss the possibility of revisional surgery being required, and the financial implications of this. I often give my patients some "homework" for this second visit: I request that my facial aesthetic patients bring in a photograph of themselves from about 15–20 years previously, that rhinoplasty patients bring in pictures from magazines of noses that they like, and breast

augmentation patients bring in any pictures they find that they like, and so forth. These help me visualize what I am trying to achieve with the surgery, and ensure that the patient and I have similar goals.

If surgery is going to go ahead, it is usually booked by the end of the second appointment. Courtiss writes of a "three strikes" rule – this means to beware the patient who requests three or more preoperative appointments with you.[13] This can be a red flag for indecisiveness or uncertainty, which indicates that this is not the ideal patient for you to operate on.

Saying "no" to a potential patient

Saying "no" to a patient can be difficult but is sometimes necessary. You should heed your intuition and be cautious. If you have concerns, do not offer the patient surgery. After all, plastic surgery is truly elective surgery, so do not undertake it if you feel that it is not in the patient's best interest.

When to say "no"

The surgeon may consider the patient unsuitable for a number of reasons. According to Gorney and Martello, the patient may be either anatomically or psychologically unsuitable for the procedure.[14] From an anatomic viewpoint, the feature that the patient wishes to have altered must be visible to the surgeon and able to be corrected. Some patients perceive with a significant degree of concern a deformity that the surgeon may consider to be minor or trivial. The ideal patient fits around the diagonal of Gorney's patient selection graph *(Fig. 1.10)*.[14,15]

However, studies on patients requesting rhinoplasty have failed to demonstrate a significant correlation between the extent of the deformity and the degree of psychological disturbance the deformity causes the patient.[16] This implies that, just because the surgeon feels that the deformity is only minor, the significance to the patient and therefore the likelihood of

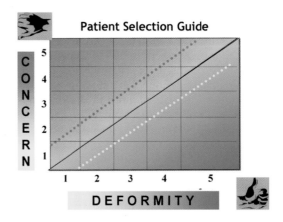

Fig. 1.10 Gorney's patient selection guide.

improving the patient's self-esteem following corrective surgery is not necessarily also minor.

Reasons for declining to operate on a patient include:

- You (or your staff) don't like the patient.
- You don't think the patient likes you.
- The patient is unreasonably demanding or has unrealistically high expectations.
- You believe the patient has a psychological problem such as body dysmorphic disorder (BDD).
- You feel that the patient has emotional instability and would not cope with the surgery.

BDD is covered in detail elsewhere in this textbook (vol. I, ch. 3), but it is suitable to discuss it briefly here as it is particularly relevant to patient selection. BDD is considered by the *Diagnostic and Statistical Manual of Mental Disorders*, fourth edition,[17] as a somatoform disorder defined by preoccupation with an imaginary defect in appearance. If a physical anomaly is present, the patient's concern is markedly excessive. To qualify as BDD the condition must be severe enough to impair the patient's social or other functioning. The incidence in the general population is unknown but is thought to be between 0.5% and 2%. Reported rates among people seeking cosmetic surgery are thought to be much higher, with studies suggesting that BDD occurs in anything from 7% to 15% of patients.[18,19] The most common symptom seen by the plastic surgeon during consultation is excessive concern or distress over a minor imperfection, manifested by spending a long time describing the defect in great detail.[18] The patient may appear to have a depressed mood and speak in a monotone. He or she may also show dissatisfaction with previous surgical procedures, or request repeated surgery. Other, less common features which may be apparent in the plastic surgeon's office include camouflaging and skin picking.

As the diagnosis of BDD requires the patient to have impaired functioning because of the defect, it is important that the plastic surgeon specifically asks the patient what effect that defect has on social or daily functioning. The importance of identifying these patients in your practice before operating on them cannot be overstated, as surgery may exacerbate the problem.[20] If surgery is performed, more than 75% will report dissatisfaction with the outcomes, and this can potentially produce a malpractice lawsuit or even violence towards the operating surgeon. Performing surgery on these patients has also been shown to lead to anything from never-ending requests for more surgery to psychosis and suicidal ideation. Unfortunately, plastic surgeons do not always identify these patients in advance. Sarwer published the results of a survey of ASAPS members in 2002, in which most respondents (84%) indicated that they had operated on a patient whom they initially believed was a suitable candidate for surgery, only to discover postoperatively that the patient suffered from BDD.[21] Of these, 43% indicated that the patient seemed to be more preoccupied with the defect after surgery than they had been before, while another 39% reported that the patient was less preoccupied with the initial defect but was now focused on a different perceived defect. Most concerningly, 40% of respondents indicated that a patient with BDD had threatened them, either legally or physically, or both. Given these risks, it is probably sensible to consider BDD to be a contraindication to plastic surgery. Referral for psychiatric consultation and treatment would be appropriate prior to reconsidering the idea of plastic surgery.[1,18]

If you are concerned about a patient's ability to cope with surgery emotionally, Sykes suggests trying less invasive procedures first.[22] For example, if the patient presents for facial rejuvenation, if it is appropriate you could trial temporary treatments such as toxins or fillers to see how well the patient tolerates these. If the patient copes well, attends regularly for follow-up, and behaves in a reasonable fashion afterward, this can help to reassure the surgeon that the patient may cope with the surgery. Similarly, poor posttreatment behavior can help unmask a difficult patient before you make the mistake of operating on this person.

How to say "no"

Once you have decided not to operate on the patient, you must be clear and honest about this. Do not be ambivalent in your wording, leaving the patient hope that you might change your mind. Do not blame the patient but instead if necessary take the blame yourself. Phrases such as, "I am not prepared to operate on you because I don't think I can achieve the result you are looking for," are most suitable.

Saying "yes": what is involved?

Managing surgical expectations

Assuming that you understand the patient's goals and desires and feel that you are able to meet them, surgery can be scheduled. Managing the patient's expectations requires full patient education. Patients should be given a clear indication of the risk-to-benefit ratio for the surgery, as well as information covering the likely time course for the operation and recovery. I tell my patients to, "Forget the word cosmetic, remember the word surgery," and that all surgery carries risk. It is helpful to show photographs of other patients at different time points following similar surgery, to provide them with an idea of what they might expect. This can be particularly relevant before procedures such as chemical peels, which can be associated with significant short-term postoperative morbidity that the patient must accept before going ahead with the procedure. I provide all my patients with written information about the procedure, as well as postoperative care instructions. They are encouraged to contact me or my patient coordinator if they have any further questions before their operation.

Managing financial expectations

Prior to any surgery going ahead, the patient receives clear documentation of all the costs involved from my patient coordinator. We make it clear that insurance coverage is unlikely for most cosmetic procedures, and that they will be responsible for the bill themselves. My practice has a policy of this bill being paid in full 14 days prior to their operation. This preoperative financial discussion also includes clear knowledge of who pays for the treatment of any complications or necessary revisions. It is also made quite clear to the patient that the bill is an estimate only. While I do not alter my surgical fee if the operation runs longer than expected, patients will be responsible for any additional operating room or anesthesia charges. While some practices offer referrals to financial lending institutes to arrange loans to pay for surgery, this is not my practice and I consider it a (relative) contraindication to perform elective plastic surgery on a patient who struggles to afford it or takes a loan to pay the bill.

Informed consent

Informed consent is a process, not a piece of paper. I clearly explain the general and specific risks in terms that the patient can understand, and I do not downplay the likely downtime postoperatively. The risks are reiterated by my surgical coordinator and by myself at the patient's second consultation. Each procedure has a specific indepth consent form *(Fig. 1.11)*. The patient is required to read and initial each page and sign on the last page. This includes the policy on paying for revisions, which must also be read and initialled, as has been suggested in the literature.[23] FIG **1.11** APPEARS ONLINE ONLY

You may wish to consider adding into your consent a restriction on the patient's ability to post information regarding you or their procedure on the internet without your written permission. While this is not my current practice, with the rapid increase in blog sites and social media, one unhappy or vindictive patient can do untold damage to your reputation with postings on the internet, reaching far more people than word of mouth alone. Legally, it can be difficult, if not impossible, to redress this situation or remove damaging posts unless you have a signed restriction, as above.

Preoperative regime for the patient

Preoperatively, I make it clear to my patients, both verbally and in the consent forms, that they must stop smoking (not just cut down) prior to their surgery. I also request that they cut down on any alcohol in the immediate preoperative period. Depending on the procedure, my nurse will discuss a skin care regime, such as starting retinoids in the preoperative period as appropriate. All my facial aesthetic patients are started on arnica and bromelain 1 week preoperatively to decrease their bruising. All patients are given a complete list of medications to avoid in the 2 weeks prior to their surgery, including aspirin, vitamin E, and analgesics containing nonsteroidal anti-inflammatories such as ibuprofen *(Fig. 1.12)*. They are also asked to stop any herbal remedies or dietary supplements. FIG **1.12** APPEARS ONLINE ONLY

Anesthesia consultation

As all cosmetic surgery is elective, in the interests of patient safety all patients are required to have clearance from their internist prior to surgery. They also meet with one of our anesthesiologists for a preoperative check-up and discussion of anesthesia care *(Fig. 1.13)*. Further investigations are ordered by the internist or anesthesiologist as required, and surgery is deferred if necessary until clearance has been received. These visits ensure that the patient is a suitable candidate for surgery, as well as confirming the patient's suitability for treatment in our office-based, credentialed operating suites. It also allows patients the opportunity to become familiar with the anesthesia plan and facilities prior to their operation. This familiarity helps avoid delays and alleviates anxiety on the day of surgery. FIG **1.13** APPEARS ONLINE ONLY

Postoperative follow-up

Following surgery, the patient may be discharged home from the recovery room or stay overnight in a private suite. Occasionally we arrange for the patient to stay at a hotel with an overnight nurse. Patients who stay overnight are reviewed in the evening by myself or a colleague and cared for overnight by qualified nursing staff. The following morning I check the patient, answer any questions, and arrange discharge. Drains may be removed prior to leaving or at a postoperative follow-up visit as suitable. All patients are given a prescription for analgesic medications and instructions on what to look out for in terms of complications *(Fig. 1.14)*. Contact details are provided prior to leaving. These calls come through to the office during working hours. After hours, an answering service takes and forwards any calls to the surgeon. If patients go home from the recovery room, they are called that evening and the next morning by myself or my nursing staff, to check on them and answer any questions. They are always given an appointment time and date for a follow-up visit prior to leaving the office. FIG **1.14** APPEARS ONLINE ONLY

Follow-up consultations

My practice has a separate internal waiting room for facial surgery patients so they do not have to spend time in the main waiting room with preoperative patients. As a matter of courtesy I always endeavor to see my patients as promptly as possible. I sit with them in the consultation room, focusing on the patient, not the clinical records, asking after recovery, comfort levels, and so forth. Then I take down the dressings and examine the wounds. I discuss progress and at this stage the patient has an opportunity to ask questions. Often the patient brings in a list of questions, and I take time to go over all these concerns.

During the first 1–2 postoperative weeks, when the swelling and bruising are maximal, the patient may have doubts about the wisdom of the surgery. After all, patients usually look worse, not better, during this period! Therefore I support them through this time by seeing them often, sometimes twice a week or more if necessary, and then space out their follow-up appointments over time. Postoperative photographs are always taken for the records. I encourage patients to continue to consult with me regularly until we can see the final outcome, perhaps 6 months to a year. Once patients have completely recovered and settled from their surgery, I offer them follow-up appointments for as long as they want to see me, usually on an annual basis.

The unsatisfactory outcome

In an ideal world, both the patient and the surgeon are happy with the results. Three unsatisfactory outcomes are possible:

1. The patient is happy, the surgeon is unhappy.
2. Both the patient and the surgeon are unhappy.
3. The patient is unhappy, the surgeon is happy.

The patient is happy

If the patient is happy, then no further treatment is indicated, even if the surgeon feels that this was far from his or her best result. A happy postoperative patient whose expectations have been met is the goal of plastic surgery. However, under these circumstances, the surgeon should suggest further follow-up to review the patient in the future, in case the patient changes his or her mind about the suitability of the outcome.

Both the patient and the surgeon are unhappy

When the outcome is unsatisfactory, you must put personal feelings aside, difficult as it may be. Do not take complications or poor outcomes personally. Accept that unhappy patients following surgery happen to everyone who practices plastic surgery.[23] Under these circumstances, further surgery is likely. During your postoperative consultations, reassure patients that you understand their dissatisfaction, that you can see what they are concerned about, that you are not happy with it either, and that you will do your utmost to fix it for them. If a complication has occurred, be upfront with the patient and explain what happened. In private, undertake an honest self-appraisal of your operative technique in your primary surgery and attempt to ascertain what produced the unsatisfactory outcome. Ask yourself, "What went wrong?" and "How will I prevent this happening again?" Next, ask yourself whether you are able to fix the problem. If you do not feel comfortable with operating again, consider referring the patient for a second opinion or to a subspecialist plastic surgeon if appropriate. The cost of further surgery should also be discussed. This conversation is easier if it has been covered preoperatively. My practice has a policy of providing free revisional surgery. Your policy may be different, but in general you should waive your surgical fee, though the patient may be liable for any facility and anesthetic fee. If you are sending the patient for a second opinion, expect to cover

(or at least contribute to) the other surgeon's fee yourself. Above all, provide patients with a clear explanation of the management plan and ensure that their concerns have been addressed.

The patient is unhappy but the surgeon is happy

This is a very bad outcome as it usually indicates a breakdown in communication between the surgeon and the patient, or poor patient selection. First, assess what went wrong. Did you have similar goals initially? Does the patient have a psychological disturbance such as BDD that you did not discover during your preoperative evaluation? Most importantly, can you see and appreciate what the patient is unhappy about? If you cannot, then you will never be able to fix it, or make the patient happy. If you can see the deformity or defect that the patient is unhappy with, further surgery may be indicated. Otherwise, it may be appropriate to refer the patient for a second opinion, to a specialist colleague, or even to a psychiatrist for further assessment.

Managing the unhappy patient

Managing the dissatisfied patient is challenging and time-consuming. It requires patience and tact on the part of the plastic surgeon. Most patient dissatisfaction is based on failure of communications and poor patient selection, rather than technical errors.[24] Obviously, improving your patient evaluation and selection skills can help limit the number of unhappy patients you deal with. However, when unhappiness occurs, underlying the dissatisfaction is normally a breakdown in rapport between the patient and surgeon.[14] This means that effective communication is the key in managing these patients. Spend time listening with empathy and compassion to patients' concerns. Try to elicit the specific reason(s) for the dissatisfaction and make sure that their issues are heard, accepted, and understood.[25]

Managing a colleague's unhappy patient

The unhappy patient could be your own or a colleague's. It is important never to criticize your colleagues on a personal or professional basis, or to criticize what took place during the previous surgery. The patient should be managed as any new patient to your practice would be, with a full history and physical evaluation. Almost always, I can explain to the patient what I find, say that I've seen it before, and explain how it can be revised. Sometimes the patient simply requires a second opinion, in which case I encourage the patient to return to the primary surgeon if they still have a rapport. If the patient insists that s/he will not return to the primary surgeon, then I will discuss the cost of the surgery. As the primary surgery was not with me, any revisional surgery will cost the patient the full fee. I explain that the patient will likely receive a lesser fee if s/he returns to the primary surgeon. If the patient wants to schedule surgery with me, I make every effort to contact the primary surgeon for information and receive old notes (including preoperative photographs) if possible. Bear in mind that you cannot contact the other surgeon or discuss the patient's care with anyone without the patient's consent.

Managing your own unhappy patient

As mentioned above, the key to improving patient satisfaction is improved communication. When a patient is unhappy or has an unsatisfactory result, I see the patient more frequently in my clinic (even though the staff and I might want to see the patient less!). I attempt to provide emotional support and reassurance to the patient. If it is appropriate to the situation, I will express regret that the outcome was not what the patient wished. Throughout these visits, any possible consultation fees are waived. It is helpful to have other staff (for example, your most senior nurse) attend all the consultations with you and develop a rapport with the patient if possible. The patient may tell the nurse information that he or she would not tell you, and if the relationship between you and the patient breaks down, the nurse can be helpful in relaying information to the patient. For similar reasons, the patient should be encouraged to bring a friend or family member along to the consultations.

For everyone's safety and to avoid later confusion, ensure that you document all visits and discussions clearly in the patient record. It can be helpful to send the patient a letter at the end of each consultation summarizing any discussions that were held and any decisions that were made.

Conclusion

Patient selection in plastic surgery is challenging. Patient evaluation can be difficult to teach during residency and unfortunately is often learnt through trial and error while in practice. Your ability to recognize patients who are unsuitable for surgery physically, or who may not cope emotionally with the surgery, is an integral part of running a successful practice. Time spent with patients preoperatively, ensuring that they understand the potential benefits, risks, and complications, pays dividends postoperatively as their expectations are more likely to be met. As plastic surgeons, our prime responsibility is to the safety of our patients, as well as their comfort and satisfaction. I will not undertake surgery that I do not feel is in the best interest of my patients. Focusing on the welfare of the patient, utilizing good communication skills, and carrying out a thorough evaluation of the patient preoperatively can prevent postoperative dissatisfaction.

Bonus images for this chapter can be found online at http://www.expertconsult.com

FIG. 1.6 Example letter to friends and family regarding surgical discount.

FIG. 1.7 (A,B) Examples of preconsultation medical questionnaires.

FIG. 1.8 Example photographic consent form.

FIG. 1.9 Example of a generic follow-up letter after consultation.

FIG. 1.11 Example surgery consent form.

FIG. 1.12 Example list of medication patient is told to avoid preoperatively.

FIG. 1.13 Example presurgery anesthesia evaluation form.

FIG. 1.14 Example discharge advice form.

 Access the complete reference list online at **http://www.expertconsult.com**

2. Bashour M. History and Current Concepts in the Analysis of Facial Attractiveness. *Plast Reconstr Surg.* 2006;118:741–756.

   Bashour provides an interesting discussion of the history of facial attractiveness with reference to the neoclassical canons, anthropology, and cephalometrics. He provides insights into social psychology and the components of facial attractiveness.

7. Perrett DI, May KA, Yoshikawa S. Facial shape and judgements of female attractiveness. *Nature.* 1994;368:239–242.

11. American Society for Aesthetic Plastic Surgery. Cosmetic surgery national data bank statistics 2010, cited 19 July 2010. Available from: http://www.surgery.org/sites/default/files/Stats2010_1.pdf.

14. Gorney M, Martello J. Patient selection criteria. *Clin Plast Surg.* 1999;26:37–40.

    The authors discuss the features of a suitable compared with an unsuitable patient for cosmetic surgery, and provide their visual representation graph of deformity vs concern level, to aid in patient selection.

15. Gorney M. Mirror, Mirror on the Wall: The Interface Between Illusion and Reality in Aesthetic Surgery. *Facial Plast Surg Clin North Am.* 2008;16:203–205.

17. American Psychiatric Association. *Diagnostic and Statistical Manual of Mental Disorders.* 4th ed. text revision. Washington, DC: American Psychiatric Association; 2000.

18. Ende KH, Lewis DL, Kabaker SS. Body Dysmorphic Disorder. *Facial Plast Surg Clin North Am.* 2008;16:217–223.

    The authors provide an excellent description of body dysmorphic disorder and how to identify it in patients presenting to a cosmetic surgery practice. Management strategies, including psychiatric referral and treatment prior to considering surgery, are covered.

21. Sarwer DB. Awareness and identification of body dysmorphic disorder by aesthetic surgeons: Results of a survey of american society for aesthetic plastic surgery members. *Aesthetic Surg J.* 2002;22:531–535.

22. Sykes JM. Managing the psychological aspects of plastic surgery patients. *Curr Opin Otolaryngol Head Neck Surg.* 2009;17:321–325.

23. Goode RL. The Unhappy Patient Following Facial Plastic Surgery: What to Do? *Facial Plast Surg Clin North Am.* 2008;16:183–186.

    Goode covers how to be a better patient selector and how to manage an unhappy patient. He clearly covers his program for dealing with a patient who has a flawed result, as well as one who has a good outcome but is still unsatisfied.

25. Sykes JM. Patient Selection in Facial Plastic Surgery. *Facial Plast Surg Clin North Am.* 2008;16:173–176.

    Sykes summarizes the process of patient selection and refusing services to plastic surgery patients with useful management suggestions and comments on the role of the plastic surgeon.

2

Nonsurgical skin care and rejuvenation

Leslie Baumann

Determining skin type

Fitzpatrick skin phototype

Dr. Thomas B Fitzpatrick first introduced his approach to categorizing skin type, now known as the Fitzpatrick skin phototype (SPT) system, in 1975 in order to evaluate a patient's response to ultraviolet (UV) exposure in preparation for treating psoriasis with light.[1] In this system, patients are assigned a skin type based on their reported ability to tan or burn. A minimum erythema dose (MED) is identified for each skin type, which the practitioner then uses as a guide for selecting doses of UV therapy for various skin conditions. Of note, this skin-typing system has evolved into a method for characterizing a patient's skin color. Currently, dermatologists may assign an SPT to a patient based on a clinical assessment of skin color and not necessarily after questions regarding the patient's history of sun tanning or burning (Table 2.1). The Fitzpatrick SPT system originally included skin types I–IV and categorized only white skin. Naturally dark pigmented skin is typically labeled as SPT IV–VI. When category V was first added, it was used to describe all skin of color (brown or dark-brown skin). The SPT VI designation was later added to classify further skin of color.[2] The correct use of the Fitzpatrick SPT is not an indicator of a patient's ethnicity or interpretation of an individual's skin color and complexion, but a measure of the skin's potential to burn or to tan.

Although the Fitzpatrick SPT is widely accepted and used in dermatology, the system does not fully address certain issues related to individuals with darker skin types. For instance, some authors have questioned the potential to predict a patient's MED based on reported ability to tan and burn. In fact, a poor correlation was observed between SPT, as obtained by self-reported tanning history, and MED in a study involving white patients. This study did reveal a better correlation between MED and skin complexion traits such as eye and hair color, freckling tendency, and number of moles.[3] A poor correlation between SPT, based on self-reported tanning history, and MED has also been found in various studies in Asian and Arab skin.[4–7] The authors of these studies have suggested that the SPT system is not applicable to non-white patients or the full range of ethnic backgrounds.

Another issue with the SPT system pertains to the correlation of visually assessed skin color with MED. Many dermatologists assign a Fitzpatrick SPT to a patient based on a clinical assessment of skin color, and rarely question a patient on skin-tanning history. Further, some authors have contended that SPT (as determined by observed skin color) does not correlate with the MED in ethnic skin. Specifically, they have suggested that, in skin of color, the constitutive pigment does not correlate with MED, as implied by the current conventional application of SPT.[8]

For example, patients of African descent are typically labeled as having Fitzpatrick SPT V (brown) or VI (dark brown). However, it has been discovered through questioning that some of these patients have reported that they do frequently burn. If categorized based on self-reported tanning history, a subset of such patients likely would be classified as having SPT III or IV. In a study that compared skin pigmentation as measured by diffuse reflectance spectroscopy of MEDs, investigators found that epidermal pigmentation was not an accurate predictor of skin sensitivity to UVB radiation.[9] These data illustrate some of the limitations of the SPT, which was originally designed to assess lighter skin types. Although the Fitzpatrick SPT remains in wide use, several other systems have been created in an attempt to depict skin type more accurately.

Baumann skin-typing system

The author has developed the Baumann skin-typing system (BSTS) in order to recognize a wider range of cutaneous variables. Four skin parameters are assessed: (1) oily versus dry;

(2) sensitive versus resistant; (3) pigmented versus nonpigmented; and (4) wrinkled versus tight (unwrinkled). These four spectra are not mutually exclusive; therefore, assessing the skin using all four parameters yields 16 potential skin-type permutations (*Table 2.2*).

The BSTS provides specific guidance to identify the most suitable skin products for individuals, and also to help standardize the discussion of skin care science. The BST is easily determined by a scientifically validated questionnaire known as the Baumann skin type indicator (BSTI), which is used to identify baseline skin type[10] (questionnaire available at no charge at www.skintypesolutions.com). Doctors and aestheticians can use this information to help identify the products and procedures most suitable for their patients. The remainder of this chapter will discuss skin care science following the format of the BSTS.

Dry skin, or xerosis, is characterized by an impaired barrier, lack of natural moisturizing factor (NMF), or reduced sebum production. Conversely, oily skin is characterized by elevated sebum production. In the BSTS, a higher score indicates increased sebum production, while a low score corresponds to diminished skin hydration. A person with a BSTI score in the middle of this parameter is considered to have "normal" skin. It is possible for a person to vacillate between oily and dry skin with climate change. These skin types are known as "combination."

Characterized by inflammation, sensitive skin manifests as acne, rosacea, burning and stinging sensations, or skin rashes. Higher scores in the "S" portion of the BSTI suggest a greater likelihood that the patient exhibits several types of sensitive skin. For instance, a patient who has symptoms of burning and stinging as well as rosacea would have a higher "S" score than a patient with rosacea only. A robust stratum corneum (SC) is typical of someone with resistant skin, which protects the skin from allergens, other environmental irritants, and water loss. Erythema and acne are rare in people with resistant skin. Stronger skin care products and in-office procedures such as chemical peels can be more safely used on patients with resistant skin than on those with sensitive skin.

The pigmented/nonpigmented parameter refers to neither skin color nor ethnicity. Rather, this designation focuses on the propensity for skin to develop hyperpigmentation under certain stresses. Examples include a history of solar lentigines, melasma, and freckles. In this system, individuals with darker skin types are more likely to be categorized as having the pigmented skin type, while individuals with light skin who do not tan easily are often categorized as the nonpigmented skin type. Knowing a patient's "P" score can alert the physician to a patient's pigmentary changes and provides helpful

Table 2.1 The Fitzpatrick skin phototypes

Skin type	Typical features/appearance	Reaction to sun exposure/tanning tendency
Type I	Very fair/pale skin; blond or red hair; light-colored eyes; freckles common	Always burns, never tans
Type II	Fair-skinned; light eyes; light hair	Burns easily, occasionally tans
Type III	Medium/darker white/fair skin; eye and hair color vary	Sometimes burns, gradually tans
Type IV	Mediterranean Caucasian skin (olive to light brown); medium to heavily pigmented	Burns minimally, tans easily
Type V	Middle Eastern skin; rarely sun-sensitive	Rarely burns, tans always
Type VI	Dark brown/black skin, rarely sun-sensitive	Never burns, always tans darkly

Table 2.2 The Baumann skin-typing system

	Oily		Dry		
	Pigmented	Nonpigmented	Pigmented	Nonpigmented	
Sensitive	OSPW	OSNW	DSPW	DSNW	Wrinkled
Sensitive	OSPT	OSNT	DSPT	DSNT	Tight
Resistant	ORPW	ORNW	DRPW	DRNW	Wrinkled
Resistant	ORPT	ORNT	DRPT	DRNT	Tight

O, oily; D, dry; P, pigmented; N, nonpigmented; S, sensitive; R, resistant; W, wrinkled; T, tight.

data for the practitioner to consider when adjusting chemical peel strengths and laser settings to prevent the development of postinflammatory hyperpigmentation.

A discussion of the fourth "wrinkled" parameter is subsumed within the following discussion on skin aging.

Skin aging

The manifestation of cutaneous aging is a result of the complex interplay between intrinsic and extrinsic factors. Intrinsic aging is attributed to individual heredity and the natural effects of the passage of time and, as such, is considered inevitable and beyond voluntary control. Extrinsic aging occurs as the result of exogenous insults, such as exposure to UV radiation, cigarette smoke, other pollution, as well as poor nutrition, and, by definition, can be avoided. Premature skin aging is evidence of extrinsic aging. In fact, 80% of facial aging is attributed to solar exposure alone.[11]

At a cellular level, UV exposure leads to skin damage through numerous mechanisms, including sunburn cell formation, thymine dimer development, collagenase production, and engendering an inflammatory response. These lead to photoaging, photocarcinogenesis, and photoimmunosuppression.[12] Interestingly, a recent paper suggests that the photoaging and melanogenesis provoked by UV exposure are linked to telomere-based DNA damage signaling that may represent a cancer avoidance protective response.[13] Telomeres, specialized chromosomal components, shorten with age; telomeric loss or erosion has thus become an important measure of cellular aging, a veritable internal aging clock.[14] The enzyme telomerase, which stabilizes or lengthens telomeres, is expressed in about 90% of all tumors but absent in many somatic tissues.[15] One of the few regenerative tissues to express telomerase, however, is the epidermis.[16] Telomerase is believed to act against excessive telomere loss in human epidermis throughout the lifelong regeneration process.[17] Interestingly, exposure to UV radiation, due to its deleterious effect on DNA and its acceleration of telomere shortening, can be characterized as influential in intrinsic as well as extrinsic aging. Signaling through p53 after telomere disruption is also typically observed in skin aging and photodamage.[18] Currently, there are no skin care products available that target telomerase.

At the macroscopic level, the development of rhytides, caused by alterations in the dermal layer of skin, is the most prominent manifestation of cutaneous aging. Because few skin care product ingredients can sufficiently penetrate the dermis to ameliorate deep wrinkles, the prevention of rhytides is the focus of dermatologic antiaging skin care.[19] Specifically, dermatologists aim to slow the degradation of or replenish the three main dermal constituents (collagen, elastin, and hyaluronic acid), all of which are known to decline with age. Reducing inflammation is key here, as inflammation can contribute to the breakdown of these structural components of the skin. Skin inflammation itself can result from the formation of free radicals, which can act directly on growth factor and cytokine receptors in keratinocytes and dermal cells.

While the exact mechanisms of growth factors and cytokines in skin aging have not been fully understood, it has been established that they function together in a complex interplay involving several types of growth factors and cytokines.[20] Better understood, however, is the influence of free radicals on the aging process. The activation of the mitogen-activated protein kinase pathways induced by free radicals has been shown to result in collagenase synthesis, paving the way for collagen degradation.[21] Using antioxidants to inhibit this pathway is believed to prevent photoaging by thwarting collagenase production. In a study on human skin, Kang *et al.* demonstrated that pretreatment with the antioxidants genistein and N-acetyl cysteine hindered the UV induction of the cJun-driven enzyme collagenase.[22] Vitamins C and E, ferulic acid, coenzyme Q10, green tea, pycnogenol, silymarin, and idebenone are among the various antioxidants featured in multiple skin care products.

Dry skin

The relative lack of moisture in the SC is indicative of xerosis, or dry skin, which is characterized by cracks and fissures when the level of water, the primary plasticizer of the skin, is low.[23] Water content in the SC must be at least 10% in order for the skin to appear and feel normal.[24] The elevation in transepidermal water loss (TEWL) that progresses to xerosis occurs when a defect in the permeability barrier permits the loss of excess water to the atmosphere. The etiology of the barrier perturbation itself is generally multifactorial and includes variables such as harsh detergents, acetone, and other contactants, as well as frequent bathing (*Box 2.1*).

Dry skin can also be engendered by changes in the epidermal lipid component of the skin. The incidence of dry skin is suspected by some dermatologists to have increased in recent years, a phenomenon that has been attributed to increased bathing and showering using hot water, foaming cleansers, fragranced bubble baths, and bath salts, all of which can denude the skin of lipids, thus impairing barrier function. In fact, soap, detergents, and hard water all have the capacity to wash off the healthy and normal barrier of the skin.

Underlying disease is not the root cause of the majority of dry-skin complaints. Most patients simply lack the ability to cope with environmental elements that adversely affect the water-binding capacity of the SC (see *Box 2.1* for environmental factors that can cause dry skin). Dry skin is more likely to occur during the fall and winter months due to lower humidity as well as excessive bathing in hot water. The condition also increases with age, as skin tends to become less oily. Indeed, xerosis has been referred to as "winter itch" because it is at its worst during that season. The areas of the body most often affected are those with comparatively few sebaceous glands, such as the arms, legs, and torso.

Box 2.1 **Exogenous factors that can lead to dry skin**	
• Hot water	• Pollution
• Detergents	• Other chemicals
• Friction from clothing	• Air conditioning
• Frequent air travel	

Clinical signs

Initial clinical signs of xerosis include a dull gray-white color and increased topographical skin markings.[25] With increased dryness, TEWL spurs a degradation in the cohesiveness between the corneocytes, while resulting in an abnormal retention of desmosomes. The loss of cohesiveness in entire sheets of corneocytes manifests in scaling, flaking, and an overall rough cutaneous texture. The resultant appearance of the skin is dull because a rough surface is less able to refract light than a smooth surface. The skin is then less pliable with stretching and bending; diminished elasticity can then yield visible cracks and fissures.

Basic skin care formulations

Xerotic symptoms can be treated by increasing the hydration state of the SC with occlusive or humectant ingredients and by smoothing the rough surface with an emollient. Moisturizers are designed to increase cutaneous hydration. Most moisturizers are oil-in-water emulsions, such as creams and lotions, or water-in-oil emulsions such as hand creams. While moisturizers are intended to enhance the hydration state of the SC, moisturizing ingredients operate in discrete ways. Occlusives coat the SC and retard TEWL; humectants draw water from the atmosphere as well as the underlying epidermis, thus hydrating the skin; and emollients soften and smooth the skin. Practitioners should understand the distinct categories of moisturizing ingredients and how various individual and combination products work. Toners were invented to remove the soap scum of cleansers. Modern cleansers do not leave this film in most cases (and when they do, it is disastrous) so toners are not really necessary in a skin care line. Cleansing agents are used by people of all skin types. Brief primers on cleansing agents and moisturizing agents follow.

Cleansers

Surfactants are the main active ingredients in cleanser products. They regulate the degree of mildness or irritancy of a formulation. Most surfactants in cleansers are anionic, because of their ideal foam and lather qualities.

Bar surfactants

Soap (alkyl carboxylate), the primary surfactant in most cleansing bars, is usually produced by saponification, involving a reaction of a triglyceride oil/fat with an alkali. Vegetable oils (e.g., palm oil, palm oil derivatives, rice bran oil, ground nut oil, and castor oil combined with coconut oil or palm kernel oil) are typical.[26] Nonvegetable ingredients in soap typically come from animal fat (e.g., tallow). Despite their effectiveness as cleansers, soaps can irritate the skin, causing erythema, xerosis, and pruritus, especially in cold weather.[27] Newer classes of soaps (i.e., superfatted soaps, transparent soaps, and combination bars) have been developed to provoke less irritancy.

Superfatted soaps

Superfatting is intended to enhance the mildness, moisturization, lather, mush value, and wear rate of a soap.[28-30] This is achieved through incomplete saponification (neutralization)

by leaving unreacted fatty acids or oils in the soap or by adding fatty alcohols, fatty acids, or esters during production.

Transparent soaps

Manufacturing with a high level of humectants intended to solubilize the soap renders a transparent, clear appearance. Transparent soaps contain high levels of active soap and an alkaline pH, qualities that typically cause irritancy. These products are usually mild, however, due to the presence of the humectant glycerin and low levels of fatty acids.[31]

Combination bars

Combination bars (combars) combine natural soaps with milder synthetic surfactants. The pH of these products is in the high range (9.0–9.5), but the synthetic surfactants seem to inhibit irritancy, leaving these products less likely to cause irritation as compared to average soaps.[32]

Synthetic detergent bars

Unlike soaps, synthetic detergent bars (syndet bars) are created through esterification, ethoxylation, and sulfonation of oils, fats, or petroleum products, and are formulated in the neutral-pH range. Alkyl glyceryl ether sulfonate, alpha olefin sulfonates, betaines, sulfosuccinates, sodium cocoyl monoglyceride sulfate, and sodium cocoyl isethionate are among the synthetic surfactants used in such bars.[33] The most commonly used synthetic surfactant is sodium cocoyl isethionate, which confers mildness on these products.

Liquid surfactants

Anionic and amphoteric surfactants are often combined in liquid cleansers. Soaps (salts of fatty acids) and synthetic surfactants such as alkyl ether sulfate, alkyl acyl isethionates, alkyl phosphates, alkyl sulfosuccinates, and alkyl sulfonates are the anionic surfactants regularly used in these products. The common amphoteric or zwitterionic surfactants used are cocoamido propyl betaine and cocoamphoacetate. Nonionic surfactants (e.g., alkyl polyglucoside) and amino acid-based surfactants (e.g., acyl glycinates, alkyl glutamates, and sarcosinates) are increasingly used as the main surfactants in liquid cleansers because they enhance mildness. Most liquid cleansers have a pH in the neutral to acidic range; however, the products that contain soap (alkyl carboxylate) as the chief active ingredient usually have an alkaline pH *(Box 2.2)*.

Moisturizers

Moisturizers increase water content in the SC by preventing water evaporation (TEWL) from the skin with the use of occlusive ingredients or by increasing the integrity of the skin

---

Box 2.2

- For patients with dry skin, suggest a nonfoaming cleanser such as a cleansing milk, oil, or cream.
- Surfactants in foaming cleansers strip necessary lipids from the skin, leaving the skin with an inability to hold on to water.
- Unpublished marketing studies show that most patients prefer the stripping foaming cleansers because they "feel cleaner," so it is crucial to educate patients with dry skin to avoid these.

barrier. The primary method of increasing the integrity of the skin barrier is delivering fatty acids, ceramides, and cholesterol to the skin and controlling the calcium gradient. Assisting the skin to hold on to water is another moisturization approach, achieved by increasing levels of NMF, glycerol (glycerin), and other humectants such as hyaluronic acid. Enhancing the ability of the epidermis to absorb important components for the circulation, such as glycerol and water through aquaporin channels, also augments skin hydration *(Box 2.3)*.

Occlusives

Typically oily substances that can dissolve fats, and therefore widely used in skin care cosmetics, occlusives coat the SC to inhibit TEWL and provide an emollient effect. Two of the best occlusive ingredients are petrolatum and mineral oil. Petrolatum, a purified mixture of hydrocarbons derived from petroleum (crude oil) and used as a skin care product since 1872, exhibits a water vapor loss resistance 170 times that of olive oil.[34] The hydrocarbon molecules present in petrolatum prevent oxidation, yielding a long shelf-life for this occlusive, considered the gold standard to which other ingredients are compared.[35] However, although also known for being non-comedogenic, petrolatum has a greasy feeling that may render it cosmetically unacceptable to patients.[36] Mineral oil, or liquid petrolatum, is derived from the distillation of petroleum in the production of gasoline; cosmetic-grade mineral oil has been available for over 100 years and is one of the most frequently used oils in skin care products.[37] In 2004, a randomized double-blind controlled trial of 34 patients with mild-to-moderate xerosis demonstrated that mineral oil and extra-virgin coconut oil were equally efficacious and safe as moisturizers, with surface lipid levels and skin hydration significantly improved in both groups.[38] However, an earlier epidemiologic review of the relationship between mineral oil exposure and cancer that revealed several associations has spawned some myths about this agent.[39] The cases of cancer that occurred resulted from prolonged exposure to industrial-grade mineral oil. Cosmetic-grade mineral oil has never been linked to cancer. Also, unlike the industrial grade, cosmetic-grade mineral oil is noncomedogenic. Significantly, occlusive agents are effective only while present on the skin; TEWL returns to the previous level once occlusives are removed.

Occlusives are typically combined with humectant ingredients in moisturizers. Other commonly used occlusive ingredients include lanolin, paraffin, squalene, dimethicone, propylene glycol, beeswax, soybean oil, grapeseed oil,[40] and other "natural" oils that have become increasingly popular, such as sunflower seed, evening primrose, olive oil, and jojoba oils.[41–45]

Lanolin

Derived from the sebaceous secretions of sheep, lanolin is a complex natural product that cannot be synthesized; its composition is very different than human sebum.[46] Nevertheless, like SC lipids, lanolin contains cholesterol, an essential component of SC lipids, and, significantly, both lanolin and SC lipids can coexist as solids and liquids at physiologic temperatures. The concern over allergic reactions to lanolin has led to the development of ultrapure medical-grade lanolin products, which have been demonstrated as effective in treating dry skin and healing superficial wounds.[47–49]

Oils

The rise in popularity of natural and organic ingredients has led to the frequent use or inclusion of essential oils in moisturizing products. Both hydrophobic and lipophilic, oil is a substance that is liquid at room temperature and insoluble in water. Oils actually contain copious lipids, which the skin requires for the proper formation and function of cell membranes to prevent TEWL. Specifically, several natural oils contain fatty acids important in maintaining the skin barrier. Linoleic acid, an omega-6 fatty acid present in sunflower, safflower, and other oils, is an essential fatty acid that must be obtained from the diet or through topical application. Several foods and oils contain linoleic acid and many of these oils are found in skin care products that supply fatty acids while functioning as occlusive agents. Linoleic acid is important because it is necessary to produce ceramide in the skin's barrier.

Humectants

Humectants are water-soluble materials with high water absorption capabilities. In low-humidity conditions, however, humectants can attract water from the deeper epidermis and dermis, thereby exacerbating xerosis.[50] Therefore, humectants are effective as intended when combined with occlusive ingredients. In cosmetic moisturizers, humectant ingredients prevent product evaporation and thickening, thereby prolonging product shelf-life. Humectants can also alter the appearance of the skin; that is, by drawing water into the skin, a slight swelling of the SC results, rendering the perception of smoother skin with fewer wrinkles. Consequently, several moisturizers are marketed as "antiwrinkle creams" even though they confer no long-term antiwrinkling benefit. Commonly used humectants include glycerin, urea, sorbitol, sodium hyaluronate, propylene glycol, alpha hydroxy acids (AHAs), and sugars. Urea, which has been included in hand creams since the 1940s,[51] is a component of the NMF and also exhibits a mild antipruritic effect.[52] It is important to note that hyaluronic acid, a humectant, does not penetrate into the dermis when applied topically.

Glycerin

A potent humectant, glycerin (glycerol) displays a hygroscopic ability comparable to that of NMF,[53] which allows the SC to retain a high water content even in a dry environment. Glycerol levels have been shown to correlate with SC hydration levels, suggesting a significant role in skin hydration for this humectant.[54] In a 5-year study comparing two high-glycerin moisturizers with 16 other popular moisturizers in 394 patients with severely dry skin, the high-glycerin products were found to be superior because they rapidly restored normal hydration to dry skin and helped to prevent the return to dryness for a longer period than other products, even those containing petrolatum.[55] Glycerin induces an expansion of the SC due to increased thickness of the corneocytes and creates expanded spaces between layers of corneocytes.[56] Therefore, it appears that glycerin generates a reservoir of moisture-holding ability that leaves the skin more resistant to drying. It is worth noting that, while glycerol can be obtained from topical preparations, it can also be transported from the circulation into the epidermis through aquaporin channels. Normal SC hydration requires endogenous glycerol according to recent studies.[57] The potential importance of endogenous glycerol for normal SC hydration has been shown by two different studies by Hara *et al.* Knockout mice, which lack the aquaporin-3 (AQP-3) water channel, cannot transport glycerol from the circulation into the epidermis and they exhibit abnormal SC hydration and decreased SC glycerol levels.[58] The topical application of glycerol remedies this defect in mice.[59]

Emollients

By filling the spaces between desquamating corneocytes and providing increased cohesion, resulting in a flattening of the curled edges of the individual corneocytes, emollients yield a smooth surface, and are added to cosmetics to soften and smooth the skin.[32,60] Many emollients act as humectants and occlusive moisturizers as well. Lanolin, mineral oil, and petrolatum are occlusive ingredients that also impart an emollient effect. Several natural ingredients also confer such benefits.

Oatmeal

Wild oats (*Avena sativa*) have been used for over 2000 years in traditional folk medicine, especially as a poultice or soak. For decades in the West, colloidal oat grain suspensions have been used as adjuvant therapy for atopic dermatitis.[61] Colloidal oatmeal has replaced rolled oats and oatmeal in skin care products, and has exhibited moisturizing and anti-inflammatory properties.[60] Further, oatmeal is one of the few botanically derived products labeled by the Food and Drug Administration (FDA) as an effective skin protectant.

Shea butter

Used widely in cosmetic formulations as a moisturizer, particularly as an emollient, shea butter (*Butyrospermum parkii*) is a natural fat derived from the African shea or karite tree that has been shown to manifest anti-inflammatory activity.[62] Shea butter is found in various skin and hair care products, especially high-end skin products, and is touted for delivering rich emollient benefits. It is also believed to confer benefits as an adjuvant moisturizer in the treatment of atopic dermatitis, dry skin, acne, scars, and striae alba.

Other ingredients

Vitamins C and E, coffeeberry, green tea, and coenzyme Q10 are among the antioxidant ingredients often found in moisturizers. These are popular ingredients because antioxidants are believed to neutralize the free radicals that assault the skin and other organs and thereby contribute to cutaneous aging. Niacinamide and soy, which are key depigmenting agents, are also popular additives in cosmetic moisturizers. Glycyl-L-histidyl-L-lysine-Cu^{2+} (GHK-Cu), a copper tripeptide complex, is also found in many moisturizers. GHK-Cu complex has been used for many years to enhance wound healing and it has also been demonstrated to augment collagen synthesis.[63,64]

Hydroxy acids

Alpha hydroxy acids

AHAs, a group of water-soluble, naturally occurring compounds so named because they contain a hydroxy group in the alpha position, function as humectants as well as exfoliants. This versatile family includes glycolic acid (derived from sugar cane), lactic acid (from sour milk), citric acid (from citrus fruits), malic acid (from apples), tartaric acid (from grapes), and phytic acid (from rice).[65] Glycolic acid and lactic acids are the most commonly used AHAs, were the first to reach the market, and will be the only ones discussed here. Topical preparations containing AHAs have long been known to influence epidermal keratinization,[66] and the use of hydroxy acids in skin care dates back to ancient Egypt and Cleopatra, who was believed to have applied sour milk to her face to foster youthfulness.

The cosmetic effects of hydroxy acids include normalization of SC exfoliation, leading to enhanced plasticization and fewer dry scales on the skin surface. AHAs and beta hydroxy acid (BHA) degrade the desmosomes and allow desquamation to proceed. They also affect corneocyte cohesion at the basement levels of the SC,[67] where they alter pH and promote desquamation. Applying AHAs and BHA in high concentrations results in the detachment of keratinocytes and epidermolysis. Application of AHAs and BHA at lower concentrations degrades intercorneocyte cohesion directly above the granular layer, which accelerates desquamation and SC thinning. A thinner SC is more flexible and compact, and better reflects light, giving the skin a more luminous and youthful appearance.[68] However, a thinner SC can confer some disadvantages, as exfoliants have been shown to reduce the MED of the skin.[69] Although one study indicated that glycolic acid delivered a photoprotective effect,[70] subsequent studies have suggested that increased photosensitivity is associated with the application of AHAs.[71,72] The FDA now requires that AHA products include a label warning that sun protection should accompany their use.

Lactic acid

Lactic acid, first used in 1943 for the treatment of ichthyosis,[73] is a popular AHA found in several at-home products as well as prescription moisturizers, and is usually not used as an in-office peel. It is unique insofar as it is an AHA as well as a component of the NMF, which plays an important role in hydration. Studies of the activity of buffered 12% ammonium lactate lotion (LacHydrin) have documented the moisturizing ability of lactic acid.[74] One study using 5% and 12% lactic acid resulted in increases in skin firmness and thickness and enhanced texture and hydration in the epidermis, but not dermis.[75] Lactic acid (particularly the L-isomer) has been shown *in vitro* and *in vivo* to augment ceramide synthesis by keratinocytes.[76] In fact, application of the L-isomer of lactic acid to keratinocytes also increased the ratio of ceramide-1-linoleate to ceramide-1-oleate, which is significant because a lower ceramide-1-linoleate to ceramide-1-oleate ratio is seen in atopic dermatitis and acne.[77,78] In addition, lactic acid imparts antiaging benefits, as implied by a double-blind vehicle-controlled study finding that an 8% L-lactic acid formula performed better than vehicle in treating photoaged skin, with statistically significant improvements in skin roughness, mottled hyperpigmentation, and sallowness.[79]

Glycolic acid

Popularly known as "the lunchtime peel" because it can be completed quickly, effectively, and discreetly within a lunch hour without obvious visible signs, glycolic acid is the AHA most commonly used in chemical peels in the offices of dermatologists and aestheticians. In 1996, Ditre et al. demonstrated that applying AHAs led to a 25% increase in skin thickness, increased acid mucopolysaccharides in the dermis, improved the quality of the elastic fibers, and increased collagen density, as determined histologically.[80] Such findings imply that AHAs reverse some of the histological signs of aging. Such data were buttressed by Moon et al., who reported that mice treated with glycolic acid exhibited a significant reduction in wrinkle score and an increase in collagen production, which typically decreases with age.[81] Increased collagen production after treatment with AHAs has been demonstrated in vivo and in vitro using fibroblast cultures. Glycolic acid treatments increased collagen synthesis as well as fibroblast proliferation in vitro in one study.[82] To prevent burning, glycolic acid, unlike many other peels, must be neutralized after use. Therefore, glycolic acid should not be used on large areas of the body, but, rather, in small areas on which application can be quickly applied and neutralized.

Beta hydroxy acid

The only BHA, salicylic acid, is a chemical exfoliant derived from willow bark, wintergreen leaves, and sweet birch, though it is also available in synthetic form.[83] Although labeled a BHA because the aromatic carboxylic acid has a hydroxy group in the beta position, the carbons of aromatic compounds are traditionally given Arabic numerals (1, 2, etc.) rather than the Greek letter designations typical for the nonaromatic structures. Salicylic acid was likely labeled a BHA at the time the peels were introduced for marketing purposes and to benefit from the popularity of AHAs. Although BHA is a newer category of chemical peels, salicylic acid has a long and versatile history of effectiveness in skin care. As a chemical peel, salicylic acid is available in over-the-counter home products (usually in 0.5–2% concentrations and often labeled as "acne washes," and suitable for treating acne, rosacea, photoaging, and hyperpigmentation) and in those used in the office (usually 20–30% concentration). It is also a component in various in-office peels using a combination of ingredients, such as the Jessner's Peel, the PCA peel by Physician's Choice, and the Pigment Plus Peel by Biomedic.

Most cosmetic dermatologists use preparations of 20% or 30% salicylic acid for in-office peels, which have been demonstrated to fade pigment spots, decrease surface roughness, and reduce fine lines,[84] comparable to AHA peels. In the early 1990s, satisfactory results were seen using 50% salicylic acid on the hands and forearms of patients with actinically induced pigmentary alterations.[85] These effects are likely a result of enhanced exfoliation and an accelerated cell cycle, as observed with AHAs. Unlike AHAs, however, BHA influences the arachidonic acid cascade and, consequently, displays anti-inflammatory activity, which may allow salicylic acid peels to be effective while causing less irritation than AHA peels. The anti-inflammatory properties of salicylic acid render it very useful in a peel for patients with acne and rosacea. BHC can also be combined with other acne treatments to accelerate the resolution of comedones and papules. In addition, salicylic acid is lipophilic, which enables it to impart a stronger comedolytic effect than AHA peels as well as penetrate the sebaceous material in the hair follicle and exfoliate the pores.

Of note, salicylic acid peels can exert a whitening effect in patients with darker skin types. A study of 24 Asian women treated with biweekly facial peeling with 30% salicylic acid in absolute ethanol for 3 months exhibited some pigmentary lightening.[86] Postinflammatory hyperpigmentation can also result from BHA peels. Unlike AHAs, BHA does not need to be neutralized and the frost is visible once the peel is complete.

Sensitive skin

Sensitive skin has been historically difficult to fully characterize. Yokota et al. as well as Pons-Guiraud offered their input on this convoluted issue by offering classification systems within the past decade; however, few agree on a typing system for sensitive skin.[87,88] Within the BSTS framework, sensitive skin is classified into four types based on clinical manifestations: type 1 (developing open and closed comedones and pimples; known as the acne type or S1 type), type 2 (facial flushing due to heat, spicy food, emotion or vasodilation of any cause; known as the flushing rosacea type or the S2 type), type 3 (burning, itching, or stinging of any cause; the S3 type), and type 4 (susceptible to developing contact dermatitis and irritant dermatitis and often associated with impaired skin barrier; the S4 type) (Table 2.3). It is important to note that patients can suffer from combinations of sensitive skin subtypes. For example, an individual may burn and sting and develop acne due to the use of particular skin care products. This person would be designated as an S1S3 sensitive skin type. The remainder of the sensitive skin discussion will focus on acne, rosacea, and the main class of topical treatments.

Acne

Acne vulgaris, characterized by open or closed comedones as well as papules and pustules, is a multifactorial process involving the pilosebaceous unit. This most commonly reported skin disorder affects more than 17 million people

Table 2.3 **Baumann sensitive skin classification**

Type 1	Pimples and comedones
Type 2	Flushing
Type 3	Burning and stinging or itching
Type 4	Impaired barrier, contact and irritant dermatitis

Box 2.4

- Acne treatment should consist of a salicylic acid cleanser, a topical antibiotic or benzoyl peroxide, a prescription retinoid and a topical anti-inflammatory serum or moisturizer.
- It is important to recommend a nonacnegenic sunscreen as well.

Box 2.5 **Topical ingredients in skin care and hair care products that may cause acne[12–14]**

- Avocado oil
- Butyl stearate
- Ceteareth 20
- Cocoa butter
- Coconut oil
- Decyl oleate
- Evening primrose oil
- Isocetyl stearate
- Isopropyl isostearate
- Isopropyl isothermal
- Isopropyl myristate
- Isopropyl palmitate
- Isostearyl neopentanoate
- Lanolin
- Laureth 4
- Lauric acid
- Myristyl myristate
- Octyl palmitate
- Octyl stearate
- Oleth-3
- PPG myristyl propionate
- Putty stearate
- Red dyes
- Soybean oil
- Stearic acid

annually in the US alone,[89] and 75–95% of all teens are affected.[90] Most patients outside this age range are adult women, who usually exhibit a hormonal aspect to their acne. Approximately 12% of women are affected by acne until the age of 44 compared to only 3% of men up to the same age.[91] Acne caused by exposure to cosmetics was dubbed "acne cosmetica" by Kligman and Mills in 1972.[92] In all cases, early and individually tailored treatment is required to achieve a satisfactory resolution and cosmetic appearance for the patient *(Box 2.4)*.

Although comedogenesis and acnegenesis are distinct processes, comedones usually precede acne. Comedogenesis is a noninflammatory follicular reaction exhibited by a dense compact hyperkeratosis of the follicle. Acnegenesis is characterized by inflammation of the follicular epithelium, which loosens hyperkeratotic material within the follicle, leading to the formation of pustules and papules. The etiology of acne varies from person to person and within individuals, and, therefore, is somewhat elusive; however, three principal factors have been identified: (1) sebaceous gland hyperactivity; (2) changes in follicular keratinization; and (3) the influence of bacteria. No topical products have been proven to decrease sebum production, although many make this claim. Retinoids and hydroxy acids normalize follicular keratinization, and antibiotics and benzoyl peroxide reduce the acne-causing bacteria *Propionibacterium acnes*.

Coconut oil and isopropyl myristate are among the numerous ingredients in skin care and hair care products that can exacerbate acne *(Box 2.5)*. Some of the more comedogenic products include blushes, lipstick, and other color cosmetics that contain drug and cosmetic red dyes, which are derived from coal tar. In addition, sunscreen ingredients have been known to provoke acneiform eruptions.[93] Another class of treatments, anti-inflammatories, will be discussed after the following section on another typical sensitive skin presentation, rosacea.

Rosacea

Known to afflict millions after the age of 30, rosacea is a chronic cutaneous disorder presenting as central facial erythema, telangiectasia, papules, pustules, flushing, and facial redness. It is often confused with acne. Rosacea is more common in fair-skinned than dark-skinned individuals. Risk factors for developing this condition include photodamage, a tendency toward facial flushing, and genetic predisposition. Aggravating factors include sunlight, heat, alcohol consumption, and spicy food *(Box 2.6)*.

The precise causal pathways of rosacea remain unknown. Several etiologic factors have been implicated, including genetic predisposition, *Demodex folliculorum* mites, *Helicobacter pylori* infection, vascular lability, response to chemical and

Box 2.6

- Rosacea treatment should combine in-office intense pulsed light treatments with an at-home regimen containing an anti-inflammatory cleanser, moisturizer, and sunscreen.
- A topical antibiotic such as metronidazole or an anti-inflammatory such as azelaic acid is added at night.
- Green tea and caffeine combinations are commonly used in serum and cream preparations.
- Avoidance of alcohol and spicy food should be stressed if these are triggers.

ingested agents, and psychogenic factors. This discussion will be limited to factors related to inflammatory pathways. While the digestive tract bacteria debate over *H. pylori* remains controversial, it has been suggested that intestinal inflammation and bacteria may induce hypersensitization of facial sensory neurons via the plasma kallikrein-kinin pathway and production of bradykinin, a well-known vasodilator.[94,95] Further, matrix metalloproteinase-9 (MMP-9), also known as gelatinase, has been implicated in the pathophysiology of rosacea as elevated levels of MMP-9 have been noted in patients with ocular rosacea.[96] An etiologic theory based on vascular response may be explained by a combination of factors such as the superficiality of cutaneous vasculature on the face,[97] greater blood flow of facial skin,[98] and vascular dysregulation via humoral and neural mechanisms causing vasodilatation.[99–101] A recent study of rosacea patients revealed the presence of vascular endothelial growth factor (VEGF) receptors on vascular endothelium in addition to the expression of both VEGF and VEGF receptors on inflammatory cells.[102] The investigators suggested that VEGF "receptor-ligand binding" may play a role in rosacea etiology. Topical antiangiogenic growth factors will likely be a target of future rosacea therapy research.[103]

In another recent study, investigators observed that individuals with rosacea express abnormally high levels of the proteins cathelicidin and SC tryptic enzyme (also called kallikrein 5), and showed that when both proteins are present in excess, aberrant enzymatic processing occurs and yields high levels of abnormal cathelicidin, which is proinflammatory, and clinically results in the erythema, inflammation, and vascular dilatation and growth characteristic of rosacea.[104] Notably, increased cathelicidins in the case of psoriasis and decreased levels in the case of atopic dermatitis have been implicated in the pathophysiologic pathways of those conditions.[105] Currently, approaches to modify cathelicidin production are under development. In the meantime, anti-inflammatories are a mainstay in multimodal rosacea therapy. (*Table 2.4* provides a wider range of rosacea treatment modalities than can be covered in this chapter.) Just as there is variability in the type of sensitive skin that patients may exhibit, there is a wide range of anti-inflammatory treatments available to treat the symptom common to all types of sensitive skin.

Table 2.4 Rosacea treatment modalities
Topical treatments
Antibiotics
Metronidazole Clindamycin Erythromycin
Anti-inflammatories
Azelaic acid Feverfew Green tea Licochalcone Licorice extract
Immunomodulators
Pimecrolimus Tacrolimus
Sulfur products
Sulfur Sodium sulfacetamide
Oral antibiotics
Tetracyclines (tetracycline, doxycycline, minocycline) Macrolides (erythromycin, azithromycin, clarithromycin) Metronidazole Ampicillin Trimethoprim/sulfamethoxazole
Other oral treatments
Isotretinoin Aspirin Beta-blockers Selective serotonin reuptake inhibitors Clonidine Hormones (oral contraceptives)
Laser and light treatments
Intense pulsed light therapy Vascular lasers (pulsed dye laser, Dornier 940 nm, KTP laser) Carbon dioxide resurfacing laser
Other treatments (for phymatous subtype)
Hot loop electrocoagulation Dermabrasion

Treatments for sensitive skin

Corticosteroids (topical)

Corticosteroids inhibit proinflammatory genes that encode cytokines, cell adhesion molecules, and other mediators interfering with the inflammatory response.[106] Specifically, they selectively induce anti-inflammatory proteins such as annexin I and MAPK phosphatase-1. Annexin I physically interacts with and blocks cytosolic phospholipase $A_2\alpha$ ($cPLA_2\alpha$).[107] Thus, corticosteroids suppress the release of arachidonic acid and its subsequent conversion to eicosanoids.[108] Bacteria, viruses, cytokines, and UV radiation are inflammatory signals that activate the MAPK cascades.[109] Although topical corticosteroids are generally well tolerated for short-term treatment of inflammatory skin diseases, long-term use can engender adverse cutaneous effects such as skin atrophy, hirsutism, folliculitis, acne, striae, telangiectasia, purpura, and unwelcome pigmentary changes.[110,111] More serious systemic side effects of chronic topical corticosteroid use have also been reported, including hypothalamic–pituitary axis suppression, hyperglycemia, avascular osteonecrosis, glaucoma, and posterior subcapsular cataracts.[112–116] Although corticosteroids work well for rosacea, they should not be used because they lead to compensatory redness when they are discontinued and can thin the skin with prolonged use.

Cyclooxygenase inhibitors (systemic)

Although their use for cutaneous conditions is somewhat limited,[117] an increasing number of nonsteroidal anti-inflammatory drugs (NSAIDs) specifically target bioactive lipids generated from arachidonic acid. Ibuprofen, for instance, has demonstrated effectiveness in treating acne, because inflammatory acne lesions are infiltrated with neutrophils and ibuprofen suppresses leukocyte chemotaxis.[118] Investigators conducted a double-blind study of 60 male and female patients 15–35 years old with acne vulgaris, randomly assigning patients to one of four groups: (1) oral ibuprofen (600 mg) plus tetracycline (250 mg) four times daily (qid); (2) ibuprofen (600 mg) plus placebo qid; (3) tetracycline (250 mg) plus placebo qid; and (4) two placebos qid. Only the combination therapy exerted a statistically better effect than the placebo in reducing total lesion count. Ibuprofen treatment alone achieved beneficial results comparable to the ones of tetracycline alone but with fewer side effects.[119] One year later, Funt performed a follow-up study, treating 22 male and female patients aged 14–25 with nodulocystic acne and a history of unsuccessful oral antibiotic treatment with a combination of minocycline (50 mg) plus oral ibuprofen (400 mg) three times daily. After 1 month, the combination therapy was associated with a 75–90% improvement in all patients.[120]

NSAIDs are also used to treat sunburn. Investigators compared ibuprofen and placebo in a randomized double-blind crossover study of 19 psoriatic patients receiving UVB phototherapy, and assessed signs and symptoms of UVB-induced inflammation. Although a statistical difference was found only in the technician's assessment of erythema, the results implied that ibuprofen was more effective than placebo in providing symptomatic relief of UVB-induced inflammation after high doses of UVB phototherapy for psoriasis. It is believed, based on the observation that dermal prostaglandins are elevated after UVB irradiation, that an NSAID that interferes with prostaglandin production may mitigate UVB-induced inflammation.[121]

Salicylic acid (topical)

Salicylates have been shown in experimental and clinical settings to exert anti-inflammatory as well as antimicrobial activity.[122] Salicylic acid, as a member of the aspirin family, truncates the arachidonic acid cascade, thus imparting analgesic and anti-inflammatory effects. Salicylates control inflammation by suppressing the expression of proinflammatory genes. Salicylic acid lowers the frequency and severity of acne eruptions by diminishing acne-associated inflammation while also conferring an exfoliating action in the pores. It is lipophilic so it is able to penetrate the sebum in the pores much better than glycolic acid can. It has therefore become a popular ingredient in over-the-counter acne products. Salicylic acid is also used in the treatment of rosacea and other superficial inflammatory conditions.

Sulfur/sulfacetamide (topical)

The medicinal use of sulfur dates back to the time of Hippocrates.[123] Although not a first-line therapy, sulfur continues to be used primarily to treat acne, seborrheic dermatitis, rosacea, scabies, and tinea versicolor.[124] Elemental sulfur and its various forms (e.g., sulfides, sulfites, and mercaptans) are thought to possess antimicrobial, antifungal, and antiparasitic properties in addition to acting as anti-inflammatory agents.[125] Sulfur is often combined with sodium sulfacetamide, a sulfonamide agent that exhibits antibacterial properties, specifically acting as a competitive antagonist to *para*-aminobenzoic acid, an essential component for bacterial growth.[126] Sodium sulfacetamide has also been shown to be active against *Propionibacterium acnes*.[127] The keratolytic and anti-inflammatory effects of sulfur and the antibacterial effect of sulfacetamide in combination yield an effective topical formulation for the treatment of acne vulgaris, rosacea, and seborrheic dermatitis.[128] This combination is available in cream, lotion, gel topical suspension, cleanser, and silica-based mask form. Many of them have a rotten egg-type smell, so this therapy is not very popular.

Natural ingredients (topical and systemic)

Botanically derived products have gained widespread usage and interest.[129] The following discussion focuses on some of the botanicals known to impart anti-inflammatory activity.

Aloe vera

Aloe vera is one of the most widely used botanical products in the world and is reputed to possess potent anti-inflammatory properties. The most likely active anti-inflammatory constituents include salicylates (delivering "aspirin-like effects"); magnesium lactate, which is thought to suppress histamine production; bradykinin and thromboxane inhibitors, which provide pain reduction; and polysaccharides, particularly acemannan, which is believed to impart immunomodulatory activity.[130,131] Of note, C-glucosyl chromone, another compound isolated from aloe, has displayed topical anti-inflammatory activity equivalent to that of hydrocortisone (200 μg/mouse ear).[132] Also, in a recent study exploring

reported antimicrobial effects of aloe, using an *in vitro* assay, investigators determined that the inner gel of aloe suppressed bacterial-induced proinflammatory cytokine production (i.e., tumor necrosis factor-α and interleukin-1β (IL-1β)) from human leukocytes stimulated with *Shigella flexneri*.[133,134]

Chamomile

Recognized for its therapeutic properties since the age of Hippocrates (circa 500 BCE), when it was used by ancient Greeks and Egyptians to treat erythema and xerosis, chamomile is a sweet-scented flower that remains one of the most used medicinal herbs.[135,136] Although Roman chamomile and German chamomile have been used for therapeutic applications, the flowers of the German variety contain a higher concentration of key active ingredients that have demonstrated anti-inflammatory activity *in vivo*: the terpenoids chamazulene and α-bisabolol.[137] Consequently, German chamomile is the official medicinal chamomile. Notably, it was found to suppress the inflammatory response and leukocyte infiltration in an animal study in which inflammation was induced by the injection of carrageenan and prostaglandin E_1.[138] Specifically, researchers have shown that chamazulene weakens the inflammatory process by inhibiting leukotriene synthesis.[139] Chamomile is also thought to improve the texture and elasticity of the skin, thus lessening the signs of photodamage. Due to reports of allergic contact dermatitis in susceptible types,[140] practitioners should caution individuals with known allergies to the compositae plant family (e.g., ragweed) about the use of topical chamomile products.

Feverfew

Feverfew, a rapidly growing small bush with citrus-scented leaves and daisy-like flowers, has been used for 2000 years to reduce fever and pain. Its use as an antipyretic led to the name "feverfew," a corruption of the Latin word *febrifugia* (fever reducer).[141,142] The feverfew extract parthenolide, a type of sesquiterpene lactone (an essential oil commonly found in members of the Asteraceae family and known for its anti-inflammatory effects) has been shown to bind to and inhibit IκB kinase β, the kinase subunit known to play a critical role in cytokine-mediated stimulation of genes involved in inflammation.[143] This may partly explain the anti-inflammatory properties attributed to feverfew. Sesquiterpene lactones also exert the major allergenic effects of the Asteraceae family. However, the anti-inflammatory properties of feverfew can still be delivered without posing the risk of contact dermatitis, as shown in a recent study using a parthenolide-depleted extract of feverfew. In this research, *in vitro* feverfew was demonstrated to attenuate the formation of UV-induced hydrogen peroxide and to blunt proinflammatory cytokine release; *in vivo*, topical feverfew diminished UV-induced epidermal hyperplasia, DNA damage, and apoptosis.[144]

Ginseng

Studies suggest that ginseng may exert chemopreventive activity against cancer. Proposed mechanisms include inhibition of DNA damage, induction of apoptosis, and suppression of cell proliferation.[145–147] Ginseng may also potently influence the inflammatory cascade and hinder the "inflammation-to-cancer sequence." For example, ginsan, a polysaccharide extracted from *Panax ginseng*, has been demonstrated to inhibit the release of proinflammatory cytokines *in vivo*.[148] Further, the ginsenoside Rg3 has been shown to block the NF-κB-mediated induction of the inflammatory process.[149] Finally, ginseng has been proven to suppress production of tumor necrosis factor-α and other proinflammatory cytokines by cultured macrophages when exposed to bacterial lipopolysaccharides.[150]

Licorice extract

Licorice (*Liquiritae officinalis*) is best known in its confectionery form of black or red candy. However, it is a botanical source of systemic or topical medications that have been used in herbal medicine for approximately 4000 years.[151] Two species of licorice, *Glycyrrhiza glabra* and *G. inflata*, have exhibited the most therapeutic actions, including anti-inflammatory effects. *G. glabra*, which grows around the Mediterranean, the Middle East, and central and southern Russia, is increasingly found in anti-inflammatory products.[152,153] Its biological active metabolite glycyrrhetic acid reportedly exhibits anti-inflammatory activity in subacute and chronic dermatoses, and therefore has been used to treat eczema, pruritus, contact dermatitis, seborrheic dermatitis, and psoriasis.[154] In fact, there is evidence that glycyrrhetic acid can exert a cortisone-like effect, thus suppressing proinflammatory prostaglandins and leukotrienes.[155] Of note, glycyrrhetic acid has not been shown to be superior to topical corticosteroids in treating acute inflammation, such as atopic dermatitis, although the combination of glycyrrhetic acid and corticosteroids has proven effective, with the addition of 2% glycyrrhetic acid enhancing hydrocortisone activity in skin in one study.[156,157] Nevertheless, in a double-blind study assessing the effects of 1% and 2% topical licorice extract preparations on atopic dermatitis in 60 patients, investigators found that the 2% topical gel was effective in reducing erythema, edema, and pruritus, which led the team to conclude that licorice extract might be a suitable agent for treating atopic dermatitis.[158] Finally, in a series of animal studies, investigators found that glyderinine, a glycyrrhizic acid derivative, exhibited anti-inflammatory, analgesic, and antipyretic activity, and concluded that glyderinine is a suitable compound for treating certain skin conditions.[159]

As for the other main medicinal licorice species, licochalcone, the primary active ingredient of Chinese licorice root, *G. inflata* has exhibited anti-inflammatory activity against arachidonic acid-induced mouse ear edema.[160,161] In a study evaluating the effects of five different chalcones, researchers found that four of the five, including licochalcone A, hindered the production of proinflammatory cytokines from monocytes and T cells. The authors concluded that licochalcone A and some of its synthetic analogs may have immunomodulatory effects, suggesting their suitability to treat infectious and other inflammatory diseases.[162]

Mushrooms

Several mushroom species have been used in traditional or folk medicine for thousands of years.[163] In particular, extracts from *Ganoderma lucidum* (lingzhi in Chinese, reishi or mannentake in Japanese), *Lentinus edodes* (shiitake in Japanese), *Grifola frondosa* (maitake in Japanese), and *Cordyceps sinensis*, among others, have been used in China, Japan, and Korea to treat a wide variety of conditions including allergies, arthritis,

bronchitis, gastric ulcer, hepatitis, hyperglycemia, hypertension, inflammation, insomnia, nephritis, neurasthenia, scleroderma, and cancer.[164] Since ancient times, *G. lucidum* has been used in China in dried powder form to treat cancer, and is now used as a home remedy to treat wounds and inflammation.[165,166] Recent research on rats and mice has suggested that the ethanol extract of the mycelium of *G. lucidum* displays significant antiperoxidative, anti-inflammatory, antimutagenic, and antioxidant properties.[167,168] *G. lucidum* is one of the most studied botanical treatments in Asia and has become a popular ingredient in topical skin care products in the West.

Oatmeal

The use of oats and oat-derived products for skin care dates back to 2000 BCE in Egypt and the Arabian peninsula. Oatmeal baths were often used to treat pruritic inflammatory skin conditions during the 19th and early 20th centuries. Further, in the late 1950s, colloidal oatmeal baths were reported to be effective in the management of pediatric atopic dermatitis.[169,170] Colloidal oatmeal, which is composed of dehulled oats ground to a fine powder, has replaced rolled oats and plain oatmeal in the modern dermatologic armamentarium. It disperses more easily in bath water and can also be added to creams and lotions in topical products. Colloidal oatmeal consists mainly of polysaccharides (60–64%), proteins (10–18%), and lipids (3–9%), but also contains enzymes (e.g., superoxide dismutase), saponins, vitamins, flavonoids, and inhibitors of prostaglandin production in a unique combination that renders it suitable for use in the care of inflammatory skin conditions, such as cleaning, moisturizing, protecting (i.e., barrier preservation), and relieving pruritus in inflamed skin as well as adjunctive therapy in atopic dermatitis, irritant and allergic contact dermatitis (including contact to poison ivy, oak and sumac), insect bites, diaper dermatitis, cercarial dermatitis, xerosis, ichthyosis, urticaria, and sunburn.[171–174] In fact, oatmeal is one of the few natural products recognized by the FDA as an effective skin protectant, and consequently colloidal oatmeal is one of the few FDA-regulated botanical ingredients.[175]

The therapeutic and cosmetic uses of oatmeal have been enhanced by the isolation and identification of avenanthramides, a newly discovered group of polyphenolic alkaloids found exclusively in oats that act as potent antioxidants, scavenging reactive oxygen and nitrogen species.[176] Further, avenanthramides reportedly inhibit prostaglandin biosynthesis almost as well as the synthetic anti-inflammatory agent indomethacin.[177] In 2007, strong anti-inflammatory activity was displayed by avenanthramides in a study in which keratinocytes were incubated with an inducer of proinflammatory IL-8 in the presence of vehicle or avenanthramides. The release of the proinflammatory cytokine IL-8 was reduced by 10–25% as a result of the inclusion of avenanthramides.[178]

Selenium

Selenium, an essential trace element in the human body, is believed to exhibit anticarcinogenic, anti-inflammatory, antioxidant, and therefore antiaging activity. Water, soil, and plant foods are the major sources of selenium. It is also found in meat, fish, Brazil nuts, shellfish, dairy products, cereals, and cereal products. Selenium is the essential antioxidant required to form glutathione peroxidase, one of the most important natural antioxidant defenses (*Box 2.7*). Glutathione peroxidase protects cell membranes from oxidative deterioration, as does vitamin E. Studies have shown that vitamin E and selenium act synergistically to impart such protection.[179] Selenium also displays anti-inflammatory activity in preventing inflammatory cytokine production, which can occur in response to UV exposure, for example, leading to a compromised immune response and photodamage.[180] Most available topical formulations contain very low concentrations of selenium, which are not well absorbed by the skin. However, recent animal and human studies have found that, when taken orally or applied topically in the form of L-selenomethionine, selenium conferred protection against daily and excessive UV damage. In one study, skin inflammation and pigmentation were reduced in treated patients; a delay in the onset and a decrease in the incidence of skin cancer were also observed.[181]

Turmeric/curcumin

Turmeric, best known as a spice used primarily in Asian cuisine, has a long history in both Chinese and Ayurvedic medicine as an anti-inflammatory agent.[182] Curcumin (diferuloylmethane), the yellow pigment corresponding to the main biologically active component of turmeric, has been shown to have more acute anti-inflammatory effects than the volatile oil fraction of turmeric,[183] and possibly even ibuprofen.[184] Curcumin has also exhibited significant wound-healing, anticarcinogenic, and antioxidant properties. At a low dose, curcumin can act as a prostaglandin inhibitor, while at higher levels it stimulates the adrenal glands to secrete cortisone.[185]

Pigmented skin

The incorporation of melanin-containing melanosomes, synthesized by the melanocytes, into the keratinocytes in the epidermis and their subsequent degradation largely account for skin color. A discussion of the various disorders of pigmentation is beyond the scope of this chapter; the focus here is on treatments for hyperpigmentations in general (*Box 2.8*).

Tyrosinase inhibitors

Considered the rate-limiting enzyme for the biosynthesis of melanin in epidermal melanocytes, tyrosinase is the enzyme that controls the synthesis of melanin. Therefore, tyrosinase activity is believed to be central in melanogenesis and is the target of several products intended to reduce melanin formation by inhibiting tyrosinase.

Hydroquinone

For many years, hydroquinone (HQ), which exerts its depigmenting effect by inhibiting tyrosinase, has been the primary treatment option for postinflammatory hyperpigmentation and melasma.[186] The use of HQ results in the reversible inhibition of cellular metabolism by affecting both DNA and RNA production. It also efficiently hinders tyrosinase, reducing its activity by 90%.[187] Although effective alone, HQ is often combined with other agents such as tretinoin, glycolic acid, kojic acid, and azelaic acid.[188] However, concerns about the safety of HQ have emerged sufficient to prompt Europe, in 2000, to ban HQ for general cosmetic purposes. Its use is permitted, but highly regulated in Asia. At the time of publication, the FDA was debating whether to ban HQ in over-the-counter formulations in the US (it was recently banned as an OTC product in Texas).

In over four decades of availability, HQ has never been etiologically linked with human cases of cancer. The most serious adverse health effect observed in workers exposed to HQ is pigmentation of the eye and, in a few cases, permanent corneal damage.[189] The FDA is primarily concerned about the side effects associated with topically applied HQ, which can engender exogenous ochronosis.[190] However, despite the prevalance of HQ, only 30 cases of ochronosis have been attributed to its use in North America.[191] Other side effects include skin rashes and nail discoloration. The safety debate about HQ within the FDA has spurred companies to research newer, less controversial skin lighteners.

Aloesin

Aloesin, a C-glycosylated chromone naturally derived from aloe vera, competitively inhibits tyrosinase by suppressing the hydroxylation of tyrosine to DOPA as well as oxidation of DOPA to DOPAchinone, and it hinders melanin production in cultured normal melanocytes.[192] Aloesin and some chemically-related chromones have been shown to inhibit tyrosinase more potently than arbutin and kojic acid.[193] Interestingly, in one study on the inhibitory effect of aloesin and/or arbutin on pigmentation in human skin after UV radiation, pigmentation was inhibited, as compared with control, 34% by aloesin, 43.5% by arbutin, and 63.3% by cotreatment with aloesin and arbutin.[194]

Arbutin

Present in the leaves of pear trees and certain herbs (e.g., wheat and bearberry), arbutin ($C_{12}H_{16}O_7$) is a naturally occurring β-D-glucopyranoside that is composed of a molecule of

HQ bound to glucose. Traditionally used in Japan, arbutin's depigmenting mechanism involves a reversible suppression of melanosomal tyrosinase activity rather than hindering the expression and synthesis of tyrosinase.[195] The effectiveness of arbutin as a depigmenting agent is uncertain, however. Deoxyarbutin, a synthetic arbutin derivative, has exhibited promising *in vitro* and *in vivo* results with a greater inhibition of tyrosinase than the plant-derived precursor.[196]

Flavonoids

Many of the 4000 flavonoid compounds manifest depigmenting activity. Several flavonoids exhibit the capacity to inhibit tyrosinase directly and act on the distal part of the melanogenesis oxidative pathway. Resveratrol, well known in recent years as an important component in red wine, also induces depigmentation by decreasing microphthalmia-associated transcription factor and tyrosinase promoter activity; the related oxyresveratrol and gnetol are more efficient tyrosinase inhibitors than resveratrol.[197,198] Ellagic acid, isolated from strawberries, green tea, eucalyptus, and geraniums, is a tyrosinase inhibitor that has been demonstrated to prevent UV-induced pigmentation. It is reportedly more effective than kojic acid or arbutin and safer than HQ as it affects melanogenesis without eliciting cytotoxic reaction.[199] Derived from gentian roots, gentisic acid has been shown *in vitro* and in cell cultures to impart an inhibitory effect on tyrosinase. Of note, methyl gentisate appears to be more effective than the free acid, and *in vitro* studies have shown methyl gentisate to be more effective and less cytotoxic to melanocytes than HQ.[200]

Hydroxycoumarins

Lactones of phenylpropanoid acid with an H-benzopyranone nucleus, hydroxycoumarins directly interact with tyrosinase. Melanogenesis and intracellular glutathione synthesis in normal human melanocytes have been demonstrated to be strongly inhibited by 7-allyl-6-hydroxy-4,4,5,8-tetramethylhydrocoumarin (hydrocoumarin 4).[201]

Kojic acid

Kojic acid (5-hydroxy-2-hydroxymethyl-gamma-pyrone or $C_6H_6O_4$) is a fungal metabolite of various species of *Aspergillus, Acetobacter,* and *Penicillium.*[202] It suppresses tyrosinase activity, chiefly by chelating copper, which results in a whitening effect on the skin.[203] Kojic acid has been used extensively in cosmetic agents, particularly in Japan,[204] and through its preservative and antibiotic activity contributes to extending product shelf-life.[205] In two separate studies, kojic acid combined with glycolic acid was more effective than 10% glycolic acid and 4% HQ for the treatment of hyperpigmentation.[206,207] Kojic acid products are typically recommended for twice-daily use for 1–2 months or until the patient achieves the desired cosmetic result. The standard concentration is 1% because kojic acid has been associated with contact allergy, with 2.5% concentrations provoking facial dermatitis, and it is considered to have a high sensitizing potential.[208,209] Sensitization to 1% creams has also been reported.[210] Of note, derivatives of kojic acid have reportedly exhibited enhanced efficiency through increased penetration into the skin.[211]

Licorice extract

Glabridin (*Glycyrrhiza glabra*), the primary active ingredient in licorice extract that affects skin, is incorporated in skin-lightening products because it inhibits tyrosinase activity in cell cultures without altering DNA synthesis. In addition, topical applications of 0.5% glabridin have been shown to inhibit UVB-induced pigmentation and erythema in guinea pig skin.[212] Clinically, *G. glabra* has demonstrated efficacy in treating melasma,[213] and glabridin has been shown in one study to exert a superior depigmenting effect as compared to HQ.[214]

Emblicanin

Emblica is an extract of the edible *Phyllantus emblica* fruit and contains the tannins emblicanin A and emblicanin B. Emblica, which is photochemically and hydrolytically stable and thus conducive to inclusion in skin care formulations, acts at several different sites in the melanogenesis pathway, as an inhibitor of tyrosinase and/or tyrosinase-related proteins (TRP-1 and -2) and peroxidase/H_2O_2,[215] as well as a broad-spectrum cascading antioxidant. Emblica is believed to be as effective as HQ and kojic acid, but has not been associated with adverse side effects.

Melanosome transfer inhibitors

Niacinamide

Niacinamide, the biologically active amide of vitamin B_3, has been shown to inhibit the transfer of melanosomes to epidermal keratinocytes. Clinical trials have revealed that niacinamide (also known as nicotinamide) inhibited melanosome transfer by up to 68% in an *in vitro* model and can improve unwanted facial pigmentation.[216] The use of a 5% niacinamide formulation twice daily for 8 weeks has resulted in significant amelioration in hyperpigmentation, as has the use of 3.5% niacinamide in combination with retinyl palmitate.[217] Of note, the pigmentation effects of niacinamide have been demonstrated to be reversible.[218]

Soy

The soybean plant provides us with tofu products as well as soybeans and soy milk. As the health benefits of soy have become known in the West, soy has been increasingly incorporated into several skin care products. In recent years, research has shown that soymilk and the soymilk-derived proteins (specifically, soybean trypsin inhibitor and the Bowman–Birk inhibitor) are able to inhibit the activation of PAR-2, a G-protein-coupled receptor found to regulate the ingestion of melanosomes by keratinocytes in culture,[219] thus inducing skin depigmentation.[220]

The lightening of pigmented spots after topical soybean extract application has been demonstrated in human trials.[221] Soy offers an excellent safety profile and side effects are negligible, because the inhibition of melanosome transfer is reversible. In a parallel, randomized, double-blind, vehicle-controlled trial, the efficacy of a novel soy moisturizer containing nondenatured soybean trypsin inhibitor and Bowman–Birk inhibitor on pigmentation, skin tone, and additional photoaging characteristics was assessed in 65 women, aged 30–61 with Fitzpatrick phototypes I–III, who had moderately severe mottled hyperpigmentation, lentigines, blotchiness, tactile roughness, and dullness. After twice-daily application of both the moisturizer and the vehicle over 12 weeks, the investigators determined by clinical observation, patients' self-assessments, colorimetry, and digital photography that the soy moisturizer conferred significant improvement in all metrics, including overall appearance, as compared to the vehicle.[222]

Wrinkled skin

Prevention is the key in managing and, ideally, avoiding wrinkled skin. Behaviors such as smoking and excessive sun exposure are best avoided. The use of broad-spectrum sunscreen (blocking UVA and UVB) and sun avoidance during the peak hours of 10 a.m. to 4 p.m. are well known to be important in preventing extrinsic photoaging. The prevention and even treatment of aging skin might be facilitated through a routine skin regimen containing retinoid application *(Box 2.9)*. Topical retinoids promote collagen production and diminish the MMPs involved in collagen and elastin degradation.[223,224] Antioxidants, which combat the oxidative stress and free radicals generated by UV irradiation, also have an important role in the armamentarium against wrinkle formation.

Retinoids

Retinoids are a family of compounds derived from vitamin A that include beta-carotene and other carotenoids, first-generation agents retinol and tretinoin, as well as third-generation agents tazarotene and adapalene. For several years, retinoids have been used topically and systemically to treat dermatologic disorders, particularly acne. Interestingly, female acne patients over a quarter of a century ago began reporting that their skin felt smoother and less wrinkled after treatment.[225] Subsequently, a clinical trial demonstrated that patients treated with tretinoin experienced improvement in sunlight-induced epidermal atrophy, dysplasia, keratosis, and dyspigmentation.[226] Numerous clinical trials have since confirmed these early observations. These data ultimately led to the FDA approval of tretinoin (brand name Renova) to treat photodamage. Currently, the only topical agents approved specifically for this purpose are Renova and Avage. Retinol, the metabolic precursor of tretinoin, is included in many over-the-counter cosmetic formulations touted as "antiwrinkle" creams.

Box 2.9

- Advise patients to use retinoids (only a pea-sized amount) every third night for the first 2 weeks.
- If they do not experience redness and flaking, they can increase to use every other night.
- After 1–2 weeks, most patients can increase to nightly usage.
- Titrating the retinoid use in this manner increases compliance by decreasing the incidence of irritation.

Mechanism of action

In 1987, investigators determined that tretinoin was a hormone as a result of the discovery of retinoic acid receptors.[227,228] The newest retinoids bear little structural resemblance to retinol but qualify as retinoids because they confer biological action through the same nuclear receptors modulated by the active natural metabolite of vitamin A called retinoic acid. Retinoids can act directly, by inducing transcription from genes with promoter regions that contain retinoid response elements, or indirectly, by inhibiting the transcription of certain genes, thus ultimately affecting cellular differentiation and proliferation.[229] The fact that early retinoids became unstable with sun exposure led to the belief that these products should be used at night, rather than in the day. Structural modifications to each successive generation of compounds have resulted in a third generation of retinoids more photostable than the first- and second-generation molecules.[230] There are now over 2500 such products.[231]

Although tretinoin has been approved for many years for the treatment of photoaging, it may also play a role in the prevention of cutaneous aging. UVB exposure significantly upregulates the production of multiple collagen-degrading enzymes known as MMPs. In turn, the activation of MMP genes leads to the synthesis of collagenase, gelatinase, and stromelysin, which fully degrade skin collagen.[232] The application of tretinoin has been shown to inhibit the induction of all three of these MMPs.[233] UV exposure has also been demonstrated to reduce collagen production. Pretreatment of the skin with tretinoin has been shown to inhibit this loss of procollagen synthesis; therefore, pretreating the skin with topical retinoids consistently may be beneficial in preventing as well as treating photodamage.[234] Retinoids have also been demonstrated to increase collagen synthesis in photoaged humans.[235] Topical application of tretinoin 0.1% to photodamaged skin partially restores levels of collagen type I.

Side effects

Xerosis, desquamation, and redness are the most common side effects of topical retinoids and appear to be related to the type and dose of the retinoid, typically occurring within 2–4 days of initial treatment.[236] Importantly, the irritation engendered by retinoids is separate from their photoaging benefits. This was shown in a study in which two different strengths of tretinoin (0.1% and 0.025%) were compared. Although equally efficacious in the treatment of photoaging, the degree of irritation differed substantially between the two treatment groups, with the 0.1% tretinoin-treated group experiencing nearly a threefold greater incidence of irritation than the 0.025% tretinoin-treated group.[237] The irritation response appears to be receptor-mediated, as suggested by findings that the topical application of tretinoin to the skin of transgenic mice deficient in retinoic acid receptors led to no detectable epidermal hyperplasia or desquamation.[238] The development of newer retinoids with specific receptor and pharmacokinetic profiles and relevant dosing may therefore result in a lower incidence of irritation, flaking, and desquamation.

Antioxidants

A full rendering of the various antioxidants useful or under investigation for dermatologic applications is beyond the scope of this chapter. The focus here will be to highlight briefly some of the most applicable antioxidants in the dermatologic armamentarium.

Vitamin C

Ascorbic acid, also known as vitamin C, is found in citrus fruits, blackcurrants, red peppers, and leafy green vegetables. Vitamin C has been demonstrated to disrupt the UV-induced generation of free radicals by reacting with the superoxide anion or the hydroxyl radical; this activity spurred its inclusion in various "after-sun" products in the 1980s.[239] The topical application of vitamin C in animal models has delivered photoprotective effects, as indicated clinically by a significant reduction in erythema and tumor formation and histologically by a decrease in sunburn cells, after both UVA and UVB irradiation.[240,241] In swine skin, the topical application of vitamin C combined with either a UVA or UVB sunscreen has improved sun protection as compared to the sunscreen alone.[242]

Most currently available topical preparations are unstable and fail to penetrate into the dermis, leaving them useless. The exposure of vitamin C preparations to UV light or air results in the molecule adding two electrons, transforming into dehydro-L-ascorbic acid, which contains an aromatic ring. This substance can be reduced back to ascorbate, but if further oxidized, the ring irreversibly opens, forming diketogulonic acid, and the vitamin C solution is rendered permanently inactive.[243] Therefore, airtight containers with UV protection are necessary and the product must be formulated at a low pH to encourage absorption. This causes many vitamin C products to sting the skin. Only a few companies have successfully developed stabilized vitamin C preparations at a low pH that are packaged so as to minimize inactivation of this easily degraded product. Other benefits of vitamin C are that it helps increase production of collagen because collagen requires ascorbic acid to be formed. In addition, vitamin C has some inhibition activity on tyrosinase, making it a useful treatment for pigmentation disorders.

Vitamin E

Vitamin E, or tocopherol, found in various vegetables such as asparagus and spinach, as well as seeds, nuts, and olives, is the universal term for eight related tocopherols and tocotrienols. Vitamin E forms are referred to as either "tocopherol" or "tocopheryl" followed by the name of what is attached to it, as in "tocopheryl acetate." Tocopherol exhibits better absorption, while tocopheryl displays a slightly longer shelf-life. The vitamin E forms used in cosmetics, usually alpha tocopheryl acetate and alpha tocopheryl linoleate, are less likely to cause contact dermatitis than D-alpha tocopheryl and are more stable at room temperature. The topical application of alpha tocopherol has been demonstrated to protect significantly against UV-induced damage to murine skin.[244]

Coenzyme Q10

Found in all cells and involved in energy production, coenzyme Q10 (CoQ10), also known as ubiquinone, is a powerful antioxidant that is easy to formulate into a topical cream. CoQ10, in addition to being an antioxidant, plays a significant role in the energy-producing adenosine triphosphate pathways in the mitochondria of each cell in the body. Topical CoQ10 has been demonstrated to penetrate the viable layers of the epidermis and lower the level of oxidation, reducing wrinkle depth, as well as inhibit the expression of collagenase in human fibroblasts following UVA irradiation.[245] Of note, most clinical work with CoQ10 has considered oral administration. Oral coenzyme Q10 has a caffeine-type effect, therefore supplements should be taken in the morning.

Grape seed extract

The extract that is prepared from the seeds of grapes (*Vitis vinifera*) is rich in polyphenolic proanthocyanidins,[246,247] members of the flavonoid family that are potent free radical scavengers found in many other foods, such as various berries (e.g., strawberry, cranberry, bilberry, and blueberry), green and black tea, red wine, and red cabbage.[248] The topical application of grape seed extract has been shown to enhance the sun protection factor in human volunteers.[249] Grape seed extract is thought to be a significantly more potent scavenger of free radicals than vitamins C and E.[250] The bioflavonoids in grape seed extract appear to foster the body's ability to absorb vitamins, thus providing a symbiotic environment for other nutrients.

Resveratrol

Highly touted for its presence in red wine, resveratrol (*trans*-3,5,4'-trihydroxystilbene) is a polyphenolic phytoalexin compound found in the skin and seeds of grapes, berries, red wine, and other foods. There are two isoforms: the more stable *trans*-resveratrol and *cis*-resveratrol. The topical application of reseveratrol before and after exposure to UVB has been shown in SKH-1 hairless mice to reduce UVB-induced tumor incidence and to produce a delay in the onset of skin tumorigenesis in long-term studies.[251] In a different study by some of the same authors, topical application of resveratrol prior to irradiation protected against UVB-mediated cutaneous damage, as manifested by a significant reduction in UVB-mediated hydrogen peroxide production and infiltration of leukocytes; skin edema was also suppressed, as was lipid peroxidation, a marker of oxidative stress.[252] Normal human keratinocytes pretreated *in vitro* with resveratrol have also demonstrated an inhibition of UVB-induced activation of the NF-κB pathway.[253] Interestingly, posttreatment with resveratrol in this study revealed equal protection to the pretreatment, implying that responses mediated by resveratrol may not be sunscreen effects. Resveratrol is incorporated into various skin care products, including antiaging creams, eye creams, facial moisturizers, supplements, and sunscreens.

Green tea

Green tea, extracted from the *Camellia sinensis* plant, is one of the most studied antioxidants, with myriad *in vitro* and *in vivo* studies investigating its effects.[254] The polyphenolic catechins of green tea, which include (–)epicatechin-3-O-gallate (ECG), (–)gallocatechin-3-O-gallate (GCG), (–)epigallocatechin-3-O-gallate (EGCG) and (–)epigallocatechin (EGC), have been shown to modulate the biochemical pathways important in cell proliferation, inflammatory responses, and responses of tumor promoters.[255] In human skin, these polyphenols from topically applied green tea have been shown to confer photoprotection, dose-dependently decreasing UV-induced erythema, the number of sunburn cells, and DNA damage while protecting epidermal Langerhans cells.[256] In addition, there is evidence from work with mice that the EGCG-induced increase of IL-12 results in augmented production of enzymes that repair UV-induced DNA damage.[257] EGCG also thwarts collagen degradation, which leads to photodamage by down-regulating UV-induced expression of AP-1 and NF-κB and inhibiting metalloproteinases in murine skin.[258] In a 2004 study, hairless SKH-1 mice were exposed to multiple doses of UVB after oral administration of green tea polyphenols, which were found to have inhibited UVB-induced protein oxidation and expression of matrix-degrading MMPs.[259] This finding, coupled with the same result seen *in vitro* in human skin fibroblast HS68 cells, suggests the antiaging potency of green tea polyphenols.

Lycopene

Lycopene is a nonprovitamin A red carotenoid found in fruits and vegetables such as tomatoes, watermelon, pink grapefruit, and apricots and responsible for their color.[260] In a 1995 study, a 31–46% reduction in skin lycopene concentration was observed following a single intense exposure (three times the MED) of solar-simulated light on a small area of the volar arm.[261] Since then, the ability of lycopene to quench singlet oxygen has been characterized as more potent than that of alpha-tocopherol or beta-carotene due to its high number of conjugated double bonds.[262] Lycopene, in synergy with other nutrients, has been demonstrated to lower biomarkers of oxidative stress and carcinogenesis.[263] While there is a wealth of literature describing the efficacy of ingested lycopene, there are few double-blind, case-controlled studies assessing the antioxidant in topical formulations. Nevertheless, lyocpene is found in various over-the-counter skin care products such as "antiaging" formulations, eye creams, facial moisturizers, eye creams, and sunscreens.

Role of noninvasive procedures

Microdermabrasion

Microdermabrasion is a painless resurfacing modality that requires no anesthesia or recuperation time and causes no side effects. It also diminishes fine wrinkles, improves skin texture, treats comedones, and eliminates excess skin oil.[264] The microdermabrasion machine propels sterile micronized aluminum oxide crystals at the skin while applying vacuum suction to remove these particles along with the desquamated skin. The depth of the treatment depends on the force at which the particles are propelled and the speed at which the device is passed over the skin. In contradistinction to traditional surgical dermabrasion, which enters the dermis, the goal of microdermabrasion is to remove the outer layer of the epidermis, promoting natural exfoliation.[265] It also appears to facilitate transdermal delivery of some medications.[266,267]

Microdermabrasion devices are classified as cosmetic rather than medical, and are therefore not regulated by the FDA. This has allowed the marketing claims of the manufacturers of these devices to go unchallenged or unproven. Typical indications include acne, acne scarring, striae distensae, and photoaging.[268] Currently, microdermabrasion is used for facial rejuvenation, in treating other dispigmented areas, in facilitating transdermal delivery of medications, as well as in selectively reducing full-thickness SC without damaging deeper tissues, thus enhancing skin permeability.[269] In 2008, microdermabrasion was among the top seven types of minimally invasive aesthetic procedures performed.[270]

Intense pulsed light

Introduced in 1995, intense pulsed light (IPL) devices are light instruments that emit noncoherent light with wavelengths between 500 and 1200 nm. They do not qualify as lasers because they lack coherent, monochromatic light. IPLs do look and act like lasers, however, and the newer systems are able to pump true laser devices in a separate handpiece, allowing for the purchase of one system for several indications. IPLs are widely available and have been used for hair removal as well as to treat acne, facial redness and telangiectasias, keratosis pilaris, lentigines, nevus flammeus, photodamage, poikiloderma, spider veins, and venous malformations.[271]

Practitioners should ascertain a patient's skin type and sun protection status prior to treatment. For instance, hypopigmentation can result from treating a recently tanned patient due to the absorption of melanin by the device. Patients should be advised to protect themselves from solar exposure before and after treatments. Practitioners should take special care in lengthening pulse widths and delays between pulses when using IPLs on patients with darker skin types (Fitzpatrick IV and V).[272,273] For patients with severe photodamage, pulses should be placed close together; far spacing can lead to striping, which can also result in any situation when higher fluences are used and pulses are not placed closely together. Additional treatment of the untreated areas resolves this complication. Fifteen minutes is the typical time elapsed for a full-face treatment. To treat photodamage successfully, three to five treatments at 1-month intervals are suggested.[274]

Topical anesthesia is not required for IPL procedures. IPLs offer the ability to treat vascular and pigmented lesions with one instrument, rapid treatment times (allowing patients to return to work after the procedure), and consistent reproducible results while causing few, if any, side effects (e.g., minimal if any downtime and perhaps mild darkening of treated lentigines, and erythema of treated areas).

Conclusion

To achieve optimal results for patients, whether they are having surgery, dermal fillers, botulinum toxin or lasers, the proper skin care must be recommended. The author's skin-typing system has proven helpful in classifying patients before choosing an appropriate regimen of skin care. The skin care regimen should be reviewed at every patient visit to increase patient compliance.

Access the complete references list online at **http://www.expertconsult.com**.

2. Fitzpatrick TB. The validity and practicality of sun-reactive skin types I through VI. *Arch Dermatol.* 1988;124:869.

After introducing his skin-typing system in the 1970s, Fitzpatrick, in this article, further clarified the categories and more firmly established the system as the pre-eminent approach to characterizing skin types.

10. Baumann L. *The Skin Type Solution.* New York: Bantam Dell; 2006.

The Skin Type Solution represents a significant advance in classifying skin and assisting practitioners and patients in selecting the most suitable skin care products. The Baumann skin-typing system, described comprehensively in this book, simultaneously considers skin type according to four different parameters that yield 16 distinct skin type permutations.

11. Uitto J. Understanding premature skin aging. *N Engl J Med.* 1997;337:1463–1465.

13. Gilchrest BA, Eller MS, Yaar M. Telomere-mediated effects on melanogenesis and skin aging. *J Invest Dermatol Symp Proc.* 2009;14:25–31.

16. Boukamp P. Skin aging: a role for telomerase and telomere dynamics? *Curr Mol Med.* 2005;5: 171–177.

Over the last 15 years, the roles of telomeres and telomerase have emerged as integral in unraveling the mechanisms of intrinsic or cellular aging. Noting that the epidermis is one of the few regenerative tissues to express telomerase, Boukamp considers the provocative question of whether epidermal telomerase can play a role in retarding or preventing cutaneous aging.

26. Abbas S, Goldberg JW, Massaro M. Personal cleanser technology and clinical performance. *Dermatol Ther.* 2004;17(Suppl. 1):35–42.

Abbas et al. comprehensively describe various types and distinguishing characteristics of the range of personal cleansing formulations. In identifying the most appropriate skin care products for a patient, as guided by the Baumann Skin Typing System, variations in cleansing agents represent one of the many areas of product expertise required of practitioners.

45. Aburjai T, Natsheh FM. Plants used in cosmetics. *Phytother Res.* 2003;17:987.

129. Baumann LS. Less-known botanical cosmeceuticals. *Dermatol Ther.* 2007;20:330.

225. Kligman L, Kligman AM. Photoaging - Retinoids, alpha hydroxy acids, and antioxidants. In: Gabard B, Elsner P, Surber C, et al., eds. *Dermatopharmacology of Topical Preparations.* New York: Springer; 2000:383.

233. Fisher GJ, Datta SC, Talwar HS, et al. Molecular basis of sun-induced premature skin ageing and retinoid antagonism. *Nature.* 1996;379:335.

It is well established that chronic sun exposure leads to the manifestation of premature or extrinsic skin aging. Fisher et al. show that retinoids, long used for treating acne as well as photoaging, can inhibit the UV induction of several collagen-degrading enzymes, suggesting that retinoids have the potential to prevent skin aging.

3

Botulinum toxin (BoNT-A)

Michael A.C. Kane

SYNOPSIS

- When properly administered to appropriately selected individuals, botulinum toxin type-A (BoNT-A) can have a rejuvenating effect on nearly the entire face and neck.
- Carefully observing the functional anatomy of each patient is the key to determining how much BoNT-A to administer and where to place each injection.
- In some facial areas, fine control can be achieved by only partially affecting muscles, causing the neighboring musculature to compensate for the ensuing weakness.

 Access the Historical Perspective section online at
http://www.expertconsult.com

Introduction

There are many components to the process of facial aging. Thinning of the dermis, elastosis, loss of facial volume, genetic factors, gravity, skeletal changes, sun damage and smoking all play a part in this process. So does facial animation. Certain rhytids are primarily caused by facial movement. Others are caused by other factors as well as a component of animation. Therefore, as long as a wrinkle or unattractive shape is as least partially caused by muscular action, it can be treated with botulinum toxin A (BoNT-A); however, how well a specific unaesthetic area responds to treatment with BoNT-A depends on how much of the unattractive area is caused by factors other than animation.

For example, a glabellar rhytid that is almost completely caused by the actions of the corrugators and procerus muscles in a relatively young patient can be totally eradicated with BoNT-A. In contrast, vertical lip rhytids in an elderly woman with thin skin, sun damage, a history of smoking, and loss of lip volume may only be partially improved by careful injection of the orbicularis oris muscle, which contributes to the accordion-like scrunching of the overlying lip skin.

BoNT-A treatment is currently the most frequently performed cosmetic procedure in the US and its importance in aesthetic plastic surgery simply cannot be overstated. In 2008, nearly 2.5 million BoNT-A procedures were performed in the US, representing approximately 30% of all non-surgical cosmetic procedures. That is more than all liposuction, breast augmentation, rhinoplasty, facelift, and blepharoplasty procedures *combined*.[1]

Although the subject of this chapter is focused on the manipulation of facial animation, the ability of the overlying skin to resist these underlying forces that would deform it, is also of paramount importance when discussing rhytids.

Key points

- The most important elements for facial rejuvenation with BoNT-A are functional anatomy, functional anatomy, and functional anatomy!
- To minimize the risk of a frozen, unnatural appearance, use the minimally effective dose of BoNT-A.
- Brow elevation depends on the relative weakness of the brow elevators versus brow depressors.
- The dose of BoNT-A used should be based on the estimated mass of the muscle being injected, not the depth of the rhytid.
- Avoiding the use of aspirin and non-steroidal antiinflammatory medications will decrease the occurrence and severity of ecchymosis.
- The lower frontalis muscle has the greatest effect on brow elevation.
- Threading the injection through the lips gives a more natural result than the near universal point technique.
- Cooling the skin before injection minimizes discomfort.
- As a general rule, injecting depressors more strongly than elevators will tend to give a more gentle lift to the area involved.
- Over-injecting the mentalis can result in a "witch's chin" deformity and oral incompetence.

Basic science

Pharmacology and pharmacokinetics

Clostridium botulinum is a Gram-positive, anaerobic bacterium that is known to produce seven serologically distinct types of toxin designated A through G, of which type A is the most potent. Botulinum toxin types A and B are used medically and are available in the US. The type-A toxin is a fully sequenced, 1296 amino acid polypeptide protein consisting of a 100-kDa heavy chain joined by a disulfide bond to a 50-kDa light chain.[6]

In the normally-functioning neuromuscular junction, the propagation of an action potential at the presynaptic neuron terminal opens voltage-dependent calcium channels. The influx of extracellular calcium ions causes vesicles containing acetylcholine to dock and fuse to the presynaptic neuron's cell membrane through the action of a 25 kDa soluble *N*-ethylmaleimide-sensitive factor attachment protein (SNAP-25). The released acetylcholine crosses the synaptic cleft, where it binds with nicotinic receptors at the motor end plate, opens sodium-potassium ion channels, depolarizes the motor endplate, and initiates the sequence of events that leads to contraction of the muscle fiber.[7]

Following the administration of botulinum toxin, the heavy chain binds to the axon terminal, which enables the toxin to enter the neuron *via* endocytosis. In the cytoplasm, the proteolytic light chain degrades SNAP-25, thereby preventing fusion of the acetylcholine containing vesicle with the cell membrane, preventing release of acetylcholine. Within a few days, the affected nerve is incapable of releasing acetylcholine, resulting in flaccid paralysis of the muscle fiber it innervates. Type-B botulinum toxin also causes flaccid paralysis but does so by inhibiting synaptobrevin, a vesicle-associated membrane protein similar to SNAP-25.[7] Unless specified, the remainder of this chapter concerns botulinum toxin type A.

Recovery begins to occur after several weeks, although the mechanism for this is not completely understood. Initially, small neuritic processes grow out of the affected neurons and establish new functional synapses, which are capable of acetylcholine release; however, these neuritic networks shrink and disappear as the original neurons regain function. The initial clinical response to botulinum toxin is usually readily apparent for 3–4 months, although 6–7 months are often required for the effects to completely disappear. BoNT-A begins to display an increased duration of action in most patients when they undergo treatment on a regular basis. When used cosmetically, the duration of action of BoNT-B is significantly less than that of type A, with an effective initial response of 2–3 months.

Commercial sources of BoNT-A

Several botulinum toxin products are currently available in the US:

- Botox® (onabotulinumtoxinA) for injection (Allergan, Inc., Irvine, CA) is supplied in vials containing 100 U of vacuum-dried *Clostridium botulinum* type A neurotoxin complex, 0.5 mg of albumin human, and 0.9 mg of sodium chloride without a preservative.[8]

- Botox® Cosmetic (onabotulinumtoxinA) for injection (Allergan, Inc., Irvine, CA) is provided in vials containing 50 U of vacuum-dried *Clostridium botulinum* type A neurotoxin complex, 0.25 mg of albumin human, and 0.45 mg of sodium chloride without a preservative, or 100 U of vacuum-dried *Clostridium botulinum* type A neurotoxin complex, 0.5 mg of albumin human, and 0.9 mg of sodium chloride without a preservative.[9]

- Dysport™ for injection (abobotulinumtoxinA) (Tercica Inc., Brisbane, CA and Medicis Aesthetics Inc., Scottsdale, AZ) is supplied in vials containing 500 or 300 U of lyophilized abobotulinumtoxinA, 125 μg human serum albumin and 2.5 mg lactose.[10]

- Xeomin for injection (incobotulinumtoxinA) (Merz) in 50 and 100 unit vials.

Commercial source of BoNT-B

- Myobloc® (rimabotulinumtoxinB) injection (Solstice Neurosciences Inc., South San Francisco, CA) is provided in 3.5 mL vials containing 5000 U of botulinum toxin type B per mL in 0.05% human serum albumin, 0.01 M sodium succinate, and 0.1 M sodium chloride.[11]

The BoNT-A in Dysport and Botox are produced by fermentation of the bacterium *Clostridium botulinum* type A (Hall Strain), while BoNT-B in Myobloc is produced by fermentation of the bacterium *Clostridium botulinum* type B (Bean strain).[12] *It is important to note that the potency of each product is specific to the preparation and assay method utilized and is not interchangeable with other preparations of botulinum toxin products.*[13,14]

While this list was comprehensive at the time it was written, there are many other toxins in clinical trials, which we will have in our armamentarium. Whether these are injectable or topically applied (RT001, Revance Therapeutics, Newark, CA) the strategy for these products remains the same; to identify the offending muscular segments and relax them to a certain extent. Dosing regimens with these products will always be in a state of flux. Good judgment, a critical eye, and an understanding of functional anatomy will never go out of style. Thus, this chapter is adaptable for neurotoxins not yet in use. New BoNT-A formulations will have different complexing proteins, different excipients, different complex sizes, different pharmacokinetics, and definitely different dosing regimens. The key to evaluating these products will be dissociation. The basic function of the lone 1296 amino acid chain is the same.

Indications

Botox is indicated for the treatment of cervical dystonia in adults to decrease the severity of abnormal head position and neck pain associated with cervical dystonia and also for the treatment of strabismus and blepharospasm associated with dystonia, including benign essential blepharospasm or VII nerve disorders in patients ≥12 years of age. Botox is also approved for the treatment of severe primary axillary hyperhidrosis that is inadequately managed with topical agents.[8] BoNT-A preparations are effective treatments for hyperhidrosis by decreasing cholinergic stimulation of eccrine glands responsible for sweat production.

Botox Cosmetic is indicated for the temporary improvement in the appearance of moderate to severe glabellar lines associated with corrugator and/or procerus muscle activity in adult patients ≤65 years of age.[9]

Dysport is indicated for the treatment of adults with cervical dystonia to reduce the severity of abnormal head position and neck pain in both toxin-naive and previously treated patients and also for the temporary improvement in the appearance of moderate to severe glabellar lines associated with procerus and corrugator muscle activity in adult patients <65 years of age.[10]

Xeomin is indicated for the treatment of adults with cervical dystonia to decrease the severity of abnormal head position and neck pain in both botulinum toxin-naïve and previously treated patients and also for the treatment of adults with blepharospasm who were previously treated with onabotulinumtoxinA (Botox) and temporary improvement in the appearance of moderate to severe glabellar lines associated with corrugator and/or procerus muscle activity in adult patients.

Myobloc (BoNT-B) is indicated for the treatment of adults with cervical dystonia to reduce the severity of abnormal head position and neck pain associated with cervical dystonia.[11]

Although the approved use of BoNT-A formulations for cosmetic use is limited to glabellar rhytids in patients under 65, it is extensively used off-label for this purpose and the author has used it to treat every muscle in the face since 1991.

BoNT-B plays a relatively minor role for cosmetic applications. It has a faster onset of action than BoNT-A, which can be beneficial, but its cosmetic usefulness is limited by greater pain on injection due to its low pH and a shorter duration of action. In isolated instances, it may be considered if a patient fails to respond to BoNT-A. It may also be useful for full face laser resurfacing and lower face scar revision as the shorter duration of action will keep the treated area relatively motionless during the early healing phase while avoiding prolonged, unattractive facial weakness.

The use of BoNT-A and BoNT-B for neurological purposes has become extensive. Its approved use for the treatment of cervical dystonia[15] has grown to include limb spasticity and dystonias, hypersecretory syndromes such as sialorrhea, headache, low back pain[16] and writer's cramp.[17]

Warnings and contraindications

The use of products containing botulinum toxin is contraindicated in the presence of infection at the proposed injection site and in individuals with known hypersensitivity to any botulinum toxin preparation or to any of the components in the formulation. The use of BoNT-A is contraindicated in patients with disorders of neuromuscular transmission, such as myasthenia gravis or Lambert–Eaton myasthenic syndrome. Dysport contains a small amount of lactose and may contain trace amounts of cow's milk protein. Dysport should not be use in patients with a known allergy to cow's milk protein.[10]

BoNT-A products should be used with caution in patients currently taking drugs known to affect neuromuscular transmission such as neuromuscular blockers, lincosamides, aminoglycosides, polymyxins, quinidine, magnesium sulfate, anticholinesterases or succinylcholine chloride as they may potentiate the effects of BoNT-A. The safety of administering botulinum toxin to pregnant women has not been established and its use in this population should be avoided.

Adverse effects

In the United States, due to reports received by the Food and Drug Administration regarding serious systemic adverse reactions including respiratory compromise and death following the use of botulinum toxins types A and B for both approved and unapproved uses,[18] the labeling of all botulinum toxin-containing products are required to containing the following boxed warning:

Postmarketing reports indicate that the effects of all botulinum toxin products may spread from the area of injection to produce symptoms consistent with botulinum toxin effects. These may include asthenia, generalized muscle weakness, diplopia, blurred vision, ptosis, dysphagia, dysphonia, dysarthria, urinary incontinence, and breathing difficulties. These symptoms have been reported hours to weeks after injection. Swallowing and breathing difficulties can be life threatening and there have been reports of death. The risk of symptoms is probably greatest in children treated for spasticity but symptoms can also occur in adults treated for spasticity and other conditions, particularly in those patients who have underlying conditions that would predispose them to these symptoms. In unapproved uses, including spasticity in children and adults, and in approved indications, cases of spread of effect have occurred at doses comparable to those used to treat cervical dystonia and at lower doses.

Adverse events reported by the manufacturers of BoNT-A and BoNT-B products include nasopharyngitis, headache, injection site pain, bleeding, bruising, edema, erythema, infection, inflammation, sinusitis, ecchymosis and nausea.[8–11] Weakness of adjacent muscles may also occur due to spread of toxin resulting in undesired effects. These types of adverse events are described in greater detail below. To minimize bruising, patients should avoid the use of aspirin and nonsteroidal antiinflammatory medications for 2 weeks prior to treatment.

Patients have rarely developed neutralizing antibodies for BoNT-A following cosmetic use. These events are more commonly associated with the use of high doses for neurologic purposes[19,20] although this has been reported following cosmetic use resulting in treatment failure.[21]

Dosing

The manufacturer of each BoNT-A product provides recommended dosing for their product, which is limited to the indicated use of treating glabellar lines. However, the facial musculature of patients is highly variable and precludes the use of standardized dosing for different aesthetic procedures. Gender also presents an obvious difference as men typically (but not always) have larger muscles requiring higher BoNT-A doses compared to women.

Using Botox for the treatment of glabellar lines as an example, the manufacturer recommends injecting 8 U in each corrugator muscle and 4 U in the procerus muscle for a total dose of 20 U; however, most practitioners inject an average of 25 U per glabella, while some advocate doses as high as 80 U and upper face doses of nearly 100 U. A median dose of 17.5 U is used by the author with a dose range of 10–27.5 U. Consequently, each clinician must gain familiarity with these products through experience and establish their own optimum BoNT-A dosing techniques.

These principles were demonstrated during a recent clinical study. Patients were stratified by demographics and randomized to receive a single treatment with different doses of BoNT-A (Dysport) or placebo.[22] Based on procerus/corrugator muscle mass, women received doses of 50, 60, or 70 U, while men were treated with 60, 70, or 80 U. Using this variable dosing technique, 85% of BoNT-A-treated patients were rated as treatment responders by a blinded evaluator after 30 days compared with 3% of placebo-treated patients ($p < 0.001$). Compared with patients in other studies who received 50 U to the glabella (the approved, on label dose), variably dosed patients tended to have improved efficacy and quicker onset without increased adverse events.

BoNT-A products are not bioequivalent and cannot be used interchangeably because of differences in unit potency and fundamental differences in how these units are measured. As randomized, double-blind, placebo-controlled clinical trials comparing the aesthetic efficacy of these products have not been performed, numerous studies have attempted to use surrogate endpoints to establish relative potency rations for these products. To date, these attempts have not been successful.[12–14,23–28] The reason for this is simple: the dose-response curves of onabotulinumtoxinA and abobotulinumtoxinA are not parallel and therefore a single dosing ratio between the two products cannot be established throughout the range of doses used.

The indicated dilution volume for the 100 unit vial of Botox Cosmetic is 2.5 mL and for the 300 unit vial of Dysport is either 2.5 mL or 1.5 mL, both with nonpreserved normal saline. In actual practice a wide range of volumes are used from 1.0 mL to 6.0 mL. Most practitioners use preserved saline (off label) for its weak anesthetic effect (benzyl alcohol is the preservative) and as a preservative if the vial is stored for a few days between uses. A recent poll of a consensus group of experts revealed that nearly all used each vial on more than one patient (also not according to the label). Smaller volumes allow for more concentrated dosing with less pain (based on volume of injection) per dosage point. Larger volumes allow for more injection points per dosage and thus, perhaps, more control. I have used 4.0 mL of nonpreserved saline for Botox 100 unit vial since 1991 and 3.0 mL of nonpreserved saline for Dysport since its introduction.

Patient selection

Decision-making details of selecting a patient for BoNT-A

The absolute key to becoming a proficient BoNT-A injector instead of a mere technician is understanding the functional anatomy of the face. Anatomy textbooks show the location of different facial muscles and their origins and insertions. While these texts allow for small and expected anatomic variations, they cannot prepare the clinician for the overwhelming differences in *functional* anatomy between individuals, or even different sides of the same face. Even though all individuals have the same mimetic muscles, their smile patterns vary depending on which muscles dominate within the group.[29] Even within a single muscle, different portions of that muscle can dominate and severely alter animation *(Fig. 3.1)*.

Therefore, it is essential that the face of each patient be carefully analyzed to determine which portions of which muscles dominate facial activity and cause wrinkles or other unaesthetic shaping of the face. These are the muscle segments that benefit from treatment with BoNT-A. The key is to take the necessary time to analyze the patient's face and discern which portions of which muscles dominate facial activity and cause unaesthetic lines or shaping of the face. This is especially important in the lower face and plastic surgeons should become highly familiar with these muscles and their possible anatomic variations. Understanding how the lower face moves is the key to using BoNT-A to improve nasolabial folds, perioral rhytids, chin dimpling, marionette's lines, and downturned oral commissures. This is not an area for the novice injector, as a few misplaced units of BoNT-A is not tolerated nearly as well as they are in the upper face.[30,31]

Treatment technique

Video 1

Treatment with BoNT-A does not need to be an all-or-nothing phenomenon. A certain amount of toxin will block a certain number of nerve terminals. Thus, fine control over the amount of denervation desired is possible. Despite the common use of the word "paralysis" when discussing the toxin, it is rare that this is actually the desired effect. Rather, a selective weakening of the musculature is performed to achieve a pleasant cosmetic effect.

Glabella

The glabella was the first area to be treated cosmetically with BoNT-A injections. Similar to other areas of the upper face, this use of BoNT-A was based on long-standing surgical procedures. During a bicoronal browlift, it was common to debulk the glabellar musculature to ease glabellar furrowing and reduce downward pull on the brow.

Even in a seemingly straightforward area of the face as the glabella, there is a great deal of variation in functional anatomy. When most people frown, they primarily bring their brows together as well as depress them; however, not everyone does this. Some people primarily frown in a vertical pattern, dramatically depressing their brows. When others frown, they may actually raise their medial brows while moving them medially, resulting in a quizzical look.

The median dose of BoNT-A used by the author for treating the corrugators and procerus muscles is 17.5–20 U of Botox for women and men, respectively, or 60–70 U of Dysport for women and men, respectively (total dose). After observing the normal animation of each patient during the consultation process, the patient is asked to frown, and relax repeatedly, and then scrunch their nose as if smelling something

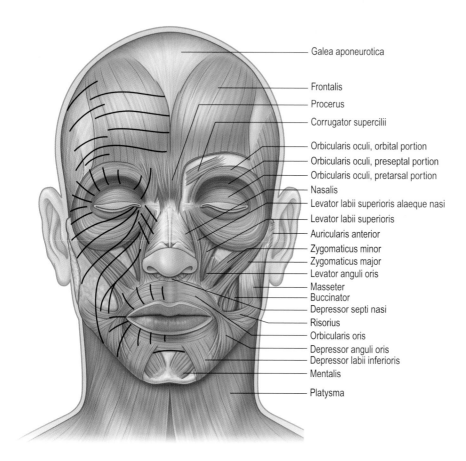

Fig. 3.1 Facial muscles.

Galea aponeurotica
Frontalis
Procerus
Corrugator supercilii
Orbicularis oculi, orbital portion
Orbicularis oculi, preseptal portion
Orbicularis oculi, pretarsal portion
Nasalis
Levator labii superioris alaeque nasi
Levator labii superioris
Auricularis anterior
Zygomaticus minor
Zygomaticus major
Levator anguli oris
Masseter
Buccinator
Depressor septi nasi
Risorius
Orbicularis oris
Depressor anguli oris
Depressor labii inferioris
Mentalis
Platysma

unpleasant, and relax repeatedly. This allows gauging which sections of which muscles dominate and which specific areas are to be targeted with BoNT-A *(Fig. 3.2)*.

To inject, the author displaces the forehead and brow cephalad and then with the noninjecting hand fixes it in position by placing pressure across the superior orbital rim. The patient is asked to frown, revealing an indentation in the skin corresponding to the site where the tail of the corrugator inserts into the dermis of the skin of the brow in a horizontal frowner. I begin injecting in this area and progress medially with small injections to the procerus, which receives little BoNT-A. The same procedure is repeated across the other brow, moving from lateral to medial. Most men have significantly longer corrugators than women with the tail extending lateral to the mid-pupillary line. Vertical frowners require much more BoNT-A to be injected into the medial (dominant) portions of the corrugators and heavy injection of the procerus. The author often does not inject the lateral tail of the corrugators in these male patients, reducing feminizing brow spread and permitting more normal animation.

Forehead

Horizontal forehead rhytids may be relieved by injecting and weakening the frontalis muscle. Using Botox, the dosing range for treating the frontalis is about 3.75–30 U, although most require 5–7.5 U. The median dose of Dysport in this area is 15 U (all total doses). The frontalis has highly variable

functional anatomy and care must be taken to not overly denervate the frontalis, which can lead to an overly smooth, artificial appearance, brow ptosis, and eyelid ptosis in patients who use the frontalis as an accessory eyelid elevator. Despite its appearance in most anatomy texts, the frontalis is usually continuous across the forehead with muscle tissue present even at the midline.

After the patient has been observed during normal animation, they are asked to raise and lower their brows repeatedly, almost to the point of exhaustion. After observing this motion, the strongest portions of the muscle, not the rhytids, are targeted. The author is unaware of any standard pattern of injection that produces reproducibly excellent results.

Crow's feet and lower eyelids

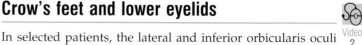
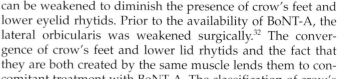

In selected patients, the lateral and inferior orbicularis oculi can be weakened to diminish the presence of crow's feet and lower eyelid rhytids. Prior to the availability of BoNT-A, the lateral orbicularis was weakened surgically.[32] The convergence of crow's feet and lower lid rhytids and the fact that they are both created by the same muscle lends them to concomitant treatment with BoNT-A. The classification of crow's feet patterns is based on the functional anatomy of this area.[33] In patients with the full fan pattern, the lateral orbicularis contracts and wrinkles the overlying skin from the lateral brow to the lower lid/upper cheek junction. It is important to

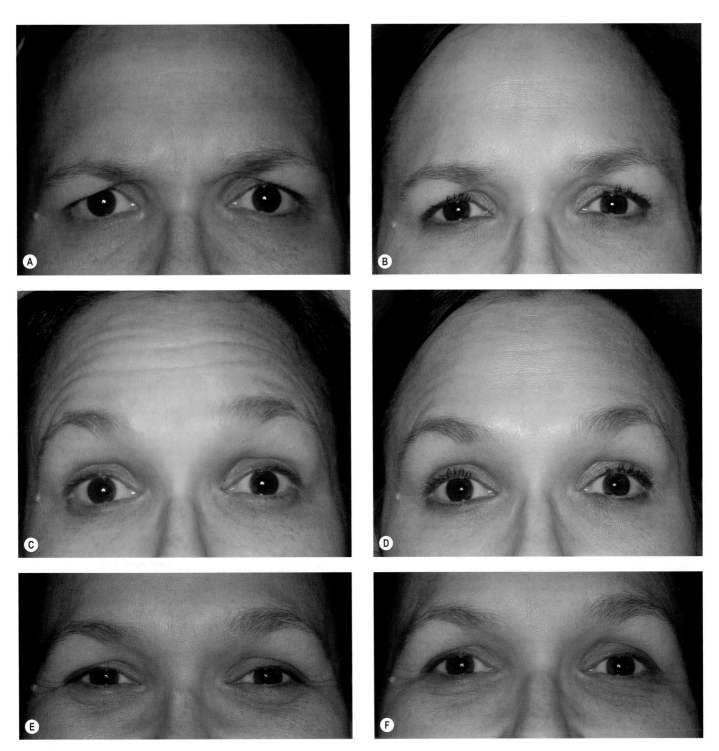

Fig. 3.2 This patient is in her late 40s. She has been injected with BoNT-A by the author for 16 years. It is 2 years since her last injection. She has shown an increasing duration of action since 3 years after her injections began. **(A)** Patient is frowning before injection. Due to long-term atrophy, she is not able to sharply fold her skin but has mild wrinkling, evidence of muscle bulge, and downward pull on her brows and upper eyelids. **(B)** Frowning after injection of 60 Dysport units to her glabellar complex. Her fine rhytids are improved, she can no longer depress her lids to fully eclipse her lateral eyelids and her muscle bulge is diminished. Note she has some recruitment of her orbicularis, greater on her right – this occasionally happens after muscle atrophy. **(C)** Patient is raising her brows before injection. She is mildly stronger on her left side. **(D)** Raising brows after 20 Dysport units were injected into her frontalis with 11 units in her left frontalis and 9 units in her right frontalis. Her forehead is smoother yet she is able to exhibit animation and emotion. Her brow asymmetry is partially corrected. Perfect symmetry is not always the goal. As long as asymmetry is not worsened, most patients are very pleased with the results, as small asymmetries are often not noticed by the patient prior to injection. **(E)** Smiling prior to injection. Note the depression of her lateral brow/upper lid mass. She also has a significant pre-tarsal orbicularis bulge that she found unsightly. **(F)** Smiling after 15 Dysport units were injected into her lateral canthal and lower eyelid area (each side received 15 units). Her crow's feet are diminished, but very importantly, not removed. No crow's feet upon smiling is a most unnatural appearance. Teenagers have crow's feet when smiling. Her lateral brow is less depressed and her orbicularis roll greatly improved without sacrificing lower lid position.

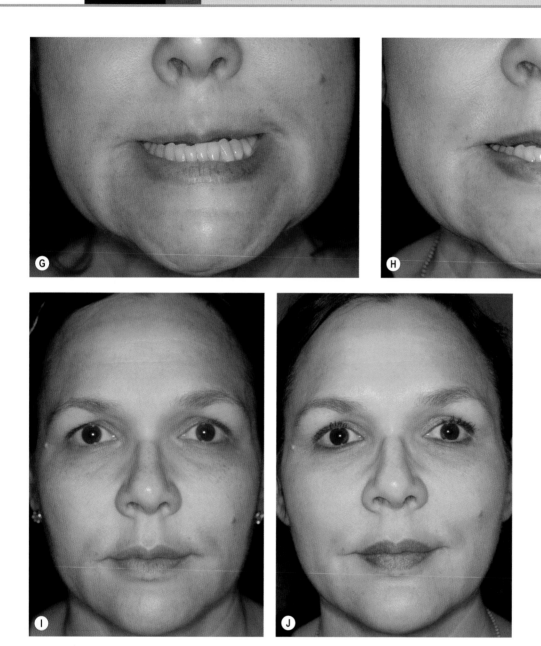

Fig. 3.2, cont'd **(G)** Showing her lower teeth prior to injection. She exhibits very little DAO activity. The DAO is the quickest muscle of the lower face to exhibit signs of atrophy in the author's experience. Note the asymmetry – the DAO is also the most asymmetric muscle in the lower face by the author's experience. **(H)** Contracting the DAO post-7 Dysport units to the left DAO and 3 units to the right. Her asymmetry is improved. Her DAO dimple on her left is also improved and her oral commissures are raised. **(I)** Repose before injection. **(J)** Repose after above injections. Her rhytids are improved and she has a slight lift of the brows with decreased upper lid heaviness. The uptick in her oral commissures is evident. Remember, this patient had less to gain than average patients due to her long-term muscle atrophy.

recognize different patterns as well as degrees of asymmetry that may occur in individual patients, and treatment is based on the functional anatomy of the orbicularis oculi.

Overly-aggressive treatment in this area can result in unpleasant results ranging from the "deer-in-the-headlights" appearance to cheek ptosis. While most plastic surgeons are aware that the upper lateral orbicularis oculi is a brow depressor, many fail to realize that the lower lateral portion of the muscle is an important accessory cheek elevator. If overly denervated in its lower lateral section, malar flattening as well as an extra "roll" of skin between the lower lid and cheek can occur.

Excessive chemodenervation of the orbicularis oculi across the lower lid can produce several unaesthetic results. In patients with a relatively lax lower eyelid, frank ectropion or lower lid retraction may result. In patients with minimal-to-borderline orbital fat prolapse, weakening the preseptal orbicularis oculi can exaggerate and hasten the appearance of fat "bags" of the lower lids. Since this sheet of muscle also functions as a pump, severe denervation can result in lymphedema.

These potential problems necessitate that these areas be injected judiciously. Although there are no standard doses or dosing patterns, the author uses between 3.75 and 5 U of Botox or 12.5 U of Dysport per side for most patients for both crow's feet and lower lid orbicularis. BoNT-A should not be wasted on relatively adynamic sections of the muscle. To do this, one must recognize that the functional anatomy of the lateral periorbita varies widely. I inject the most dynamic area of the muscle first, followed by smaller injections radiating out from this point. The idea is to create a gentle gradient of decreased muscle activity and avoid sharp extremes between total muscle immobility and adjacent areas of compensatory hypermotility. Care must also be taken when injecting the lower lateral orbicularis as it is an important accessory cheek elevator.

Brow elevation

The use of BoNT-A injections to achieve brow elevation was once considered controversial. Publications in the plastic surgical and dermatologic press claimed that BoNT-A could only depress the brows or at best create the illusion of a browlift by dropping the medial brow; however, the author routinely uses BoNT-A to easily and reliably lift the brows in excess of 6 mm. The concept is remarkably easy.

To lift the brows, concentrate on injecting muscle segments that depress the brows actively and at rest, allowing the brows to rise. On the other hand, the concept of increasing browlift by weakening the only muscle that lifts them is not well understood. The explanation for this seeming paradox is that the nonweakened sections of muscle react by increasing their pull in compensatory fashion. This explains why when the lateral orbicularis is strongly injected, lower lid rhytids will increase.

This is not simply an illusion due to smoothing of the skin laterally but the result of increasing the resting tone of the noninjected portion of the muscle across the lower lid. This also explains why the lateral brows often peak in an unattractive "Mr Spock" appearance with worsening of lateral supra-brow rhytids when only the central frontalis is injected with a high dose of BoNT-A. Weakening portions of the frontalis causes other portions of the frontalis to lift more strongly. To maximize browlift, injecting the portions of the frontalis not responsible for raising brows will induce the frontalis responsible for brow elevation to pull harder. Usually, this means injecting the frontalis more strongly centrally in the zone above and medial to the brows. The frontalis lateral to the brows is also injected causing the frontalis directly over the brows to lift more strongly.

There are 11 muscle segments which can depress the medial brow: the procerus, transverse heads of the corrugator, oblique heads of the corrugator, depressor supercilii, medial orbicularis oculi, and in some patients, the nasalis muscles. In most patients, the effect of the nasalis on brow position is negligible; however, injecting the other medial brow depressors has occasionally resulted in disappointing brow elevation. With the other muscle segments, completely nonfunctional, these patients depress their brows by wrinkling their nasalis. Subsequent nasalis injection gave the brows additional elevation.

The lateral brow is depressed by the cephalad portion of the lateral orbicularis oculi. The dynamic of this action differs widely among patients and there is no single point that can be injected to reliably elevate the lateral brow. Some patients who do not depress their brows when smiling will not achieve reliable brow elevation by simply injecting the upper lateral orbicularis. The key is individualized treatment, based on the functional anatomy of each patient.

There is no standard BoNT-A injection pattern for brow elevation. For a more medial brow elevation, denervate the medial depressors and weaken the frontalis over the lateral brow, leaving the medial frontalis strong. For a more lateral elevation, weaken the lateral depressor and the medial frontalis. For a peaked and arched brow, weaken the lateral depressor and leave the frontalis over the junction of the middle and lateral third of the brow strong. For men, leave a wider band of frontalis working to raise the brows uniformly, while keeping them flat, avoiding feminized, peaked brows. For a unilateral browlift (in addition to the zones not directly over the brows), weaken the frontalis slightly over the higher brow, inducing the frontalis over the lower brow to pull harder.

Neck

Platysmal bands are another area where BoNT-A injections can yield excellent results.[34] The key to evaluating the neck as a potential site for cosmetic improvement involves determining the relative contributions of the skin and the platysma to banding. The best patients have minimal skin excess and relatively strong bands *(Fig. 3.3)*. Patients with lax neck skin are poor candidates for BoNT-A injection because the lax skin will continue to hang even when the bands are completely paralyzed.

Using Botox, the dosing range is approximately 15–30 U, with most patients requiring about 20 U. The typical dose of Dysport is about 50 U. By asking the patient to show their lower teeth with their teeth clenched, the platysma band becomes apparent and may be grasped between the thumb and index finger of the noninjecting hand. The patient is then asked to relax and the muscle is injected starting just below the mandibular border and progressing inferiorly to the point at which the band is visible during normal animation. The horizontal "necklace" rhytids can also be very mildly improved by injecting toxin just above and below them.

Good candidates for the treatment of platysmal bands with BoNT-A include the following: relatively young (35–45 years) patients with strong bands and minimal skin laxity are excellent candidates; similarly, patients of any age who have undergone surgical removal of excess skin and which have recurrent bands are also good candidates. A smaller but more frequently seen group includes young patients following an aggressive fat removal via liposuction in the neck, who subsequently develop visible platysmal bands.

Nasolabial folds

The nasolabial fold is an excellent area for BoNT-A injections in properly-selected patients who have been instructed in what to expect.[35,36] The levator labii superioris alaeque nasi is the muscle primarily responsible for the medial nasolabial fold and the final 3–4 mm of central upper lip elevation.[35] Weakening this muscle smoothes the medial nasolabial fold and changes the smile pattern of the patient. The three major smiling patterns were described by Rubin.[29] The most common or "Mona Lisa" smile pattern is dominated by the zygomaticus muscle, which elevates the oral commissures to the highest point of the smile. The "canine smile" is caused by a dominant levator labii superioris and the highest part of the smile is the

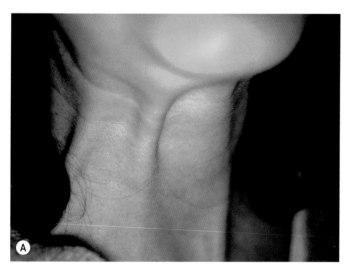

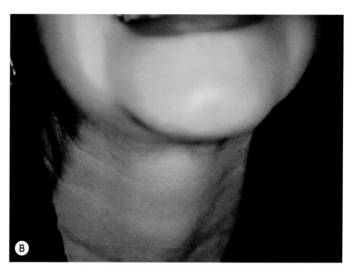

Fig. 3.3 This patient is in her mid-30s and requested neck rejuvenation. **(A)** Straining prior to injection. She has minimal excess skin or fat and prominent platysmal bands. Her platysma is thick on palpation, she has a greater than normal muscle mass. **(B)** Straining post-injection of Botox 20 units to her right primary (medial) band and 7.5 units to her right secondary (lateral) band as well as treatment of her left platysma.

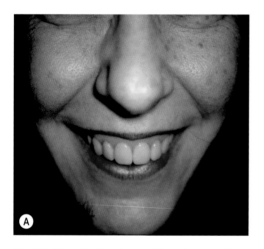

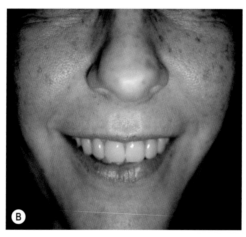

Fig. 3.4 This patient is in her mid-30s and requested improvement of her gummy smile. **(A)** Prior to injection, smiling. **(B)** After injection of 750 units of Myobloc (BoNT-B) to her levator labii superioris alaeque nasi muscles and 500 units into her upper orbicularis oris. Note the softening of her nasolabial folds as well as the lowering of her central greater than her lateral lower lip. This illustrates how all toxins can be used for cosmetic improvement. The cosmetic use of the currently available BoNT-B is limited however by its increased pain on injection (lower pH), potential for greater spread, and decreased duration of action compared to current BoNT-A preparations.

central upper lip. This pattern occurs in 35% of the population and they are the potential candidates for this procedure. Since injecting this muscle results in a drop of the central upper lip when smiling, it converts "canine" smilers into "Mona Lisa" smilers. Injecting patients with the Mona Lisa smile results in an exaggerated Mona Lisa smile that most patients find unattractive.

Patients with "gummy smiles" are basically extreme canine smile pattern patients *(Fig. 3.4)*. This group benefits the most from BoNT-A injection of the levator labii superioris. Gummy smilers often smile asymmetrically, requiring asymmetric injection. They also tend to have deeper medial nasolabial folds, which are the area of primary improvement with this technique. The resulting drop of the upper lip hides the gingiva and results in a more pleasing smile.

The technique for this injection is relatively straightforward once the patient has been determined to be a suitable candidate. Before injection, the patient can be given a preview of the proposed change: the patient smiles into a mirror held at eye level. Pushing the upper lip down 3–4 mm with a cotton applicator stick gives the patient a rough approximation of the change to be expected to the smile as well as the nasolabial fold.

During injection, use the index finger of the noninjecting hand to firmly press against the inferior portion of the nasal bone where it meets the maxilla. Thus, half of the finger is falling into the pyriform aperture while the other half lies in the groove between the nasal bone and maxilla. Then ask the patient to smile strongly – the levator labii superioris alaeque nasi can usually be felt just lateral to this groove. It is injected once on each side, just above the periosteum. The dosing range for this muscle is about 5–15 U of Botox with most patients requiring 5–7.5 U in total. The usual total dose of Dysport is about 15–20 U.

Perioral lines

BoNT-A is an excellent adjunct for rejuvenating the lower face; however, excellent control and familiarity with the drug is essential before injecting these rewarding but technically demanding areas of the face *(Fig. 3.5)*. Perioral rhytids, dimpled chin, and downturned oral commissures are all amenable to improvement by BoNT-A injection. Once again, fully understanding the functional anatomy of each patient is the key to achieving reproducibly good results and avoiding the disastrous consequences of a few misplaced units of BoNT-A. When first beginning to inject the lower face, lower doses of BoNT-A and more frequent touch-ups are better than larger initial doses and severe complications.[30,31]

The perioral rhytids are a common area of complaint for many patients. Radially-oriented rhytids are caused by intrinsic aging of the skin (dermal thinning, sun damage, smoking), a loss of volume over time, and forced wrinkling of the skin caused by its densely adherent underlying muscle, the orbicularis oris. The most common rejuvenative procedure for this area is the use of dermal fillers. Injecting hyaluronic acid-containing products into the vermilion and cutaneous lip improves the rhytids, restores lost volume, and offers immediate results with negligible recovery time; however, BoNT-A is an increasingly effective rejuvenative modality for some patients. First, there are those who are already undergoing BoNT-A treatment into other areas of the face and wish to also improve their lip lines. Others want to improve their wrinkles but are adamant about not increasing the size of their lips for fear of looking "done". The third and largest group of patients receive concomitant BoNT-A and filler injections. The dermal filler restores volume and fills wrinkles while the BoNT-A relieves some of the contracting force applied to the skin by the underlying orbicularis oris.

To judge the relative strength of the sphincter muscle, the patient is asked to repeatedly purse, then relax the lips. The

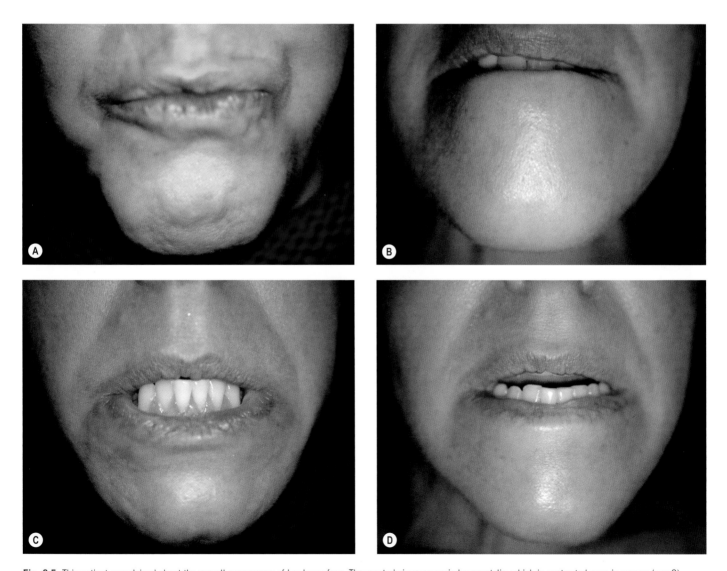

Fig. 3.5 This patient complained about the overall appearance of her lower face. The most obvious cause is her mentalis, which is contracted even in repose (see G). **(A)** Patient contracting her mentalis prior to injection by pushing her lower lip up. **(B)** Her mentalis after 5 Botox units were injected across its surface. The irregularities are greatly improved. **(C)** Depressing her lower lip reveals her gingival and bilateral rhytids across her labiomental area (her "DAO dimple"). **(D)** Depressing her lower lip after 7.5 Botox units were injected to her DAO muscles symmetrically. She is unable to show her gingival or even the lower half of her dentition. Her DAO dimples are greatly improved.

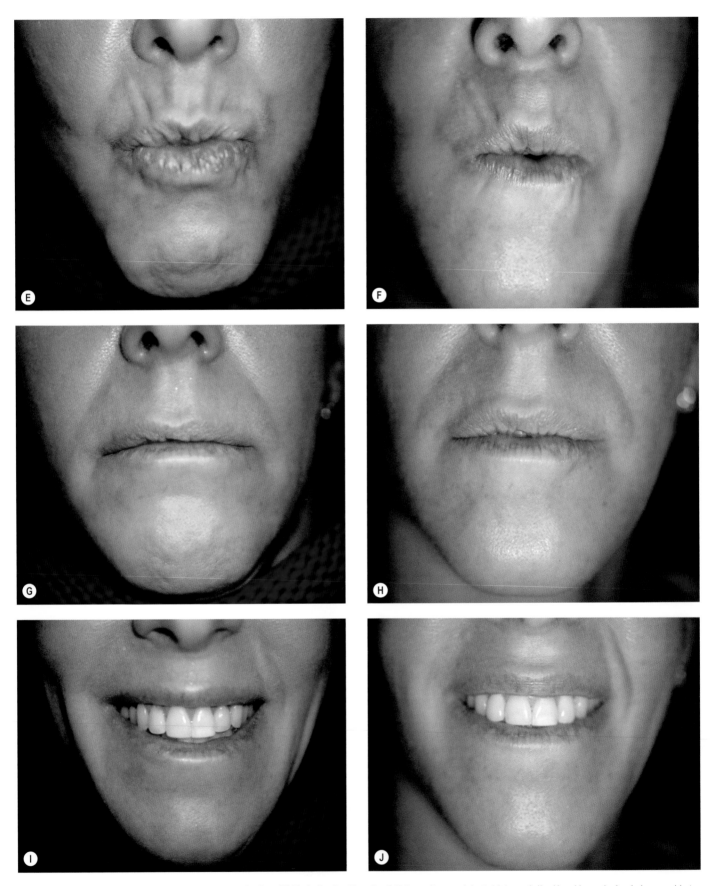

Fig. 3.5, cont'd (E) Patient puckering her lips prior to injection. **(F)** Puckering her lips after 2 Botox units were injected into each lip. Her skin puckering is improved but not gone. Threading toxin injections across the lip can improve this appearance. **(G)** Repose prior to injection. **(H)** Repose after the above injections. Her chin is less wide and more refined from mentalis injection. Her commissures are raised and her apparent volume deficit below the commissures is gone, due to relaxation of the DAO. Her lips appear more full and without rhytids from her orbicularis oris injection. The horizontal width of her mouth appears diminished and the overall shape of the lower face has been improved. **(I)** Smiling prior to injection. **(J)** After injection, the patient exhibits a natural smile. Her lower lip is slightly raised, which helps protect her oral competence and is also more youthful. When injecting many areas of the lower face simultaneously, the patient can experience a feeling of weakness.

dosing range for Botox is about 2–7 U per lip (5–15 U for Dysport), although most patients will require only about 3 U per lip (7.5 U Dysport). In contrast with other areas of the face where small, precise doses of BoNT-A are injected, this area is more broadly injected to achieve a diffuse, general weakening of the sphincter muscle. The philtrum is almost never injected, as it rarely contains strong rhytids. The addition of normal saline into the syringe containing the appropriate BoNT-A dose allows more even placement of the drug.[31] The needle is inserted parallel to and a few millimeters above the vermillion border and the BoNT-A is injected as the needle is withdrawn. The upper and lower lips can be treated in the same session. Complications can easily result in this area and are usually due to over-injection. Excessive weakening of the upper lip leads to problems, first with plosive sounds followed by general speech and finally oral competence. Over-injection of the lower lip is more likely to result in drooling and competence problems. Beware the elderly patient with severe rhytids and decreased muscle mass.

Slightly weakening the superficial fibers of the orbicularis oris can help alleviate the overlying rhytids caused by this sphincter with or without concomitant filler injection. In 1998, the author abandoned the more popular injection point technique and began using the method of threading the injection a few millimeters above the vermilion border. This results in a more even appearance and avoids compensatory areas of hypermotility.

Mentalis

Many patients form an unattractive, dimpled pattern on their chin during active speech or repose with the lips closed. This appearance results from contraction of the underlying mentalis muscle, which is connected to the overlying dermis by dense fibrous septae. These septae transmit the forces and contours of the superficial mentalis to the skin. Dimpling and occasional ridging of the skin in patients with hypertrophy of the mentalis can result.

Using Botox as an example, the dosing range for the mentalis is about 2.5–12.5 U, with most patients requiring 5–7.5 U. Similar results may be achieved using 10–20 U of Dysport (all doses total). Weakening the mentalis must be done cautiously, as this muscle raises the chin pad and lower lip and is critical for oral competence. Care must be taken to inject only the superficial mentalis, leaving the deep mentalis fully functional. The injection needle is threaded cephalad, parallel to the skin surface, aiming for the plane between the superficial muscle and its overlying fascia. It is important to remember that patients who have an underlying problem with oral competence can exhibit mentalis hypertrophy from constant use and present with dimpling. These patients must be injected with caution and told of the possible risks this treatment entails. Consequently, injection of the mentalis is often paired with depressor anguli oris injection to maintain the height of the lower lip.

Depressor anguli oris

The depressor anguli oris is a triangularly-shaped muscle which depresses the oral commissures. This action contributes to the formation of marionette lines and often creates a distinct horizontal rhytid below the commissure. Injecting this muscle with BoNT-A raises the oral commissures and decreases the show of the lower dentition when smiling. It also helps to improve marionette lines and the horizontal crease below the commissure.

Using Botox as an example, the dosing range is about 2.5–12.5 U, with most patients requiring 5–7.5 U (10–15 U of Dysport). All doses are total for both sides. The patient is repeatedly asked to show their lower teeth with their dentition occluded. This usually creates a horizontal rhytid below the commissure. Each muscle is injected twice with the point of the first injection at the level of the horizontal rhytid. The second injection point is midway between the first point and the lower border of the mandible, and in the direction that the muscle pulls the commissure when contracting. Most patients pull their commissures down and laterally when contracting; however, some patients will pull their commissures down and medially. It is along this axis of motion that the second injection is placed.

Once again, the key to success is to know the functional anatomy of each patient. Also, care must be taken not to inject the cephalad portion of this muscle. First, there is very little muscle activity in the cephalad portion as the muscle tapers and becomes aponeurotic. Second, the existing muscle (lower orbicularis oris) does not tolerate concentrated injections laterally, which can easily result in oral incompetence and drooling. When properly injected, the depressor anguli oris is one of the safest muscles to inject in the lower face. Even if it is slightly over-injected, it does not lead to oral incompetence but an actual rising of the lower lip. In fact, patients with oral competence problems caused by the lower orbicularis oris or mentalis weakening or a facial nerve injury, may obtain relief by injecting the depressor anguli oris. Injection of the lower lip with a viscous hyaluronic acid product at the same time can also add some static support.

Repair of surgical complications

Many complications from aesthetic surgical procedures can be effectively treated with BoNT-A:

- *Browlift*: Excessive downward muscle pull on the brows observed during the early postoperative period caused by incomplete corrugator or procerus resection can be treated with BoNT-A, maintaining brow elevation. Overly-elevated brows can be dropped by aggressively injecting the frontalis muscle.
- *Chin augmentation*: Surgical misadventures leading to mentalis disinsertion and dimpling of the chin can be effectively treated with careful injection of the superficial mentalis.
- *Breast augmentation*: Prolonged spasm of the pectoralis major can be treated by injecting the lower pectoralis major.
- *Surgery or trauma*: Facial nerve injuries can often be effectively masked by weakening the unaffected muscle on the other side of the face. For marginal mandibular nerve injury after facelift, this usually entails injecting the contralateral depressor anguli oris muscle and possibly the depressor labii inferioris and mentalis.

Hyperhidrosis

BoNT-A injections have been used for the treatment of palmar,[37] plantar,[38] facial[39] and axillary[40,41] hyperhidrosis (excessive sweating). Injections of the soles and palms may be very painful unless some of analgesia is used[42] and care must be taken not to inject and weaken hand and foot muscles. Results for this application typically last somewhat longer, approximately 6 months.

Postoperative care

There is wide disagreement regarding postoperative care during the first 24 h following treatment with BoNT-A. Recommendations range from no bending for 6 h, to avoiding airline travel for the first 24 h after treatment, although evidence for these is lacking. Nevertheless, the author believes it may be beneficial for patients to avoid heavy exertion for 90 min following treatment with BoNT-A. That is approximately the time most believe it takes for the toxin to bind to the neuron cell membrane.

Outcomes, prognosis, complications

Potential adverse reactions

Adverse events happen with every procedure and BoNT-A is no exception. Complications, however, tend to be mild, infrequent, and temporary. Most adverse events related to treatment arise from proximity spread of the toxin into adjacent musculature. Difficulty in assessing muscle mass also may play a part as there is no definite method to measure muscle mass prior to injection.

Ecchymosis and tenderness are common adverse events which can occur with any percutaneous procedure. The most frequent adverse events from toxin in the upper face are brow and lid ptosis. Occasionally, these may be improved with additional weakening of depressor musculature, leaving the elevating musculature (frontalis) dominant. Alpha agonist drops may also help to ameliorate lid ptosis by stimulating Mueller's muscle.

Lower face complications from BoNT-A administration include asymmetry, dysphagia, and oral competence issues. For example, adverse events associated with the treatment of vertical lip rhytides include eating and drinking difficulties or difficulty making certain plosive sounds.

Secondary procedures

Treating patients who had the procedure but desire improved results

The most common secondary procedure associated with BoNT-A injection is concomitant filler injection. The use of BoNT-A and fillers is highly synergistic. They attack unaesthetic areas via their different causes, often with outstanding results. While BoNT-A attacks the underlying mimetic cause, the filler addresses volume and structural causes of facial and neck aging.

Laser resurfacing is another procedure that benefits from treatment with BoNT-A. In many ways, the mechanism is similar to the improved results seen with BoNT-A and scar revision. It appears that the relative decrease in motion improves wound healing and results in less apparent scar tissue. In addition, it has been apparent that BoNT-A has several direct dermal effects, which are now being studied.

 Access the complete references list online at **http://www.expertconsult.com**

1. American Society for Aesthetic Plastic Surgery. Cosmetic Surgery National Data Bank: 2008 Statistics. Online. Available at: http://www.surgery.org/sites/default/files/2008stats.pdf (accessed February 2, 2010).

2. Scott A, Rosenbaum A, Collins C. Pharmacologic weakening of extraocular muscles. *Invest Ophthalmol Vis Sci.* 1973;12(12):924–927.

3. Scott A. Botulinum toxin injection into extraocular muscles as an alternative to strabismus surgery. *J Pediatr Ophthalmol Strabismus.* 1980;17(10):21–25.

4. Scott A, Kennedy R, Stubbs H. Botulinum A toxin injection as a treatment for blepharospasm. *Arch Ophthalmol.* 1985;103(3):347–350.

5. Carruthers J, Carruthers J. Treatment of glabellar frown lines with Clostridium botulinum A exotoxin. *Dermatol Surg.* 1992;18:17–21.

6. Sharma S, Zhou Y, Singh B. Cloning, expression, and purification of C-terminal quarter of the heavy chain of botulinum neurotoxin type A. *Protein Expr Purif.* 2006;45(2):288–295.

7. Huang W, Foster J, Rogachefsky A. Pharmacology of botulinum toxin. *J Am Acad Dermatol.* 2000;43(2 Pt 1): 249–259.

8. Botox® (onabotulinumtoxinA) for injection. Prescribing Information. Irvine, CA: Allergan, Inc.; July, 2009.

9. Botox® Cosmetic (onabotulinumtoxinA) for injection. Prescribing Information. Irvine, CA: Allergan, Inc.; July, 2009.

10. Dysport™ for injection (abobotulinumtoxinA). Prescribing Information. Brisbane, CA: Tercica, Inc., and Scottsdale, AZ: Medicis Aesthetics Inc.; May, 2009.

11. Myobloc® (rimabotulinumtoxinB) injection. Prescribing Information. South San Francisco, CA: Solstice Neurosciences Inc.; July, 2009.

12. Wenzel R, Jones D, Borrego J. Comparing two botulinum toxin type A formulations using manufacturers' product summaries. *J Clin Pharm Ther.* 2007;32(4):387–402.

13. Wohlfarth K, Sycha T, Ranoux D, et al. Dose equivalence of two commercial preparations of botulinum neurotoxin type A: Time for a reassessment? *Curr Med Res Opin.* 2009;25(7):1573–1584.

14. Karsai S, Raulin C. Current evidence on the unit equivalence of different botulinum neurotoxin A formulations and recommendations for clinical practice in dermatology. *Dermatol Surg.* 2009;35(1):1–8.

15. Truong D, Duane D, Jankovic J, et al. The efficacy and safety of botulinum type A toxin (Dysport) in cervical dystonia: Results of the first US randomized double-blind, placebo-controlled study. *Mov Disord.* 2005;20(7):783–791.

16. Ney J, Joseph K. Neurologic uses of botulinum neurotoxin type *A. Neuropsychiatr Dis Treat.* 2007;3(6):785–798.

17. Wissel J, Kabus C, Wenzel R, et al. Botulinum toxin in writer's cramp: objective response evaluation in 31 patients. *J Neurol Neurosurg Psychiatry.* 1996;61(2):172–175.

18. Food and Drug Administration. *Update of Safety Review of OnabotulinumtoxinA (marketed as Botox/Botox Cosmetic), AbobotulinumtoxinA (marketed as Dysport) and RimabotulinumtoxinB (marketed as Myobloc).* Department of Health and Human Services; April, 2009. Online. Available at: http://www.fda.gov/Drugs/DrugSafety/PostmarketDrugSafetyInformationforPatientsand Providers/DrugSafetyInformationforHeathcare Professionals/ucm174959.htm.

19. Borodic G, Johnson E, Goodnough M, et al. Botulinum toxin therapy, immunologic resistance, and problems with available materials. *Neurology.* 1996;46(1):26–29.

20. Dressler D, Adib Saberi F. New formulation of Botox: complete antibody-induced treatment failure in cervical dystonia. *J Neurol Neurosurg Psychiatry.* 2007;78(1):108–109.

4

Soft-tissue fillers

Trevor M. Born, Lisa E. Airan, and Dimitrios Motakis

SYNOPSIS

- The availability of multiple safe soft-tissue fillers today offers a unique tool in the correction of facial wrinkles and in the restoration of the volumetric loss that appears with aging.
- Reversibility is more often than not an advantageous property of fillers, allowing adjustments that may be needed due to technical errors or changes in the tissues that may occur with aging.
- Inexperienced injectors should always opt for rapidly resorbable fillers such as hyaluronic acid (HA). This allows for faster resolution of any technical errors that may occur. Hyaluronidase can be used to dissolve the filler.
- With respect to the treatment of deep folds and tear troughs, it is important to undercorrect these deformities. This results in a more natural appearance, and leaves room for further correction in the future if that is desirable. Overcorrection of these areas can result in visible abnormalities.
- "Off-label" use of synthetic materials is technically possible but does carry some risk. The plastic surgeon is vulnerable from a liability standpoint, and should use discretion when using products in an "off -label" manner. The patient must be informed of "off-label" use.
- In cases where slight correction is required, patients often forget their preoperative appearance. It is imperative to use photography and point any asymmetries prior to injection.
- Complications of dermal fillers can be avoided by the use of proper technique (small aliquots, appropriate level and quantity of injection, undercorrection, massaging with some fillers).

Access the Historical Perspective section online at
http://www.expertconsult.com

Introduction

There has been historical interest in the use of injected material to modify the contour of skin and underlying soft tissue. However, effective and safe tools to accomplish such a goal have become available only in recent decades. The plastic surgeon now has access to numerous fillers to soften the stigmata of aging or correct the contour deficits that occur with many disease processes. In order to use the soft tissue optimally, one has to understand the nature of each product and its mode of integration and adsorption.

The goal of this chapter is to present the different classes of fillers and the indications and techniques for their use. Particular attention is paid to the correction of common areas in the face. Furthermore, we will present possible contraindications and complications of fillers and how to avoid or treat them. Prior to mastering the use of soft-tissue fillers, it is important to understand how wrinkles form.

The pathophysiology of wrinkles

Aging is a complex process, which is the result of both intrinsic factors (soft-tissue maturation, skeletal change/atrophy, and muscular hyperactivity) and extrinsic factors (gravity and solar damage). As a consequence, the smooth confluent appearance of the face is slowly replaced by sharp angles, fine and deep wrinkles, and abrupt hollows and bulges. The anatomy of facial aging is thoroughly reviewed in Chapters 6 and 11.

With aging, skeletal changes occur with an overall decrease in facial height and a moderate widening and deepening of the facial structure. The decrease in maxillary height and the increase in orbital volume result in sunken eyes, and less space for attachment of the available soft tissue. The cheeks descend, the nasolabial folds become deeper, the upper lip complex appears bulkier and tear troughs as well as perioral rhytides appear. If teeth are lost, alveolar height decreases and the chin atrophies. Apart from the decrease in overall bone volume, the ligamentous attachments of the soft tissue and skin become lax and further contribute to the appearance of furrows and creases.

With chronological aging, all cells divide more slowly; this includes keratinocytes, fibroblasts, and melanocytes. The epidermis thins out and the epidermal–dermal junction becomes flatter, while the integrity of the stratum corneum decreases and the basal cells acquire more atypia. As a result of this decreased integrity, water loss through the skin is increased, leading to skin which is drier, more fragile, and more prone to shearing. The dermis becomes thinner and contains fewer but thickened elastic fibers and fewer loosely woven collagen fibers. Sebaceous glands become hypertrophic, but are less numerous and less active, thus contributing to skin dryness. All the above changes lead to a drier, less elastic, coarser, more fragile skin that is susceptible to gravitation forces and thus wrinkling.

Chronic sun exposure is probably the most significant environmental factor impacting skin maturation, leading to dyschromia, lentigines, telangectasias, and the loss of the youthful pink hue. Skin texture becomes coarser. The epidermis is actually thicker in photoaged skin than in normal skin. Overall collagen amount decreases. However, in the superficial dermis there is an area of increased normal collagen production (grenz zone) representing a chronic inflammatory process known as heliodermatitis. Solar elastosis is pathognomonic of photoaged skin with abundant, degraded, thickened elastic fibers. Lastly, sun exposure contributes to a reduction in ground substance, contributing to deeper folds and wrinkles.

Microscopically all wrinkles appear like thinned breaks in the dermis. Even though the terms wrinkles, folds, creases, furrows, and rhytides are often used interchangeably, specific features can be used to distinguish between different types of rhytides. Fine wrinkles refer to changes in the texture of the skin that involve the superficial aspect of the dermis. Mimetic wrinkles can extend down to the middle level of the dermis (lines) or down to its full thickness (furrows). These are due to the repeated folding of the skin secondary to the contraction of the facial muscles. As a result they are perpendicular to the direction of these muscles and occur in locations such as the glabella, periorbita, forehead, and lips. These dynamic wrinkles eventually become static, remaining visible even when the underlying muscle is relaxed.

Folds refer to larger grooves with some level of skin overlap. These are the result of soft-tissue descent secondary to gravity, decreased support, and loss of skin elasticity. Examples include upper eyelid dermatochalasis, nasolabial folds, jowls/marionette lines, and horizontal neck lines. The tear trough is an infraorbital groove that results from soft-tissue tethering along the arcus marginalis between bulging orbital fat above and descending soft tissue below.

The importance of being able to classify wrinkles is central to being able to direct treatment.[1] Superficial lines that course at the upper level of the dermis are amenable to dermabrasion, chemical peels, and lasers. On the other hand, mimetic wrinkles respond to muscle inactivation with Botox or myectomy/myotomy. Mimetic wrinkles can also be improved with the concomitant use of dermal fillers. Dermal fillers are also useful in the treatment of folds during their early stages,

Table 4.1 Biological fillers approved by the Food and Drug Administration (FDA) in the United States

FDA-approved biological filler	Type
Cymetra	Human dermis
AlloDerm	Human dermal matrix
Dermalogen	Human collagen matrix
Surgisis	Porcine collagen matrix
Fascian	Human tensor fasciae latae
Zyderm/Zyplast	Collagen (bovine)
CosmoDerm/CosmoPlast	Collagen (human-based)
Restylane/Perlane	Hyaluronic acid (bacterial)
Elevess	Hyaluronic acid (bacterial)
Juvederm	Hyaluronic acid (bacterial)

Box 4.1 **Ideal filler characteristics**

- Nontoxic
- Biocompatible
- Long-lasting (if not permanent)
- Reversible
- Off the shelf
- Autologous
- Easy to use
- Safe
- Produces positive, natural, discernible change
- Minimal downtime
- Level of placement (could be placed through dermis at subcutaneous, intramuscular, or periosteal levels)
- Predictable (permanence, bulk, and behavior)
- Performs well as a person ages
- Not discernible by touch/appearance

or as an adjuvant modality to surgery, during their more advanced stages. Several classification systems have appeared over the years. The Lemperle classification is based on wrinkle depth and is helpful in guiding treatment and assessing change/improvement *(Table 4.1)*.

Classification of fillers

Soft-tissue fillers are an ideal option for patients seeking facial rejuvenation with minimal downtime. For the young patient not requiring surgery, these materials offer a viable option, while for older patients, surgery can be combined with fillers and other surface treatments to create an optimal result.[8,9]

The number and variety of products available are impressive.[10–12] Yet the ideal filler has not been found; neither have we agreed on the properties that would be appropriate for all fillers. For example, although permanence would clearly be a virtue, it could also be a negative if the filler used did not age appropriately as the patient's soft tissues became ptotic and attenuated.[13,14] Therefore reversibility is an important characteristic. Despite these reservations, there are certain basic qualities that are sought in the ideal filler material *(Box 4.1)*.

Worldwide research for the ideal soft-tissue filler continues, although a balance is needed between embracing new products and ensuring the patient safety. In order to understand better the properties of each product that is either already available or in the pipeline, fillers can be classified under the following categories:

- autologous materials
- biologic materials
- synthetic materials.

Autologous fillers

Autologous materials are derived from the patient's own tissue.[15–18] They come closest to matching the description of the ideal soft-tissue filler in terms of safety, but they are not as convenient to use. They have to be harvested from another site on the body, which may produce a scar, and the process of harvesting and then inserting these materials elsewhere requires a two-step procedure. Toxicity, allergenicity, immunogenicity, carcinogenicity, and teratogenicity are not issues, but there can be problems with infection, migration, inflammatory reactions, loss of persistence, and reproducibility. Autologous fillers include:

- dermis, fascia, cartilage, superficial musculoaponeurotic system (SMAS), breast implant capsule
- fat grafts
- platelet-rich fibrin matrix (PRFM)
- cultured fibroblasts.

Dermal, fascial, and cartilage grafts have a long history of use in plastic surgery, and with careful handling and placement in an appropriate recipient bed these grafts may have very good, long-lasting results. Less volume survives when lipodermal grafts are used because it is the dermal surface that must derive the blood supply from the host and serve as a vascularizing carrier for the fatty elements. Similarly, fascial grafts from the fascia lata of the thigh, the temporalis, and the SMAS can be used. In a good recipient bed, fascia is permanent and persists through a combination of creeping replacement by host fibroblasts and continued viability of fascial fibroblasts.

Fat grafts as free en bloc transfers of tissue have the disadvantage of losing at least one-half of their bulk after transplantation, and they develop cysts, calcifications, and necrotic lumps. However, this is not the case with injectable fat grafting: small intact packets of fatty tissue are harvested as atraumatically as possible and injected in tiny amounts along multiple tracts. The purpose is to keep the injected fat cells near a blood supply for survival and integration. The great advantage of injectable fat grafting is that it is permanent if the fat survives. The disadvantage is the unpredictability of the survival, the need for a donor site, and the time required to process and inject the tissue.[15–17,19]

Selphyl (Aesthetic Factors, Princeton, NJ) is a patented system that allows the extraction of PRFM from the patient's own blood.[20,21] This novel technology allows processing of blood in the office in a three-step process that takes approximately 20 minutes. The collected PRFM is then injected into the patient's wrinkles. The collection of a 9-cc blood sample allows the collection of 4 cc of PRFM. The development of collagen and dermal matrix increases over a period of 3 weeks

and there is early evidence to suggest long-lasting wrinkle correction (up to 20 months). Possible applications include correction of nasolabial folds, glabellar lines, and panfacial rejuvenation, as well as acne and other scar treatments. Selphyl has been cleared for use in the US (FDA) and Europe (CE mark). Although additional long-term data are still required to prove its efficacy, this product represents the first practical modality for autologous wrinkle collection.

More recently, LAVIV or Azficel-T (Fibrocell Science, Exton, PA: www.fibrocellscience.com; FDA approval June 2011) became approved for the correction of moderate to deep nasolabial folds. LAVIV is an autologous cellular product composed of fibroblasts harvested from postauricular skin (www.mylaviv.com/pdf/LAVIV-prescribing-info.pdf). The fibroblasts obtained from the skin biopsy are aseptically cultured and expanded until sufficient cells for three consecutive injections are obtained. The treatment sessions are spaced 3–6 weeks apart. Although the mechanism of action of LAVIV is unclear, a two-point improvement in the Lemperle classification scale was achieved in up to 57% of subjects treated. The longevity of this correction beyond 6 months remains to be shown.

Biologic fillers

Biologic materials derived from organic sources (humans, animals, or bacteria) offer the benefits of ready "off-the-shelf" availability and ease of use, but introduce issues of sensitization to foreign animal or human proteins, transmission of disease, and immunogenicity.[22–26] Biologics provide only a temporary effect and typically do not correct the wrinkles or creases completely. The three major types of biologic tissue fillers are acellular soft-tissue matrix, collagen, and HA products (*Table 4.1*).

Fascian (Fascia Biosystems, Beverly Hills, CA) is a preserved particulate human fascial graft that is marketed in syringes and is prepared from prescreened human cadaver fascia lata. It is injected intradermally, subdermally, or in deep tissue, depending on the application and it is reported that Fascian particles tend to last two or three times longer than bovine collagen products.

AlloDerm (LifeCell, Branchburg, NJ) is an acellular, structurally intact sheet of human dermal graft that was first used clinically in the treatment of full-thickness burns. Processed from prescreened human cadaver skin, the cells responsible for immunogenicity are removed while the matrix structure and biochemical components are left intact. The grafted material then acts as a template for recipient cell repopulation resulting in soft-tissue regeneration. Some of its cosmetic-related applications include lip augmentation, nasolabial fold correction, glabellar wrinkle softening, rhinoplasty (dorsum and tip) as well as septal perforation, Frey syndrome, liposuction defect, and scar treatments. Complications include infection, persistent palpability or lumpiness, and variable "take" of the grafted material. Reports of volume diminution in mobile graft areas range from 30% to 40% at 1 year to 70% retention after 18 months.

Cymetra (LifeCell, Branchburg, NJ) is also a lyophilized acellular collagen matrix derived from human cadaver dermis, but in a particulate form. It is FDA-approved for subcutaneous injection and is used for lips, nasolabial folds, and deep

Table 4.5 Filler characteristics

Filler	Category	Composition	Viscosity*	Level of placement†	Advantages	Disadvantages and complications
Zyplast	Biologic	Bovine collagen	+ +	Superficial to deep dermis	Less swelling (~24 hours) Easy to use	Skin test More inflammatory Correction very short-term
Zyderm I and II	Biologic	Bovine collagen	+	Dermoepidermal junction	Less swelling (~24 hours) Easy to use	Skin test More inflammatory Correction very short-term
CosmoPlast	Biologic	Human collagen	++	Superficial to deep dermis	Less swelling (~24 hours) Less inflammatory Easy to use	Length of correction variable
CosmoDerm	Biologic	Human collagen	+	Dermoepidermal junction	Less swelling (~24 hours) Less inflammatory Easy to use	Short- and long-term correction
Perlane/ Juvederm Ultra Plus/ Puragen	Biologic	HA (bacterially derived) HA (bacterially derived) HA (bacterially derived)	+++	Deep dermis	Long-lasting Can be used in deep tissue and along bone Minimal reactions No skin test	More swelling – up to 3–5 days
Restylane/ Juvederm Ultra/ Elevess/ Hylaform	Biologic	HA (bacterially derived) HA (bacterially derived) HA (bacterially derived) HA (avian culture-derived)	++	Superficial dermis	Long-lasting Can be used in deep tissue and along bone Minimal reactions No skin test	More swelling – up to 3–5 days
Restylane Fine Lines	Biologic	HA (bacterially derived)	+	Dermoepidermal junction	Great for glabellar region and fine lines Do not use along bone	Shorter-term longevity than Restylane or Perlane
ArteFill (ArteColl)	Synthetic/ biologic	Polymethylmethacrylate (PMMA) beads covered with bovine collagen	+++	Deep dermis or subcutaneous	Long-lasting in deep folds and acne scars	Bumps, which may require treatment with steroids or surgery to remove Risk of granuloma Collagen reactivity Requires skin test
Radiesse	Synthetic	Calcium hydroxyapatite	+ + +	Deep dermis or subcutaneous	Long-lasting Can be used in deep tissue and along bone Minimal reactions No skin test	More swelling – up to 3–5 days Irregularities (technically dependent)
Sculptra	Synthetic	Poly-L-lactic acid (PLLA)	+ +	Deep dermis or subcutaneous	Long-lasting Can be used in deep tissue and along bone Minimal reactions No skin test	More swelling – up to 3–5 days Irregularities (technically dependent) Inflammatory reactions Multiple treatments required

HA, Hyaluronic acid.

*Viscosity is not measured by most companies in terms of flow: + least thickness, easiest/best flow; ++ in between; +++ most thickness, more difficult flow.

†Level of placement is also dependent on amount/type of desired correction.

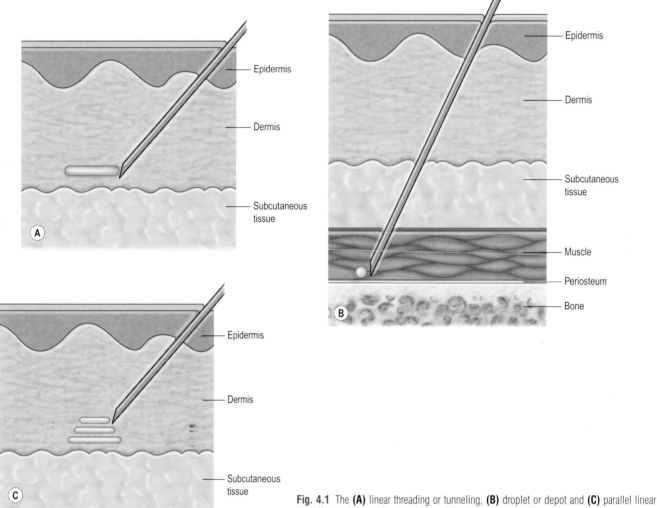

Fig. 4.1 The **(A)** linear threading or tunneling, **(B)** droplet or depot and **(C)** parallel linear threading techniques for dermal filler injection.

threading is most commonly used to correct wrinkles and furrows. However, when deeper creases are treated, multiple parallel linear threads at different levels have to be used to accomplish the desired volumetric augmentation *(Fig. 4.1C)*. Examples of where this technique is commonly used include the glabellar lines, the nasolabial folds, the lips and the tear trough, among others.

Radial fanning is a variation of the linear threading technique *(Fig. 4.2A)*. Just before the needle is completely withdrawn from the skin, it is reinserted in a different direction and the product is again injected in a retrograde fashion. This process is repeated multiple times in different directions until adequate correction is accomplished. This approach is particularly useful in malar augmentation, but it is also used in the correction of the prejowl sulcus and the nasolabial fold.

Cross-hatching is often used in the correction of large surface areas such as the marionette lines/prejowl sulcus or the hollowing of the lower cheek *(Fig. 4.2B)*. Two independent radial fanning injections oriented perpendicular to each other constitute also a form of cross-hatching, and are commonly used in cheek augmentation.

Frequently the needle is inserted deep into the tissue and an aliquot of product is laid down; this is known as the depot or droplet technique *(Fig. 4.1B)*. Large volumes deposited in this fashion can lead to palpable nodules and irregularities. Usually multiple small droplets are deposited in a serial fashion; this is known as the serial puncture technique. These aliquots have to be close together to prevent irregularities. If any irregularities appear they can be managed by massage until flat. This technique is frequently used in the tear trough correction and in lip augmentation, but also in the treatment of all other wrinkles and creases. Experienced injectors normally use all of these techniques in combination.

Indications and applications

There are multiple indications for the use of dermal fillers. Below is a list of the most common areas of the aging face usually addressed with injectables. The appropriate types of fillers that should be used to treat each of these areas, as well as some of the technical nuances for their optimal application, are also described. For the purpose of this discussion, low-viscosity HA (LVHA) fillers refer to Restylane Fine Lines, medium-viscosity HA (MVHA) fillers refer to Restylane/Juvederm Ultra/Eleveess, while high-vicosity HAs (HVHA) include Perlane/Juvederm Ultra Plus/Puragen.

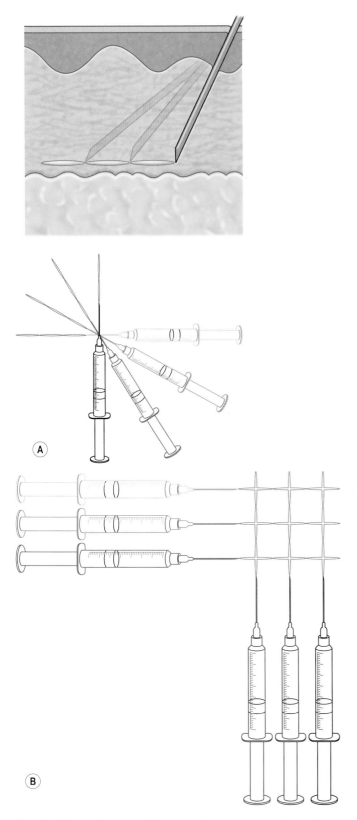

Fig. 4.2 (A) Radial fanning and **(B)** cross-hatching techniques of derma filler injection.

Glabellar lines

The folds of the glabella are ideally treated in combination with botulin toxin. Often Botox may soften the fold on its own. The glabellar fold may be a fairly superficial line with a deeper etched component that is best treated with Restylane Fine Lines at the dermal–epidermal junction; the product is placed in a serial droplet or serial linear threading fashion. Threading can be done in a parallel or in a crisscross manner. Either technique undermines the line while placing the filler. If the fold is broader, then an MVHA filler may be used; this is placed at the mid to superficial dermis. Small amounts must be injected to avoid tissue necrosis. When combined with Botox, the effect can last from 8 months to much longer. Layering of these fillers may be needed on occasion. Care should be taken in the patient with very thin skin as the filler may cause lumps or bumps.

Forehead lines

The injection technique in this area is similar to that used for the glabellar lines. If the patient has a very dynamic forehead, then Botox will be very helpful in achieving a better result and increasing its longevity. If Botox is not used, then the filler may only last for a short period of time. Caution with Botox should be exercised in patients with moderate to severe brow ptosis. More commonly, Restylane Fine Lines or collagen is used, and these are placed at the dermal–epidermal junction in a serial droplet or in a linear threading technique *(Fig. 4.3C)*.

Eyebrows

The eyebrows may be elevated 1–2 mm by the addition of an MVHA filler such as Restylane to the deep tissue layer of the lateral eyebrow. The volume of the temples generally decreases with age and the placement of approximately 1 cc of HA on the deep layer can help restore the youthful contour and raise the eyebrow. Moreover, the surgical removal of the fat of the upper eyelid is sometimes to such a degree that it results in a hollow or skeletonized orbital rim. The same hollowing may be seen in some individuals as a consequence of the aging process. This cadaveric appearance may be corrected with placement of HA on the inferior aspect of the supraorbital rim. This also gives the illusion of raising the eyebrows while restoring a more youthful appearance to the upper lid and eyebrow region.

Care must be taken to inject small volumes with each pass to prevent emboli and injury to the sensory nerves. The filler is placed at a level that is not mobile. Caution is necessary in the central eyebrow as the supraorbital nerve emerges here. MVHA fillers are good deep fillers in this case. HVHAs, such as Perlane, are a longer-lasting alternative and can be used in a similar fashion.

Tear troughs

Tear troughs can be corrected with fillers to give a rested and more youthful appearance. The infraorbital rim hollowing and nasojugal groove can be filled by injecting product deep

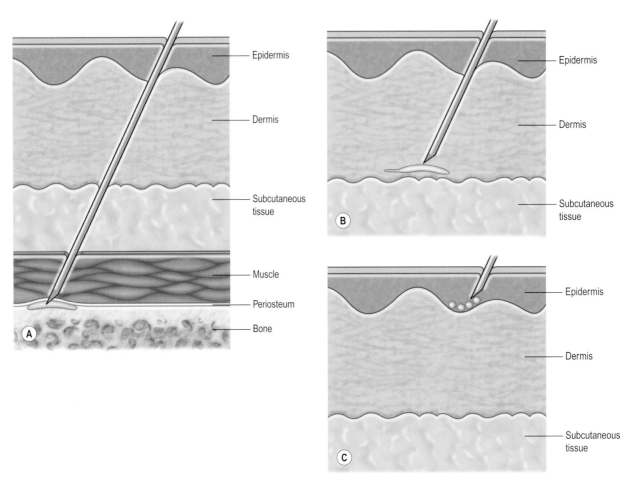

Fig. 4.3 Injection of dermal filler into the deep tissue/periosteal level **(A)**, more superficial into the subcutaneous tissue **(B)**, and into the most superficial epidermal-dermal junction **(C)**.

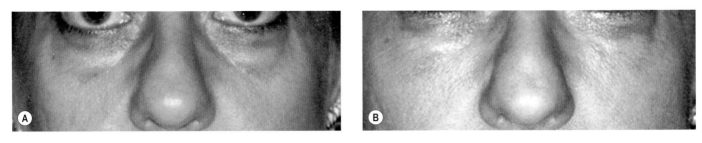

Fig. 4.4 Tear troughs. **(A)** This 48-year-old woman presented with significant tear troughs that made her appear tired. Perlane was placed at the depth of the periorbital hollow on the bone and on the malar bone to augment cheek projection and minimize the negative vector. A total volume of 1.1 cc was placed per side; it was placed mainly in the periorbital hollow, but a smaller amount was placed on the malar bone to increase cheek projection relative to the globe. **(B)** The patient is seen 6 months after treatment.

on the bone and periosteum *(Fig. 4.4)*. This ensures that the product is not palpable or visible, especially with animation. Various fillers have been used for this purpose but the most commonly applied are Restylane, Juvederm, or Perlane. Collagens have very low longevity so they are not practical for this use. Other long-term fillers such as Radiesse, Sculptra, and ArteFill can have a devastating outcome in case of visible nodular/granulomatous formation, and should be avoided for this use.[45,56–58]

Usually 0.5–1.5 cc of filler is used per side depending on the severity of the tear trough and the desired projection of the malar prominence. The area to be corrected should be marked before the injection of local anesthetic and adequate time should be given to maximize the effect of the epinephrine and minimize bruising. The filler is applied in a retrograde fashion by the serial droplet or serial threading techniques, always feeling for the orbital rim with the free hand. Once injected the product can be massaged to smoothen its distribution over the bone and the hollow. If swelling and bruising are noticed immediately after filler injection, pressure and cold compresses should be applied. In case of overcorrection the product can be massaged down for up to 2–3 weeks. If the overcorrection persists, the HA filler can be partially dissolved with hyaluronidase.

Nasolabial folds

The nasolabial folds may be of different shapes, lengths, and depths. In addition, some patients have pre-existing telangiectasia in this area that can be made worse with injections. The gradation system, as described by Dr. Lemperle *(Table 4.6)*, is useful in evaluating and discussing with patients their goals.

The amount of change in the average case should be approximately 50% correction of the depth of the fold *(Fig. 4.5)* Care must be taken not to overfill the fold because this will give patients an odd appearance when they animate or smile. Fillers can be used to soften the broader portion of the fold, which is usually the upper two-thirds down to the lateral oral commissure. Choices here include all types of fillers.[32] MVHAs and collagens can be placed at the level of the mid- to deep dermis. With HVHA fillers such as Perlane, as well as the semipermanent or permanent fillers (Radiesse, Sculptra, ArteFill) the product should be placed in the deep subcutaneous tissue *(Fig. 4.3C)*.[37,56,59,60] The filler is placed at angles to the fold, and layering may be done to enhance longevity *(Fig. 4.4B)*. Also, for very deep folds, more viscous products (Perlane, Cosmoplast, Zyplast) or permanent/semipermanent (Radiesse, Sculptra, ArteFill) products may be placed deep under less viscous fillers such as Restylane, Juvederm, and Cosmoderm. This may increase longevity of the correction and give a more polished appearance. If the nasolabial fold

has a superficial line etched into it, this can be softened with Restylane Fine Lines. As with all repeated injections of HA, the product lasts longer and less volume of product is needed to achieve the same volume and contour change. Taping of the fold after the injection for a few days may help the product bind into place with scar tissue and can prevent the lateral displacement of the product to the nasolabial fold when the patient smiles.

Malar augmentation

Malar augmentation can be achieved with most fillers available.[61] In the case of semipermanent and permanent fillers, care must be taken for the product to be injected deep in the tissue *(Fig. 4.3A)*. With HA fillers, the product can be applied from the deepest layers to the most superficial *(Fig. 4.3A–C)*. MVHAs such as Juvederm and Restylane can be used in this manner applying the product over bone, into deep tissue and in the dermis. Alternatively, more durable fillers such as HVHAs, Radiesse, Sculptra, or ArteFill can be used deep, with MVHAs placed more superficial to obtain further refinement if necessary. This approach leads to a more durable result. The most appropriate technique for malar augmentation is the radial fanning technique with entry points first lateral and then inferior to the malar prominence *(Fig. 4.4A)*. Nevertheless, any other technique can probably yield adequate results. Pressure over the augmented area should be avoided over the first week posttreatment. When used appropriately, dermal fillers can replace the use of an implant for malar augmentation.

Marionette lines

Marionette lines extend from the oral commissure in a downward oblique fashion, giving a sad appearance. Usually there is a volume deficit medially extending to the level of the jawline, creating what is known as the prejowl sulcus. Therefore, correction of the marionette lines is often combined with correction of the prejowl sulcus. Most fillers available today can be used for correction of the marionette lines. The

Table 4.6 **The Lemperle nasolabial fold classification**

Class	Description
0	No wrinkles
1	Just perceptible wrinkle
2	Shallow wrinkles
3	Moderately deep wrinkles
4	Deep wrinkle, well-defined edges
5	Very deep wrinkle, redundant fold

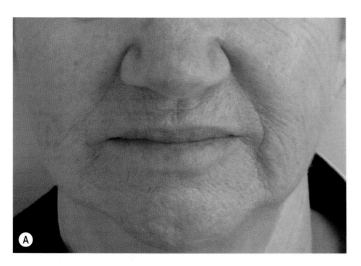
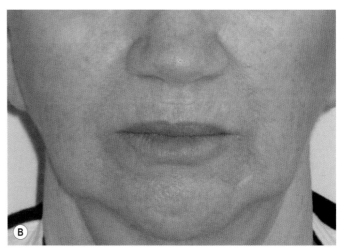

Fig. 4.5 Nasolabial folds and marionette lines. **(A)** This 64-year-old woman presented with perioral lines and significant jowls. However, she was not interested in surgical rejuvenation and wanted just to soften the appearance of her perioral wrinkles and folds. Approximately 0.4 cc of Restylane was used for each nasolabial fold and 0.3 cc to address the marionette lines on each side. **(B)** The patient is shown 1 month posttreatment.

principles mentioned earlier for other sites apply here too. More permanent viscous fillers are used for deeper correction with less viscous, finer products such as Restylane for more superficial correction.[62] The area to be filled is actually triangular, extending from the marionette line to the lower lateral lip vermilion to the superolateral aspect of the chin *(Fig. 4.6)*. Usually a radial fanning technique from two independent injection sites, superior and inferior, can lead to a smooth correction of the area *(Fig. 4.4C)*. One should be aware of the fact that this is a very dynamic area, where only partial correction is often possible. Overcorrection can lead to lumps that are visible or felt intraorally under the oral mucosa, as well as a strange appearance upon animation.

Jawline augmentation

In the areas along the jawline (filling the hollow anterior to the jowl) filler is best placed on the very deep plane on the bone (ideally beneath the periosteum) to allow augmentation of the soft tissues similar to a solid implant *(Fig. 4.3A)*. HVHAs or MVHAs may be used. Jawline augmentation is usually combined with marionette/prejowl sulcus correction. HA is placed in the deepest point of the hollow. This will correct most of the deformity. Placement of the material in the deep dermis may be required for complete correction of the jowl deformity.

Panfacial volumetric augmentation

With aging, soft-tissue descent and atrophy make the appearance of hollows and creases more pronounced. Reconstitution of the overall facial volume, including correction or the temporal hollowing, lifting of the brow, filling of the periobrital hollowing, malar, jawline and perioral enhancement, can result in a markedly rejuvenated appearance *(Figs 4.7, 4.8)*. This nonsurgical facelift can be achieved with Scultra or Radiesse injected in the deep tissues and HA or collagen fillers used to obtain more superficial refinement. Because both Radiesse and Sculptra show a delay in the appearance of the final result and because multiple injections may be required, the use of more viscous HA fillers in the deep tissues may be used instead for an immediate effect. The advantage of using Radiesse and Sculptra is that they last for 1 and 2–3 years, respectively. Alternatively, fat can be used for panfacial volumetric augmentation, with "finer" fillers such as Restylane or Restylane Fine Lines used to obtain a more superficial correction.

Facial lipoatrophy

HVHAs or MVHAs are ideal fillers to soften the appearance of lipoatrophy associated with antiretroviral therapy for HIV. Other options include Sculptra, Radiesse, ArteFill, and fat.[63,64] The areas that are best treated are the concavities adjacent to the zygomatic-temporal bone, the zygomatic arch, and less so for the inframalar hollow. In the temple and adjacent to the arch, it is important to place the filler deep within or under the periosteum and take care to inject slowly to be sure of even placement and to minimize bruising. The product is easily massaged, but if the massage is too aggressive the entire effect will be minimized. The idea is not to fill the entire area of

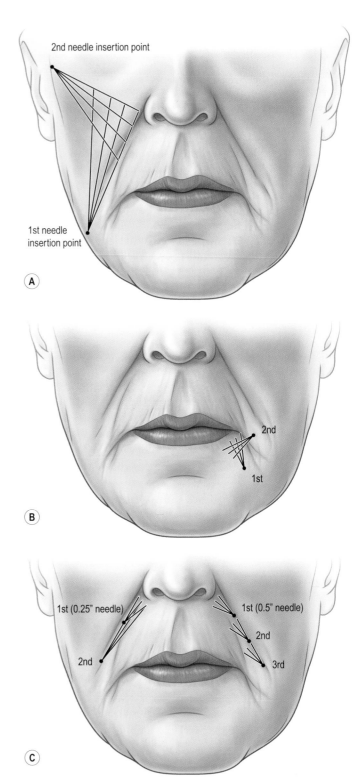

Fig. 4.6 Technique used **(A)** for malar augmentation, **(B)** for marionette lines, and **(C)** for nasolabial folds.

atrophy completely but to soften the contours so that the wasting does not appear too severe. In the inframalar hollow, the goal should be to correct one-third to one-half of the hollow. Linear threading or a fanning technique may be used, and a gradual and consistent result can be achieved.

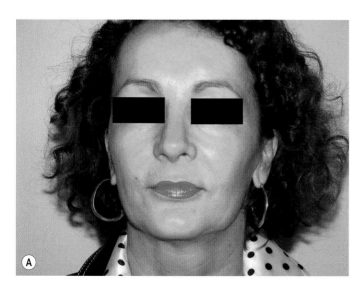

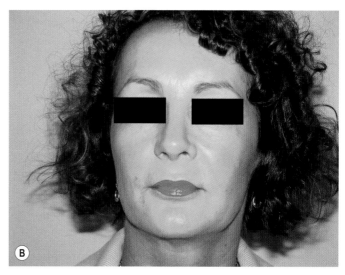

Fig. 4.7 Sculptra. **(A)** Preoperative and **(B)** 1-year postoperative results after augmentation to the brow, cheeks, and jawline with three sessions of Sculptra (two vials per session) in a 51-year-old female. The dilution of each vial of Sculptra consisted of 7 cc of sterile water and 3 cc of 1% Xylocaine with epinephrine.

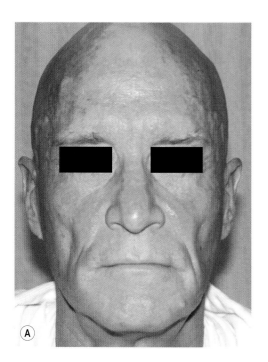

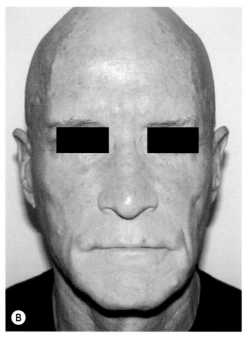

Fig. 4.8 Fat grafts. **(A)** Preoperative and **(B)** 1-year postoperative results after microfat grafrting to the temples, cheeks, and jawline and bilateral upper blepharoplasty in a 50-year-old male.

Volumes of 0.5–1.5 cc per area may be used, on average. This will vary among individuals, depending on their requested goals. Repeated injections on a 2–4-week basis may help to contour areas that have a large volume deficiency.

Lips

Contouring of the lips may be accomplished with several kind of fillers *(Fig. 4.9A, B)*.[65,66] Ideally, patients have a good shape to their lips at the start. In these patients, just augmenting the vermilion is enough to produce an excellent result. Often the left and right sides of the lips differ in length and thickness, and this must be demonstrated to the patient prior to augmentation.

The injection process generally starts with augmentation of the vermilion border of the lip to enhance its definition and provide increased projection. The philtral columns may also be augmented with filler placed in the mid dermal level. Palpation of the tissue as the filler is injected is important. Injection of the lip proper from the wet–dry junction to the vermilion border may also be carried out just deep to the mucosa within the orbicularis oris muscle. If it is placed immediately beneath the mucosa, it will be seen as a blue color. Placement posterior to the wet–dry junction along the wet mucosa may enhance the lip volume as well as the projection. Variation in the placement of the product must be done, depending on the desires of the patient and the starting shape of the lips.

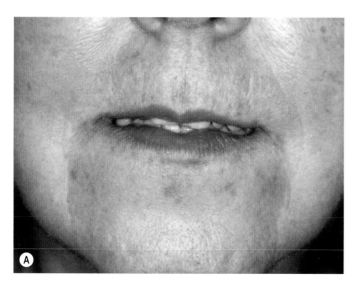
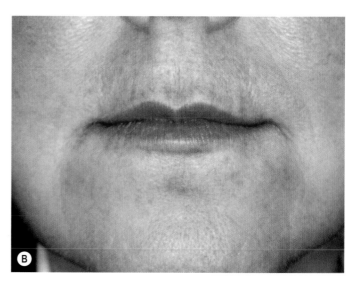

Fig. 4.9 Lips. **(A)** This 51-year-old woman requested lip augmentation. Restylane was injected into the vermilion border and philtral columns to achieve a narrower appearance. Restylane was injected from the inside of the lip from the vermilion border to the wet–dry junction. **(B)** She is shown 3 months after injection with good persistence of filler.

The cupid's bow becomes wider with age and should be made narrower. The depth of the mental fold increases with age and may require softening. Frequently the upper lip is atrophied above the vermilion border, particularly the lateral aspects, and restoration is done with MVHA placed at the mid dermal level to improve volume and projection of the upper lip. One should use minimal volume in the upper lip above the vermilion border as any added volume may cause lengthening of the upper lip. Care must also be taken to limit the amount of filler placed in the upper lip skin adjacent to the nasolabial fold because this will result in an awkward animation of the upper lip and nasolabial fold, particularly during smiling, and can give the appearance of a "joker-type" upper lip or create an unusual fold at the lateral edge of the upper lip.

Patients with long, thin lips and very broad smiles may get limited results because of tissue tension. Often patients complain that their lips are too thin when they smile. This is a dynamic change and cannot be corrected with fillers or implants. Patients with lips that are tight to the dentition or a class II occlusion should be augmented with conservative volumes, since irregularities of dentition may be reflected in the upper lip appearing too prominent or "duck-like."

Approximate volumes for augmentation of the lips may range from 0.5 to 1.0 mL per lip. MVHAs should last for a period of 4–6 months; however, when it is repeated, the results may last for 8 months up to 1 year. Collagens have a shorter half-life. HVHAs may be used as an alternative to MVHAs for lip augmentation. They are best suited for patients with lips that are not very mobile. Care must be taken in persons with soft, supple lips that move a lot with animation; these patients may not respond well to HVHAs and their lips may appear too stiff. When injecting HVHAs one must avoid the formation of lumps or bumps as they are difficult to massage out of the tissue. Radiesse and Sculptra should not be used for lip augmentation due to their high incidence of nodule formation. ArteFill is an option for permanent augmentation, but can result in visible nodularity.

If the patient has lip implants, then the filler may be added around the implant. HA fillers can also be combined with other tissue fillers. Collagen or less viscous HAs may first be injected along the vermilion border, which provides augmentation of the white roll. MVHAs may also be placed in areas where ArteFill has been placed previously after a minimum waiting period of 2–3 months. Lastly, patients with a history of herpes should be given prophylaxis because the treatment may cause a herpetic outbreak and scarring.

Nasal reshaping

Many fillers have been used in the correction of minor nasal deformities *(Fig. 4.10A, B)*.[48,67] More commonly, HA fillers and calcium hydroxyapatite have been used for nonsurgical rhinoplasty. Radiesse, even though it may provide more support than HA fillers, can also become visible if placed in large amounts or too superficial. In general, permanent fillers have a higher risk of becoming visible or palpable. If a permanent filler such as ArteFill is to be used, it is probably preferable to attempt correction with a resorbable filler first. Injection can be by either serial threading or tunneling techniques. The product should be placed in the subcutaneous/sub-SMAS tissue, especially in patients with thin skin, to avoid visibility. Irregularities over the dorsum or the tip can be corrected in this manner. Despite several anecdotal reports of alar skin and nasal tip necrosis, the occurrence of this complication is rare. Nevertheless, injections over the dorsum and nasal side walls appear to be somewhat safer, especially shortly after open rhinoplasty, when blood supply to the nasal tip may be tenuous. Care should be exercised to inject small amounts (<0.1 cc) with each pass and to assess continuously for blanching to avoid any skin compromise. The advantage of using HA fillers lies in the fact that the product can be melted out with hyaluronidase in case of blanching postinjection. Nitropaste and warm compresses can also help prevent or limit skin necrosis in such cases.

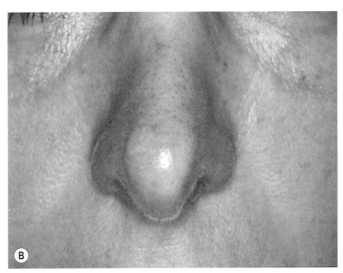

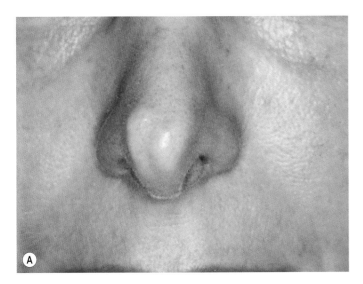

Fig. 4.10 Nose. **(A)** This 30-year-old woman had concerns about the irregular appearance of her nasal tip cartilage. Restylane was used to fill in the hollows and shape the tip of her nose. Restylane, 0.4 cc, was used to soften the appearance of the nasal cartilage. The patient had inquired initially about rhinoplasty with tip alteration. She had not had previous surgery, and the nasal tip had not changed other than the irregularity becoming more noticeable with time. The skin at the tip of the nose was very thin, and any slight surgical irregularity may have been noticeable; additionally, the skin may have been compromised by an open rhinoplasty. The new tip contour was achieved under a block with local anesthetic and 0.4 cc of Restylane. **(B)** She is seen here 5 months after injection.

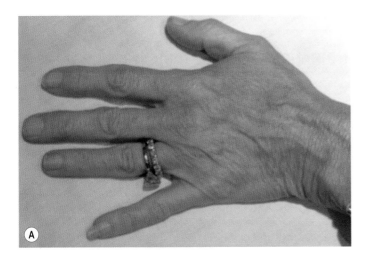

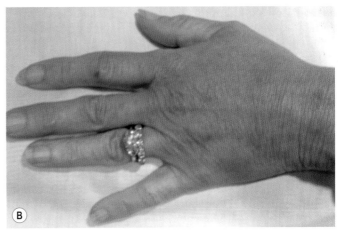

Fig. 4.11 Hand. **(A)** Preoperative and **(B)** 6-month postoperative results after injection of 1.3 cc of Radiesse to the left hand in a 60-year-old female.

Scars and deformities

Many soft-tissue deformities can be corrected with HA fillers (Restylane/Juvederm), collagens, or permanent fillers (ArteFill, fat). The choice somewhat depends on the depth and extend of the scar. It is important that the scar tissue be soft and distensible. The product should not be placed under high pressure as this may result in tissue necrosis. More than one treatment may be required for full correction, but often the correction is permanent. Excellent results can be achieved in acne, chickenpox, and traumatic scars, and these can be long-lasting. Simultaneous release of the scar with an 18G needle may improve the results. The use of Restylane Fine Lines in steroid atrophy is helpful but may result in incomplete correction. Botox is helpful in scars located in mobile areas such as the glabella, forehead, and chin where the

mimetic action may be reduced. This may increase the longevity of the filler placed.

Hand rejuvenation

Even though the primary use of dermal fillers is in facial rejuvenation, increasing attention has been paid to their application in hand rejuvenation *(Fig. 4.11A, B)*.[68–70] Fat has been shown to be an excellent autologous filler for this purpose. although this requires the harvesting of fat. HA fillers, Radiess and Sculptra can be used to plump up the soft tissues over the dorsum of the hand and up to the level of the metacarpophalangeal joints. This soft-tissue augmentation decreases the appearance of veins, extensor tendons, and bony prominences, which become pronounced with aging. Multiple fanning subcutaneous injections can be used, making sure to avoid the vessels, tendons, and nerves of the dorsal hand.

Contraindications and considerations

There are not many strict contraindications to the use of dermal fillers. Probably the most important is unrealistic patient expectations. The use of fillers is not a substitute for surgery in cases where tissue descent and skin laxity are advanced. In such cases, the patient should be advised of the adjuvant role that fillers can play in relation to the more dramatic improvement that could be achieved surgically. Furthermore, some of the creases of the face are present from a young age and they are a result of animation. Obliteration can result in an unnatural mask-like appearance. This should be pointed out to the patient who wants some folds completely erased.

In patients who are prone to form keloids and hypertrophic scars, the risk should be stressed to the patient.[13] It is best to try first with a small amount of filler and possibly test the product in an inconspicuous area. The presence of infection, foreign-body reaction, or inflammation is a contraindication to filler use. If a known allergy to collagen exists, then the use of collagen fillers is contraindicated. ArteFill also contains collagen and should not be used under these circumstances. With all collagen-containing fillers skin testing prior to use is required.

The use of blood thinners (coumadin, nonsteroidal anti-inflammatories, heparin) or natural products with similar effects (fish oils, vitamin D, garlic), can lead to significant ecchymoses. The patient should be informed of this fact and should preferably stop taking such substances several weeks prior to injection. Nevertheless, if that is not possible, dermal fillers can be used as long as the patient is willing to accept the possible downtime secondary to bruising.

In patients with telangectasias, it is possible that the injection of filler will make their appearance and size worse. Even though this is not a strict contraindication, the patient has to be informed before treatment. The use of lasers can help diminish the appearance of these superficial vascular malformations.

The use of lasers does not affect deep fillers such as Radiesse or ArteFill. This is due to the fact that the product is deep and the melting point of these compounds is much higher than the heat generated by the laser. However, the injection of more superficial HA and collagen fillers should be done at a later date following laser treatment, if possible.

There are no data to suggest adverse effects of dermal filler use during pregnancy, breastfeeding, and in patients younger than 18 years old. Despite the fact that such side-effects are unlikely, it is prudent to avoid the use of fillers in these groups of patients.

Viscous and longer-lasting compounds such as Radiesse, Sculptra, ArteFill, and Perlane/Juvaderm Ultra Plus are contraindicated for use in the superficial dermis because of palpable/visible nodule formation. Specifically, Radiesse should be avoided in the lips since there is a significant percentage of early nodule formation (up to 20%).

Because the use of fillers may result in an undesirable appearance, it is always more prudent that a temporary filler is used the first time. If the effect is indeed that anticipated by the patient, a more permanent correction may be pursued the next time.

Fillers have not been associated with any autoimmune disease. Moreover, autoimmune and connective tissue diseases such as scleroderma are not a contraindication to the use of dermal fillers, since wound healing is normal. There is some evidence to suggest that certain conditions such as sarcoidosis may predispose to a more pronounced inflammatory reaction (extensive granuloma formation and facial edema) with Sculptra injection, but it is anecdotal. Similarly, these products can be used in patients with diabetes, HIV, or immunosuppression, without a significantly higher incidence of infection.

Patients with very thin skin have a higher risk of palpability or visibility; deep injection of small amounts of filler is important. Sebaceous skin camouflages irregularities better, but product can escape through pores and even form pustules.

Lastly, there have been no reports of adverse reaction with the layering of different types of fillers. However, it would be prudent only to inject a second type of filler in the same locale several months after the primary injection. This way, in case of an adverse reaction, it would be possible to identify which product is responsible for the adverse reaction.

Complications and their treatment

All fillers have possible side-effects. Common complications that may occur are lumps, bumps and irregularities, pain, ecchymoses or hematoma, and overcorrection. Uncommonly the patient may experience intermittent swelling in the region treated. This usually resolves by 2–6 weeks. The occasional individual will have massive swelling in response to the injection and may consider using oral steroids to alleviate this immediate swelling.[71–80]

Rarely, individuals may develop erythema of the overlying skin for the first several weeks. Clinically it does not behave like an allergy and cellulitis has to be ruled out. A light topical steroid may be used as an initial treatment. In general, this reaction resolves without therapy over a short period of time. HA fillers have an incidence of allergic reaction of approximately 1 in 3000.[81] Bovine collagen (Zyplast and Zyderm) has been associated with severe local or regional allergic reactions that can become chronic and difficult to treat (incidence 1–3%).[82] Again, if these reactions are unresponsive or minimally responsive to local steroid injection, they may require oral steroid treatment. Allergic reactions can result in long-term scarring. Such hypersensitivity reactions are rare with human-derived Cosmoderm/Cosmoplast or other fillers.[83]

With Sculptra and Radiesse inflammatory nodules or papules can develop and are usually associated with superficial injection. Skin discoloration can accompany such superficial nodules. The role of massage is critical in preventing such inflammatory nodule formation. With Radiesse complications occur most often in the lips, where there can be a 10–20% early nodularity rate. If a lump, bump, or irregularity occurs, it may be treated with a dilute steroid injection and massage. However, irregularities may require excision if they persist and do not respond to steroids.

Other early reactions to fillers include sterile abscess and telangiectasia.[84–86] If the patient has pre-existing telangiectasia, this should be noted prior to injection. Additionally, the patient should be informed that there is a possible risk of formation of telangiectasia and that pre-existing telangiectasias may become more severe and require treatment after injection. When larger volumes of filler are used at one time, a sterile abscess may occur that will require drainage. This may occur up to 2 weeks after the initial injection. This is treated with local incision and drainage using an 18G needle. Immediate drainage of clear fluid mixed with yellow-white debris resolves the problem, with rapid resolution of the symptoms.

ArteFill can result in local granulomatous reactions.[71,87,88] The instances reported to date in North America are low (0.02–1%). There have been more extensive reports of granulomas in Europe (perhaps due to the earlier generations of the product). These may present as localized bumps, nodules that are tender to the touch. Giant cells and multinuclear giant cells are present in the nodules on histologic examination of the tissue with an accompanying inflammatory response. If the product is placed too superficial in the dermis, the resultant tissue formation may lead to a white coloring of the skin. This is similar to the bluish discoloration (Tyndall effect) that may occur with any of the HA fillers when placed in the superficial layer of the dermis. If ArteFill is not placed in small amounts with each pass, nodules can occur. These may be treated with local excision, massage, or dilute steroid injection (0.2 mg Kenalog/mL). Stronger Kenalog concentration (up to 40 mg/mL) may be needed to control the inflammation. If granuloma occurs, treatment options include direct steroid injection, excision, systemic treatment with oral steroids, or a combination of these treatments depending on the severity of the granuloma.[71,79,88]

Soft-tissue necrosis and embolic phenomenon have been reported but are rare.[89–92] The area mostly implicated is the glabella, rarely upon injection with Restylane and more commonly collagen. An algorithm for treatment of blanching postinjection, including warm compresses, nitroglycerine, epinephrine, hyaluronidase, and heparin has been proposed to reverse/minimize such ischemic events.

The injection of all filling substances may result in a herpetic outbreak if the patient has a predisposition. It must be noted that patients with a previous history of herpes simplex outbreak should receive prophylactic treatment with an appropriate antiviral medication.

Complications of fat transfer are similar to those of any other injection or surgical technique. Fat transfer is covered in Chapter 14.

Conclusion

The development of numerous fillers has armed the plastic surgeon with an invaluable tool in the area of minimally invasive facial rejuvenation. Diagnosis, proper technique, and choice of fillers are the keys to creating a natural appearance and avoiding iatrogenic problems.

Access the complete references list online at **http://www.expertconsult.com**

1. Lemperle G, Holmes RE, Cohen SR, et al. A Classification of Facial Wrinkles. *Plast Reconstr Surg.* 2001;108:1751–1752.

   The authors offer a standard classification for the assessment of facial rhytids. This system is based on wrinkle depth and can be a useful guide in the treatment of wrinkles, including nasolabial folds.

2. Kontis TC, Rivkin A. The history of injectable facial fillers. *Facial Plast Surg.* 2009;25:67–72.

17. Coleman SR. Structural fat grafts: The ideal filler? *Clin Plast Surg.* 2001;28:111–119.

   In this article, Coleman first presents microfat grafts as an ideal autologous filler. Structural fat grafts have become a unique tool in permanent soft-tissue augmentation with applications that span all areas of plastic surgery.

20. Sclafani AP. Platelet-rich fibrin matrix for improvement of deep nasolabial folds. *J Cosmet Dermatol.* 2010;9:66–71.

55. Arian LE, Born TM. Nonsurgical lower eyelid lift. *Plast Reconstr Surg.* 2005;116: 1785–1792.

   In this publication the authors present for the first time a means of correcting the tear trough and the infraorbital rim hollow. They offer a nonsurgical alternative to a lower blepharoplasty by camouflaging the infraorbital fat bulge. This is ideal in the case of the nonsurgical candidate.

63. Sturm LP, Cooter RD, Mutimer KL, et al. A systematic review of permanent and semipermanent dermal fillers for HIV-associated facial lipoatrophy. *AIDS Patient Care STDS.* 2009;23:699–714.

72. Sclafani AP, Fagien S. Treatment of injectable soft tissue filler complications. *Dermatol Surg.* 2009;35(suppl 2): 1672–1680.

   Even though rare, complications of dermal fillers can be devastating. The authors present a thorough review of all possible complications of dermal fillers and their causes in order to prevent them. The author also offers an algorithm of how to treat such complications once they occur.

85. Sherman RN. Avoiding dermal filler complications. *Clin Dermatol.* 2009;27:S23–S32.

5

Facial skin resurfacing

Steven R. Cohen, Ryan C. Frank, and E. Victor Ross

SYNOPSIS

- Non-surgical facial rejuvenation relies on matching the presenting skin pathology to an appropriate intervention that reverses that aspect of aging.
- Laser-based interventions rely on precise skin injury based on either selective photothermolysis, precise deposition of layered heating, or fractional wounding.
- Facial rejuvenation procedures that work at the skin surface can be complemented by neurotoxins and fillers.
- Fractional lasers achieve their rejuvenative effect with decreased risks of infection, pigment dyschromia, pain, as well as shorter recovery times versus their nonfractional counterparts.
- Vascular dyschromias can be reduced by a wide range of visible light and near infrared technologies.
- Hyperpigmented lesions can be treated by selective photothermolysis, repeated fractional procedures, or by precise ablative approaches that confine heating based on short laser tissue interaction times.

Access the Historical Perspective section online at
http://www.expertconsult.com

Introduction

Laser, chemical peeling, and other energy-based technologies have increasingly been applied in facial rejuvenation.[1] A logical approach to rejuvenation follows an understanding of skin anatomy and physiology, as they relate to skin aging. Any assessment of the face should include the surface, where sun and aging result in pigment inhomogeneities, wrinkles, and telangiectasia. Epidermal changes include basilar hyperpigmentation, hyperkeratosis, and thinning of the "living" portion of the epidermis. Another component of skin aging derives from changes in the dermis, where decreased glycosaminoglycans (GAGs), decreased elastin fibers, and changes in the character of collagen result in fine lines, sallowness and

eventually in cobblestoning of the skin. Microscopically, the changes present as solar elastosis. Also, weakened blood vessels dilate and present as telangiectasia. In some patients, hyperpigmentation results from both dermal and epidermal pigment dyschromias. The third component of aging skin results from bone regression, weakening of connections from the hypodermis to the surface, and volume loss.[1,2]

Most energy-based interventions address one or more of these components of skin aging. Epidermal pigmentation can be addressed by pigment-specific lasers or laser peels. In the first case, visible (VIS) light is used to selectively heat the epidermis. Proper parameter selection allows for preferential targeting of the hyperpigmented lesion, whereas the normal background "innocent" bystander skin is unharmed. Traditional "nonfractional" laser peels, on the other hand, target water and therefore heat a confluent "slab" of the uppermost skin. The depths of ablation of heating are determined by wavelength, power density, fluence, and pulsewidth.[1]

Blood vessels are heated by three broad categories of devices: (a) visible light technologies (520–600 nm); (b) near infra red (NIR I) technologies (755, 800 nm); and (c) NIR II (940, 980, 1064 nm). The former is associated with very strong HgB and melanin heating, the second by moderate HgB and melanin heating, and the third by moderate HgB heating but relatively weak melanin heating. Deep heating devices have included laser, halogen lamps, xenon flash lamps with long wavelength cut-off filters, RF, US, and combination technologies.[3]

The use of light as a medical treatment has grown considerably since the advent of the medical laser in the 1960s. The word laser is an acronym for the term: light amplification by stimulated emission of radiation. The device itself consists of an energy source, a laser medium and a resonating tube. The medium can be a gas, liquid, or solid, and this will often be used to name the type of laser. (Examples: ruby laser and CO_2 laser). The light emitted is composed of photons that travel in the same direction, making laser light highly directional. Laser light is monochromatic, which means that all photons have the same wavelength. By contrast, intense pulse light (IPL) consists of many different wavelengths. The specific wavelength of each laser will determine how the laser beam interacts with tissue. The light can be reflected by tissue, scattered by the tissue, or it can transmit through tissue. The intention is that the laser light be absorbed by a specific target tissue (the "chromophore"). The mechanism by which lasers are used to target specific tissue is called selective photothermolysis (photo = light, and thermolysis = decomposition by heat).[4]

Lasers can be broadly broken into two categories, ablative and nonablative. Until recently, ablative (means "to remove"), lasers have been the "gold standard" of care for wrinkle reduction. The carbon dioxide laser with a wavelength of 10 600 nm and the Er:YAG with a wavelength of 2940 nm are mainstays of ablative laser treatment. A relative newcomer is erbium YSGG at 2790 nm.[5] With each of these lasers, an intense burst of energy is delivered onto the skin. The energy heats water in the skin and causes both the water and tissues to vaporize. With each pass of the laser, a controlled depth of skin is vaporized and/or coagulated. In response to the injury and subsequent healing, new layers of collagen are produced. While ablative nonfractional lasers can be very effective and have a firm place in laser skin rejuvenation, each can be associated with risks of infection, scarring, hypopigmentation and unnatural alterations in the texture and sheen of the skin. Moreover, complex aftercare is required until the skin is fully healed. Resolution of erythema may take months. Outside of fractional approaches (vide infra), these lasers are also limited to the thicker skin of the face rather than the thinner skin of the neck and hands.[3]

Nonablative nonfractional treatments are safer than their ablative counterparts, but require epidermal cooling, which may reduce efficacy of the treatment. Generally, small therapeutic windows are associated with nonablative treatments and outside of dyschromia reduction with visible light approaches, only modest cosmetic enhancement is achieved. The Nd:YAG 1320 nm pulsed laser (e.g., Cooltouch) is an example of a nonablative laser in wide clinical use. IPL (intense pulsed light), monopolar radiofrequency skin tightening, LHE (light heat energy) and LED (light emitting diode) are all examples of nonablative treatments.[1–3]

Skin rejuvenation with fractional photothermolysis represents a newer class of therapy *(Fig. 5.1)*. Thousands of microscopic wounds surrounded by viable tissue permit rapid healing and are made with a variety of laser wavelengths and delivery systems. Immediate and delayed therapeutic results are seen through a combination of epidermal coagulation for surface enhancement and dermal heating for deeper remodeling. Unlike selective photothermolysis, in which targets are damaged based on color contrast, fractional photothermolysis only damages specific zones based on the pattern of the micro-beams, leaving other zones completely intact. Fractional laser techniques began with a 1550 nm wavelength. The concept of a fractional laser can be applied, however, to almost any wavelength of light and can be used with both ablative laser resurfacing and nonablative laser rejuvenation. With increasingly aggressive densities and depths of injury, the fractional approach may achieve comparable results to non fractional approaches, without the associated side-effects.[4]

Fractional photothermolysis was introduced in 2003 as the Fraxel™ SR by Reliant Technologies of Palo Alto, California, now Solta Medical, Hayward, California.[4,5] Their fractional laser was cleared by the FDA for periorbital wrinkles (2004), skin resurfacing (2005), melasma (2005), pigmented lesions,

Conventional Selective Photothermolysis (SP)

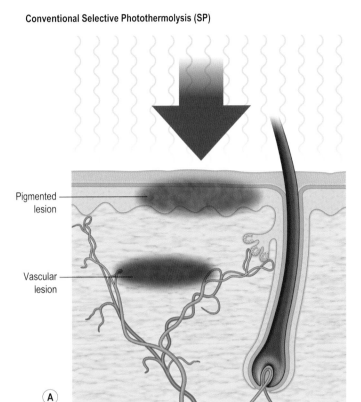

Pigmented lesion

Vascular lesion

(A)

Fractional Photothermolysis (SP)

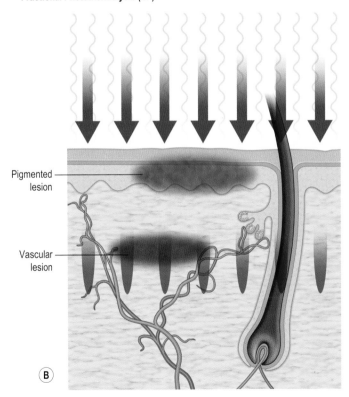

Pigmented lesion

Vascular lesion

(B)

Fig. 5.1 (A) Conventional selective versus **(B)** fractional photothermolysis.

freckles, age spots (2004), acne (2006). Since then, a number of other companies have introduced lasers capable of delivering fractionated light. Herein, we review the various laser devices available and discuss our clinical experience with fractional photothermolysis.[4,5]

Chemical peelings represent accelerated exfoliation or skin damage induced by caustic agents that cause controlled damage, followed by the release of cytokines and inflammatory mediators, resulting in thickening of the epidermis, deposition of collagen, reorganization of structural elements, and increases in dermal volume. This process decreases solar elastosis and replaces and reorients the new dermal connective tissue. The result is an improved clinical appearance of the skin, with fewer rhytides and decreased pigmentary dyschromia.[1,3]

Basic science of resurfacing procedures

Biology of wound healing following chemical peeling

The aim of most forms of chemical peeling is to provide a controlled injury to the target skin, such that healing potential is maximized while scarring is minimized.[18,19] The three main forms of wound healing include re-epithelialization, scar formation, and wound contraction.[20]

In superficial insults to the skin, the basal layer of epidermis is intact and is capable of proliferating and repopulating the epidermis. This form involves minimal involvement of the underlying dermis and thus no scar formation ensues. Following deeper injuries to skin, wound healing relies on keratinocytes from the wound edge and skin adnexa to migrate and proliferate. Collagen within the dermis is affected and undergoes some change. The migration of keratinocytes from the wound edge begins within hours of injury and involves four phases: (1) *Mobilization:* epithelial cells immediately adjacent to the wound enlarge, flatten, and detach from neighboring cells and the basement membrane; (2) *Migration:* as marginal cells migrate, the cells immediately behind them also tend to flatten, break connections, and drift along. Epithelial stream continues until advancing cells contact cells from other side, whereupon motion stops abruptly – a process called contact inhibition; (3) *Proliferation/mitosis:* fixed basal cells away from the wound edge begin mitosis to replace the migrating cells. The cells that have migrated in turn start to divide and multiply; (4) *Differentiation:* once the wound gap is bridged by advancing cells from the perimeter, normal differentiation of basal cells occurs. The stimuli for keratinocyte migration and proliferation include loss of cell-to-cell contact, growth factors (EGF, TGF-α, KGF, TGF-β), loss of contact with normal components of a basement membrane (type IV collagen and laminin), and contact with proteins of the provisional matrix (fibrin, fibronectin, type I collagen).[19,20]

The re-epithelialization is facilitated by a moist environment (the proper dressing), debridement of scabs (fibrin, dead neutrophils and other debris), growth factors, and high concentration of skin adnexa (the face and scalp).[19,20]

Once contact of keratinocytes occurs and contact inhibition is achieved hemidesmosomes re-form, cells become more basaloid, and cellular proliferation generates a multilaminated neo-epidermis that is slightly thinner.[19,20]

Wound healing that occurs following deeper insults to the skin (deeper chemical peels) result in the scar formation pathway of wound healing. The phases of this process include inflammation, proliferation, and remodeling and are described below.

Inflammation

Tissue injury leads to parenchymal cell damage and the extravasation of blood constituents. The blood clot that forms re-establishes hemostasis and provides a provisional matrix for cell migration. Vasoactive and inflammatory mediators are then generated by platelets (PDGF), the coagulation cascade, the activated complement pathway (C3a and C5a), and injured or activated parenchymal cells.[10] Vasoconstriction begins within seconds of the injury and lasts 10–15 min and occurs as a result of epinephrine being release in to peripheral circulation, stimulation of the sympathetic nervous system and release of norepinephrine. Vasodilatation and capillary leak are mediated by a variety of factors including leukotrienes, prostaglandins, kinins, histamine, and complement factors C3a and C5a. Leukocyte migration is stimulated by components of the extracellular matrix and several inflammatory mediators. Neutrophils cleanse the wound of foreign particles and bacteria and are then extruded with the eschar or phagocytosed by macrophages. In response to specific chemoattractants, monocytes infiltrate the wound and become activated macrophages that contribute to the coordination of wound healing. Specifically, angiogenesis, fibroblast migration and proliferation, collagen production, and wound contraction are all directed by macrophages.[19,20]

The wound healing process is regulated, in a large part, by the ordered production of cytokines that control gene activation responsible for cellular migration and proliferation and synthetic activities.[20]

Proliferation

This phase includes epithelialization, angiogenesis, granulation tissue formation, and collagen deposition. Epithelialization was discussed above, in the previous section. Angiogenesis, stimulated by TNF-α, is marked by endothelial cell migration and capillary formation. The migration of capillaries into the wound bed is critical for proper wound healing.[19,20] Much of the angiogenesis occurs during the early phase of wound healing and involves the sprouting of endothelial cells from post-capillary venules. The granulation phase and tissue deposition require nutrients supplied by the capillaries, and failure of this to occur results in a chronically unhealed wound. The final part of the proliferative phase is granulation tissue formation. Fibroblasts migrate into the wound site from the surrounding tissue, become activated, and begin synthesizing collagen and proliferate. Platelet-derived growth factor (PDGF) and EGF are the main signals to fibroblasts and are derived from platelets and macrophages. PDGF expression by fibroblasts is amplified by autocrine and paracrine signaling.[19,20] Fibroblasts already located in the wound site (termed "wound fibroblasts") will begin synthesizing collagen and transform into myofibroblasts for wound contraction (induced by macrophage-secreted TGF-β1); they have less proliferation compared with the fibroblasts coming in from the wound periphery. In response to PDGF, fibroblasts begin synthesizing a provisional matrix composed of collagen type III, glycosaminoglycans, and fibronectin.[20]

Remodeling

This phase is comprised of both wound contraction and collagen remodeling.

Wound contraction is the result of specialized fibroblasts that express α-actin (myofibroblasts) and their interaction with cytokines and the ECM. During the 2nd week of healing, fibroblasts assume a myofibroblast phenotype characterized by large bundles of actin-containing microfilaments along the cytoplasmic surface of the cell membrane. Fibroblasts maintain contact with collagen matrix by integrin receptors.[19,20] Contraction requires stimulation by TGF-β, PDGF and myofibroblast-ECM interaction via integrin receptors. As myofibroblasts contract they exert force on the ECM and subsequently the wound margin. Scar remodeling predominates after ~21 days. There is no net increase in collagen content despite an increase in tensile strength. Collagen production continues although at a slower rate, and there is an equal rate of collagen breakdown by collagenases. As the wound matures disorganized fine collagen fibres are replaced with thicker fibres arranged parallel to skin stresses. The percentage of type III collagen gradually decreases, as does the quantity of water and proteoglycans. The duration of the maturation process varies depending on how long the wound remains open.[19,20]

The edge of migrating epithelium marks transition between inflammation and fibroproliferation. In the center, where the wound is open, chronic bacterial invasion provides persistent stimulus for inflammation. This tissue contains inflammatory cells, a high concentration of immature vessels and the components of a provisional matrix (collagen type I, fibrin and fibronectin).[19,20] When the inflammatory response is prolonged, this tissue looks like 'granulation tissue'. Once epithelium covers the wound, the inflammatory stimulus is eliminated and fibroblasts predominate. Farther behind the migrating epithelium, there are fewer fibroblasts indicating a more mature wound. Epithelial cells appear to be the source of a stimulus for inflammatory cells to undergo apoptosis. However, if the inflammatory phase continues longer than 2–3 weeks, then this stimulus may be lost and hypertrophic scarring may result.

Deeper chemical peels will activate this inflammatory and proliferative reaction, with subsequent collagen remodeling. However, if the peel is performed in a controlled environment under optimal conditions, scarring tends to be minimized as the collagen is re-organized. This reorganization results in skin tightening and can help to diminish the presence of fine wrinkles.[17,18]

Laser tissue interactions and properties of lasers

An understanding of light-tissue and electrical-tissue interactions allows physicians to expand their laser repertoire and optimize outcomes. Lasers as light sources are useful because they allow for exquisite control of where and how much one heats.[21] However, tissue reactions are not intrinsically specific to the heating source. In principle, a large number of nonlaser devices (i.e., intense pulsed light) can be used for heating skin.[21] In many cases, laser is simply a way to convert lamplight to a more powerful monochromatic form. With respect to lasing media, there are diode lasers, solid-state lasers, and gas lasers.[1] An example of a solid-state laser is the erbium glass laser. These lasers have a solid rod that is pumped by a flash lamp. Miniaturized diode lasers have become popular. Some diode lasers are housed separately from the handpiece and delivered by fiberoptics. Others are configured with the laser diodes in the handpiece. Intense pulsed light devices are increasingly comparable to lasers that emit millisecond (ms) domain pulses. Absorption spectra of skin chromophores are broad, and therefore a broadband light source is a logical approach for certain cosmetic applications.[1]

Basic parameters for any procedure using light are power, time, and spot size for continuous wave lasers; and for pulsed lasers, the energy per pulse, pulse duration, spot size, fluence, and repetition rate.[22] All of these parameters should be considered in characterizing a laser procedure. Energy is measured in joules (J). The amount of energy delivered per unit area is the fluence, sometimes called the dose or radiant exposure, given usually in J/cm^2. The rate of energy delivery is called power, measured in watts (W). One watt is one joule per second ($W = J/s$). The power delivered per unit area is called the irradiance or power density, usually given in W/cm^2. Laser exposure duration (called pulse-width for pulsed lasers) is the time over which energy is delivered.[1]

Fluence is equal to the irradiance times the exposure duration.[23] Other important factors are the laser exposure spot size (which for wavelengths from 400 to 1200 nm greatly affects intensity inside the skin), whether the incident light is convergent, divergent, or diffuse, and the uniformity of irradiance over the exposure area (spatial beam profile). The pulse profile, that is, the character of the pulse shape in time (instantaneous power versus time), is another feature that can impact the tissue response.[22–24]

Molecular basis of light-tissue interaction (LTI)

In any light-tissue interaction, the thermal or photochemical effects depend on the local absorbed energy density at the target. Spatial localization of temperature elevation is possible when: (1) the absorption coefficient of the target exceeds that of surrounding tissue (selective photothermolysis); (2) when the "innocent bystander" tissues are cooled so that their peak temperatures do not exceed some damage threshold;[24] or (3) by applying very small (usually <500 μm in diameter) beamlets or microbeams (i.e., fractional methods – *vide supra*). Localized heating, for example, in telangiectases and lentigines, follows from the relative excess of HgB and melanin, respectively, in the lesions versus surrounding skin. In contrast, "nonfractional" mid-IR lasers spatially confine temperature elevation by using heating and cooling schemes that allow for selective dermal heating.[25]

Targeting discrete chromophores offers advantages over targeting tissue water, especially where the ratio of light absorption between the chromophore and surrounding tissue is large, (i.e., >10).[24–26] For example, at least in lighter-skinned patients, targeting dermal Hgb can be achieved with minimal surface cooling. Whereas cooling is desirable even in these cases, the primary indication is analgesia rather than epidermal protection. Also, the risk of a severe injury to the skin is lessened, as there is no bulk heating. Lastly, because temperature elevations are localized, there is often less pain than with devices targeting ubiquitous tissue water. Thermal injury is determined by time/temperature combinations. Protein denaturation is dependent linearly on exposure time and exponentially on temperature. That is, cell death is more sensitive to temperature than time.[24] Most devices for rejuvenation are based on photothermal or "electrothermal" mechanisms, that is, the conversion of light or electrical energy to heat. More recently, ultrasound devices have been applied to tighten the skin.[27] Two processes govern all interactions of light with matter: absorption and scattering. The absorption spectra of major skin chromophores dominate laser tissue interactions. If tissues were clear, then only absorption would be required to characterize light propagation in skin. However, the dermis is white because of light scatter (milk is a reasonable model for the dermis with regard to scattering). Scattering is responsible for much of the light's behavior in the skin (beam dispersion, spot size effects, etc.). The main scattering wavelengths are between 400 and 1200 nm (those where tissue water absorption is poor).[1]

There are three chromophores of interest in skin (water, blood, and melanin). Water makes up about 65% of the dermis and lower epidermis. There is some water absorption in the UV. Between 400 and 800 nm, water absorption is quite small (which is consistent with our real world experience that visible light propagates quite readily through a glass of water). Beyond 800 nm, there is a small peak at 980 nm, followed by larger peaks at 1480 and 10600 nm. The water maximum is 2940 nm (erbium YAG).[1]

Selective photothermolysis (SPT)

With the exception of cases where water is heated, rejuvenation of the skin is based on discrete heating by chromophores of relatively low concentration (i.e., melanin, hemoglobin). Anderson described the concept of selective photothermolysis more than 25 years ago.[4] He noted that extreme localized heating achieved with selective photothermolysis relies on: (a) a wavelength that reaches and is preferentially absorbed by the desired target structures; (b) an exposure duration less than or equal to the time necessary for cooling of the target structures; and (c) sufficient energy to damage the target.[4] The heterogeneity of the skin with respect to HgB and melanin allows for very selective injury in thousands of microscopic targets.

The *thermal relaxation time* is the time it takes for a target to cool to a certain percentage of its peak temperature (after laser exposure). Larger targets take longer to cool and therefore spatial selectivity is preserved with a wider range of pulse durations. Even so, as a general rule, assuming adequate fluences are applied, longer pulse durations will result in greater collateral damage. In laser scenarios, we assume instantaneous heating of the target, so that τ is usually thought of as the time for cooling *after* the pulse.[4]

Reaction types

Photothermal

Most laser applications rely on heating. Photothermal approaches depend on the type and degree of heating, from coagulation to vaporization. There is a range of effects on tissue based on temperature. Below 43°C, the skin remains unharmed, even for exposures as long as 20 min. Thus, one can exceed body temperature by about 5°C without a measurable change in the skin. The first change is a conformational change in the molecular structure. These typically occur at temperatures from 42–50°C. At higher temperatures, very short times (seconds or in extreme cases (>100°C) less than 1 ms) can induce cell death.[1,4]

Photochemical

Photochemical reactions are governed by specific reaction pathways, and the most common photosensitizer (PS) in skin is PpIX. This PS is formed by skin cells by the pro-drug, aminolevulinic acid (ALA).[1,4]

Biostimulation

Biostimulation (*aka* low level laser therapy) belongs to the group of photochemical interactions. Most biostimulation studies involve low-power lasers and this field continues to be a subject of controversy. Home use devices that use LEDs (light emitting diodes) are now available in a wide range of wavelength ranges. Typical fluences are in the range of 1–10 J/cm², and normally there is no acute temperature elevation, nor any clinical endpoint.[1,4]

Cooling

Before the addition of surface cooling, fluence thresholds for efficacy and epidermal damage were often close. Visible light technologies, (especially green–yellow light sources such as IPL, KTP laser, and PDL) are the wavelength ranges where epidermal damage is most likely. The epidermis is an innocent bystander in cutaneous laser applications where the intended targets, such as hair follicles or blood vessels, are located in the dermis.[1,4]

Beyond visible light (green, yellow, and red) sources, surface cooling also has been employed in NIR and MIR lasers. With NIR lasers, surface cooling is important, but not only because of dermal/epidermal-junction derived epidermal heating. In addition, deep beam penetration may cause catastrophic bulk heating. With MIR lasers (1.32, 1.45, and 1.54 μm), the chromophore is water. It follows that with even very low fluences, surface cooling is imperative. Without cooling or a fractional design, water's ubiquitous nature in the skin causes a laser-induced top to bottom injury. All techniques are susceptible to operator error and device failure. It follows that as physicians rely more heavily on cooling devices, any lack of their proper deployment unveils the dark side of cooling. Fractured sapphire windows, disabled cryogen spray apparatus, and crimped forced air chiller tubes have all contributed to unintended epidermal injury.[1,4]

Nonablative facial skin rejuvenation (NSR)

The original concept of NSR was wrinkle reduction by selective dermal heating.[28,29] Deeply penetrating mid-IR lasers coupled with surface cooling were designed to "bypass" the epidermis. A slab-like dermal injury was created. Unfortunately, "CO₂-like" results were never replicated because dermal heating was either too deep or too mild. Superficial severe dermal heating was almost always associated with epidermal damage. It followed that all of these devices "bypassed" the solar elastosis ultimately responsible for most static wrinkles of the face.[1,4]

The "nonablative" term has now evolved to include any electrical, light, or ultrasound based intervention with "relative" epidermal preservation.[30] In addition to wrinkle reduction, new outcome measures include acne scar improvement, telangiectasia resolution, homogenization of pigment, pore size reduction, skin tightening (jowls, neck, and some extrafacial sites) and "improved" skin tone.[28–30]

Sadick developed a classification scheme for NSR based on photodamage type. In his paper, type I photodamage consisted of surface irregularities, of which there were three subtypes. Type 1a included rosacea and telangiectases; 1(b) was comprised of pore size and skin roughness; and type 1c included pigmentation changes. Type II rejuvenation included deeper wrinkles and volume loss.[30]

Fractional resurfacing

Resurfacing with fractional photothermolysis represents a newer class of therapy *(Fig. 5.1)*. When wavelengths of around 1500 nm are used, the stratum corneum is left largely intact as thousands of microscopic wounds surrounded by viable tissue are made with a variety of laser wavelengths and delivery systems. Immediate and delayed results are seen through a combination of epidermal coagulation for resurfacing effect and dermal heating for deeper remodeling.

As mentioned above, fractional laser resurfacing first became commercially available in 2003.[31] The initial fractional laser uses an erbium-doped fiber to deliver 3000 infrared (1550 nm) laser pulses per second and targets water as a chromophore. The Fraxel™ SR (Solta Medical, Hayward, CA) creates an array of microscopic treatment zones (MTZs) measuring 50–150 μm in densities ranging from 400 to 6400 MTZ/cm².[31] Each MTZ forms a column of thermally denatured collagen from the epidermis to mid-dermis. In contrast to ablative lasers, fractional lasers coagulate only 20% of the treated skin, sparing islands of viable epidermis and untreated dermis that maintain the skin's barrier function while speeding re-epithelialization *(Fig. 5.2)*.[1,31]

Diagnosis and clinical evaluation

Adequate evaluation and photographic documentation of the patient prior to peeling or laser treatment is essential.[17,18,31] This assessment includes consideration of the severity of actinic damage, depth and number of rhytides, and need for any additional resurfacing procedures. The patient with deep rhytides and excessive facial skin laxity is likely a better candidate for traditional rhytidectomy. The patient with moderate photodamage and medium rhytides may be a more optimal candidate for one of the many types of resurfacing procedures. Some patients may benefit from both procedures because rhytidectomy typically addresses skin quantity and soft tissue malposition, whereas resurfacing addresses skin quality.[17,18] It should be noted, however, that great care should be undertaken when both rhytidectomy and resurfacing are performed concurrently. If rhytidectomy is performed, it is recommended to avoid any resurfacing of the undermined facial skin, as wound healing issues may ensue.[17,18]

An important tool of the evaluation of the patient for a resurfacing procedure is Fitzpatrick's scale of sun-reactive skin types. This scale describes patients' reactions to ultraviolet radiation and existing degree of pigmentation. Type I patients always burn and never tan. Type II patients tan only with difficulty and usually burn. Type III patients tan but sometimes burn. Type IV patients rarely burn and tan with ease. Type V patients tan very easily and very rarely burn. Type VI patients tan very easily and never burn.[32] Patients with lighter skin types can expect to undergo peeling or laser treatments with minimal concern for abnormal pigment changes, whereas individuals with darker skin are at higher risk for unwanted hyperpigmentation or hypopigmentation.[32] Another helpful classification system is the Glogau[33] photodamage scale. Type 1 patients have little wrinkling, no keratoses, no scarring, and require no make-up. Type 2 patients

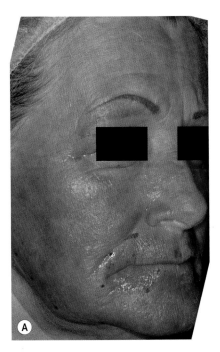
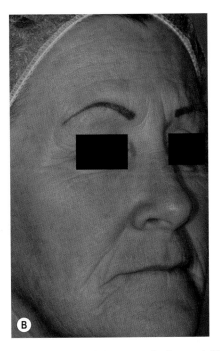
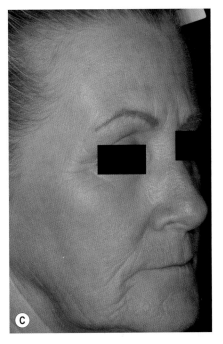

Fig. 5.2 Fractional resurfacing patient – set at 2940 nm: **(A)** immediately, **(B)** at 3 days after laser, and **(C)** 3 months after laser.

have early wrinkling, early actinic changes, minimal scarring, and require a small amount of make-up. Type 3 patients have wrinkles present at rest, moderate actinic keratoses, moderate scarring, and always require make-up. Type 4 patients have severe wrinkling, actinic keratoses, and scarring that even large amounts of make-up does not cover.

A thorough medical history and review of systems should be completed in concert with the physical examination, as part of a thorough patient work-up.[17,18] Pre-existing cardiac, hepatic, and renal disease may influence the treatment decision and choice of chemical peel or alternative resurfacing method. The use of exogenous estrogens, oral contraceptives, and other photosensitizing medications have been shown to predispose patients to unpredictable pigment changes.[17,18] Therefore, such agents should be avoided several weeks before and after treatment. For any procedure that includes epidermal compromise the physician should provide antiviral prophylaxis several days before and after the treatment for those patients with a history of herpes simplex infection. Prophylaxis will help minimize chances of unwanted viral reactivation as the re-epithelialization process occurs. It is also advisable to allow any existing viral-type lesion to heal completely before proceeding with a resurfacing procedure.[17,18]

Patient cooperation and compliance with the post-treatment regimen is required to ensure normal wound healing and to avoid complications.[17,18] It is ill advised to treat patients likely to be noncompliant or unable to avoid sun exposure because of occupation. Men are considered less optimal candidates because of thicker, oilier skin that risks uneven penetration of the peeling agent or laser. Men are also less likely to be willing to use camouflage make-up in the event of pigmentary disturbances. Patients with a decreased number of epithelial appendages from prior radiation treatment or current isotretinoin (Accutane) use are also poor candidates because healing will proceed more slowly and scarring is more likely. Consider recent use of Accutane an absolute contraindication to medium and deep peels, or certain types of laser resurfacing. One should wait at least 12 months after stopping Accutane to allow sufficient regeneration of epithelial appendages prior to treatment.[17,18] For nonablative treatments, the role of isotretinoin (Accutane) in wound healing is unclear. Most likely healing will proceed unimpeded and no special precautions are necessary. Still treatments during an actual course of Accutane should only be undertaken if the benefits outweigh the potential risks.

Patient selection and treatment

For chemical peels

Video 1

There are many indications for performing a chemical peel on a patient. These include: pigmentary disorders (melasma, post-inflammatory hyperpigmentation, freckles, lentigines); acne (superficial acne scars, post-acne dyspigmentation, comedonal acne); aesthetics (photoaging, fine superficial wrinkling, dilated pores, superficial scars); and epidermal growths (seborrheic keratoses, actinic keratoses, warts, milia, sebaceous hyperplasia). Typically, the more superficial the pathology or target issue, the more superficial the peel that is required.[17,18]

The real challenge of chemical peeling technique and application lies in proper patient and peeling agent selection.[1,17,18] In general, the more severe the actinic damage or advanced the aging changes, the more aggressive the treatment that is required to produce the desired result. Once the patient is appropriately selected to undergo a chemical peel, informed consent, including a thorough discussion of possible complications, should be obtained.[1,17,18] Preconditioning the skin can be a useful adjunct to improving overall results. The most common agent used for preconditioning is trans-retinoic acid (Retin-A, Renova), an exfoliative agent, which is believed to facilitate uniform penetration of the peeling agent and promote more rapid re-epithelialization. This may be applied nightly or every other night for several weeks prior to peeling, depending on the degree of skin irritation caused and patient tolerance. Preconditioning promotes a thinning of the stratum corneum with shedding of keratinocytes while fibroblasts are stimulated.[1,17,18] Prior to application of the peel, the patient should thoroughly cleanse the face with soap on the evening before, as well as the morning of the procedure. The skin should be cleansed immediately prior to the procedure with acetone or isopropyl alcohol to remove any remaining traces of makeup or oils. This step is absolutely essential to perform even penetration of the peeling agent.[17,18]

Superficial chemical peels are typically accomplished with use of alpha hydroxy acids (AHA). This group of chemicals is largely comprised of naturally occurring fruit acids, including glycolic, lactic, citric, tartaric, and malic acid.[1,17,18] One of the most popular physician grade AHA used is glycolic acid, which is derived from sugar cane. Most formulations include concentrations of 50% glycolic acid or higher.[34] After application subsequent exfoliation occurs over the next several days. Over-the-counter AHA products usually contain 3–10% glycolic acid, but they can also contain one of the many other milder fruit acids.[1,17,18] These formulations cause slow exfoliation over several weeks, but can also be used as a pre-peel primer to potentiate the effects of a higher concentration peel. Unlike other peeling agents, penetration of glycolic acid is time dependent. The agent is therefore applied for a specific amount of time and then neutralized. The systematic application of glycolic acid with a sponge is typically performed from one facial region to another, dividing the face into 6–8 regions and treating each in succession. The length of time that glycolic acid is left on the skin relates to its concentration, with increasing concentrations creating the desired effect in less time.[1,17,18] The agent is removed by washing the face with water or neutralizing it with an alkaline solution such as sodium bicarbonate. Erythema is present following application, which is often accompanied by edema. White patches slowly begin to develop, indicating epidermolysis of the epidermis from the underlying dermis. Development of a frost indicates deeper depth of destruction into the dermis and is not desirable during procedures which are meant to be superficial treatments. Exfoliation will occur over the next several days, and re-epithelialization is complete within 7–10 days.[1,17,18] Multiple treatments may be required to achieve the desired results. These repeat treatments should be spaced several weeks apart. Glycolic acid peels are meant to be superficial in nature and therefore will produce the least profound results. The trade-off, however, is that these peels are also associated with the lowest frequency of complications. Another agent used for superficial peeling is Jessner's solution. This solution is comprised of 14 g of resorcinol, 14 g of salicylic acid, and 14 mL of 85% lactic acid mixed in enough 95% ethanol to bring the quantity to 100 mL. The Jessner's solution is usually applied evenly with one or more coats to achieve a light but uniform frost.[1,17,18] It is likely that 2–4 coats may be necessary in some cases to achieve the desired level of resurfacing. The frosting achieved with Jessner's solution typically results in the subjective feeling of heat with a mild discomfort that is easily controlled with a fan. A mild erythema appears after several minutes, with only faint evidence of scattered frosting over the skin surface.[1,17,18]

Medium depth peels are usually performed with trichloroacetic acid (TCA) in concentrations ranging from 20% to 35%.[17,34] Depth of penetration is directly proportional to concentration, with formulations of 50% having a well-documented ability to penetrate into the reticular dermis. Concentrations approaching 50% are not recommended because of the extremely high risk of scarring associated with this depth of penetration. For this reason, 35% TCA is considered the high end of a medium-depth peel formulation. Trichloroacetic acid works as a keratocoagulant that produces a frost or whitening of the skin, which is dependent on the concentration used.[17,18,34,35] Vigorous rubbing of the agent yields a deeper penetration, and must be performed cautiously. This technique is not time-dependent, and the agent does not require neutralization. Combination use of TCA along with other peeling agents has been demonstrated to provide more effective skin resurfacing in some cases. Coleman has reported improved results with application of 70% glycolic acid prior to a 35% TCA peel. The systematic application of TCA with a sponge also involves treating the face in a succession of 6–8 regions. TCA application is associated with an intense burning that usually resolves within 30 min.[17,18,34] Nerve blocks with lidocaine can often help the patient better tolerate the procedure. Patient comfort may also be improved by having a fan to cool the face and by applying sponges soaked in iced saline prior to moving from one facial region to another. If the frosting is not uniform or complete during the procedure, reapplication may be performed until frosting of a desired level is reached. Once completed, exfoliation proceeds for several days, and re-epithelialization is complete within 10–14 days.[17,18,34]

Deeper chemical resurfacing procedures are typically performed using phenol. Phenol peels may be performed with various formulations, such as pure phenol (which is really 88%) or phenol mixed with soap, water, croton oil, and sometimes olive oil.[36] These formulas have such names as Baker-Gordon, Venner-Kellson, Maschek-Truppman, and Grade. The classic Baker-Gordon formula is composed of 3 mL of United States Pharmacopeia (USP) phenol, 2 mL of tap water, 8 gtt of liquid soap, and 3 gtt of croton oil. Phenol causes keratolysis and keratocoagulation.[17,18,36] In contrast to other agents, increasing the concentration of phenol actually decreases the penetration up to a point, because the ensuing destruction forms a barrier to further penetration of the chemical. Pure phenol does not penetrate as deeply as the various formulations. Occlusion with a waterproof mask is reported to deepen the level of the peel, which increases the time required to fully re-epithelialize and increases post-treatment erythema. Following the peel, application of a thick layer of petroleum jelly or other equivalent agent is used to increase predictability and decrease penetration. Similar to

trichloroacetic acid (TCA), the time spent applying the agent and the amount of sponge strokes used will be proportional to the depth of penetration. The addition of croton oil to the various formulations as a skin irritant also allows deeper penetration. Although phenol produces the most remarkable resolution of actinic damage and wrinkling among the various chemotherapeutic agents, it also possesses some of the more significant morbidities. Many have abandoned phenol in favor of other agents or laser resurfacing.[17,18,36] Marked hypopigmentation may result following the use of phenol and is correlated with the depth of penetration, use of the Baker-Gordon formula, and addition of croton oil. Hypopigmentation may occur in all skin types, noticeably lightening the skin of patients with darker skin and making lighter-skinned patients appear waxy or pale. A clear line of demarcation may be present between treated and untreated skin. Phenol causes an intense burning upon application that may last 4–6 h, which is much longer than other agents. Patients should be provided with sufficient oral analgesics and anxiolytics for use at home following the peel. Phenol is absorbed through the skin, metabolized by the liver, and subsequently excreted by the kidneys. Some practitioners preload the patient with fluids to facilitate renal clearance. Due to the toxicity of phenol, overdoses may injure the liver and kidney and may lead to myocardial irritability, including arrhythmias. For this reason, patients should be monitored with telemetry during the procedure and in the immediate recovery period. The face is again divided into 6–8 regions, but 20 min must be allowed to elapse between treating subsequent regions. This allows for some degree of ongoing metabolism and helps avoid a toxic systemic dose.[17,18,36]

For laser treatments

Video 2

For wavelengths from 520 to 800 nm, the primary absorbers are hemoglobin and melanin, so that improvement of pigmentation and vascularity is achieved by direct heating of melanosomes and HgB (either by a single wavelength or flash lamp).[37] While devices targeting HgB/vessels are confined to pulse-widths (pw) ranging from 0.45 to 100 ms, melanosome heating is achieved by either Q-switched ns pulses, or gentler heating with ms domain pulses. For discrete smaller (0.1–0.6 mm) telangiectases, pulsed dye laser (PDL), potassium titanium oxide phosphate (KTP) laser, or intense pulsed light (IPL) can be applied (Fig. 5.3).[37] For larger vessels (>1 mm) and/or darker skin, the Nd:YAG laser is preferred, but care must be taken to apply the smallest fluence and smallest spot sufficient for closure. An alternative is the Cynegry™ laser (Cynosure, Chelmsford, MA), which combines 595 nm and 1064 nm sequential pulses that can simultaneously address both smaller and larger telangiectases.[38]

If a patient presents with telangiectases confined to very small areas, we typically use a small spot size (1–4 mm) and the long pulsed KTP laser or PDL.[1,37] Alternately, we use non-purpuric settings with an IPL. The specific type of PDL determines the spot size, fluence range, and cooling type, and pulse-width. Modern PDLs can generate effective fluences with 10–12 mm spots; moreover, the macropulses (pulse envelopes) are comprised of 6–8 micropulses, allowing for greater efficacy without a high risk of purpura. However, the most popular modern pulsed dye laser requires two passes for complete rejuvenation, one for treatment of pigmented

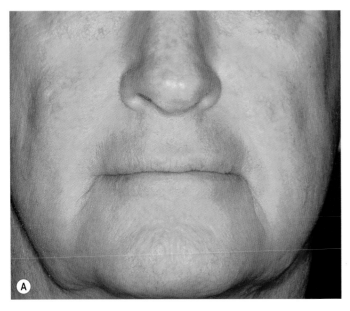

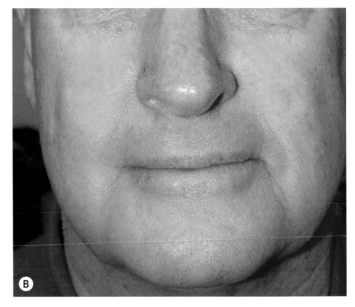

Fig. 5.3 **(A)** Pre- and **(B)** post-KTP laser treatment (8 J/cm²–20 ms).

lesions (with a dedicated pigmented lesion "compression" handpiece) or the cooling device disabled, and another for treatment of vascular lesions.[1,37] More recently, the alexandrite laser has been used for medium diameter blood vessels. The depth of penetration permits coagulation of vessels as large as 1–2 mm, but the high melanin absorption limits its usefulness to lighter patients unless very aggressive cooling is applied.[39]

If a lighter patient presents with a few discrete lentigines, we use the Q-switched alexandrite laser. The endpoint is frosty whitening. The only exception to our Q-switched approach for isolated dyschromias is when a patient has a pressing engagement where "robust" crusting is intolerable. In these cases, despite the better one-time treatment clearance with ns pulses, we apply ms devices as the delayed "coffee-ground" crusts tend to be less obvious.[1,37,38]

On the other hand, in darker skinned groups, we usually observe some persistence of pigment after Q-switched 532, 755, and 694 nm applications. In this scenario, it is sometimes difficult to determine after a short interval, whether the pigment represents residual melanin in the treated lesion or PIH. As patients usually report almost complete clearance of the lesions after 3–7 days, we suggest, at least for thinner lentigines, that most persistent pigmentation is post-inflammatory. We therefore delay repeat treatments for 8–12 weeks, allowing for at last partial resolution of any PIH. Unfortunately, this period is poorly accepted by patients, who, with the exception of exophytic seborrheic keratoses, are disappointed or angry that the lesions are darker than on initial presentation. Clearing of PIH can be accelerated by use of creams containing hydroquinone, tretinoin, and/or topical steroids of various strengths and combinations. Pre-treatment with these agents might decrease the risk of PIH. Sun protection is essential. For lighter, thinner seborrheic keratoses, one can apply multiple 532 nm ns pulses. For some thicker darker seborrheic keratoses, the long pulsed diode laser or long pulsed alexandrite can be used to clinical endpoint of graying. Care must be taken to mask any darker perilesional background skin.[1,40] A recent article suggests that longer pulse visible light technologies

are less likely to cause PIH in darker patients.[41] However, for lighter lentigines or somewhat tanned skin, whether one applies PDL with compression, IPL, or KTP laser, selective lesional heating is compromised because there is often insufficient color contrast. For these so-called "low contrast" lesions, the "therapeutic index" is dangerously small.

For diffuse hyperpigmentation (*aka* actinic bronzing), we apply the long pulsed variable spot KTP laser (Gemini, Iridex, Mountain View, CA) with contact cooling as a first choice. This laser enjoys a low rate of side-effects, will not damage the hair bulb (important for male patients), and the handpiece is light and manoeuvrable. When confronted with a combination of darker and lighter lentigines in Caucasian patients, we use the Q-switched alexandrite laser for the lighter lentigines first, followed by pan-facial treatment with IPL or KTP laser in the same session. We use the pulsed CO_2 laser or erbium YAG laser for some lighter lentigines, particularly if they are evolving into a seborrheic keratosis (SK).[1,37–40] More exophytic, lighter seborrheic keratoses must be treated with ablative lasers, or as an alternative, so long as there is at least minimal color contrast. We focus the Q-switched alexandrite beam to a very small spot (1–2 mm) and vaporize smaller flatter SKs by repeated pulses (the Q 532 nm laser can be used as well). Sometimes slight bleeding is observed, but this technique is associated with rapid healing. Alternatively, the long pulsed diode laser (810 nm) or long pulsed alexandrite laser can used for some pigmented seborrheic keratoses.[1,20] High fluences must be applied, and in darker patients, one should mask the normal surrounding skin with a plastic "guard".[40]

We have recently applied the long pulse alexandrite laser for pan facial rejuvenation (see *Fig. 5.6*), both with and without cooling. With cooling, both vessels and pigment can be treated, however, only light skinned patients are appropriate candidates, as the ratio for melanin to Hgb heating is high for 755 nm. For treatment of exclusively pigmented lesions, no cooling is necessary. Like the IPL, one must be careful to avoid darker beard areas to decrease the risk of alopecia.[1,37–40]

For flashlamp systems, filters placed between the lamp and skin are configured to optimize heating of specific targets. In choosing a laser or IPL for pan facial rejuvenation of the face or neck, the pulse configuration should achieve maximal differential heating between the epidermis and the dermal vessels. Models show that longer pulses (or pulse trains) favor vessel heating over epidermal heating.[1,40]

Melasma is a challenging condition to treat via lasers, most likely due to its dynamic and inflammatory nature (compared with the static nature of lentigines).[42] Ablative lasers sometimes improve the condition, however the ablation normally has to be carried out deeply (or *very* superficially – just involving the upper epidermidis), or post-inflammatory hyperpigmentation may outweigh any achievement gains. On the other hand, longer pulsed visible light laser technologies, Q-switched Nd:YAG lasers, and fractional approaches can sometimes achieve gradual improvement in melasma so long as the settings are not too high.[43,44] If the patient presents exclusively with melasma and no discrete "static" pigmented lesions (i.e., lentigines), we start with topical hydroquinone and retinoids before considering interventional therapy. Use of the Q-switched Nd:YAG laser, treating every 1–2 weeks for approximately eight sessions, oftentimes clears some of the pigment; however, there is a high relapse rate. Also, recently guttate hypomelanosis has been reported after multiple treatments with Q-switch Nd:YAG laser.[45,46] We have not found Q-switched alexandrite, Q-switched ruby or Q-switched 532 nm lasers helpful in melasma.[1,40] In all cases, although there is nice resolution within 1 week, worsening of the melasma follows (see *Fig. 5.7*).

Small nevi can be lightened by repeated Q-switched Nd:YAG and Q-switched alexandrite laser sessions; we reserve these treatments for Asian patients with small discrete uniformly colored lesions on the face. Long pulsed alexandrite lasers can be used. Red scars and traumatic tattoos can be treated by a combination of PDL and Q-switched YAG laser.[1,37–44] Banal appearing flesh colored nevi in Caucasians can be treated by ablative CO_2 or erbium YAG lasers. Optimally, a shave of the lesions is performed to debulk the lesions (at last one of which should be submitted for pathologic interpretation as a representative sample if all of the lesions are clinically similar), after which the laser can be used with a small spot (1–2 mm) to vaporize the lesions "flush" with the surrounding skin. Recurrence is not uncommon; also even in cases where flattening has been achieved, surface darkening can occur. Q-switched alexandrite or ruby laser treatments are then applied until the pigment remains clear.

Improvement in wrinkles can be performed by primary heating of vasculature (low fluence PDL, low fluence KTP, or low fluence 1064 nm). These technologies depend solely on a cascade effect, i.e., release of inflammatory mediators after capillary heating for wrinkle reduction. Short pulsed (0.3–50 ms) low fluence Nd:YAG lasers have been used for rejuvenation. The principle is that gentle sequential heating over a large volume (or either possibly through focal heating of microvessels) might stimulate new collagen deposition, tighten skin, reduce inflammation, and even reduce pore size.[47–49] One example is the "Genesis" procedure (Cutera, Brisbane, CA) where 5000–12 000 pulses are painted over the face at 5–7 Hz with a 5 mm spot at 12–15 J/cm². The endpoint is localized transient skin warming just below the pain threshold. No anesthetic is applied, thus ensuring that the patient will provide feedback regarding excessive temperatures. A newer version of this laser includes a real-time temperature feedback option.[50]

Improvement in skin can be performed by heating of dermal tissue water (1.32, 1.54, and 1.45 μm devices). These lasers heat tissue water. It follows that, without surface cooling, unless very small fluences or microbeams (<0.4 mm) are applied, a top to bottom broad thermal injury is observed. All of these wavelengths can be made to heat the reticular dermis with the proper mixture of fluences, repetition rates, epidermal cooling, and pulse duration.[51–54]

Acne scars are common and can be improved via nonablative techniques. Jacob *et al.*[55] proposed a three-type scar system: ice pick, rolling, and boxcar. Ice-pick scars are narrow, deep, sharply demarcated "holes" that extend into the deep dermis or subcutaneous layer. Rolling scars are usually wider than 4–5 mm and stem from the tethering of otherwise normal looking skin. Boxcar scars are depressions with sharply demarcated vertical edges. Another classification scheme includes other scar designations, including macular scars (erythematous, white, or brown), elastolytic scars (like ministriae), papular scars, and hypertrophic scars.[56]

A rational approach considers the microscopic anatomy of the scar. Rolling scars occur deep in the follicle and are the end-product of inflammation that causes destruction of the subcuticular fat. A number of "dedicated" skin tightening procedures can be applied (i.e., Thermage, Hayward CA, or Titan, Cutera, or Fractional IR, Palomar). Although sometimes helpful, predictable improvement is lacking, and the intervention should only be reserved for rolling scars or others with volume loss (atrophy). For boxcar scars, fractional technologies should be considered first (nonablative or ablative), depending on the patient's expectations and tolerance for downtime. The best results are achieved with high densities (20–30% surface area per treatment) and "deeper" holes.[1,30,31]

Long pulse and ms domain Nd:YAG devices have been applied to acne scars.[57] The Q-switched Nd:YAG laser beam is typically delivered at 2–4 J/cm² with a 4–6 mm spot and three passes per region. The endpoint is erythema and occasionally petechiae. The treatments are only mildly uncomfortable with the exception of male patients, where pulses over hair-bearing areas can be more painful. In applying the longer pulse systems, multiple passes (usually three) are delivered at 10–50 J/cm². Endpoints are mild erythema and edema.[57] Care should be taken to avoid black-haired areas in male patients to avoid potential hair reduction. Fillers can complement the aforementioned procedures, particularly when there is marked volume loss associated with rolling type scars.

First proposed as a means for treating individual AKs, photodynamic therapy (PDT) is now being used with blue and red light for "photo" peels. In one configuration, 20% liquid aminolevulinic acid (ALA) solution (Levulan, DUSA, Tarrytown, NJ) is spread lightly over the skin for 0.5–2 h, after which the entire cosmetic unit is irradiated with a wide array of light sources (*Fig. 5.4*). ALA has been shown to enhance the pulsed light responses for dyschromias and vascular lesions.[58] We use ALA in the following manner: if a patient presents with AKs, telangiectases, and dyschromias, we combine ALA with a pulsed visible light source followed by 5–10 min of a CW red light source (Omni-LUX, Carlsbad, CA). In this scenario, immediately after an acetone scrub, the solution is applied, and 30 min later, a 5% lidocaine cream is applied. After an additional 30 min the pulsed light source is used,

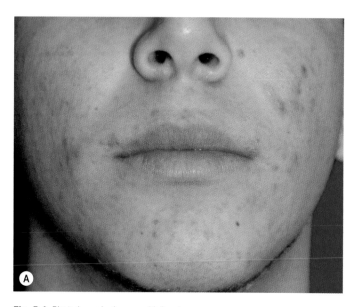
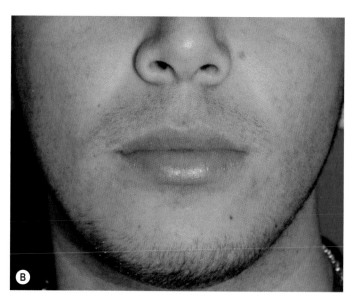

Fig. 5.4 Photodynamic therapy with levulan.

immediately followed by the CW light source. Refrigerated air is applied for anesthesia. We shorten the ALA application period with numbing cream, as we have found it accelerates the ALA absorption and enhances the PDT effect. If the patient presents solely with AKs and few dyschromias and telangiectases (and if the patient desires insurance coverage for the entire procedure), we apply ALA (without anesthesia) for 1–2 h, followed by application of red CW light. Although ALA-PDT has been recommended for sebaceous hyperplasia,[59] we have only found it helpful with longer incubation times and CW red light.

Deeper heating long pulse skin tightening procedures

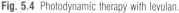

There are a number of deep heating handpieces for skin tightening. The six main approaches are: (1) monopolar RF; (2) deep heating halogen lamps; (3) bipolar RF combined with light; (4) xenon flashlamp with rapid repetition rates and filtering that features 800–1200 nm portion of the output spectrum; (5) fractionated ultrasound; and (6) fractionated RF. Most deep heating strategies are based on time-temperature dependent heating of collagen, which can produce focal "fractional" fibril damage.

Monopolar radiofrequency uses a controlled radiofrequency pulse to selectively heat zones of the lower dermis and sub-dermis, while avoiding injury to the superficial dermis through use of a cryogen spray.[13] One of the most popular monopolar radiofrequency devices is the ThermaCool Radiofrequency device (Thermage, Inc.). It was approved by the FDA in 2005, for full-body skin tightening treatments. Some studies have revealed high patient satisfaction with the device when proper technique and patient selection are employed.[13] Treatment typically involves 1–3 applications of the radiofrequency to the affected areas, depending on the severity of the deformity. Pain and downtime are minimal. Most patients are able to resume all normal activities immediately after treatment. Appropriate patients include those with mild to moderate rhytids who understand the limitations of the device *(Fig. 5.5).*[13]

Deeper penetration halogen lamps heat the upper 1–2 mm of the dermis. Pulses typically last 2–6 s and are accompanied by surface cooling. Xenon flash lamp devices have been electronically modulated to deliver rapid pulse trains with surface cooling. Like their halogen counterparts, the goal is sustained elevation of the dermal temperature. Low cost IR (temperature) meters are used during treatment to maintain surface temperatures of 38–41°C. A newly introduced ultrasound system (Ulthera) coagulates small dermal zones about 3–5 mm deep in the dermis. The depth is dependent on the transducer configuration. The goal is brow, cheek, and neck elevation/tightening. Also, an RF device (e-prime, Syneron) achieves skin tightening by coagulating deeper dermal zones (2–3 mm deep). This device deploys five pairs of needle electrodes into the skin for each "pulse". Temperatures of about 70°C are sustained for about 4 s, 1–3 mm beneath the skin surface in the most common application.

Fractional photothermolysis

A broad array of fractional lasers have appeared on the market since the introduction of the Fraxel™ SR *(Table 5.1).*

Here, we will attempt to present each of the above listed lasers and their relative benefits, as well as any scientific information available. There will likely be some lasers not covered (i.e., the Fraxel™ Fine Lines, etc.) Also, the reader will note there is a dearth of comparative data, but we will attempt to summarize comparative scientific data if available. Lastly, the authors' primary experience has been with the Fraxel™ devices by Solta. That is not to say the other devices are not comparable, or perhaps in some cases better. Wherever possible, we have tried to highlight the relative advantages and disadvantages of each laser. In general, the critical determinant for long-term skin resurfacing results is not the degree of immediate skin tightening, but the production of new collagen – a biological process that is highly dependent upon the depth of damage.[1,60,61]

The Fraxel™ SR laser (Solta Medical Inc., Palo Alto, CA) penetrates deeply into the skin dermis with thousands of tiny microthermal treatment zones, employing a technique called fractional photothermolysis.[31,60,61]

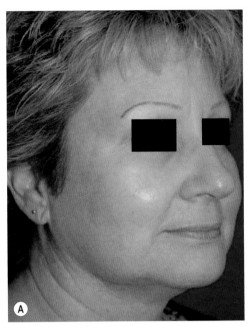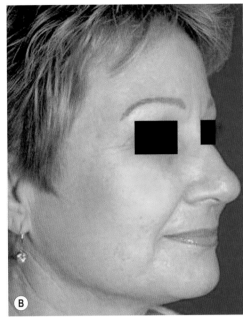

Fig. 5.5 (A) Pre- and **(B)** 6 months post-treatment with Thermage.

Table 5.1 **Fractional laser devices**

Laser	Manufacturer
Fraxel (Re:store, Re:pair)	Reliant Technologies Inc. (Mountain View, CA) now Solta Medical (Hayward, CA)
Affirm	Cynosure Inc. (Westford, MA)
Harmony^{XL}; Pixel CO$_2$ Omnifit	Alma Lasers Inc. (Buffalo Grove, IL)
PROFractional	Sciton Inc. (Palo Alto, CA)
ActiveFX; DeepFX	Lumenis Inc. (Santa Clara, CA)
Lux 1540 Fractional nonablative laser; Lux 2940 Fractional ablative laser	Palomar Medical Technologies Inc. (Burlington, MA)
Juvia CO$_2$ Fractional	Ellipse Inc. (Horsholm, Denmark)
Mosaic	Lutronic U.S.A. (Princeton Junction, NJ)

Solta Medical's approach is based upon the evolving science of fractional photothermolysis. This has been developed in part by Drs Rox Anderson and Dieter Manstein of Harvard's Wellman Laboratories, in collaboration with Dr Scott Herron and Len DeBenedictis, of Reliant Technologies (now Solta).[31,60,61]

Treating the skin fractionally with patterns of microscopic laser spots, each of which is 70–100 μm in diameter, results in a unique wound healing process. This is aided by the fact that each laser spot (known as a MicroThermal Zone, or MTZ) is surrounded by healthy tissue. Many of the stem cells and melanocytes in the papillary dermis are spared. Fractional wound healing results in both rapid re-epithelialization of the epidermis as well as collagen remodeling to depths of 400–700 μm.[31,60,61]

Clinical studies[4,5,9] suggest that 4–6 treatments spaced about 1 week apart produce a gradual remodeling of dermal matrix components, firming collagen and elastin. A topical anesthetic and a blue dye were used prior to treatment, which takes about 60 min. Laser treatment itself takes another 45 min. With the newer Fraxel™ 1500 (Re:store) laser (see below) the blue dye is no longer needed.

Side-effects are generally minimal. A mild sunburn sensation occurs for approximately 1 hour after the treatment. The skin has a pinkish tone for 1–3 days *(Fig. 5.4)*. This is a normal sign of healing. Swelling is minimal. Within 24 h, new epidermal skin begins to emerge. This process of skin repair involves flaking and bronzing. The use of sunscreen throughout the process is absolutely necessary. Optimal improvement may take 3–6 months.[4,5,9]

Fractional laser treatment appears to be effective in reduction of fine wrinkles; rejuvenation of sun damaged skin on the face, neck, shoulders, hands and arms; reduction of age spots, blotches and dyschromia; acne scars; hyperpigmentation and in some patients, coarse and deeper wrinkles, may demonstrate considerable improvement.[31,60,61]

Recently, our group published the results of the Fraxel™ SR laser (Reliant Technologies Inc., Palo Alto, CA) in 59 patients undergoing 202 treatments for a variety of skin conditions.[31] Some 75% of patients were very satisfied (4 or 5 rating) with the experience. Significantly more treatments were administered to those with higher satisfaction scores. The average number of treatments per patient was 3.4. Those with satisfaction scores of 4 or 5 had an average of 3.6 treatments; while those with satisfaction scores of ≤3, had an average of 2.8 treatments ($p = 0.029$).

Of the 44 patients with a concern of dyschromia, 33 (75%) had a satisfaction score of 4 or 5. All 14 patients (100%) with a scarring concern had a satisfaction score of 4 or 5 with the Fraxel laser. And, 74% of patients (42/57) with a texture concern had a satisfaction score of 4 or 5.

Logistic regression found that the number of treatments was an important factor in the patient's concern. The odds of giving a satisfaction score of 4 or 5 increased approximately two-fold for each additional treatment a patient received.

The Fraxel™ 1500 Re:store (Solta Medical, Inc., Palo Alto, CA) laser replaced the earlier SR version and combines proprietary advancements in optical technology with medical software offering physicians a treatment option that penetrates up to 30% deeper than the Fraxel™ SR laser, delivering consistent dosage control and optimizing lesion depths. This leap in technology provides patients a safe and effective, noninvasive treatment option for skin conditions ranging from mild sun damage to severe acne scarring.[31,60,61]

With the newly designed optical zoom hand control system, physicians can penetrate up to 1.0 mm below the skin surface with precise dosage control. Deeper penetration provides a greater catalyst for natural generation of new collagen to promote self healing and remodeling.[31,60,61]

In designing the Fraxel™ 1500 Re:store laser, Solta attempted to accomplish two goals, First, they wanted to achieve maximum efficiency in dosage control. Second, they wanted to optimize the lesion characteristics delivered. These changes enabled physicians to deliver both consistent dosage control and optimal lesion depth resulting in a predictable treatment for every patient every time.[31,60,61]

After 2–3 years of study, Solta Medical, Inc. released a Fractional CO_2 in December of 2007. *The Fraxel™ Re:pair* is a fractionally ablative microscopic CO_2 laser with a 10 600 nm wavelength. The Re:pair approaches the efficacy of fully ablative lasers, but with markedly less downtime, less risk of adverse events and no reports of delayed hypopigmentation. A single treatment is carried out for most patients, although the treatment may be repeated 3–6 months later. There are 2–3 days of real downtime with severe erythema and oozing followed by marked redness fading to a lighter shade by day 6 or 7. Over the next month, the redness gradually fades. The primary clinical targets are wrinkle removal; skin tightening, severe photodamage, acne and surgical scars. Whereas the Re:store Fraxel™ 1500 coagulates the epithelial and dermal tissue in the microthermal zone of injury, the Re:pair vaporizes the tissue centrally, leaving a rim of coagulation necrosis on the periphery of the injury and produces immediate skin tightening and wrinkle reduction. As pulse energy is increased penetration depth also increases. As density is increased, more surface area is treated. With experience and carefully chosen parameters, varying both energy and density, one can safely treat virtually all skin types. The Re:pair delivers the deepest injury of any of the nonablative and ablative fractional lasers. Although the injury is pronounced, reepithelialization occurs within 48 h.[31,60,61]

In terms of the laser itself, the laser interface is similar to that of the Fraxel™ 1500 Re:store. The cart is integrated with a smoke evacuator, which is a unique feature that is space saving and efficient. There are two tips: a 7 mm and 15 mm, the smaller being useful for the periorbita, the nose and upper lip and the larger for the cheeks, neck, forehead, chest and larger surface areas. The cartridge captures debris. Both the tips and cartridges require replacement, which adds some cost. Energy varies from 5 to 70 mJ and density from 5% to 70%. Both can be dialed in to customize treatment to the skin type and skin condition. The delivery system is thought to be faster then any other device on the market and has the deepest penetration, up to 1.6 mm. In addition, it provides a very versatile range of fractionally ablative treatments. The handpiece is a continuous motion scanning handpiece like the Fraxel™ 1500 Re:store laser and provides optimal, uniform delivery of energy for greater safety, speed and efficacy.[31,60,61]

The Affirm™ (Cynosure, Westford, MA) is a 1440 nm Erbium:glass laser, which is nonablative. It has some unique features that, in essence, delivers fractionated treatments to the skin surface. The unique aspect of this laser is the combined apex pulse (CAP) technology, which employs diffractive elements to bend the wavelength to treat larger surface areas. The laser also delivers both high and low energy light to the selected treatment areas, which "fractionates" the treatment. The CAP array in the 1440-nm Nd:YAG Affirm laser system was developed to combine both mechanisms in a single treatment, using high fluence regions surrounded by low level heating. This micro-thermal rejuvenation approach creates apices of high-fluence regions for collagen remodeling surrounded by a collagen-stimulating, low-fluence treatment zone. The CAP array is a special lens construction that consists of approximately 1000 diffractive elements affecting more surface area per single pulse. The high-fluence "apices" create a pattern of coagulated columns, while the background fluence gently heats the intervening uncoagulated tissue. Histologically, the high-fluence CAP columns are limited to approximately 300 μm in depth, constraining treatment to the zone of superficial photodamage. This combination of mechanisms is proposed to improve treatment efficacy, while maintaining the side-effects profile of existing methods. The laser light is delivered via a stamping technology with a spot size of 300 μm, which is five times the spot size relative to repair. It is delivered with a pulsed technique. The handpiece must be replaced with each treatment and is the only consumable.[31,60,61]

Bene and colleagues[62] studied 20 subjects under an IRB-controlled protocol, presenting with either superficial photoaging, including facial wrinkles, textural and/or pigmentary changes; or presenting with mature, white scars (including acne scars) on the face or body. Subjects were evaluated and photographed prior to the initiation of treatment, prior to each subsequent treatment, and 1 and 3 months following the final treatment. Subjects received at least three treatments at 4-week intervals. As many as six total treatments were permitted for subjects who requested additional treatments. Prior to treatment, the skin was cleaned and any make-up was removed. Subjects were treated using the Affirm laser system at 1440-nm wavelength, 3-ms pulse duration, and 10 mm diameter CAP array. Treatment fluences range from 3 to 7 J/cm^2, and 1–2 Hz pulse repetition rate. Treatment areas received between one and three treatment passes, with areas of greater visual defects receiving more passes. All treatments were delivered in conjunction with only SmartCool™ (Cynosure, Inc., Westford, MA) cold-air cooling, with fans speed of between 2 and 4. No additional anesthesia was required. The CAP array requires full contact with the skin for appropriate treatment. Subjects could resume normal activities immediately following treatment. Biopsies of periauricular test spots were conducted within 3 h of treatment in those who consented to determine the acute affects of treatment.

Some 90% of patients completed at least five treatments, with 78% of the subjects achieving observer graded improvements of at least 26–50% (on a quartile scale).[60]

Treatments were well tolerated, with subjects reporting an average discomfort of 2.3 (moderate discomfort) on a 0 (none) to 5 (worst) scale. The CAP technology provides a denser pattern of energy distribution creating a uniform treatment. This allows treatment with fewer passes and shortens treatment time. Typical initial response to treatment was mild to moderate erythema and edema which resolved within hours to a few days. In rare or one patient case, the treated areas became tan or dusky 36–48 h after treatment.

This transient discoloration resolved within 3 weeks in affected subjects. There were no scars, hyper or hypopigmentation observed. Histology showed that the CAP enabled 1440-nm Nd:YAG laser creates localized regions of injury with limited epidermal damage (no denudation of epidermis). Depth of treatment was limited to the zone of photoaging, and was self-limited to approximately 300 µm depth. According to the author, the new 1440-nm Nd:YAG with CAP technology found in the Affirm laser showed an exciting new development in nonablative devices for the treatment of wrinkles and scars. The micro-thermal injury CAP ability shows promise of many different ways to achieve efficacy, though it is still early in developing best parameters. In addition, clinical applications are expanding to other scar types, wrinkles, and pigmentation. The Affirm laser has proved to be a good compromise between full ablative and previous nonablative infrared resurfacing devices.

The Harmony[XL] (Alma Lasers, Buffalo Grove, IL) is a fractional 2940 nm wavelength Er:YAG laser that is part of a platform system that offers multiple applications including 10 distinct technologies that treat a wide array of problems ranging from vascular lesions to photoaging. The 2940 nm Er:YAG, micro-optic lens creates 49 (7 × 7) or 81 (9 × 9) pixel size ablation dots on the skin with an 11 × 11 mm treatment zone. The spot size is three times larger then the Fraxel[TM] Re:pair and has a fixed density of 20%. The Harmony[XL] delivers energy to a depth of 20–50 µm when using the fractional handpiece. The pulse duration is 1, 1.5, or 2 ms. Delivery of the laser is pulsed. Maximum coverage rate ranges from 98 mm²/s or 121 mm²/s. The handpiece must be replaced for each treatment. The laser is touted as providing the patient with the effectiveness of an ablative approach with the comfort level and convenience of a nonablative treatment. The laser can safely be used on the face, neck, chest, arms and hands.[31,60,61]

The Pixel CO$_2$ Omnifit[TM] (Alma Lasers, Buffalo Grove, IL) is a fractionated CO$_2$ adapter that can be fitted to a number of different CO$_2$ lasers, including CO$_2$ laser from Coherent®, Lumenis®, Sharplan® (Medical Tech Co., Ltd.) and others upon request. The operational mode is superpulsed and the spot size is 10 mm. Coverage is about 15–20% of the treatment area. The Pixel CO$_2$ Omnifit[TM] may make good financial sense for those who would like to convert a pre-existing CO$_2$ laser into a fractionated device. No studies were found comparing this solution to other fractional laser devices, which makes it difficult to assess its treatment efficacy.[31,60,61]

The PROfractional[TM] (Sciton Inc., Palo Alto, CA) is also a fractional 2940 nm Er:YAG laser that employs a scanned stamping technology for delivery with a spot size of 250–430 µm that is up to four times as large as the Fraxel[TM] Re:pair. The laser is delivered as a pulse. There are no consumables. There is a separate smoke evacuator included in the purchase price of the laser.

The combined scanning and stamping method of delivery of laser light is less painful. Penetration of the laser is thought to range from 25 to 1500 µm. The density within each treatment zone can be varied from 1.5–60%. Like most erbium YAG fractional lasers, as depths exceed 500 µm, punctate bleeding is observed.[31,60,61]

Both the ActiveFX[TM] and DeepFX[TM] (Lumenis Inc., Santa Clara, CA) use a scanned stamping technology for laser delivery. Both use ultrapulse delivery of a 10 600 nm CO$_2$, which is similar to the Fraxel[TM] Re:pair. The system injures the skin in a bridge fashion, leaving small bridges of normal skin intact. The spot size for the ActiveFX[TM] is 89 times the size of the spot size of the Fraxel[TM] Re:pair, but the spot size for the DeepFX[TM] is clinically equivalent to the Re:pair. Density ranges from 55–100% for the ActiveFX[TM] and 5–25% for the DeepFX[TM]. Energy ranges from 80 to 100 mJ for the ActiveFX[TM] and 5–50 mJ for the DeepFX[TM]. Depth of tissue damage, which is an important component in the degree of injury and subsequent skin shrinkage and collagen remodeling, is from 80 to 100 µm for the ActiveFX[TM] and up to 1500 µm for the DeepFX[TM]. Maximum coverage rate for the DeepFX[TM] is 98 mm²/s, which is the same as the Pixel CO$_2$ Omnifit[TM], but slower than the Re:pair. Cost is an important advantage of the ActiveFX[TM], in that there are no consumables necessary for the ActiveFX[TM]. Tips and lenses are necessary to purchase for the DeepFX[TM]. A separate smoke evacuator comes with both devices. One of the nice features of the ActiveFX[TM] is that the system can also be used to perform surgical incisions for blepharoplasty and browlift as well as treat rhinophyma. The ActiveFX favors high coverage rates and superficial injuries, and the deep FX achieves narrower lower density deeper injuries. It follows that the active FX device achieves excellent reduction of pigment dyschromias and fine lines whereas the deep FX handpiece favors treatment of deeper wrinkles and acne scars. In any fractional application, the provider should match the skin's pathology to the laser wound type.[31,60,61]

The Lux 1540 nm (Palomar Medical Technologies, Burlington, MA) is a fractional erbium:glass fiber laser that delivers tiny microbeams up to a depth of 1 mm. It cools the skin surface with a sapphire window and is nonablative. Some improvement in superficial wrinkles and dyschromia can be expected. The Lux 2940 (Palomar Medical Technologies) is a fractional ablative, Er:YAG laser that uses a stamping technology to deliver a wavelength of 2940 nm. It has a spot size of 100 µm, which is clinically equivalent to the Repair. It is a pulsed delivery system with a nonconsumable handpiece and no built-in smoke evacuator. Wound depths normally range from 100–500 µm depending on the pulse-width and pulse energy. Impressive changes in skin texture without concern for adverse changes in pigmentation have been noted in Fitzpatrick level I–III patients. Improvement at 2 years may be similar to that seen with ablative CO$_2$ according to one study.[11]

The micro-fractional technology of the erbium:YAG laser (Lux 2940) enables practitioners to potentially treat several-fold deeper than traditional CO$_2$ and Er:YAG lasers and evoke a dramatic healing response. The Lux 2940 laser uses fractional photothermolysis to generate an array of micro-columns of ablation that are bordered by residual layers of slight tissue coagulation (abut 20–30 µm ring of coagulation versus 60–80 µm with narrow cylinder fractional CO$_2$ lasers). Reepithelialization of the epidermis can be observed in as little as 12 h.[1]

Practitioners using the Lux 2940 can select different pulse widths for varying amounts of adjacent thermal damage and, therefore, tailor a subject's treatment to meet the individual's expectations of results and downtime. The Lux 2940, in addition to a short-pulse ablative mode, has a long-pulse coagulative mode and a dual pulse mode that combines short and long-pulses. Combining the two modes allows for increased depth of ablation together with increased coagulation zones for improved hemostasis and clinical efficacy. Subjects desiring only a short downtime (≤2 days) can be treated with less energy and/or fewer passes to achieve mild improvements in wrinkles, skin texture, and tone. For those seeking more robust wrinkle reduction, the higher settings of the Lux 2940 deliver deeper ablation and wider coagulation with about 3–5 days of downtime.

The Juvia (Ellipse, Horsholm, Denmark) is a fractional CO_2 laser with a wavelength of 10600 nm. Its spot size is fairly large at 500 μm and the laser is delivered by a scanned stamping technique. Energy ranges from 5 to 15 mJ and penetration into the skin is shallow at 30 μm. The laser is a superpulse. There is a handpiece that requires no consumables. The handpiece is among the lightest and smallest of any of the fractional lasers.[1,31]

The Mosaic (Lutronic US, Princeton Junction, NJ) is an Er:glass laser that employs a microfractional technique, delivering an energy of 4–40 mJ. They utilize a special stamping technique with the microfractional injuries laid down in a chaotic fashion, hence the term 'controlled chaos technology' has been used to describe their technique. This eliminates the need for multiple linear passes and the clinical disadvantages of unavoidable overlap. The Mosaic's automatic total density counter also gives precise control over all aspects of energy delivery, which is thought to result in a more uniform treatment of the target area, reduced treatments times and more rapid healing. The advantage of the laser seems to be that using the controlled chaos technology permits more rapid treatment at varying depths. Unlike traditional lasers and light-based technologies that achieve homogenous thermal damage at a particular depth, Mosaic's exclusive patented technology sprays multiple arrays of randomized microscopic laser beams to the skin. These beams selectively coagulate a small proportion of the collimated micro necrotic columns (MNCs) that reach as far down as the reticular dermis

while sparing the surrounding tissue. Re-epithelialization occurs within 24 h and like the Fraxel™ Re:store, the stratum corneum is not disrupted. Multiple treatments are usually needed to achieve improvement in certain conditions such as acne scars.

There are two modes of delivery, dynamic and static, which allow both rapid treatment (full face in 15 min) and static mode's stamp-like approach, which is suitable for smaller treatment areas. In this mode, the Mosaic has the ability to deliver 50–300 spots per square centimeter for virtually pain free treatment. There is a choice of four different tip sizes, which permits treatment to be tailored to treat areas of different sizes without damage to the surrounding tissue. According to the company's web site, one of the key features of the Mosaic system is its ability to track and record the total number of MNCs delivered to the skin. In conjunction with their patented Skin Sensor Tip system, which will only deliver treatment when in contact with the skin, the automatic total density counter allows for precise control over both the density and depth of the MNCs delivered, by tracking the number and site of each MNC.[1,31]

Clinical experience with fractional resurfacing procedures

Peri-oral wrinkles *(Fig. 5.6)* are most difficult to treat with all fractional lasers and require 4–6 treatments, 2–4 weeks apart, depending on severity of the wrinkles. They are slow to respond and often require skin fillers. Higher energy is usually needed (3–4 passes). That said, for deeper peri-oral wrinkles, we generally recommend a CO_2 fractional device or CO_2 laser *(Fig. 5.7)*. For acne scarring, one must be patient and allow time for collagen remodeling *(Fig. 5.8)*. With the 1550 Erbium:glass fractional laser (The Re:store, Solta Medical) 4–6 treatments, 3–4 weeks apart is usually required. As aggressive as the skin type allows, higher energy is used.[1,31] Analgesic pre-medication may be needed. Hyperpigmentation is improved as well. Patients with melasma and dyschromia are pre-treated with hydroquinone. Generally, 4–5 treatments are used, spaced 10–14 days apart. Lower energy is used with more passes. Good results may be seen in Asian skin, although melasma may be very difficult to treat and eradicate. Treatment

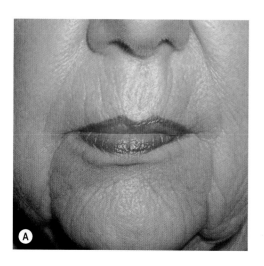
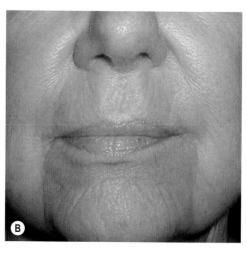

Fig. 5.6 1550 nm Erbium:glass laser in a 65-year-old woman for perioral wrinkles. **(A)** Before and **(B)** 6 months after six treatments.

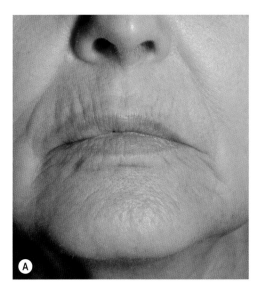 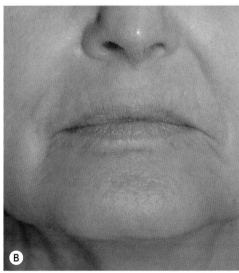

Fig. 5.7 Treatment of perioral wrinkle lines with fractional CO_2 laser, single treatment, **(A)** before and **(B)** 6 months after treatment.

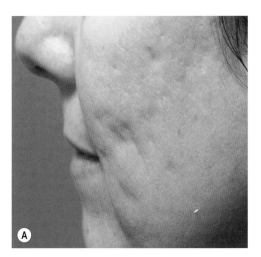 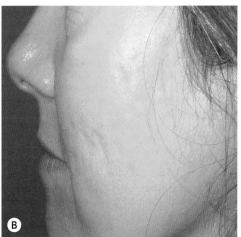

Fig. 5.8 Acne treatment with 1550 nm Erbium:glass fractional laser. **(A)** Before and **(B)** 6 months after three treatments.

failures with melasma are not uncommon and may be disappointing. Realistic expectations must be set with the patient and patient education is necessary to insure they understand the limitations of treatment.[1,31,60,61]

Although infrequent, complications do occur. Post-inflammatory hyperpigmentation (PIH) can occur and can take 3–6 months to resolve. It is managed with hydroquinone and tretinoin (0.05% or 0.10%). We use the Obagi skin care system consisting of hydroquinone, tretinoin, vitamin C and sunscreen. Patients with a history of herpes may experience an outbreak if not pre-treated with Zovirax or a similar medication. If this history is known, we treat the patient for 48 h prior to fractional laser therapy.[1,31]

Over time, the patient can expect lessening of hyperpigmentation then improvement of "crepey" skin tone followed by lessening of fine lines and then deep lines. Changes in deep lines can be a delayed phenomenon and can take months to occur due to the collagen remodeling process. Significant tightening of the skin may result as a secondary response and appears to be cumulative. The tightening is particularly evident in the nasolabial folds and glabella. Results with the

use of the 1550 Erbium:glass fractional laser have been more consistent than those obtained with other nonablative systems. No comparative clinical outcome data for the other fractional lasers in this class are available, so it is difficult to assume equivalency, especially if lasers do not penetrate as deeply or if similar numbers of treatments are not delivered.[1,31,60,61]

Patients tolerate the 1550 Erbium:glass fractional laser as well as the other Er:YAG or Er:glass laser treatments very well when used with the Zimmer Cooler, Benadryl, and Tylenol (or similar medications). Men tolerate it less well than women and lower energy may need to be used. Women's skin may be more sensitive around their menstrual cycle.[1,31,60,61]

The best response is in solar damaged skin, fine lines and "crepey" skin. Very good outcomes may also be seen with periorbital lines. Using a lower setting and a higher density (6–8 mJ/cm^2; 250) results in a good response. Fractional photothermolysis can be utilized as an adjunct to surgery as well, but safety parameters have not been fully studied. Fractional laser of undermined skin flaps during facelift is unknown *(Fig. 5.9)*.[1,31,60,61]

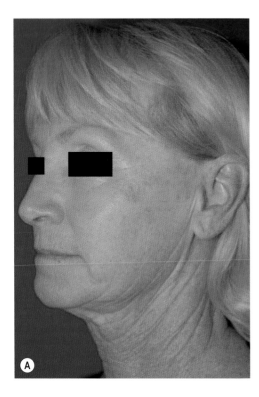

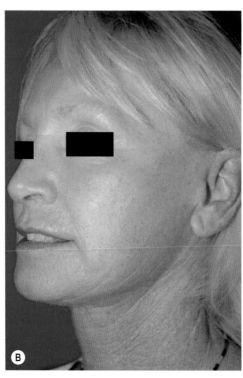

Fig. 5.9 Fractional CO_2 resurfacing done sequentially – SMAS facelift followed by fractional CO_2 3 months later. **(A)** Before and **(B)** 6 months after treatment.

In patients undergoing fractional CO_2 therapy, our pre-laser skin care regimen is similar to the less invasive, 1550 nm Er:glass fractional laser. Patients are prepped with topical anesthetic ointment for 1 hour prior to the laser. Metal eye shields are routinely used. Many require an oral pain medication and some require nerve blocks to divisions I–III of the trigeminal nerve for facial anesthesia. Full-face laser takes around 20 min. The energy and density are selected based on the patient's skin type and condition being treated. Lower energies and densities are used for darker Fitzpatrick skin types and higher energies and densities are used for acne and deep wrinkles, depending on skin type. In general, lower energies and densities are used on the neck and chest as well.[1,31,60,61]

Contraindications

Laser and chemical resurfacing have common contraindications. These include active bacterial, viral, fungal, or herpetic infection; open wounds; history of drugs with photosensitizing potential; pre-existing inflammatory dermatoses; uncooperative patients; patients with unrealistic expectations; history of abnormal or keloid-type scarring.[17,18]

Post-procedure care

Postoperative care is aimed at providing an ideal environment for moist wound healing. Initially, a generous amount of bland ointment (white petrolatum, A&D ointment) is applied to the entire treated area. Crisco vegetable shortening historically had been used quite successfully but has been reformulated and now actually may be irritating to patients. Patients are instructed to reapply the ointment throughout the day, any time the face feels tight or dry. As the outer layers begin to shed, the patient is allowed to shower and gently wash the face with nonresidue soap using fingertips only. After showering, the face should be patted dry and a new coating of ointment applied. Instruct patients not to pick at the face during the recovery period.[17,18] Following chemical peeling, some practitioners use topical agents that contain platelet products or growth factors. While these products have been reported to improve wound healing in other clinical situations, no randomized controlled clinical trials presently support their use in this setting. This is an area in which further research is ongoing. Understanding the process of re-epithelialization and the importance of compliance with the prescribed post-treatment regimen is essential information for every patient. This includes awareness of likely facial edema that may contribute to symptoms such as diplopia. If antiviral therapy is instituted, continue therapy until re-epithelialization is complete. In the early stages of wound healing, re-examine the patient within 48 h and again every several days. Instruct patients to refrain from trans-retinoic acid, sunscreen, or make-up, until the face is healed to the satisfaction of the treating physician.[17,18]

Post-laser treatment generally consists of gauze and ice packs immediately after treatment followed by vinegar and H_2O soaks every 3–4 h when awake for the first 2–3 days depending on exudate and crusting. Benedryl® capsule is recommended each evening for the first 3 days. Aquaphor® ointment dressing is used for the first 3 days, then Cetaphil® lotion for the duration of the healing process. Healing takes place over the first few days with re-epithelialization nearly complete by 48 h. Redness subsides over the next 3–4 days and gradually disappears over the next 3–4 weeks. Early results have been impressive.[17,18]

Complications

Pigmentary change

Pigmentary change is not an uncommon complication, especially with the deeper peeling agents, or deep penetration laser therapy. Taking proper precautions (as described earlier) can help prevent undesirable pigmentary changes. Usually, patients with lighter complexions have a lower risk of hyperpigmentation than darker skinned individuals. Skin priming using a combination of hydroquinone and tretinoin cream (Kligman formulation) before a superficial or medium-depth peel and early introduction of this preparation after deep peels reduces the rate of this complication.[17,18]

Scarring

Scarring remains the most feared complication of facial resurfacing. The contributing factors are still not well understood. By employing the most appropriate resurfacing procedure for any given patient, the risk of scarring can be decreased. In addition, to further decrease the risk of scarring, the patient should be advised to refrain from touching or picking at the healing skin. Patients with a history of keloids should absolutely not undergo medium or deep treatments because of the risk of scarring. Weaker superficial treatments that only exfoliate the stratum corneum or superficial epidermis can be used for these high risk patients.[17,18]

Infection

By using bacitracin for the medium and deep treatments and cleaning the face with a povidone wash, the risk of infection is decreased. Cold sores can be prevented with acyclovir (400 mg PO bid), beginning 2 days prior to the treatment and continuing 7 days after the treatment. *Candidiasis* infection also can develop, for which a short course of fluconazole can be used. Cultures need to be taken, and appropriate antibiotics should be administered.[17,18] More recently, atypical mycobacterial infections have been reported after ablative fractional procedures.[63] Most likely, the penetrating nature of fractional approaches allows these opportunists to thrive. Measures to decrease the risk include thorough cleansing before treatment and avoidance of tap water at the wound site during and immediately after treatment.

Prolonged erythema

Patients usually do not report erythema because it generally subsides in 30–90 days, but sometimes erythema continues. Prolonged erythema is usually not permanent, and topical hydrocortisone can be used to speed the healing process.[17,18]

Acne

Some patients develop acne after a facial resurfacing procedure. This usually occurs between days 3–9. Cultures should be taken, and an antibiotic that covers Gram-positive bacteria should be prescribed. If it is a true acne occurrence, then the appropriate topical treatment also should be started. If severe enough, isotretinoin may be initiated.[17,18]

Milia

Small inclusion cysts, sometimes called milia, can appear in the healing process after a treatment. These usually appear about 2–3 weeks after re-epithelialization and may be aggravated by ointments, owing to occlusion of the sebaceous glands.[17,18]

Disclosures

Drs Cohen and Frank have no financial relationships with any commercial laser company discussed in this chapter. Dr Ross receives honoraria from Palomar, Lumenis, Candela, and Cutera; Dr Ross receives research support from Candela, Palomar, Sciton, Cutera, and Syneron.

 Access the complete references list online at **http://www.expertconsult.com**

7. Goldman L, Rockwell RJ. Laser action at the cellular level. *JAMA*. 1966;198(6):641–644.

11. Fitzpatrick RE, Goldman MP, Satur NM, et al. Pulsed carbon dioxide laser resurfacing of photo-aged facial skin. *Arch Dermatol*. 1996;132(4):395–402.

    This is a blinded assessment of CO_2 laser efficacy for periorbital and perioral rhytids. CO_2 laser was found to be useful in this setting.

14. Manstein D, Herron GS, Sink RK, et al. Fractional photothermolysis: a new concept for cutaneous remodeling using microscopic patterns of thermal injury. *Lasers Surg Med*. 2004;34(5):426–438.

    A novel method for skin resurfacing is presented. Microscopic treatment zones are targeted for thermal injury.

26. Ross E, Anderson R. Laser tissue interactions In: Goldman M, ed. *Cutaneous and cosmetic laser surgery*. Philadelphia: Elsevier; 2006.

30. Sadick NS. Update on non-ablative light therapy for rejuvenation: a review. *Lasers Surg Med*. 2003;32(2): 120–128.

    A review of nonablative skin resurfacing modalities is presented.

34. Dinner MI, Artz JS. The art of the trichloroacetic acid chemical peel. *Clin Plast Surg*. 1998;25(1):53–62.

    The authors highlight the continued importance of chemical peels in facial rejuvenation. All aspects of the TCA technique are described.

56. Goodman G. Post acne scarring: a review. *J Cosmet Laser Ther*. 2003;5(2):77–95.

    The acne scar is a historically difficult problem with pathology that varies considerably within and between patients. The authors emphasize the necessity of applying lesion-specific techniques in their review of evolving technologies to address acne scars.

6

Anatomy of the aging face

Bryan Mendelson and Chin-Ho Wong

SYNOPSIS

- Aging of the face is a multifactorial process that can be explained on an anatomical basis.
- The face is constructed of five basic layers that are bound together by a system of facial retaining ligaments.
- To facilitate the mobility needed for facial expression independent of the basic functions of the face, particularly of mastication, a series of soft tissue spaces are incorporated into the architecture of the face.
- This arrangement, most clearly seen in the scalp, also exists in the rest of the face, although with significant compaction and modifications.
- This chapter will describe, in detail, the five-layered construct of the face, including the spaces and retaining ligaments, and will highlight the relevance of these structures in the aging face.
- In addition, the profound impact of aging of the facial skeleton should be appreciated.
- Understanding these principles will help not only in understanding the aging process but also in designing procedures that are logical and effective in reversing the stigmata of the aging face.

Introduction

Facial aging is a complex process that is the cumulative effect of simultaneous changes of the many components of the face as well as the interaction of these components with each other. An understanding of the anatomical changes associated with aging is required in order to design effective procedures to rejuvenate various aspects of the aging face. Fundamental to understanding these changes is a firm grounding in the principles on which the facial soft tissue layers are constructed.[1] This is important because the pathogenesis of facial aging is explained on an anatomical basis, particularly the variations in the onset and outcome of aging seen in different individuals. Understanding the principles on which the facial soft tissues are constructed is the basis for an accurate and reliable

intraoperative map for the surgeons to safely navigate to the area of interest to correct aging changes. This is most important in addressing the overriding concern, being the course of the facial nerve branches. An anatomical approach to surgical rejuvenation of the face provides the way to obtaining a "natural" result that is lasting and with minimal morbidity.

Regions of the face

The traditional approach to assessing the face is to consider the face in thirds (upper, middle, and lower thirds).[2] While useful, this approach limits conceptualization, as it is not based on the function of the face. From a functional perspective, the face has an anterior aspect and a lateral aspect. The anterior face is highly evolved beyond the basic survival needs, specifically, for communication and facial expression. In contrast, the lateral face predominantly covers the structures of mastication.[3] A vertical line descending from the lateral orbital rim is the approximate division between the anterior and lateral zones of the face. Internally, a series of facial retaining ligaments are strategically located along this line to demarcate the anterior from the lateral face (*Fig. 6.1*). The mimetic muscles of the face are located in the superficial fascia of the anterior face, mostly around the eyes and the mouth. This highly mobile area of the face is designed to allow fine movement and is prone to develop laxity with aging. In contrast, the lateral face is relatively immobile as it overlies the structures to do with mastication, the temporalis, masseter, the parotid gland and its duct, all located deep to the deep fascia. The only superficial muscle in the lateral face is the platysma in the lower third, which extends to the level of the oral commissure.

Importantly, the soft tissues of the anterior face are subdivided into two parts; that which overlies the skeleton and the larger part that comprises the highly specialized sphincters overlying the bony cavities.[4] Where the soft tissues overlie the orbital and oral cavities they are modified, as there is no deep

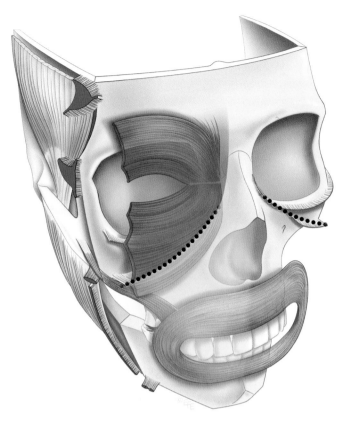

Fig. 6.1 Regions of the face. The mobile anterior face is functionally adapted for facial expressions and is separated from the relatively fixed lateral face (shaded), which overlies masticatory structures. A vertical line of retaining ligaments (red) separates the anterior and lateral face. These ligaments are, from above: temporal, lateral orbital, zygomatic, masseteric, and mandibular ligaments. In the anterior face, the mid-cheek is split obliquely into two separate functional parts by the mid-cheek groove (dotted line) related to two cavities: the periorbital part above (blue) and the perioral part below (yellow). (© Dr Levent Efe, CMI.)

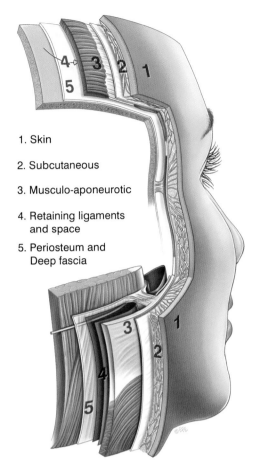

1. Skin

2. Subcutaneous

3. Musculo-aponeurotic

4. Retaining ligaments and space

5. Periosteum and Deep fascia

Fig. 6.2 The face is constructed of five basic layers. This five-layered construct is most evident in the scalp but exists in the rest of the face, with significant modification and compaction for functional adaptation. Layer 4 is the most significantly modified layer, with alternating facial soft tissue spaces and retaining ligaments. Facial nerve branches also transition from deep to superficial in association with the retaining ligaments through layer 4. (© Dr Levent Efe, CMI.)

fascial layer for support. Accordingly, support does not come from within the cavity beneath, but from the rim of the cavities. The transitions between these areas, while not seen in youth, become increasingly evident with aging.

Surgical anatomy of the face, SMAS, facial spaces and retaining ligaments

The soft tissue of the face is arranged concentrically into the five basic layers[5,6]: (1) skin; (2) subcutaneous; (3) musculo-aponeurotic layer; (4) areola tissue; and (5) deep fascia. This five-layered arrangement is most clearly seen in the scalp and forehead as a result of evolutionary expansion of the underlying cranial vault necessary to accommodate the highly developed frontal lobe in humans. Accordingly, the scalp is an excellent place to study the principles of the layered anatomy (*Fig. 6.2*). Layer 4 (the loose areolar tissue) is the layer that allows the superficial fascia (defined as the composite flap of layers 1 through 3) to glide over the deep fascia (layer 5). The simplified anatomy over the scalp gives the basic prototype of layer 4. There are not any structures crossing this plane, which is essentially an avascular potential space. At the boundaries of the scalp along the superior temporal line and

across the supraorbital rim, the scalp and the forehead are firmly anchored by ligamentous attachments. Vital structures, the nerves and vessels are always located in close proximity to the retaining ligaments. In the face proper, while the principles of construction remain the same, there is considerably greater complexity. This is due to the compaction resulting from the absence of forward projection of the midface, as occurs in other species, and the predominance of the orbital and oral cavities that limit the availability of a bony platform for attachment of ligaments and muscles. To secure the superficial fascia to the facial skeleton, a system of retaining ligaments bind the dermis to the skeleton, and the components of this system pass through all layers (*Figs 6.3, 6.4*).[7,8]

The structure and composition of each of the 5 layers will now be described in turn.

Layer 1: skin

The epidermis is a cell-rich layer composed mainly of differentiating keratinocytes and a smaller number of pigment producing melanocytes and antigen-presenting Langerhans cells. The dermis is the outer layer of the structural superficial fascia and comprises predominantly the extracellular matrix secreted

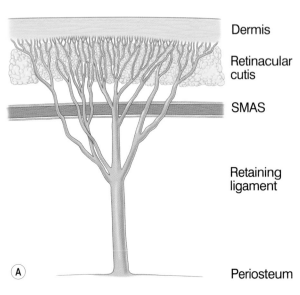

Dermis

Retinacular cutis

SMAS

Retaining ligament

Periosteum

(A)

(B)

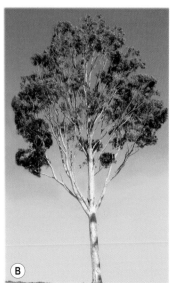

Fig. 6.3 The retaining ligaments of the face can be likened to a tree. The ligaments attach the soft tissues to the facial skeleton or deep muscle fascia, passing through all five layers of the soft tissues. It fans out in a series of branches and inserts into the dermis. At different levels of dissection, it is given different names, such as the retinacular cutis in the subcutaneous layer and ligaments in the subSMAS level. (© Dr Levent Efe, CMI.)

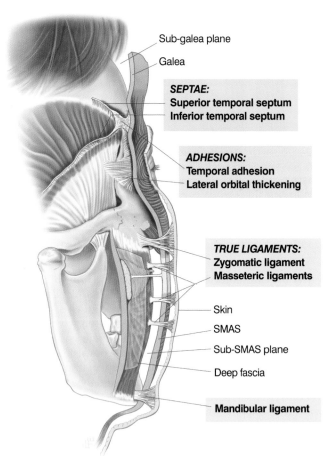

Sub-galea plane

Galea

SEPTAE:
Superior temporal septum
Inferior temporal septum

ADHESIONS:
Temporal adhesion
Lateral orbital thickening

TRUE LIGAMENTS:
Zygomatic ligament
Masseteric ligaments

Skin

SMAS

Sub-SMAS plane

Deep fascia

Mandibular ligament

Fig. 6.4 Three morphological forms of retaining ligaments of the face. (© Dr Levent Efe, CMI.)

by fibroblasts. Type I collagen is the most abundant protein. Other collagen types (III, V, VII), elastin, proteoglycans and fibronectins are present in smaller quantities. A rich vascular plexus is an important component of the dermis. The thickness of the dermis relates to its function and tends to be inversely proportionate to its mobility. The dermis is thinnest in the eyelids and thickest over the forehead and the nasal tip.

The thinner the dermis, the more susceptible it is to qualitative deterioration aging changes.

Layer 2: subcutaneous tissue

The subcutaneous layer has two components: the subcutaneous fat, which provides volume, and the fibrous retinacular cutis that binds the dermis to the underlying SMAS.[9] Of note, the retinacular cutis is the name given to that portion of the retaining ligament that passes through the subcutaneous tissues. The amount, proportion and arrangement of each component vary in different regions of the face. In the scalp, the subcutaneous layer has uniform thickness and consistency of fixation to the overlying dermis. In contrast, in the face proper, the subcutaneous layer has significant variation in thickness and attachments. In specialized areas such as the eyelids and lips, this layer is significantly compacted such that fat may appear non-existent. In other areas, such as the nasolabial segment, it is very thick.[4] In areas with thick subcutaneous tissue, the retinacular cutis lengthens significantly, predisposing its fibers to weakening and distension with aging. Within the subcutaneous tissue, the overall attachment to the overlying dermis is stronger and denser than the attachment to the underlying SMAS.[9] This is a result of the tree-like arrangement of the retinacular cutis fibers *(Fig. 6.3)*, with fewer but thicker fibers deep as its rises through the SMAS that progressively divide into multiple fine microligaments as they reach the dermis. This explains why it is easier to perform subcutaneous dissection in the deeper subcutaneous level (just on the surface of the underlying SMAS) than more superficially nearer the dermis, as there are fewer retinacular cutis fibers and the subcutaneous fat here does not attach directly to the outer surface of the underlying SMAS.

Furthermore, the retinacular cutis fibers are not uniform across the face, but vary in orientation and density according to the anatomy of the underlying deeper structures. As will be apparent when the anatomy of the underlying Layer 4 is described, at the location of the retaining ligaments, the vertically oriented retinacular cutis fibers are the most dense and are the most effective in supporting for the overlying soft tissues and in so doing, forms boundaries that

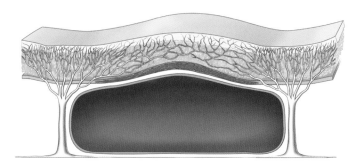

Fig. 6.5 The density and strength of the retinacular cutis fibers in the subcutaneous layer varies in different areas of the face. Where it overlies the retaining ligaments, the fibers are denser and oriented more vertically. In these areas, sharp release is usually necessary to raise a subcutaneous flap. In contrast, in areas overlying a space, the fibers are less dense and oriented more horizontally. Here, it is relatively easy to elevate a subcutaneous facelift flap. (© Dr Levent Efe, CMI.)

compartmentalize the subcutaneous fat. These areas, such as the so-called McGregor's patch over the body of the zygoma, often require sharp release to mobilize. In between these retaining ligaments in layer 4 are located the soft tissue spaces of the face, that facilitate the mobility of the superficial fascia over the deep fascia. Where the subcutaneous fat overlies a space, the retinacular fibers are less dense and orientated more horizontally, as a result of which, the tissues tend to separate with relative ease, often with just simple blunt finger dissection *(Fig. 6.5)*. This variation in the density and orientation of the retinacular cutis fibers in the subcutaneous fat is the anatomical basis for the compartmentalization of the subcutaneous fat into discrete compartments, described in detail in Chapter 11.1.[10,11]

Layer 3: musculo-aponeurotic layer

The muscles of facial expression are unique and fundamentally different from skeletal muscles beneath the deep fascia because they are situated within the superficial fascia and they move the soft tissues of which they are a part. All muscles of facial expression have either all or the majority of their course within layer 3 and they are predominantly located over and around the orbital and oral cavities. In the prototype scalp, the occipital-frontalis moves the overlying soft tissue of the forehead, while its undersurface glides over the subaponeurotic space (layer 4). Layer 3 is continuous over the entire face, although for descriptive purposes, different names are given to certain parts according to the superficial muscle within. It is called the galea over the scalp, the temporoparietal (superficial temporal) fascia over the temple, the orbicularis fascia in the periorbital region, the superficial musculoaponeurotic system (SMAS) over the mid- and lower face and platysma in the neck.[5,12]

Within layer 3, the facial muscles themselves have a layered configuration, with the broad, flat muscles forming the superficial layer that covers the anterior aspect of the face. The frontalis covers the upper, orbicularis oculi, the middle and the platysma, and lower thirds, respectively. The muscles of this layer have minimal direct attachment to the bone, stabilized to the skeleton at their periphery indirectly by the vertically orientated retaining ligaments as noted earlier. The frontalis is fixed along the superior temporal line by the superior temporal septum, the orbicularis oculi laterally by the

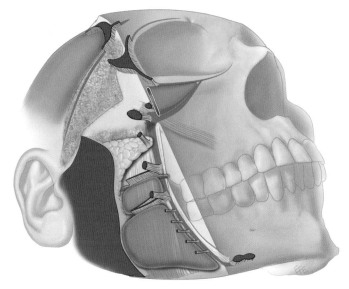

Fig. 6.6 Topographical anatomy of layer 4 over the lateral face. Spaces (blue), ligaments (red) and the areas of important anatomy (stippled). The largest area of ligamentous attachment, the platysma-auricular fascia (PAF), dominates the posterior part of level 4 at the least mobile part of the face. The lateral face transitions into the anterior face at the vertical line of retaining ligaments. Immediately above and below the arch of the zygoma are the triangular-shaped areas that contain the important anatomy proceeding from the lateral into the anterior face. (© Dr Levent Efe, CMI.)

lateral orbital thickening and the main zygomatic ligament at its inferolateral border and the platysma at its upper border by the lower masseteric ligament. The deeper muscles in layer 3 provide greater functional control of the sphincters over the bony cavities. For the upper third, these are the corrugators and procerus, and around the oral cavity, the elevators (zygomaticus major and minor, levator labii superioris, *levator anguli oris*), and the depressors (*depressor anguli oris*, depressor labii inferioris) around the oral sphincter and the mentalis.

Layer 4

Layer 4 is the plane in which dissection is performed in subSMAS facelifts. It is an area of significant complexity and contains the following structures: (1) soft tissue spaces; (2) retaining ligaments; (3) deep layers of the intrinsic muscles passing from their bone attachment to their more superficial soft tissue origin; and (4) facial nerve branches, passing from deep to superficial. Functionally, a series of soft tissue spaces exist in layer 4 to allow independent movement of the periorbital and perioral muscle of facial expressions over the deep fascia responsible for mastication directly beneath the muscles of facial expression.[13] The retaining ligaments of the face are strategically placed within the boundaries between the soft tissue spaces and functions to reinforce the boundaries *(Fig. 6.6)*. In the lateral face, immediately in front of the ear, extending 25–30 mm forward of the ear cartilage to the posterior border of the platysma, is a diffuse area of ligamentous attachment, described by Furnas as the platysma auricular fascia (PAF).[7] As no facial expression occurs here, the dermis, subcutaneous tissue, SMAS and the underlying parotid capsule (layers 1–5) are bound together as an area of retaining ligament. Layer 4 is reduced to a layer of fusion here, without a soft tissue space. The ligamentous character of this immobile area makes it surgically useful for suture fixation. Furnas had originally described the lower part of the PAF, the platysma auricular ligament,[7] also named by Stuzin and colleagues, the parotid cutaneous ligament[5] and this ligament was subsequently named the tympanoparotid fascia.[14] The part of the PAF immediately in front of the lower tragus has been labeled, Lore's fascia.[14]

In contrast, in the anterior face where there is considerable movement over and around the bony cavities, the ligaments are significantly compacted and arranged around the edges of the bony cavities. These boundaries provide the last position where there is underlying deep fascia for the mobile shutters of the lids and lips to be supported. Importantly for the surgeon, the retaining ligaments also act as transition points for the facial nerve branches to pass from deep to superficial, on their way to innervate their target muscles.

Soft tissue spaces of the face are in two forms: (1) those overlying bony cavities, such as the preseptal space of the eyelid over the orbit and the vestibule of the oral cavity, under the lips and the lower nasolabial segment of the cheek and (2) those overlying the bone, where soft tissue spaces allow the overlying superficial fascia to glide freely over the bone.

Layer 5

The deep fascia, the deepest soft tissue layer of the face, is formed by the periosteum where it overlies bone. Over the lateral face, where the muscle of mastication (temporalis and masseter) overlie the bone, the deep fascia is instead the fascial covering of the muscles, the deep temporal fascia above the zygomatic arch, and masseteric fascia below the arch. The parotid fascia is also part of the deep fascia. The investing deep cervical fascia is the corresponding layer in the neck where it covers the supraomohyoid muscles and splits to form the submandibular space that contains the submandibular gland. The deep fascia, although thin, is tough and unyielding and gives attachment to the retaining ligaments of the face. In the mobile shutters over the bony cavities, the deep fascia is absent, being replaced by a mobile lining derived from the cavities, that of the conjunctiva or oral mucosa.

Anatomy over the cavities in the skeleton

The general pattern of the five-layered anatomy is modified where the soft tissues overlie the orbital, oral and nasal cavities over the anterior face *(Fig. 6.7)*. Only the outer three layers of the composite continue from the periphery as the soft tissue over the cavities. The SMAS layer within this composite includes the sphincteric orbicularis muscles that extend right to the free edge of the soft tissue aperture of the eyelids and lips. The retaining ligaments, which are such a key feature of the five-layered anatomy, are not present over the cavities. There are thus anatomical variations associate with thee functional transitions from the relative stability of the "fixed" areas to the high mobility of the soft tissue shutters over the cavities. At the transition, to support the shutters, the retaining ligaments are condensed along the bony orbital rim *(Fig. 6.8)*. This is the anatomical basis for the periorbital ligament around the orbit, of which the lower lid part is the orbicularis

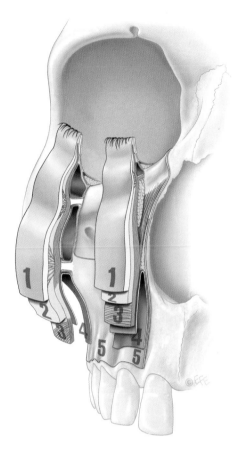

Fig. 6.7 The anatomy over the skeleton and over bony cavities (1–5), showing the relationship of the soft tissue spaces to bony cavity spaces. (© Dr Levent Efe, CMI.)

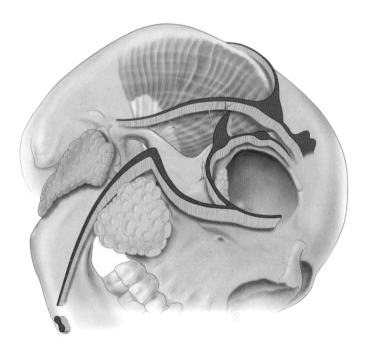

Fig. 6.8 The system of retaining ligaments situated around the bony cavities stabilizes the soft tissue over the cavities. (© Dr Levent Efe, CMI.)

retaining ligament, which stabilizes the orbicularis oculi to the orbital rim periosteum. Around the oral cavity where the boundary is less distinct, the ligaments arise mainly from the platform of the body of the zygoma, and from the deep fascia over the masseter.[15–17]

The deeper component of the eyelid and lips are derived from the origin of the cavity and are not an extension of the facial soft tissues. In the eyelid, the deeper lid muscles with their related aponeurosis (levator and capsulopalpebral fasciae) and fat are retained by the fascial system of the septum orbitale. The free edges of the upper and lower eyelids obtain their ligamentous support from the tarsal plates, with their canthal tendon attachments to the medial and lateral orbital rims. In the pretarsal area, the superficial and deep lid structures, the anterior and posterior lamellae, merge. But between the pretarsal area of the lid and the orbital rim the lamellae remain quite separate, i.e., the preseptal orbicularis does not have an attachment to the septum orbitale. This is the anatomical basis for the, surgically significant, preseptal space of the lower lid. In the upper lid, there is not an equivalent space as the submuscular fat pad over the superior orbital rim continues on the outer surface of the septum orbitale where it is adherent to the overlying fascia on the underside of the orbicularis almost down to where the levator crosses into the orbicularis.

The extent of the vestibule of the oral cavity covering the maxilla and the mandible has a major impact on the susceptibility to aging of the overlying soft tissue. The skeleton underlying the space is not available to provide ligamentous attachment for support of the soft tissues that cover this large area. The extreme mobility of the lip and adjacent part of the cheek renders it susceptible to aging changes and the indication for a lower facelift is largely to correct aging changes in this unsupported tissue.

Facial spaces

A large part of the subSMAS layer 4 consists of soft tissue "spaces." These spaces have defined boundaries that are strategically reinforced by retaining ligaments.[18] Significantly, these areas are by definition anatomically "safe spaces" to dissect, as no structures crosses within and all branches of the facial nerve are outside these spaces. As the roof of each space is the least supported part, it is more prone to developing laxity with aging, compared with the ligament-reinforced boundaries. This differential laxity accounts for much of the characteristic changes that occur with aging of the face. Once a space has been surgically defined to its boundaries, the retaining ligaments in the boundary can then be precisely released under direct vision to achieve the desired mobilization, while preserving the vital structures closely associated with the ligaments. A brief description of surgically significant facial soft tissue spaces is given below.

Upper temporal space

The upper temporal space separates the temporoparietal fascia (superficial temporal fascia) from the (deep) temporal fascia and is separated from the forehead by the superior temporal septum (STS) along the superior temporal line *(Fig. 6.9)*. Anteroinferiorly, the upper temporal space is separated from

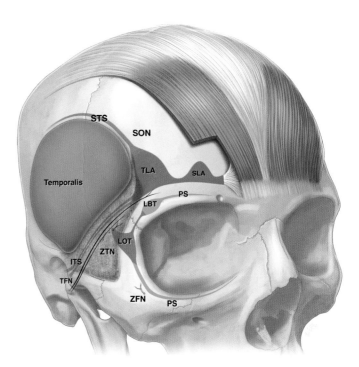

Fig. 6.9 The upper temporal space and the retaining ligaments of the temple. The boundaries of the space are the superior temporal septum (STS) and the inferior temporal septum (ITS), which are extensions of the temporal ligament adhesion (TLA). No structures cross the temporal space. The TLA continues medially as the supraorbital ligamentous adhesion (SLA). Inferior to the temporal space is the triangular-shaped area of important anatomy (stippled). Crossing level 4 in this area are the medial and lateral branches of the zygomatic temporal nerve (ZTN) and the sentinel vein. The temporal branches of the facial nerve (TFN) course on the underside of the temporal-parietal fascia over the area immediately inferior to the inferior temporal septum. The periorbital septum (PS, green) is on the orbital rim at the boundary of the orbital cavity. The lateral orbital thickening (LOT) and the lateral row thickening (LBT) are parts of the periorbital septum. SON, supraorbital nerve; ZFN, zygomaticofacial nerve. (© Dr Levent Efe, CMI.)

the lower triangular shaped temporal area that contains important anatomy, by the inferior temporal septum (ITS). These septi merge at the triangular-shaped zone of adhesion called the temporal (orbital) ligament.[15] The upper temporal space provides safe surgical access to the lateral brow and upper mid-cheek. The space can be readily opened by blunt dissection to its boundaries. Once identified, the boundaries are then released by precise sharp dissection. The superior temporal septum can be released sharply, taking care only to preserve the lateral (deep) branch of the supraorbital nerve, which runs parallel to the septum about 0.5 cm medial to it.[19] The inferior temporal septum provides a marker to the important anatomy here as the temporal branches of the facial nerve are located parallel to and immediately inferior to this septum. To release the inferior temporal septum, the roof of the space is gently lifted off the deep temporal fascia floor, which three-dimensionalizes the septum in preparation for its gentle release at the level of the floor, bearing in mind the frontal branches are located under the roof of the lower temporal area where they travel in the ceiling within the layer of fat suspended on the underside of the temporoparietal fascia. Once released, the sentinel vein comes into view. The sentinel vein is not a good landmark for locating the temporal branches as they course cephalad to the vein, that is, inferior to the inferior temporal septum. This anatomy is also reviewed in Chapter 7.

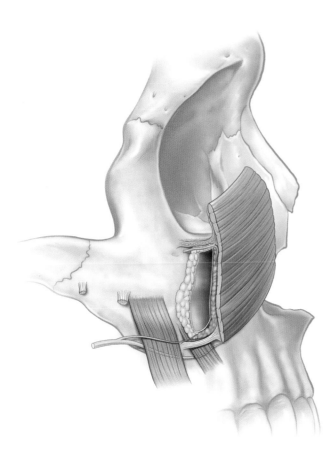

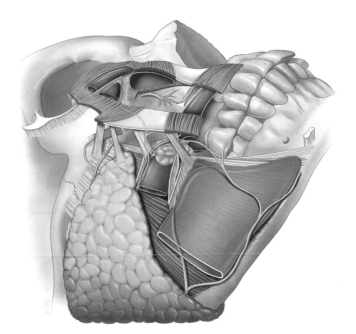

Fig. 6.10 The prezygomatic space overlies the body of the zygoma. The origin of the zygomatic muscles extends under the floor. The roof is formed by the orbicularis oculi line by the suborbicularis oculi fat (SOOF). The upper ligamentous border formed by the orbicularis retaining ligament is not as strong as the zygomatic ligament reinforced lower border. (© Dr Levent Efe, CMI.)

Fig. 6.11 The rhomboidal-shaped premasseter space overlies the lower half of the masseter. The roof of the space is formed by the platysma. The posterior border is defined by the anterior edge of the strong PAF and the anterior border is reinforced by the masseteric ligaments near the anterior edge of the masseter. The inferior boundary is mesenteric-like and does not contain any ligament. Weakness of attachment of the platysma roof at the inferior boundary leads to the formation of the jowl directly behind the strong mandibular ligament. The buccal space containing the buccal fat is anterior to the upper masseteric ligaments. All facial nerve branches course around and outside the space. The surgically important mandibular branch, after leaving the fixed PAF, courses under the inferior boundary of the space, then rises onto the highly mobile outer surface of the mesenteric inferior border before reaching the mandibular ligament. (© Dr Levent Efe, CMI.)

Prezygomatic space

This triangular-shaped space overlies the body of the zygoma, its floor covering the origins of the zygomatic muscles. The space allows the independent displacement of the orbicularis oculi (pars orbitale) in the roof from the zygomatic muscles under the floor. Contraction of the overlying orbicularis elevates the prezygomatic soft tissues, which results in zygomatic smile lines (below the crow's feet) *(Fig. 6.10)*. With the laxity of aging the roof of the space rests at a lower level than in youth. As a result, there is a now a greater amplitude of movement on orbicularis contraction that has the effect of exaggerating the zygomatic lines with aging.[13,16] This aging of the prezygomatic space, with bulging over its roof accentuated by its well-supported boundaries, is the anatomical basis for the clinical entity variously described as malar mounds, bags or malar crescent. These deformities indicate the presence of significant laxity and the treatment is directed to tightening the laxity of the roof and upper ligamentous boundary.

Premasseter space

This space overlies the lower half of the masseter and is analogous to the temporal space, in that it overlies the deep fascia of a muscle of mastication *(Fig. 6.11)*.[18] This gliding soft tissue plane allows opening of the jaw without restriction and avoids excessive distortion of the overlying soft tissues. The roof of this space is formed by the platysma. The lower premasseter space has profound clinical significance, as it is the anatomical basis for the development of jowls with aging. Laxity in the roof of the space, particularly where it has a weakened attachment to the anterior masseter by the masseteric ligaments and its inferior boundary where there is no ligament, manifests as the labiomandibular fold and jowl, respectively. The relatively stable fixation at the anteroinferior corner of the premasseter space provided by the mandibular ligament accounts for the dimple that is commonly seen separating the labiomandibular fold above and the jowl below.

Buccal space

This is one of the deep facial spaces, being, like the submandibular space (which contains the submandibular gland), deep to the deep fascia (layer 5). The buccal space is located in the anterior face, medial to the anterior border of the masseter above the level of the oral commissure in youth.[20,21] The space and its contents, the buccal fat, facilitates movement of the overlying nasolabial segment of the mid-cheek as well as buffering this area from excessive motion from jaw movement. Aging and attrition of the boundaries, particularly of the masseteric ligaments inferiorly result in the platysma being less firmly bound to the masseter. This allows the space to enlarge and also allows the buccal fat to prolapse inferiorly, below the level of the commissure into the lower face. As the buccal fat comes to overlie the anterior border of the lower masseter it results in increased prominence of the labiomandibular fold and jowl.

Facial nerve branches

The danger zone for facial nerve injury has been well described in the literature, but is of limited value to the surgeon due to the two-dimensional perspective that gives the expected course of the nerve relative to surface landmarks.[22-24] Confidence when approaching the nerve surgically comes from an understanding the three-dimensional course of the nerve relative to the layered anatomy as described above and visually identifying the nerves in relation to defined landmarks (Fig. 6.12). The facial nerve branches exit the parotid gland and remain deep to layer 5 in the lateral face. As they approach the anterior face, the branches traverse layer 4 to reach the underside of mimetic muscles of the face. It is at these transition points across layer 4 that the nerves are at greatest risk of injury.[1,25] The transitions occur at predictable locations, in close association with retaining ligaments that provide stability and protection for the nerves. The surgical release of these ligaments to gain the needed mobility should be performed with extreme care on account of the proximity of the nerves.

The surface marking of the temporal branch of the facial nerve is along the Pitanguy line, from a point 0.5 cm below the tragus to a point 1.5 cm lateral to the supraorbital rim.[26,27] It is traditional teaching that once the temporal branch exits the parotid, it immediately runs superficially from the deep fascia and comes to lie just deep to the SMAS as it crosses the arch of the zygoma.[5,28,29] Because of its superficial location,

surgical transection of the SMAS here, so-called high SMAS transection (i.e., at or above the arch) has been generally discouraged. It is now apparent that the nerve is deeper than was previously thought as it crosses the zygomatic arch.[30] A histological study confirmed that the frontal branches are in transition from where they exit the parotid below the zygomatic arch, to where they enter the underside of the temporoparietal fascia some 2 cm above the arch. They course in a tissue layer (layer 4), just deep to the temporoparietal fascia (layer 3) and immediately superficial to the periosteum and above that, the temporalis fascia (layer 5), all along protected by a fascial, fatty layer, which is an upward prolongation of the parotid-masseteric fascia and named the parotid-temporal fascia.[27] Another study noted the temporal branch to transition to under the temporoparietal fascia (layer 3) at a distance of 1.5–3 cm above the zygomatic arch.[31] The temporal branch completes the transition to the underside of the temporoparietal fascia well before the nerve crosses cephalad to the sentinel vein.[15] Accordingly, once the sentinel vein is visualized from the temporal aspect, the temporal branches would already be located in the roof of the lower temporal area.

The zygomatic branch exits the parotid gland deep to the deep fascia just below the zygoma and cephalad to the parotid duct. It travels horizontally on the masseter with the transverse facial artery.[32,33] At the lateral border of the origin of zygomaticus major muscle is the substantive zygomatic retaining ligament (that attaches to the body of the zygoma). At the lateral border of zygomaticus major, after a branch is given off to supply the orbicularis oculi, entering the muscle at its inferolateral corner, the zygomatic nerve continues medially and then transitions to the underside of the muscles it innervates zygomaticus major and minor, and supplies them from the deep aspect in close association with the zygomatic ligaments. Careful dissection by vertical spreading of the scissors is crucial to avoid damaging this branch here.[16,24,34]

The upper buccal trunk exits the parotid, about in line with, but superficial to, the parotid duct and continues deep to the investing masseter fascia. Approaching the anterior edge of the masseter, this branch leaves the floor under the masseter fascia in close association with the upper key masseteric ligament.[5,35] The lower buccal trunk leaves the parotid lower down, at about the level of the earlobe and remains under the masseter fascia as it crosses under the floor of the premasseter space . Similarly, upon approaching the anterior edge of the masseter, in the upper membranous boundary of the premasseter space, the lower buccal trunk transitions from deep to gain the underside of the SMAS in close association with the upper surface of the lower key masseteric ligament.[18] After the nerves reach level 3, the zygomatic, upper and lower buccal trunks, and mandibular branch connect with each other before continuing their course to innervate the mimetic muscles. This accounts for the overlap in muscles innervated by these nerves.

The temporal and mandibular branches are the most significant in terms of surgical risks because of the lack of cross innervation of their target muscle. The marginal mandibular nerve is at risk where it is fixed by its close association with the retaining ligaments. Early in its course, around the angle of the mandible, this is within the PAF, and then well anteriorly by the mandibular ligament. Over most of its course, the mandibular branch is mobile, being in relation to the inferior

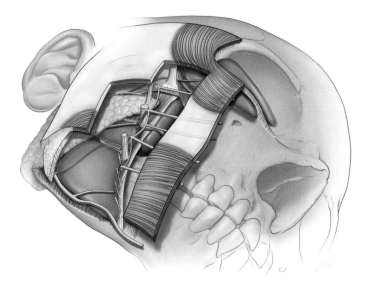

Fig. 6.12 The relationship between facial nerve branches, spaces and retaining ligaments. The nerves stay deep to and outside of the spaces at all times in the lateral face. In the boundary between the lateral and anterior face, the facial nerve branches transition from under layer 5 to enter layer 3, always in close association with the retaining ligaments of the face. (© Dr Levent Efe, CMI.)

boundary of the premasseter space. It is not necessary to dissect in the vicinity of the nerve because of the inherent mobility of the platysma where it overlies the jaw and sub-mandibular area. The mobility of the nerve as it travels within the inferior membranous boundary of the lower premasseter space accounts for the reported variability of the location of this part of its course (occasionally below the mandible).[36–38]

Aging changes of the face

The youthful face has the general appearance of high rounded fullness, while the aging process is characterized by a look of depletion and sagging, suggestive of tiredness. Changes with aging occur at every level of the facial anatomy, starting with the facial skeleton. A key unresolved question is how much of the change at each level is intrinsic aging and how much is secondary to the changes from adjacent layers. This is not easy to quantitate due to the difficulties of measurement of a single layer in the context of the complicated and interrelated layered structure.

Current understanding of the aging process remains largely empirical, given that it is based on the effectiveness of treatments designed to satisfy the requirements of patients for a younger appearance. Historically, stretching of loose facial skin (traditional facelift), removal of apparent tissue excess (traditional blepharoplasty), tightening the dermis and evening the complexion (early phenol peels and CO_2 laser resurfacing) and, in recent years, soft tissue volume augmentation (lipofilling and soft tissue fillers) have all had a positive impact on rejuvenating appearance. The success of each is attributed to having reversed a cause of facial aging. Yet, when each of these modalities is continued as the sole treatment, to further reverse the aging appearance, the results tend to be bizarre, leading to the conclusion that multimodal therapy is required to further reverse, what must be, multiple components of the aging process.

An understanding of the changes that occur in the layered anatomy forms the basis for logical treatment. Changes of the skin are readily observable and changes in the skeleton effecting layer 5 can also be observed radiologically. Because the changes within the superficial fascia (layers 2 and 3) are not directly measurable, empiricism has remained prevalent. A correlation of the surface anatomy changes of aging with the anatomy of layers 2, 3, and 4 indicates that bulging occurs over the roof of soft tissue spaces, which stand out in contrast to the absence of bulging of the adjacent cutaneous grooves. The grooves reflect the restriction imposed by the dermal insertions of the retaining ligaments at the boundaries of the spaces. The degree to which the bulging reflects true elongation from primary tissue degeneration and laxity and how much it is 'apparent' laxity secondary to loss of volume (skeletal and soft tissue) remains unanswered.

Skin

Skin aging is influenced by genetics, environmental exposure, hormonal changes and metabolic processes.[39–41] With aging, the supple skin of youth becomes thinned and flattened, with loss of elasticity and architectural regularity. Atrophy of the extracellular matrix is reflected by the decreased number of fibroblasts and decreased levels of collagen (especially types I and III) and elastin in the dermis. While chronological skin aging and photo-aging can be readily distinguished and considered separate entities, both share important molecular features, that of altered signal transduction that promote matrix-metalloproteinase (MMP) expression, decreased pro-collagen synthesis and connective tissue damage. Oxidative stress is considered of primary importance in driving the aging process, resulting in increased hydrogen peroxide and other reactive oxygen species (ROS) and decreased anti-oxidant enzymes.[42,43] These changes result in gene and protein structure alterations. Other environmental factors notably smoking accelerates skin aging, by between 10 and 20 years.[44] Increased collagenase and decreased skin circulation has been suggested as possible mechanisms. The muscles of facial expression flex the skin in a specific pattern. As the underlying collagen weakens and the skin thins, the dermis loses its capacity to resist the constant force of the muscles and these lines become etched in the skin and ultimately even at rest.

Subcutaneous tissue

The fibrous and fat components in the subcutaneous tissue are not a uniform but arranged in discrete compartments.[10] Over specific sites, due to the prominence of the subcutaneous fat it has been given specific names such as the malar fat pad and nasolabial fat. The boundary of these subcutaneous compartments corresponds to the location of the retaining ligaments, which pass superficially to insert into the dermis. In youth, transition between compartments is smooth and non-discernible. With aging, a series of concavities and convexities develop which separates these compartments. These changes have been attributed to a number of causes including fat descent, selective atrophy and hypertrophy and attenuation of the retaining ligaments that causes fat compartments malpositioning.[9,10,45,46] It is now apparent that fat descends minimally with aging.[47] As noted the subcutaneous fat is not a confluent layer that can descend with aging. Distinct compartmentalization by the retaining ligaments holds the fat in its relative positions.

Muscle aging

Skeletal muscles, in general, have been noted to atrophy up to 50% with age.[48] This may be applicable to the muscle of mastication such as the temporalis and masseter (compounded by the decreased demand and deterioration of the dentition with aging) although no specific study on the effect of aging on these muscles has been done to date. The mimetic muscle of the face, in contrast to skeletal muscles, may not undergo the same degree of degeneration with aging because of their constant use with facial expression. The orbicularis oculi has been noted to remain histologically unchanged with no loss of muscle fibers aging.[49] The upper lip elevators, zygomaticus major and levator labii superioris were also noted to remained unchanged with aging, based on magnetic resonance imaging (MRI) of their length, thickness and volume.[45] In contrast, the upper lip orbicularis atrophies with aging, with decreased muscle thickness, smaller muscle fascicles and increase in surrounding epimysium.[50]

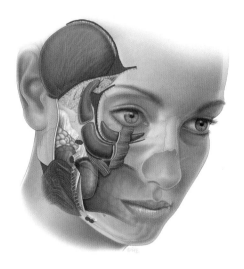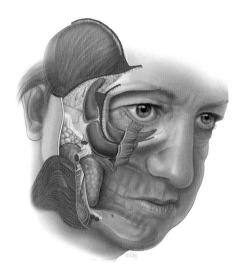

Fig. 6.13 In youth, the spaces are tight. The retaining ligaments are stout and the transition between spaces is not discernible. With aging, spaces expand to a greater extent than the laxity that develops in ligaments within their boundaries, resulting in bulges between areas of relative fixations. These spaces open with relative ease with blunt dissection. (© Dr Levent Efe, CMI.)

Facial spaces and retaining ligaments

The multi-linked fibrous system attenuates with aging, with decreasing strength of the ligaments and increasing laxity. The spaces expand with aging as well, to a greater extent than the laxity that develop in the ligaments within their boundaries, resulting in bulges between areas of relative fixations.[18] Accordingly, the spaces dissect easily in older patients, and the boundaries widen as the ligaments weaken.[13] In young people, the spaces are more potential that real and do not open quite so easily with blunt dissection *(Fig. 6.13)*.

Bone changes

The facial skeleton changes dramatically with aging *(Fig. 6.14)* and this has a profound impact on the appearance of the face with aging *(Fig. 6.15)*. At birth, the facial skeleton is under-developed and rudimentary. This explains why infants and toddlers often transiently have distinct mid-cheek segments (despite excellent tissue quality), which disappear as they grow older with the expansion of the mid-cheek skeleton.[51] Peak skeletal projection is probably attained in early adult-hood. Thereafter, while certain areas continue to expand,[4,52–55] selective areas of the facial skeleton undergoes significant resorption. Areas with strong predisposition to resorption include the superomedial and inferolateral aspects of the orbital rim, the midface skeleton, particularly that part contributed by the maxilla including the pyriform area of the nose and also the prejowl area of the mandible.[56–64] The resultant deficiencies in the skeletal foundation have a significant effect on the overlying soft tissues. In the mid-cheek in particular, retrusion of the maxilla causes increased prominence of the tear-trough and the nasolabial folds.[59] The retrusion of the facial skeleton causes the origin of the multi-linked fibrous retaining ligaments to be displaced posteriorly. This pulls the skin inwards, exaggerating the concavity between the areas of relative convexity that develop with aging. Retrusion of the mid-cheek with loss of projection gives the visual impression

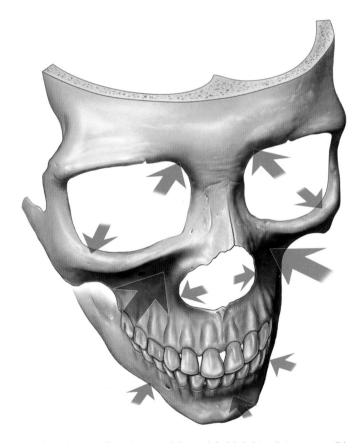

Fig. 6.14 Arrows indicate the areas of the craniofacial skeleton that are susceptible to resorption with aging. (© Dr Levent Efe, CMI.)

of tissue descent with aging. Some patients have a congeni-tally weak or inadequate skeletal structure. In such cases, the skeleton may be the primary cause of the manifestations of premature aging. Accordingly, patients who suffer premature facial aging, a weakness of the relevant part of the underlying skeleton is immediately suspect and should be addressed in order to obtain better aesthetic results.

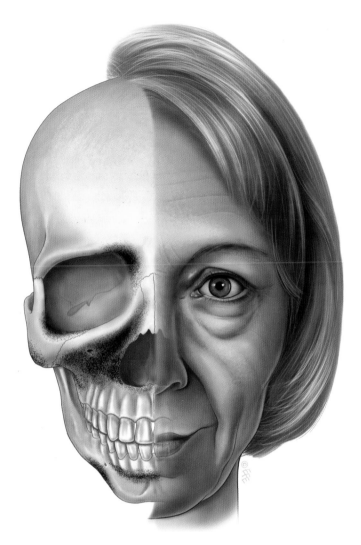

Fig. 6.15 The darker areas denote areas of greatest bone loss. Note how the stigmata of aging as manifested by the facial soft tissues correspond to the areas of weakened skeletal support due to bone loss. (© Dr Levent Efe, CMI.)

Regional changes observed with the aging face

Temple and forehead

The skin of the temple differs from that of the forehead, being thinner and less firmly supported to the underlying layers. The loose attachment reflects the underlying temporal space, which is extensive, and the nature of the surrounding temporal ligaments that are septal like and do not continue through the thin, loose subcutaneous layer over the temple to fix to the dermis as do facial ligaments elsewhere. This explains why deep layer procedures in the temple are not as effective in toning the overlying skin as they are, for example, in the cheek.

Corrugator muscle contraction is associated with the emotional states of grief and sadness.[65] The transverse head of corrugator supercilii moves the eyebrow medially and produce vertical glabella lines. The oblique head of the corrugator, the depressor supercilii and the medial fibers of the

orbicularis oculi act in concert to depress the medial brow and produce oblique glabella frown lines. The procerus, also a brow depressor causes transverse nasal skin lines. Laterally, the action of the lateral fibers of the orbicularis oculi with the transverse head of the corrugator supercilii promotes lateral brow ptosis. The ptosis of the lateral brow together and to a lesser extent, the laxity of the skin with aging produces a pseudoexcess of the upper eyelid skin. Frontalis muscle hypertonicity from lateral brow skin hooding and its reaction to the action of antagonistic muscles (corrugator supercilii, orbicularis oculi and procerus) results in the development of transverse forehead skin lines.[18,65] The medial brow in contrast, seldom descends with aging and in fact, may rise.[66,67] The mechanism responsible for this includes the chronic activation of the frontalis muscle. This may either be to elevate the brow/eyelid complex associated with clinical or subclinical levator system weakness or to relieve visual field obstruction due to excess lateral upper eyelid skin.[65] Anatomically, the frontalis muscle ends at approximately the temporal fusion line (superior temporal septum). Lateral to this, there is no upward vector to counteract the downward pull of brow depressors and gravity on the lateral brow. This may explain why descent preferentially occurs at the lateral brow.

The mid-cheek

The mid-cheek is the anterior part of the midface.[4] It is triangular in shape and bounded superiorly by the pretarsal part of the lower eyelid, medially by the side of the nose and the nasolabial groove below, and laterally around the lateral cheek where the arch of the zygoma meets the body. A smooth rounded mid-cheek is a powerful image of youth and gives a certain freshness to the face. With aging, the three mid-cheek segments become clearly discernible, as they become separated by the three cutaneous grooves of the mid-cheek; the nasojugal, palpebromalar and mid-cheek grooves.[4] This 'segmentation' of the mid-cheek has a profound impact on appearance that is responsible for giving the 'tired' look we associate with aging.

The soft tissues of the mid-cheek are structurally composed of three segments or "modules", with each overlying a specific part of the mid-cheek skeleton *(Fig. 6.16)*. The lid-cheek segment overlies the prominence of the inferior orbital rim, the malar segment overlies the body of the zygoma and the nasolabial segment overlies the anterior surface of the maxilla. The skeletal foundation of the mid-cheek borders the three bony cavities of the anterior face, the orbital, nasal and oral cavities. Because of the many spaces and limited bony support available, the mid-cheek has some intrinsic structural weaknesses. Three factors make the mid-cheek susceptible to aging changes. These are: (1) the wedge shape of the soft tissue of the mid-cheek, which are thin above and thicker below; (2) the natural posterior incline of the mid-cheek skeleton, from the relative prominence of the infra-orbital rim; and (3) the significant retrusion as a result of resorption of the maxilla with aging. This is not uniform, as the maxilla recedes more medially and inferiorly.[58–61] With early aging, the retrusion of the maxilla, along with a slight descent of the wedge shaped cheek soft tissue results in an appreciable reduction of volume of the upper cheek. The result is that the small amount of orbital fat over the prominent edge of the infraorbital rim, (originally concealed by the volume of the upper

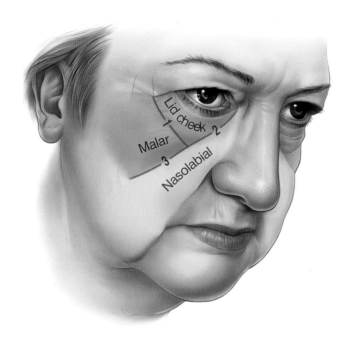

Fig. 6.16 The mid-cheek has three segments, the lid-cheek segment (blue) and the malar segment (green) are within the periorbital part and are adjacent to the nasolabial segment (yellow) in the perioral part, which overlies the vestibule of the oral cavity. The three grooves define the boundaries of the three segments and interconnect like the italic letter *Y*. The palpebromalar groove (1) overlies the inferomedial orbital rim and the nasojugal groove (2) which overlies the inferolateral orbital rim, then continues into the mid-cheek groove (3). (© Dr Levent Efe, CMI.)

cheek), now becomes revealed, especially the underside of the lid fat bulge over the middle part. The visual impression is of a 'lengthened' lower lid.[47] At the same time, the increased thickness of the soft tissue mass over the lower cheek tends to conceal the degree of maxillary resorption and gives the profound visual impression that the soft tissue mass has descended into the lower part of the mid-cheek.

Of the three segments of the mid-cheek, the lower lid segment changes the most dynamically with aging. It has two distinct grooves across its surface, which vary in their expression during the aging process, often co-existing. The upper is the infratarsal groove at the junction of the pretarsal and preseptal parts of the eyelid. The groove is defined by the lower boundary of the pretarsal muscle bulge. The pretarsal bulge in youth is the visual separation of the lid above and the cheek below. This so-called "high lid-cheek junction" is located well above the infraorbital rim and is a characteristic of youth. The infratarsal groove location does not change with aging, although its contour usually fades. The lower groove is the lid-cheek junction that relates to the lower edge of the preseptal part of the lid. It is not usually present in youth and appears with aging and then progressively deepens and descends slightly over time. Its shape when it first appears is a gentle C contour but as it "descends", particularly in its central portion, its shape changes to a progressively more angulated V shape with the medial side being formed by the developing nasojugal groove and the lateral side by the palpebromalar groove. The center of the V, the lowest and deepest part has the nasojugal groove continuing down the cheek as the mid cheek groove that separates the cheek into the malar and nasolabial segments. The reason why this contour demarcation changes while the skin itself does not descend is

explained by difference in the tissue layers. In level 4, the orbicularis retaining ligament is not rigid where it is over the center of the inferior orbital rim, so distension results in relative sliding between it and layer 3, the orbicularis oculi. As the lid-cheek junction becomes more prominent, it visually takes over from the infratarsal groove and becomes the new separation between the lower eyelid and the cheek. This is the basis for the commonly used but misleading phrase "lengthening of the lid cheek junction with aging", which is in fact the result of a visual shift from the prominence of the infratarsal groove in youth to the lid-cheek junction with age. Correction of the aging of the lid cheek segment of the mid-cheek, the visibly descended contour of the lid cheek junction and long lower lid, has gained the colloquial name of "blending the lid cheek junction."

Lower face

The jowl and the labiomandibular fold in the lower face are not present in youth, and develop with aging. With the description of the concept of soft tissue spaces of the face, and specifically the premasseter space, the mechanism for the formation of the jowl can now be understood on an anatomical basis.[68] With the onset of aging, laxity develops in the roof of the premasseter space associated with attenuation of the anterior and inferior boundaries. The major retaining ligaments (the key masseteric and mandibular) in contrast remain relatively strong and at these locations the superficial fascia remains firmly fixed to the underlying deep fascia. Distension of the weaker masseteric ligaments at the anterior border of the lower premasseter space (below the key masseteric ligament) and inferior displacement of the buccal fat (within the buccal space) is the anatomical basis for the development of the labiomandibular fold. The mandibular ligament demarcates the transition from the labiomandibular fold above and the jowl below. The jowl develops as a result of distension of the roof of the lower premasseter space with resultant descent of the tissues below the body of the mandible. The more prominent the jowl, the more apparent will be the cutaneous tethering provided by the mandibular ligament. Accordingly, the anatomical solution to correcting these aging changes is to reduce the inferiorly displaced buccal fat and to tighten the roof of the premasseter space.

Considerations for correcting aging changes of the face based on the anatomy of the aging face

Dissection planes

The subcutaneous plane of dissection (*level 2*) is the most commonly used plane in facelifts, either in isolation or more commonly with some form of SMAS management from the superficial aspect (*Fig. 6.17*).[69–71] A distinction should be drawn between subcutaneous dissection over the lateral face from that over the anterior face. This plane of dissection is perceived to be "safe" as dissection remains superficial to the facial nerve branches at all times and is the main appeal of level 2 dissection. The subcutaneous dissection can be

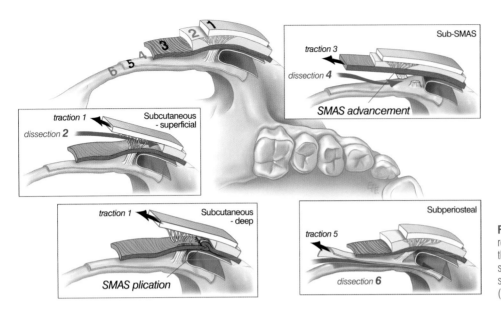

Fig. 6.17 Alternative levels for dissection and redraping in facelifts. Dissection can be performed through any one of three alternative layers, namely subcutaneous (level 2), subSMAS (level 4) and subperiosteal for the upper two-thirds of the face. (© Dr Levent Efe, CMI.)

performed either in the superficial subcutaneous or deep subcutaneous level. In the former, there is more density of the retinacular cutis fibres as the multi-linked ligaments branches out before inserting into the dermis. In the latter on the outer surface of the SMAS, there are fewer fibres, which tend to be thicker and stronger. The deep subcutaneous layer is not uniform in its tenacity: some areas, as over the facial spaces are inherently easier to dissect, while others that overlie the ligament are more adherent and require sharp release.[7,72] For example, over the malar eminence at McGregor's patch, where the zygomatic ligaments are located, sharp release is often needed as is required over the mandibular ligament. In contrast, in the lower face over the premasseter space, the subcutaneous layer separates quite readily, requiring only blunt finger dissection.

SubSMAS dissection (*level 4*): in the scalp, this is the preferred tissue plane for dissection as the scalp readily separates from the underlying periosteum (level 5) through the avascular areolar tissue with ease and inherent safety. Bruising and swelling is kept to a minimum because of this anatomy. In the face proper, while the anatomical principles remain the same, level 4 is potentially the most risky plane to dissect because of the facial nerve branches which transition through this level, from level 5, to supply the facial muscles in level 3. However, it should be noted that similar to the situation in the scalp where raising the flap at level 4 gives a robust and structurally integrated composite flap that can be effectively tightened, subSMAS dissection in the face has the same advantages and potential benefits.[73,74] Dissection can be performed safely in level 4 by applying the understanding of the three-dimensional anatomy of the face described earlier; the key being the facial spaces, which provide safe access through this layer. Because these spaces are 'pre-dissected', access is quick, atraumatic, and easy. An example of this is the lower premasseter space. Subcutaneous dissection is performed to approximately 30 mm anterior to the tragus through the zone of fixation, the platysma auricular fascia (PAF), where the SMAS is fused to the deep fascia including the parotid capsule. Because the objective of the surgery is to correct laxity in the mobile anterior face, the level of dissection used in the lateral face is of secondary importance. A further benefit of leaving

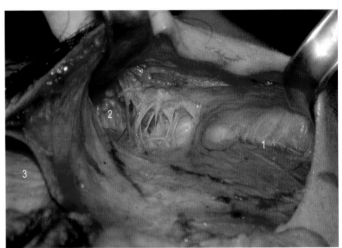

Fig. 6.18 Using the facial spaces for safe and anatomical access to subSMAS dissection in facelifts. (1) Premasseter space. (2) Prezygomatic space. (3) Upper temporal space.

the PAF intact is that it is strong and can be used for suture fixation.[75] Once dissection has proceeded beyond the PAF (indicated by the posterior border of the platysma), the SMAS should then be incised to gain direct access into the lower premasseter space. The space can then be opened by gentle blunt dissection only, to define the boundaries of the space. The premasseter space below and the prezygomatic space above form a series of spaces in the anterior face *(Fig. 6.18)*. The boundaries of the spaces, reinforced by retaining ligaments, are where the important anatomy is located. These need to be precisely released to eliminate their tethering effect on the soft tissues,[76] which is more difficult in younger patients as the ligaments are denser and stronger. Clear visualization, optimized by lifting the opened adjacent facial spaces, is beneficial. When blunt scissors are used with gentle vertical spreading of the blades the surrounding fat and areolar tissue separate to reveal the ligaments and the facial nerve branches in relation to them. With further lifting, the ligaments become more certainly defined as they tighten further, at which time they can be safely released while the nerves, being obliquely orientated, dislodge out of the way, unaffected by the controlled stretching. The subSMAS spaces can be used to safely and atraumatically access various part of the face, the deep temporal space to the lateral brow,[13] the preseptal space to the lower eyelid, and the prezygomatic space to the mid-cheek.[15,16]

Level 5: subperiosteal "lifts" have the appeal of safety as far as the facial nerve risk is concerned as they are superficial and the remote nerves never cross this plane.[77–79] However, there are inherent limitations to subperiosteal lifts.. The accumulated aging changes across all five layers are elevated as part of the subperiosteal lift. Overcorrection is required to effect the desired changes of soft tissue shape and skin tone, to compensate for the "lift-lag" phenomenon, which is in proportion to the soft tissue thickness and laxity. Accordingly, subperiosteal lifts work best in areas where the layers are more compacted as the lift-lag is minimized. An example being in the brow where subperiosteal lifts are effective and popular.[80] Where the layers are thicker, such as the nasolabial segment of the mid-cheek, the lift-lag phenomenon significantly limits the improvement that can be achieved. Because of the unyielding nature of the periosteum, extensive undermining beyond the target area is needed or alternatively a "periosteal release" immediately beyond the area that requires lifting to isolate the area to a limited island of periosteum

Placement of sutures

While adequate surgical release is needed for mobility, it is the surgical fixation that achieves the desired effect by holding the mobilized soft tissue in its new position.[76] The strength and tenacity of the superficial fascia is not uniform. The areas where the retaining ligaments are located have inherent ligamentous reinforcement, making them ideal for suture placement. It is also the location in which traction gives the most natural appearance, as these are the natural suspension sites of the face. Accordingly, the suture fixation should be placed where the retaining ligaments are located. Where fixation sutures are placed in the anterior face in subSMAS surgery, they function as replacements for the retaining ligaments that have weakened or have been divided in order to mobilize the composite flap. Accordingly, the replacement sutures should replicate the quality of support provided by the original ligaments as the "mobile" spaces remain. In this respect braided permanent sutures are advantageous as they stimulate collagen and elastic deposition within the suture similar to a ligament.[81] The platysma auricular fascia, a diffuse ligamentous area on the lateral face, provides an ideal area both anatomically and physically to fix the facelift flap, due to its inherent strength.

Summary

This chapter has been structured to assist the reader to develop a conceptual understanding of facial anatomy and how it changes with aging. It is the framework that unifies the detailed anatomical information now available in the literature. Once understood, this knowledge provides the anatomical foundation for the logical and sound selection of surgical techniques for rejuvenation of the aging face.

 Access the complete references list online at **http://www.expertconsult.com**

4. Mendelson BC, Jacobson SR. Surgical anatomy of the mid-cheek; facial layers, spaces, and mid-cheek segments. *Clin Plast Surg.* 2008;35:395–404.

5. Stuzin JM, Baker TJ, Gordon HL. The relationship of the superficial and deep facial fascias: relevance to rhytidectomy and aging. *Plast Reconstr Surg.* 1992;89(3): 441–449.

   A discussion of the concept of facial soft tissue being arranged in concentric layers, and the SMAS as the "investing" layer of the superficial mimetic muscles of the face. The relationship between the deep and superficial fascias is described, with acknowledgement of "areola" planes and areas of dense fibrous attachments, including true osteocutaneous ligaments and other coalescences representing the retaining ligamentous boundaries of the face. Age-associated laxity of the retaining ligament was noted to be a key component of facial aging.

7. Furnas DW. The retaining ligaments of the cheek. *Plast Reconstr Surg.* 1989;83:11.

10. Rohrich RJ, Pessa JE. The fat compartments of the face: anatomy and clinical implications for cosmetic surgery. *Plast Reconstr Surg.* 2007;119(7):2219–2227.

13. Muzaffar AR, Mendelson BC, Adams WP Jr. Surgical anatomy of the ligamentous attachments of the lower lid and lateral canthus. *Plast Reconstr Surg.* 2002;110(3): 873–884.

14. Moss CJ, Mendelson BC, Taylor GI. Surgical anatomy of the ligamentous attachments in the temple and periorbital regions. *Plast Reconstr Surg.* 2000;105(4): 1475–1490.

   A thorough description of the retaining ligaments of the temporal and periorbital regions is given. The term "ligamentous adhesion" is introduced to increase the understanding of the system, and there is emphasis on the relations of the temporal branch of the facial nerve and the trigeminal branches to structures visualized in surgery rather than to less useful landmarks which are not. A discussion of age related changes to the region compliments one of surgical approach with respect to the anatomy described.

16. Mendelson BC, Muzaffar AR, Adams WP Jr. Surgical anatomy of the mid-cheek and malar mounds. *Plast Reconstr Surg.* 2002;110(3):885–911.

18. Knize DM. Anatomic concepts for brow lift procedures. *Plast Reconstr Surg.* 2009;124(6):2118–2126.

68. Mendelson BC, Freeman ME, Wu W, et al. Surgical anatomy of the lower face: the premasseter space, the jowl, and the labiomandibular fold. *Aesthetic Plast Surg.* 2008;32 (2):185–195.

   Introduces the concept of the "premasseter" space, age-related changes, and utility for safe subSMAS dissection. Distinction is made between this space, over the lower part of the masseter, and another space overlying the upper part of the masseter where the neurovascular structures, the accessory lobe of the parotid gland and duct are located. The true shape of the anterior border of the masseter muscle is described, with the border ending anteroinferiorly at the mandibular ligament. This description completes the picture of the retaining ligaments as a continuous border separating the anterior and lateral parts of the face. The relations of the facial nerve branches, particularly that of the lower buccal trunk, to the masseter and its fascia is described.

75. Mendelson BC. Surgery of the superficial musculoaponeurotic system: principles of release, vectors and fixation. *Plast Reconstr Surg.* 2001;107(6): 1545–1552.

This article highlights the importance of adequate release of retaining ligaments of the SMAS in repositioning of the composite flap. Inadequate release can lead to suboptimal advancement of the flap, and worse, distortion of the flap if the direction of pull is incorrect, due to unwanted rotation about the parts of the retaining ligamentous system which have been left intact. The biomechanical function of the retaining ligaments is described as "quarantining" sections of the SMAS with less substantial fixation (areas now appreciated as subSMAS facial soft tissue spaces), preventing unwanted traction on areas of the face distant to the desired action in facial expression. There is discussion on the advantage of extensive SMAS mobilization in allowing multiple and varied force vectors to be applied, which allows proper anatomical repositioning of the soft tissue of the face.

7

Forehead rejuvenation

Richard J. Warren

SYNOPSIS

- Detailed knowledge of forehead anatomy is the basis for rejuvenation strategies of the forehead region.
- Eyebrow position is the net result of forces which depress the brow, forces which raise the brow and the structures which tether the eyebrow in place.
- Brow depression is caused by glabellar frown muscles, the orbicularis and gravity. Frontalis is the only effective brow elevator.
- Attractiveness of the periorbital region is intimately related to eyebrow shape and eyebrow position as it relates to the upper eyelid and the upper lid sulcus.
- Aging causes enlargement of the orbital aperture as well as changes in eyebrow shape. In a subset of individuals there is ptosis of the entire forehead complex.
- Key elements of forehead rejuvenation are the attenuation of frown muscle action and the repositioning of ptotic eyebrow elements. The lateral eyebrow is often the only portion requiring elevation.
- Forehead rejuvenation can be accomplished using a combination of surgical and non-surgical techniques.
- If surgical elevation of the brow complex fails early, it is usually due to lack of soft tissue release. If it fails late, is usually due to failure of fixation.
- Many methods of soft tissue fixation and bony fixation have been proven effective in maintaining the position of the surgically elevated brow.

 Access the Historical Perspective section online at
http://www.expertconsult.com

Introduction

The periorbital region is the most expressive part of the human face. The eyes are central, framed above by the eyebrows, and below by the cheek. Alteration in components of the orbital frame, as well as the eyelids themselves, will profoundly affect facial appearance. The aesthetic balance created by surgery can project strong human emotions, ranging from joy to sadness and from restfulness to fatigue.

In the younger individual, aesthetic alteration of the forehead is generally limited to the nonsurgical alleviation of glabellar frown lines and lateral orbital wrinkles. These issues are discussed in Chapters 3 and 4. Occasionally, surgery is indicated to change the basic shape of a youthful eyebrow. In the older individual, the forehead typically becomes ptotic laterally, while in the orbit, there is a relative loss of orbital fat together with an accumulation of loose eyelid skin. Understanding the interplay between these complex anatomical changes is critical in choosing an appropriate surgical strategy to rejuvenate the upper third of the face.

Anatomy

The frontal bone is crossed laterally by a curved ridge called the temporal crest (also called the temporal ridge or the superior temporal fusion line of the skull). This is a palpable landmark which separates the temporal fossa and the origin of the temporalis muscle from the forehead portion of the frontal bone *(Fig. 7.1)*. It also marks a change in nomenclature as tissue planes transition from lateral to medial. The deep temporal fascia covering the temporalis muscle attaches along the temporal ridge and continues medially as the periosteum which covers the frontal bone. Similarly, the superficial temporal fascia (also known as the temporal parietal fascia) continues medially as the galea aponeurotica which encompasses the frontalis muscle.

The surgical significance of the temporal crest line is that all fascial layers are tethered to bone in a band approximately 5 mm wide immediately medial to the palpable ridge. This has been called the zone of fixation.[22,23] Where this zone approaches the orbital rim at its inferior end, the fascial attachment widens and becomes more dense, forming the orbital ligament *(Fig. 7.2)*. All fascial attachments in this region must

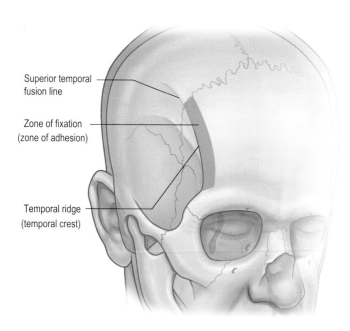

Fig. 7.1 Bony anatomy of the forehead and temporal fossa. The palpable temporal ridge separates the temporal fossa from the forehead. The zone of fixation (*aka* zone of adhesion, superior temporal septum) is a 5 mm wide band along the temporal ridge where all layers are bound down to periosteum.

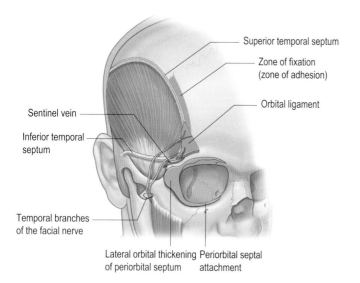

Fig. 7.2 Fascial attachments around the orbital rim. The inferior end of the zone of fixation is the orbital ligament. The lateral orbital thickening is a lateral extension of the septum which extends across the lateral orbital rim onto deep temporal fascia.

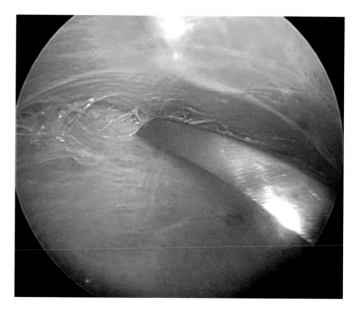

Fig. 7.3 Endoscopic view of the inferior temporal septum, right side.

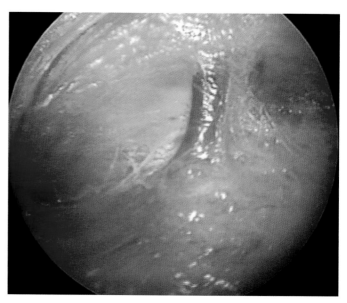

Fig. 7.4 Endoscopic view of the medial zygomaticotemporal vein (sentinel vein), right side.

be released from bone when a full thickness forehead flap is being repositioned.

Some fascial structures in this area have been named by different authors, generating some confusion. The superior temporal septum[24] and the zone of adhesion[16] are alternate terms used to describe the zone of fixation. The temporal ligamentous adhesion[24] describes the lower portion of the zone of fixation and the orbital ligament. The inferior temporal septum[24] and the orbicularis-temporal ligament[25] both describe the criss-crossing white fibers which loosely attach the superficial to the deep temporal fascia.

The inferior temporal septum is a useful landmark during endoscopic dissection from above, because it separates the safe upper zone containing no vital structures from the lower zone where facial nerve branches travel in the cavity's roof. The medial zygomatic temporal vein (sentinel vein) is also present in this lower zone, adjacent to the lateral orbital rim. The temporal branches pass immediately superior to this vein (*Figs 7.3, 7.4*).

Galea

Knize has described galeal anatomy in detail.[26] In the forehead, the galea aponeurotica splits into a superficial and deep

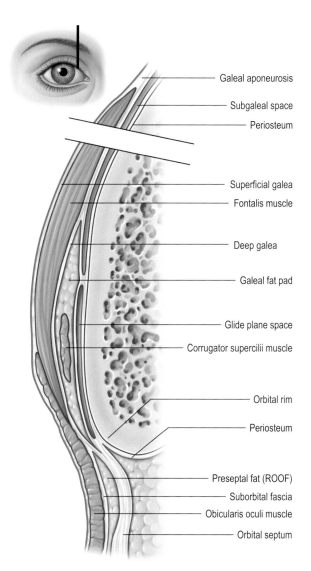

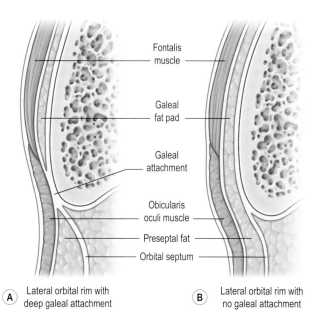

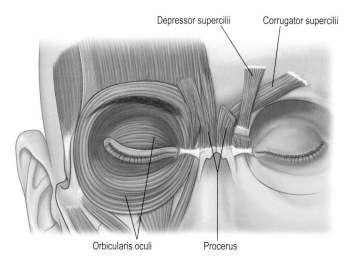

Fig. 7.5 Relationship of galea to surrounding tissue as it splits to encompass the frontalis muscle, the galeal fat pad, and the glide plane space. The corrugator supercilii traverses through the galeal fat pad as it courses from its deep bony origin to its superficial insertion in the orbicularis and dermis.

Fig. 7.6 Lateral orbital rim variation. On the left, galeal attachment tethers the overlying brow. On the right, the galeal fat pad is contiguous with retro orbicularis oculi fat, potentially making the lateral brow prone to ptosis.

Fig. 7.7 Glabellar frown muscles.

layer encompassing the frontalis muscle *(Fig. 7.5)*. Inferiorly, the deep galea layer separates further into three separate layers: one layer immediately deep to the frontalis forming the roof of the galeal fat pad, a second layer forming the floor of the galeal fat pad but not adherent to bone, and a third layer adherent to periosteum. The two deepest layers define the glide plane space between the galeal fat pad and the skull. Inferiorly, the septum orbitale divides orbital fat from PreSeptal fat (also known as retro orbicularis oculi fat or ROOF).

When the eyebrow is raised by frontalis contraction, the soft tissue slides over the glide plane space. The galeal fat pad extends across the entire width of the lower 2 cm of the forehead; medially it surrounds the supra orbital and supra trochlear nerves as well as portions of the frown musculature. The galeal fat pad is separated from the preseptal fat (ROOF) by a reflected layer of galea. Laterally, this separation is thought to be variable, with some individuals having a continuous layer of fat from galeal fat pad to the preseptal fat *(Fig. 7.6)*.[26]

Muscle

Eyebrow level is the result of a balance between the muscular forces which elevate the brow, the muscular forces which depress the brow, and the universal depressor: gravity *(Fig. 7.7)*.

Brow depressors in the glabella originate from bone medially, inserting into soft tissue. The procerus runs vertically, the depressor supercilii and orbiculars run obliquely, and the corrugator mostly runs transversely. The transverse corrugator

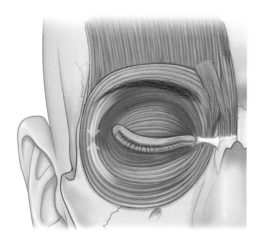

Fig. 7.8 Lateral orbicularis acts like a sphincter, depressing the lateral brow.

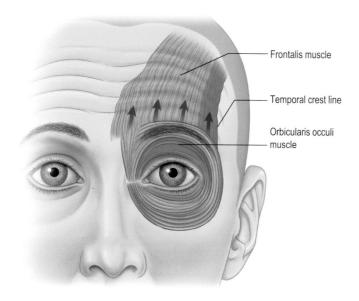

Frontalis muscle

Temporal crest line

Orbicularis occuli muscle

Fig. 7.9 Frontalis acts to raise the eyebrow complex. On contraction, most movement occurs in the lower third of the muscle, and action is strongest on the medial and central eyebrow.

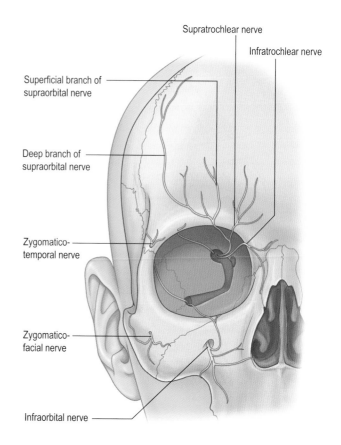

Supratrochlear nerve

Infratrochlear nerve

Superficial branch of supraorbital nerve

Deep branch of supraorbital nerve

Zygomatico-temporal nerve

Zygomatico-facial nerve

Infraorbital nerve

Fig. 7.10 Sensory nerves.

Sensory nerves

Innervation to the upper periorbita is supplied by the supraorbita and supratrochlear nerves, as well as two lesser nerves, the infratrochlear, and zygomaticotemporal (*Fig. 7.10*).

The infratrochlear nerve exits the orbit medially supplying sensation to the nasal dorsum and medial orbital rim. It is seldom damaged and rarely a cause of postoperative concern.

The zygomaticotemporal nerve exits posterior to the lateral orbital rim piercing the deep temporal fascia just inferior to the sentinel vein. In brow lifting, with complete release of the lateral orbital rim, it is often avulsed. Consequences of this are minimal and temporary.

The supratrochlear nerve usually exits the orbit superomedially although this is variable, and it occasionally will exit near the supraorbital nerve. It immediately divides into 4–6 branches which can pass superficial (anterior) to the corrugator, or more frequently, directly through the substance of the corrugator. These branches then become more superficial, innervating the central forehead.

The supraorbital nerve exits the superior orbit either through a notch in the rim, or through a foramen superior to the rim. Much variation occurs with foramina present about 20% of the time.[28] The location of the notch or foramen is between 16 and 42 mm from the midline, with a mean of 25 mm. A useful landmark for this is a palpable notch, or failing that, the mid-papillary line. When a foramen is present, it has been found as far as 19 mm above the rim. Because of such variation, blind dissection from above should be discontinued at least 2 cm above the orbital rim.

supercilii is the largest and most powerful of these muscles. It originates from the orbital rim at its most supero-medial corner, with the large transverse head later passing through galeal fat becoming progressively more superficial until it interdigitates with the orbicularis and frontalis at a skin dimple which is visible when the patient frowns.[27]

The orbicularis encircles the orbit acting like a sphincter. Medially and laterally the orbicularis fibers run vertically and act to depress brow level. Laterally, orbicularis is the only muscle which depresses brow position (*Figs 7.8, 7.9*).

Frontalis is the only elevator of the brow. It originates from the galea aponeurotica superiorly, and interdigitates inferiorly with the orbicularis. Contraction raises this muscle mass, and in so doing, lifts the overlying skin which contains the eyebrow. Due to its deficiency laterally, the primary effect of frontalis contraction is on the medial and central portions of the eyebrow.

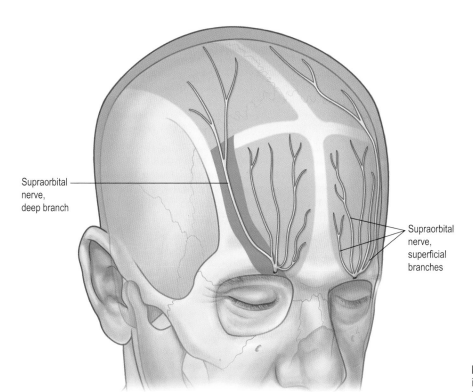

Supraorbital nerve, deep branch

Supraorbital nerve, superficial branches

Fig. 7.11 The deep branch of the supraorbital nerve travels in a 1 cm wide band between 5 and 15 mm medial to the temporal ridge.

The supraorbital nerve immediately divides into two distinct segments: superficial and deep. The superficial branch pierces orbicularis and frontalis, dividing into several smaller branches which travel on the superficial surface of the frontalis to innervate the central forehead as far posteriorly as the first 2 cm. of hair. The rest of the scalp, as far back as the vertex, is innervated by the deep branch. The deep branch courses superiorly in a more lateral location, remaining between the periosteum and the deepest layer of galea. As it travels superiorly, it becomes more superficial, piercing frontalis to innervate the skin.

It is a double branch approximately 60% of the time.[29] An important fact during endoscopic brow lifting is that the deep branch runs in a 1 cm wide band, which is between 5 mm and 15 mm medial to the palpable temporal ridge *(Fig. 7.11)*.

Motor nerves

The temporal branch of the facial nerve is the only motor nerve of concern in this area. Loss of this branch would result in a brow ptosis and asymmetry due to impaired frontalis action *(Fig. 7.12)*. The anatomy of this nerve has been well described.[30–33]

The temporal branch enters the temporal fossa as multiple (2–4) fine branches which lie on the periosteum of the middle third of the zygomatic arch. Between 1.5 cm and 3.0 cm above the arch, these branches become more superficial, entering the superficial temporal fascia (temporoparietal fascia), traveling on to innervate the frontalis, superior orbicularis and glabellar muscles.[34]

A number of different landmarks are commonly used to predict the course of the temporal branches. These include:

1. The middle third of the palpable zygomatic arch

2. 1.5 cm lateral to the tail of the eyebrow

Facial nerve, temporal branch

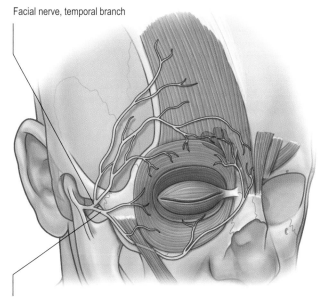

Facial nerve, zygomatic branch

Fig. 7.12 Facial nerve branches in the periorbital region. Note the corrugator has dual innervation from the temporal branch and the zygomatic branch. The temporal branch crosses the middle third of the zygomatic arch as 2–4 branches.

3. Parallel and adjacent to the inferior temporal septum

4. Immediately superior to the sentinel vein (medial zygomaticotemporal vein).

In all forehead lift procedures, dissection planes are designed to protect the temporal branches. This can be done by staying deep to them, which requires dissecting directly on deep temporal fascia in the temple and in the subgaleal or subperiosteal planes over the frontal bone. Alternatively, dissection can be kept superficial to the frontalis, the orbicularis, and the superficial temporal fascia.

Patient presentation

Forehead aging

Historically, the visible signs of forehead aging have been described in two ways. First, and most obvious are the furrows caused by the repetitive action of underlying muscles: transverse lines are due to the eyebrow lifting action of the frontalis, while glabellar frown lines are due to the corrugator, depressor supercilii, and the procerus. The corrugator, being the most transverse of these muscles causes vertical frown lines, the depressor supercilii, being oblique, causes oblique folds which cut across the orbital rim, and the vertically running procerus causes transverse lines at the radix (*Figs 7.13, 7.14*).

Second, it has been assumed that the forehead/eyebrow complex becomes ptotic with age, encroaching on the orbit, causing a pseudo-excess of upper eyelid skin. While consistent with the age-related ptosis of most other body parts, the

facts are not so clear. Some studies actually suggest that eyebrows may rise with age, at least in the medial and central portions (*Figs 7.15, 7.16*).[35–37]

Logically, the medial and central eyebrows could rise over time through the action of frontalis. This may be caused by a subconscious reaction to excess upper lid skin or to early eyelid ptosis caused by senile levator disinsertion. Both phenomena will stimulate frontalis contraction to open the line of sight. Also at play is personal habit, exhibited by the brow elevation seen when most individuals are confronted with a mirror, or on facing a camera. Closing the eyes will usually, but not always, relax the frontalis, causing the eyebrows to drop. Frontalis paralysis due to facial nerve injury or botulinum toxin will always drop the level of the eyebrow, indicating that some resting tone is normal.

A final factor is the shape of the orbital aperture which appears to enlarge with age, the superomedial brow rising, and the inferolateral orbital rim dropping and receeding.[38,39] This could contribute to a rising medial brow, because of soft tissue attachment and the soft tissue support provided by the trunk of the supraorbital nerve (*Fig. 7.17*).

As described earlier, the level and shape of the eyebrow is the result of a balancing act between the many forces of brow depression and the only elevator, which is the frontalis muscle. The lateral portion of the brow is particularly sensitive to this interplay because frontalis action is attenuated laterally.[40] Against the unrelenting force of gravity and the lateral orbicularis oculi, the principle resistance to lateral brow decent is soft tissue attachment. This attachment is variable and may be absent, leaving the lateral brow free to move.[41] The result is often a gradual ptosis of the lateral third of the brow, relative to the medial brow. This effect will be accentuated if a patient also has a rising medial brow. The resulting downturned lateral brow imparts a look of sadness, tiredness and age.

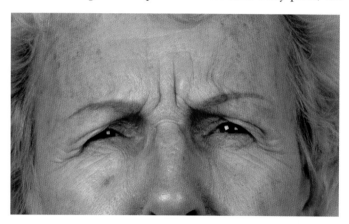

Fig. 7.13 Patient frowning. The paired vertical folds are caused by the corrugator supercilii and the transverse lines at the nasal radix are caused by the procerus. The paired oblique lines are caused by the depressor supercilii and the medial orbicularis oculi. Laterally the "crow's feet" lines are caused by the vertically running fibers of the orbicularis oculi.

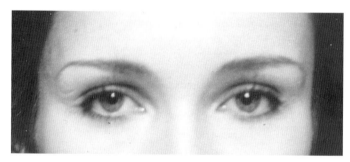

Fig. 7.15

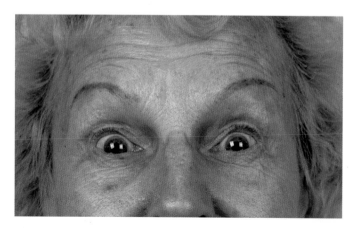

Fig. 7.14 Patient raising eyebrows. The transverse forehead lines are caused by the frontalis.

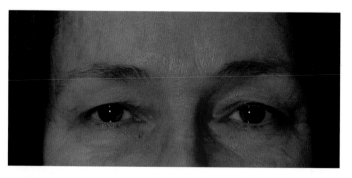

Fig. 7.16 From age 25–50, photographs demonstrate a 3–4 mm rise in the medial and central brows.

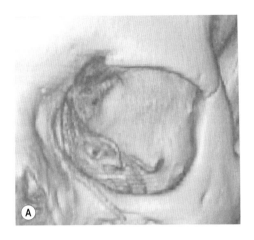

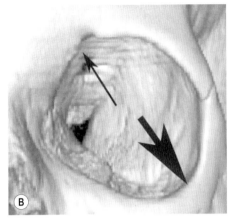

Fig. 7.17 Orbital changes with age: orbital volume expands, most marked superomedial and inferolateral. (With permission from Kahn DM, Shaw RB. Aging of the bony orbit. A three-dimensional computed tomographic study. Aesthet Surg J 2008; 28(3):258–264.)

Another effect of a dropping lateral brow is a bunching up or a pseudoexcess of lateral upper eyelid skin. In response to this, Flowers and Duval have described the phenomenon of compensated brow ptosis where patients subconsciously contract the frontalis to open their line of sight.[42] This further exacerbates the appearance of a downturned lateral brow.

Many patients recognize these changes and treat themselves to eyebrow plucking, make-up or tattooing in order to make the lateral brow appear higher. Alternatively, they may seek blepharoplasty to deal with lateral soft tissue hooding, unaware that the ptotic lateral brow is the most significant factor. The unsuspecting surgeon who performs blepharoplasty in this circumstance will see the frontalis relax, unmasking the compensated brow ptosis, causing the medial and central brow to fall.

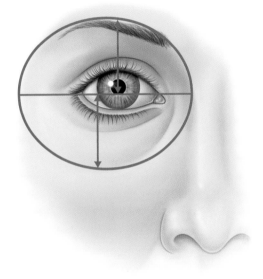

Fig. 7.18 An oval formed by the eyebrow above, and the nasojugular fold below, should have the pupil at its equator. (Adapted from: Gunter J, Antrobus S. Aesthetic analysis of the eyebrows. Plast Reconstr Surg 1997; 99:1808–1816.)

Aesthetics

Traditional teaching has been that the correct eyebrow position is at or above the supra orbital rim. While usually true, this axiom is overly simplistic, because eyebrow height is only one of many variables. In many individuals, the lateral brow becomes more ptotic than the medial brow, altering brow shape. Studies have demonstrated that our impression of people can be affected by altering the shape of their eyebrows, implying that the shape of the brow is more important than its absolute height.[43,44] Also, age related changes in eyebrow position do not occur in isolation. The upper lid sulcus may become more hollow as fat is lost, upper lid skin may become more redundant, and there may be a modest degree of senile eyelid ptosis. As mentioned earlier, reflex brow raising is often the result, with a rising medial brow in relation to the lateral brow (Fig 7.16).

Gunter observed that the eyebrow and naso-jugular fold create an oval shape, and that in an attractive eye, the pupil will lie at the equator of that oval (Fig. 7.18).[45] Applying this analysis is a useful exercise to determine if brow position is an issue (Fig. 7.19).

Ovals which are vertically wide look aged, while vertically narrow ovals look youthful.

There is an intimate relationship between eyebrow position and the eyelid. The ratio of the visible eyelid from the lashes to the palpebral fold should be one-third, and at most one half the distance from the lashes to the lower border of the

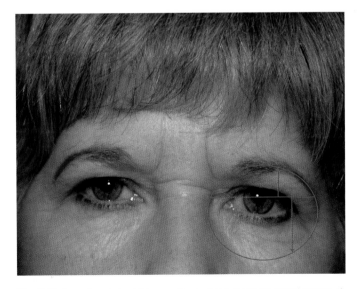

Fig. 7.19 On oval analysis of this case, the pupil lies above the natural equator of the oval. This confirms a low lying eyebrow plus or minus a low lying nasojugular fold.

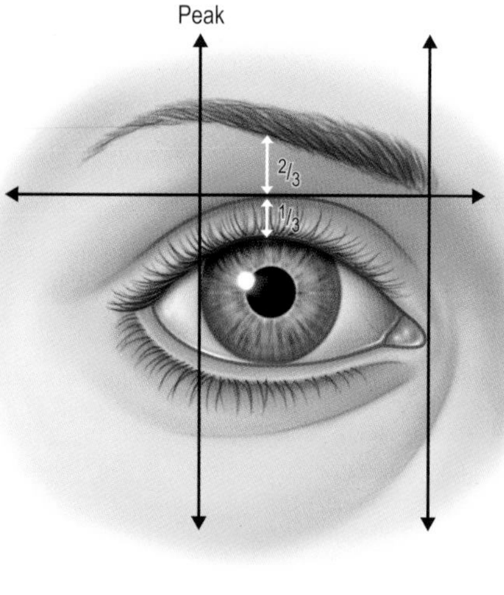

Fig. 7.20 The modern ideal brow/upper eyelid complex.

eyebrow *(Fig. 7.20)*.[45] A number of different factors may change this ratio:

- Changing eyebrow height
- Lid ptosis or lid retraction
- Redundant upper eyelid soft tissue
- Loss of upper sulcus fat.

Any one of these issues can be treated independently or in conjunction with a brow lift. Brow repositioning is a powerful tool but it must be considered in the context of other possibilities such as ptosis repair, blepharoplasty, and fat grafting to the upper lid sulcus.

Individualization is a key component to any periorbital rejuvenation. Gender, ethnicity, eye prominence and overall facial proportions must be considered. For example, Oriental faces look attractive with higher eyebrows than would seem appropriate for the Caucasian face. Complicating matters, the "ideal" eyebrow has also changed over time. Renaissance painters tended to portray their subjects with normal eyebrows and relatively hollow upper sulci, while in the 1950s, eyebrows became very high and arched.[44] Individual variation aside, there are certain themes which define "the ideal eyebrow" *(Fig. 7.20)* in the era when this text is being written:

1. The medial eyebrow level should lie over the medial orbital rim
2. The medial border of the eyebrow should be vertically in line with the medial canthus
3. The eyebrow should rise gently, peaking slightly at least two-thirds of the way to its lateral end; typically this peak lies vertically above the lateral limbus
4. The lateral tail of the brow should be higher than the medial end
5. The male brow should be lower and less peaked.

Patient selection

Most patients are not aware of the many variables involved in periorbital rejuvenation, and they may not want the multiple procedures required to treat all of these components. For that reason, identifying the main component of every patient's periorbital aging is important. Old photographs are very helpful in determining which aging changes predominate. Such a review will also help to focus patients' perspectives on exactly how they have aged, and what, if any, rejuvenation they would like to undergo.

Assessment of the patient should be done with the patient's head in the vertical position; the patient will be sitting or standing. The following issues are evaluated: visual acuity; eyebrow and orbital symmetry; position of anterior hairline; thickness of scalp hair; transverse forehead lines; glabellar frown lines; thickness of eyebrow hair; eyebrow height; axis of the eyebrow (downward or upward lateral tilt); shape of the eyebrow (flat or peaked); passive and active eyebrow mobility, and the presence of old scars or tattoos. The upper eyelids should be assessed for soft tissue redundancy, for hollowness and for lid level (ptosis versus lid retraction). The patient should be examined with eyes open and eyes closed. With the eyes closed, the frontalis can usually be made to relax, revealing the true position and shape of the eyebrows. If the brow is held in this position when the patient opens their eyes, the eyebrow/eyelid relationship without frontalis effect will be revealed. The surgeon can then manually reposition the eyebrows, experimenting with various positions and different vectors of mobilization.

Patients may be a candidate to have their entire brow complex lifted, or more commonly to have only part of the eyebrow raised, thus improving eyebrow shape. Occasionally, this may involve raising the medial brow only, but most typically it involves raising the lateral third to half of the brow, with little or no lift of the medial portion. Weakening or eliminating the glabellar frown muscles is a useful parallel objective. Numerous methods are available, ranging from botulinum toxin, to surgical techniques which may weaken, or completely eliminate the glabellar frown muscles.

Surgical techniques

Surgical rejuvenation of the forehead has changed dramatically from the one-size-fits-all approach of an earlier era. As our understanding of anatomy and aging has improved, our available surgical techniques have also evolved. Alongside this evolution, the introduction of botulinum toxin for aesthetic indications has changed many of our fundamental concepts.

Open coronal approach

The coronal approach was long considered the "gold standard" against which other techniques must be measured. Many surgeons still consider it to be the most effective method for modification of the forehead. The principal advantage of this approach is the unparalleled surgical exposure which facilitates release and mobilization of brow soft tissues, as well as the modification of glabellar muscles under direct vision. Surgical results are stable, and long lasting.

The technique involves an incision over the top of the head, classically about 6–8 cm behind the anterior hairline, although this incision can be placed almost anywhere in the hair-bearing scalp *(Fig. 7.21)*. An incision as far back as the vertex

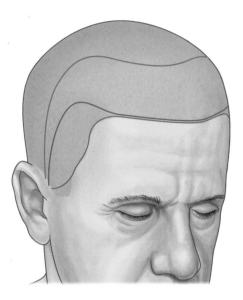

Fig. 7.21 Coronal and anterior hairline approaches.

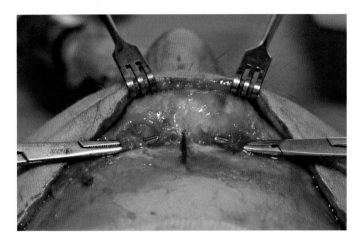

Fig. 7.23 Coronal approach showing corrugator muscles.

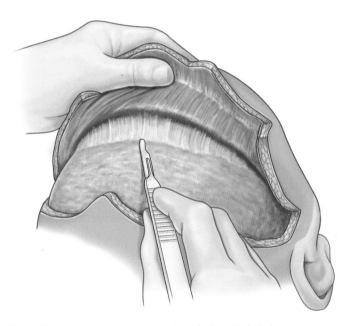

Fig. 7.22 Open coronal flap dissection shown in the subgaleal plane.

will be at the watershed between posterior and anterior running sensory nerves, thus reducing scalp numbness. However, a more anterior incision involves less scalp dissection, better visibility, and a closer point of traction on the eyebrows *(Figs 7.21–7.23)*.

The incision is made full-thickness down to periosteum, and the anterior flap can then be raised in either the subperiosteal, or more commonly, the subgaleal plane. Under direct vision, the flap is elevated down to the orbital rim. If glabellar muscles are to be exposed, the galea must be breached on its deep surface, entering the galeal fat pad for access to the muscles *(Fig. 7.22)*. The frown muscles, corrugator, depressor supercillii and procerus can be removed or weakened as necessary *(Fig. 7.23)*. Typically, resection of the corrugator requires dissection of the supratrochlear nerve branches which course through the substance of this muscle. It is often advantageous

to leave some galeal attachment medially to prevent over-elevation of the medial scalp. Otherwise, for proper brow elevation, there must be a thorough release of the galeal attachments along the central and lateral orbital rims. The zone of fixation will be released as dissection progresses laterally over the deep temporal fascia. The trunk of the supraorbital nerve is identified and preserved. To reposition the brows, the flap is drawn supero-laterally, and a full-thickness strip of scalp is excised. Laterally, scalp excision will range from 1 to 3 cm, but centrally, little or no scalp is excised. The scalp is closed directly, approximating galea and skin. Although deeper fixation can be added, the classic open coronal lift relies on scalp excision alone to maintain brow position.

Disadvantages of the open coronal approach include scalp numbness, which may be permanent, a long scar, disruption of hair follicles, and scalp dysesthesia. Inevitably, the anterior hairline will be raised and some hair-bearing scalp will be sacrificed. This technique should be used cautiously or not at all in patients with a high anterior hairline, with thin hair, or in patients who may eventually lose their hair.

Anterior hairline approach

This incision is usually placed along the anterior hairline, until it reaches the hairline laterally, where it transitions into the hair-bearing temporal scalp. Alternatively, it can follow the hairline over its entire extent *(Fig. 7.21)*. Certain technical details help minimize scar visibility. These include placing the incision within or just posterior to the fine hair of the anterior hairline, and beveling the incision parallel to the hair follicles. Alternatively, the principle of cutting across the hair follicles may be used in order to promote growth of hairs through the resulting scar.[46] The incision, when made as a slightly wavy line, tends to create a less visible scar. Skin tension is minimized by approximating the galea, and doing a meticulous skin closure.

From the anterior hairline incision, dissection of the forehead flap can be done in one of three different planes: subperiosteal, subgaleal, and subcutaneous. Regardless of the plane being used, the anterior hairline approach offers the same advantage as the coronal approach, namely excellent surgical exposure, without the disadvantage of moving the anterior

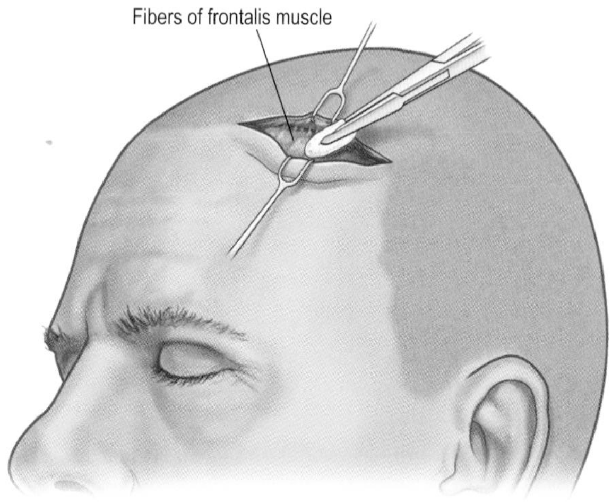

Fibers of frontalis muscle

Fig. 7.24 Limited hairline subcutaneous approach.

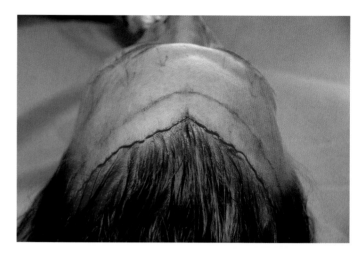

Fig. 7.25 Anterior hairline incision to lower the anterior hairline.

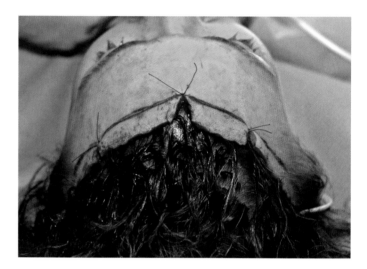

Fig. 7.26 Hairline lowering.

hairline posteriorly. In addition, there are two unique advantages.

Because there is no undermining of hair follicles, the surgeon has the option of a subcutaneous dissection plane which is done on the superficial surface of the frontalis muscle. This allows brow elevation without the need to divide any sensory nerves, and also provides a potential effacement of deep transverse forehead lines. A popular modification of this method is a short incision in the widow's peak, which is used to target only the lateral brow *(Fig. 7.24)*.[47]

The anterior hairline approach can also be used to lower an excessively high anterior hairline or to lower overly high eyebrows. These problems may be congenital but often are the result of previous brow lift surgery. Hairline lowering involves a posterior dissection past the vertex of the skull, in order to extensively mobilize the scalp. Releasing incisions are made in the galea, and the scalp is advanced, utilizing bony fixation to maintain the new hairline position *(Figs 7.25, 7.26)*. If the anterior approach is used to lower the eyebrows, bony fixation is done at the supraorbital rim *(Figs 7.25, 7.26)*.[48–50]

The main disadvantage of the anterior hairline incision is the presence of a permanent scar along the anterior hairline. In addition, if the scalp incision is full-thickness, the resulting scalp denervation will be worse than with the coronal approach because the posterior running sensory nerves are transected closer to their origin. Lastly, a full dissection of forehead skin may compromise cutaneous blood flow leading to partial skin necrosis.

Endoscopic approach

More than any other innovation, the introduction of endoscopy to facial aesthetic surgery stimulated the quest for better understanding of forehead and temple anatomy. Basic anatomic principles are integral to the theory of endoscopic brow lifting. Laterally, brow lifting is accomplished by releasing all galeal attachments and relying on some method of mechanical fixation to maintain the scalp in a higher position. Medially, brow lifting happens passively by removing muscular depressors, and allowing the frontalis to lift unopposed.

The principle advantages of the endoscopic brow lift are a very good surgical exposure, magnification of the surgeon's

view, and short, undetectable incisions. In addition, the scalp denervation associated with the open coronal approach is largely avoided *(Fig. 7.27)*.

Access for the procedure is through 3–5 small (1–2 cm) incisions placed within the hair-bearing scalp. Forehead flap dissection is done to the same extent as with the open coronal lift. Medial to the zone of fixation, the dissection plane can be subgaleal, or the more popular subperiosteal approach. Flap dissection can be done blindly at first, but is completed under endoscopic control when approaching the orbital rim in order to avoid damaging the supraorbital nerve. Lateral to the zone of fixation, dissection is done against the deep temporal fascia, with the inferior temporal septum and the sentinel vein used as landmarks for the position of the overlying temporal nerve branches. The medial and lateral dissection pockets are then joined by going from lateral to medial. Soft tissue attachments along the lateral orbital rim and the supraorbital rim are then visualized and released. Dissection down the lateral orbital rim may be preperiosteal or subperiosteal. The supraorbital nerve is visualized during orbital rim release. If glabellar musculature is to be removed, the supratrochlear nerves are visualized as they pass through the substance of the corrugator

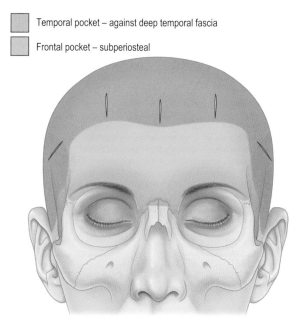

Temporal pocket – against deep temporal fascia

Frontal pocket – subperiosteal

Fig. 7.27 Five port endoscopic approach.

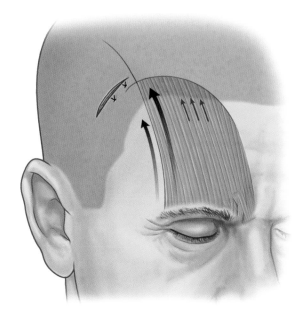

Fig. 7.28 Temple approach.

supercilii. Care is taken to avoid excessive release of the flap medially to prevent over-elevation medially and to avoid separation of the eyebrows. Once dissected, the forehead flap is drawn superiorly and somewhat laterally. Specific vectors have been described in this regard,[51] but the surgeon can make an artistic decision during preoperative planning, with appropriate vectors customized for each individual patient. While some authors have suggested that no fixation is necessary,[17] two methods of fixation are usually employed: suture fixation in the lateral dissection pocket from the superficial to the deep temporal fascia, and bony fixation in the medial dissection pocket. In an attempt to make the operation more predictable, a wide variety of fixation devices and techniques have been described.[52]

The main disadvantages of endoscopic brow lifting are: the technical demands of using endoscopic equipment, the potential of overly elevating or separating the medial eyebrows, and some uncertainty about maintaining adequate fixation.[15]

Temple approach

A temple approach involves a full-thickness scalp incision in the temple, lateral to the temporal crest line.[53] Knize improved and popularized this approach with dissection on the deep temporal fascia, releasing of the lateral orbital rim, the supraorbital rim, and the zone of fixation with using an endoscope *(Fig. 7.28)*.[14] After flap mobilization, fixation is done with sutures between the superficial and deep temporal fascia. If surgical modification of glabellar frown muscle modification is desired, a transpalpebral approach can be used.

Disadvantages of this method include limited visibility of the central and medial supraorbital rim, and the fact that the fixation vector applied to the lateral eyebrow is oblique, rather than vertical, which may be inappropriate for some patients *(Fig. 7.28)*.

Transpalpebral approach – muscle modification

Using the upper lid blepharoplasty approach, the glabellar frown muscles can be approached directly.[54,55] This is an excellent method to attenuate glabellar frown lines in patients who do not require a forehead lift. It can also be used as an adjunct to the patient undergoing an isolated elevation of the lateral third of the brow. The advantage of this method is a hidden incision, which may be used for two purposes, blepharoplasty and frown muscle ablation.

Through an upper blepharoplasty incision, dissection proceeds superiorly deep to the orbicularis oculi, but superficial to the orbital septum. Over the supraorbital rim, the transverse running fibers of the corrugator supercilii will be found. The muscle becomes more superficial as it coursed laterally through the galeal fat pad, eventually combining with the orbicularis oculi and the lower frontalis. The muscle can be removed, although care must be taken to protect supra trochlear nerve branches which travel through the substance of the muscle or around its inferior border. Medially in the wound, the depressor supercilii can be seen coursing almost vertically, and the orbicularis oculi courses obliquely. Portions of these muscles are removed. The procerus can be transected by dissecting across the root of the nose.

The main disadvantages of this approach include potential damage to sensory nerves (supraorbital and supratrochlear), and increased bruising and edema compared to an isolated upper lid blepharoplasty *(Fig. 7.29)*.

Lateral brow approach

The lateral brow approach utilizes a more medial incision than the temple approach. Its location is based on the observation that the most effective vector for lateral brow lifting seems to be directly along the temporal crest line *(Fig. 7.30)*.

Video 1

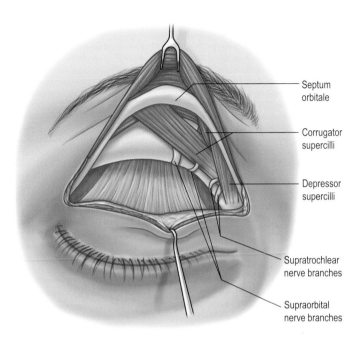

Fig. 7.29 Transpalpebral exposure of the frown musculature.

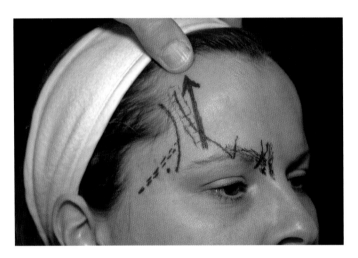

Fig. 7.30 Preoperative marking for modified lateral brow lift. The planned vector of pull is marked. Laterally, the purple dashed lines mark the expected course of the facial nerve temporal branches. The purple dot represents the sentinel vein. The curved purple line marks the temporal crest line which is accentuated when the patient clenches her teeth, contracting the temporalis. Medial to the crest line, the black cross hatched band is the expected course of the deep branch of the supraorbital nerve, in purple. The corrugator supercilii, depressor supercilii and procerus are marked in black.

A variety of fixation methods can then be used including simple scalp excision, deep temporal sutures, or fixation to bone.[56] The modified lateral brow lift is a hybrid procedure utilizing a 5–6 cm incision in the scalp, approximately 1 cm behind the hairline.[16] Because the desired vector is directly along the course of the deep branch of the supraorbital nerve, this procedure is designed to be nerve sparing. Orbital rim release can be done with or without an endoscope. A full-thickness excision of scalp is done (like an open coronal lift), but nerve branches are preserved as a neurovascular bundle. Fixation is accomplished with deep temporal sutures and by

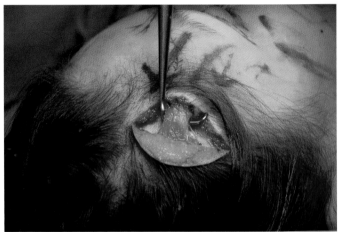

Fig. 7.31 The neurovascular bundle of the deep branch of the supraorbital nerve. The subperiosteal pocket has been developed medially and the temporal pocket against the deep temporal fascia has been developed laterally. The two pockets are joined along the temporal crest line. When the lateral brow is raised, the neurovascular bundle will telescope up under the scalp closure.

galeal closure. The main advantages of this method are those of the endoscopic approach, plus the same strength of fixation provided by a coronal lift. The main disadvantage, compared with the pure endoscopic approach, is a slightly longer incision *(Fig. 7.31)*.

Direct suprabrow approach

Because the eyebrow is a cutaneous structure, the most effective method to lift it would theoretically be a subcutaneous approach done adjacent to the eyebrow itself. This simple technique was described almost a century ago. An excision of full-thickness skin is done along the upper margin of the eyebrow, or alternatively within a deep forehead crease. On closure, there is initially a 1:1 relationship between the amount of skin removed and brow elevation, but the surgeon should plan for a 50% relapse in the first few months following the procedure. The closer the incision is to the eyebrow, the less will be the relapse. The principle advantages of this technique are: the surgery is easy; it is well tolerated by the patient; there is no scalp denervation; there is no risk to motor nerves, and the result is relatively predictable.

The principle disadvantages of this method are the visible scar it creates and that fact that over time, brow depressing forces will once again stretch out the skin, causing a recurrence of brow ptosis. Certain individuals, especially older men with deep forehead creases, or thick eyebrows may be good candidates for this procedure, which can easily be repeated if necessary.

Transpalpebral browpexy

During upper lid blepharoplasty, the ptotic lateral brow can be addressed through the same upper lid incision.[57,58] The lateral portion of the superior orbital rim is easily exposed, and dissection proceeds superiorly over the frontal bone, superficial to the periosteum. Dissection should continue for 2–4 cm above the orbital rim, or at least 1 cm above the level of planned fixation. Several sutures are then used to tether the mobilized brow in a more superior position, fixating the underside of the orbicularis to the periosteum. Alternate methods of fixation to bone can also be used. Overly tight sutures must be avoided because of suture dimpling in the eyebrow. A more modest pexy is achieved if the cut edge of orbicularis oculi is simply suture to the orbital rim, with no superior dissection at all.[59] Advantages of transpalpebral browpexy are the ease of the procedure and a hidden scar. The principle disadvantage is the limited effect achieved and questionable longevity.

Suture suspension browpexy

A number of methods have been developed to elevate the brow only using sutures, with no dissection at all. Methods include barbed sutures or suture loops which are placed blindly through subcutaneous tunnels. The obvious advantage of these methods is extreme simplicity and relative safety, while the principle drawback is their limited effect, and poor longevity.[60]

Postoperative care

Postoperative care for minor brow procedures is limited to head elevation, cold packs, ointment application, and analgesics.

More extensive procedures (e.g., open coronal lift, endoscopic lift) will require dressings and the possibility of drains for 24 h. Use of bupivacaine to block the supraorbital and supratrochlear nerves is very helpful in decreasing the incidence of postoperative headache. Patients can shower after 48 h, with scalp suture removal in 7–10 days.

After initial healing, measures can be adopted to prevent relapse of lateral brow ptosis. The use of botulinum toxin in the lateral orbicularis is helpful, as is the use of sunglasses and sun avoidance to prevent squinting in the first postoperative month.

Outcomes and complications

The surgical result of forehead rejuvenation depends on the type of deformity, the procedure done and the quality of its execution.

Lesser procedures generally produce lesser results, but for the individual patient with appropriate expectations, this may be adequate.

More involved procedures afford the opportunity for greater anatomic intervention, more dramatic results and potentially greater longevity. However, as our understanding of the aging brow has progressed, it is clear that brow ptosis is not as significant a factor as was once thought, and therefore, overly aggressive surgery can produce an exaggerated, un-aesthetic result. Historically, the main problems encountered by surgeons performing browlift procedures have been aesthetic – in some cases overdoing the surgery and in other cases, failing to achieve a predictable long term result.

Every patient presents with a different set of challenges, the most important of which is to first make a proper aesthetic

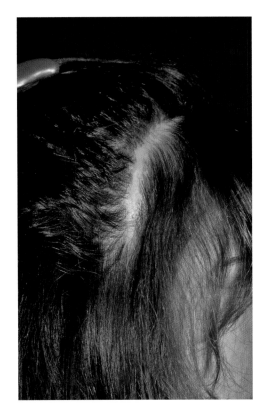

Fig. 7.32 Scar alopecia after coronal brow lift.

diagnosis. Once the decision has been made to raise all or part of the brow complex, a myriad number of surgical procedures are available. No one method can be considered best, but rather, the surgical procedures must be chosen based on the individual patient's needs. In addition, every surgeon will have greater comfort with some procedures compared with others, and it is incumbent on surgeons to carefully analyze their results in order to give patients a realistic idea of what can be expected.

In addition to the aesthetic issues mentioned above, surgical complications of brow rejuvenation include scar alopecia, hematomas, infections, contour deformities, and nerve damage *(Fig. 7.32)*.

Significant problems with brow positioning and shape may be treated with secondary procedures. Alopecia due to hair follicle damage may be temporary, but if permanent can be treated with scar excision or hair grafting.

Hematomas are uncommon, but if they occur, are treated with drainage. Infections are rare, consistently reported at less than 1%, and are treated with wound care and appropriate antibiotics.[18] Contour deformities can occur in areas of muscle excision; these problems are ideally prevented by the intraoperative utilization of filling material such as fat or temporal fascia. If identified late, similar tissue can be added at a separate procedure.

Sensory nerve damage is a common problem, and is universal with some types of procedures. With coronal incisions, all posterior running sensory nerves are routinely transected. The resulting scalp denervation will extend to the vertex, but will gradually improve, sometimes over several years. With limited incisions, sensory nerves may be traumatized

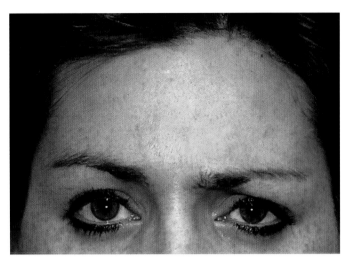

Fig. 7.33 Temporary neurapraxia of left temporal branch after coronal brow lift.

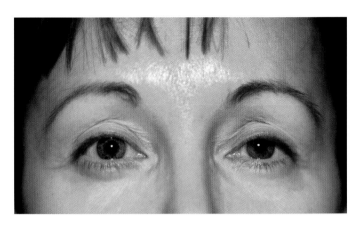

Fig. 7.34 Over elevated medial brow after endoscopic brow lift.

due to traction, cautery, or instrumentation. Temporary neurapraxia of the supratrochlear nerves after frown muscle ablation is almost universal, with sensory return typically appearing by 2–3 weeks. Similarly, temporary neurapraxia of the supraorbital rim is very common after a thorough release of the supraorbital rim.

The only motor nerve in the forehead is the temporal branch of the facial nerve, and damage to this nerve is the most worrisome complication. Temporary neurapraxias are relatively common, but permanent damage to the temporal branch is fortunately very rare. Should a neurapraxia develop, watchful waiting is a must *(Fig. 7.33)*.

Secondary procedures

As mentioned above, minor issues such as areas of alopecia and contour deformities in the glabella, can be treated with simple procedures.

The most common reason for revision surgery after brow surgery is to correct aesthetic deformities. Not infrequently,

overly aggressive brow lift surgery can create an unaesthetic eyebrow shape, most frequently an over-elevation of the medial brow *(Fig. 7.34)*.

Minimal deformities can be corrected with botulinum toxin in the central frontalis. If the medial brow has been aesthetically over-elevated, but the lateral brow remains unelevated, the lateral brow can be elevated as a separate maneuver.

Alternatively, the medial brow can be lowered, a procedure which involves a full release of the scalp's attachment to the underlying skull, lowering of the medial brow, and bone anchoring to the medial orbital rim.[50]

If there is simply a loss of effect from brow lift surgery, the situation can often be resolved to the patient's satisfaction with a conservative upper lid blepharoplasty. However, if the loss of effect is significant, repeat brow lifting may be necessary, preferably using a different technique and a different dissection plane.

In the case of a temporal branch palsy which does not improve with time, treatment options include applying botulinum toxin to the normal side, or alternatively, performing another brow lift on the affected side.

Access the complete references list online at **http://www.expertconsult.com**

1. Paul, MD. The evolution of the brow lift in aesthetic plastic surgery. *Plast Reconstr Surg.* 2001;108(5): 1409–1424.

   In this paper, the author thoroughly reviews the published history of brow lift surgery, from 1919 to 2001.

14. Knize DM. Limited incision foreheadplasty. *Plast Recontstr Surg.* 1999;103:271–284.

16. Warren RJ. The modified lateral brow lift. *Aesthetic Surg J.* 2009;29(2):158–166.

20. Guyuron B, Kopal C, Michelow BJ. Stability after endoscopic forehead surgery using single-point fascia fixation. *Plast Reconstr Surg.* 2005;116: 1988.

22. Knize DM. An anatomically based study of the mechanism of eyebrow ptosis. *Plast Reconstr Surg.* 1996;97(7):1321–1333.

   In this paper, the author presents the results of careful anatomic dissections to delineate the fascial structures which govern eyebrow stability. Surgical implications are described in the second paper in the same journal.

24. Moss CJ, Mendelson BC, Taylor I. Surgical anatomy of the ligamentous attachments in the temple and periorbital regions. *Plast Reconstr Surg.* 2000;105:4: 1475–1490.

   The authors describe a different way of describing fascial structures surrounding the orbit and creating structural layers in the temple. A number of anatomic terms are introduced for the first time.

26. Knize DM. Galea aponeurotica and temporal fascias. In: Knize DM, ed. *Forehead and temporal fossa: anatomy and technique.* Philadelphia: Lippincott Williams & Wilkins; 2001:45.

    This text thoroughly presents the anatomy of the temporal fossa, the forehead and the soft tissues which relate to the eyebrows. Knize combines several anatomical studies to summarize this anatomy, while several additional authors contribute to the technique portions of the book.

36. Matros E, Garcia JA, Yaremchuk MJ. Changes in eyebrow shape and position with aging. *Plast Reconstr Surg.* 2009;124(4):1296–1301.

41. Knize DM. Muscles that act on glabellar skin: A closer look. *Plast Reconstr Surg.* 2000;105:350.

45. Gunter J, Antrobus S. Aesthetic analysis of the eyebrows. *Plast Reconstr Surg.* 1997;99:1808–1816.

    The authors analyze the features of periorbital attractiveness. They conclude that eyebrow aesthetics must be considered in concert with the entire periorbital area, including the eyelids. They describe novel ways to analyze eyes for attractiveness and identify eight features of attractive eyes.

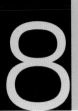

Blepharoplasty

Julius Few Jr. and Marco Ellis

SYNOPSIS

■ Blepharoplasty is a vital part of facial rejuvenation. The traditional removal of tissue may or may not be the preferred approach when assessed in relation to modern cosmetic goals.

■ A thorough understanding of orbital and eyelid anatomy is necessary to understand aging in the periorbital region, and to devise appropriate surgical strategies.

■ Preoperative assessment includes a review of the patient's perceptions, assessment of the patient's anatomy, and an appropriate medical and ophthalmologic examination.

■ Surgical techniques in blepharoplasty are numerous and should be tailored to the patient's own unique anatomy and aesthetic diagnosis.

■ Interrelated anatomic structures including the brow and the infraorbital rim may need to be surgically addressed for an optimal outcome.

 Access the Historical Perspective section online at
http://www.expertconsult.com

Introduction

Properly performed aesthetic periorbital surgery is one of the most rejuvenating of all facial surgeries performed today. Properly conceived and executed, it proves a tremendous source of joy for both surgeon and patient. Done poorly, it can lead to a lifetime of disfigurement and functional problems for the patient, sleepless nights for the surgeon, and dissatisfaction for both participants. The problem is magnified because aesthetic periorbital surgical procedures are among the most commonly performed in plastic surgery practices.

Traditional methods of aesthetic periorbital surgery often produce suboptimal results. A departure from the standard techniques of the past is recommended. Most plastic surgeons know there is a better way, and those who persist with

traditional techniques may soon be deviating from a new standard of surgical care. It is this new standard that is advocated in this chapter. When they are understood and adopted, these new standards eliminate the classic complications and risks associated with traditional techniques.

Instead of the common practice of excising precious upper and, to a somewhat lesser degree, lower eyelid tissue, it is preferable to focus on restoration of attractive, youthful anatomy. To expect that the simple removal of tissue will always result in beautiful or youthful eyes is unrealistic because this may not fully correct the aging eye deformity.

One should first conceptualize the desired outcome, then select and execute procedures accurately designed to achieve those specific goals. For this task to be accomplished, several important principles are advocated (*Box 8.1*). Enthusiastically embraced, this approach is likely to result in excellent aesthetic quality of surgical outcomes.

Basic science/disease process

Essential and dynamic anatomy

It is an absolute necessity that the surgeon understands the essential and dynamic periorbital anatomy to effect superior aesthetic and functional surgical results. No surgeon should perform surgery without fully understanding the aesthetic and functional consequences of the choices.[2–5]

Osteology and periorbita

The orbits are pyramids formed by the frontal, sphenoid, maxillary, zygomatic, lacrimal, palatine, and ethmoid bones (*Fig. 8.1*). The periosteal covering or periorbita is most firmly attached at the suture lines and the circumferential anterior orbital rim. The investing orbital septum in turn attaches to the periorbita of the orbital rim, forming a thickened perimeter known as the arcus marginalis. This structure reduces the

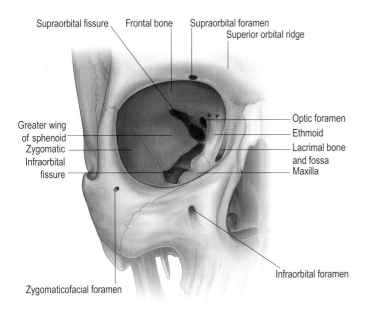

Fig. 8.1 Orbital bones. Frontal view of the orbit with foramina.

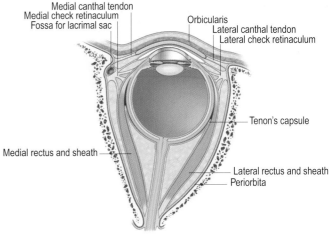

Fig. 8.2 Horizontal section of the orbit showing the lateral retinaculum formed by the lateral horn of the levator, lateral canthal tendon, tarsal strap, the Lockwood suspensory ligament, and lateral rectus check ligaments.

<hr>

Box 8.1 Principles for restoration of youthful eyes

- Control of periorbital aesthetics by proper brow positioning, corrugator muscle removal, and lid fold invagination when beneficial.
- Restoration of tone and position of the lateral canthus and, along with it, restoration of a youthful and attractive intercanthal axis tilt.
- Restoration of the tone and posture of the lower lids.
- Preservation of maximal lid skin and muscle (so essential to lid function and aesthetics) as well as orbital fat.
- Lifting of the midface through reinforced canthopexy, preferably enhanced by composite malar advancement.
- Correction of suborbital malar grooves with tear trough (or suborbital malar) implants, obliterating the deforming tear trough (bony) depressions that angle down diagonally across the cheek, which begin below the inner canthus.
- Control of orbital fat by septal restraint or quantity reduction.
- Removal of only that tissue (skin, muscle, fat) that is truly excessive on the upper and lower lids, sometimes resorting to unconventional excision patterns.
- Modification of skin to remove prominent wrinkling and excision of small growths and blemishes.

perimeter and diameter of the orbital aperture and is thickest in the superior and lateral aspects of the orbital rim.[6]

Certain structures must be avoided during upper lid surgery. The lacrimal gland, located in the superolateral orbit deep to its anterior rim, often descends beneath the orbital rim, prolapsing into the postseptal upper lid in many persons. During surgery, the gland can be confused with the lateral extension of the central fat pad destined for removal during aesthetic blepharoplasty. The trochlea is located 5 mm posterior to the superonasal orbital rim and is attached to the periorbital. Disruption of this structure can cause motility problems.[7]

Lateral retinaculum

Anchored to the lateral orbit is a labyrinth of connective tissues that are crucial to maintenance of the integrity, position, and function of the globe and periorbital. Understanding how to effectively restore these structures is key to periocular rejuvenation by canthopexy. These structures, known as the lateral retinaculum, coalesce at the lateral orbit and support the globe and eyelids like a hammock *(Fig. 8.2)*.[8–10] The lateral retinaculum consists of the lateral canthal tendon, tarsal strap, lateral horn of the levator aponeurosis, the Lockwood suspensory ligament, Whitnall's ligament, and check ligaments of the lateral rectus muscle. They converge and insert securely into the thickened periosteum overlying the Whitnall tubercle. Controversy exists surrounding the naming of the components of the lateral canthal tendon. Recent cadaveric dissections suggest that the lateral canthal tendon has dual insertions. A superficial component is continuous with the orbicularis oculi fascia and attaches to the lateral orbital rim and deep temporal fascia by means of the lateral orbital thickening. A deep component connects directly to the Whitnall tubercle is classically known as the lateral canthal tendon *(Fig. 8.3)*.[11]

In addition, the tarsal strap is a distinct anatomic structure that inserts into the tarsus medial and inferior to the lateral canthal tendon.[12] In contrast to the canthal tendon, the thick tarsal strap is relatively resistant to laxity changes seen with aging. The tarsal strap attaches approximately 3 mm inferiorly and 1 mm posteriorly to the deep lateral canthal tendon, approximately 4–5 mm from the anterior orbital rim. It shortens in response to lid laxity, benefiting from release during surgery to help achieve a long-lasting restoration or elevation canthopexy *(Fig. 8.4)*. Adequate release of the tarsal strap permits a tension-free canthopexy, minimizing the downward tethering force of this fibrous condensation. This release along with a superior reattachment of the lateral canthal tendon is key to a successful canthopexy.

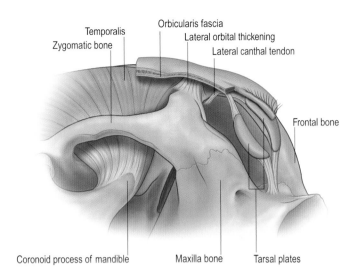

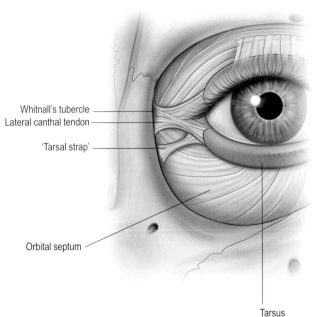

Fig. 8.3 Lateral canthal tendon has separate superficial and deep components. The deep component attaches inside the orbital rim at Whitnall's tubercle. The superficial component passes from the tarsal plates to the periosteum of the lateral orbital rim and lateral orbital thickening. Both components are continuous with both superior and inferior lid tarsal plates. (Adapted from Muzaffar AR, Mendelson BC, Adams WP Jr. Surgical anatomy of the ligamentous attachments of the lower lid and lateral canthus. Plast Reconstr Surg 2002; 110(3):873–884.)

Fig. 8.4 The deep portion of the lateral canthal tendon inserts securely into the thickened periosteum overlying Whitnall's tubercle. The tarsal strap is a distinct anatomic structure that suspends the tarsus medial and inferior to the lateral canthal tendon to lateral orbital wall, approximately 4–5 mm from the orbital rim.

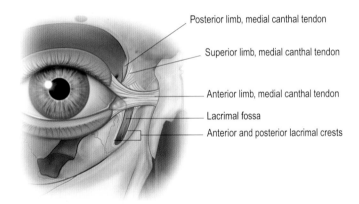

Fig. 8.5 The medial canthal tendon envelops the lacrimal sac. It is tripartite, with anterior, posterior and superior limbs. Like the lateral canthal tendon, its limbs are continuous with tarsal plates. The components of this tendon along with its lateral counterpart are enveloped by deep and superficial aspects of the orbicularis muscle. (Adapted from Spinelli HM. Atlas of Aesthetic Eyelid and Periocular Surgery. Philadelphia: Saunders; 2004:13.)

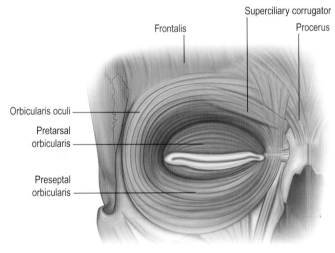

Fig. 8.6 Facial muscles of the orbital region. Note that the preseptal and pretarsal orbicularis muscles fuse with the medial and lateral canthal tendons.

Medial orbital vault

A hammock of fibrous condensations suspends the globe above the orbital floor. The medial components of the apparatus include medial canthal tendon, the Lockwood suspensory ligament and check ligaments of the medial rectus. The medial canthal tendon, like the lateral canthal tendon, has separate limbs that attach the tarsal plates to the ethmoid and lacrimal bones.[13] Each limb inserts onto the periorbital of the apex of the lacrimal fossa. The anterior limb provides the bulk of the medial globe support *(Fig. 8.5).*

Forehead and temporal region

The forehead and brow consist of four layers: skin, subcutaneous tissue, muscle, and galea. There are four distinct brow muscles: frontalis, procerus, corrugator superciliaris, and orbicularis oculi *(Fig. 8.6).* The frontalis muscle inserts predominately into the medial half or two-thirds of the eyebrow *(Fig. 8.7),* allowing the lateral brow to drop hopelessly ptotic from aging, while the medial brow responds to frontalis activation and elevates, often excessively in its drive to clear the lateral overhand. Constant contraction of the frontalis will

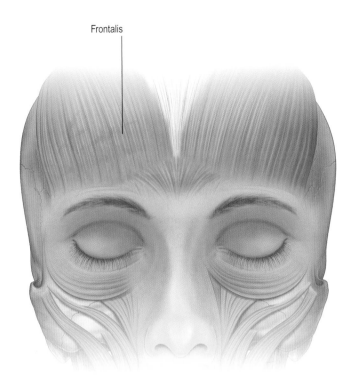

Frontalis

Fig. 8.7 The frontalis muscle inserts predominantly into the medial half or two-thirds of the eyebrow. The medial brow responds to frontalis activation and elevates, often excessively, in its drive to clear lateral overhang.

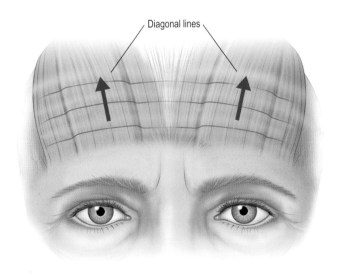

Diagonal lines

Fig. 8.8 Frontalis action. The frontalis muscle inserts into the medial two thirds of the brow. Exaggerated medial brow elevation is required to clear the lateral overhang and to eliminate visual obstruction. Constant contraction of the frontalis will give the appearance of deep horizontal creases in the forehead. This necessarily means that when the lateral skin is elevated or excised, the over-elevated and distorted medial brow drops profoundly.

give the appearance of deep horizontal creases in the forehead *(Fig. 8.8).*[3]

The vertically oriented procerus is a medial muscle, often continuous with the frontalis, arising from the nasal bones and inserting into the subcutaneous tissue of the glabellar region. It pulls the medial brow inferiorly and contributes to

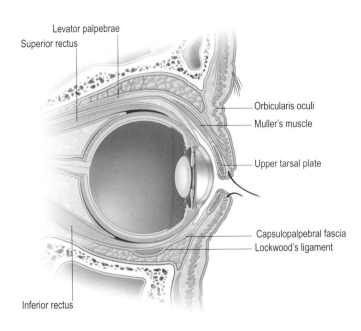

Levator palpebrae
Superior rectus
Orbicularis oculi
Muller's muscle
Upper tarsal plate
Capsulopalpebral fascia
Lockwood's ligament
Inferior rectus

Fig. 8.9 Eyelid anatomy. Each eyelid consists of an anterior lamella of skin and orbicularis muscle and a posterior lamella of tarsus and conjunctiva. The orbital septum forms the anterior border of the orbital fat.

the horizontal wrinkles at the root of the nose. More commonly, these wrinkles result from brow ptosis and correct spontaneously with brow elevation.

The obliquely oriented corrugators muscle arises from the frontal bone and inserts into the brow tissue laterally, with some extensions into orbicularis and frontalis musculature, forming vertical glabellar furrows during contraction. Wrinkles from procerus and corrugators contraction can worsen significantly after upper lid tissue excision as a result of the frontalis muscle's relaxing after being relieved of the need to clear the obstructing lid skin.[14]

Eyelids

The eyelids are vital, irreplaceable structures that serve to protect the globes. Their shutter-like mechanism is essential to clean, lubricate, and protect the cornea. Any disruption or restriction of eyelid closure will have significant consequences for both the patient and the surgeon.

There is much similarity between upper and lower eyelid anatomy. Each consists of an anterior lamella of skin and orbicularis muscle and a posterior lamella of tarsus and conjunctiva *(Fig. 8.9).*[15]

The orbicularis muscle, which acts as a sphincter for the eyelids, consists of orbital, preseptal, and pretarsal segments. The pretarsal muscle segment fuses with the lateral canthal tendon and attaches laterally to Whitnall tubercle. Medially it forms two heads, which insert into the anterior and posterior lacrimal crests *(Fig. 8.6).*

Upper eyelid

The orbital septum originates superiorly at the arcus and forms the anterior border of the orbit. It joins with the levator aponeurosis, just superior to the tarsus. The sling formed by the union of these two structures houses the orbital fat.

The levator palpebrae superioris muscle originates above the annulus of Zinn. It extends anteriorly for 40 mm before becoming a tendinous aponeurosis below Whitnall's ligament.[7,16] The aponeurosis fans out medially and laterally to attach to the orbital retinacula. The aponeurosis fuses with the orbital septum above the superior border of the tarsus and at the caudal extent of the sling, sending fibrous strands to the dermis to form the lid crease. Extensions of the aponeurosis finally insert into the anterior and inferior tarsus. As the levator aponeurosis undergoes senile attenuation, the lid crease rises into the superior orbit from its remaining dermal attachments while the lid margin drops.

Müller's muscle, or the supratarsal muscle, originates on the deep surface of the levator near the point where the muscle becomes aponeurotic and inserts into the superior tarsus. Dehiscence of the attachment of the levator aponeurosis to the tarsus results in an acquired ptosis only after the Müller's muscle attenuates and loses its integrity.[14]

In the Asian eyelid, fusion of the levator and septum commonly occurs at a lower level, allowing the sling and fat to descend farther into the lid.[15,16] This lower descent of fat creates the characteristic fullness of their upper eyelid. In addition, the aponeurotic fibers form a weaker attachment to the dermis, resulting in a less distinct lid fold *(Fig. 8.10)*.

Septal extension

The orbital septum has an adhesion to the levator aponeurosis above the tarsus. The septum continues beyond this adhesion and extends to the ciliary margin. It is superficial to the preaponeurotic fat found at the supratarsal crease. The septal extension is a dynamic component to the motor apparatus, as traction on this fibrous sheet reproducibly alters ciliary margin position *(Fig. 8.11)*. The septal extension serves as an adjunct to, and does not operate independent of, levator function, as mistaking the septal extension for levator apparatus and plicating this layer solely results in failed ptosis correction.[17]

Lower eyelid

The anatomy of the lower eyelid is somewhat analogous to that of the upper eyelid. The retractors of the lower lid, the capsulopalpebral fascia, correspond to the levator above. The capsulopalpebral head splits to surround and fuse with the sheath of the inferior oblique muscle. The two heads fuse to form the Lockwood suspensory ligament, which is analogous to Whitnall's ligament. The capsulopalpebral fascia fuses with the orbital septum 5 mm below the tarsal border and then inserts into the anterior and inferior surface of the tarsus.[18] The inferior tarsal muscle is analogous to Muller's muscle of the upper eyelid and also arises from the sheath of the inferior rectus muscle. It runs anteriorly above the inferior oblique muscle and also attaches to the inferior tarsal border.

The combination of the orbital septum, orbicularis, and skin of the lower lid acts as the anterior barrier of the orbital fat. As these connective tissue properties relax, the orbital fat is allowed to herniate forward, forming an unpleasing, full lower eyelid. This relative loss of orbital volume leads to a commensurate, progressive hollowing of the upper lid as upper eyelid fat recesses.[19]

The capsulopalpebral fascia and its overlying conjunctiva form the posterior border of the lower orbital fat. Transection of the capsulopalpebral fascia during lower lid procedures, particularly transconjunctival blepharoplasty, releases the retractors of the lower eyelid, which can reduce downward traction and allow the position of the lower lid margin to rise.

Retaining ligaments

A network of ligaments serves as a scaffold for the skin and subcutaneous tissue surrounding the orbit. The orbital retaining ligament directly attaches the orbicularis at the junction of its orbital and preseptal components to the periosteum of the orbital rim and, consequently, separates the prezygomatic space from the preseptal space. This ligament is continuous with the lateral orbital thickening, which inserts onto the lateral orbital rim and deep temporal fascia. It also has attachments to the superficial lateral canthal tendon *(Figs 8.3, 8.12, 8.13)*.[20] Attenuation of these ligaments permit descent of orbital fat onto the cheek. A midfacelift must release these ligaments to achieve a supported, lasting lift.[21]

Blood supply

The internal and external carotid arteries supply blood to the orbit and eyelids *(Fig. 8.14)*. The ophthalmic artery is the first intracranial branch of the internal carotid; its branches supply the globe, extraocular muscles, lacrimal gland, ethmoid, upper eyelids, and forehead. The external carotid artery branches into the superficial temporal and maxillary arteries. The infraorbital artery is a continuation of the maxillary artery and exits 8 mm below the inferomedial orbital rim to supply the lower eyelid.[22]

The arcade of the superior and inferior palpebral arteries gives a rich blood supply to the eyelids. The superior palpebral artery consists of a peripheral arcade located at the superior tarsal border – the area where surgical dissection occurs to correct lid ptosis and to define lid folds. Damage to a vessel within this network commonly results in a hematoma of Müller's muscle, causing lid ptosis for 2–8 weeks postoperatively. Likewise, on the lower lid, the inferior palpebral artery lies at the inferior border of the inferior tarsus.

The supratrochlear, dorsal nasal, and medial palpebral arteries all traverse the orbit medially. Severing these arteries during fat removal, without adequately providing hemostasis, may lead to a retrobulbar hematoma, a vision-threatening complication of blepharoplasty.

Innervation: trigeminal nerve and facial nerve

The trigeminal nerve along with its branches provides sensory innervations to the periorbital region *(Fig. 8.15)*. The ophthalmic division enters the orbit and divides into the frontal, nasociliary, and lacrimal nerves. The terminal branch of the nasociliary nerve, the infratrochlear nerve, supplies the medial conjunctiva, and lacrimal sac. The lacrimal nerve supplies the lateral conjunctiva and skin of the lateral upper eyelid. The frontal nerve, the largest branch, divides into the supraorbital and supratrochlear branches. The supraorbital nerve exits through either a notch or a foramen and provides sensory innervations to the skin and conjunctiva of the upper eyelid and the scalp. The supratrochlear nerve innervates the skin of the glabella, forehead, medial upper eyelid, and medial conjunctiva. A well-placed supraorbital

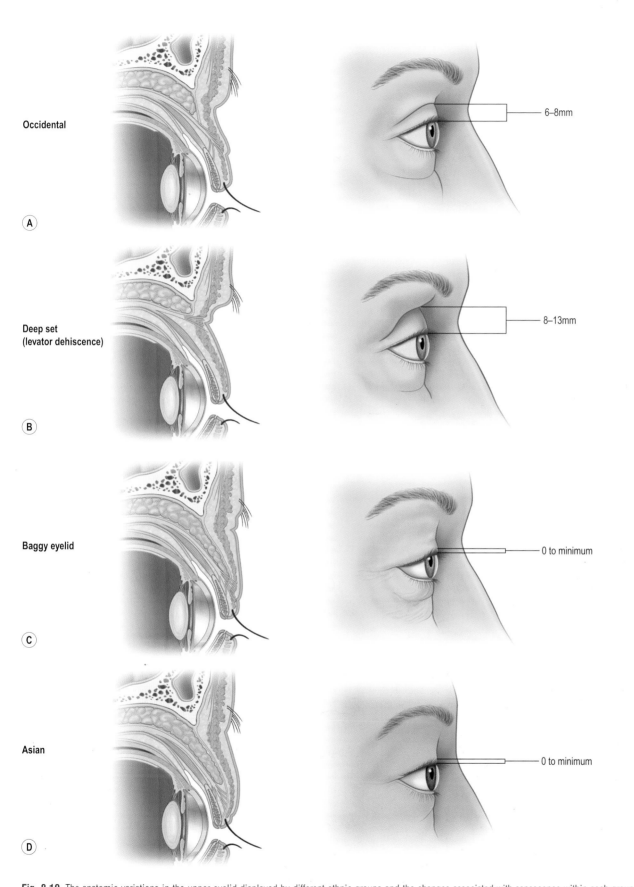

Fig. 8.10 The anatomic variations in the upper eyelid displayed by different ethnic groups and the changes associated with senescence within each group allow for a convergence of anatomy. **(A)** The occidental upper eyelid has levator extensions inserting onto the skin surface to define a lid-fold that averages 6–8 mm above the lid margin. The position of the levator-skin linkage and the anteroposterior relationship of the preaponeurotic fat determine lid-fold height and degree of sulcus concavity or convexity (as shown on the right half of each anatomic depiction). **(B)** In the case of levator dehiscence from the tarsal plate, the upper lid crease is displaced superiorly. The orbital septum and preaponeurotic fat linked to the levator are displaced superiorly and posteriorly. These anatomic changes create a high lid crease, a deep superior sulcus, and eyelid ptosis. **(C)** In the aging eyelid, the septum becomes attenuated and stretches. The septal extension loosens, and this allows orbital fat to prolapsed forward and slide over the levator into an anterior and inferior position. Clinically, this results in an inferior displacement of the levator skin attachments and a low and anterior position of the preaponeurotic fat pad. **(D)** The youthful Asian eyelid anatomically resembles the senescent upper lid with a low levator skin zone of adhesion and inferior and anteriorly located preaponeurotic fat. The characteristic, but variable, low eyelid crease and convex upper eyelid and sulcus are classic. (Adapted from Spinelli HM. Atlas of Aesthetic Eyelid and Periocular Surgery. Philadelphia: Saunders; 2004:59.)

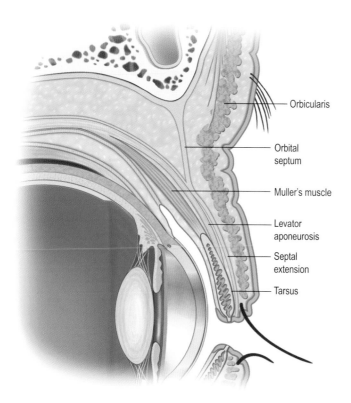

Fig. 8.11 The orbital septum has an adhesion to the levator aponeurosis above the tarsus. The septal extension begins at the adhesion of the orbital septum to the levator and extends to the ciliary margin. It is superficial to the preaponeurotic fat found at the supratarsal crease. (Adapted from Reid RR, Said HK, Yu M, *et al.* Revisiting upper eyelid anatomy: introduction of the septal extension. Plast Reconstr Surg 2006; 117(1):65–70.)

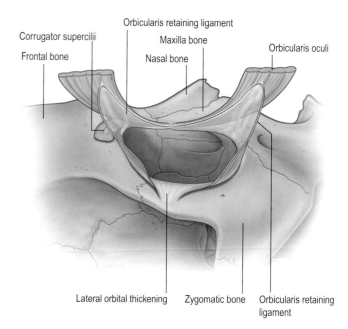

Fig. 8.12 The orbicularis muscle fascia attaches to the skeleton along the orbital rim by the lateral orbital thickening (LOT) in continuity with the orbicularis retaining ligament (ORL). (Adapted from Ghavami A, Pessa JE, Janis J, *et al.* The orbicularis retaining ligament of the medial orbit: closing the circle. Plast Reconstr Surg 2008; 121(3):994–1001.)

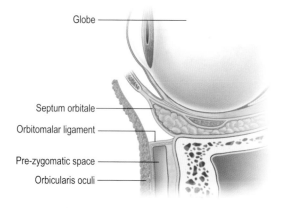

Fig. 8.13 The orbital retaining ligament (ORL) directly attaches the orbicularis oris (OO) at the junction of its pars palpebrarum and pars orbitalis to the periosteum of the orbital rim and, consequently, separates the prezygomatic space from the preseptal space. (Adapted from Muzaffar AR, Mendelson BC, Adams WP Jr. Surgical anatomy of the ligamentous attachments of the lower lid and lateral canthus. Plast Reconstr Surg 2002; 110(3):873–884.)

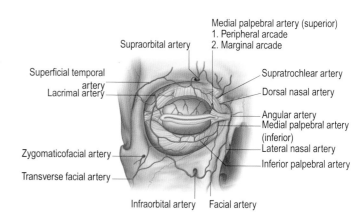

Fig. 8.14 Arterial supply to the periorbital region.

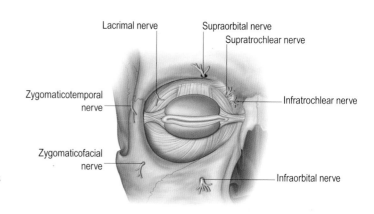

Fig. 8.15 Sensory nerves of the eyelids.

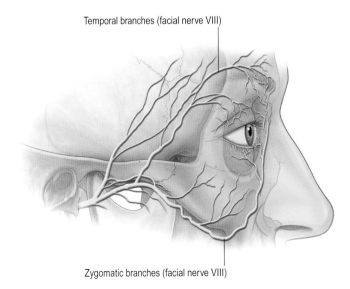

Temporal branches (facial nerve VIII)

Zygomatic branches (facial nerve VIII)

Fig. 8.16 Anatomy of the brow and temporal region. The light green opaque area denotes the deep temporal fascia and the periosteum where sutures may be used to suspend soft tissue. Wide undermining, soft tissue suspension and canthopexy are safely performed here.

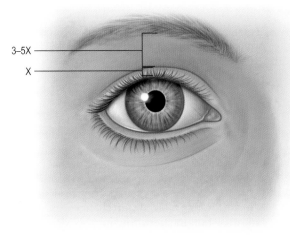

3–5X

X

Fig. 8.17 On relaxed forward gaze, the ideal upper lid should rest approximately 2 mm below the upper limbus. The lower lid ideally covers 0.5 mm of the lower limbus. The ratio of distance from the lower edge of the eyebrow to the open lid margin to the pretarsal skin ratio should be greater than 3.

block will anesthetize most of the upper lid and the central precoronal scalp.[6,14,23]

The maxillary division exits the orbit through one to three infraorbital foramina. It provides sensation to the skin of the nose, the lower eyelids, and the upper lid. Dissection is necessary lateral to the infraorbital nerve for successful midface-lifting and around the nerve for placement of tear trough implants.

The facial nerve exits the stylomastoid foramen and divides in the substance of the parotid gland into the superior temporofacial and inferior cervicofacial branches *(Fig. 8.16)*. The temporofacial nerve divides into the frontal, zygomatic, and buccal nerves; the cervicofacial nerve divides into the buccal, mandibular, and cervical nerves. There are significant variations in the branching of the facial nerve, which is responsible for facial expression. Innervation of facial muscles occurs on their deep surfaces. Interruption of the branches to the orbicularis muscle from the periorbital surgery or facial surgery may result in atonicity due to partial denervation of the orbicularis with loss of lid tone or anomalous reinnervation and possibly undesirable eyelid twitching.[15]

The frontal branch of the facial nerve courses immediately above and attached to the periosteum of the zygomatic bone. It then courses medially approximately 2 cm above the superior orbital rim to innervate the frontalis, corrugators, and procerus muscles from their deep surface. A separate branch travels along the inferior border of the zygoma to innervate the inferior component of orbicularis oculi.[24] The surgeon should take great care when operating in this area to avoid damaging this nerve during endoscopic and open brow lifts.

Youthful, beautiful eyes

The characteristics of youthful, beautiful eyes differ from one population to another but generalizations are possible and provide a needed reference to judge the success of various surgical maneuvers. Attractive, youthful eyes are bright eyes. Bright eyes have globes framed in generously sized horizontal apertures (from medial and lateral), often accentuated by a slight upward tilt of the intercanthal axis *(Fig. 8.17)*. The aperture length should span most of the distance between the orbital rims. In a relaxed forward gaze, the vertical height of the aperture should expose at least three-quarters of the cornea with the upper lid extending down at least 1.5 mm below the upper limbus (the upper margin of the cornea) but no more than 3 mm. The lower lid ideally covers 0.5 mm of the lower limbus but no more than 1.5 mm.[4,15]

In the upper lid, there should be a well-defined lid crease lying above the lid margin with lid skin under slight stretch, slightly wider laterally. Ideally, the actual pretarsal skin visualized on relaxed forward gaze ranges from 3 to 6 mm in European ethnicities. The Asian lid crease is generally 2–3 mm lower, with the distance from lid margin diminishing as the crease moves toward the inner canthus. Patients of Indo-European and African decent show 1 to 2 mm lower than European ethnicities. The ratio of distance from the lower edge of the eyebrow (at the center of the globe) to the open lid margin to the visualized pretarsal skin should never be less than 3–1 *(Fig. 8.1)*, preferably more.

Scleral show is the appearance of white sclera below the lower border of the cornea and above the lower eyelid margin. In general, sclera show is contradictory to optimal aesthetics and may be perceived as a sign of aging, previous blepharoplasty, or orbital disease (e.g., thyroid disease). More than 0.5 mm of sclera show beneath the cornea on direct forward gaze begins to confer a sad or melancholy aura to one's appearance. However, in some youthful persons, the largeness of these apertures gives dramatic emphasis to the eyes and may be considered a strong and positive feature.

The intercanthal axis is normally tilted slightly upward (from medial to lateral) in most populations. Exaggerated tilts are encountered in some Asian, Indo-European and

African-American populations. Such upward tilt of the lateral canthal axis may give the eye a youthful appearance, which is aesthetically pleasing in any ethnic group. The lower lid that droops in its lateral aspect and the eye with a downward tilt generally convey to the viewer an aging, ill-health distortion or unattractiveness.[25]

Etiology of aging

In the upper lid, excessive skin due to loss of elasticity and sun damage is one of the major causes of an aged appearance in the periorbital area. If there is an excess of skin that hangs over the lid or the upper eyelid appears to have multiple folds, it is difficult to have a rejuvenated appearance with cosmetics alone. In addition to relaxed skin changes, excessive fat herniation can cause bulging, resulting in a heavy appearance to the upper lid area. Although this fat is normal orbital fat, it appears to be protruding outward because of the laxity of the orbital septum, which holds the fat in place. Theoretically, replacement of the fat into a position that maintains a normal level of fat in the orbital area seems an optimal solution. However, this is not easily accomplished and may result in complications that are difficult to correct. Therefore, the skin and fat that seem to be in apparent excess should be treated accordingly.

The etiology of aging changes in the lower lids is similar in some ways but quite different in others. Aging changes include relaxation of the tarsal margin with scleral show, rhytides of the lower lid, herniated fat pads resulting in bulging in one or all of the three fat pocket areas, and hollowing of the nasojugal groove and lateral orbital rim areas. Hollowing of the nasojugal groove area appears as dark circles under the eyes, mostly because of lighting and the shadowing that result from this defect *(Fig. 8.18)*.[26] It is clear that evaluation of all aspects of aging changes in the lids is important so the surgeon can plan the most effective operative procedure.

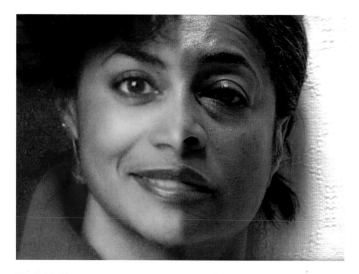

Fig. 8.18 Morphed digital photography (split right half = current preoperative photograph, split left half = photograph 20 years ago), demonstrating descent of periorbital fat and skin during the aging process. (From Odunze MO, Reid RR, Yu M, *et al*. Periorbital rejuvenation and the African-American patient: a survey approach. Plast Reconstr Surg 2006; 118:1011–1018.)

Diagnosis/patient presentation

Evaluation basics

The first essential step is to look at the patient carefully, thoroughly, and critically. The surgeon should be seated directly in front of the prospective patient with the patient's eyes at his or her eye level. Note the general impression and feeling generated from looking at this person *(Fig. 8.19)*.

One should also look for areas of symmetry or asymmetry. Notice the shape of the eye; the prominence or asymmetry of the globes; and evidence of exposure, dryness, or injection of vessels. Look for evidence of decreased tone and dropped posture of the lower lids. What is the posture of the upper lid? Are the upper lids symmetric? Is there lid ptosis? At what level does the upper lid traverse the globe? What levels do the upper and lower lids sit in relation to the limbus?

Next, have the patient relax the brow and close the eyes. Do the lids close? Then ask the patient to open the eyes. Is it necessary to raise the brows to effect comfortable forward vision? Does the corrugator frown increase in prominence with the eyes closed and the forehead relaxed? Is there transverse brow wrinkling? Is one brow lower? Which one and how much? Is there a prominent frown?

Assess the lower lid tone by pulling the lid away from the globe and releasing, making sure the patient does not blink (modified snap test). Does each lid spring back immediately, reluctantly, or not at all? Is it held against the globe by only the tear seal? Most people presenting for blepharoplasty have a significant decrease in their lower lid tone, often asymmetric.

What, if anything, would improve the aesthetic appearance of the eyes and periorbital region? Are there festoons or deep grooves (i.e., nasojugal grooves or tear trough deformities)? Is there excess skin, muscle, or fat? Quantitate any excess soft tissue on a simple eye diagram. Does restoration of lateral canthal posture correct the illusion of excess skin on the lower eyelid? Does it diminish it? Does the orbital septum appear to be excessively relaxed? Note the tilt of the intercanthal axis or lack thereof.

The "four-finger lift" is performed by encircling the outer orbit with the tips of the index, middle, ring and little fingers on one hand. With the index and middle fingers above the lateral brow, place the ring finger lateral to the canthus and little finger beneath the lateral canthus just lateral to the malar prominence. Gently move the four fingers posteriorly and superiorly to lift the lateral brow, canthus, and cheek. If this test restores youthfulness and attractiveness, a canthopexy, brow lift, and midfacelift may be beneficial.

Medical and ophthalmic history

A thorough history and physical examination should be performed before surgery *(Box 8.2)*. In addition, an adequate eye history encourages positive outcomes and reduces eye complications.

Contact lens wear poses particular risks when eyelid surgery is performed. The natural progression of aging dries the eyes out, and long-term contact lens wearing hastens this process considerably. Traditional blepharoplasty techniques

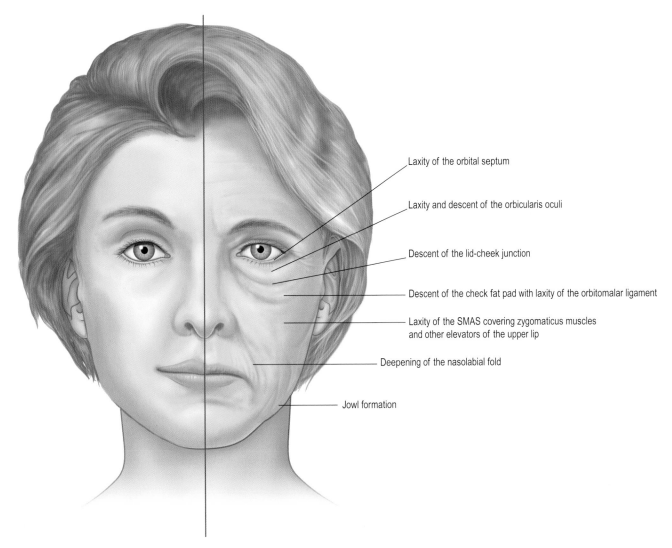

Laxity of the orbital septum

Laxity and descent of the orbicularis oculi

Descent of the lid-cheek junction

Descent of the check fat pad with laxity of the orbitomalar ligament

Laxity of the SMAS covering zygomaticus muscles and other elevators of the upper lip

Deepening of the nasolabial fold

Jowl formation

Fig. 8.19 Mid cheek deflation due to loss of superficial and deep fat. SMAS, superficial musculoaponeurotic system. (Adapted from Rohrich RJ, Pessa JE. The fat compartments of the face: anatomy and clinical implications for cosmetic surgery. Plast Reconstr Surg 2007;119(7):2219-2227.)

Box 8.2 Important information to obtain during history and physical examination

- Medication use: particularly anticoagulants, anti-inflammatory and cardiovascular drugs, and vitamins (especially vitamin E).
- Herbal supplement use: herbs represent risks to anesthesia and surgery, particularly those affecting blood pressure, blood coagulation, the cardiovascular system, and healing.
- Allergies: medication and type.
- Past medical history: especially hypertension, diabetes, cardiovascular and cerebrovascular disease, hepatitis, liver disease, heart disease or arrhythmias, cancer, thyroid disease, and endocrine disease.
- Bleeding disorders or blood clots.
- Psychiatric disease.
- Alcohol and smoking history.
- Recreational drug use, which may interact with anesthesia.
- Exposure to human immunodeficiency virus and hepatitis virus.
- Any history of facial herpes zoster or simplex.

---

consistently produce vertical dystopia with increased scleral exposure, making the lens wear difficult if not dangerous. Ptosis and canthopexy surgery may alter the corneal curvature and require that contacts be refitted. The patient should discontinue contact lens wear in the perioperative period to allow healing without the need to manipulate the eyelids. Levator dehiscence or attenuation commonly accompanies long-term hard contact lens wear, caused by the mechanical stresses posteriorly from the rigid lens rubbing against the posterior lamella of the lid.[27]

The same population that seeks aesthetic surgery also gravitates toward refractive surgery, such as LASIK (laser-assisted *in situ* keratomileusis). A history of such surgery is necessary information because periorbital surgery particularly canthopexies and levator surgery, can affect the refractive characteristics, cause mechanical irritation of the conjunctiva and cornea, or affect the corneal flap.[28] Ptosis repair or debulking of heavy upper lids can change the corneal curvature, resulting in the need for a new prescription for eyeglasses. Canthopexy normally raises the contact point of the lid with the globe and can increase the tension of the lid with the globe and can increase the tension of the lid against the cornea, affecting corneal curvature. It can cause conjunctival chemosis or produce corneal erosion early postoperatively. Dry eye exposure problems are most prevalent in patients who have undergone LASIK surgery because the flap disrupts corneal innervations, forming an anesthetic effect that suppresses tear production. When in doubt, such patients should be reviewed by their refractive surgeon before undergoing blepharoplasty.

One should check for a history of other eye procedures, including glaucoma surgery (forms a bleb of conjunctival tissue on the superior limbus), retinal, strabismus, and cataract surgery. Evaluate carefully for a history as well as physical evidence of facial muscle weakness, extraocular muscle imbalance, Bell palsy, or trauma in addition to orbicularis hyperactivity such as blepharospasm or hemifacial spasm. Any ocular condition may affect the type or result of eyelid surgery.[29]

Superior or lateral visual field loss suggests functional ptosis or pseudoptosis. A 12–20 degree or a 30% improvement of the superior visual field, between a taped and untaped upper lid, may qualify for medical necessity.

Chronic eye irritation, such as tearing, dryness, excessive blinking, discharge, eyelid margin inflammation, crusting, burning, or itching, must be brought under control before any surgery. Dry eyes should be aggressively sought out and treated before surgery.

Dry irritated eyes before surgery will lead to irritated eyes after surgery, and the surgeon may be blamed. On questioning, most patients will rarely admit to dry eyes, although it is known that the eyes dry out considerably throughout our lifetime. Treatment options include artificial tears, ointment, anti-inflammatory drops, and punctal plugs or punctal closure.[29,30]

Exophthalmos, unilaterally or bilaterally, associated with a thyroid disorder should be completely stabilized for approximately 6 months before elective aesthetic surgery. However, there may be an urgent requirement in active Graves' disease to perform procedures to protect the globe or the vision.[13]

Ocular examination

An ocular examination before elective periorbital aesthetic surgery should include all of the elements covered in the following sections (*Fig. 8.20*).

Visual acuity

The most essential preoperative test is assessment of visual acuity, by the surgeon or ophthalmic colleague. Document the vision with patient wearing glasses or contact lenses if they are needed. Note any vision deficits and have them evaluated before surgery. The most common cause of unrecognized loss of vision is amblyopia (lazy eye), which is present in 2% of the general population. A patient may often be unaware of the unilateral amblyopia (or any loss of vision) until the eyes are tested individually.

External examination

The periorbital skin and tissues are examined for benign or malignant lesions, including xanthelasma, syringoma, basal cell carcinoma, benign moles, skin tags, and chalazia. Marked anesthetic improvement results from removal of benign lesions about the eyes, especially those that rise above the lid margin. Any cancerous (or precancerous) lesions must be removed before any aesthetic procedure is performed to preserve eyelid skin for reconstruction, if needed.

Eyelid measurements are documented for use during ptosis surgery and, if necessary, for insurance purposes. In the eyelid of the white individual, the aperture (distance between the upper and lower eyelids) average 10–12 mm. The margin reflex distance (MRD), measured from the light reflex on the center of the cornea to the upper eyelid margin, ranges from 3 to 5 mm. True blepharoptosis is defined by the degree of upper lid infringement upon the iris and pupil. As the MRD decreases towards zero, the severity of blepharoptosis increases. Before method selection, the levator function must be determined by measuring the upper eyelid excursion from extreme downward gaze to extreme upward gaze; it generally ranges from 10 to 12 mm. If ptosis exists, the type of repair depends upon the severity of the ptosis and the reliability of the levator to recreate smooth, upper lid elevation. A deep upper lid sulcus with a high lid fold in the presence of a droopy eyelid usually indicated a levator dehiscence, which is often unilateral or asymmetric.[31,32]

Pseudoptosis occurs when excess upper lid skin covers the eyelid, depressing the eyelashes, forming hooding and simulating ptosis. It is easily differentiated from true ptosis by simply elevating the brow or the hooded skin itself to determine the true resting lid level.[33] Photographic evidence of this is often necessary for insurance purposes when a levator aponeurosis repair or a excisional blepharoplasty is planned. When the hooded skin hangs over the lashes, the lashes turn downward and sometimes interfere with vision or rub against the cornea. True trichiasis (misdirected lashes) may also exist, but inward-turning lashes can be trained to return to their natural posture after eyelid repair with lash rotation.

Brow ptosis is a common aspect of facial aging. It adds weight and volume to the upper eyelid to develop, or exacerbate, eyelid ptosis. The more ptotic brow is often selectively elevated or over-elevated by frontalis muscle contraction, which may confuse the surgeon as to whether eyelid ptosis or retraction exists. The ability to differentiate the causes of droopy eyelids – brow ptosis (brow weight resting on the eyelids), dermatochalasis (excess skin), and blepharoptosis (levator attenuation or dehiscence) – will enable the surgeon to select the proper correction.

Unilateral as well as bilateral upper eyelid retraction is commonly associated with prominent globes, which are often asymmetrically proptotic. Most commonly, it is the result of Graves' ophthalmopathy, which can lift the lid above the superior limbus. A thyroid evaluation is appropriate before any surgery to correct retraction. If it is stable for more than 6 months, levator recession surgery can be combined with fat reduction blepharoplasty, but lid skin should rarely if ever removed.

Long-term soft contact lens wear is also a common cause of lid retraction that raises the lid to the superior limbus or above. Congenitally shallow or traumatically small orbits are also a cause of lid retraction, as is idiopathic retraction.[27] If the retraction persists in spite of taping the brow or lid tissue out of the way of vision, the surgery to correct the retraction must either precede or accompany the eyelid or brow surgery. Retraction can also be accompanied contralateral blepharoptosis according to Hering's Law.

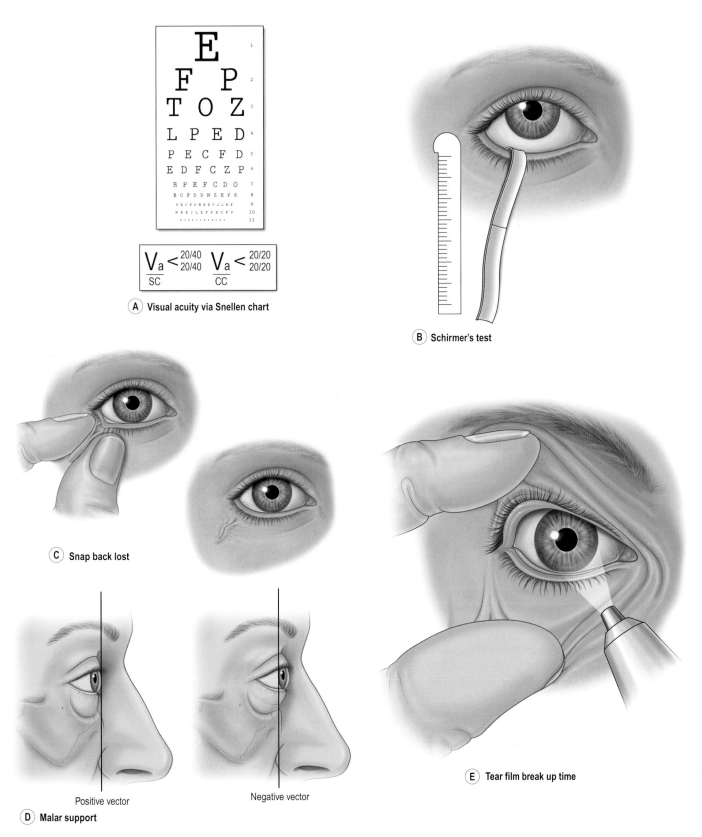

A Visual acuity via Snellen chart

B Schirmer's test

C Snap back lost

D Malar support

Positive vector

Negative vector

E Tear film break up time

Fig. 8.20 (A–E) Evaluation of the patient should include an appreciation of visual acuity (with and without correction), baseline tear production, intrinsic lid tone, lower eyelid support, and tear film quality. The tests performed and their interpretation should be tailored by the clinician within the context of each patient and applied on an individual basis. (Adapted from Spinelli HM. Atlas of aesthetic eyelid and periocular surgery. Philadelphia: Saunders; 2004:31.)

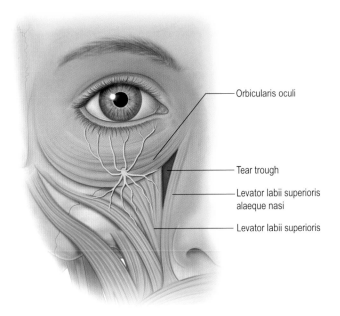

Fig. 8.21 The anatomy of the tear trough deformity demonstrates the muscular triangle formed by the orbicularis oculi, levator labii superioris, and levator labii superioris alaeque nasi. (Adapted from Hirmand H. Anatomy and nonsurgical correction of tear trough deformity. Plast Reconstr Surg 2010; 125(2):699–708.)

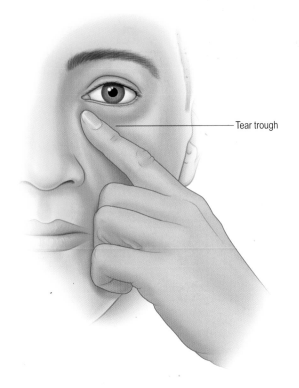

Fig. 8.22 Tear trough test. The ability to place the side of a finger into the bony furrow under the nasojugal groove suggests a potential benefit from tear trough augmentation.

Orbits and malar eminence

The relative position of the globe to orbital anatomy greatly influences appropriate surgical technique. There is a normal 10–12 mm projection of the globe seen in a lateral, as measured from the lateral orbital rim at the level of the canthal tendon to the pupil. Proptosis and enophthalmos are relative anterior and posterior displacement of the globe, respectively. Hertel exophthalmometry can be used to quantitate the degree of relative projection for documentation purposes.[15,24]

The tear trough is at the inferior orbital rim most medially, triangulated by the orbicularis, levator labii superioris alaeque nasi and levator labii superioris muscles *(Fig. 8.21)*. The indentation is at the junction of the thin eyelid skin above and the thicker and different nasal and cheek skin below, with attenuated subcutaneous tissue overlying the maxillary bone. It is the deepening of this groove that leads to true indentation and significantly impacts facial appearance. The relative lack of subcutaneous tissue in this area is subject to worsening concavity with aging. The cause of the deformity is due to a combination of orbital fat herniation, skin laxity and malar volume loss and ptosis of skin and subcutaneous tissue.[26] The ability to place the side of the finger into the bony furrow under the nasojugal grooves suggests a potential benefit from a tear trough implant or the addition of soft tissue augmentation *(Fig. 8.22)*.[34]

Pupils

The pupils are evaluated for direct and consensual response to light. An abnormal result indicates a problem behind the globe (i.e., the optic nerve or brain). Refractive errors, amblyopia, and corneal or retinal problems will not present with an abnormal papillary response.

Extraocular muscles

The extraocular muscles are tested for deviations, motility problems, or restrictions. Eye deviations often present with amblyopia unilaterally and corresponding reduced vision. One should examine the patient for the presence of an intact Bell's phenomenon, an upward and outward rotation of the cornea with lid closure. This can be accomplished by gently forcing the upper eyelids open during closure. The presence of an intact Bell reflex affords protection for the eye and cornea in the event of incomplete eyelid closure. If the eyelid fails to close during sleep, the cornea may remain uncovered and dry out. Thus, the absence of Bell phenomenon raises the risk for postoperative problems, especially in those with preexisting problems or dry eyes.[29]

Globe

The globe is examined for clarity of the cornea, iris, and lens. The corneal light reflex should be sharp and no lesions noted anywhere on the globe. If there is any question of a corneal defect, a slit-lamp examination is needed, either by a surgeon or by an ophthalmologist on referral. Any whitening of the cornea is possibly an infectious infiltrate and should be treated aggressively with antibiotics.

Tear film

Assessment of tear production is a necessary but unreliable task. Schirmer testing consists of placing filter paper strips in the lateral third of the lower eyelid. The irritation of any foreign object against the globe stimulates reflex tearing, possibly yielding a deceptively good test result. A topical anesthetic (tetracaine or proparacaine) eases discomfort and reflex tearing, giving a better assessment of basal tear secretion. After 5 min, normal tear production should be greater than 15 mm; 5–10 mm indicates borderline tear secretion, and below 5 mm is hyposecretion.

Basal tear production diminishes with age in all persons to a degree that usually becomes symptomatic by 50 years of age. In contact lens wearers, allergy sufferers, arthritics, and people with autoimmune diseases, this process accelerates and often becomes symptomatic in their 30s. It is important for patients to be aware of this age-related decrease in tear production preoperatively.

Photographic documentation

No other area of cosmetic surgery is more dependent on accurate photography than the periorbital region *(Box 8.3)*. It is essential in documenting existing anatomy and pathologic changes. Accurate photography assists in surgical planning, intraoperative decision-making, and documentation of results, and it may be necessary for legal protection.[35]

Unintentional deception in eye appearance

There is a natural phenomenon that prevents surgeons from fully appreciating the potential adverse effects of the surgery. Women, and some men to whom appearance is important, subconsciously and automatically modify their appearance when they are confronted with a mirror, a camera, or someone carefully examining their appearance. They lift the chin, tilt the head backwards, elevate the eyebrows, and smile slightly. This gives the illusion of elevated lower eyelids (although it alters the intercanthal axis, turning it downward), and it cleans the upper lids. These unintentional changes simulate a brow lift, although the medial brow is typically disproportionately elevated. This disguises from the surgeon, both on direct inspection and in photographs, the accurate preoperative appearance and true outcome of the surgery. When the mirror and camera disappear, the brow drops, the corrugators contract, and the lower lids drop to their natural posture. This then, is the face the real world is seeing.

Patient selection

Operative planning

Before surgical planning, one must have a meaningful conceptualization of the desired result. Only then can the surgical

maneuvers required be organized in a meaningful way *(Box 8.4)*.[35] Preoperative planning should take place with the patient upright under good lighting and with complete facial relaxation. It is also important to document the brow, canthus, and upper and lower eyelid posture and position and all other desired alterations preoperatively. The preoperative photographs and surgical plan should be easily visible to the surgeon during the entire surgery.

Skin and muscle are quantified for excision in millimeters or any standardized system comfortable to the surgeon. Fat excision is measured in terms of cubic centimeters (cc) or milliliters (mL). A pea-sized amount is roughly equivalent to 0.5 ccs or 0.5 mL. Determination of fat excision should be approximated in multiples of this standard measure. Measurements should be consistent with the patient in a vertical position to avoid lid hollowness or concave depressions. In proptotic patients, more aggressive fat excision offers the possibility of reduction of globe projection, but skin removal, of any quantity, is most likely contraindicated.

Anatomic-directed therapy

Upper eyelid position

In the typical person with the brow in an aesthetically pleasing position, 20 mm of upper lid skin must remain between the bottom of the central eyebrow and the upper lid margin to allow adequate lid closure during sleep, a well-defined lid crease, and an effective and complete blink.

Lower eyelid tonicity

The presence of atonic lower lids and lateral canthal laxity may give the impression that there is excess skin requiring removal. However, lower lid posture and optimal lateral canthal position should be restored manually before determining the amount of skin and other tissues to be removed. Lid and canthal restoration frequently eliminates skin excess. When skin removal is indicated, the surgeon will often need to remove skin more centrally than laterally.[9,36]

Eyelid ptosis or retraction

In patients with unilateral eyelid ptosis, one may be tempted to operate on the normal eye, which may appear to be retracted, instead of the "disguised" ptotic eye. As a consequence of Hering's law, both levators are energized equally in an attempt to clear the visual axis of the ptotic lid, thereby making the normal lid appear retracted. Covering each eye separately and observing the lid position often lead to the discovery of the ptotic eye as the pathologic source. The retracted eye will drop to its normal position once the ptotic eye is covered, only to have the ptotic eye rise when it is uncovered. Symmetric elevation of the brow is similarly helpful in patients in whom asymmetric brow pseudoptosis obstructs peripheral vision.

It is easy to correct existing true ptosis, or true retraction, at the time of blepharoplasty surgery. Even when ptosis is mild, correction avoids the probable worsening of the ptosis by the additional insults of a weakened levator due to surgical trauma, an edematous or bruised lid, a hematoma in the levator muscle, a cicatrix associated with even the smallest amount of orbital bleeding, or a simple asymmetric surgical rendering.[37,38]

Globe position and malar prominence

The position of the globe greatly affects the procedural choices and quality of outcome in periorbital surgery. The high frequency of asymmetry in globe prominence is often not appreciated in aesthetic periorbital surgery. Unless it is recognized and treated appropriately, unfortunate outcomes are almost inevitable.

In patients with infraorbital malar hypoplasia or tear trough deformity, it is not possible to achieve optimal aesthetic results without some contour correction. If the globe extends anteriorly past the inferior orbital rim, lower lid surgery will increase scleral show and lid deformity unless the lid and canthal posture are raised, the orbital rim-malar complex is enhanced, or the prominent globe is retropositioned. This bone deficit of the lower orbit, which occurs most commonly in men, creates an exophthalmos of the lower half of the globe. The patients can be described as vector-negative or having hemiexophthalmos. A youthful, vector-positive profile consists of an inferior orbital rim and malar soft tissue that are in the same plane of the globe (see *Fig. 8.20*).[39]

When a vector-negative profile exists, there is a relative scarcity of lower eyelid skin. Lids must not be shortened either by blepharoplasty. To do so causes the lid margins to ride down the globe surface, resulting in more scleral show and pathologic exposure. Similar to proptotic patients, suspension canthopexy must be placed more superiorly and anteriorly to prevent scleral show. This relative lack of lower lid skin can also increased with lower lid spacers, canthal tendon elongation or orbital fat reduction.

In exophthalmos, tightening the lower lid, even when it is repositioned with a canthopexy or a lid shortening, may cause some severe potential problems. When it is horizontally tightened, the lid takes the course of least resistance and migrates under the proptotic globe, especially when the canthal attachment is not lifted. To overcome this, the canthopexy attachment commonly needs to be placed higher than is aesthetically most desirable. In addition, the canthal fixation must be placed more anteriorly to accommodate the proptotic globe, and occasionally the canthus needs an extension to reach the bone or augmentation of the orbital rim.

Tear trough deformities

The tear trough deformity is a type of relative infraorbital malar hypoplasia, where there is an asymmetric bony depression along the medial infraorbital rim. Tear trough implants *(Fig. 8.19)* are reserved for severe deformities where the volume of surgical fat repositioning is inadequate and cost of filler exceptional.[34,40]

If the surgeon can place the side of his or her finger into this diagonally recessed bone, augmentation of the concavity should be considered. Factors such as age, skin quality and severity of the hollowing dictate the appropriate procedure. Young patients with good skin quality will benefit from hyaluronic acid fillers placed between the deep dermis and orbicularis oculi fascia. This outpatient procedure can be performed concomitantly or weeks after blepharoplasty once perioperative swelling subsides *(Fig. 8.23)*. Older patients require orbital fat repositioning from the medial and central compartments during a transconjunctival blepharoplasty. Alternative soft tissue injectables include autogenous fat, hydroxyapatite and micronized acellular dermis.

Optimal brow positioning

Aesthetic surgery of the forehead is thoroughly reviewed in Chapter 7. Brow positioning is a cornerstone of blepharoplasty surgery. The majority of aesthetic improvement of the upper orbital region comes from proper brow positioning and canthopexy. When advocating periorbital rejuvenation, it is therefore appropriate to consider repositioning the resting brow position when considering blepharoplasty.[41]

A low resting brow is extremely common and occurs in people of all ages. The lateral overhang of the eyebrow, upper eyelid and juxtabrow skin can cause visual field obstruction. These tissues progress downward from degenerative changes resulting in stretching of the forehead and brow tissues. The recurring pull of the orbicularis, corrugator, and procerus muscles contributes to descent of the brow. Many adults presenting for aesthetic surgery have significant – but often undetected – "resting" brow ptosis. This phenomenon has been termed "compensated brow ptosis", where brow ptosis remains undetected because of the compensatory activation of the frontalis muscles to clear the obstructing lid overhang.[42]

If the brow is simply elevated to its proper position, the seemingly elevated upper lid tissue either disappears or diminishes dramatically, leaving most if not all of the irreplaceable eyelid skin. Furthermore, any scars resulting from skin excision, when it is required, remain short and need not extend beyond the orbital rim.

If a blepharoplasty alone is performed in these patients, the visual incentive to elevate the brow disappears. The frontalis relaxes and the brow drops – exaggerating the aged, tired look that the blepharoplasty was supposed to correct *(Fig. 8.24)*. In addition, the weakened frontalis now fails to oppose the corrugators and relaxes its pull on the glabellar and interbrow skin, thereby accentuating the glabellar crease and frown – a heavy price to pay for an aesthetic procedure designed to rejuvenate the face. These features can be prevented by a concomitant or preceding temporal brow lift that restores the eyebrows to their proper position and checks against a profound drop in the resting posture of the brow after blepharoplasty.

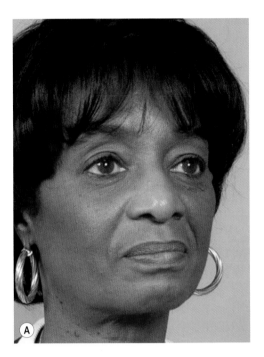
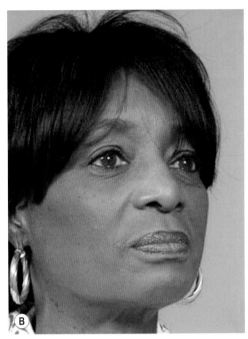

Fig. 8.23 **(A)** Preoperative and **(B)** postoperative photograph demonstrating tear trough augmentation with fillers.

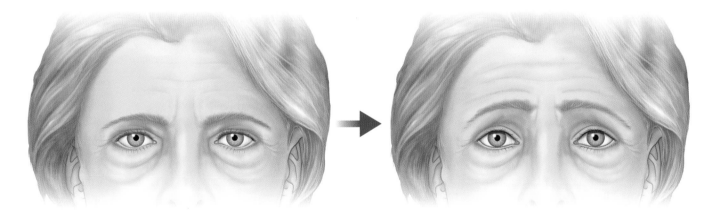

Fig. 8.24 Compensated brow ptosis – continuous obligatory frontalis muscle contraction to clear the periorbital tissues (and to affect comfortable and unobstructed forward vision).

Treatment/technique

Continuum of aesthetic enhancement

The goal of the eyelid surgeon when evaluating patients is to develop an individualized treatment plan for the classic symptoms of periorbital aging. While surgical techniques deliver the most dramatic and lasting results, these procedures are not without inherent risks and postoperative recovery. Surgery is not always the first and immediate response. Patients in their 30s and 40s will frequently benefit from office-based, nonsurgical care. Chemodenervation can minimize the early appearance of brow ptosis and fine-line rhytides along the lateral orbital rim. Fillers, which range in cost and resorption rates, can augment the infraorbital rim in negative vector patients. Photodynamic and laser therapy are alternatives to treat minor skin excess. It is prudent to develop lasting relationships with patients and provide the least invasive, targeted procedure needed for rejuvenation.

Upper eyelid surgery

Video 1

The most common approach to upper blepharoplasty has been the *en block* excision of skin, muscle, and fat in an attempt to debulk the eyelid. However, traditional blepharoplasty may not always fulfill the promise of producing youthful, aesthetically pleasing eyelids. In particular, aggressive upper lid skin excision performed as standard procedure is both a functionally and aesthetically harmful form of upper eyelid blepharoplasty.

Simple skin blepharoplasty

Preserving orbicularis muscle and preaponeurotic fat has been shown to enhance aesthetic outcomes for a variety of presentation. Many who present for upper blepharoplasty hope for a result that is aesthetically enhancing yet avoids a "surgical appearance" or hollowed upper periorbital. Volume-maintaining methods by preserving the orbicularis muscle can be used to preserve or restore a youthful convexity of the upper eyelid-brow junction. Excessive skin and facial soft-tissue descent may rest more on the deflationary effects of regional volume loss rather true, gravitational descent.

A youthful appearance is gained with maintenance or enhancement of volume, and a shorter pretarsal fold. Closure of the skin ellipse after skin resection and orbicularis preservation can improve supratarsal and infrabrow volume. The effects of muscle preservation can be similar to results achieved by soft-tissue filler. Muscle resection should be reserved for patients with orbicularis redundancy or relative hypertrophy. The primary indication for selective myectomy is upper eyelid fold disparities and mild lid ptosis.

When skin-only excision is elected, it should occur above the supratarsal fold or crease, leaving that structure intact. This retains most of the definition of an existing lid fold. If eyelid skin containing the crease is part of the excision, the lid fold becomes ill-defined, indistinct, and irregular. The supratarsal fold is located approximately 7–8 mm above the ciliary margin in women and 6–7 mm in men. The upper marking must be at least 10 mm from the lower edge of the brow and should not include any thick brow skin. The use of a pinch test for redraping the skin is helpful.

The shape of the skin resection is lenticular in younger patients and more trapezoid-shaped laterally in older patients. The incision may need to be extended laterally with a larger extension, but extension lateral to the orbital rim should be avoided if possible, to prevent a prominent scar *(Fig. 8.25)*. Similarly, the medial markings should not be extended medial to the medial canthus because extensions onto the nasal side wall result in webbing. At the conclusion of the case, the patient should have approximately 1–2 mm of lagophthalmos bilaterally. *Figure 8.26* displays the predictable, restorative outcomes that can be achieved with skin excision alone.

Anchor (or invagination blepharoplasty)

Anchor blepharoplasty involves the creation of an upper eyelid crease by attaching pretarsal skin to the underlying aponeurosis. The advantage of an anchor blepharoplasty is a crisp, precise, and well-defined eyelid crease that persists indefinitely. Such lids are more desirable in women than in men because they tend to glamorize the orbital region. The disadvantage is that it is more time-consuming, requires greater surgical skills and expertise, and encourages greater frontalis relaxation as a result of more effective correction of the overhanging pseudoptotic skin. It accomplishes that task while minimizing upper lid skin removal.[43]

Key components of the anchor blepharoplasty include minimal skin excision (2–3 mm) extending cephalad from the tarsus. A 1–2 mm sliver of orbicularis must be removed in proportion to the amount of skin removed. A small pretarsal skin and muscle flap are dissected from the aponeurosis and septum adhesion. After sharply disinserting the aponeurosis from the tarsus, pretarsal fatty tissue can be removed to debulk the pretarsal skin. Key components of the anchor blepharoplasty include minimal skin excision (2–3 mm) extending cephalad from the tarsus. A 1–2 mm sliver of orbicularis must be removed in proportion to the amount of skin removed. A small pretarsal skin and muscle flap are dissected from the aponeurosis and septum adhesion. After sharply detaching the septal extension from the tarsus, pretarsal fatty tissue can be removed to debulk the pretarsal skin. Mattressed anchor sutures are placed connecting the tarsus to the aponeurosis and pretarsal skin *(Fig. 8.27)*. Finally, a running suture approximates the preseptal skin incision.

Orbital fat excision

A relative excess of retroseptal fat may be safely excised through an upper eyelid blepharoplasty incision. A small septotomy is made at the superior aspect of the skin excision into each fat compartment in which conservative resection of redundant fat has been planned. The fat is teased out bluntly and resected using pinpoint cautery. This fat usually includes the medial or nasal compartment, which contains white fat. Yellow fat in the central compartment is usually more superficial and lateral. Gentle pressure on the patient's globe can reproduce the degree of excess while the patient lies recumbent on the operating room table *(Fig. 8.28)*. Overall, undercorrection is preferred to prevent hollowing, which can be dramatic and recognized as an A-frame abnormality.

The attenuated orbital septum may be addressed by using selective diathermy along the exposed caudal septum. Inflammation-mediated tightening can enhance septal integrity. Septal plication aid is unnecessary and may induce a brisk, restrictive inflammatory response.

Blepharoptosis

During upper blepharoplasty, with the septum open and the aponeurosis and superior tarsus exposed, there is an ideal opportunity to adjust the level of the aperture. Inappropriate aperture opening can be due to upper lid ptosis or upper lid retraction. It is not uncommon for there to be ptosis of only the medial portion or retraction of only the lateral portion. A surgeon should not hesitate to take advantage of this opportunity for repair. True ptosis repair involves reattachment of the levator aponeurosis to the tarsus, with or without shortening of applicable structures (e.g., aponeurosis, Müller's muscle, and tarsus).[32,33]

Approximately half of all patients presenting for periorbital aesthetic surgery have one brow that is several millimeters lower than the other. Half of those have significant unilateral ptosis on the side of the lower brow from the "mechanical weight" of the excess skin. Half of those patients' ptosis will be corrected by manually raising the brow on the affected side. The other half have true ptosis, which most likely has gone undiagnosed because of overhanging tissue.

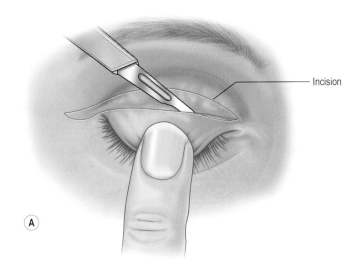

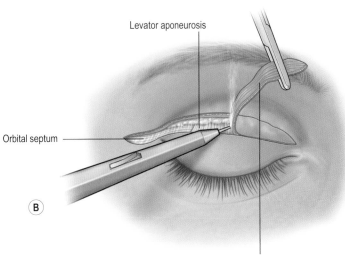

Incision

Levator aponeurosis

Orbital septum

Skin and orbicularis muscle resection

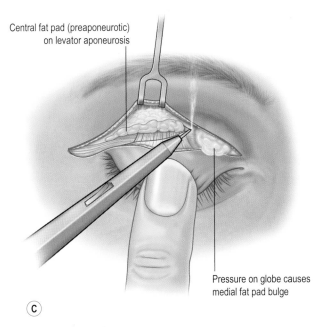

Central fat pad (preaponeurotic) on levator aponeurosis

Pressure on globe causes medial fat pad bulge

Fig. 8.25 Simple skin excision blepharoplasty. **(A)** Digital traction and light pressure by the surgeon allow smooth quick incisions. **(B)** The skin may be elevated with the orbicularis muscle in one maneuver, proceeding from lateral to medial. **(C)** The orbital septum is then opened, exposing the preaponeurotic space. The underlying levator aponeurosis is protected by opening the septum as cephalad as possible. (Adapted from Spinelli HM. Atlas of Aesthetic Eyelid and Periocular Surgery. Philadelphia: Saunders; 2004:64.)

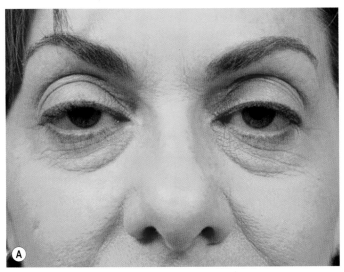

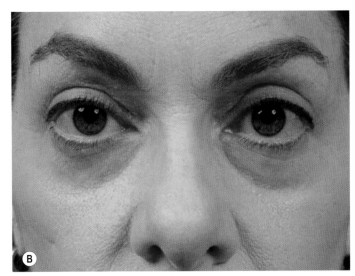

Fig. 8.26 (A) Preoperative and **(B)** postoperative photograph depicting predictable results with simple skin excision blepharoplasty anchor technique in addition to levator advancement with reinsertion into tarsus.

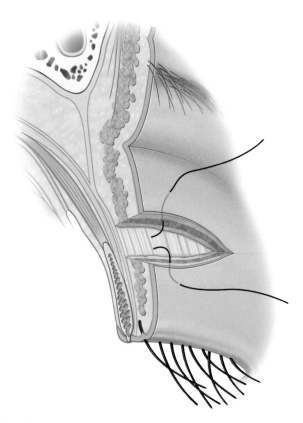

Fig. 8.27 Anchor blepharoplasty technique. Attaching the dermis of the pretarsal skin flap to the superior aspect of the tarsus and to the free edge of the aponeurosis. (Adapted from Spinelli HM. Atlas of Aesthetic Eyelid and Periocular Surgery. Philadelphia: Saunders; 2004:69.)

Surgical technique

There are a variety of techniques to address blepharoptosis but they are outside the scope of this chapter. We will thus present our preferred technique for uncomplicated involutional ptosis. A ptosis repair may be undertaken in combination with a skin excision upper blepharoplasty. The difference is adjusting (or advancing) the point of attachment of the levator aponeurosis to the tarsus. There is a significant learning curve to performing a ptosis repair, and even then, the ability to get perfect symmetry is elusive.

In the setting of mild upper eyelid ptosis (approx. 1 mm), where the decision has been made to avoid a formal lid ptosis procedure, selective myectomy of the upper eyelid orbicularis can be performed to widen the lid aperture. The amount of muscle to be resected depends on a host of factors, including the severity of relative lid ptosis, brow position, and fold disparity *(Fig. 8.29)*. The orbicularis muscle is then resected selectively using cautery that strips orbicularis muscle from the underlying orbital septum. The amount of resection is titrated depending on the amount of effect desired. For 1 mm or less of relative upper lid ptosis, resection of at least 3–4 mm of orbicularis is required. The effects are more powerful the closer the resection is to the inferior edge of the elliptical wound. No attempt is made to close orbicularis muscle in this resection, which could increase the risk of lagophthalmos. On the opposite side, which is likely retracted, a slight ptosis can be induced by resecting a larger degree of orbicularis

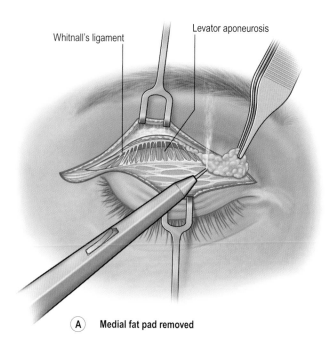

Ⓐ **Medial fat pad removed**

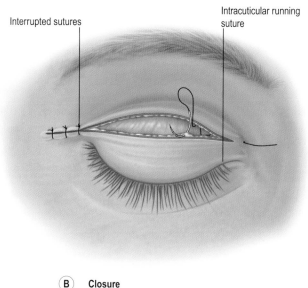

Ⓑ   **Closure**

Fig. 8.28 Simple skin excision blepharoplasty. **(A)** The medial fat pad may require digital pressure to expose and grasp; however, care should be taken not to overly resect fat when using digital pressure techniques. **(B)** Closure may then be performed with a combination of interrupted and running intracuticular sutures. (Adapted from Spinelli HM. Atlas of Aesthetic Eyelid and Periocular Surgery. Philadelphia: Saunders; 2004:65.)

and/or lowering the upper eyelid margin. Placing the upper eyelid incision and crease 2 mm or higher on the relatively retracted side can also reduce the need for formal lid retraction surgery.[38]

The key components of formal lid ptosis correction include correct identification of the distal extensions of the aponeurosis and the orbital septal extension.[12] The superior edge of the tarsus is freed from any dermal or tendinous extensions. Leaving a small cuff of filmy connective tissue (approx. 1 mm) on the tarsus will minimize bleeding from the richly vascularized area. Ensure that there is complete hemostasis by use of

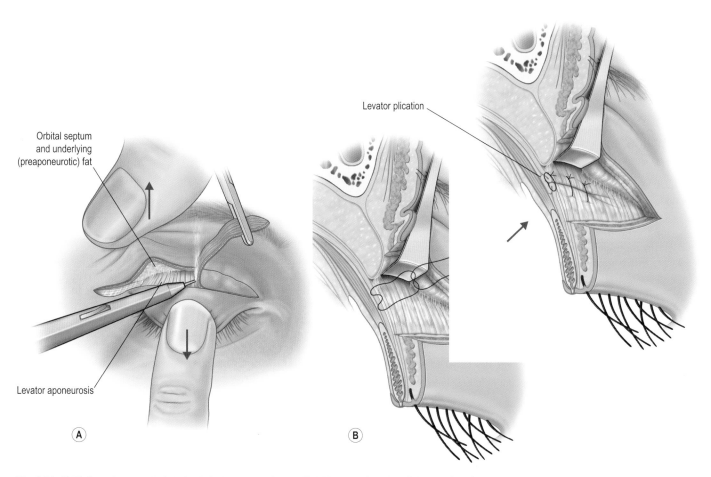

Fig. 8.29 (A,B) Once the upper lid is incised, the levator may be modified (shortened/lengthened) in a number of ways, including simple plication. A suborbicularis skin flap can also be developed allowing access to preaponeurotic fat. (Adapted from Spinelli HM. Atlas of Aesthetic Eyelid and Periocular Surgery. Philadelphia: Saunders; 2004:69.)

a fine forceps cautery, lifting all lid tissues away from the cornea and globe before cauterizing. Anchor the upper third of the tarsus to the remaining levator with 5–0 silk suture, placed as a horizontal mattress. The lid should be flipped to ensure that the suture is not exposed posteriorly on the tarsus, which could cause a troublesome corneal abrasion. The level should be checked by having the patient open the eye. Some coaxing helps the patient open the eye gently rather than maximally, which the patient has been used to doing consistently to compensate for ptosis. The patient should blink frequently and look superiorly to ensure that the lid never rises above the superior limbus. For cases under general anesthetic, one should attempt to create one to two times the amount of lagophthalmos relative to the preoperative ptosis.

If there is any medial or lateral retraction or ptosis, the central suture should be repositioned medially or laterally as many times as needed, with adjustment to a pleasing lid height and contour. Both sides should be completed before the suture is permanently tied. Once the desired lid height and contour of both eyes are achieved, the patient should be asked to open and close the eyes to ensure symmetry. Anchoring the tarsus, dermis, and aponeurosis at the right level keeps the pretarsal skin taut and flat, prevents lash eversion, and forms a neat, crisp lid crease that will persevere for many years.

Lower lid blepharoplasty

Lower blepharoplasty has evolved substantially. There are two trends in blepharoplasty, one towards more aggressive techniques to maximize the aesthetic outcome and the other towards more conservative techniques to minimize the risk of complications. Although excellent aesthetic results can be achieved with transcutaneous lower blepharoplasty, lid retraction and ectropion are concerning complications. Conservative excisional techniques center on the concept of fat preservation. Transconjunctival lower blepharoplasty, although more conservative, does not eliminate the risk of lid malposition. An effective, lasting procedure should address the extrinsic and intrinsic support of the eye, which is weakened during the aging process.

In the classic concept of lower lid blepharoplasty, the concern of the surgeon who resects lid fat is the difficulty of estimating the correct amount of fat to remove.[44] If this is not done correctly, this miscalculation may lead to asymmetry, hollowing, or a sunken lid appearance. Relative enophthalmos is an obvious sign of aging because the volume of fat decreases due to involution and herniation within the bony orbit. By extension, rejuvenation proceeds by maintaining the fatty volume and strengthening the globe's extrinsic support by canthopexy and orbicularis and midface suspension.

Transconjunctival blepharoplasty

Transconjunctival blepharoplasty is the preferred procedure for fat reduction in patients without excess skin and with good canthal position. A transconjunctival approach is less likely to lead to lower lid malposition than is a transcutaneous approach. It minimizes but does not eliminate postoperative lower lid retraction; transection of the lower lid retractors can cause a temporary rise in the lid margin, especially if they are suspended during the healing period. Previously suspected septal scarring through transconjunctival fat excision has not been shown to significantly alter lid posture or tonicity.[45]

The lower lid retractors (capsulopalpebral fascia and inferior tarsal muscle) and overlying conjunctiva lie directly posterior to the three fat pads of the lower lid. A broad and deep transconjunctival incision severs both conjunctiva and retractors but typically should not incise the orbital septum, orbicularis, or skin. The conjunctival incision is made with a monopolar cautery needle tip at least 4 mm below the inferior border of the tarsus – never through the tarsus (*Fig. 8.30*). A preseptal approach is obtained by entering the conjunctiva above the level of septal attachment to the capsulopalpebral fascia. A retroseptal approach involves a 1.5–2 cm incision lower down in the fornix, and is typically used to excise fat. There are differences of opinion about whether to leave the transconjunctival incision open or to close it; however, it is preferable to leave it open. Suturing the wound may trap bacteria or cause corneal irritation. Conjunctival closure, when it is elected, is simplified by a monofilament pull-out suture that enters the eye externally, closes the conjunctiva, and exits through the skin and is taped.

The incision through the conjunctiva and retractors gives excellent access to the orbital fat. A 6–0 silk traction suture passed through the inferior conjunctival wound and retracted over the globe gives wide access to the orbital fat, even helping to prolapse the fat into the wound. The thin film of synovium-appearing capsule encasing the orbital fat is opened, releasing the fat to bulge into the operative field (*Fig. 8.31*).

Once fat is removed or repositioned through a transconjunctival incision, excess skin can be removed through a subciliary position. Fat reduction may leave skin excess, leading to wrinkling. A conservative "skin pinch" can be done to estimate skin removal, or alternatively, skin can be tightened by skin resurfacing with chemical or laser peels (*Fig. 8.32*). One should be careful not to incise the orbital septum, which leads to increased postoperative retraction. This procedure works particularly well when there is an isolated fat pad, especially medially, accessed through a single stab incision through the conjunctiva.

Transcutaneous blepharoplasty

A subciliary incision can be used to develop a skin flap or a skin-muscle flap. With either method, pretarsal orbicularis fibers should remain intact. For the skin-muscle flap, skin and preseptal orbicularis are elevated as one flap, while with a skin flap, the muscle and its innervation can be preserved.[14] Periorbital fat, muscle, and skin can be addressed with either approach. Once the plane deep to the orbicularis is entered, dissection continues between the muscle and the orbital septum down to the level of the orbital rim. Periorbital fat can

be excised through small incisions in the septum. The fat can also be retropositioned using capsulopalpebral fascia placation, or it can be transferred into the naso-jugular fold. Orbicularis muscle fibers and skin can be excised at closure. However, care must be taken with muscle excision, which can lead to orbicularis denervation and lid malposition.

Orbital fat

The relative excess of orbital fat may be handled in several ways. Most commonly, surgeons choose to excise the herniated fat with meticulous attention to hemostasis. Additional techniques exist to reposition the fat to create periorbital harmony.

Orbital fat transposition

An alternative to excising prominent orbital fat is to redrape the pedicled fat onto the arcus marginalis. Patients with tear trough deformities who have prominent medial fat pads are excellent candidates.[46] Access to the medial and central fat pads is by the subciliary or transconjunctival incision.[47] The minor degree of lateral fat pad prominence is generally insufficient to affect any change with repositioning. A supraperiosteal or a subperiosteal dissection for 8–10 mm caudal to the inferior orbital rim permits tension-free placement. The fat can be secured in place with interrupted absorbable sutures. This technique can be used as an alternative to fat grafting or filler injection. Patients must be warned that various degrees of fat loss and hardening are possible. There is also a rare but described possibility of restrictive strabismus related to aggressive fat mobilization and fixation.

Plication techniques

The fundamental agreement among surgeons who practice plication is that bulging of orbital fat is the major component in most cases of eyelid aging deformity. The conclusion is that most cases of baggy eyelids occur from a true herniation of the orbital fat out of the bony orbit. Consequently, rejuvenation centers on re-establishing the normal position of the globe orbital fat. Plication offers the advantages of prevention of depletion of the orbita, achievement of a homogeneous and natural eyelid, avoiding local hollowing and sunken lid appearance, and no risk of infraorbital hematomas. Access is through a transcutaneous approach, which gives superior exposure.

Orbital septum plication

In this procedure, the herniated septum is plicated and repositioned to its normal anatomic site within the orbit. The fat is replaced in the retroseptal position to regain its original anatomic integrity (*Fig. 8.33*). Three to four 5–0 polyglycolic acid sutures are placed in a vertical fashion from medial to lateral. The protruding fat pads are invaginated and the integrity of the thin, flaccid septum is restored. Additional support may be gained with septo-orbitoperiostoplasty variation.[48] This technique plicates the flaccid septum and secures it to the periosteum of the inferior orbital rim. Because of no disruption of the eyelid anatomy occurs, complications of related to lid malposition such as lid retraction, scleral show, and ectropion are reduced.[49]

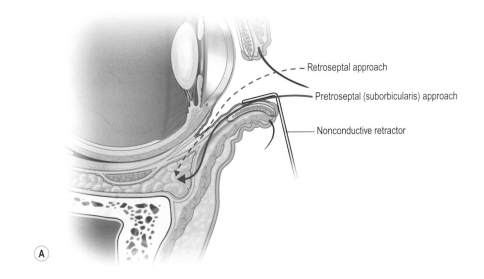

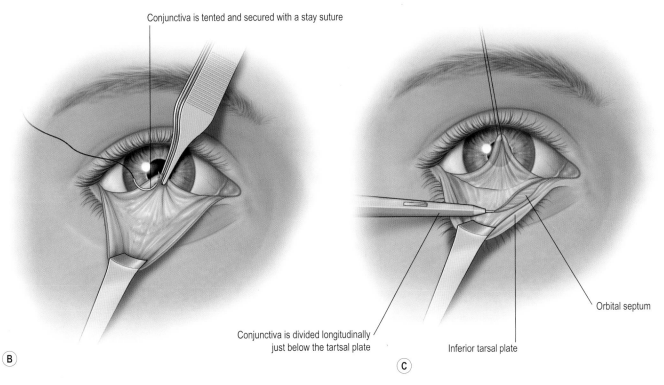

Fig. 8.30 (A) The transconjunctival approach to the retroseptal space may be in one of two ways: preseptal or retroseptal. The preseptal route requires entry into the suborbicularis preseptal space above the fusion of the lower lid retractors and the orbital septum. This will allow direct visualization of the septum, and each fat pad can be addressed separately in a controlled fashion. **(B)** A conjunctival stay suture is placed deep in the fornix and traction is applied superiorly while the lid margin is everted. This causes the inferior edge of the tarsal plate to rise toward the surgeon. **(C)** The conjunctiva and lower lid retractors are incised just below the tarsal plate entering the suborbicularis preseptal space. This plane is developed to the orbital rim with the assistance of the traction suture and a nonconductive instrument. (Adapted from Spinelli HM. Atlas of Aesthetic Eyelid and Periocular Surgery. Philadelphia: Saunders; 2004:86.)

Capsulopalpebral fascia plication

Anatomical dissection suggests that the Lockwood suspensory ligament descends with aging that leads to relative enophthalmos and fat herniation. Moreover, simply plicating the orbital septum, which is an acellular membrane with little tensile strength, will not restore the globe's position. The capsulopalpebral fascia can be plicated to the orbital rim either through a transcutaneous or a transconjunctival approach. In the transcutaneous method, dissection is carried out between the orbicularis and the septum down to the orbital rim; the capsulopalpebral fascia is then sutured to the orbital rim. In the transconjunctival method, the capsulopalpebral fascia is divided from the tarsus, and orbital fat is retroplaced, its position maintained by suturing the capsulopalpebral fascia to the periosteum of the orbital rim using a continuous running

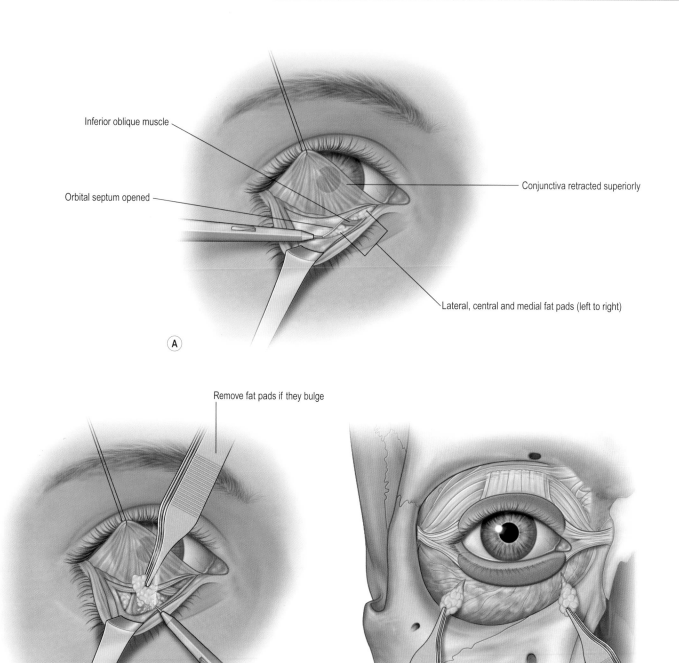

Inferior oblique muscle

Orbital septum opened

Conjunctiva retracted superiorly

Lateral, central and medial fat pads (left to right)

(A)

Remove fat pads if they bulge

(B)

Reposition fat pads transconjunctivally

Fig. 8.31 (A) The orbital septum may then be punctured and the inferior oblique muscle identified and preserved. **(B)** The fat pad may be addressed individually in-keeping with preoperative plans with either resection, repositioning, conservation or any combination of the these techniques. (Adapted from Spinelli HM. Atlas of Aesthetic Eyelid and Periocular Surgery. Philadelphia: Saunders; 2004:87.)

6–0 nonabsorbable suture. The conjunctival gap of a few millimeters is allowed to reepithelialize *(Fig. 8.34)*.[50–52] One advantage of the transconjunctival approach is the division of lower eyelid depressors, which helps maintain the lower eyelid at an elevated level due to the unopposed action of the pretarsal orbicularis. Several series have shown this disruption does not interfere with lower eyelid or globe function.[48,50]

Orbicularis suspension

Orbicularis repositioning can be used to eliminate hypotonic and herniated orbicularis muscle, soften palpebral depressions, and shorten the lower lid to cheek distance. The main steps include elevation of a skin muscle flap, release of the orbicularis retaining ligament and resuspension of the orbicularis – frequently after lateral canthopexy. Along the entire

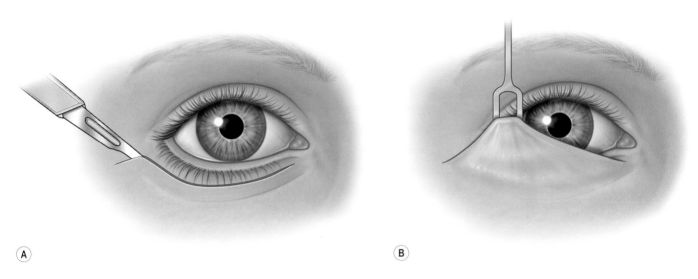

Fig. 8.32 (A) Simple skin excision lower eyelid blepharoplasty. **(B)** Typical removal of redraped skin or skin-muscle from the lower lid, which can be the shape of an obtuse triangle, with the largest amount sacrificed laterally.

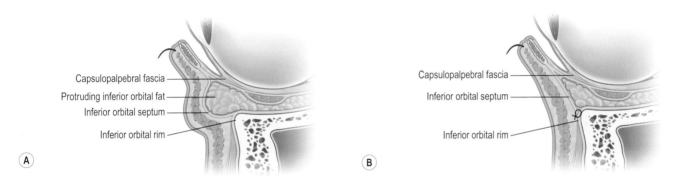

Fig. 8.33 (A,B) Schematic representation of procedure for lower eyelid. Note that only the inferior orbital septum is plicated and sutured to the inferior orbital rim. (Adapted from Sensöz O, Unlu RE, Percin A, *et al.* Septoorbitoperiostoplasty for the treatment of palpebral bags: a 10-year experience. Plast Reconstr Surg 1998; 101(6):1657–1663.)

infraorbital rim, the orbicularis retaining ligament is divided. Additional medial dissection is performed to release the levator labii when a tear trough deformity is present.

The skin muscle flap is draped in a superior lateral vector rather than a pure vertical vector. Excision of skin and muscle are performed by removing a triangle of tissue lateral to the canthus, thereby minimizing the amount of tissue removed along the actual lid margin. The lateral suspension of the orbicularis is to the orbital periosteum. Lower lid support is gained by resuspension of the anterior (skin and muscle) and posterior lamellae (tarsus by canthopexy).

This technique is best suited for patients with scleral show, lid laxity, and a negative vector, which put them at risk for lid malposition in the postoperative period. Its drawback is that it inherently disrupts the orbicularis, which may lead to denervation. Mobilization of the levator labii muscles also may put the buccal branch of the facial nerve at risk.

Canthopexy

As the lateral canthal tendon lengthens, it shortens the aperture and allows the lid posture to drop to give the illusion of excess lower lid skin as the tissues accordion inferiorly. With restoration of the normal intercanthal axis tilt, lid tone, and septal integrity, the appearance of excess skin and herniated fat disappears with minimal tissue excision and, in many patients, without the need for any muscle, skin, or fat excision *(Fig. 8.35)*.[37,53]

A lateral canthopexy can establish an aesthetically and functionally youthful eyelid *and* reduce the incidence of lower lid malposition and scleral show *(Fig. 8.36)*. It has become an integral part of a lower lid blepharoplasty and midface-lifting.[36] It is increasingly appreciated that good and long-lasting surgical results in lower lid surgery are rarely possible without an *effective* canthopexy.

A lasting canthopexy involves more than a simple stitch into the periosteum. A properly executed canthopexy restores the tone, posture, and tilt to the lower lid and serves as the fulcrum point for rejuvenation of the entire midface. In addition, it raises the Lockwood suspensory ligament (and the entire retinacular complex), lifting orbital structures upward, reducing lower lid fat herniation, and reducing upper lid hollowing – all an essential part of a youthful periorbital restoration.

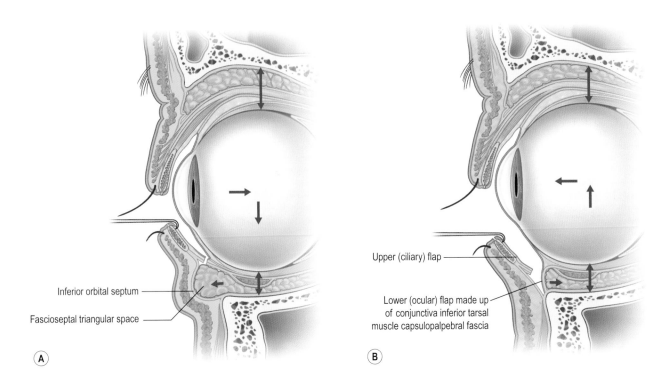

Inferior orbital septum

Fascioseptal triangular space

(A)

Upper (ciliary) flap

Lower (ocular) flap made up of conjunctiva inferior tarsal muscle capsulopalpebral fascia

(B)

Fig. 8.34 (A,B) Suturing the lower capsulopalpebral flap to the arcus marginalis to reduce and contain the herniated fat. (Adapted from Camirand A, Doucet J, Harris J. Anatomy, pathophysiology, and prevention of senile enophthalmia and associated herniated lower eyelid pads. Plast Reconstr Surg 1997; 100(3):1535–1538.)

The degree of laxity predetermines the type of lateral canthal support. A lateral canthopexy is recommended for moderate lid laxity, which is considered <6 mm of lid distraction away from the globe. This technique takes advantage of a bluntly dissected tunnel extending from the lateral upper lid blepharoplasty incision into the lateral aspect of a lower lid incision. Next, the lateral retinaculum and tarsal strap are bluntly dissected off the periosteum 5 mm in both directions *(Figs 8.4, 8.37)*.

A double-armed 4–0 Prolene or Mersilene is used to suture the tarsal plate and lateral retinaculum to the inner aspect of the lateral orbital rim periosteum above the Whitnall tubercle. Periosteum is thickest at the superior and lateral orbital rim, making it a secure suture site. The mattress suture is placed through the periosteum within the lateral orbital rim to maintain the posterior position of the lid margin against the globe.

Bone canthopexy is technically possible through upper and lower lid incisions but is technically demanding. Wide exposure through a coronal brow lift provides the ideal environment and access. Bone fixation gives a profoundly longer lasting result than does periosteal fixation. Drill holes (1.5 mm drill bit) are placed 2–3 mm posterior to the lateral orbital rim. The inferior and superior holes are separated by 5–10 mm to allow suture separation and ligation *(Fig. 8.38)*.

The vertical position of the lateral canthal suture is dependent on eye prominence and preexisting canthal tilt. Patients with prominent eyes and negative vector morphology are at higher risk for lid malposition and require additional vertical

support of the lateral canthus. While the standard position of the lateral canthopexy suture is most commonly at the lower level of the pupil, patients with prominent eyes or negative vectors require additional vertical positioning of the lateral canthal support suture at the superior aspect of the pupil.

Lateral canthoplasty, which includes surgical division of the lateral canthus, is recommended for more significant lower lid laxity, defined by lid distraction >6 mm away from the globe. Lateral canthotomy, cantholysis of the inferior limb of the lateral canthal tendon, and release of the tarsal strap are performed. This dissection is followed by a 2–3 mm full-thickness lid margin resection, depending on the degree of tarsoligamentous laxity. The lateral commissure is carefully reconstructed by aligning the anatomical grey line with 6–0 plain gut. Final fixation to the lateral orbital periosteum can be as described above.

Midfacelifting

Patients will frequently complain that they would like the lower skin to be smoother and tighter, the fatty pads to be eliminated, and the tissues of the malar eminence to be fuller. Midface descent occurs in the spectrum of periorbital aging, clinically apparent in the 4th decade *(Fig. 8.39)*. The orbicularis muscle and suborbicularis oculi fat (SOOF) descend in an inferonasal direction and, in conjunction with descent of the malar fat pad, results in the fullness of the nasolabial fold frequently seen with the aging face. This inferonasal vector of aging also creates a visual lengthening of the lower

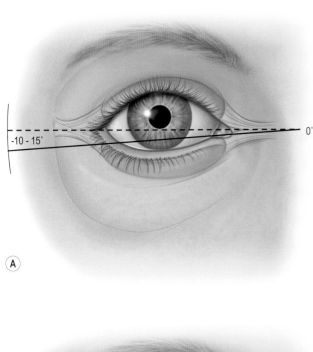

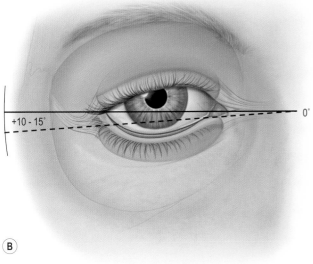

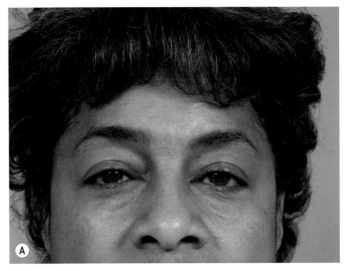

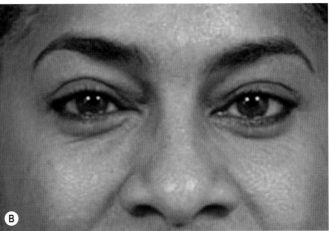

Fig. 8.36 (A) Preoperative and **(B)** 5-year postoperative photograph of a patient with a lower lid blepharoplasty and canthopexy.

Fig. 8.35 (A) Attenuation with aging produces a descent of the lateral canthus. **(B)** The end result is a lateral canthus that is linear or declined compared with the medial canthus. As the lateral canthus sags, the intercommissure distance shortens and the lower lid and inferior lateral septum become lax. This produces sclera show, lid malposition and orbital fat prominence laterally and tear drainage problems. With restoration of the normal intercanthal axis tilt, lid tone, and septal integrity, the appearance of excess skin and herniated fat disappears with minimal tissue excision and, in many, without the need for any muscle, skin, or fat excision. (Adapted from Spinelli HM. Atlas of Aesthetic Eyelid and Periocular Surgery. Philadelphia: Saunders; 2004:35.)

lids beyond the orbital margin. Lastly, relative loss of soft tissue secondarily skeletonizes the inferior orbital rim and zygoma, deepening the tear trough and diminishing the malar prominence.[54,55]

The middle third of the face, or midface, lies between the lateral canthal angle and the top of the nasolabial fold. It includes the lateral canthal tendon, the medial canthal tendon, the skin, fat, and orbicularis oculi muscle of the lower eyelids, the sub–orbicularis oculi fat pad, the malar fat pad, the orbito-malar ligament (orbicularis ligament), the orbital septum, and origins of the zygomaticus major and minor muscles and levator labii superioris. When evaluating the midface for aesthetic surgery, all the structures listed above must be considered.

The author's preferred technique includes approaching the midface through a transconjunctival incision. After repositioning or resection of orbital fat, the midface is elevated in a supraperiosteal plane. The attachment of the orbicularis oculi muscle to the orbital septum is preserved. Adequate release of the remaining, lax orbitomalar ligament then permits malar fat pad suspension in a superolateral vector to the lateral orbital rim and temporoparietal fascia *(Fig. 8.40)*. Canthopexy is then performed to redrape lower eyelid skin and recreate a youthful intercanthal angle. Finally, a skin only resection of the lower lid may be necessary to address any redundancy.

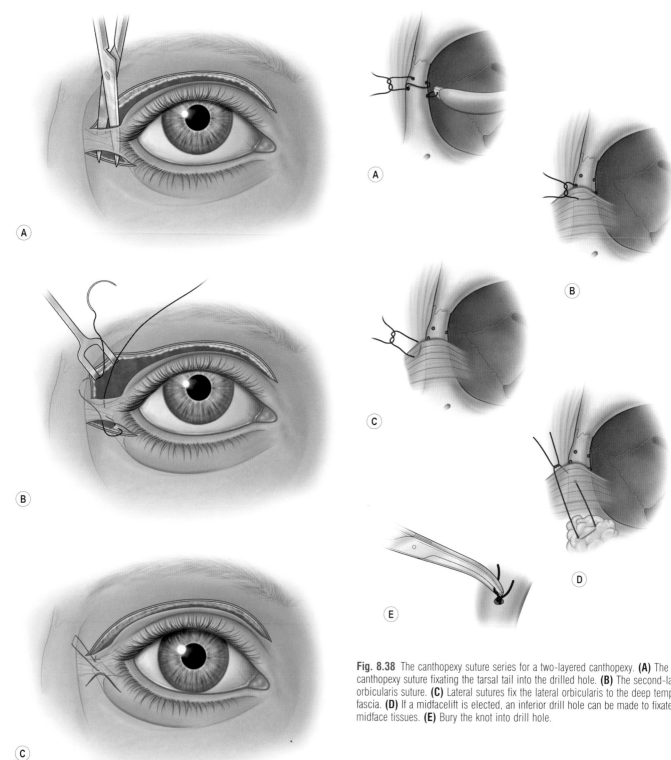

Fig. 8.38 The canthopexy suture series for a two-layered canthopexy. **(A)** The canthopexy suture fixating the tarsal tail into the drilled hole. **(B)** The second-layer orbicularis suture. **(C)** Lateral sutures fix the lateral orbicularis to the deep temporal fascia. **(D)** If a midfacelift is elected, an inferior drill hole can be made to fixate the midface tissues. **(E)** Bury the knot into drill hole.

Fig. 8.37 (A–C) Periosteal canthopexy. The inferior ramus of the lateral canthal tendon is secured and elevated to a raised position inside the orbital rim. Tension free suspension occurs with release of the tarsal strap and lateral orbital thickening.

Postoperative care

All patients are advised to expect swelling, bruising, some degree of ptosis, and tugging sensation on gazing upward. Although complete recovery takes months, patients generally look presentable approximately 2–3 weeks after surgery.

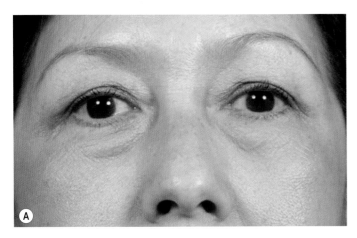

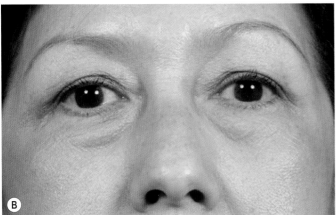

Fig. 8.39 (A) Preoperative and **(B)** postoperative photograph demonstrating the benefit of midfacelift in the setting of blepharoplasty.

Surgical literature has not advocated compression bandaging of the eyes after surgery. The concern is an undetected retrobulbar hemorrhage that results in vision loss. However, the reality is that the risk for hemorrhage, chemosis, and other problems is more likely in an eye that has no compression. Retrobulbar hemorrhage is likely to induce orbital pain, which should never be ignored, alerting the surgeon to the potential vision-threatening complication. If one chooses not to use gently compressive bandages, postoperative edema can be reduced with cool compresses for up to 20 min intermittently during the initial 36 hours postoperatively. Patients are advised against using frozen compresses directly over their face in the setting of previous anesthetic use and pain medication.[29]

Additional recommendations include having the patient lie in a semi-recumbent position while resting and to avoid bedrest. Prescriptions for rewetting drops, Lacri-Lube® and antibiotic ophthalmic ointment can be given to reduce the incidence of exposure keratoconjunctivitis and dry eye symptoms in the immediate postoperative period. Patients are permitted to shower the next day and use antibiotic ointments as needed, for routine incisional care. Avoiding direct sun exposure with sunglasses may reduce the severity of sunburn and the formation of irregular, darkened pigmentation. It is also suggested that patients refrain from using contacts and to minimize the use of prescription eyeglasses.[30]

When no canthopexy is performed, half-inch Steri-Strips, retracted superiorly, are applied as a "cast" (with benzoin or Mastisol for security). This treatment tends to reduce lid retraction. Alternatively, a Frost suture placed in the lower lid margin and fixed to the brow suspends the lid during early healing. Temporary medial or lateral limbus tarsorrhaphies were previously popular after aggressive skin excision blepharoplasty techniques. These sutures were primarily used to minimize chemosis during the first 48 h. Discomfort, restricted vision and secondary office visits for suture removal have led to their limited use today. However, the best support during healing is a secure extended canthopexy.[45]

Complications

Even the most carefully planned procedures will have a small percentage of complications. The possibility of such complications and a realistic appraisal of likely outcome should be discussed with the patient before surgery.

Asymmetry is common postoperatively and can be caused by edema, bruising, and asymmetric sleep posture, but it also predictably follows undiagnosed preoperative asymmetry, including mild ptosis, made worse by the weight of postoperative edema. Patients should be advised that no reoperations are indicated before 8 weeks, and then only if the lids have stabilized and no edema or bruising is seen. The need for reoperations is infrequent, but when ptosis or exophthalmos is involved, incidence increases significantly to 10–30%.[45]

Retrobulbar hemorrhage is the most feared complication of eyelid surgery. Any complaint of severe orbital pain needs to be examined immediately, especially that of sudden onset. Acute management involves immediate evaluation, urgent ophthalmologic consultation and a return to the operation for evacuation of the hematoma. Medical treatments, in addition to operative exploration, include administration of high flow oxygen, topical and systemic corticosteroids and mannitol. Acute loss of vision mandates bedside suture removal and decompressive lateral canthotomy. Hospitalization with head elevation and close observation may be necessary to supplement the described measures.[29] Peribulbar hematoma, in contrast, does not threaten vision. It usually results from bleeding of an orbicularis muscle vessel. Small hematomas may resolve spontaneously, though larger hematomas can be evacuated in the office.

Visual changes, including diplopia, are generally temporary and can be attributed to wound reaction, edema and hematoma. Any damage to the superficial lying oblique muscles can be permanent and lead to postoperative strabismus. Conservative management is recommended; refractory cases should be referred to an ophthalmologist.

The most common complication after blepharoplasty is chemosis. Disruption of ocular and eyelid lymphatic drainage leads to development of milky, conjunctival and corneal edema. Chemosis can be limited by atraumatic dissection, cold compresses, elevation and massage. It is usually self-limited and resolves spontaneously, though prolonged chemosis can be treated with topical steroids.

Dry eye symptoms are also frequently cited in the post operative phase. Patients may complain of foreign body sensation, burning, secretions and frequent blinking. Preexisting

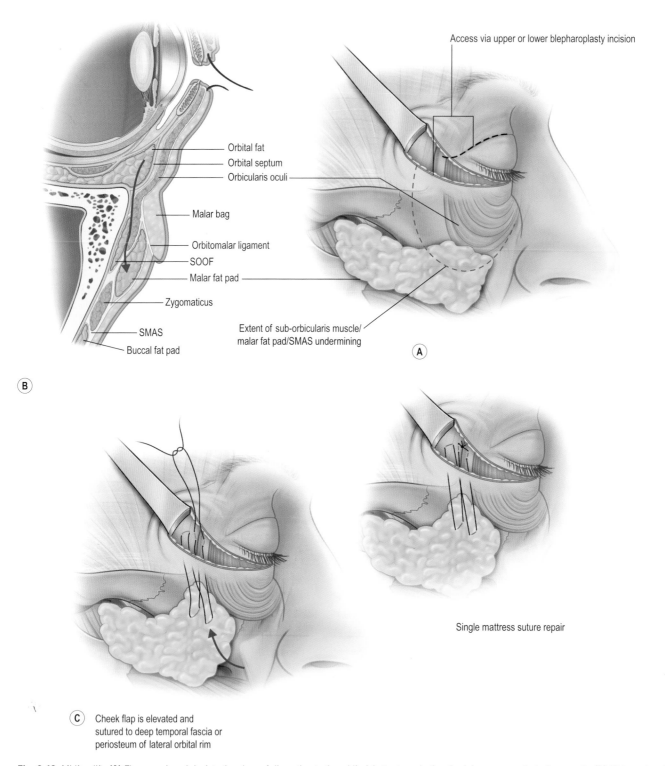

Access via upper or lower blepharoplasty incision

Orbital fat
Orbital septum
Orbicularis oculi

Malar bag

Orbitomalar ligament
SOOF
Malar fat pad

Zygomaticus

SMAS
Buccal fat pad

Extent of sub-orbicularis muscle/
malar fat pad/SMAS undermining

(A)

(B)

Single mattress suture repair

(C) Cheek flap is elevated and
sutured to deep temporal fascia or
periosteum of lateral orbital rim

Fig. 8.40 Midfacelift. **(A)** The arrow in red depicts the plane of dissection to the midfacial structures in the cheek in a supraperiosteal approach. **(B)** Wide undermining of the periorbital ligamentous structures and lateral retinaculum may be transconjunctival or through the upper blepharoplasty incision. **(C)** Canthopexy and cheek suspension then proceed sequentially. (Adapted from Spinelli HM. Atlas of Aesthetic Eyelid and Periocular Surgery. Philadelphia: Saunders; 2004:129.)

dry eyes may be aggravated by postoperative lagophthalmos. Ocular protection can achieved medically with liberal use of corneal lubricants.

Additional complications such as lower lid malposition, lagophthalmos, undercorrection, asymmetry, and iatrogenic ptosis all require careful observation and photographic documentation. Reoperation should be performed no earlier than 3 months later. Secondary blepharoplasty can range from simple office-based procedures to extremely challenging interventions.

Special considerations

Male blepharoplasty

In the United States, 16% of blepharoplasties are performed on men, and blepharoplasty is the second most common cosmetic surgery performed on male patients.[56] Men tend to seek out blepharoplasty more for functional reasons than women, but this difference has become less and less distinct in recent years. A more natural look is preferred, and the "operated look" will not be tolerated well by most male patients. Men typically do not use cosmetics, so all scars must be carefully concealed. This also makes male patients suboptimal candidates for laser resurfacing. The lateral incision should rarely be extended beyond the later orbital rim. In men with heavy brows, resection of upper eyelid skin only will result in profoundly ptotic brows. Therefore, one should consider combined brow surgery with upper blepharoplasty. Many men are reluctant to have cosmetic surgery to correct brow ptosis, so careful preoperative counseling is needed to prevent a dissatisfied patient with worse brow ptosis postoperatively.[30,57] Often, conservative eyelid resection is all that is required.

Blepharoplasty in people of color

Patients who identify themselves other than Caucasian now account for 27% of all cosmetic procedures. Hispanics, African-Americans and Asian-Americans have seen a steady rise in their market share over the last 10 years. According to the American Society for Aesthetic Plastic Surgery, there was a 293% increase in the number of African-American patients who underwent cosmetic plastic surgery from 1997 to 2004.[58] The awareness of the benefits of cosmetic plastic surgery is becoming ever-present to a patient population which transcends cultural and racial boundaries.

African-American patients pursuing eyelid rejuvenation have preconceived notions and concerns distinct from their Caucasian counterparts, thereby demanding a different surgical strategy. African-Americans are twice as likely as Caucasians to be afraid of losing their ethnic identity and 10 times as likely to choose a surgeon with special interests in ethnic plastic surgery. There are several features that make the African-American eye ethnically unique. The lateral canthus is cephalad to the medial canthus in great frequency. In addition, there is a tendency for a more oval, Asian-like palpebral aperture, as opposed to the more rounded Caucasian palpebral fissure. The supratarsal fold distance tends to be shorter than in the Caucasian eyelid but longer than the Asian eyelid. The lateral orbit and cheek skin is more sebaceous, and there is a decreased tendency toward rhytid formation. Finally, African-Americans tend to be poor candidates for lower eyelid resurfacing because of pigmentation risk. The preferred surgical approach includes canthopexy to restore lateral canthal position, preservation of the majority of orbicularis to restore supratarsal contour and avoidance of cephalad malposition of the upper eyelid incision to preserve limited pretarsal show. These subtleties are discussed preoperatively, often with the aid of youthful photographs, to appropriately plan surgery.[25,59]

The unique characteristics of the Asian blepharoplasty will be thoroughly discussed in Chapter 10.

 Access the complete references list online at **http://www.expertconsult.com**

12. Flowers RS, Nassif JM, Rubin PA, et al. A key to canthopexy: the tarsal strap. A fresh cadaveric study. *Plast Reconstr Surg*. 2005;116(6):1752–1758.

    Flowers and colleagues detail the anatomy of the lateral orbital retinaculum and highlight the importance of full dissection to achieve a tension-free canthopexy.

14. Spinelli HM. *Atlas of aesthetic eyelid and periocular surgery.* Philadelphia: Saunders; 2004.

15. Zide BM. *Surgical anatomy around the orbit: the system of zones.* ed 2. Philadelphia: Lippincott, Williams & Wilkins; 2006.

17. Reid RR, Said HK, Yu M, et al. Revisiting upper eyelid anatomy: introduction of the septal extension. *Plast Reconstr Surg*. 2006;117(1):65–70.

    This cadaveric and histologic study identifies an extension of the orbital septum that must be identified and spared when performing a levator advancement for blepharoptosis.

21. Muzaffar AR, Mendelson BC, Adams Jr WP. Surgical anatomy of the ligamentous attachments of the lower lid and lateral canthus. *Plast Reconstr Surg*. 2002;110(3):873–884.

26. Hirmand H. Anatomy and nonsurgical correction of tear trough deformity. *Plast Reconstr Surg*. 2010;125(2):699–708.

30. Rohrich RJ, Coberly DM, Fagien S, et al. Current concepts in aesthetic upper blepharoplasty. *Plast Reconstr Surg*. 2004;3:32e–42e.

    This continuing medical education article provides a concise description of upper eyelid aging and a step-by-step guide to popular rejuvenation techniques.

36. Flowers RS. Canthopexy as a routine blepharoplasty component. *Clin Plast Surg*. 1993;20(2):351–365.

44. Mendelson BC. Fat preservation technique of lower-lid blepharoplasty. *Aesthet Surg J*. 2001;21(5):450–459.

    Results shown in Mendelson's article demonstrate the safe, reproducible outcomes of a skin-only blepharoplasty and help swing the pendulum away from aggressive, fat excisional techniques.

45. Codner MA, Wolfi J, Anzarut A. Primary transcutaneous lower blepharoplasty with routine lateral canthal support: a comprehensive 10-year review. *Plast Reconstr Surg*. 2008;121(1):241–250.

59. Few JW. Rejuvenation of the African American Periorbital Area: Dynamic Considerations. *Semin Plast Surg*. 2009;23(1):198–206.

    Few's survey-based study shows that one must prioritize a patient's ethnic identity and heritage when approaching the periorbital area in African-Americans.

9

Secondary blepharoplasty: Techniques

Glenn W. Jelks, Elizabeth B. Jelks, Ernest S. Chiu, and Douglas S. Steinbrech

SYNOPSIS

- Serious complications of primary blepharoplasty surgery are rare, but should they occur, can be difficult to correct and be potentially disastrous.
- Some serious complications which develop early, such as corneal exposure, require aggressive treatment, but lesser complications such as minor lid malpositions should be dealt with after time has passed to allow for scar maturation.
- The eyelids can be divided into four anatomic zones.
- Upper eyelid problems include ptosis and lid retraction. An understanding of Herring's law is necessary to diagnose the problem responsible for lid level asymmetry.
- Lower lid malposition is a common problem after primary blepharoplasty, and is due to an interplay between the patient's unique orbital and eyelid anatomy, and the cicatricial forces. There are a number of predisposing factors.
- Lower lid evaluation should address the presence of cicatricial contraction, a vector analysis of the globe in relation to the malar eminence, a soft tissue to bone distance at the lateral canthus, tarsoligamentous integrity (distraction and snap tests), lower lid eversion, and the level of the malar fat pad.
- Lower lid malposition can be treated with various methods, including a wide variety of canthopexy and canthoplasty procedures, vertical spacer grafts and midface elevation. In severe cases, a combination of modalities is often indicated.

Introduction

Each year, over 200 000 people in the United States have a blepharoplasty operation.[1] These operations are generally very successful with a high level of patient satisfaction. Successful operations are the result of thorough preoperative evaluation, skillfully performed customized surgical procedures, uneventful anesthesia, proper surgical venue and individualized postoperative management. Although rare, complications and unfavorable results may occur following blepharoplasty. It has been estimated that the complication rate following blepharoplasty is 2%.[2-21] Minor complications are temporary and self-limiting with minimal visual disturbance or aesthetic consequence (Table 9.1). Major complications are definitely undesirable and potentially disastrous. They include visual loss, fixed eyelid deformities, corneal decomposition, and significant aesthetic compromise (Table 9.2). In addition, an apparent technically successful operation may produce a very unhappy patient.

Once the complication is discovered, a careful and thorough evaluation of the patient's anatomical deformity and its prognosis is essential. If impending visual compromise is apparent, early emergent intervention may be warranted. Most lid malpositions are temporary and resolve within 4–6 weeks postoperatively. It is important to protect the cornea during this time. If the lid malpositions aggravate and contribute to corneal decompensation, they should be corrected as soon as possible. However, lid malpositions that do not compromise visual function may be corrected after scar maturation. In general, a delay in secondary surgical procedures to address the problem is recommended. Secondary surgery is more predictable in a surgical environment that is less inflammatory. Better results are obtained if secondary surgery can be postponed for at least 6 months and preferably 1 year following the initial surgery.

The effect of blepharoplasty procedure complications on patient and physician can be profound. When the results of an elective aesthetic surgical procedure are suboptimal, the patient usually becomes more difficult to manage. It is easier to manage a dissatisfied patient when there has been a thorough preoperative discussion of risks resulting in a signed informed consent to the procedure. It is imperative to have a handwritten note by the operating surgeon in the patient's chart documenting the explanation of the proposed surgical procedures including any risks or complications to their surgery. In addition, the alternatives to surgery should be discussed.

Table 9.1 Minor blepharoplasty complications

Retrobulbar hemorrhage without visual loss	Eyelid malposition
	  Upper eyelid
	    Ptosis
	    Retraction
	    Contour change
	    Marginal rotation
	  Lower eyelid
	    Scleral show
	    Lid retraction
	    Lid paresis
	    Marginal rotation
	    Ectropion or entropion

Pupil changes	
Glaucoma	
Extraocular muscle disorder	

Corneal changes
  Exposure
    Keratitis
    Erosion
    Ulcer
  Refractive
    Astigmatism
    Edema
    Tear film abnormality
  Basement membrane disorder
	Eyelid deformities
	  Hematoma
	  Epicanthal folds
	  Cysts
	  Wound separation
	  Eyelid numbness
	  Eyelid discoloration
	  Scars
	  Loss of eyelashes

Lacrimal disorder
  Dry eye
  Epiphora
    Tear film abnormality
    Reflexly stimulated tears
    Tear distribution abnormalities
      Lid margin eversion
      Lid retraction
      Lid ectropion
      Lid entropion
      Lid paresis
    Tear drainage abnormalities
      Punctal eversion
      Obstruction of nasolacrimal system
      Lid paresis
  Dacryocystitis
	Inflammatory conditions
	  Infectious
	    Cellulitis
	    Abscess
	    Hordeolum
	    Chalazion
	    Blepharitis
	  Noninfectious
	    Allergic
	    Chemical
	    Blepharitis

Conjunctival changes
  Chemosis
  Prolapse
  Incarceration
  Hemorrhage	

From Jelks GW, Jelks EB. Blepharoplasty. In: Peck GC, ed. Complications and problems in aesthetic plastic surgery. New York: Gower Medical Publishing; 1992.[27]

Once a complication occurs, more time and effort by the physician and his support staff will be required. This often translates into arranging for more frequent office visits. The physician must devote more time to help the patient through this disappointing situation. Reassurance by the surgeon in the face of temporary complications will aid in patient acceptance of prolonged healing.

The easiest complication to avoid is failure to recognize a pre-existing condition that would increase the likelihood of an unfavorable result from standard blepharoplasty (*Table 9.3*).[22–25] The pre-existing conditions include: (1) medical or ophthalmological conditions that may increase the risk of visual impairment; (2) morphological variants that predispose the patient to post-blepharoplasty eyelid malpositions;

(3) anatomical variations that may be accentuated after eyelid skin, muscle; and fat removal and, most importantly, (4) the psychological status of the patient and assessment of their expectations of surgery. The presence of a pre-existing condition does not preclude cosmetic blepharoplasty; however, the surgical timing, venue, and technique may have to be altered.

The following discussion contains relevant information regarding anatomical zones of the eyelids as well as prevention, diagnosis, and management of complications in the post-blepharoplasty patient. Although malposition of both the upper and lower eyelid are presented, a particular emphasis is placed on unnatural distortion of the lower eyelid as these are the most common types of defects encountered.

Table 9.2 Major blepharoplasty complications

Visual loss or alteration	Contour changes
Globe penetration	Margin abnormalities
Retrobulbar hemorrhage	Lower eyelid
Glaucoma	Scleral show
Extraocular muscle disorder	Retraction
Corneal	Laxity
Exposure	Paralysis
Ulcer	Margin abnormalities
Filaments	Ectropion
Scar	Entropion
Neovascularization	Eyelid deformities
Refractive	Palpebral aperture asymmetry
Astigmatism	Unveiled pre-existing condition
Tear film abnormality	Iatrogenic
Contact lens intolerance	Upper eyelid fold
Basement membrane disorder	Asymmetric
Permanent eyelid deformities and functional disorders	Absent
Lacrimal disorders	High
Dry eye	Low
Epiphora	Multiple
Tear film abnormalities (reflexly stimulated)	Epicanthal folds
Tear distribution abnormalities	Cicatrix
Lid eversion	Inadequate fat removal
Lid retraction	Excessive fat removal
Ectropion	Suture tunnels
Entropion	Dermal pigmentary changes
Tear drainage abnormalities	Festoons
Lid paralysis	Malar pads
Medial punctal eversion	
Obstruction of nasolacrimal system	
Eyelid malpositions	
Upper eyelid	
Ptosis	
Retraction	

From Jelks GW, Jelks EB. Blepharoplasty. In: Peck GC, ed. Complications and problems in aesthetic plastic surgery. New York: Gower Medical Publishing; 1992.[27]

Anatomical zones

To facilitate complete and thorough anatomical analysis, the eyelids are divided into zones *(Fig. 9.1)*.[22,26] Zone 0 includes the ocular globe and orbital structures behind the arcus marginalis, posterior lacrimal crest, and lateral retinaculum. Zones I and II include the upper eyelid and lower eyelid, respectively, from the lateral commissure to the temporal aspect of canalicular puncti. Zone III is the medial canthus with the lacrimal drainage system. Zone IV is the lateral retinaculum. Zones I–IV are further subdivided into structures that are anterior (preseptal) or posterior (postseptal) to the orbital septum. Zone V includes the contiguous periorbital structures of nasal, glabella, brow, forehead, temple, malar, and nasojugal regions which merge with zones I–IV *(Fig. 9.2)*. The diagnosis and management of upper eyelid (zone I) and lower eyelid (zone II) complications that occur as a result of blepharoplasty procedures will be discussed in detail.

Corneal protection

In both primary and secondary surgery of the eyelids and orbital region, protection of the cornea is essential. Specially designed, protective contact lenses should be routine *(Fig. 9.3)*.[27] Colored lenses are preferred as they filter bright operating light if the procedure is performed under local anesthesia, and they are also less often inadvertently left on the cornea postoperatively. The contact shell prevents desiccation and inadvertent corneal injury by an instrument or gauze. In order to avoid postoperative corneal abrasions, deep sutures on or near the conjunctival surface should be placed in such a manner that the knots are buried in the tissue or placed externally. A continuous buried suture that may be pulled out after healing is particularly useful in the approximation of tissue over the cornea. Skin grafts should not be placed in the conjunctival sac if they are to be in contact with the cornea; only conjunctival or other mucosal tissue is tolerated by the cornea.

Table 9.3 **Prevention of blepharoplasty complications: preoperative evaluation**

Pre-existing conditions
  Medical conditions
    Hypertension
    Diabetes
    Bleeding disorders
    Inflammatory skin condition
    Asthma
    Sulfite allergy
    Venous thrombosis
    Cardiac disorders
    Atherosclerosis
    COPD
    Emphysema
    Sleep apnea
  Ophthalmological conditions
    Amblyopia
    Diplopia
    Strabismus
    Glaucoma
    Corneal disease
    Eyelid disorder
    High myopia
    Contact lens wearer
    Retinal disorders
    Uveitis
    Dry eye
    Tear film dysfunction
    Refractive surgery
	Morphology
	  Negative vector
	    Malar hypoplasia
	    High myopia
	    Small orbital volume
	  Horizontal lid laxity
	    Involutional
	    Cicatricial
	    Ectropion
	    Entropion
	
	Anatomical variations
	    Tear trough deformity
	    Malar pads
	    Festoons
	    Cheek-lid interface deformity
	    True ptosis
	    Look ptosis
	    Frontalis spasm
	    Corrugator hyperactivity
	    Crow's feet
	    Punctal eversion
	    Ectropion
	    Entropion
	
	Psychological
	    Realistic outcome expectations
	    Ability to deal with vision loss, deformity
	    Body dysmorphic disorder
	    Body image

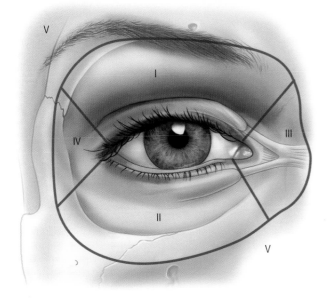

Fig. 9.1 Surgical zones of the eyelids and periocular structures. Zone I, upper eyelid; zone II, lower eyelid; zone III, medial canthal structures including the lacrimal drainage system; zone IV, lateral canthal area; zone V, periocular contiguous area-glabella, eyebrow, forehead, temple, malar, nasojugal and nasal areas. (From Spinelli HM, Jelks GW. Periocular reconstruction: a systematic approach. Plast Reconstr Surg 1993;91:1017.)

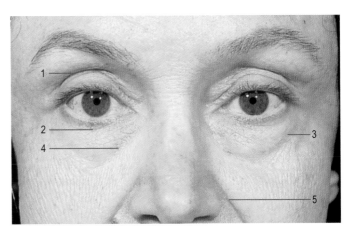

Fig. 9.2 Topographic anatomy of the eyelids and cheeks. (1) Superior eyelid fold; (2) inferior eyelid fold; (3) malar fold; (4) nasojugal fold; (5) nasolabial fold. (Modified from Jelks GW, Jelks EB. Blepharoplasty. In: Peck GC, ed. Complications and problems in aesthetic plastic surgery. New York: Gower Medical Publishing; 1992.)

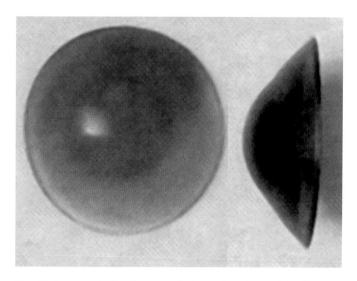

Fig. 9.3 Corneal protective shields manufactured with a steep central radius of curvature and a flat peripheral radius of curvature. This configuration prevents direct contact. Colored lenses are preferred as they filter bright operating light if the procedure is performed under local anesthesia, and they are also less often inadvertently left on the cornea postoperatively. (From Jelks GW, Jelks EB. Blepharoplasty. In: Peck GC, ed. Complications and problems in aesthetic plastic surgery. New York: Gower Medical Publishing; 1992.)

Upper eyelid

Upper eyelid malposition: evaluation and management

A thorough evaluation of the upper eyelid (zone I) level is facilitated by dividing the structure into anterior, middle, and posterior lamella (*Table 9.4*). The anterior lamella is composed of upper lid skin and orbicularis muscle. The middle lamella is composed of the tarsus, levator mechanism, orbital septum, and fat. The posterior lamella consists of the conjunctiva. The palpebral aperture is primarily influenced by the upper eyelid levels (*Fig. 9.4*). The palpebral aperture usually varies in shape, size, and obliquity due to hereditary, racial, traumatic, or other acquired situations. The surrounding bony orbital anatomy, the internal orbital volume, and the integrity of the eyelids, with their muscular and tarsoligamentous supports, are some of the factors that influence the palpebral aperture (*Figs 9.5, 9.6*). It is also influenced by the relative amount of associated periorbital skin, fat, and soft tissues. Unique individual combinations of eyelid and orbital anatomy can cause variations in the palpebral aperture (*Fig. 9.4*).[28]

The eyelid fold position should also be evaluated. In the occidental patient, the upper eyelid fold is normally 8–10 mm above the lid margin. This corresponds to the superior attachments of the levator aponeurosis to the subcutaneous tissue of the eyelid. Above the lid fold, the aponeurosis does not attach to the preseptal or orbital subcutaneous tissue, and the overhanging skin forms a fold. Inferior to the lid fold there

Table 9.4 Secondary blepharoplasty candidate evaluation: upper eyelid				
Anterior lamella	Lagophthalmos	Absent	Present	
	Skin	Normal	Abnormal	Over-resection Excess
	Scars	Normal	Abnormal	Position Quality
	Lid fold position	Normal	Abnormal	High Low Absent Multiple
	Lash position	Normal	Abnormal	
	Palpebral aperture	Symmetric	Asymmetric	
Middle lamella	Lid levels	Equal	Ptosis Unilateral Bilateral Cicatricial Mechanical Involutional	Retraction Physiologic Thyroid Bell's Cicatricial
	Levator function (measurement)	0–3 mm	3–10 mm	>10 mm
	Fat	Normal	Abnormal	Excess removal Retention
Posterior lamella	Palpebral conjunctiva	Normal	Abnormal	

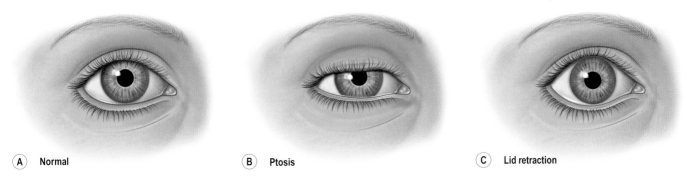

(A) Normal   **(B)** Ptosis   **(C)** Lid retraction

Fig. 9.4 (A) Normal palpebral aperture. The upper eyelid is normally 1–2 mm below the superior corneal limbus. **(B)** Ptosis is seen when the upper eyelid level is below that seen in (A), interfering with the superior visual field. **(C)** Lid retraction is seen when the elevation of the upper lid is at or above the superior corneal limbus. (Modified from Jelks GW, Jelks EB. Blepharoplasty. In: Peck GC, ed. Complications and problems in aesthetic plastic surgery. New York: Gower Medical Publishing; 1992.)

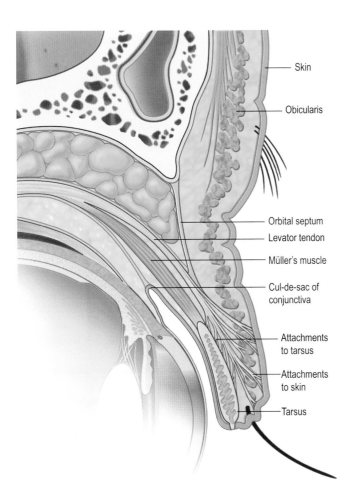

Skin

Obicularis

Orbital septum

Levator tendon

Müller's muscle

Cul-de-sac of conjunctiva

Attachments to tarsus

Attachments to skin

Tarsus

Fig. 9.5 Sagittal section through the upper eyelid showing the relationship of the orbicularis oculi muscle, septum orbitale, levator palpebrae superioris, and Mueller's muscle. (Modified from Jelks GW, Smith BC. Reconstruction of the eyelids and associated structures. In: McCarthy JG, ed. Plastic surgery. Philadelphia: WB Saunders; 1990:1671.)

are levator attachments to the subcutaneous tissue overlying the tarsus. In the Asian patient, the orbital septum inserts more inferiorly onto the distal expansion of the levator aponeurosis, which allows more preaponeurotic fat to descend into the upper eyelid and the resultant lower eyelid crease. Blepharoplasty in Asians requires the identification of suborbicular fat. Dissection through this fat layer provides access to the orbital septum and the retroseptal (preaponeurotic) fat.

Ptosis and lid retraction are conditions that alter the palpebral aperture by affecting the anatomic position of the upper eyelid. Localization of any major eyelid pathology facilitates the delineation of corrective procedures. The most commonly seen upper eyelid complications requiring secondary correction are ptosis and lid retraction.

Ptosis

Ptosis is the abnormally low level of the upper eyelid.[28–31] Ptosis of the upper eyelid can result from damage to the levator complex during retroseptal dissection by direct trauma, hematoma, edema, or septal adhesions.[28,32–38] The normal upper eyelid level covers 2–3 mm of the superior limbus or lies at the level midway between the superior edge of a 4 mm pupil and the superior corneal limbus *(Fig. 9.4)*. Preoperative variations in upper eyelid levels may result from the level of alertness, pharmacologic agents, direction of gaze, size of the ocular globe, orbital volume, visual acuity, and extraocular muscle balance.[28] Occasionally, unrecognized ptosis manifests itself in the postoperative blepharoplasty patient. Review of the preoperative examination records and medical photography usually reveals the etiology. When no presenting condition can be documented, a surgical misadventure is implicated in the etiology.

Mechanical ptosis due to postoperative edema is symmetric and transient and usually resolves spontaneously within 48–72 h. A hematoma in the retroseptal space can cause impairment of levator muscle function, maintaining the upper eyelid in a ptotic position. Resorption of the hematoma may produce secondary fibrosis of the levator with persistent ptosis. Attempts to create high upper eyelid supratarsal folds involve fixing the skin muscle edges to the levator aponeurosis. This can lead to tractional ptosis if the lid fold is

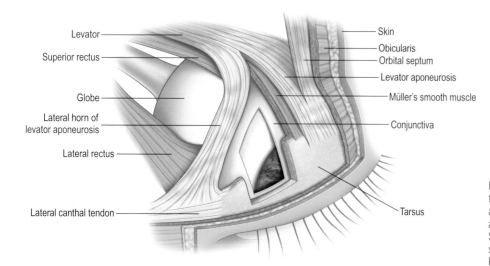

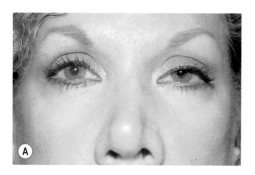

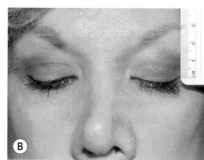

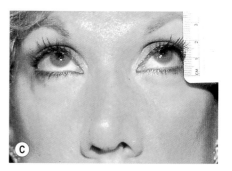

Fig. 9.6 Sagittal section illustrating the structures of the upper eyelid, including the levator muscle, its aponeurosis, and its relationship with Mueller's muscle and the septum orbitale. (Modified from Jelks GW, Smith BC. Reconstruction of the eyelids and associated structures. In: McCarthy JG, ed. Plastic surgery. Philadelphia: WB Saunders; 1990:1671.)

Fig. 9.7 (A) Patient with acquired ptosis of the left upper lid. **(B,C)** Levator function of 15 mm was measured with a ruler from down gaze to up gaze while manually blocking brow elevation of the upper eyelid. Levator function >10 mm is considered good. (From Jelks GW, Jelks EB. Blepharoplasty. In: Peck GC, ed. Complications and problems in aesthetic plastic surgery. New York: Gower Medical Publishing; 1992.)

placed too high. The medial and lateral retinaculae become tense and lower the upper lid level. Treatment consists of observation and massage of the upper eyelid. If ptosis persists more than several weeks, removal of the supratarsal fixation sutures is necessary. Ptosis may also occur when adhesions develop between the orbital septum and the levator aponeurosis at a level higher than the original septal origin.

Ptosis is classified as mild at 1–2 mm, moderate at 2–3 mm, and severe at ≥4 mm.[4,22,28] The amount of ptosis is documented by measuring the vertical dimensions of the palpebral apertures at the midpupillary line. The amount of levator function in millimeters is measured whenever ptosis is diagnosed in order to plan a surgical correction. The test is performed by examining the upper eyelid excursion from complete down gaze to up gaze, while blocking any contribution to upper eyelid elevation by the eyebrow *(Fig. 9.7)*. Asymmetric or absent lid creases must be identified, because asymmetry can be accentuated with standard blepharoplasty techniques. The vertical dimensions of the palpebral apertures at the midpupillary line are also measured.[23]

Aponeurosis disinsertion, or dehiscence, is the most common form of acquired ptosis. The typical clinical presentation is a mild (1–2 mm) to moderate (2–3 mm) case of ptosis associated with thin upper eyelids, high lid folds, and good levator excursion *(Figs 9.8, 9.9)*.[28] The levator muscle originates from the apex of the orbit and passes anteriorly, becoming aponeurotic at the superior orbital margin to insert onto the anterior two-thirds of the anterior tarsal surface. Some fibers of the aponeurosis extend to the orbicularis fascia to attach to the dermis of the upper eyelid, forming the upper lid crease. The anterior orbital fat removed during upper blepharoplasty lies posterior to the septum and anterior to the levator aponeurosis. Inadvertent penetration or detachment injury to the levator aponeurosis can occur during removal of the preseptal orbicularis oculi muscle or retroseptal fat *(Fig. 9.9A)*.

The condition is repaired by levator exploration and advancement of the aponeurotic structures to the anterior tarsus.[32–38] Patients with levator detachment should be repaired by levator advancement to the anterior tarsus. The

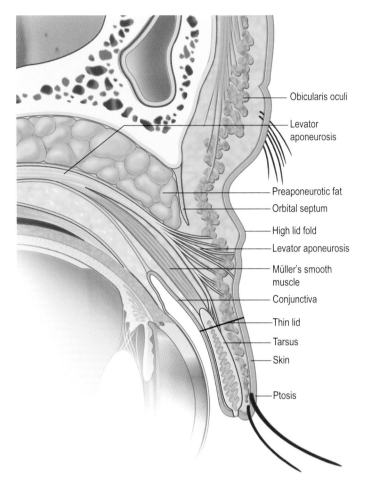

Fig. 9.8 Levator aponeurosis dehiscence produces a high upper lid fold, thin upper eyelid, and ptosis. (Modified from Jelks GW, Jelks EB. Blepharoplasty. In: Peck GC, ed. Complications and problems in aesthetic plastic surgery. New York: Gower Medical Publishing; 1992.)

Fasanella–Servat[38] technique and its various modifications *(Fig. 9.10)*, or variations of a tarso-mullerectomy are also excellent approaches to correct minimal ptosis.

Retraction

Lid retraction of the upper eyelid is an elevation of the upper eyelid margin above the superior corneal limbus. Lid retraction may be unilateral or bilateral, giving the patient a staring appearance and the illusion or accentuation or exophthalmos. Excessive skin removal from the upper eyelid may result in lagophthalmos and lid retraction which prevents complete closure of the eyelids *(Fig. 9.11A)*. Varying amounts of lid margin eversion may also be present *(Fig. 9.11B)*. Surgical correction requires release of the retraction through application of a retro- or preauricular full-thickness skin graft *(Fig. 9.11C,D)*.[37–42]

Adhesion, fibrosis, and foreshortening of the mid-lamellar structures of the upper lid (levator aponeurosis, orbital septum, and tarsus) can cause upper eyelid retraction *(Fig. 9.12A)*. Treatment requires surgical release of the adhesion, levator aponeurosis recession, interpositional fascial grafts, and lid traction sutures, which should establish a minimal amount of ptosis of the involved lids *(Fig. 9.12B)*.[27,37–42] Subsequent ptosis correction by a levator aponeurosis advancement or partial tarso-mullerectomy usually produces an acceptable result *(Fig. 9.12C)*.[27,37]

Herring's law

Retraction in the upper eyelid may also present as a result of ptosis in the contralateral eye *(Fig. 9.13)*. This type of retraction can be explained by Herring's law of equal innervation,[43] which states that both the levator palpebrae muscles receive the same level of innervation (for motor power), regardless of whether they are asymmetric. Therefore, if one eyelid is ptotic, when the body produces a reflex action to overstimulate the eyelid to improve the ptotic eyelids position, the contralateral eye will then appear retracted. Herring's law is an important consideration in both ptosis repair and lid retraction repair. By covering each eye independently during evaluation, the true amount of retraction may be revealed. Treatment consists of repair of the ptotic eyelid which should ultimately correct the asymmetry *(Fig. 9.13)*.

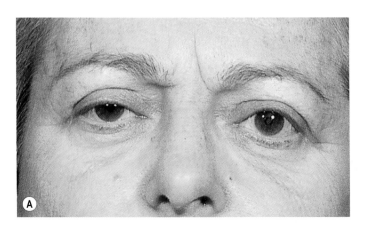

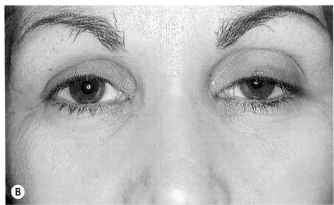

Fig. 9.9 (A) Patient who underwent cosmetic blepharoplasty with inadvertent disinsertion of the right levator aponeurosis during orbicularis oculi and retroseptal fat removal resulting in a right upper eyelid ptosis. **(B)** Patient following cosmetic blepharoplasty with a left upper eyelid ptosis from inadvertent levator aponeurosis detachment.

Labels in Fig. 9.8:
- Obicularis oculi
- Levator aponeurosis
- Preaponeurotic fat
- Orbital septum
- High lid fold
- Levator aponeurosis
- Müller's smooth muscle
- Conjunctiva
- Thin lid
- Tarsus
- Skin
- Ptosis

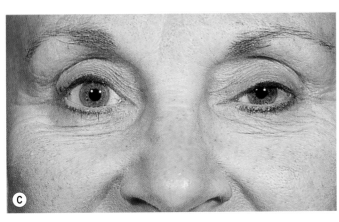
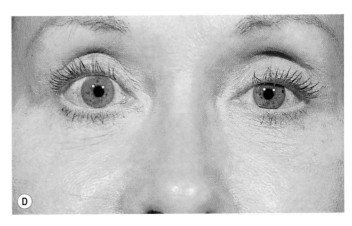

Fig. 9.9, cont'd (C,D) Patients with left upper eyelid cicatricial ptosis due to adhesions between the levator aponeurosis, orbital septum, and skin. (From Jelks GW, Jelks EB. Blepharoplasty. In: Peck GC, ed. Complications and problems in aesthetic plastic surgery. New York: Gower Medical Publishing; 1992.)

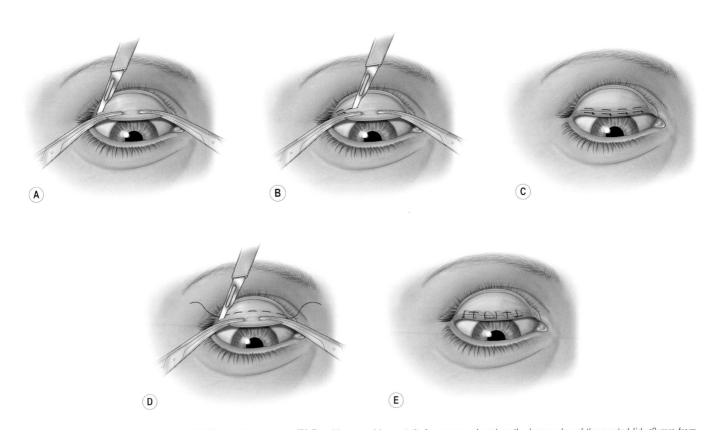

Fig. 9.10 The Fasanella–Servat technique. **(A)** The eyelid is everted. **(B)** Two thin, curved hemostatic forceps are placed on the lower edge of the everted lid ≤3 mm from the upper border of the tarsus. The first of the interrupted incisions is made. The interrupted incisions are extended in steps of 4–5 mm. A mattress suture is placed after each incision. **(C)** The sutures are tied so as to hold the tissues firmly yet allow the lid to be returned to its normal position at the end of the procedure. **(D)** Fasanella's alternative method of suturing a running continuous or "serpentine" fashion. **(E)** The running continuous or "serpentine" suture is returned, and the suture is tied on the temporal side. (Modified from Jelks GW, Smith BC. Reconstruction of the eyelids and associated structures. In: McCarthy JG, ed. Plastic surgery. Philadelphia: WB Saunders; 1990:1671.)

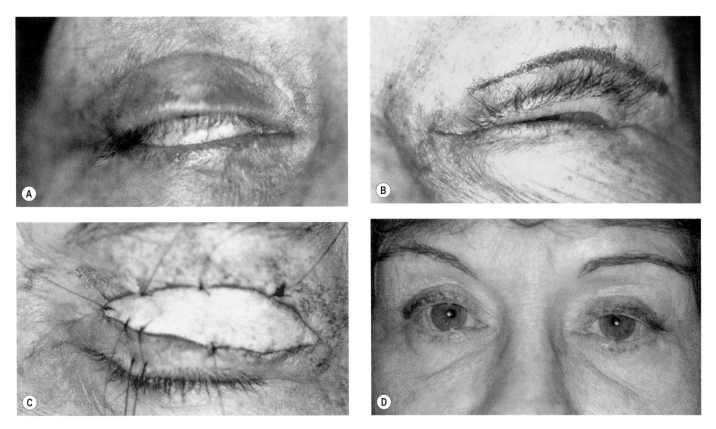

Fig. 9.11 (A) Patient with excessive skin removal from the upper eyelid and lagophthalmos. Bell's reflex is fair. **(B)** Patient with upper eyelid retraction, lid margin eversion, and exposure keratopathy due to excessive upper eyelid skin excision. Note the surgical marking for the proposed incision to release the scar and establish a wide defect. **(C)** Retroauricular full-thickness skin graft sutured to the defect. **(D)** Patient 9 months postoperatively. (From Jelks GW, Jelks EB. Blepharoplasty. In: Peck GC, ed. Complications and problems in aesthetic plastic surgery. New York: Gower Medical Publishing; 1992.)

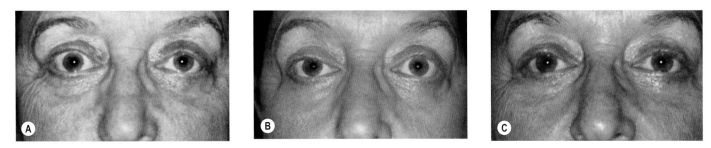

Fig. 9.12 (A) Patient 2 months postoperatively with right upper eyelid cicatricial retraction of the midlamellar structures (tarsus, orbital septum, and levator aponeurosis. **(B)** Patient 6 months after the release of lid adhesions and a levator recession of the right upper eyelid. Minimal ptosis of the right upper eyelid was deliberately produced. **(C)** Patient 6 months after ptosis correction by tarso-mullerectomy. (From Jelks GW, Jelks EB. Blepharoplasty. In: Peck GC, ed. Complications and problems in aesthetic plastic surgery. New York: Gower Medical Publishing; 1992.)

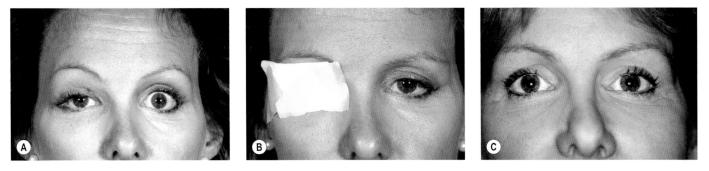

Fig. 9.13 (A) Patient presents with left t upper lid retraction and right lid ptosis secondary to purulent granulation tissue in the right upper eyelid. **(B)** By covering the right ptotic eye, the retracted eye exhibits a normal lid level due to Herring's law of equal innervation. **(C)** Following excision of granulation tissue and correction of ptosis, the patient exhibits normal lid levels bilaterally.

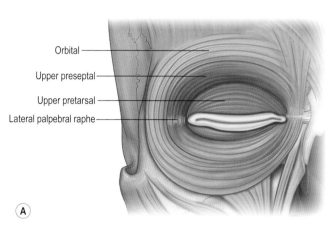

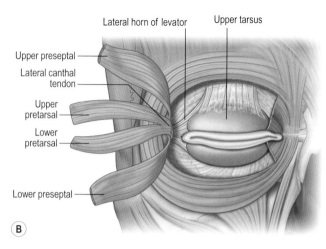

Fig. 9.14 **(A)** The lateral palpebral raphe. **(B)** The lateral canthal tendon and the anatomy of the structures of the lateral canthus. (Modified from Jelks GW, Smith BC. Reconstruction of the eyelids and associated structures. In: McCarthy JG, ed. Plastic surgery. Philadelphia: WB Saunders; 1990:1671.)

Lower eyelid

Lower eyelid malposition

Evaluation

The complications of primary blepharoplasty have been described in Chapter 6. Asymmetry is a common problem and distortion of lower lid position is a common contributor to this phenomenon.[2-4,7-10,13,18-21]

This malposition is often due to an interplay of the patient's unique periorbital anatomy with mechanical distraction due to gravitational and cicatricial forces of the skin, muscle, and septum displacing the lid inferiorly following blepharoplasty procedures.[22,23] Canthal and eyelid laxity, edema, hematoma, excessive resection of skin and fat, or impaired orbicularis oculi muscle function may also contribute to the disruptive forces.

The lower eyelids (zone II) extend from the lid margin to the cheek area *(Fig. 9.1)*. The medial canthus zone (zone III), is a complex region containing the origins of the orbicularis oculi muscle, the lacrimal collecting system, and associated neurovascular structures. The lateral canthus (zone IV) is an integral anatomic unit of the temporal aspects of the eyelids. The lateral canthus zone, which is more correctly termed lateral retinaculum, consists of: (1) the lateral horn of the levator palpebrae superioris muscle; (2) the continuation of the preseptal and pretarsal orbicularis oculi muscle (the lateral canthal tendon); (3) the inferior suspensory ligament of the globe (Lockwood's ligament); and (4) the check ligaments of the lateral rectus muscle *(Fig. 9.14)*.[22,23,26,27] The lateral retinaculum structures attach to a confluent region of the lateral bony orbital wall on a small promontory just within the lateral orbital rim known as Whitnall's tubercle *(Figs 9.2, 9.15)*.[23,27]

Similar to the upper lid, the lower lid is also divided into structural layers, consisting of the anterior, middle, and posterior lamella. The anterior lamella is composed of the lower lid skin and orbicularis muscle. The middle lamella (or midlamellar) structures include the tarsus, capsulopalpebral

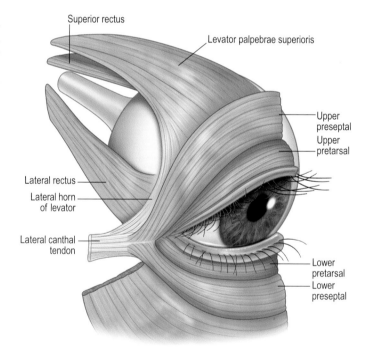

Fig. 9.15 The lateral extension or horn of the levator aponeurosis (upper arrow) splits the lacrimal gland into its orbital **(O)** and palpebral **(P)** lobes and extends inferolaterally to join the lateral retinaculum. The lateral portion of Whitnall's ligament **(W)** inserts into the orbital lobe of the gland by way of the interglandular fascial septa. The inferolateral pole of the palpebral lobe of the lacrimal gland usually rests at the level of the lateral retinaculum (lower arrow). The lateral retinaculum is a confluence of the lateral horn of the levator, the lateral canthal tendon, Lockwood's suspensory ligament of the globe, and check ligaments from the lateral retinaculus muscle. (Modified from Jelks GW, Smith BC. Reconstruction of the eyelids and associated structures. In: McCarthy JG, ed. Plastic surgery. Philadelphia: WB Saunders; 1990:1671.)

Table 9.5 **Secondary blepharoplasty candidate evaluation: lower eyelid**

Anterior lamella	Pretarsal orbicularis oculi function	Absent	Present	
	Scars	Absent	Present	Position Severity
	Skin	Normal	Abnormal	Over-resection Excess
	Lid margin eversion	Absent	Present	LME I LME II (w/scleral show) LME III (w/lash rotation) Ectropion
	Lagophthalmos	Absent	Present	
Middle lamella	Vertical cicatricial midlamellar retraction	Present	Absent	
	Fat	Normal	Abnormal	Excess removal Retention
Posterior lamella	Palpebral conjunctiva	Normal	Abnormal	

Table 9.6 **Lateral canthal zone evaluation**

Anatomical morphology			
Vector analysis	Positive	Neutral	Negative
Soft tissue: bone distance	<1 cm	<1 cm	>1 cm
Tarsoligamentous integrity			
Distraction test	Normal	Abnormal (>8 mm)	
Snap test	Normal	Abnormal	
Lateral canthal laxity	No	Yes	
Medial canthal laxity	No	Yes	
Medial to lateral canthal position	Equal	Abnormal	High
Palpebral aperture	Symmetric	Asymmetric	

fascia, and orbital septum. The posterior lamella is the conjunctiva.

Anatomical analysis, especially of the lateral canthal region, and a thorough understanding of lower eyelid malposition etiology are required to choose and perform the appropriate, corrective secondary blepharoplasty procedure in the lower lid *(Tables 9.5, 9.6)*. Predisposing factors for post-blepharoplasty eyelid malposition include: hypotonicity/involutional changes, malar hypoplasia, shallow orbit, thyroid ophthalmopathy, unilateral high myopia, and patients undergoing secondary blepharoplasty.[3,22]

A thorough clinical assessment should include evaluation of: (1) pretarsal orbicularis oculi muscle function; (2) presence of vertical midlamellar cicatricial lid retraction/excessive skin resection; (3) morphology: vector analysis and soft tissue to bone distance; (4) tarsoligamentous integrity; (5) presence of lower margin eversion; (6) posterior lamellar integrity; and (7) presence of malar fat pad descent.

Significant deformities may occur when excess skin and muscle are excised during a blepharoplasty procedure.

Scarring of the pretarsal orbicularis oculi muscle to the middle lamella can result in lower lid malposition and scleral show. Denervation of the orbicularis oculi muscle leads to flattening of this area resulting in an aged, unnatural look. More importantly, denervation or damage to orbicularis oculi muscle can lead to an incomplete blink mechanism, lack of tone, laxity of the lower lid and scleral show.

During the evaluation of the patient with lower eyelid malposition it is important to determine if there is any element of midlamellar (tarsus, capsulopalpebral fascia, orbital septum) cicatricial retraction *(Fig. 9.16)*. If lid retraction is present, then surgical management may require lysis of the adhesions, interpositional grafts (cartilage, palatal mucosal), and other grafts, flaps, and procedures for correction. Ordinarily, when upward traction is placed on the lower eyelid, it is easily displaced to the level of the mid-pupil or above. When midlamellar retraction is present, the eyelid will have restricted upward mobility *(Fig. 9.17)*.

The lateral view reveals the vector relationship of the (1) ocular globe to (2) the lower lid and (3) the malar eminence *(Fig. 9.18)*.[22,44–46] A *positive vector* relationship is when the most anterior projection of the globe lies behind the lower eyelid margin, which lies behind the anterior projection of the malar eminence. It is a favorable anatomic situation because there is good bony, eyelid, and tarsoligamentous support with normal eyelid contours and levels. A *neutral vector* relationship is when the most anterior projection of the globe is in a vertical relationship with the lower lid and malar eminence. Like the positive vector relationship, it has minimal risk for lower eyelid malposition following aesthetic blepharoplasty. The *negative vector* relationship is when the most anterior projection of the globe lies anterior to the lower lid and malar eminence These patients often have scleral show. They have a hypoplastic malar relationship which increases the risk for an unfavorable result, and requires alteration in the aesthetic blepharoplastic procedure to prevent postoperative lower eyelid malposition *(Fig. 9.19)*.

The soft tissue to bone distance is measured from the lateral canthus to orbital rim *(Fig. 9.20)*. This distance is important for determining what type of lower lid support procedure is necessary to deliver acceptable results. If the distance is <1 cm,

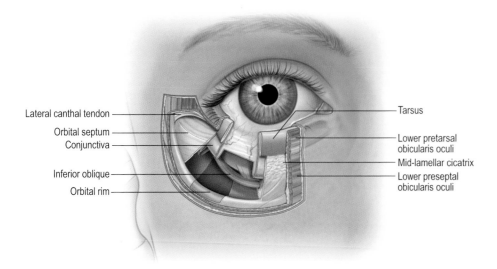

Lateral canthal tendon

Orbital septum

Conjunctiva

Inferior oblique

Orbital rim

Tarsus

Lower pretarsal obicularis oculi

Mid-lamellar cicatrix

Lower preseptal obicularis oculi

Fig. 9.16 Midlamellar cicatricial retraction is one of the most common indications for secondary blepharoplasty. Correction requires lysis of adhesions in conjunction with lateral canthoplasty with or without spacer grafts.

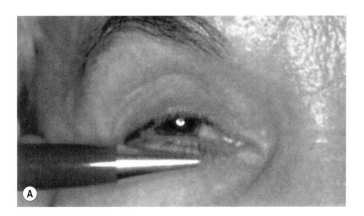

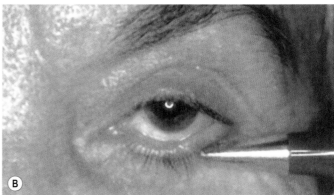

Fig. 9.17 (A) Patient with vertical displacement of the right lower eyelid demonstrates movement of the eyelid to the mid-pupillary level. **(B)** Same patient with displacement of the left lower eyelid demonstrating midlamellar cicatricial changes preventing movement of the lid (lid retraction). (From Jelks GW, Jelks EB. Blepharoplasty. In: Peck GC, ed. Complications and problems in aesthetic plastic surgery. New York: Gower Medical Publishing; 1992.)

the patient usually presents with deep set eyes (i.e., *positive/ neutral vector*). Tarsal strip lateral canthoplasty and inferior retinacular lateral canthoplasty/canthopexy are effective procedures to address this problem. If the distance is >1 cm and the patient presents with prominent eyes (i.e., *negative vector*), inferior retinacular lateral canthoplasty, dermal orbicular pennant lateral canthoplasty, and midfacial elevation are effective procedures in the surgical armamentarium to correct lower lid malposition in these patients.

The tarsoligamentous integrity is determined by three components: lower lid laxity, medial canthal laxity, and lateral canthal laxity. Horizontal lower lid laxity is diagnosed by "distraction" and "snap" test *(Fig. 9.21)*.[3,22,37] In the distraction test, the lower lid is grasped with the thumb and index finger and displaced anteriorly. In the post-blepharoplasty patient, when the lower lid can be distracted laterally >8 mm, there should be concern for compromised tarsoligamentous integrity. The snap test is performed by pulling the eyelid inferiorly to the level of the inferior orbital margin and then releasing it to judge the speed at which it returns to a normal level. A lid

with a slow snap back or a persistent eversion may have eyelid and canthal laxity requiring correction *(Fig. 9.22)*. If the lateral canthus is higher than or equal to the level of the medial canthus, one may elect to perform horizontal lid shortening with a wedge resection alone or in combination with lateral canthoplasty. If, however, the lateral canthus is lower than the medial canthus, a lateral canthoplasty procedure is necessary for optimal correction.

Another component of the evaluation of the secondary blepharoplasty patient involves lower lid eversion, which is divided into four subtypes. The four types of lower lid eversion are as follows: (I) lid margin eversion (LME) with scleral show; (II) LME with scleral show and horizontal lid laxity; (III) LME with lash rotation; and (IV) ectropion – involutional or cicatricial *(Fig. 9.23)*. The term ectropion denotes an outward turning or eversion of the eyelid. Ectropion may be classified as either involutional or cicatricial.[5,22,37] A common factor in all forms of ectropion is conjunctival hyperemia or keratinization, punctual occlusion, and inflammatory changes that become progressively worse. Involutional ectropion (*aka,*

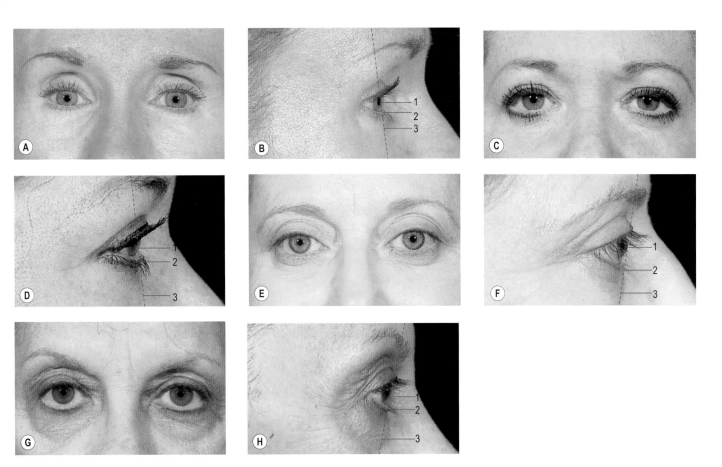

Fig. 9.18 Comparison of the variable anatomic relationships of the orbital region that influence the palpebral aperture. (1) Ocular globe; (2) lower lid; (3) malar eminence. Cosmetic blepharoplasty may have to be combined with other surgical procedures to prevent complications. **(A,B)** Young woman with high lid folds, deep set eyes (large, bony orbital volume with small ocular globes), and well-developed malar eminences. The most anterior projection of the ocular globe lies behind the lower eyelid margin and the malar eminence. This positive vector relationship is a favorable anatomic situation as there is good eyelid and tarsoligamentous integrity with normal eyelid contours and levels. **(C,D)** Woman presenting for cosmetic blepharoplasty with prominent ocular globes and increased periorbital skin and fat. The most anterior projection of her ocular globes are posterior to the lower eyelid margin and inferior orbital margin (malar eminence). This is a neutral vector relationship with a minimum risk for lower eyelid malposition. **(E,F)** Woman with prominent ocular globes, slight scleral show, and malar hypoplasia. The lateral view demonstrates the influence of the globe on the lower eyelid position and the lack of eyelid support from the inferior orbital rim. This patient has a negative vector relationship with the most anterior portion of portion of the globe anterior to the lower lid and malar eminence. This negative vector relationship requires alterations in the cosmetic blepharoplastic procedure to prevent lower eyelid malposition. **(G,H)** Middle-aged woman with excess eyelid skin and fat, normal ocular globe position, marked inferior scleral show, lower eyelid laxity, and malar hypoplasia. This woman has a negative vector relationship and is at risk for an unfavorable result from lower eyelid surgery. A lower eyelid and lateral canthal tightening with repositioning (lateral canthalplasty) should be combined with the cosmetic blepharoplasty. (From Jelks GW, Jelks EB. Blepharoplasty. In: Peck GC, ed. Complications and problems in aesthetic plastic surgery. New York: Gower Medical Publishing; 1992.)

senile ectropion) is caused by horizontal lid laxity of the eyelid supportive structures and usually begins with scleral show *(Fig. 9.24)*. Cicatricial ectropion is caused by a deficiency of the skin or skin and muscle of the lid. In secondary blepharoplasty patients, cicatricial ectropion is seen following excess skin removal and/or multiple previous blepharoplasty procedures and resultant scarring *(Fig. 9.24)*.

Patients with lower lid retraction often have a descent of the malar fat pad.[7,9] A procedure such as a subperiosteal midface suspension techniques may be required to elevate the malar fat pad to a position that will assist in supporting the lower eyelids. A transblepharoplasty subperiosteal midface elevation in conjunction with lateral canthoplasty (with or without a spacer graft) may be required in patients who present with lagophthalmos from multiple procedures and excessive skin resection to obviate or reduce a full

thickness skin grafting requirement. This is partially covered in Chapter 11.1.[22,47]

Finally, examination of the inner component of the posterior lamella should be conducted to determine if fibrosis, infection, inadequate blood supply, etc., is present.

Management

Several surgical procedures are available to provide excellent lower eyelid function and contour in the secondary blepharoplasty patient requiring correction of lower lid deformities.[2,3,8,9,16,48–57] As mentioned previously, careful evaluation of the etiology of the lower eyelid defect as well as a thorough morphological anatomical examination will assist the surgeon in determining the optimal procedure(s) to perform to best address the defect or defects *(Fig. 9.25, Table 9.7)*.

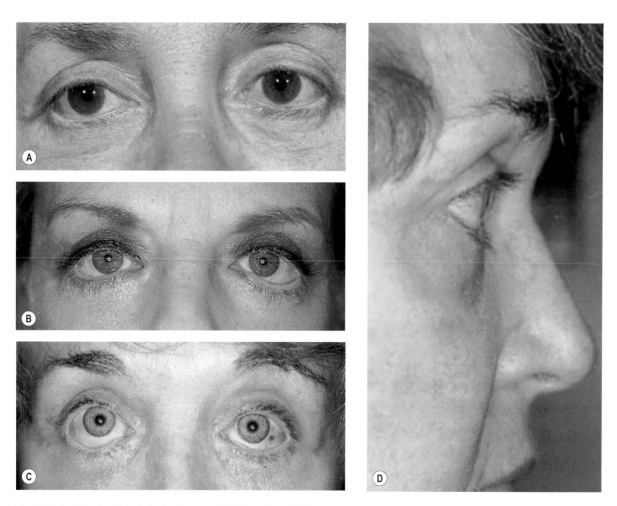

Fig. 9.19 Eyelid malpositions following lower eyelid blepharoplasty. **(A)** Patient with bilateral lid margin eversion, round of the lateral canthi, and scleral show. **(B)** Patient with lower eyelid horizontal laxity as well as the findings shown in **(A)**. Note the malar hypoplasia. **(C,D)** Patient with marked lower eyelid malpositions and corneal exposure. Note the malar hypoplasia with inadequate bony support to the lower eyelid and ocular globe. (From Jelks GW, Jelks EB. Blepharoplasty. In: Peck GC, ed. Complications and problems in aesthetic plastic surgery. New York: Gower Medical Publishing; 1992.)

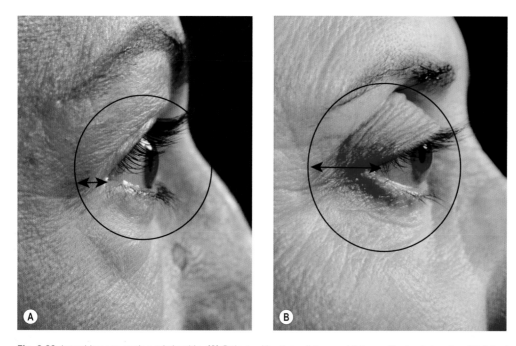

Fig. 9.20 Lateral bone to canthus relationship. **(A)** Patients with <1 cm distance exhibit a positive/neutral vector. **(B)** Patients with >1 cm exhibit an negative vector.

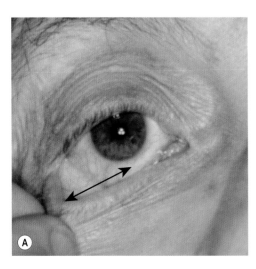
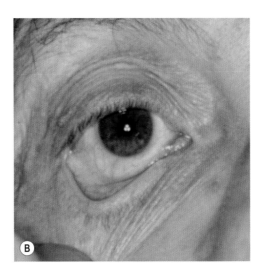

Fig. 9.21 Distraction and snap test. **(A)** In the distraction test, the lower lid is grasped with the thumb and index finger and displaced anteriorly. In the post-blepharoplasty patient, when the lower lid can be distracted laterally >8 mm there should be concern for compromised tarsoligamentous integrity. **(B)** The snap test is performed by pulling the eyelid inferiorly to the level of the inferior orbital margin and then releasing it to judge the speed at which it returns to a normal level. A lid with a slow snap back or a persistent eversion may have eyelid and canthal laxity.

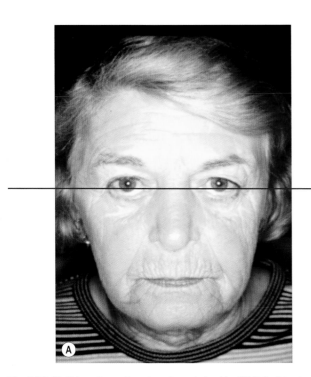
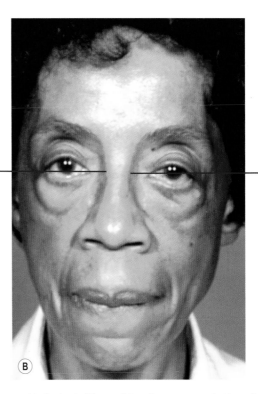

Fig. 9.22 Medial canthus to lateral canthus relationship. **(A)** If the lateral canthus is higher than or equal to the level of the medial canthus, one may elect to perform horizontal lid shortening with a wedge resection alone or in combination with lateral canthoplasty. **(B)** If, however, the lateral canthus is lower than the medial canthus, a lateral canthoplasty procedure is necessary for optimal correction.

The lateral canthoplasty and its various modifications are useful in addressing lower eyelid malposition.[48–57] The procedures described in the following text require a precise knowledge of the orbital anatomy and the desire to preserve the external commissure. There are key surgical points that should be kept in mind when performing a lateral canthoplasty to achieve symmetric lateral canthal repositioning. The lateral canthal and lower eyelid incision should be horizontal *(Fig. 9.26A)*. After selective release of the lower eyelid with its portion of lateral retinaculum, the lid is elevated far enough to cover 1–2 mm of the inferior limbus *(Fig. 9.26B)*. The level of fixation to the inner aspect of the orbital rim should correspond to a point level with the superior aspect of the pupil in primary position *(Fig. 9.26C)*. Finally, upon closure of the lateral canthal skin incisions, the angle of the divergence from the original horizontal orientation must be equal and symmetric from one side to the other to ensure lateral canthal and lower eyelid symmetry *(Fig. 9.26D)*.

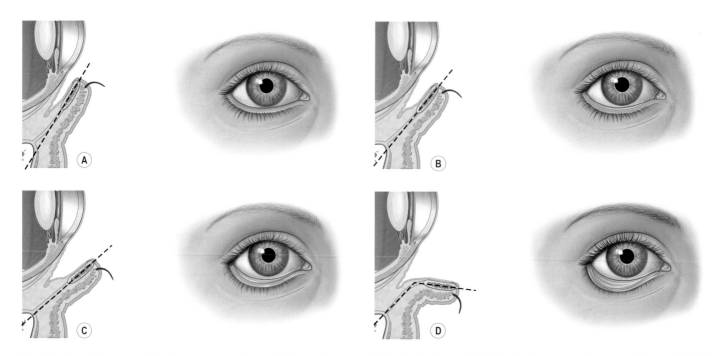

Fig. 9.23 Lower lid eversion divided into four types subtypes: **(A)** lid margin eversion (LME) with scleral show; **(B)** LME with scleral show and horizontal lid laxity; **(C)** LME with lash rotation; **(D)** ectropion – involutional or cicatricial.

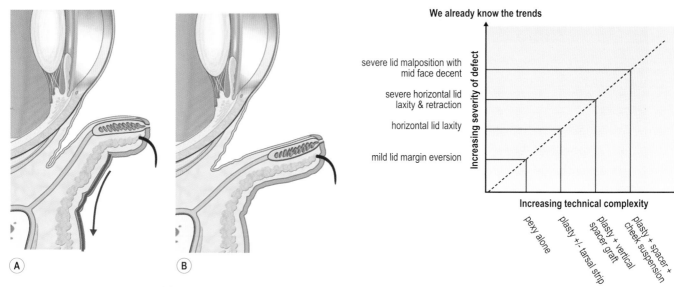

Fig. 9.24 Classification of ectropion: **(A)** cicatricial or **(B)** involutional. (Modified from Jelks GW, Smith BC. Reconstruction of the eyelids and associated structures. In: McCarthy JG, ed. Plastic surgery. Philadelphia: WB Saunders; 1990:1671.)

Fig. 9.25 Etiology of the lower eyelid defect versus the optimal procedure to address the defect.

It is not advisable to rely on horizontal lid shortening with simple wedge resections for lower lid support or to preserve the lateral canthal anatomy. Pentagonal resection of the lower eyelid only addresses one aspect of the lower lid malposition, namely excess horizontal length. Optimal correction should address all aspects of the pathology, in particular the restoration/preservation of canthal anatomy to maximize postoperative success.

Fixation of a lateral canthoplasty or canthopexy may be accomplished by directly suturing the lateral canthus to the lateral orbital rim periosteum. However, in some patients, the soft, connective tissue of the periosteum has lost its integrity due to damage from scarring or trauma. In patients with milder damage, the fixation may be supplemented with a local periosteal flap[58–60] or a fascial graft.[61] However, patients who have undergone multiple procedures with extensive damage to the orbital rim periosteum may require drill hole fixation.[52,62] Drill hole fixation of the lateral canthus is accomplished by determining the desired point of fixation in the lateral orbital rim. The point of fixation is determined by tucking the lateral canthus against the orbital rim until it corresponds with the vertical level of the superior aspect of the pupil. This position is marked with surgical ink, and a single drill hole with is made no less than 1 mm and generally approximately 4 mm posterior to the lateral orbital rim. A double-armed 4–0 Mersilene (ME-2) suture is used for fixation. In a canthopexy procedure (no lysis of the lateral canthus) the suture is double-looped into the canthal tissue and both suture arms are brought through the single hole *(Fig. 9.27)*. In

a canthoplasty procedure (lysis of the lateral canthus) a single loop of suture is brought through the canthal edges of the lids, and the arms are brought out through the single hole. Both arms of the suture are secured to the deep temporal fascia.[62]

Tarsal strip lateral canthoplasty and vertical spacer grafts

Early in the senior author's experience, the procedure of choice for post-blepharoplasty lower lid malposition was the tarsal strip lateral canthoplasty[48–51,54] combined with horizontal lid shortening and lateral support with or without vertical spacer grafts of skin, cartilage, or mucosa *(Fig. 9.28)*. The tarsal strip lateral canthoplasty procedure divides the lateral palpebral commissure and selectively releases the lower lid. The amount of horizontal lid shortening can be varied with the suture placement and fixation in the orbital periosteum. The tarsal strip procedure, and its many variations is useful for secondary correction of the lax lower eyelid, however, this technique produces a decrease in the horizontal dimension of the palpebral aperture which may cause deformities of the lower lid and a rounding of the external commissure *(Fig. 9.29)*.

If midlamellar cicatricial retraction is present, then surgical correction may only require incising the midlamellar cicatricial adhesion. However, if the vertical lid defect is excessive, an interpositional graft composed of palatal mucosa, cartilage, or a flap of de-epithelialized lateral canthal dermis (dermal pennant flap) may be required *(Fig. 9.30)*.[3,53,54] The preferred graft is palatal mucosa.[3,27,37] The graft donor site is between the gingival and the midline which is a location of well-defined submucosa for easy separation of the graft from the fat and periosteum. When performing bilateral retraction repair, it is preferable to take two grafts from both sides of the mouth rather than one large graft; this will encourage more rapid healing. Once the graft has been thinned and all

Table 9.7 Canthoplasty techniques and indications

Canthoplasty technique	Indications
Tarsal strip lateral canthoplasty	Lower lid canthal malposition without lid laxity or ectropion
Tarsal strip lateral canthoplasty with horizontal lid shortening	Lid laxity or ectropion
Dermal-orbicular pennant lateral canthoplasty	Bone to soft tissue distance of >1 cm
Inferior retinacular lateral canthoplasty	Bone to soft tissue distance of <1 cm
Inferior retinacular lateral canthopexy	Bone to soft tissue distance of <1 cm, minimal distraction, + snap test
Vertical spacer graft	Vertical deficiency from release of midlamellar cicatrix or skin deficiency
Subperiosteal midface elevation	Multiple previous procedures – recruitment of skin and tissue

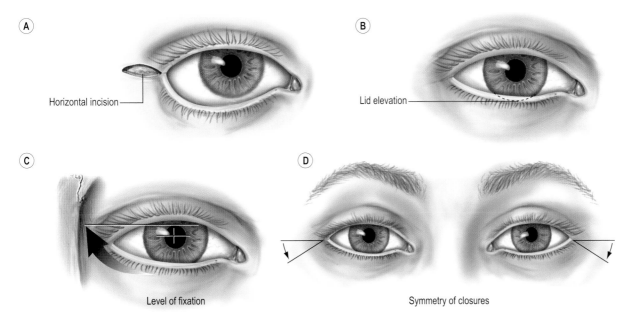

Fig. 9.26 Key points to achieve symmetric lateral canthal repositioning. **(A)** The lateral canthal and lower eyelid incision should be horizontal. **(B)** The lid is elevated to cover 1–2 mm of the inferior limbus. **(C)** The level of fixation to the lateral orbital periosteum is at a level corresponding to the superior aspect of the pupil in primary position. **(D)** On closure of the lateral canthal skin incisions, the angle of divergence from the original horizontal orientation must be equal and symmetric to ensure lateral canthal and lower eyelid symmetry. (Modified from Jelks GW, Smith BC. Reconstruction of the eyelids and associated structures. In: McCarthy JG, ed. Plastic surgery. Philadelphia: WB Saunders; 1990:1671.)

remaining fatty tissue excised, it is sutured into the lower eyelid. A 6–0 mild chromic suture is used to attach the graft(s) to the inferior tarsal edge and the recessed conjunctiva and capsulopalpebral fascia.

Dermal orbicular pennant lateral canthoplasty

The *dermal orbicular pennant lateral canthoplasty* (DOPLC) was developed to reduce the incidence of tarsal strip lateral canthoplasty contour complications *(Fig. 9.31)*.[3,54] This procedure uses an extension of the lower lid in the form of a deepithelialized pennant of skin and underlying orbicularis muscle, but it does not divide the lateral palpebral commissure *(Fig. 9.32)*. This method maintains the horizontal dimension of the palpebral aperture while allowing for tightening of the lower lid as well as lateral suspension *(Fig. 9.33)*.

The DOPLC is useful in post-blepharoplasty patients with lower lid malposition, especially in patients with a bone to soft tissue relationship *(Fig. 9.20)* of >1 cm. However, because the incision between the upper and lower lids has a very narrow skin bridge, persistent edema between the upper and lower lids may occur laterally with this technique.

Inferior retinacular lateral canthoplasty/canthopexy and midface elevation

The inferior retinacular lateral canthoplasty/canthopexy (IRLC) was developed for secondary blepharoplasty patients requiring correction of lower lid malposition and lateral canthal deformities without the problems associated with the tarsal strip lateral canthoplasty and DOPLC *(Fig. 9.34)*.[55] The IRLC is indicated in the secondary or primary blepharoplasty patient with a negative vector analysis, but with a

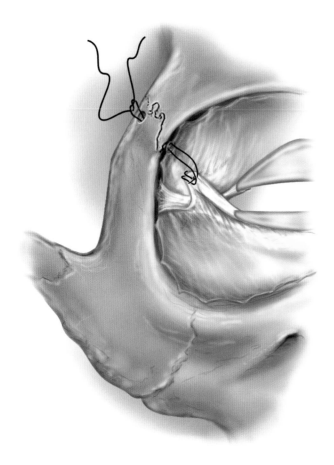

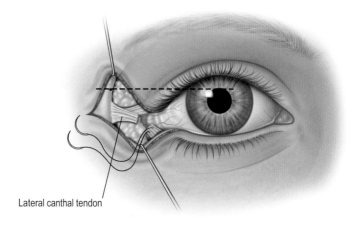

Lateral canthal tendon

Fig. 9.27 Drill hole fixation of a lateral canthopexy. Following determination of the proper point of fixation, a single drill hole is made no less than 1 mm and generally approximately 4 mm posterior to the lateral orbital rim. A double-armed 4–0 Mersilene (ME-2) suture is used for fixation. In a canthopexy procedure (no lysis of the lateral canthus) the suture is double-looped into the canthal tissue and both suture arms are brought through the single hole. (From Aston, Aesthetic Plastic Surgery, 2009, Saunders.)

Fig. 9.28 Tarsal strip lateral canthoplasty. The lower portion of the lateral retinaculum is divided and development of a tarsal element for fixation is formed by excising the temporal lid margin, cilia, conjunctiva, and skin. The tarsal strip is then fixed in position to the lateral orbital periosteum with sutures. (Modified from Jelks GW, Smith BC. Reconstruction of the eyelids and associated structures. In: McCarthy JG, ed. Plastic surgery. Philadelphia: WB Saunders; 1990:1671.)

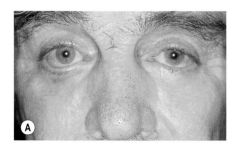
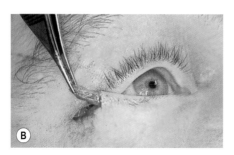
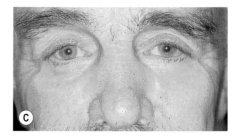

Fig. 9.29 (A) Patient exhibiting post-blepharoplasty complications of scleral show, temporal bowing, and mild ectropion that is greater on the right side than on the left. **(B)** The tarsal strip ready for periosteal fixation. **(C)** At 6 months after bilateral tarsal strip procedures. (From Jelks GW, Jelks EB. Blepharoplasty. In: Peck GC, ed. Complications and problems in aesthetic plastic surgery. New York: Gower Medical Publishing; 1992.)

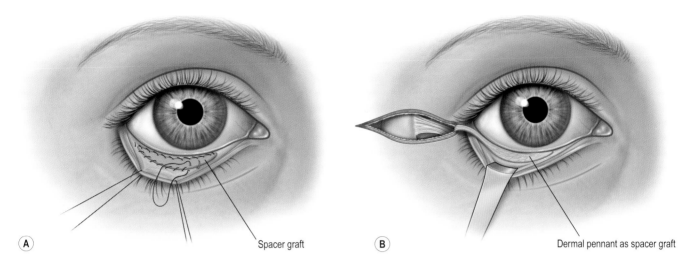

(A)   Spacer graft   (B)   Dermal pennant as spacer graft

Fig. 9.30 Lower eyelid spacer grafts. **(A)** A spacer graft of autogenous palatal mucosal or auricular cartilage, or a **(B)** vascularized, de-epithelialized lateral canthal dermal pennant flap may be used to increase vertical height of the retracted or deficient lower eyelid in conjunction with a lateral canthoplasty. Spacer grafts are useful in enhancing the results in post-blepharoplasty patients with defects secondary to cicatricial retraction or excessive skin resection.

favorable bone to soft-tissue relationship (<1 cm discrepancy) *(Figs 9.18, 9.20)*.[3,54–57]

The IRLC is performed through the lateral aspect of the upper eyelid blepharoplasty incision. A skin-muscle flap is elevated along the lateral orbit extending onto the lateral aspect of the inferior orbital rim. This maneuver exposes the lower lid lateral fat pad that lies behind the orbital septum. The inferior aspect of the lateral retinaculum lies immediately superior to this fat. The lateral fat pad can be removed to better expose the lateral retinaculum. Following removal of the fat pad, the suborbicularis plane will be elevated to the level of the lateral retinaculum. The lower lid component of the lateral retinaculum may then be identified.

In the canthoplasty procedure, the lateral retinaculum is released completely from all lateral attachments to the orbit and allows free movement of the lower orbit. A canthopexy procedure is a non-lysis canthoplasty in which the lower lid component of the lateral retinaculum is plicated and anchored to the lateral orbital rim. A canthopexy is only appropriate for those patients with minimal distensibility and a firm snap test.

Both needles of a 4–0 Polydek suture are then passed into a *hitching* stitch. The suture is passed through the lateral orbital rim periosteum at a level corresponding to the superior edge of the pupil with the globe in primary gaze. The Polydek suture is adjusted and tightened so that the lower lid covers 1–2 mm of the inferior cornea. The lower lid component of the lateral retinaculum is fixed in its newly elevated position on the lateral orbital rim. The position of the lateral canthus will appear over-corrected, and there may be some initial bunching of the soft tissue at the lateral canthal region. This relaxes to a normal contour over 2–4 weeks postoperatively as the lateral canthus settles inferiorly.

Midface elevation and fixation

Transblepharoplasty subperiosteal midface elevation is useful in conjunction with lateral canthoplasty with or without spacer grafts for patients who have undergone multiple cosmetic procedures who present with lower eyelid and midface malposition with a deficiency of lower lid skin.[9,47,56,63] Proper midface fixation and canthoplasty prevent lower lid descent in the first critical weeks of postoperative healing.

Subperiosteal midface elevation is achieved through a lower blepharoplasty incision. A skin-muscle flap is dissected down to the infraorbital rim. Periosteum at the anterior margin of the infraorbital rim is elevated with a subperiosteal pocket. The periosteum is released laterally over the inferior lateral rim followed by release of the entire subperiosteal flap so it can be mobilized superiorly. The midfacial flap is suspended with using two 4–0 Vicryl sutures on half-circle cutting needles that are used to purchase the suborbicularis oculi fat and the malar fat pad. The sutures are then tied to a titanium screw placed on the anterior surface of the lateral orbital bone (zygomatic bone) *(Fig. 9.35)*. The screw is tightened until the head is flush with the bone surface. Alternate methods which can be used to elevate the midface include a preperiosteal dissection from the lower lid,[64] the concentric malar lift,[65] and the endoscopic, subperiosteal approach from the temple (covered further in Chapter 11.8).

The elevated and stabilized structures support the repositioned lower lid and the recruited and elevated cheek skin and tissue help replace deficient posterior lamella.

Choosing the appropriate technique(s)

Careful evaluation of specific indications in regard to the patient's anatomy as well as their specific defect, enable the surgeon to choose the optimal lateral canthoplasty procedure *(Table 9.7)*. In patients with a bony (lateral orbital rim) to soft-tissue (external commissure) distance of ≥1 cm, the dermal orbicular pennant lateral canthoplasty has become the procedure of choice for correction of lower lid malposition. The dermal orbicular pennant lateral canthoplasty (DOPLC) allows for correction of the lateral canthal angle, while preserving the external commissure.[54] Lid laxity or ectropion are indications for canthoplasty, however, it is still preferable to utilize some form of horizontal lid shortening (usually with a tarsal strip). This maneuver allows for correction of the laxity while allowing for canthal resuspension.

Scratch through dermis

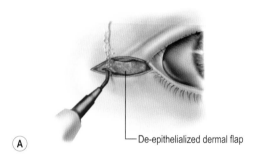

Protective contact lens

Strumming inferior retinaculum
with Colorado needle to release lower lid

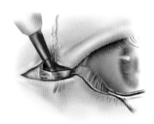

Suture fixation is to lateral rim corresponding to the upper
level of the pupil with the patient in the primary gaze

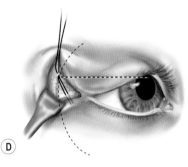

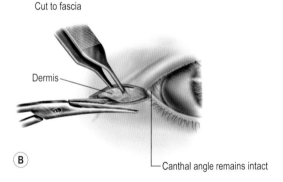

De-epithelialized dermal flap

(A)

(D)

Cut to fascia

Spacer graft

Dermis

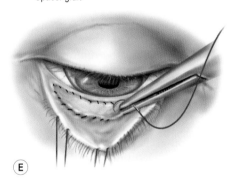

Canthal angle remains intact

(B)

(E)

Mobilize flap to pretarsal muscle

Orbicularis muscle

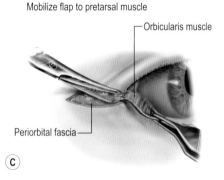

Periorbital fascia

(C)

Fig. 9.31 Dermal-orbicular pennant lateral canthoplasty (DOPLC). **(A)** Patient is illustrated with a protective, colored contact lens in place. The dermal-orbicular flap is outlined at the lateral canthus. Note the horizontal alignment and the maintenance of the external commissure. An incision is made through the superficial layers. **(B)** The flap is de-epithelialized preserving the underlying dermis. The superficial border of the flap is incised to the suborbicularis muscle plane. **(C)** The inferior border of the dermal-orbicular pennant is elevated to the external commissure, which remains intact. The lower lid component of the lateral retinaculum is divided by "strumming" the structure with a Colorado needle. **(D)** The fixation of the suture is to the lateral orbital rim corresponding to the upper level of the pupil with the patient in primary gaze. **(E)** A spacer graft can be added as necessary. (Modifed from Jelks GW, Jelks EB. Repair of lower lid deformities. Clin Plast Surg 1993; 20:417–421.)

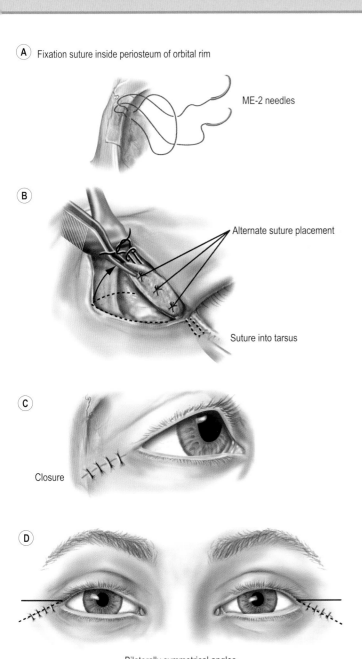

(A) Fixation suture inside periosteum of orbital rim

ME-2 needles

(B)

Alternate suture placement

Suture into tarsus

(C)

Closure

(D)

Bilaterally symmetrical angles

Fig. 9.32 Dermal-orbicular pennant lateral canthoplasty (DOPLC) fixation and closure. **(A)** Both arms of an ME-2 4–0 Polydek suture are passed through periosteum from the inner to the outer aspect of the orbital rim. The needles are passed through the loop, and cinched tightly down, hugging the inner aspect of the orbital rim. **(B)** Most commonly, periosteal fixation is to the lateral edge of the tarsus. Fixation of the lower lid to the orbital rim should result in an over-correction such that the lower lid covers 1–2 mm of the inferior cornea. **(C)** Upon closure, elevation causes inferior angulation of the original horizontal incision. **(D)** When bilateral procedures are performed, care is taken to obtain symmetry of closure. (Modifed from Jelks GW, Jelks EB. Repair of lower lid deformities. Clin Plast Surg 1993; 20:417–422.)

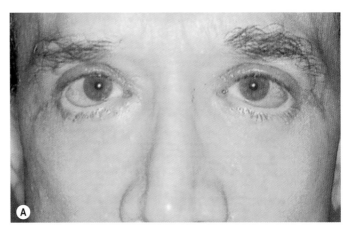

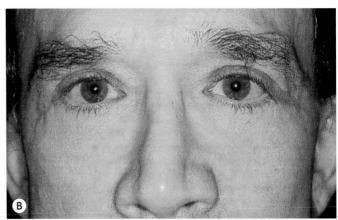

Fig. 9.33 **(A)** Patient with bilateral lower eyelid malposition after blepharoplasty. **(B)** The patient is seen 9 months following bilateral dermal-orbicular pennant lateral canthoplasties. (From Jelks GW, Jelks EB. Blepharoplasty. In: Peck GC, ed. Complications and problems in aesthetic plastic surgery. New York: Gower Medical Publishing; 1992.)

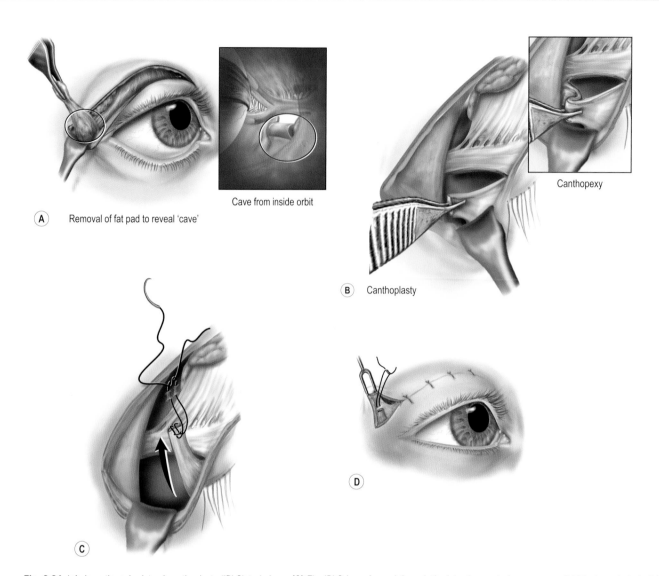

Fig. 9.34 Inferior retinacular lateral canthoplasty (IRLC) technique. **(A)** The IRLC is performed through the lateral aspect of an upper eyelid blepharoplasty incision. A skin-muscle flap is elevated along the lateral orbit exposing the lower lid lateral fat pad. The inferior aspect of the lateral retinaculum lies immediately superior to this fat. The lateral fat pad can be removed to better expose the lateral retinaculum. Inset: following removal of the fat pad, a "cave" is revealed superior to the lateral retinaculum. The illustration reveals this area as it would be visualized from inside the orbit. **(B)** Canthoplasty procedure with lysis of the lateral retinaculum. Inset: canthopexy, or non-lysis procedure in which the lower lid component of the lateral retinaculum is plicated and anchored to the lateral orbital rim. **(C)** Both needles of 4–0 Polydek suture have been passed into a *hitching* stitch. The suture has been passed through the lateral orbital rim periosteum (as denoted by the arrow) at a level corresponding to the superior edge of the pupil with the globe in primary gaze. **(D)** The Polydek suture is adjusted and tightened so the lower lid covers 1–2 mm of the inferior cornea. The lower lid component of the lateral retinaculum is then fixed in its elevated position to the lateral orbital rim. (Modifed from Jelks GW *et al*. The inferior retinacular lateral canthoplasty: a new technique. Plast Reconstr Surg 1997; 100:1262–1265.)

In patients with lid retraction, a DOPLC may be sufficient to correct the problem if there is associated soft-tissue to bony disparity. If release of midlamellar (orbital septum, lid retractors) cicatricial retraction is the cause of the vertical deficiency, the use of autogenous palatal mucosal or auricular cartilage as a spacer graft is recommended. Spacer grafts should also be utilized when release of the posterior lamella (conjunctiva) produces a vertical deficit. In patients with multiple previous procedures presenting with deficient lower eyelid skin and tissue, midface elevation techniques may also be necessary for an optimal result. Finally, for secondary or primary blepharoplasty patients with negative vectors and favorable bony to soft-tissue relationships (<1 cm), the inferior retinacular lateral canthoplasty/canthopexy (IRLC) is recommended.[22,44,45,54–57] The IRLC procedure avoids the pitfalls of horizontal lid shortening and the edema associated with DOPLC.

Miscellaneous complications

Excessive fat resection is a most disturbing problem, especially when associated with lower eyelid malposition. Autogenous fat pad sliding, fat grafting *(Fig. 9.36)*, and fat injection have been utilized to correct this deformity with variable

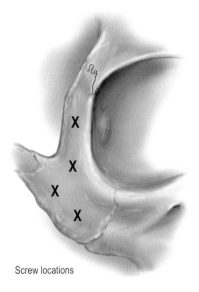

Screw locations

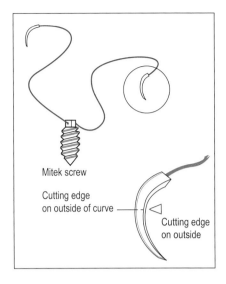

Mitek screw

Cutting edge
on outside of curve

Cutting edge
on outside

Fig. 9.35 Mitek screw fixation in subperiosteal midface elevation. Following elevation of the subperiosteal midface flap, fixation is achieved by suspending the flap using two 4-0 Vicryl sutures on half-circle cutting needles. The sutures are then tied to a titanium screw placed on the anterior surface of the lateral orbital bone (zygomatic bone). The screw is tightened until the head is flush with the bone surface. The elevated and stabilized structures support the repositioned lower lid and the recruited and elevated cheek skin and tissue help replace deficient posterior lamella. (From Aston, Aesthetic Plastic Surgery, 2009, Saunders.)

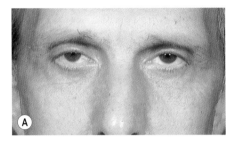
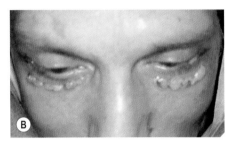
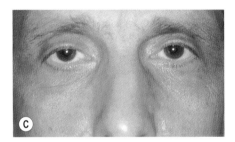

Fig. 9.36 (A) Patient with excessive lower lid fat resection with associated lower eyelid malposition. **(B)** The supplementary submental autogenous fat grafts are shown before their placement into a retroseptal position through a lateral canthal incision. Lateral canthoplasties were also performed. **(C)** Patient seen one year postoperatively. (From Jelks GW, Jelks EB. Blepharoplasty. In: Peck GC, ed. Complications and problems in aesthetic plastic surgery. New York: Gower Medical Publishing; 1992.)

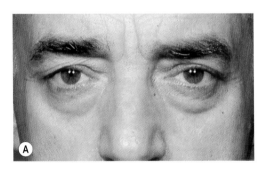
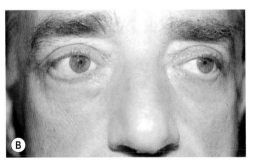
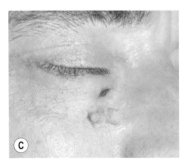

Fig. 9.37 (A) Blepharoplastic patient preoperatively. **(B)** At 2 months postoperatively with evidence of inadequate resection of fat from the right lower eyelid medial compartment. **(C)** The fat is removed via a small stab incision through skin, muscle, and orbital septum. (From Jelks GW, Jelks EB. Blepharoplasty. In: Peck GC, ed. Complications and problems in aesthetic plastic surgery. New York: Gower Medical Publishing; 1992.)

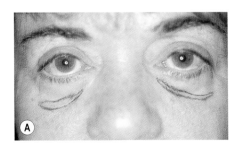
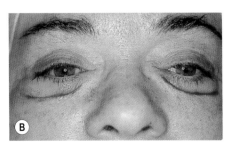
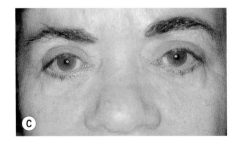

Fig. 9.38 (A) Patient seen following blepharoplasty with persistent malar excess skin. **(B)** Immediately after direct excision. **(C)** A satisfied patient seen 9 months postoperatively. (From Jelks, GW, Jelks EB. Blepharoplasty. In: Peck GC, ed. Complications and problems in aesthetic plastic surgery. New York: Gower Medical Publishing; 1992.)

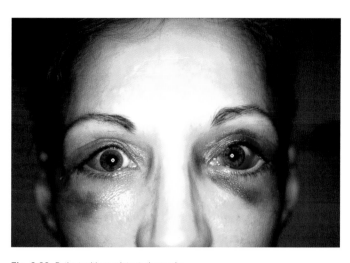

Fig. 9.39 Patient with persistent chemosis.

results.[66–72] A lateral canthoplasty should be performed at the time of fat augmentation.

Inadequate fat resection most commonly occurs in the upper and lower medial and lower lateral compartments. A small stab incision through the skin, muscle, and septum can be utilized to deliver the residual fat for excision *(Fig. 9.37)*.[27] In the lower lid, the transconjunctival approach may also be used.

Persistent malar bags, or excess skin that presents without lower lid cicatricial retraction can be directly excised and carefully closed to produce acceptable results *(Fig. 9.38)*.[27]

Chemosis is a milky edema of the subconjunctival tissues. It results from obstruction of the lymphatic drainage channels of the periorbital area *(Fig. 9.39)*. Repositioning the eyelids over the chemotic conjunctiva and patching usually resolve the situation. If the chemosis becomes more marked or there is actual incarceration by the eyelids, temporary suture tarsorrhaphy may be required.[3,27,37]

Access the complete references list online at http://www.expertconsult.com

3. Jelks GW, Jelks EB. Repair of lower lid deformities. *Clin Plast Surg.* 1993;20:417.

5. Jelks GW, Jelks EB. Preoperative evaluation and treatment of lower lid ectropion following blepharoplasty. *Plast Reconstr Surg.* 1990;85: 971.

   Preoperative identification of a predisposition to ectropion is the first step in preventing this complication after blepharoplasty. The authors discuss surgical techniques to avoid this common adverse outcome and address procedures designed to reverse ectropion if it does occur.

7. Patipa M. The evaluation and management of lower eyelid retraction following cosmetic surgery. *Plast Reconstr Surg.* 2000;106:438.

   Causes of lower eyelid retraction are discussed from an anatomical perspective. The author then presents etiology-based corrective procedures.

12. Lisman RD, Hyde K, Smith B. Complications of blepharoplasty. *Clin Plast Surg.* 1988;15:309.

24. Zide BM, Jelks GW. Surgical anatomy of the orbit. *Plast Reconstr Surg.* 1984;74:301.

43. Carraway JH. The impact of Herring's law on blepharoplasty and ptosis surgery. *Aesthetic Surg J.* 2004;24:275.

45. Pessa JE, Desvigne LD, Lambros VS, et al. Changes in ocular globe-to-orbital rim position with age: implications for aesthetic blepharoplasty of the lower eyelids. *Aesthetic Plast Surg.* 1999;23(5):337–342.

   The authors present findings from CT scans assessing the relationship of the globe to surrounding anatomy throughout the aging process. Their findings inform recommendations for lower lid blepharoplasty and are incorporated into a model of craniofacial aging.

51. Rees TD. Prevention of ectropion by horizontal shortening of the lower lid during blepharoplasty. *Ann Plast Surg.* 1983;11:17.

57. Fagien S. Algorithm for Canthoplasty. The lateral retinacular suspension: a simplified suture canthopexy. *Plast Reconstr Surg.* 1999;103:2042.

   Methods to provide canthal support and avoid lower lid malposition in midface/lower eyelid rejuvenation are presented. The author describes his novel transpalpebral lateral retinacular suspension in this context.

61. McCord CD Jr, Ellis DS. The correction of lower lid malposition following lower lid blepharoplasty. *Plast Reconstr Surg.* 1993;92:1068.

   Methods to correct lower lid malposition are presented based on the underlying anatomical pathology.

10

Asian facial cosmetic surgery

Kyung S. Koh, Jong Woo Choi, and Clyde H. Ishii

SYNOPSIS

- The Asian's concept of beauty has changed over time. Currently, most Asians want to improve their appearance while preserving their ethnic identity.
- Asian cosmetic surgery is not simply Western cosmetic surgery applied to Asians. Rather, cosmetic surgery in Asians must account for the underlying differences in anatomy and aesthetic proportions between Asians and Caucasians.
- Asian blepharoplasty and augmentation rhinoplasty are two of the most popular facial cosmetic procedures in Asia today. Facial bone contouring and aesthetic orthognathic surgery are also becoming more common in certain parts of Asia.
- Since there is no perfect way to define beauty, one must use both subjective and objective tools for analyzing facial profiles according to ethnic standards.

Everything is in the face

(Cicero)

Introduction

The face, while only a single part of the body, is the icon of self-identity and can be easily recognized among hundreds of thousands of faces. Asian and Caucasian faces each have unique features. It is generally accepted that Asians have small, puffy eyes with an epicanthal fold, shallow orbits, a low profile nasal dorsum with thick skin, flat faces with large cheekbones and broad width. This is especially true for East Asians, including people from China, Japan, Mongolia, North Korea, South Korea and Taiwan.[1] Asia is the largest continent, and has numerous ethnic groups.[1,2] Southern Asians have darker, thicker skin, larger eyes with double folds and smaller, narrower facial skeletons compared to northern Asians, whereas western Asians have quite different facial features

from other Asians. Although there are some constants, the standard of beauty varies among countries. Anatomic characteristics and cultural differences, including trends in each ethnic group, should be considered before performing facial cosmetic surgery.

Much controversy surrounds the concept of universal beauty. Humans, even babies, have an innate affinity for beautiful people.[3] Symmetry and a healthy, young-looking appearance make a face more attractive, regardless of ethnic background. A key feature of beautiful faces is the quality known as youthfulness.[4] In Caucasian women, high cheekbones are an important factor, whereas Asian women with round or oval-shaped faces are considered more beautiful. When Asians see facial photographs of themselves alongside Caucasians, they, especially younger individuals, are sometimes disappointed with their appearances. In general, Asian faces tend to look broader with a flatter contour to their eyes, nose, and face. We live in a three-dimensional world, and the faces we observe directly are three-dimensional. Facial cosmetic surgery is a three-dimensional procedure, and more emphasis is being placed on facial contour changes.

Over the past two decades, many countries in East Asia, including South Korea, China, Taiwan, and Japan, have emerged as strong economies. More people in these countries can now afford to spend money on items that are not considered basic necessities, including cosmetic and luxury items. These items usually come from wealthier countries with well-established economies, mostly located in Europe and North America. People in East Asia have adopted Western habits, as "westernization" has progressed into these countries. Among the items brought to East Asia is a new concept of beauty for young female adults and teenagers. Due to globalization, Western and Eastern cultures interact to a greater degree than ever before, indirectly or directly. Thus, people from both cultures have become familiar with each other's looks.

Young female Asians have become acutely interested in their appearance, creating a boom in cosmetic surgery. This phenomenon has created a new standard of beauty. Females in East Asia seek larger eyes, a higher nose, and a smaller face, which are not traditional to "Asian" beauty but have been influenced by Western countries. It is incorrect to simply assume that Asians seek to "westernize" their faces. Although westernization of the Asian face seemed to be a goal in the past, most patients now want to preserve their ethnic identity, while at the same time improving their appearance.[1,2,5] This has reached a point where people wonder if the concept of traditional beauty no longer exists in these Asian countries and traditional beauty is no longer deemed beautiful. Some patients in cosmetic surgery clinics want to look like celebrities in their respective countries. These celebrities have beautiful and attractive faces that are popular not only in their own countries but in neighboring countries. Patients seeking cosmetic surgery must be properly counseled in order to avoid disappointment from unrealistic expectations.

Following the introduction of Western medicine in Asia, aesthetic surgery was disorganized and sporadic. Although the history of aesthetic surgery in Japan has been described, the exact details are not known due to lack of documentation. This is also true in other Asian countries. Modern concepts of facial cosmetic surgery, including double fold and augmentation rhinoplasty, began and were developed in Japan in the late 19th and 20th centuries. In South Korea, facial cosmetic surgery flourished following the Seoul Olympics in 1988. With economic development, cosmetic surgery in China has grown rapidly. Due to the increased scientific knowledge and training of board-certified plastic surgeons in East Asia, facial cosmetic surgery has advanced rapidly. These plastic surgeons have also played a key role in introducing new ideas and techniques about Asian facial plastic surgery.

Double eyelid surgery and augmentation rhinoplasty are two of the most popular facial cosmetic procedures throughout Asia. Facial bone contouring is also becoming another common procedure in East Asia. Experience with orthognathic surgery/craniofacial surgery initiated facial bone operations like mandible angle contouring and zygoma reduction. Development of special bone surgery tools, such as a variety of electrical saws and burrs has expanded the scope of cosmetic facial bone surgery, with favorable results.

Some Asians have attractive facial traits, including large eyes, a well-balanced nose with a good profile, and small lower faces.[6] Individuals who regard their facial features as falling short of the mainstream ideals of beauty are willing to undergo facial cosmetic surgery. Younger individuals, for example, wish to undergo facial bone contouring to make their faces smaller. These individuals do not have "below average faces".[1] Rather, they want to look above average, sometimes chic and stylish, not merely natural. Most patients who want facial cosmetic procedures like double eyelids and augmentation rhinoplasty are women, but these cosmetic procedures are also requested by men.

Asian blepharoplasty

Introduction

Few young Caucasians undergo cosmetic procedures for their upper eyelids. Most of these individuals have large eyes with crisp, tall upper lid creases. In contrast, Asians are described by westerners as having puffy, small eyes, epicanthal folds,

and lack of supratarsal folds. However, this is not true of all Asians. About 50% of women in East Asia have these features.[1,2] Many Asian women wish to enhance their appearance but they do not want Caucasian eyelids.[1,2,7] Asian blepharoplasty or "double eyelid" surgery is the most common cosmetic operation in Asia, with some reports suggesting that 30–60% of Asians undergo this procedure.[8] If these women have deep-set, large eyelids with high folds like Caucasians, they look unnatural, as such eyelids do not match the shape of their faces. Therefore, ethnic differences should be considered.

The first procedure to create a supratarsal fold or "double eyelid" was described by Mikamo in 1896.[9] The procedure was performed on a patient who lacked a fold in one of her upper eyelids. Shirakabe *et al.* made a historical review of 32 surgical techniques reported in Japan.[10] In the western countries, Sayoc reported anatomic differences of upper eyelids between Caucasians and East Asians. The anatomic differences and their implications regarding double eyelid surgery were discussed.[11] Fernadez and Flowers in Hawaii, where East meets West, published papers about double eyelid surgery for Asians.[4,12] Newer techniques seeking to be more refined and less invasive while imitating the natural fold are being reported.[13]

Anatomic considerations

Multiple theories exist regarding the formation of the supratarsal crease or fold *(Fig. 10.1)*. First, Sayoc explained the presence of double fold based on anatomic differences between Caucasian and East Asian eyelids. Expansions of the levator palpebrae superioris muscle penetrating through the septum and orbicularis oculi muscle to the overlying dermis were thought to be present in Caucasian eyelids and less so in Asians *(Fig. 10.2A)*.[14] The presence of such attachments between the levator aponeurosis and skin was established by Cheng and Xu through scanning electron microscopy studies.[15] Another concept is the role of fibrous septa between the tarsal plate and pretarsal skin. The adherence between the tarsal plate and pretarsal skin is loose in the single eyelid and tight in the double eyelid.[4,16] Therefore, both explanations focus on the connection between the levator mechanism and the pretarsal skin.

An important factor contributing to supratarsal crease formation is the level of fusion of the orbital septum and the levator aponeurosis. The supratarsal crease is formed by the dermal insertion at the confluence of the septum and levator aponeurosis.[13] The level of adhesion between the orbital septum and levator aponeurosis defines the superior palpebral crease in most Caucasian eyelids,[17] whereas lower fusion of the orbital septum to levator aponeurosis results in a low lying or absent crease in the Asian eyelid *(Fig. 10.2B)*. Asians with naturally occurring superior palpebral folds have a relatively higher fusion of the orbital septum and levator aponeurosis *(Fig. 10.3)*.[18] The preaponeurotic orbital fat present in the pretarsal space eliminates the formation of double fold in Asians. Among Asians, it is not unusual for the upper lids to vary, being double and single in the same individual, depending on such variables as fatigue, diurnal variations of eyelid swelling, and weight change.

The epicanthal fold is also a characteristic feature of Asian upper lid. It hides the medial part of eye, including the

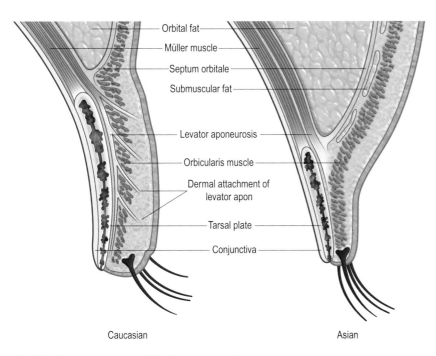

Orbital fat
Müller muscle
Septum orbitale
Submuscular fat

Levator aponeurosis

Orbicularis muscle

Dermal attachment of
levator apon

Tarsal plate

Conjunctiva

Caucasian

Asian

Fig. 10.1 Anatomy of upper eyelid in Caucasians and Asians.

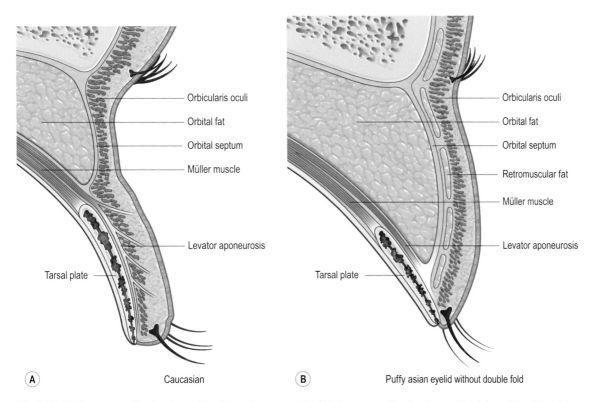

Orbicularis oculi

Orbital fat

Orbital septum

Müller muscle

Levator aponeurosis

Tarsal plate

Orbicularis oculi

Orbital fat

Orbital septum

Retromuscular fat

Müller muscle

Levator aponeurosis

Tarsal plate

A Caucasian

B Puffy asian eyelid without double fold

Fig. 10.2 (A) The cross-sectional anatomy of the Caucasian upper eyelid. **(B)** The cross-sectional anatomy of the Asians with puffy eyelid.

caruncle and lacrimal lake and increases the intercanthal distance. In East Asians, at least 50% of adults have epicanthal fold. If slight traces are included, almost all East Asians retain epicanthal folds, and a mild epicanthus is not an unusual feature for them.[1] There has been a recent trend to eliminate or loosen the epicanthal fold as part of the double eyelid operation. This medial epicanthoplasty will decrease the wide intercanthal distance and increase the horizontal width of the palpebral apertures. However, surgeons should be very cautious about total elimination of epicanthal folds, because this can leave a noticeable scar and result in loss of ethnic identity.

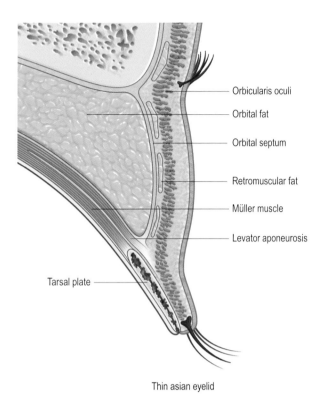

Orbicularis oculi

Orbital fat

Orbital septum

Retromuscular fat

Müller muscle

Levator aponeurosis

Tarsal plate

Thin asian eyelid

Fig. 10.3 The cross-sectional anatomy of the Asians with thin eyelid.

Preoperative considerations and diagnosis

Most Asian patients desiring double eyelids no longer want a westernized appearance, but rather an appearance more appropriate for Asians. Because the anatomy of the orbit differs greatly between Asians and Caucasians, Asian blepharoplasty should be performed in accordance with the orbital anatomy of Asians. Previously, most young Asians seeking upper blepharoplasty have done so only for double fold formation. More recently, Asians have undergone upper blepharoplasty to achieve a more attractive eyelid shape by reducing the puffiness in their eyelids, obtaining a double fold, and increasing the palpebral fissure length.[18] These patients also prefer a flat upper eyelid which looks young and stylish, not sunken or deflated.[4]

The height of double eyelid is an important issue. In young Caucasians, the superior palpebral fold is small and the height of the pretarsal skin exposure is similar to te height of the superior palpebral crease.[18] In contrast, the Asian lid crease is generally 2–3 mm lower, and a large superior palpebral fold hangs over the pretarsal skin.[7] Thus, exposure of pretarsal skin is less than in Caucasians. The lower border of the fold is called the double eyelid line, and the distance between this line and the margin of the lid at primary gaze is pretarsal exposure *(Fig. 10.4)*. After blepharoplasty, the pretarsal exposure is determined by several factors, such as the height of incision, the amount of pretarsal skin excision, the height of

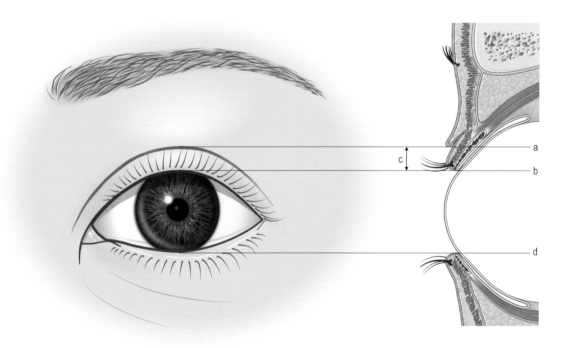

Fig. 10.4 The mechanism of double eyelidplasty in North-East Asians. a, Double eyelid line, lower border of fold; b, upper lid margin; c. pretarsal exposure; d, lower lid margin.

fixation, and levator function.[18] Currently, the preference for most Asians is a pretarsal exposure <3 mm, and as little as 1 mm.[7] These desires have geographical variation *(Fig. 10.4)*.

Another preoperative consideration is the shape of the desired crease. Caucasians typically have a semilunar shaped crease where the central third of the crease lies farther from the lash line than the medial and lateral thirds.[19] Most Asians are uncomfortable with this configuration, since it appears unnatural to them. They prefer a fold that for most part is parallel to the lid margin. Laterally, the crease may have a slight flare, in that the crease lies farther from the lash line than the central third. Medially, the crease may taper toward the medial canthus ("inside fold") or run outside the epicanthus ("outside fold") *(Fig. 10.5)*.[20]

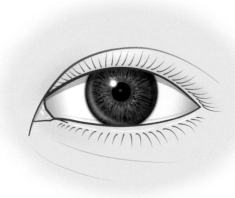

Inside fold

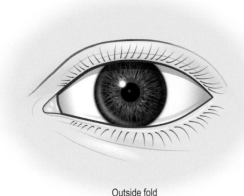

Outside fold

Fig. 10.5 "Inside" vs "outside" fold in Asian blepharoplasty.

Treatment/surgical technique

Although procedures for blepharoplasty in Asians have a number of similarities to those in Caucasians, it is important to recognize that upper blepharoplasty in Asians is not a westernization procedure. Thus, surgical techniques should differ in some respects from a Caucasian blepharoplasty.

Incisional versus nonincisional methods

Generally, surgical techniques for double fold formation can be categorized as incisional and nonincisional methods, although some authors have advocated partial incisional methods.

Nonincisional methods

Numerous nonincisional methods have been described.[21–26] These methods are used primarily for young people who do not require skin excision and for patients with thin upper eyelid tissue who do not have an excess of fat. The advantages of these minimally invasive techniques must be balanced against the knowledge that the fixation may not be as durable over time when compared with the incisional methods. Nonincisional methods can be categorized as single stitch and multiple stitch methods, both of which have advantages and disadvantages.

Video 1

In these techniques, stitches are simply inserted through the skin at the level of the preferred lid crease, traversing the full thickness of the lid tissues down to and including either the levator aponeurosis or the tarsal plate. The stitches are tied in such a way that the knots are buried.

- Single stitch nonincisional methods have many modifications.[21] *Figure 10.6* shows a nonincisional single stitch method. Fixation through the levator aponeurosis can result in a more natural appearance and minimal

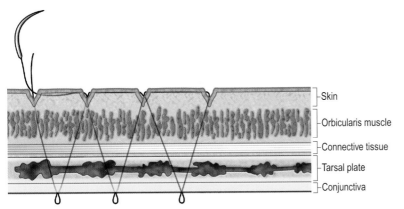

—Skin
—Orbicularis muscle
—Connective tissue
—Tarsal plate
—Conjunctiva

Fig. 10.6 Nonincisional double eyelidplasty (single stitch method).

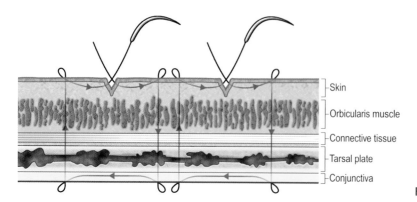

Skin
Orbicularis muscle
Connective tissue
Tarsal plate
Conjunctiva

Fig. 10.7 Nonincisional double eyelidplasty (multiple stitch method).

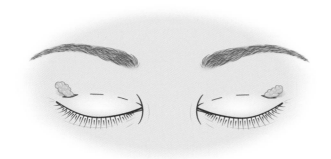

Fig. 10.8 Partial incisional double eyelidplasty with fat removal.

postoperative edema, but relapse can sometimes occur. Fixation through the upper portion of the tarsal plate can result in a more definite eyelid crease with minimal relapse, but postoperative edema can occur more frequently than in levator fixation methods.

- Multiple stitch nonincisional methods can be performed, usually with 3–5 stitches on each side *(Fig. 10.7)*.[27]

Several factors should be considered when performing nonincisional double fold formation. First, the conjunctival side of the stitches should not be exposed, since this exposure can result in corneal damage postoperatively and second, the possibility of relapse should be considered and mentioned preoperatively to all patients.

Video 2

Partial incisional methods

Partial incisional methods *(Fig. 10.8)* are being used more frequently.[28,29] These procedures have evolved to overcome disadvantages of the above two methods. Partial incisional methods can result in moderate tissue adhesions, preventing the early relapse observed using nonincisional methods. Moreover, partial incision can result in a more natural appearance, minimizing scarring of the upper lid. Using the partial incisional approach, preaponeurotic fat can be easily removed to correct puffy eyelids.

In the partial incision method, one or more small stab incisions can be made in the planned upper eyelid crease, and after going through orbicularis, the preaponeurotic fat is removed. A permanent suture material is then placed between the skin edges and the underlying aponeurosis or superior edge of the tarsal plate. The lid should be inverted to confirm that the suture has been placed to catch the upper border of the tarsal plate, and to ensure that the suture has not pierced the conjunctiva.

Incisional methods

For double fold formation in the upper lid, traditional tarso-dermal fixation through incisional methods *(Fig. 10.9A,B)* has been an effective standard method.[30] In patients with redundant eyelid skin, the incisional approach is unavoidable. There are as yet no definite standards for incisional blepharoplasty, but the common procedures will be described. The placement of the double fold on the upper lid should be decided preoperatively according to each patient's appearance and preference utilizing forceps or a probe.

The skin incision marking tapers closer to the lash line as it progresses medially towards the epicanthal fold. Some patients may prefer that the medial portion of the crease lies outside the epicanthus. The superior incision is marked such that the skin to be excised will also taper, usually measuring 1 mm medially, 2 mm centrally, and 3 mm laterally. The skin incision is then made and the strip of skin excised. A strip of orbicularis oculi wider than the skin strip is then removed in order to create a sharp lid crease. Leaving excess orbicularis can result in a puffy appearance. The septum is then entered, and a variable amount of retroseptal fat may be either excised or released, allowing it to ride up superiorly. The levator aponeurosis is exposed as it approaches the tarsal plate. The Asian tarsal plate typically measures 6–7 mm in height. Fixation of the new upper lid crease is then done. Various methods of suture fixation involving internal buried sutures have been described. One method is to use 3–7 sutures passing through the aponeurosis and the dermis-muscle of the inferior skin edge. The skin is thus anchored to the levator mechanism, creating the new lid crease, which will be hidden by the overhanging tissue of the palpebral fold. Alternatively, fixation can be done to the superior edge of the tarsal plate, a procedure which is thought to create a more static and defined upper lid crease *(Fig. 10.9B–D)*.

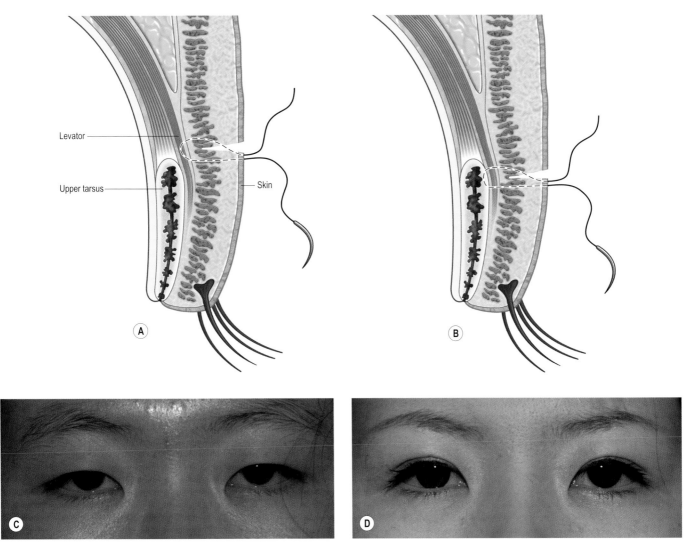

Fig. 10.9 (A) Incisional method: skin–aponeurosis. **(B)** Incisional method: skin–tarsus. **(C)** Double eyelidplasty: preoperative view. **(D)** Double eyelidplasty: postoperative view.

Subclinical ptosis repair

Many Asian people who want more attractive looking eyelids are not satisfied with the creation of a simple double crease.[31] They may have a low resting level of their eyelids, which if corrected will give them a more open and attractive palpebral fissure.[32] These patients have a tendency for upper eyelid ptosis, and are defined as having "subclinical ptosis". They may be candidates for the same procedures utilized in cases of mild ptosis, including Müllerectomy, or levator aponeurosis plication or advancement.[33–35]

Medial epicanthoplasty

Medial epicanthoplasty *(Figs 10.10–10.12)* is a very important component of Asian eyelid surgery.[36] Various methods were originally introduced for the correction of blepharophimosis in Western countries. In Asia, however, these procedures have been used for the correction of average Asian medial epicanthal folds. Although traditional methods, including the Mustarde technique,[37,38] have been used, these procedures may result in bad scars on the medial canthal area. These problems may be overcome by the half Z-plasty technique.[37,39,40] Nevertheless, the amount of release is limited and a moderate scar remains. Many Asian patients have complained about these scars. New methods, including skin redraping methods, have therefore been developed to eliminate the possibility of scarring of the medial canthal area.[36,41] These skin redraping methods, which have become very popular in Asia, include a medial subciliary incision on the lower eyelid which makes a nonvisible scar and resection/releaser of medial epicanthal adhesions, procedures that can minimize medial epicanthal scars and correct medial epicanthus quite well *(Figs 10.11 and 10.12)*.

These methods, however, can also have side-effects, including unnatural dimpling at the releasing points of medial epicanthal adhesions.

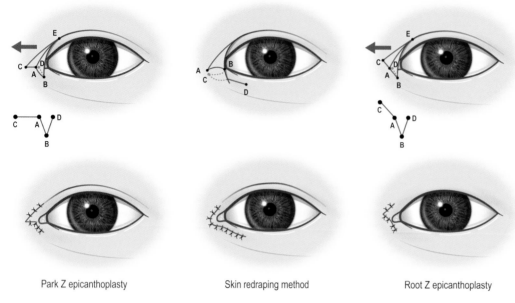

Park Z epicanthoplasty   Skin redraping method   Root Z epicanthoplasty

Fig. 10.10 Various methods of medial epicanthoplasty.

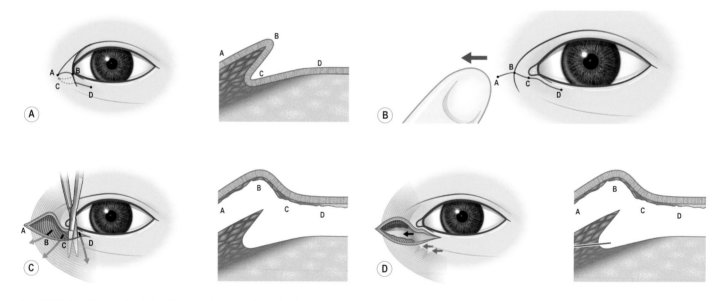

Fig. 10.11 Medial epicanthoplasty with skin redraping method: planning.

Lateral canthoplasty

Lateral canthoplasty *(Figs 10.13, 10.14)* may increase the horizontal length of the palpebral fissure and result in a more natural appearance around the lateral canthus.[42] Although currently controversial, these procedures are being used for these purposes.

Postoperative care

Postoperative care for Asian blepharoplasty patients is similar to that for Caucasians. Scarring is generally not a problem, although excessive swelling can result in a higher crease height than is desired. Postoperative instructions are as follows:

1. Cold compresses, as tolerated, for 24 h
2. Antibiotic ointment for the suture lines
3. Cleanse the wound with clean water
4. The external sutures may be removed in 4–5 days.

Outcomes, prognosis, and complications

Complications are similar to those observed during routine blepharoplasty procedures. These complications include

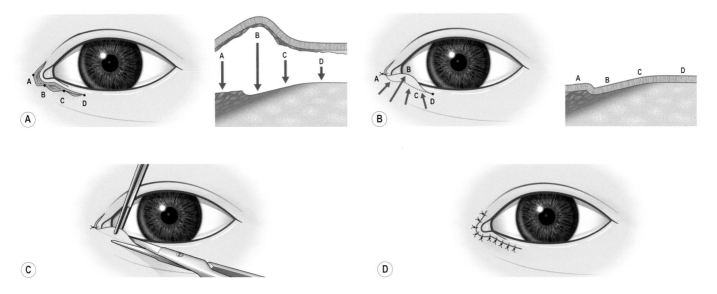

Fig. 10.12 Medial epicanthoplasty with skin redraping method: completion.

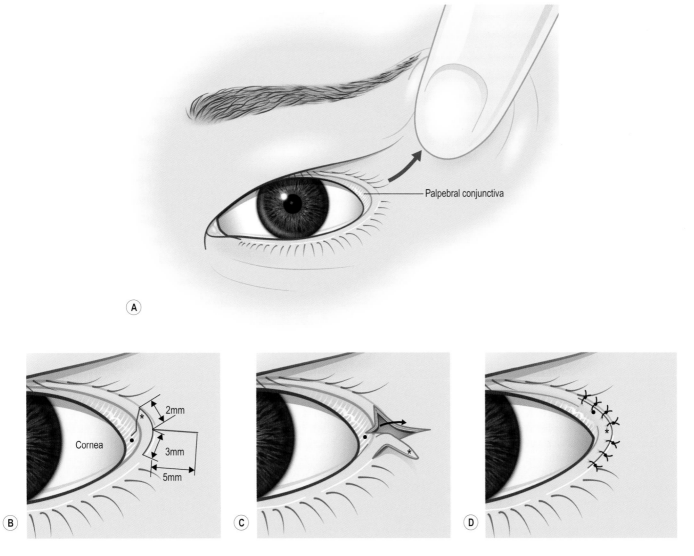

Fig. 10.13 Lateral canthoplasty technique.

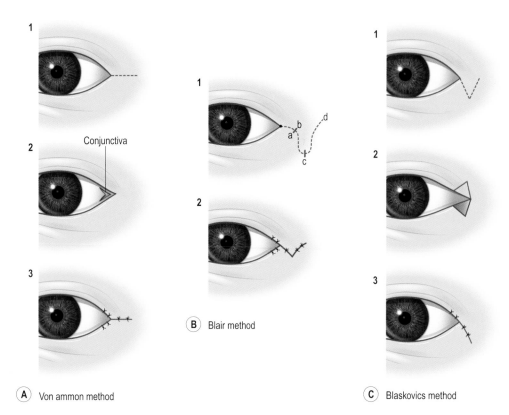

Conjunctiva

(A) Von ammon method

(B) Blair method

(C) Blaskovics method

Fig. 10.14 Lateral canthoplasty: other techniques.

asymmetry, prolonged swelling, multiple folds, infection and hematoma.

Asymmetry is the most common problem after Asian blepharoplasty, especially when combined with levator plication or advancement. Revision surgery may be required for patients with major and persistent asymmetry. Patients should be informed of this preoperatively.

Asian rhinoplasty

Introduction

Augmentation rhinoplasty is one of the most common aesthetic plastic surgery procedures in Asian countries. Whereas most Western literature addresses issues related to rhinoplasty in Caucasians, such as reduction and corrective rhinoplasty procedures, augmentation of the nasal dorsum and tip remain key issues for Asian plastic surgeons.[43] In the past, most of these operations consisted of simple augmentation rhinoplasty. More recently, however, the needs of patients have become more complex, requiring more meticulous preoperative diagnosis and more involved surgical techniques. Ideally, rhinoplasty should enhance the harmony between the nose and face, thus requiring general evaluation of the entire face. For this purpose, the entire face must be evaluated. The general principles for rhinoplasty in Asians are quite similar to those in Caucasians. However, rhinoplasties in Asians and Caucasians have different characteristics. This section will describe various aspects of rhinoplasty in Asians, as well as commonly encountered problems and solutions.

Differences in nasal soft tissue and skeletons between Asian and Caucasian noses

The nasal profile of Asians is quite different from that of Caucasians. The Asian nose has a shorter height, less tip projection, and a wider nasal base when compared to the Caucasian nose. The Asian nose has a similar height and narrower width than the African nose.[44] The overlying soft tissue enveloping Asian noses consists of a dense fibromuscular layer along with a fatty layer, especially over the alar lobule. The linear dimensions of the nose are smaller in Asians than in Caucasians, but their noses are wider, although their nostril floor widths are quite similar. These findings can be attributed to the thicker, flaring alar lobule in Asians.[45] A comparison of the aesthetic proportions of Asian and Caucasian noses found that Asian noses projected less from the face and were broader at the intercanthal level and alar base, but not at the bony base. Moreover, Asian noses projected less at all levels, including the nasion projection and tip projection.[46]

Although there are racial variations among Asians, nasal skeletons are generally smaller and weaker in Asians than in Caucasians.[47] The shape of the nasal bone in Germans has been classified into eight types, whereas the width of the nasal bones was shorter and the width of the pyriform aperture was wider in Asians than in Germans. The nasal base width in Asians is greater than in Caucasians but less than in Africans. Asian noses have been found to be wider at the nasal base, but similar or shorter in the height of the nasal base (tip projection), than in Caucasians.[48] Contrary to popular thought, the alar cartilage in Asians is not markedly smaller than in Caucasians, although there are differences in the

Capsular contracture around implants

Capsular contractures may occur around any alloplastic implant and cause deformity and possible implant extrusion. Treatment of this complication is similar to that advocated for implant exposure.

Secondary procedures

Forehead augmentation (Fig. 10.15)

Augmentation rhinoplasty can make the lateral profile more attractive. However, patients with a flat forehead profile may benefit from a simultaneous forehead augmentation. Traditionally, custom-made silicone or Gore-Tex® implants have been used for forehead augmentation despite the possibility of seroma or infection of the implant.[73] This may be due to the ease of the technique and the more natural contour of the forehead resulting from the use of these implants. Microfat grafting with the Coleman technique or augmentation with various cements may also be used to improve the forehead profile.

Paranasal augmentation

In Asia, augmentation rhinoplasty combined with paranasal augmentation has become quite popular. Paranasal augmentation is performed using PTFE (Gore-Tex®), silicone or polyethylene (Medpor) implants. Since this procedure can result in inflammation or chronic infection, patients should be informed preoperatively. Microfat grafts with the Coleman technique may also be used for paranasal augmentation.

Alar base surgery

Many Asians are also concerned about the width of their nasal base. The very real risk of visible scarring must be carefully discussed with the patient before proceeding with any modification of the alar base.

Genioplasty

As in Caucasian patients, chin projection should always be considered in relation to nasal tip projection and the overall profile of the face. Osseous genioplasty or augmentation genioplasty with alloplastic materials are both successful in Asian patients.

Asian facial bone surgery

Introduction

Although the standards of facial beauty have changed over time, certain features remain constant. Many studies have shown that symmetry and averageness could be the overall standards for beauty profiles.[74] Throughout history, humans have attempted to define beauty objectively. Beauty can be measured by various methods, including artistic standards, cephalometric standards and anthropometric analysis.[75]

By using the golden ratio, Leonardo Da Vinci employed artistic standards to try and explain facial beauty mathematically. The golden ratio, which was originally used in architecture, geometry and other areas is defined by a line divided into two unequal segments, where the ratio of the entire line to the longer segment is identical to the ratio of the longer to the shorter segment, or 1.618.[76] The golden ratio has been used in planning correctional surgery for a facial deformity, creating a line drawing of a mask outlining ideal facial proportions.[77] Although others have claimed that this mask does not describe an ideal facial shape, the facial golden mask has been used as an objective index for facial analysis, with some correlation to the degree of facial attractiveness.[78] In view of artistic standards, the Asian is known to have a relatively wider mid and lower face, based on the golden ratio. These findings may explain why many Asians request facial reduction procedures, including the malar reduction, mandible angle reduction and maxillomandibular setback procedures. In addition, Asian people have smaller noses and greater bizygomatic and bigonial widths, according to the golden ratio.[79] Reduction of the mandible angle and/or zygoma reduction is regarded by many Asian women as a means of becoming more attractive.

The second tool for measuring the facial profile is cephalometric analysis.[75] This method, along with other analytic methods, has been the standard until now for facial analysis. However, these analytic methods have their shortcomings. Thus, it has been concluded that clinical aesthetic evaluations are more valuable than cephalometric standards, and that strict adherence to cephalometric standards does not lead to either harmonious or more beautiful faces. Despite these controversies, cephalometric analysis has been the standard tool for analysis of facial growth and orthognathic surgery. McNamara *et al.* reported a study of the lateral profile of 60 Koreans and 42 European–American adults with normal occlusion.[80] Their study showed that the Koreans had a lower angle of nasal inclination and a higher degree of lip protrusion, whereas the slope of the forehead did not differ significantly. Dentoalveolar protrusion is another characteristic of Asian people. Thus, many of orthognathic procedures in Asia are done to setback of dentoalveolar complex and maxillomandibular complex.[81]

Anthropometry, a method by which direct measurements are taken on live subjects, offers numerous advantages: these measurements are easy to take, noninvasive, and inexpensive, as well as being suitable for a wide variety of purposes. In order to be meaningful, there must be an adequate number of subjects representing all ethnic groups and different social backgrounds. In addition, well-trained examiners should use sophisticated measurement tools. Honn and Goz used this method to investigate differences between female Korean-Americans and Caucasian–Americans.[75]

The above discussion suggests that there is no perfect way to define beauty. Therefore, it would be wise to use the both subjective and objective tools for analysis of facial profiles according to the ethnic standards.

History

Malar reduction

Reduction malarplasty, first reported at 1983 by Onizuka and colleagues, was based on underpositioning of the osteotomized zygoma through an intraoral approach.[82] In 1988,

Baek *et al.* reported 94 cases using a technique involving the coronal approach followed by either an *in situ* transposition osteoplasty or the removal of the malar complex and contouring of the bone with replacement as a free bone graft.[83] In 1991, Uhm and Lew classified zygoma prominence into three categories, including true zygoma protrusion, pseudozygomatic protrusion and combination.[84] Yang and Park reported, in 1992, an infracture technique for the zygomatic body and arch reduction, which he postulated could minimize the age-related ptosis of soft tissues of the cheek. Surgical procedures for zygomatic reduction in Orientals have also been described, as has an "infracture technique for zygomatic osteotomy and arch reduction."[85] In 1993, Satoh and Watanabe showed the results using the tripod osteotomy via the coronal approach and simultaneous frontoperiorbital lifting in oriental patients.[86] Cho compared the results of the intraoral and bicoronal approaches.[87] Baek and Lee showed that intraoral malar reduction could result in cheek drooping. Thus, the combination of reposition malarplasty and facelift proved to be a satisfactory method.[88] Many reports for simultaneous mandibular contouring and zygoma reduction have been reported for balanced facial contours.

Mandible angle reduction

The presence of prominent mandibular angles in Asians suggests a harsh and masculine appearance. This led to the design of procedures for aesthetic contouring of the mandible. The square facial appearance in Asians is not only due to masseteric hypertrophy but also to a posterior projection and lateral flaring of the mandibular angle. In 1989, Baek *et al.* reported the mandible angle ostectomy in 42 Asian patients.[89] In 1994, technical refinements were reported,[5] which classified the prominent mandible angle according to the anatomic type of mandibular angle: lateral bulging in frontal view and posteroinferior projection in lateral view, or a combination of these types. Curved and/or tangential osteotomy of the lateral flaring was performed based on the category. Mandible contouring surgery could be performed with an oscillating saw, and multiple mandible angle ostectomy was found to result in a smoother contour of the mandible angle postoperatively. In 1994, Kyutoku *et al.* invented the gonial angle stripper for treatment of prominent gonial angle.[90] Satoh reported mandibular contouring surgery by angular contouring combined with genioplasty in orientals.[91] In 1997, Deguchi *et al.* reported angle-splitting ostectomy for reducing the width of the lower face.[92] In 2005, Gui and colleagues reported intraoral one-stage curved osteotomy in 407 cases.[93] Among the methods described to reduce the bigonial width were external corticotomy with a sagittal split which involved removal of the external cortex of the mandibular ramus, thus reducing the bigonial angle. Han and Kim reported reduction mandibuloplasty, which he described as ostectomy of the lateral cortex around mandibular angle.[94] Lo *et al.* showed the high satisfaction rates after zygoma and mandible reduction surgery in outcome assessments. He also showed the significant volume change in osseous mandible and masseter muscle after the mandibular contouring surgery.[95] Hong and colleagues three-dimensionally analyzed the relationship among lower facial width, bony width, and masseter muscle volume in prominent mandible angles.[96] Long curved osteotomy was recently introduced in Korea to reduce the mandibular body as well

as the mandibular angles. Sometimes, these procedures are performed simultaneously with narrowing genioplasty, resulting in a smaller lower face.

Orthognathic surgery and anterior segmental ostectomy

Profiloplasty of the lower face by maxillary and mandibular anterior segmental osteotomies (ASO) was first described in 1993.[97] Taiwanese plastic surgeons YuRay Chen, Philip Chen, and LunJou Lo have played important roles in developing orthognathic surgery suitable for Asians. Recently in Korea, orthognathic surgery is being performed for purely aesthetic reasons. Although maxillo-mandibular complex clockwise rotation has been found quite helpful for skeletal class III patients, the true indications for these procedures have not yet been clarified.

Diagnosis and indications

Mandible angle

Many Asian people want to improve their square face appearance by reducing the size of their prominent mandible angles. Therefore, mandibular angle reduction is a popular procedure in Asia. An acute gonial angle can be corrected by mandible angle ostectomy (bone removal). Mandible angle reduction results in a narrower bigonial distance. Moreover, the lateral flaring in frontal view can be corrected with external corticotomy and angle reduction. If, in addition, a patient has masseteric hypertrophy, it can be corrected with Botox injection, but only with temporary effects. Thus, an alternative in such patients is to combine an osseous mandibular angle reduction and resection of the masseter muscle. These combined procedures are still controversial.

Zygoma

Most Asian people have prominent cheekbones. Prominent cheekbones are considered attractive in Western women. This is not true in eastern societies, where prominent cheekbones are indicative of strength and considered undesirable in Asian women. Thus, most Asian women want less prominent zygomas. However, in performing zygoma reduction surgery, the bitemporal widths should be considered. Overcorrected zygoma widths can result in an unnatural appearance, removing the soft contour of the face. Moreover, the anterior part of the zygoma should be preserved in most patients. Without this protrusion, patients tend to look older. Therefore, to preserve a youthful appearance, only the anterolateral and lateral parts of the zygoma should be reduced.

Chin

Genioplasty in Asian people, either for setback or advancement, is a similar procedure to that in Caucasians. Recently, a narrowing genioplasty has been introduced in Korea. This is often done in conjunction with mandible angle reduction. Park reported the narrowing genioplasty, either as a single procedure or in combination with mandible reduction, making the lower face appear slender and produces a more feminine chin contour. Trapezoid or broad chins can be reduced by narrowing genioplasty.

Dentoalveolar protrusion

Anterior segmental setback ostectomy (ASO) is indicated in Asians with bimaxillary protrusions. Many Asian people have a tendency towards dentoalveolar protrusion, which may require orthodontic treatment or ASO. The latter procedure, however, should be limited to patients with large protrusions. Mild dentoalveolar protrusion might be better treated with orthodontic treatment alone. Excessive dentoalveolar setback with ASO can result in an unnatural appearance in Asians.

Facial profiles

Orthognathic surgery was originally designed to correct dentofacial deformities in patients with angle classification II or III. In Asia, the indications for orthognathic surgery have recently been extended to patients with almost normal occlusion and mild skeletal dentofacial disharmony. Although standard protocols have not yet been defined, orthognathic surgery has been found to change the facial proportions more ideally and reduce the size of the face. Since many Asian people have a mild skeletal class III pattern, many orthognathic surgery procedures in Asia involve class III corrections. Moreover, recent trends in facial bone surgery in Asia include the reduction of the facial contour, making it smaller than Asian average. In 2006, Jin *et al.* showed that orthognathic surgery for correction of occlusal class I in skeletal class III cases is effective in some patients. This report showed that it is possible to enhance the aesthetic outcome in this subset of Asians by changing skeletal characteristics so that the facial measurements more closely approach normal values.[98] However, the indications for orthognathic surgery in this group of patients remain controversial.

Surgical techniques and treatments

Facial contouring surgery

Mandible angle ostectomy *(Figs 10.20, 10.21)*

Traditionally, mandible angle ostectomy has been performed with an oscillating saw. An external approach was previously used because it allowed direct access to the mandibular angle. However, this procedure is now usually performed using an intraoral approach. In the latter, meticulous subperiosteal dissection is important to minimize bleeding and postoperative edema. Mandible angle ostectomy with an oscillating saw requires the somewhat blind removal of the mandible angle area. In patients with inwardly curved angles, ostectomy may be facilitated by burring on the ramus area or by the use of indirect mirrors. Important anatomical structures must be respected. In women, the average distances of the inferior alveolar nerve from the mandibular angle are 23.69 mm for square faces versus 20.66 mm for normal faces. In men, these distances are 27.30 mm and 23.28 mm, respectively.[99] During this procedure, the facial artery and the retromandibular vein are the most vulnerable vessels and should therefore be avoided. Following ostectomy, the secondary angle should also be manipulated by burring or doing multiple ostectomies

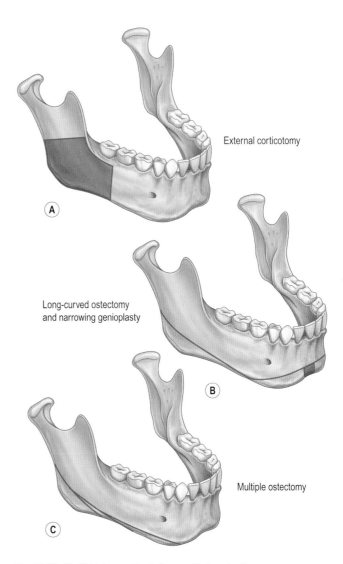

External corticotomy

Long-curved ostectomy and narrowing genioplasty

Multiple ostectomy

Fig. 10.20 (A–C) Various methods for mandibular reduction.

on the mandible body area. If not, patients may complain of irregular mandibular contours postoperatively. Three different ostectomy patterns may be performed:

- *Curved ostectomy with an oscillating saw*: This procedure is indicated in most patients with prominent mandible angles. It especially helps in reducing posteroinferior flaring in the lateral view.
- *Tangential ostectomy with a reciprocating saw*: With this procedure, the external cortex of the mandibular ramus is removed. Tangential ostectomy is performed to narrow the bigonial distance in mandibles with lateral flaring in the frontal view. This procedure alone, however, may not make the lateral contour smooth.[100]
- *Long-curved ostectomy*: This procedure is indicated in patients with a prominent mandible angle and wide mandibular body. Simultaneous reduction of the mandibular angle and body can result in a much smaller lower facial contour. Recently in Korea, this procedure is often performed along with narrowing genioplasty.

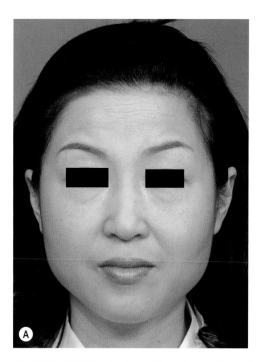
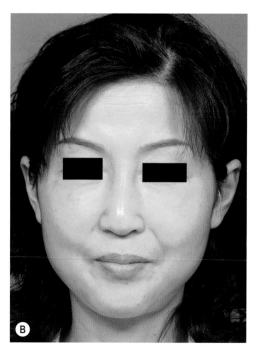

Fig. 10.21 (A,B) Prominent mandible angle: mandible angle ostectomy and external corticotomy with microfat graft in older ages.

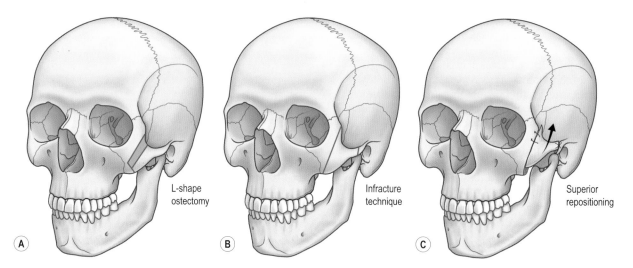

Fig. 10.22 (A–C) Various methods for malar reduction. **(A)** Typical L-shape ostectomy. **(B)** Green stick fracture. **(C)** Superior repositioning of malar complex via the bicoronal approach.

Malar reduction surgery

Malar reduction *(Fig. 10.22)* was first performed in the early 1980s to reduce the bizygomatic width. While the malar complex can be approached through intraoral, bicoronal, or preauricular incisions, the intraoral approach is often preferred. This approach to malar reduction begins with an oral incision and subperiosteal dissection. The osteotomy line is usually between the most concave line to the maxillary buttress, but may vary according to the preference of the surgeon. A higher position on the upper osteotomy site can result in greater malar reduction. Exposure of the maxillary sinus does not usually lead to infection, but avoiding an excessive anterior osteotomy is important in order to achieve good bony contact. Intraoral malar reduction has some pitfalls, the

first of which is soft tissue ptosis. Wide periosteal dissection involves detachment of the zygomatico-cutaneous ligaments. Postoperatively, soft tissue tends to displace downwards. The implication is that minimal dissection over the maxilla is preferred. The second pitfall is nonunion. With the intraoral approach, high fixation of the zygomatic segments is not easy. The masseteric power is quite great so postoperative downward displacement of the zygomatic bone may occur. Without bone union, the masseter muscle tends to displace the zygomatic complex. These problems may be overcome by using a bicoronal approach, an infracture technique with incomplete osteotomy, or by minimizing dissection during malar reduction. For osteotomy of the zygomatic arch, a small incision around the hairline is usually made, allowing for use of a reciprocating saw or a small osteotome. Use of the former may sometimes involve a temporal approach with a small incision. Some surgeons perform intraoral osteotomy on the zygomatic arch area without making any incision on the preauricular area. The optimal procedure for malar reduction in Asians has not been determined, but may depend primarily on each patient's condition and the surgeon's preferences *(Fig. 10.22)*. Possible approaches to malar reduction include the following.

Intraoral L-shaped ostectomy

This is the traditional method of malar reduction *(Fig. 10.22A)*. Segmental resection of the malar bone decreases the bizygomatic width and often results in an unnatural appearance.

Intraoral infracture technique with incomplete osteotomy

To overcome the limits of intraoral malar reduction, this procedure may be useful *(Figs 10.22B)*. Infracture with green stick fracture of the malar bone can minimize the incidence of postoperative soft tissue ptosis and malar nonunion. Additional burring is often needed to decrease the bony step in the malar area. Also, secure zygomatic arch fixation may be needed.

Bicoronal approach

For purely aesthetic reasons, this procedure is not well-accepted. However, in complicated cases, malar reduction via bicoronal approach can give the best results in fixation and precise correction of the malar complex. This approach may be advantageous in middle age or older patients because a forehead lift can be done simultaneously without additional incisions.

Narrowing genioplasty

Narrowing genioplasty *(Fig. 10.23)*, either as a single procedure or in combination with mandible reduction, makes the lower face appear slender and produces a more feminine chin contour. Soft tissue attachment of the chin is maintained to produce a maximum narrowing effect and maintain the blood flow to bony segments. Horizontal osteotomy and two vertical osteotomies are designed as shown in figure. The amount of resection in the central segment is determined preoperatively, depending on the width of chin and the patient's desire. The two segments are approximated centrally and fixed with microplates and screws. Advancement of the two segments is also possible if correction of the profile is required. The resection of the central strip has ranged from 6 to 12 mm.

Orthognathic surgery and anterior segmental ostectomy

Lip and chin profiles differ considerably between Asian and Western populations. Asians tend to have bimaxillary protrusion and a class III skeletal pattern, which have made ASO setback and class III correction with orthognathic surgery quite popular in Asian countries.

Orthognathic surgery: jaw rotation

The standard approach in management of class III dentofacial deformity in Caucasian patients is simultaneous maxillary advancement and mandibular setback. This procedure is indicated when maxillary hypoplasia exists relative to

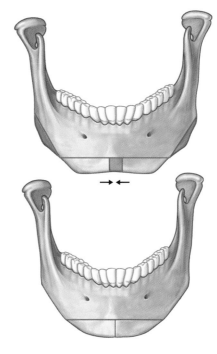

Narrowing genioplasty

Fig. 10.23 Narrowing genioplasty for the correction of the chin width.

mandibular prognathism in class III dentofacial deformities. However, many Asian patients have a varying degree of dentoalveolar protrusion which makes the Asian face look different from their Caucasian counterparts. In Asians, the maxillary advancement procedures may sometimes cause the aggravation of dentoalveolar protrusion or widening of alar base, both of which would be detrimental to their facial appearance. Moreover, Asian females tend to have a flat occlusal plane and a prominent mandibular angle which results in a square appearance. For these reasons, a posterior maxillary impaction without any maxillary advancement would be the preferable in some Asian class III patients *(Figs 10.24–10.27)*. However, caution must be exercised because excessive posterior impaction of maxilla along with the mandibular set back may impair the airway or change the shape of the smile.

In some cases, total maxillary setback is needed for simultaneous correction of a dentoalveolar protrusion. The vascular plexus should be avoided during this procedure and the total amount of total maxillary setback is limited compared to that with ASO *(Fig. 10.27)*.

Bimaxillary protrusion: anterior segmental setback ostectomy

This procedure is designed to osteotomize the anterior portions of the Lefort I segment and mandible and move them posteriorly. Preoperatively or intraoperatively, the first or second premolar is extracted for ASO setback. For anterior segmental ostectomy of the maxilla, two different pedicles can be used, with the palatal pedicle commonly used with the buccal approach. This approach provides improved exposure and easier performance of surgery. During these procedures, care must be taken to preserve the palatal mucosa. Preoperative

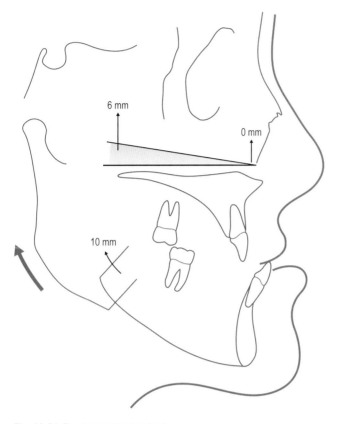

Fig. 10.24 Two jaw rotational setback.

and postoperative orthodontic treatment is mandatory to obtain predictable results.

Outcomes, prognosis, and complications

Zygoma reduction

Intraoperative complications are rare. However, long-term complications include drooping of cheek tissues and malar bone nonunion. Excessive wide dissection can release the zygomatico-cutaneous ligaments leading to soft tissue ptosis. Poor fixation of the osteotomy can lead to nonunion. Unfortunately, intraoral fixation of the malar complex in the superior-medial direction is not easy. The bicoronal approach can solve this problem by providing access for secure fixation. Alternatively, an infracture technique with a green stick fracture can be done. Finally, in order to minimize complications, less invasive approaches with minimal dissection are being introduced.

Mandible angle reduction

Many complications from mandible angle reduction have been reported.[101] The most critical complications include the condyle fracture caused by a wayward osteotomy, massive bleeding from the retromandibular vein or facial vessels and damage to the mental nerve. During angle reduction, precise ostectomy around the mandible posterior border is important in order to avoid a condylar fracture. When using the oscillating saw, adequate periosteal dissection is needed to allow visualization of the posterior mandibular border. If the retromandibular vein is torn during the procedure, direct coagulation or other means of hemostasis is not easy. Therefore, manual compression for at least for 30 min can help. The facial artery is sometimes injured during periosteal dissections. This problem can be addressed by manual compression or direct ligation of vessel. Fortunately, damage to the facial nerve is rare.

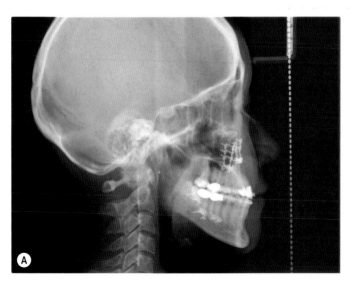
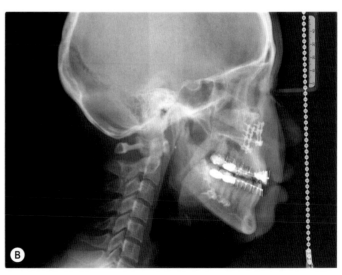

Fig. 10.25 (A,B) Preoperative and postoperative lateral cephalometry. The lateral cephalometry shows the rotational movements of maxilla and mandibular complex (MMC). In these cases, the maxillary advancement procedures may cause aggravation of dentoalveolar protrusion or widening of alar base and these changes are harmful to the aesthetics of Asian face. Moreover, Asian females tend to have a flat occlusal plane and a prominent mandibular angle which causes their faces to look square. For these reasons, a large amount of posterior maxillary impaction without any maxillary advancement would be the preferable in Asian class III patients.

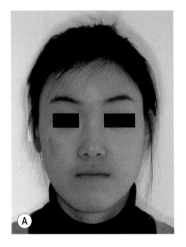
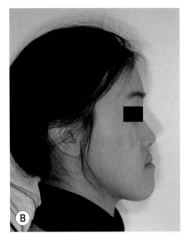
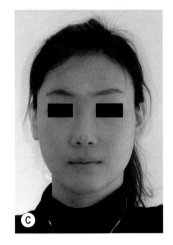
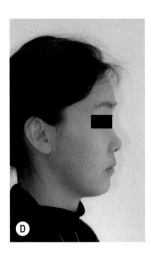

Fig. 10.26 **(A,B)** Class III dentofacial deformity: preoperative view. **(C,D)** Postoperative view. Two jaw surgery with jaw rotational setback procedure.

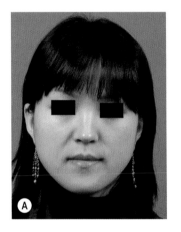
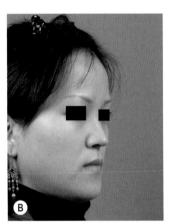
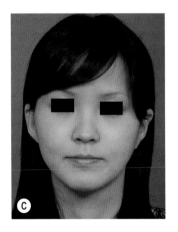
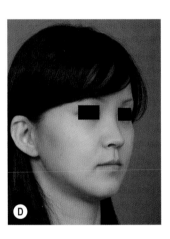

Fig. 10.27 **(A,B)** Preoperative view. Jaw rotation in skeletal class III profiles. Combined maxillary posterior impaction and mandibular rotation. **(C,D)** Postoperative view. Jaw rotation in skeletal class III profiles. Combined maxillary posterior impaction and mandibular rotation.

Access the complete references list online at **http://www.expertconsult.com**

4. Flowers RS. The art of eyelid and orbital aesthetics: multiracial surgical considerations. *Clin Plast Surg.* 1987;14(4):703–721.

   Basic and original article for orbital aesthetics.

28. Lam SM, Kim YK. Partial-incision technique for creation of the double eyelid. *Aesthet Surg J.* 2003;23(3):170–176.

41. Oh YW, Seul CH, Yoo WM. Medial epicanthoplasty using the skin redraping method. *Plast Reconstr Surg.* 2007;119(2):703–710.

   This technique has changed the concept of medial canthoplasty.

43. Toriumi DM, Swartout B. Asian rhinoplasty. *Facial Plast Surg Clin North Am.* 2007;15(3):293–307.

50. Han SK, Lee DG, Kim JB, et al. An anatomic study of nasal tip supporting structures. *Ann Plast Surg.* 2004;52(2):134–139.

64. Rohrich RJ, Deuber MA. Nasal tip refinement in primary rhinoplasty: the cephalic trim cap graft. *Aesthet Surg J.* 2002;22(1):39–45.

85. Yang DB, Park CG. Infracture technique for the zygomatic body and arch reduction. *Aesthetic Plast Surg.* 1992;16(4):355–363.

89. Baek SM, Kim SS, Bindiger A. The prominent mandibular angle: preoperative management, operative technique, and results in 42 patients. *Plast Reconstr Surg.* 1989;83(2):272–280.

   The pioneer article for Asian mandible angle ostectomy.

97. Baek SM, Baek RM. Profiloplasty of the lower face by maxillary and mandibular anterior segmental osteotomies. *Aesthetic Plast Surg.* 1993;17(2):129–137.

   First article for Asian profiloplasty.

100. Jin H, Park SH, Kim BH. Sagittal split ramus osteotomy with mandible reduction. *Plast Reconstr Surg.* 2007;119(2):662–669.

   New concept of mandible angle ostectomy.

11.1

Facelift: Principles

Richard J. Warren

SYNOPSIS

- Age-related changes occur in all layers of the face, including skin, superficial fat, SMAS, deep fat, and bone.
- Patients presenting for facial rejuvenation surgery are usually middle aged or older, thus increasing the chance of underlying medical problems. Risk factors such as hypertension and smoking should be dealt with prior to facelift surgery.
- A careful preoperative assessment will provide the surgeon with an aesthetic diagnosis regarding the underlying facial shape, the age related issues which predominate and the appropriate surgical procedures for every individual patient.
- Almost all facelift techniques begin with a subcutaneous facelift flap. Careful incision placement, tissue handling, and flap repositioning are important in order to avoid the obvious stigmata of facelift surgery.
- Volume augmentation, and in some locations volume reduction, should be considered in all cases of facelift surgery.
- Facial aging is usually a pan-facial phenomenon. Therefore, in order to obtain a harmonious result, patients will often benefit from surgery to other components of their face.
- The most common complication of facelift surgery is hematoma. This problem should be dealt with promptly.

Access the Historical Perspective section online at
http://www.expertconsult.com

Introduction

A complete discussion of facial rejuvenation would involve the periorbital region, forehead, cheek, neck, and perioral region. (The periorbital zone is reviewed in Chapter 8 and the forehead in Chapter 7.) In this chapter, we will be dealing with the middle and lower thirds of the face – the cheek and neck. Terminology for procedures which address these areas include rhytidectomy, rhytidoplasty, meloplasty and

facialplasty, although in this text, the more common term, "facelift" will be used.

Facelift surgery was originally conceived as a method of placing traction on the aging face by excising skin in the periphery of the face and closing the resulting defect under tension. Since that simple beginning over 100 years ago, the procedure has evolved to encompass a wide range of techniques which lift, augment, and rearrange facial tissues in an attempt to rejuvenate the aging face.

Despite the development of many less invasive technologies, nothing can match a facelift in its ability to globally treat the face, returning its basic architecture to a more youthful configuration.

Anatomy and patient presentation

The classic stigmata of the aging face include:
- Visible changes in skin, including folds, wrinkles, dyschromias, dryness and thinning
- Folds in the skin and subcutaneous tissue created by chronic muscle contraction: glabellar frown lines, transverse forehead lines, and crow's feet over the lateral orbital rim.
- Deepening folds between adjoining anatomic units: the nasojugular fold (tear trough), nasolabial folds, marionette lines and submental crease
- Ptosis of soft tissue, particularly in the lower cheek, jowls and neck
- Loss of volume in the upper two-thirds of the face which creates hollowing of the temple, the lateral cheek and the central cheek. The result is a more skeletal appearance in the temple, the periorbita and the malar region
- Expansion of volume in the neck and lateral jaw line which leads to the formation of jowls and fullness of the neck *(Fig. 11.1.1)*.

The driving force behind our ability to explain these many changes has been an improved understanding of facial anatomy and the way this anatomy changes over time. Aging

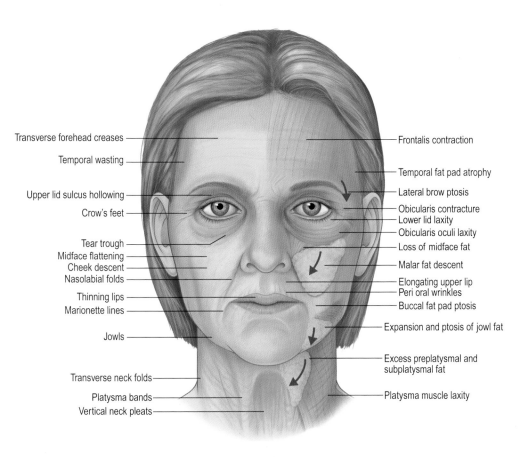

Transverse forehead creases

Temporal wasting

Upper lid sulcus hollowing

Crow's feet

Tear trough
Midface flattening
Cheek descent
Nasolabial folds

Thinning lips
Marionette lines

Jowls

Transverse neck folds

Platysma bands
Vertical neck pleats

Frontalis contraction

Temporal fat pad atrophy

Lateral brow ptosis

Obicularis contracture
Lower lid laxity
Obicularis oculi laxity

Loss of midface fat

Malar fat descent

Elongating upper lip
Peri oral wrinkles

Buccal fat pad ptosis

Expansion and ptosis of jowl fat

Excess preplatysmal and
subplatysmal fat

Platysma muscle laxity

Figure 11.1.1 The aging face exhibits changes in the skin, superficial wrinkles, deeper folds, soft tissue ptosis, loss of volume in the upper third and middle third and increased volume in the lower third.

of the face occurs in all its layers, from skin down to bone; no tissue is spared. For the purposes of this discussion, the face will be viewed as a five-layer structure as described in Chapter 6: skin, subcutaneous fat, the superficial musculoaponeurotic system (SMAS) and muscles of facial expression, fascial spaces, and deep fascia. Underlying everything is bone, except over the oral cavity. The surgical significance of this concentric layer arrangement is that dissection can be done in the planes between the layers. Also, anatomical changes in each of the layers can be addressed independently, as required to treat the presenting problem.

Skin

Normal skin is directly adherent to underlying fat via the retinacular cutis system. In certain predictable areas the skin is tethered to bone or underlying muscle by condensed areas of connective tissue. In some places, these are string-like cutaneous ligaments, and in other areas, these are ribbon-like septae. Because nerves and vessels often reach the skin adjacent to these vertically running fibrous structures, dissection of skin is more difficult and bloody where the skin is tethered; McGregor's patch is such an area because of its association with the zygomatic cutaneous ligaments and a perforating

branch of the transverse facial artery. Changes in the skin of the face are some of the most obvious signs of aging. Skin aging over time is both intrinsic and extrinsic. Intrinsic aging is the result of genetically determined apoptosis. The skin becomes thinner; there is a decrease in melanocytes, a reduced number of fibroblasts and a loss of skin appendages. In the dermal matrix, there is fragmentation of the dermal collagen and impairment of fibroblast function.[61,62] As the skin weakens and thins, the underlying contraction of facial muscles creates permanent skin folds in predictable locations (see *Fig 11.1.5*).

Extrinsic forces include sun exposure, cigarette smoke, extreme temperatures and weight fluctuations. The net result is that facial skin loses its ability to recoil, a condition called elastosis. This has surgical implications, because firm tight skin is youthful, and to varying degrees, the tightening of loose facial skin is part of a good surgical result. However, a facelift does not appreciably improve the quality or texture of the skin. Therefore, patients with good quality skin are likely to enjoy a better result from facelift surgery than the patient with poor quality skin. Alternatively, when skin quality is poor, other options such as injectable fillers and skin resurfacing may be more important for rejuvenation than facelift surgery. In most cases of facial rejuvenation, medical and surgical therapies can work in concert for a more complete result.

(These complementary therapies are reviewed in Chapters 4 and 5.)

Facial fat: ptosis, volume loss and volume gain

The face is carpeted in a layer of superficial fat which lies immediately deep to the dermis. Between individuals, there is much variability in the thickness of the superficial fat layer. This has surgical implications, because a heavier patient will have thicker, heavier tissues to reposition, but the dissection of the facelift skin flap will be easier. Conversely in a thin patient, facial layers are packed closely together, like an onion, necessitating greater care if the surgeon wishes to separate skin from SMAS and SMAS from underlying structures. Superficial facial fat also varies in thickness depending on the area of the face. The most important area of thickened subcutaneous fat is the malar fat pad.[54] This is a triangular shaped mass of fat bordered by the nasolabial fold, the infraorbital arch and a diagonal line across the mid-cheek. Its apex is over the malar eminence. The malar fat pad is present throughout life *(Fig. 11.1.2)*.

One study looked at fat volume in the cheek area and found 56% of the fat superficial to the SMAS and 44% was deep to the SMAS and the muscles of facial expression.[63] The superficial fat is separated by vertical septae into five distinct compartments: nasolabial, medial cheek, middle cheek, lateral temporoparietal, and the inferior orbital fat *(Fig. 11.1.3A)*.[64]

The two central fat compartments (medial and middle) are the primary components of the Malar Fat Pad.

The deep fat is also divided into compartments *(Fig. 11.1.3B)*. The most significant is the deep medial fat compartment, which lies directly against bone and is bordered above by the orbicularis retaining ligament, laterally by the zygomaticus major and buccal fat pad and medially by the pyriform aperture[65] *(Fig. 11.1.3C)*.

The authors who identified this compartment propose that age related deflation of deep medial fat compartment leads to "pseudoptosis" of the overlying superficial fat and skin – ptosis which is real, but which is caused by lack of underlying support.[65]

This in turn is thought to cause deepening of the nasolabial fold and development of the "inverted V deformity" inferior to the infraorbital rim.[66] Adjacent and lateral to the deep medial fat is the suborbicularis oculi fat (SOOF), which itself is divided into a medial and lateral component.

Generally in youth, facial fat is tightly packed, creating surface contours which undulate smoothly from convexity to concavity. Cosmetic highlights rise above areas of depression. The malar fat pad which extends over the body of the zygoma creates the principle cosmetic highlight zone in the youthful face, immediately above the normal depression overlying the buccal recess. Make-up artists accentuate this zone by highlighting the apex and simulating a depression immediately below. In the aging face, fat is less tightly packed, and facial contours become more abrupt. In areas of tight ligamentous attachment, such as the preparotid area, the anterior jowl border and the zygomatic ligament insertions, there appears to be an acceleration of volume loss with indenting of the surface contour.[67] With more advanced aging, there is malar fat atrophy, leading to a more skeletal appearance of the

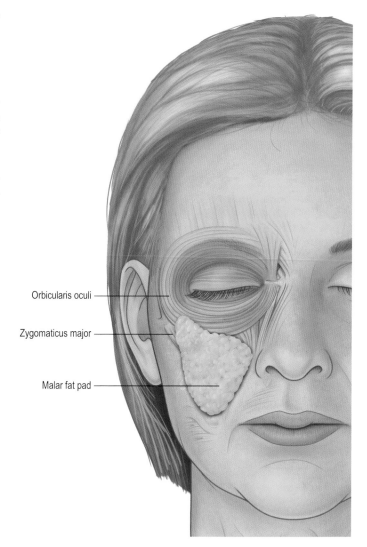

Figure 11.1.2 The malar fat pad is a triangular area of thickened superficial fat with its base along the nasolabial fold, and its apex over the superolateral malar prominence.

zygoma. Simultaneously there is an apparent ptosis of the malar fat pad which causes bunching of fat and deepening of the nasolabial fold. Surgeons have traditionally viewed superficial fat in the cheeks as a ptotic layer which requires correction for facial rejuvenation to occur. In support of this theory, it has been demonstrated that the primary muscles of facial expression in the mid-cheek (zygomaticus major and minor) do not change in length, while the overlying fat appears to migrate inferiorly.[68] Another study, using CT scans, confirmed the presence of facial fat compartments and identified age related inferior migration of the midfacial fat compartments as well as inferior volume shift within the individual compartments.[68a]

At the time of writing, it is unclear whether the cause of superficial fat ptosis is gravitational due to relaxed fixation, or if it relates to pseudoptosis caused by the loss of volume in the deep fat compartments. Also, it is uncertain whether volume of facial fat is lost equally from the deep and

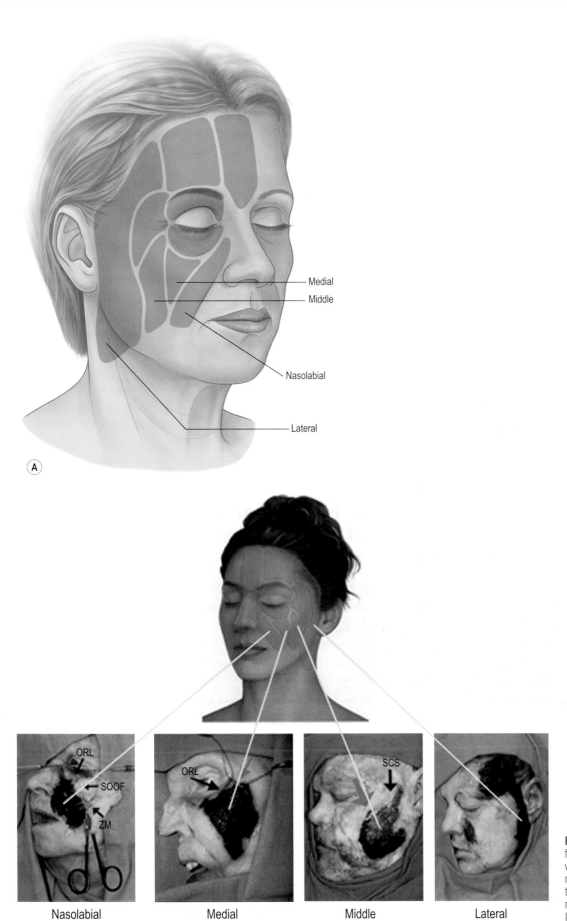

Medial

Middle

Nasolabial

Lateral

(A)

ORL

SOOF

ZM

ORL

SCS

Nasolabial

Medial

Middle

Lateral

Figure 11.1.3 (A) Superficial facial fat is compartmentalized by vertically running septae. In the mid-cheek, from medial to lateral, these compartments are the nasolabial, medial, middle, and lateral compartments.

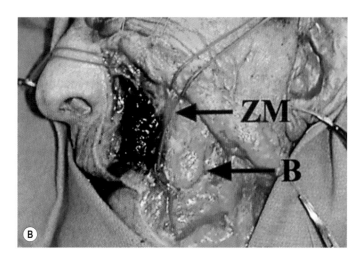

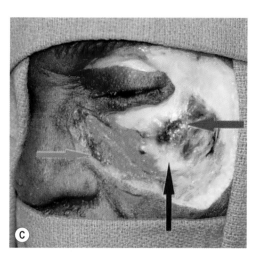

Fig. 11.1.3, cont'd The nasolabial and medial compartments make up the malar fat pad. **(B)** The deep facial fat is also compartmentalized by septae. The deep medial fat pad (here stained blue) is bounded above by the orbicularis retaining ligament, medially by the pyriform aperture, and laterally by the zygomaticus major (labeled ZM) muscle and the buccal fat pad (labeled B). **(C)** Over the body of the zygoma, the sub orbicularis oculi fat (SOOF) is deep fat. It is seen here with a medial portion (yellow) and a lateral portion (stained blue). It is bounded medially by deep medial fat pad (stained red). (A, Courtesy of Rohrich RJ, Pessa JE. The fat compartments of the face: anatomy and clinical implications for cosmetic surgery. Plast Reconstr Surg. 2007;119:2219–2227; B,C Courtesy of Rohrich RJ, Pessa JE, Ristow B. The youthful cheek and the deep medial fat compartment. Plast Reconstr Surg. 2008;121(6):2107–2112).

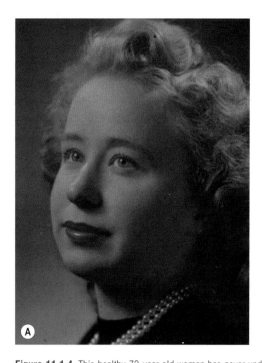

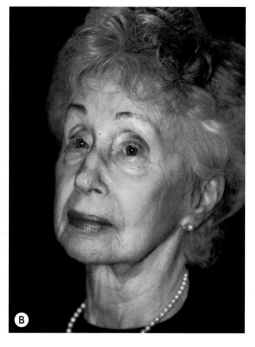

Figure 11.1.4 This healthy 72-year-old woman has never undergone facial surgery, has gained 10 pounds, but has aged 50 years. She appears to have lost fat in the periorbital region and middle third of her face, revealing underlying bone. The orbit seems to have enlarged. Overall volume has been lost in the middle third of the face. The soft tissues which remain appear to be ptotic, flattening her cheeks, and widening her jaw line. The heart-shaped face of youth has become more rectangular.

superficial fat layers, or if it lost equally or differentially from the various fat compartments which have been identified.[65]

In the lower face, the area of the jowl just posterior to the marionette lines appears to become thicker with age, making the mandible appear wider. This phenomenon has been called "radial expansion" (Lambros, pers. comm. 1999).[69] This may be due to fat accumulation, or it may be caused by soft tissue ptosis within the premasseteric space, a natural glide plane.[69a] Below the mandible, a similar expansion occurs in the neck as soft tissue falls away from deep tissue attachments and fat tends to accumulate.

Change in facial shape

The loss of facial volume is an important phenomenon which surgeons recognized much later than the more obvious ptosis of soft tissue. To arrive at this conclusion, astute observations were made about changes in surface contours which lead to inferences about internal volume loss.[65,67,70,71]

The combination of volume loss in some areas, volume gain in others, and soft tissue ptosis creates a cascade effect which results in the loss of natural youthful curves *(Fig. 11.1.4)*.

Gradually, there is a reversal of facial shape as the cheek prominence of youth gives way to the jowl prominence of age. Effectively, in youth, the cheeks are full, but with age, the jowls and neck become full. The face changes from a heart shape to a more rectangular shape, or from an egg sitting on its narrow end to an egg resting on its broad end. This change has been called losing the "inverted cone of youth", and has been likened to a reversal of the "Ogee" curve, a natural S-shaped curve seen in architecture.[60,72]

Superficial musculoaponeurotic system

Immediately deep to the subcutaneous fat is the superficial musculoaponeurotic system (SMAS), described by Mitz and Peyronie in 1976.[73] The SMAS, or its analogues can be thought of as a continuous fascial sheath which encompasses the entire face and neck. Superiorly, it continues into the temple as the superficial temporal fascia (temporoparietal fascia) and then into the scalp as the galea aponeurotica.[74] Inferiorly, into the neck, the SMAS becomes the superficial cervical fascia which envelopes the platysma muscle. Clinically, the thickness and strength of the SMAS varies between patients, and also varies in every individual face, being thicker and adherent over the parotid, and thinner anteriorly. The SMAS is most tenuous under the malar fat pad where it splits to encompass the zygomaticus major and the orbicularis oculi.[53,75] The SMAS has important surgical implications because its fibrous attachments to skin allow it to act as a carrier for overlying subcutaneous fat; also it has been shown to be much more resistant to stretch than skin.[76] Furthermore, below the zygomatic arch, all branches of the facial nerve are deep to the SMAS.

The relationship of the SMAS (superficial fascia of the face) to the deep fascial structures of the face, involves areas of mobility interspersed between areas of attachment. The superficial fascia is tethered to the deep fascia by retaining ligaments in the following locations: over the parotid gland, at the inferior border of the zygomatic body, and along the anterior edge of the masseter. (These ligaments are described in Chapter 6 and are reviewed later in this chapter.) Between areas of fixation the SMAS is free to move over the underlying deep fascia. These are the suprazygomatic zone where superficial temporal fascia slides over the deep temporal fascia, the mid-cheek, where SMAS rides over the parotid masseteric fascia (premasseteric space), and the neck where the platysma overlies the underlying strap muscles.

Facial muscles

The muscles of facial expression are found in a superficial layer and a deep layer. The superficial muscles are orbicularis oculi, orbicularis oris, zygomaticus major, zygomaticus minor, levator labii superioris, risorius, and depressor anguli oris. All of these muscles are innervated on their deep surface by branches of the facial nerve (VII). Consequently, surgical dissection on the superficial surface of these muscles will not endanger their innervation. The only facial muscles innervated on their superficial surface are the muscles in the deep layer: levator anguli oris, mentalis and buccinator. The three facial muscles which are most important to surgeons are orbicularis oculi and platysma, because they are often manipulated during facelift surgery, and zygomaticus major

because it is used as a landmark in certain facelift techniques (*Fig. 11.1.5*).

Most muscles of facial expression take their origins from bone and insert into the dermis thus allowing for voluntary and involuntary movement of facial soft tissues. The platysma is a purely subcutaneous muscle which takes its origin from the fascia of the pectoralis, and inserts into soft tissue of the face, with a small bony insertion on the anterior mandible. The platysma interdigitates with the depressor labii inferioris which in some individuals, gives it some effect on the depression of the lower lip. In the neck the platysma is thicker, forming visible bands; superiorly the platysma thins dramatically as it crosses the mandibular border, but continues superiorly, often visible during surgical dissection well into the mid-cheek, at times approaching the lower fibers of the orbicularis oculi.

While most muscles of facial expression do not change appreciably with age, the orbicularis oculi and the platysma are thought to undergo age-related changes. Both of these muscles have a large surface area but are relatively thin – a configuration which lends them to potential redundancy if they lose tone or if there is attenuation of their deep tissue attachment. For example, in some individuals redundancy develops in the lower half of the orbicularis, a condition which has been speculated to cause lower eyelid festoons.[77] Some have suggested that it is the loss of support of the orbicularis through attenuation of the orbicularis retaining ligament (orbitomalar ligament), which contributes to deformities of the lower eyelid/cheek junction.[66] Similarly, the paired platysma muscles, which are encased by SMAS, appear to gradually fall away from their deep cervical attachment carrying the overlying fat and skin. The net result is a more obtuse cervico-mental angle and the development of visible platysma bands at the anterior platysmal border. Another issue common to orbicularis oculi and platysma is that these are the only facial muscles which are undermined during certain surgical procedures, thus imperiling some of their motor innervation. Fortunately, the orbicularis has multiple motor nerve branches which provide a level of collateral innervation.[78] There is a less elaborate innervation to the platysma; two or three cervical branches can be identified just inferior and anterior to the angle of the mandible in the plane between the deep cervical fascia and the undersurface of the platysma. Preservation of these branches is potentially important because the platysma acts as a support structure and also influences lower lip depression, especially in those individuals with a "full dentition" smile.[79]

Retaining ligaments

Facial soft tissue and skin is held in place by retaining ligaments which run from underlying fixed structures through facial fat, inserting into the dermis.[45,48,80] Effectively, these ligaments attach the superficial fascia (SMAS) and the overlying skin to the underlying deep fascia and bone (*Fig. 11.1.6*).

There are two ligament systems. The first group is true osteocutaneous ligaments, which tether skin to bone: the orbital, zygomatic and the mandibular ligaments. The orbital ligament is found at the junction of the superior and lateral orbital rims and constitutes the inferior thickening of the temporal crest line zone of fixation (zone of adhesion). (This area

gland, where it is called the parotid fascia or capsule; the combined complex is called the parotid masseteric fascia (parotidomasseteric fascia). When the SMAS is raised surgically, just anterior to the parotid gland in the premasseteric space, the parotid masseteric fascia can be seen as a thin shiny membrane – an important landmark, because in the cheek (unlike the neck and temple), all branches of the facial nerve are deep to this deep fascial layer. Superficial to this layer, but deep to the SMAS, there is often an additional thin layer of fat, the sub – SMAS fat, which adds further protection to the underlying nerves when the SMAS is raised. In the neck along the posterior border of the platysma, the SMAS becomes fused with the deep cervical fascia where the deep fascia covers the sternocleidomastoid muscle. This is important, because a surgeon planning to mobilize a platysma flap to address the neck, will have to release the platysma's attachment to the deep cervical fascia in this area.[87]

Video 1

Bone

The bony skeleton of the face was once thought to be quite stable in volume and shape as the body aged. However, there is ample evidence that atrophy in certain portions of the facial skeleton is a significant factor in facial aging.[88–93]

Computed tomography of young and old skulls has shown a retrusion of the infraorbital rim as well as recession of the maxillary face below the infraorbital rim (*Fig. 11.1.8*).[90]

This has been confirmed by others who have demonstrated an enlarging orbital aperture (*Fig. 11.1.9*).[94]

The loss of bone has surgical implications because it contributes to an overall loss of volume, and more specifically, to loss of soft tissue support in critical areas such as the infraorbital rim. This contributes to development of the tear trough deformity and age related flattening of the anterior midface. Following the principle of replacing like with like, bone loss can be replaced with solid objects such as facial implants (Ch. 15), or with soft tissue volume enhancement such as with fat grafting (Ch. 14).

Nerve anatomy

Facial nerve

The facial nerve exits the stylomastoid foramen, and separates into an upper and lower division within the parotid glad. Classically, there are five branches which arise and exit the cover of the superficial lobe of the parotid: temporal, zygomatic, buccal, marginal mandibular, and cervical. There are typically 2–3 temporal branches; 4–5 zygomatic branches; 3 buccal branches; 2–3 mandibular branches, and 2–3 cervical branches.

In fact, there is considerable variation in the anatomy of facial nerve branches. One study identified up to eight branches exiting the parotid, with multiple connections between these branches.[95–97]

The temporal branches exit the parotid superiorly, coursing obliquely and superiorly across the middle-third of the zygomatic arch. Like all other facial nerve branches, the temporal branches start out deep to the deep fascia of the mid-cheek (parotid masseteric fascia), but unlike all other facial nerve branches in the cheek, they become more superficial. At

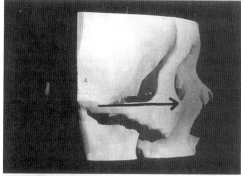

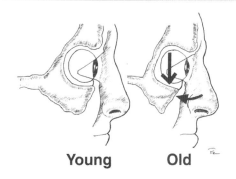

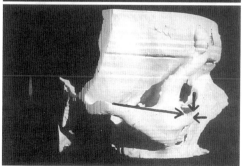

Young   Old

Figure 11.1.8 Computed tomography of young and old skulls has demonstrated a retrusion of the infraorbital rim. (Courtesy of Pessa JE. An algorithm of facial aging: verification of Lambros's theory by three-dimensional stereolithography, with reference to the pathogenesis of midfacial aging, scleral show, and the lateral suborbital trough deformity. Plast Reconstr Surg. 2000;106:479.)

a point 1.5–3.0 cm superior to the zygomatic arch, the temporal branches transition from deep to superficial, travelling at first on the undersurface and then within the superficial temporal fascia (temporoparietal fascia), staying there until they terminate in the frontalis muscle, upper orbicularis and frown musculature. The surgical implication is that a SMAS flap can be safely raised from a point just superior to the zygomatic arch providing that surgical dissection does not extend superiorly to the level where the temporal branch transitions superficially.[98]

A classic external landmark for the course of the temporal branch has been along a line drawn from a point 0.5 cm below the tragus to a point 1.5 cm lateral to the lateral eyebrow.[99]

More recent studies have found that the temporal branch actually consists of 2–5 individual branches which do not adhere completely to this landmark. One study found that these branches cross the middle-third of the zygomatic arch, with a posterior safe zone 1 cm anterior to the acoustic meatus, and an anterior safe zone 2 cm posterior to the lateral orbital rim. Once above the zygomatic arch, these branches were

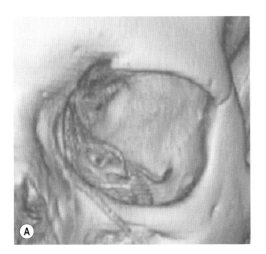

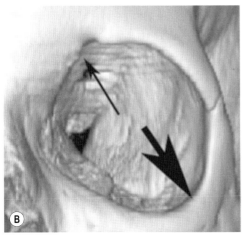

Figure 11.1.9 Computed tomography scan of (A) a male patient in the young age group and (B) a male patient in the older age group. The image from the older age groups shows significant bony remodeling (arrows) both superomedially and inferolaterally. (Courtesy of Kahn DM, Shaw RB. Aging of the bony orbit: a three-dimensional computed tomographic study. Aesthetic Surg J. 2008;28:258.)

consistently found anterior and inferior to the anterior branch of the temporal artery, a palpable landmark in the temple.[100]

The zygomatic and buccal branches, all exit the parotid gland deep to the parotid masseteric fascia. As they travel anteriorly, they often arborize with each other. Zygomatic branches course parallel to the transverse facial artery. When they reach the area of the zygomatic retaining ligament, they travel to the undersurface of the muscles which they innervate: zygomaticus major, zygomaticus minor, and orbicularis oculi. Deep to the parotid masseteric fascia, within the premasseteric space, the parotid duct courses anteriorly along an imaginary line from the tragus to the corner of the mouth. Accompanying the duct is normally a buccal branch. Beyond the anterior border of the masseter, a buccal branch can normally be seen crossing the buccal fat pad (fat pad of Bichat). At this level, the portion of buccal fat seen is the buccal extension, which is the most inferior portion of the buccal fat pad.[101]

The mandibular branches exit the parotid approximately near the angle of the mandible. They then travel anteriorly near the border of the mandible, until they encounter the facial artery and vein, crossing those vessels and then turning

more superiorly. In Chapter 6, facial spaces are described, with the mandibular branches coursing at the lower border of the premasseteric space, which displaces inferiorly with age. Consequently, in elderly patients in the supine position, they have been found coursing well inferior to the mandibular border.[102]

The cervical branches are the most inferior, exiting the parotid at its inferior border and always coursing below the mandibular border. The cervical branches innervate the platysma. There are usually two or three branches with considerable variation in branching patterns. A contribution from the sensory transverse cervical nerve has also been described.[79]

Because the buccal and zygomatic branches are multiple and interconnected, there is a reserve capacity in the event of a single branch injury; therefore, permanent injury is uncommon. However, the temporal and marginal mandibular branches enjoy less collateral innervation making permanent loss much more likely if these branches are injured. Damage to the cervical branches can lead to a "pseudo paralysis" of the lower lip because in some patients the platysma contributes to depression of the corner of the mouth *(Fig. 11.1.10)*.[103]

Sensory nerves

The great auricular nerve, a branch of the cervical plexus, is sensory to the earlobe and lateral portion of the pinna. This nerve wraps around the posterior border of the sternocleidomastoid, and courses obliquely across the muscle in a superior direction. The classic landmark for this nerve is at the mid portion of the sternocleidomastoid, 6.5 cm. below the external auditory canal *(Fig. 11.1.11)*.

It runs parallel and about 1 cm posterior to the external jugular vein which also crosses the sternocleidomastoid roughly along the same vector. The nerve is deep to the superficial cervical fascia, but the platysma is usually absent over the posterior sternocleidomastoid. Hence, the nerve is at risk of injury during surgical dissection along the posterior border of the sternocleidomastoid, because with lack of fascial cover, it is technically subcutaneous.[104,105]

The auriculotemporal nerve, a branch of the trigeminal is sensory to the preauricular skin and the lesser occipital nerve is sensory to the retroauricular scalp. The zygomaticofacial nerve exits through its foramen in the body of the zygoma, piercing the malar fat pad to provide sensation to the skin of the malar prominence; this nerve is often transected when the malar fat pad is surgically mobilized *(Fig. 11.1.12)*.

Patient selection

Like any elective surgical procedure, a prerequisite is to confirm that a patient's physical status and mental status are appropriate to withstand the rigors of surgery, the recovery phase and any potential complications. The patient's expectations must be explored to determine if they are realistic, and if they are technically achievable. The quality of surgical result will be affected by many patient related factors including the facial skeleton, the weight of facial soft tissue, the depth and location of folds, and the quality of the skin.

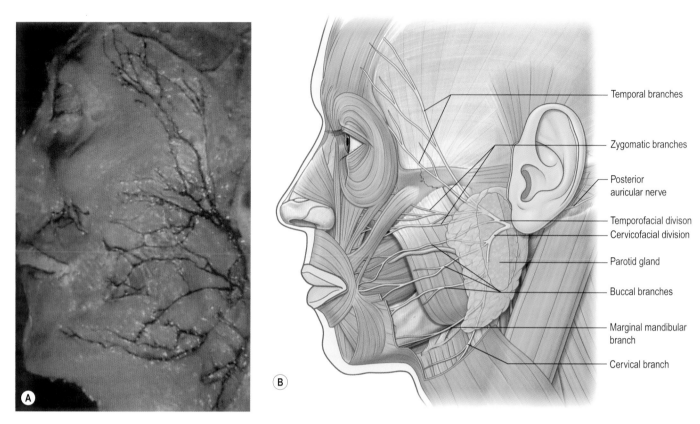

Figure 11.1.10 (A) A cadaveric dissection of the facial nerve. Note three temporal branches crossing the middle third of the zygoma, the arborization between zygomatic and buccal branches, the marginal mandibular branch running along the mandibular border, and two cervical branches innervating the platysma. (Courtesy of Dr Julia Terzis). (B) Diagram of the facial nerve. The facial nerve exits the stylomastoid foramen and normally divides within the parotid gland into a superior and inferior division. Classically, five groups of branches are seen: temporal, zygomatic, buccal, mandibular, and cervical. There is arborization between branches, particularly between the zygomatic and buccal branches.

Some issues can be reversed, others attenuated, and some may not be correctable at all.

The patient presenting for facial rejuvenation will usually be middle age or older, thus increasing the chances of underlying medical problems. In an otherwise apparently healthy individual, specific issues which must be addressed are blood pressure, smoking history and the use of medications or supplements which can promote surgical bleeding.

Incipient hypertension is common in the general population and can promote postoperative hematomas if it is not identified prior to surgery. Hematoma is by far the commonest complication in facelift surgery. Uncontrolled hypertension is a contraindication for surgery, while controlled hypertension is not a contraindication. The labile hypertensive can be the most insidious situation; if possible it should be identified preoperatively and controlled. If patients have intermittent hypertension (the white coat syndrome), or they are simply type A individuals who are easily excitable, perioperative treatment with medications such as Clonidine should be considered

Smokers have been shown to exhibit delayed wound healing due to microvasoconstriction and abnormal cell function.[106] One study reported a 12.5 times greater chance of having skin flap necrosis in a smoking patient compared with a non-smoker.[107] Long-term smokers have a reduction in

arteriole function, which may never return to normal. Nevertheless, there are significant short-term effects which can be reversed by abstaining from tobacco use for 2–3 weeks prior to surgery. Tests for the metabolites of nicotine in the blood are available to confirm abstinence from smoking.

Commonly used non-steroidal anti-inflammatory medications (NSAIDs) and the consumption of certain dietary supplements may promote intraoperative and postoperative bleeding based on platelet function inhibition. Patients should avoid these medications for 3 weeks prior to surgery.

Female patients in the facelift age group may be on hormone replacement and are therefore at increased risk for developing postoperative deep vein thrombosis (DVT) and a potentially lethal pulmonary embolism. For these patients, in addition to all recognized preventative measures, consideration should be given to stopping hormonal replacement 3 weeks prior to surgery.

With respect to the surgical objectives in facelift surgery, aging causes fundamental anatomical changes in all parts and in all tissues of the face. However, patients will typically present with specific concerns about specific areas – often the ptosis of soft tissue in the neck or jowls, or the visible wrinkles and folds in the cheek and neck. Patients are usually unaware of the underlying anatomic changes which are causing the problems they can see in the mirror. Nevertheless,

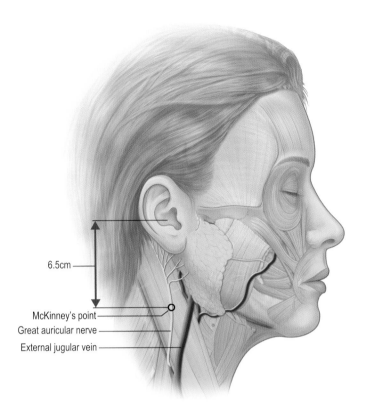

Figure 11.1.11 The great auricular nerve crosses the midportion of the sternocleidomastoid at McKinney's point, which is 6.5 cm inferior to the external auditory canal. It usually travels about 1 cm posterior to the external jugular vein. Anterior to McKinney's point, the nerve is covered by the superficial cervical fascia and the platysma (SMAS), but at the posterior border of the sternocleidomastoid, the nerve is effectively subcutaneous. The most common point of injury is at the posterior border of the sternocleidomastoid muscle.

it is important to recognize what the patient can see is the patient's primary concern. To help focus the discussion, old photographs are very useful in determining which aging changes predominated and what features the patient would most like corrected. This will help improve patients' understanding of exactly how they have aged, and what, if any, rejuvenation they would like to undergo. They will also gain a better understand of the magnitude of surgery which may be required to accomplish what they desire.

Prior to surgery, the entire face should be properly assessed. This examination is conducted in a well lit room with the patient sitting vertically in a comfortable position. Examination should proceed in an orderly fashion so that nothing is missed. The face is examined with the patient in repose as well as in animation. In doing so, facial nerve function is clinically assessed. The face should be assessed as a whole – looking for the equality of facial thirds, the degree of symmetry, and the overall shape (round, thin, wide). Underlying skeletal form will potentially influence the choice of surgical procedure; for example, a wide full face will not be as amenable to malar fat pad repositioning as a narrow, long face. Conversely, a thin face will require the preservation of all soft tissue, overlapping it rather than excising it, and potentially adding

additional volume. Any asymmetry should be pointed out to the patient because facelift surgery will make some asymmetries more obvious.

Surgeons should develop an organized way to examine all the zones of the face: forehead, eyelids, cheeks, the perioral area, and the neck. In certain individuals, the appropriate procedure will be a correction of only one of these areas, but more commonly, all or most or the zones should be addressed in order to achieve a harmonious result. Assessment of the forehead and orbital area are discussed in Chapters 7 and 8. In the cheeks, the surgeon should assess the shape and prominence of the underlying skeleton, the volume and distribution of facial fat, the degree of soft tissue atrophy and ptosis and the relative mobility of the subcutaneous (superficial) fat. Any significant hollowing or flattening should be noted, and conversely, any radial expansion in the jowl and neck should be noted. With the diversity of surgical techniques available, a surgeon should think like a sculptor – considering the face in three dimensions with a view to adding tissue in some areas, removing tissue in other areas, and repositioning tissue where indicated. In the perioral area, the plumpness of the lips should be assessed, and any elongation of the upper lip should be noted. On smiling, the amount of dental show is observed. The skin should be assessed, with its quality noted, along with the depth of wrinkles and folds, including the nasolabial fold and the marionette lines.

Assessment of the neck is discussed in Chapter 13, but in general, the neck should be examined in various positions: neutral, flexion, and turning side-to-side. The patient is asked to contract the platysma by clenching the teeth and grimacing. This will help identify the degree of platysma laxity, the strength of platysma bands and the amount of subcutaneous fat superficial to the platysma. The amount of subplatysma fat is also estimated. Ptosis of the submandibular gland should be noted and pointed out to the patient preoperatively; this condition, if untreated, will be more obvious after facelift surgery than before.

The ear should be examined with a thought to the potential placement of incisions. Important factors include the size and orientation of the earlobe, the angle of attachment of the tragus, the difference in character of the cheek skin and tragal skin, and the size of the tragus. Also influencing the choice of incisions are the density of the hair surrounding the ear and the location of the hairline in the temple, the sideburn, and posterior to the ear.

A careful assessment of the overlying skin is also important to determine if anything of a non-surgical nature is indicated either before, during or after facelift surgery. Assessment will include skin type, skin quality, skin excess, the depth of folds, the degree of fine wrinkling and the amount of photo-aging. In particular, perioral rhytides should be examined as they are often a significant concern for the patient. Issues with the skin should be pointed out to the patient, and options discussed because facelift surgery itself will not improve the texture and quality of the skin – a common misconception.

Excellent photographic documentation of the preoperative face is very important, and should include frontal, oblique, and profile views. Other optional views include the smile and close up views of the neck in repose and with platysma contracture. Changes in the face from facelift surgery may be more subtle than other aesthetic procedures, so a reliable record of the surgical starting point is imperative.

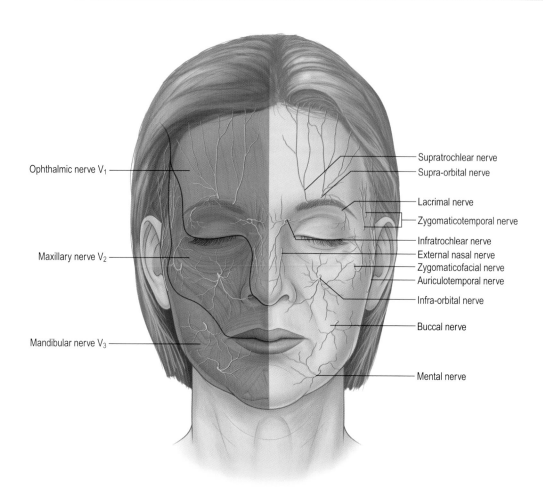

Ophthalmic nerve V₁

Maxillary nerve V₂

Mandibular nerve V₃

Supratrochlear nerve
Supra-orbital nerve
Lacrimal nerve
Zygomaticotemporal nerve
Infratrochlear nerve
External nasal nerve
Zygomaticofacial nerve
Auriculotemporal nerve
Infra-orbital nerve
Buccal nerve
Mental nerve

Figure 11.1.12 Major sensory nerves of the face.

Surgery

A facelift is a significant operation. It should be done under excellent conditions with appropriate medical staff, appropriate equipment and adequate back up. Anesthesia can be safely done with many different approaches, including local anesthetic with different levels of intravenous sedation and with varying levels in the spectrum of general anesthesia. An anesthesiologist, if involved, can decide in consultation with the surgeon what form of anesthesia is preferred for an individual patient. There should be proper intraoperative patient positioning, intraoperative monitoring, intraoperative warming, and intraoperative DVT prophylaxis.

Technique

Historically, surgeons have been guided by the empirical finding that people look younger when soft tissue of the lower

cheek is shifted into the middle and upper cheek. Patients see the same thing in a mirror when they manually lift their cheek or if they lie on their back. Effectively, by shifting lower facial fat superiorly, volume is restored to the midface while simultaneously, ptotic tissue is lifted. As we have seen, changes in volume are a significant part of facial aging. Surgeons have been able to improve the lower third of the face and neck by removing excess volume, and in recent years, surgeons have demonstrated that people may look younger with volume augmentation alone.[108,109] By combining these approaches – adding volume in some areas, subtracting volume in others, and by repositioning ptotic tissue, the surgeon has the ability to sculpt facial shape and more accurately restore the contours of youth.

The repositioning of ptotic tissue is the principle objective which has interested surgeons since facelift surgery began. Many methods have been described. The choice of technique will depend on the individual patient's aesthetic diagnosis, the patient's desires, and the surgeon's comfort level with a certain procedure. While differences between surgical techniques can be significant, many commonalities exist. In this section, the classic subcutaneous facelift will be described and the fundamental issues which pertain to all facelift techniques will be reviewed. (The various methods specifically designed to manipulate the deep tissues of the face will be described later, in Chapters 11.2–11.8.)

Subcutaneous facelift

The first facelift, which dates from the early 20th century, was a simple skin incision at the temporal hairline and anterior to the ear; several authors lay claim to this innovation.[9–11] This method soon evolved into a subcutaneous dissection of a large random pattern skin flap which was shifted in a superior-lateral direction.[24,26] Still used today, this classic procedure tightens excess skin, and relies completely on skin tension to shift underlying facial soft tissue against the force of gravity. The advantages of the subcutaneous facelift are that it is relatively safe, it is easy to do, and patient recovery is rapid. For the thin patient with excess skin, and minimal ptosis of deep soft tissue, this procedure is effective. However, the reverse, namely a heavier patient with significant ptosis of deep tissue, is a poor candidate. The inherent disadvantage of the "skin-only" facelift is that skin placed under tension to support heavy underlying soft tissue will stretch, leading to a loss of surgical effect. An attempt to overcome this problem with excess skin tension may lead to distortion of facial shape, abnormal re-orientation of wrinkles, and local problems at the incision line including stretched scars and distorted earlobes.

Facelift incisions

The purpose of a facelift incision is two-fold. First, the incision allows elevation of a flap which provides access for surgical manipulation of the deep tissues of the face. Second, the resulting skin flap can be repositioned with excess skin being removed along the incision line; this is the primary goal of a skin-only subcutaneous facelift. Generally, the incision is hidden by the hair and by contours of the ear.

In the temple area, the incision can be placed in the hair, at the anterior hairline, or a hybrid of the two, with an incision in the hair plus a transverse extension at the base of the sideburn (*Fig. 11.1.13A,B*).

The advantage of the incision in the hair is that it is hidden, but when the flap is drawn up, the anterior hairline and sideburn will shift, the degree of this depending on skin laxity. If the incision is placed at the anterior hairline, the scar is potentially more visible, but there will be no shift of the hairline. A transverse incision at the base of the sideburn is a compromise solution, which ameliorates much of the hairline shift, while preserving a largely hidden scar. Other compromises have been described.[110] Several factors should be assessed before committing to an incision within the temple hair. First, a preoperative estimate of skin redundancy will give the surgeon some sense of how far the skin flap will move. The distance between the lateral orbital rim and the temporal hairline should be assessed. In youth, this distance is generally <4–5 cm, while in older patients, the distance increases.[111] If the distance is already excessive, or if the expected movement of the temporal hairline will create a distance over 5 cm, then an incision in the hair should be avoided (*Fig. 11.1.13C*). On the other hand, patients must be

informed that the alternative incision along their temporal hairline may result in a more visible scar. Because of this problem a number of solutions have been devised along the temple hairline including beveling the incision to encourage growth of hair through the scar and the use of zig-zag incisions.[112,113] In any circumstance, the anterior hairline incision should be meticulously sutured under minimal tension. Also, the patient's wishes should be taken into consideration prior to surgery, because the location of the incision in the temple is inevitably a compromise and the patient may have preferences which will influence the surgeon's choice.

Anterior to the ear, the incision can be pre-tragal, or along the tragal edge (*Fig. 11.1.13D,E*). The advantage of the tragal edge incision is that it is hidden, but care must be taken to thin the flap covering the tragus in order to simulate a normal tragal appearance. Furthermore, as pointed out by Connell,[111,114] the tragus looks like a rectangle, with a top and a bottom, and to preserve a distinct lower border, a short transverse cut at the inferior end of the tragus (the incisura) should be done. Before committing to a tragal edge incision, the quality of tragal skin and that of facial skin must be compared; if the difference is too great, drawing thick cheek skin onto the tragus may be problematic because the skin covering the tragus will not be anatomically appropriate. Therefore, in certain cases, a pretragal incision is preferred. For example, in men, the pretragal approach may be beneficial if it appears that thick-bearded skin will be drawn up onto the tragus and the surgeon is concerned that removing hair follicles and thinning the flap will not ameliorate the appearance of cheek skin on the tragus. Elsewhere in front of the ear, the superior portion of the incision should follow a curved line along the helix, and a slightly straighter curve along the anterior attachment of the earlobe; a long, straight line incision in front of the ear should be avoided.

Video 2

Around the earlobe, the incision can be place either in the cleft of earlobe attachment or 1–2 mm distal to the cleft, leaving a cuff of skin along the earlobe. This cuff will ease the process of insetting the earlobe on skin closure.

In the retroauricular sulcus, the incision can be placed directly in the conchal groove as it courses superiorly. Various landmarks have been described to determine how high to carry this incision. These include the level of the external auditory canal, or slightly higher, at the level of the antihelix.

A significant surgical decision is whether to extend the postauricular incision across the non hair baring skin into the occipital region. Generally speaking, the occipital incision should be made when there is a need to remove excess redundant neck skin. A "short scar" facelift is one which avoids the occipital incision, and will suffice for many patients.[115] If the incision is kept short, the lateral neck is accessed from the earlobe and retroauricular incision, and any bunching of skin is redistributed within the retroauricular sulcus. Disadvantages of the short scar technique are that access to deep tissues is somewhat limited, there is a tendency to draw the skin flap in a more superior direction possibly requiring a pre-hairline incision in the temple, and the fact that excess neck skin, if there is any, must be gathered up in the retroauricular sulcus, often creating pleats.

If the decision has been made to extend the incision beyond the retroauricular sulcus, many variations are described, ranging from an incision which goes vertically into the scalp[116] to an incision which courses inferiorly along the hairline of

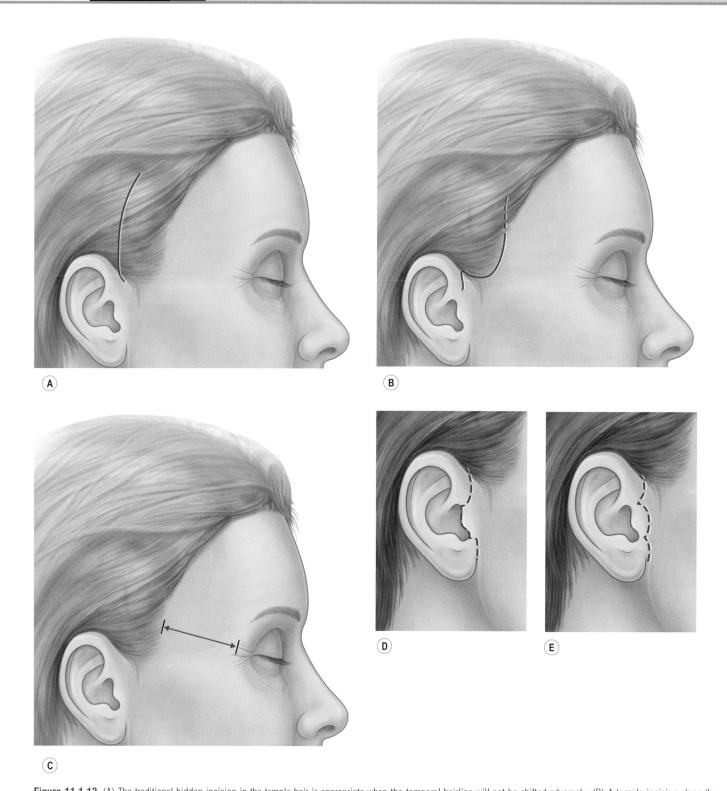

Figure 11.1.13 (A) The traditional hidden incision in the temple hair is appropriate when the temporal hairline will not be shifted adversely. (B) A temple incision along the hairline is used if a hidden incision will adversely shift the hairline. (C) The distance from the lateral orbital rim to the temporal hairline should not exceed 5 cm (D) The retrotragal incision follows the edge of the tragus. (E) The pretragal incision is placed in the pretragal sulcus.

the neck. Most commonly, surgeons use an incision which is between these two extremes. The principle objectives for the occipital incision are to gain access to the neck in order to take up redundant neck skin, while making the incision as invisible as possible with little or no distortion of the occipital hairline. If a small amount of skin is going to be removed,

the retroauricular incision can curve posteriorly into the occipital hair from the retroauricular sulcus. If more skin from the neck is going to be removed, this approach could create a notch in the posterior hairline, so a called "lazy S" pattern can be used, where the incision follows the occipital hairline for 1–2 cm, before angling more posteriorly into the scalp. A

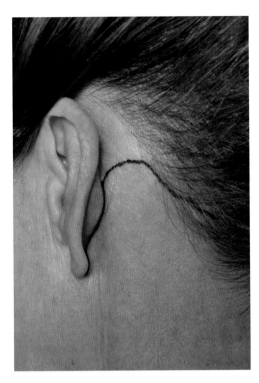

Figure 11.1.14 When there is minimal skin shift expected, the incision is limited to the retro-auricular sulcus only ("short scar" technique). When more skin shift is expected, especially from the neck, the incision is extended across nonhair-baring skin into the occipital hair. A wide range of patterns for this extension have been described, ranging from a vertical incision down to an incision that follows the hairline. Most surgeons follow a course somewhere in between, as in this photo where a "lazy S" follows the occipital hairline for 1 or 2 cm before entering the occipital hair.

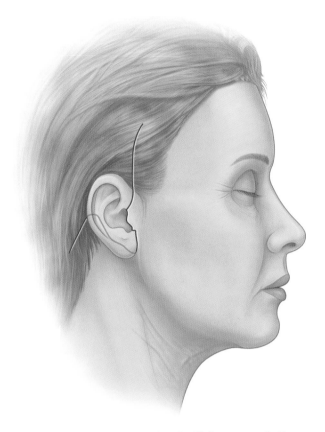

Figure 11.1.15 The traditional incision for a facelift flap curves vertically or slightly anteriorly in the temple, follows the contours of the ear, both anteriorly and posteriorly, and then angles into the posterior scalp.

rough guide is to use the lazy S approach if 2 cm or more of neck skin is to be removed at the incision line.[117] This approach allows an adequate excision of skin without a stair-step deformity, while hiding the lower, potentially most visible part of the scar in the wispy hair of the lower occipital scalp (*Figs 11.1.14, 11.1.15*).

Either the temple dissection or the post-auricular dissection can be done first, depending on surgeon preference. The dissection is usually begun with a scalpel, for the first 1–2 cm, at which point many surgeons switch to scissors. In the post-auricular area, the flap is firmly attached to the deep cervical fascia of the sternocleidomastoid and the mastoid. Also, this is the most common location to see skin flap necrosis, so the flap should be raised sharply under direct vision, keeping the dissection against the underlying deep fascia in order to maintain flap thickness. As the dissection continues inferior to the earlobe level, the surgeon must be cognizant of the great auricular nerve, where it is most at risk over the posterior border of the sternocleidomastoid. By keeping the dissection in the subcutaneous plane, the great auricular nerve will be protected.

In the temple, if the incision has been made along the anterior hairline, dissection is begun directly in the subcutaneous plane. If the incision has been made in the hair baring scalp of the temple, dissection can be carried out in one of two planes: superficial to the superficial temporal (temporoparietal fascia) which will continue directly into the subcutaneous facelift plane, or between the superficial temporal fascia and the deep temporal fascia. If the deeper approach is used, the dissection proceeds quickly against deep fascia, but at the

anterior hairline, the dissection plane must transition into the subcutaneous facelift plane. This change of plane results in a narrow ribbon of superficial temporal fascia which will contain the superficial temporal artery and vein and branches of the auriculotemporal nerve. This is known as the "mesotemporalis", and must be divided, often requiring ligation of the superficial temporal vessels. The argument in favor of the deeper dissection is to protect temporal hair follicles, although vessels and a nerve must be sacrificed (*Fig. 11.1.16A*). The superficial plane has the reverse attributes: vessels and nerves within the superficial temporal fascia are preserved, but the hair follicles can be injured during the dissection unless care is taken (*Fig. 11.1.16B*).

Anterior to the anterior hairline, the subcutaneous plane is then developed. Commonly referred to as the "facelift plane", the level of dissection normally leaves about 2 mm of fat on the dermis. This results in a large random pattern skin flap the survival of which will entirely depend on the subdermal plexus. In the upper face, this dissection continues anteriorly until the orbicularis oculi is encountered where it encircles the lateral orbital rim. Depending on the type of deep plane surgery planned, the mid-cheek dissection may stop short of the malar fat pad (see Ch. 11.7), or alternatively, carry on over the fat pad, freeing it from the overlying skin in the temple and cheek (see Ch. 11.6). Lower in the cheek, immediately anterior to the ear and the earlobe, the skin is tethered to underlying structures by secure fascial attachments (variously named: platysma auricular fascia, parotid cutaneous ligament, and Lore's fascia). Beyond this area, the subcutaneous

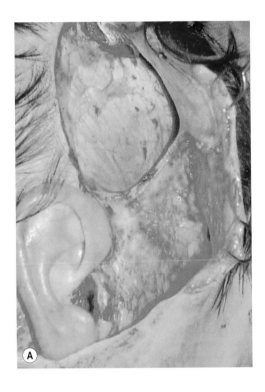

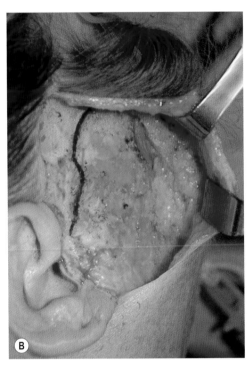

(A)

(B)

Figure 11.1.16 (A) Facelift flap has been raised in two different planes, initially deep to the superficial temporal fascia, against the deep temporal fascia (seen as an oval window), with a change of planes near the anterior temporal hairline into the subcutaneous plane. The "mesotemporalis" is a bridge of tissue which develops between these two planes. In order to unify the planes, it has been divided with ligation of the superficial temporal artery. (B) Facelift flap has been raised in a single subcutaneous plane, with dissection directly on the superficial temporal fascia and deep to the hair follicles of the scalp. The purple line outlines the course of the anterior branch of the superficial temporal artery.

dissection proceeds relatively easily. Once the skin flaps anterior and posterior to the ear have been raised, the two dissections are joined. The extent of the facelift flap dissection into the cheek and neck will depend on the type of deep tissue technique being employed (see Ch. 11.2). When a submental incision is done with midline platysma muscle plication (Ch. 13), there will be traction on the cervical skin toward the midline of the neck. In that circumstance it is important to widely mobilize the cervical skin from the underlying platysma in order to allow the cervical skin to be redraped along a vector opposite to that in which the platysma is being moved. If, on the other hand, there is no submental incision, the neck dissection can be more limited *(Figs 11.1.17, 11.1.18)*.

Deep tissue surgery

The subcutaneous facelift flap does two things – it allows for reposition and removal of excess facial skin, and it provides access to the deep tissues of the face. Techniques to address the deep tissues of the face will be reviewed in Chapters 11.2–11.8. These will include: SMAS plication, loop sutures (MACS lift), SMASectomy, subSMAS with skin attached, sub SMAS with separate skin flap, and subperiosteal.

Video 4

Skin flap mobilization and closure

Once the deep tissues have been managed, skin flap mobilization and closure must be done accurately and with care. Despite masterful deep tissue surgery, errors made on skin closure can create some of the most obvious of facelift deformities. At all times, the skin should be considered a covering layer, not a structural one. Therefore, skin flap repositioning should be seen as a removal of redundancy rather than a method to hold up ptotic soft tissue. Most techniques advance

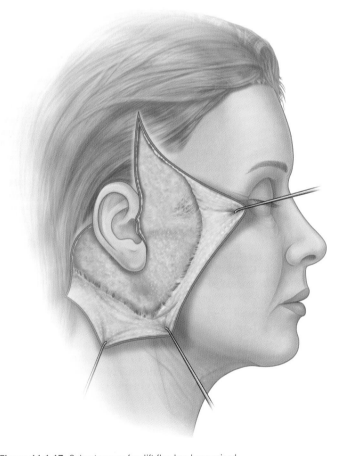

Figure 11.1.17 Subcutaneous facelift flap has been raised.

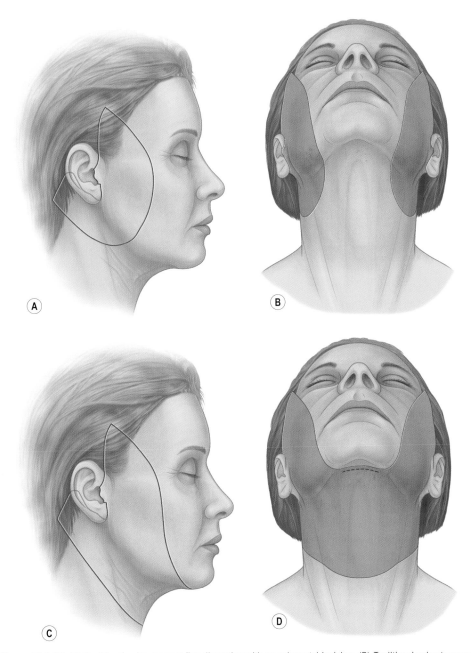

Figure 11.1.18 (A) Traditional subcutaneous flap dissection with no submental incision. (B) Traditional subcutaneous flap dissection with submental incision.

the skin flap along an oblique vector which is slightly less vertical than the vector for repositioning deep tissues. In certain techniques, surgeons employ a nearly vertical vector to the skin flap (Ch. 11.4). One concept is to place the skin flap "where it lies", using the vector which facial skin naturally assumes when the patient is lying in the supine position. This is based on the theory that we all look better lying on our back with facial skin redraping itself in a natural direction (Fogli, pers. comm.). A common guide is to advance the skin flap toward the temple along a vector which is perpendicular to the nasolabial fold. This is also approximately along the line of the zygomaticus major muscle. A skin flap marker can be very useful in determining where the skin should be incised. The anterior anchor point is immediately adjacent to helix of the ear at the junction of the hair baring scalp. This will be the

first of two anchor points; it can be held in place with a half buried mattress suture in order to minimize the chance of a visible suture mark *(Fig. 11.1.19)*.

Posteriorly, the skin flap should be drawn along a vector which roughly parallels the body of the mandible. The second anchor point will be at the superior most extent of the postauricular sulcus at the point where the incision starts to transition posteriorly. Once again, a half buried mattress suture can be used. At this point, trimming of the overlapping flap and suturing can be done in the temple and in the occipital region; the order is based on surgeon's preference. During this process, the facelift flap is redraped in the desired direction with gentle tension. Attention is then turned to trimming excess skin around the ear, with absolutely no tension on the closure. If a tragal edge incision is used, the tragal flap is

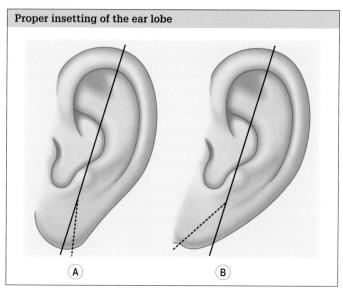

Proper insetting of the ear lobe

Ⓐ   Ⓑ

Figure 11.1.20 The earlobe should be inset with the long axis of the earlobe (dotted line) about 15° posterior to the long axis of the ear itself. If the earlobe is pulled forward, an unnatural appearance results.

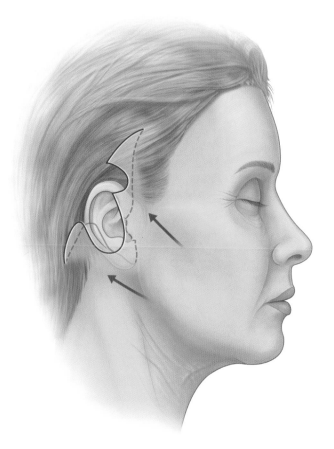

Figure 11.1.19 Diagram shows typical skin flap redraping along an oblique direction which is slightly less vertical than the vector along which deep tissues are moved. There is considerable variation in this however; some techniques involve a more horizontal vector (dual plane extended SMAS, see Ch. 11.6), while other techniques utilize a nearly vertical vector (MACS, see Ch. 11.4).

thinned and hair follicles are removed. In the retroauricular sulcus, there is normally little or no skin to be trimmed if the posterior flap has been correctly positioned. Earlobe inset is done last and is designed to angle 15° posterior to the long access of the ear *(Fig. 11.1.20)*.[114,117]

Skin trimming around the ear should be guided by having no tension on the sutures when the wound is closed. Tension on the earlobe can lead to distortions such as the pixy ear deformity and the malpositioned earlobe, both of which are difficult to correct (see Ch. 12).

Neck surgery

The basic principles of neck surgery will be covered here. (Surgical rejuvenation of the neck is reviewed in Chapter 13.) Like the face, the layers of the aging neck must be assessed independently in order to devise an appropriate surgical plan.

Superficially, the skin of the neck is typically thinner and less elastic than facial skin. With age, further skin laxity develops, causing vertical wrinkles and pleats. These can be corrected by tightening the skin in a posterior oblique direction. Some surgeons believe that such a correction should be accompanied by superior oblique repositioning of the underlying platysma.[118,119] With age, subcutaneous fat usually

accumulates in the anterior neck, although this is highly variable; in some thin individuals, there may be little or no subcutaneous fat in the neck. If subcutaneous fat is the only problem, and the skin is firm, or will be surgically tightened, the fat can be simply removed with closed liposuction.[120]

Deep to the fat, the paired platysma muscles have well recognized variations in their anatomy. The majority (roughly 75%) of necks exhibit interdigitation of the platysma muscles in the submental region for the first 1–2 cm behind the chin.[121,122] The remaining 25% either overlap extensively, or do not overlap at all *(Fig. 11.1.21)*.

With age, there appears to be a loss of tethering of the platysma muscles to the deep cervical fascia, analogous to the loss of tethering of the orbicularis oculi along the infraorbital rim. As a result, the platysma seems to fall away from the cervical mandibular angle and the sharp angle of youth gives way to the obtuse angle of age. The visible bands, which develop with age, are normally the leading edge of the paired platysma muscles, but clinical experience has demonstrated these visible bands may also represent pleats in the redundant muscle just posterior to their leading edge. Bands are considered either static (present at rest), or active (only present on animation). There are two different surgical options to deal with platysma bands in the anterior neck. One approach involves mobilizing the posterior borders of the paired platysma muscles, drawing them in a superior oblique direction and fixating the muscle to firm fascia (platysma auricular fascia, or the Lore's fascia component).[83,118]

Alternatively, the paired platysma muscle can be drawn medially, and approximated in the midline of the neck.[28,123] Access for this is through a 2–3 cm incision placed adjacent to or in the submental fold. Through this submental incision, several anatomical structures can be addressed directly: subcutaneous fat, subplatysma fat, the platysma muscles, digastric muscles, and the submandibular glands. A common approach is to remove excess subcutaneous and subplatysma fat, to approximate the anterior platysma muscle edges

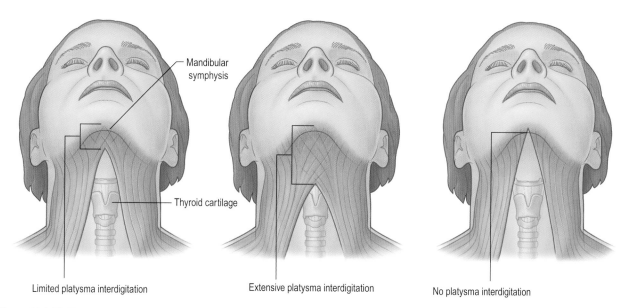

Limited platysma interdigitation   Extensive platysma interdigitation   No platysma interdigitation

Mandibular symphysis

Thyroid cartilage

Figure 11.1.21 Three types of platysma anatomy.

centrally and to do a partial transaction of the muscle inferiorly. Some surgeons advocate multiple rows of sutures to aggressively advance the platysma muscles medially: the corset platysmaplasty.[124] Deep to the platysma, excess subplatysmal fat may be removed, hypertrophic digastric muscles can be thinned and ptotic submandibular glands can be corrected by repositioning or by partial excision.[125,126]

In some facelift cases, only minimal correction of the neck is required and a facelift with deep tissue advancement will supply adequate correction. Conversely, in patients concerned only with the neck, this can be treated as an isolated procedure utilizing a number of different techniques: isolated liposuction, liposuction plus platysma plication and transection, or a retroauricular approach to tighten the platysma posteriorly.[127] If after submental surgery, there is skin laxity, it can be tightened with an isolated retroauricular incision, or with a full subcutaneous facelift.

In some older males, the preferred procedure may be a direct neck excision of excess skin, leaving a scar in the midline. This can be done with a zig-zag pattern or with a vertical ellipse broken up with two or more Z-plasties.[128]

In the typical case of the aging neck, there is usually a combination of factors (skin laxity, excess fat, and lax platysma muscle). In such a scenario, there is controversy as to how aggressive to be with surgical treatment. While most surgeons agree that a youthful neck contour is one of the principle objectives of facelift surgery, many fear the possibility of creating the "overdone" neck. And while some surgeons feel that any platysma banding warrants open surgery, others virtually never do an open neck procedure, relying instead on liposuction and posterior-superior platysma traction. Some surgeons feel that ptotic submandibular glands should always be addressed while others feel it need never be done. The implication of these opposing opinions is that a perfect, universal procedure for the neck probably does not exist, and surgeons must individualize their approach to variations in anatomy and patient expectations.

Ancillary techniques

Browlift surgery and blepharoplasty

Facial aging rarely occurs in a regional fashion, and is typically a pan-facial phenomenon. Therefore, a comprehensive approach to facial rejuvenation is normally required to achieve a harmonious result. For many patients, surgery for the brow (Ch. 7) and the eyelids (Ch. 8) are critical components of a global approach for which a facelift would be only part of the solution.

Volume removal

With radial expansion of the lower third of the face, many patients require fat removal. Subcutaneous fat can be removed either by direct excision or with liposuction. In the cheek, this is often done on a limited basis for the jowls, especially in cases where jowls cannot be corrected by soft tissue elevation alone. Removal of deep fat can be done by partially removing the buccal fat pad, which can be approached through a facelift dissection or through an incision in the upper buccal sulcus. In the neck, superficial fat can be removed using liposuction or by direct excision through a submental or a facelift incision. Fat deep to the platysma can be removed using direct excision through the submental approach. In all cases of fat removal, caution is advised because of the potential defects which can be produced when too much fat is removed.

Volume augmentation

Long-term experience with elevating deep facial tissues has shown this approach to add some fullness to the middle third of the face (see Chs 11.2–11.8). However, a more complete result can be obtained if specific volume augmentation is done. The addition of volume can be accomplished with a number of different methods including: synthetic implants (cheek implants, submalar implants, orbital rim implants), injectable synthetic fillers, hydroxy appetite granules or injected fat (all of which are reviewed in Chs, 4, 14, and 15). In particular, the harvesting, processing and injection of micro-droplet fat grafts (lipofilling) have undergone great technical improvements.[70,129]

This technology is now reproducible, and for many surgeons is a major component of their facelift technique.[130,131] There is a high rate of fat graft take after fat injection in the middle third and upper third of the face; in fact significant over-grafting should be avoided in the periorbital area because of the propensity for visible ridges and lumps if excess fat grafting has been done. Fat grafting is less reliable around the vascular, mobile lips. Specific areas which are commonly grafted in conjunction with facelift surgery fat are the periorbita (orbital rim, upper lid sulcus, and the tear trough), the mid-facial groove, and the malar prominence. The depth of injection can be in the superficial fat layer (superficial to SMAS), or in the deep fat layer. As mentioned above, it has been proposed that the deep medial fat compartment may play a unique role in support of soft tissue in the mid face, suggesting the benefits of fat grafting this zone.[64] Fat injection can be done independently, or in combination with facelift surgery. When done in conjunction with facelifting, it is usually done first, before the facelift flap has been raised.

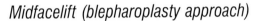
Video
5

Midfacelift (blepharoplasty approach)

In an attempt to lift the tissue immediately inferior to the infraorbital rim (the midface), an approach through the lower lid was developed.[132] This involves a subciliary or a transconjunctival blepharoplasty type incision followed by a dissection down over the face of the maxilla. This procedure can be done in the subperiosteal plane, which requires an inferior periosteal release, or it can be done in a supraperiosteal plane.[133] After mobilization of the cheek mass the soft tissue is fixated superiorly, either laterally along the lateral orbital rim,[132] or more vertically with anchoring to the bone of the infraorbital rim.[134] Disadvantages have included the learning curve necessary for surgeons to feel comfortable with this approach and a significant incidence of revisions for malposition of the lower eyelid.[135] An alternative approach to the midface is endoscopically through the temple. This procedure is described in detail in Ch. 11.2.

Lip procedures

The aging face often develops changes in the perioral region, but a facelift will not affect the perioral region to any appreciable degree. Common changes include elongation of the upper lip as measured from Cupid's bow to the base of the columella, a thinning of the vermillion, and the development of perioral rhytides.

Elongation of the upper lip is highly variable, but if present, tends to hide the upper teeth, in some cases almost eliminating the normal upper dental show on smiling. It has been estimated that the ideal distance from Cupid's bow to the base of the columella is 15 mm.[136,137]

The upper lip can be shortened by performing a skin excision along the contours of the base of the nose (bull horn pattern). Skin is excised, with the direct approximation of skin acting as a subcutaneous lift. Disadvantages include a

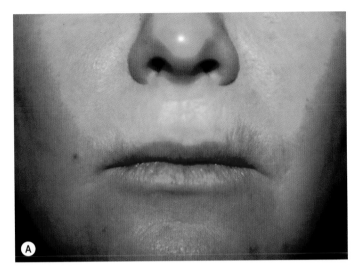

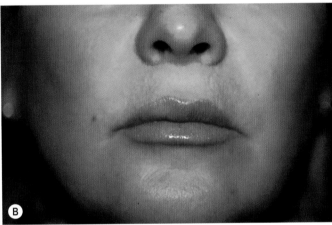

Figure 11.1.22 Pre- and postoperative photographs of a lip-shortening procedure using a bullhorn-shaped incision along the nostril sill.

potentially visible scar and a certain degree of relapse making revisions common *(Fig. 11.1.22)*.

Alternatively, a strip of skin can be removed along the vermillion border, advancing the vermillion superiorly. This has the advantage of immediately increasing the apparent width of the vermillion lip, but the disadvantages that the white roll is eliminated and a permanent scar will be left along the vermilion border. Women can deal with this by using lipstick, but this is usually a life-long commitment when the scar is visible.

Lip augmentation can be done with many different techniques. Commonly used methods include: injectable fillers (Ch. 4), injected fat, dermal fat graft, acellular dermis and SMAS grafts. Many different human tissues, and many synthetic materials have been used to thicken lips. Depending on the technique used, problems have included resorption and loss of effect, permanently over filled lips, distorted shaped lips, immobile lips, and in some cases tissue necrosis from vascular compromise. Attempts to augment the lip along the vermillion border lead to a duck like appearance, while augmentation along the wet dry junction is more likely to achieve a normal appearing lip.

Perioral rhytides are a common finding in the facelift age group. They can be effectively treated at the time of surgery with resurfacing procedures. Options include chemical peel, surgical dermabrasion or laser treatment. (These techniques are discussed in Chapter 5.) The most common problem is permanent depigmentation when the resurfacing has been overly aggressive.

Dressings

Some surgeons feel that dressings after facelift surgery are not necessary, but most surgeons use light dressings to protect the incisions and to act as an absorbent for wound drainage. Dressings should not be tight or constrictive, but rather soft and comfortable. The initial dressing is normally removed on the first postoperative day.

Postoperative care

In the initial postoperative period, the patient is kept still and blood pressure is monitored closely. Any signs of blood pressure increase should be taken very seriously; the patient is examined for possible causes (pain, anxiety, urinary retention) and appropriate measures taken. If the increase in blood pressure is endogenous, it should be treated pharmacologically. If the surgical procedure has been long (>3 h), sequential compression devices are kept on the legs in recovery room until the patient can ambulate normally. The patient is then encouraged to get out of the bed with assistance, in order to walk to the bathroom. The patient's positioning involves keeping the head of the bed elevated, but avoiding flexion of the neck. Avoiding the use of a pillow for 10–14 days will help keep the patient's head in a neutral, non-flexed position. Cool packs to the face will increase comfort and help decrease swelling. Analgesics and antinauseants are used as necessary. In some jurisdictions, patients are discharged home, but in other settings, patients are kept under the care of a medically trained individual for the first night after surgery. On the first postoperative day, the patient is reviewed, paying particular attention to the possibility of a hematoma, the dressings are changed or removed, and drains are removed. After the first day, options include another light dressing, a commercially available "chin strap", or no dressing at all. Patients are usually permitted to have a shower and wash their hair when the incisions are sealed from the environment – usually 2–4 days postoperatively. Subsequently, patients are seen for dressing changes, suture remove and wound inspection, at intervals up to 7–9 days when the final sutures are removed. Typically, there is a return visit at 2–3 weeks and then again between 6 and 8 weeks. Photographic documentation of the surgical result should be deferred for at least 6 months to allow for all postoperative swelling to settle completely.

Surgical complications

Hematoma

Postoperative hematoma is the most common facelift complication, and has a reported incidence of 2–3% in women. The incidence in men has been reported up to 8%, although this can be decreased to 4% through meticulous surgery and postoperative blood pressure control.[138,139] Numerous variables

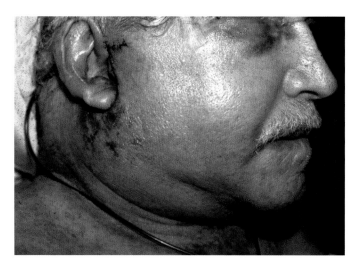

Figure 11.1.23 Postoperative hematoma in a hypertensive male. Note the ineffective suction drain.

have been explored, including dressings, drains, fibrin glue, and platelet gel. A positive association has been found when simultaneous open neck surgery is done, with patients taking platelet inhibitors such as Aspirin and anti-inflammatories, with hypertension in the postoperative period, and with the rebound effect when the epinephrine wears off postoperatively.[140,141] Hematoma prevention involves avoiding these variables as much as possible. Hematomas typically develop in the first 12 h after surgery. If an expanding hematoma is identified it should be promptly drained. If skin flap compromise is suspected and there is a delay in returning to the operating, a temporary solution can be the removal of sutures in order to relieve pressure (*Fig. 11.1.23*).

Sensory nerve injury

The terminal branches of sensory nerves to a facelift flap are routinely divided when the flap is raised. The consequence is a self-limiting paresthesia which usually recovers completely in 6–12 months. The great auricular nerve is the major sensory nerve at greatest risk for damage during facelift surgery. Transection will lead to numbness of the lateral portion of the external ear as well as skin anterior and posterior to the ear. A painful neuroma can also develop. If knowingly transected during facelift surgery, either partial or complete, it should be repaired intraoperatively. A portion of the zygomaticofacial nerve is often transected when the malar fat pad is lifted; this will lead to numbness of the lateral cheek, which will continue to improve for over a year. In this area, some permanent numbness is possible.

Motor nerve injury

Damage to a facial nerve branch can easily go unnoticed by the surgeon until muscle paralysis is identified postoperatively. Immediately after surgery, in the recovery room setting, facial nerve paresthesias are extremely common and are usually caused by the lingering effects of local anesthetic. Once the temporary anesthetic effects are gone (approx. 12 h for bupivacaine), persisting dysfunction may be due to

11.2

Facelift: Introduction to deep tissue techniques

Richard J. Warren

SYNOPSIS

- In its pure form, the subcutaneous, skin-only facelift has a limited effect on the position of heavier deep tissue.
- In SMAS plication, a skin flap is created with suture manipulation of the superficial fat and the underlying SMAS/platysma.
- In loop suture techniques (MACS lift), a skin flap is created with long suture loops taking multiple bites of superficial fat and platysma – fixed to a single point on the deep temporal fascia.
- The supraplatysma plane creates a single flap of skin and superficial fat mobilized and advanced along the same vector.
- SMASectomy involves a skin flap plus excision of superficial fat and SMAS from the angle of the mandible to the malar prominence, with direct suture closure of the resulting defect.
- A SMAS flap raised with skin attached (deep plane) creates a flap of SMAS/platysma, superficial fat and skin, all mobilized and advanced along the same vector.
- A separate SMAS flap (dual plane) creates two flaps, the skin flap and the superficial fat/SMAS/platysma, which are advanced along two different vectors.
- The subperiosteal lift involves dissection against bone, with mobilization and advancement of all soft tissue elements.

Introduction

In the previous chapter, the generic subcutaneous "skin-only" facelift was described. However, as reviewed in Chapter 6, the anatomy of facial aging is a complex process involving all layers of the face from the skin through to the bone. Logically, surgical rejuvenation of the aging face should address all or most of these tissue layers. To this end, rejuvenation of the skin is reviewed in Chapter 5. Within the soft tissue of the face, the two principle age-related changes are loss of midface volume and soft tissue descent. (Surgical methods to add volume are described in Chapters 14 and 15.) With regard to soft tissue descent, a host of surgical approaches have been

described. In this chapter the standard methods available to elevate and rearrange the deep soft tissues of the face are outlined; in the coming chapters, they will be described in detail by authors who developed these techniques, or by authors who use them routinely. The subcutaneous facelift is included here for comparison purposes, although in its classic form, there is no attempt to address the deeper tissues of the face.

Subcutaneous facelift

The "skin-only" facelift *(Fig. 11.2.1)* is used to tighten loose facial skin by advancing a random pattern skin flap and removing the excess. By definition, there is nothing done to the deep facial tissues. A tried and true technique, this method can be effective when the only significant problem is loose skin. For example, some patients with very thin faces and little or no subcutaneous fat may present with loose skin only. It is also useful in secondary or tertiary situations where deep tissues have previously been repositioned and the presenting problem is a recurrence of skin laxity. In that setting, a short scar approach will often suffice. Advantages of the skin-only facelift include its simplicity, a rapid postoperative recovery, and the use of a dissection plane which does not risk damage to the facial nerve or other deep structures. Disadvantages include: a minimal effect on underlying facial shape and the inherent disadvantage that skin is an elastic structure which will stretch when tension is applied. Therefore, the longevity of effect is in question, especially when the skin is used to reposition heavy facial tissues. Unfortunately, if the surgeon increases skin tension in a misguided attempt to reposition ptotic deep tissue, the shape of the face can be distorted. Skin tension will flatten facial shape, negating the rounded contours of youth. Also patients in the facelift age group have usually lost elasticity in their skin and therefore, with tension, are prone to a stretched look with wrinkles re-oriented in abnormal directions. Lastly, excess skin tension at the incision

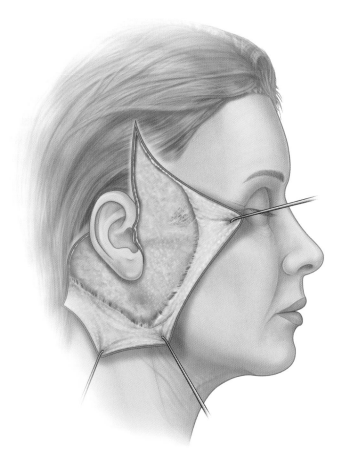
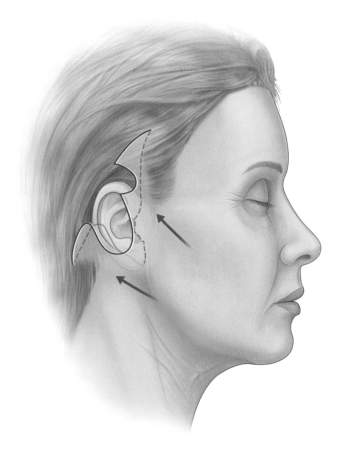

Fig. 11.2.1 Subcutaneous facelift.

line can cause malposition of the hairline, alopecia, distorted earlobes, widened scars, and the potential for skin flap necrosis.

SMAS plication

After surgeons learned to raise a large random pattern skin flap, it became apparent that facial shape could be changed by using sutures to manipulate the underlying soft tissue.[1]

Suture plication creates an infolding of the superficial fat, drawing fat from the lower in the face up to the point where the sutures are placed. Areas of fixed tissue, such as the fixed SMAS (*Fig. 11.2.2*) over the parotid gland are less movable, and can act as an anchoring point; anterior to the parotid, mobile tissues can be easily manipulated.[2] Multiple sutures with customized vectors can be used allowing reshaping of the superficial facial fat. The technique is relatively easy to master; it can be customized for the individual case, and can be modified intraoperatively by removing and replacing sutures as necessary. The superficial fat can be shifted in a different direction than the skin. When plication sutures are placed properly, there is little or no risk to branches of the facial nerve. Proponents of plication claim long-lasting results without the need for invasive and potentially dangerous dissections.[3] The primary concern with plication is the potential loss of effect if sutures cut through the soft tissue (the "cheese wire" effect). Another concern is that the degree of improvement may be limited by the tethering effect of the retaining ligaments which in this technique are not released. When the subcutaneous fat is fragile, suture fixation may fail, and plication may have a limited effect in patients with heavy jowls and ptotic tissues in the neck.

Loop sutures (MACS lift)

A variation of suture plication is the loop suture method (*Fig. 11.2.3*), for which the main variant is the MACS lift (minimal access cranial suspension). This procedure, which itself was derived from the "S-lift", relies on long suture loops which take multiple small bites of soft tissue.[4,5] Some of these bites are strategically placed into the SMAS and platysma. The loop sutures are fixated to the deep temporal fascia at a point just superior to the zygomatic arch and anterior to the ear. The theoretical explanation for the efficacy of this technique relates to the use of multiple bites of tissue which the developers of the technique feel creates "microimbrications" of the superficial fat and SMAS.[5] Anteriorly, a third suture can be placed to advance the malar fat pad, although the fat pad is not surgically released and its repositioning depends on its own intrinsic mobility. Treatment of the neck usually involves closed liposuction. Proponents of this technique recommend a nearly vertical vector for the skin flap, with a short scar incision. The advantages with this technique are similar to those of plication, although proponents point to the added benefit of using a more firm point of fixation (deep fascia) and the

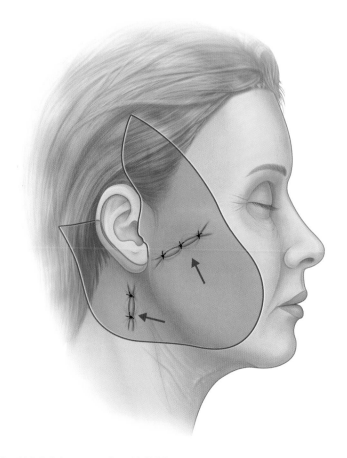

Fig. 11.2.2 Subcutaneous flap with SMAS plication.

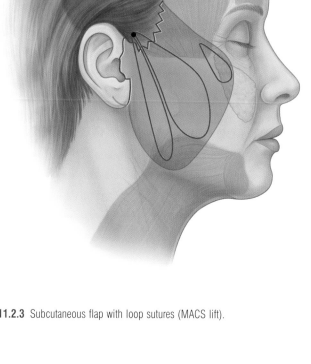

Fig. 11.2.3 Subcutaneous flap with loop sutures (MACS lift).

improved effect of micro-imbrications. Disadvantages are the same as SMAS plication: potential loss of effect if the sutures pull through, the lack of ligamentous release and concerns about the effectiveness of sutures holding heavy jowls and ptotic neck tissues against gravity. Lastly, surgeons must address the tendency for loop sutures to cause fat to bunch up, potentially leaving bulges which can be visible through the skin.

Supra-platysmal plane facelift

The supra-platysmal plane facelift *(Fig. 11.2.4)* involves a deep subcutaneous dissection carried out immediately superficial to the SMAS and platysma. Originally described as the extended supra-platysmal (ESP) dissection plane, this procedure raises the superficial fat and skin as a single layer, leaving the SMAS layer untouched. The zygomatic ligaments are released as dissection of the superficial facial fat extends over the malar prominence as far forward as the nasolabial folds. The theory behind this technique is the belief that the superficial fat is a ptotic structure, but the underlying SMAS and platysma are not.[6] After the flap has been raised, the fat on the underside of the flap can by contoured and sutures can also be placed from this fat to underlying fixation points. This technique provides good mobilization because ligaments are

released, and it produces a thick very robust flap. Also, with no surgical penetration of the underlying SMAS, there is theoretically no risk to branches of the facial nerve. Concerns about this method are that the flap is unidirectional (the skin and fat move en bloc), and the fact that repositioning the weight of this flap depends primarily on skin tension at the suture line.

Subcutaneous facelift with SMAS removal (SMASectomy)

In the SMASectomy procedure *(Fig. 11.2.5)*, a strip of SMAS and overlying fat is removed with direct suture closure of the resulting defect.[7] The excised strip angles obliquely across the cheek from the angle of the mandible to the lateral malar eminence at the edge of the malar fat pad. The procedure has been described after using either a conventional facelift incision or a short scar approach. Advantages include the fact that the location of traction is close to the ptotic lower facial tissues, and therefore potentially more effective than a SMAS flap raised at a higher level. The technique allows for skin and SMAS to be moved along different vectors. By suturing two opposing freshly cut edges, fixation is potentially more secure than plication alone. The cut edges being sutured have not been undermined, potentially making them more viable, and the resulting fixation more secure than undermined flaps.

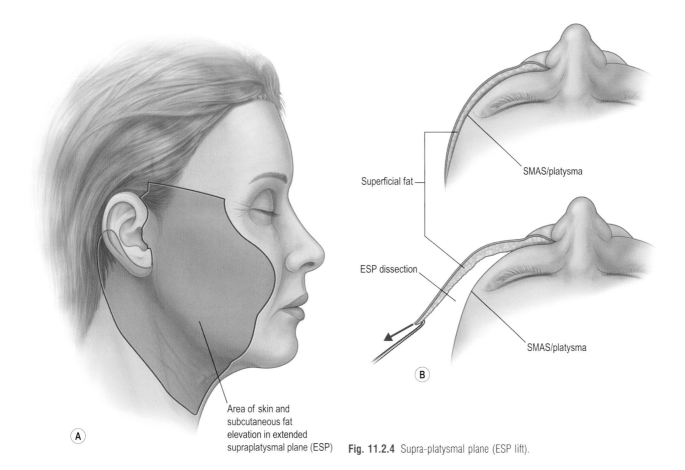

Superficial fat

SMAS/platysma

ESP dissection

SMAS/platysma

(B)

(A)

Area of skin and subcutaneous fat elevation in extended supraplatysmal plane (ESP)

Fig. 11.2.4 Supra-platysmal plane (ESP lift).

Compared with a SMAS flap, the procedure is more rapid, with less theoretical risk to the facial nerve because there is no deep plane dissection. Proponents feel that fixation is effective because the location of the SMASectomy resection is roughly at the junction of the mobile SMAS, which allows mobile tissue to be sutured to the fixed SMAS. Disadvantages include the possibility of injuring a facial nerve branch (if the SMAS removal is done too deeply) and the lack of any ligamentous release, which may limit the movement of certain tissues such as the malar fat pad.

SMAS flap with skin attached (deep plane facelift)

Tord Skoog, in 1974, published his method of raising skin, subcutaneous fat, and the SMAS as a single layer which created a thick robust flap with excellent blood supply. It also contained a stretch-resistant structure (the SMAS), with the promise of a long-lasting result.[8] Originally, there was limited improvement in the anterior face with little or no change to the nasolabial fold. This lack of anterior movement was later found to be due to tethering of the SMAS to the lip elevators: zygomaticus major and minor, and levator labii superioris.[9] In order to overcome some of these shortcomings, multiple variations have been developed (Barton: high SMAS; Hamra: deep plane) *(Fig. 11.2.6)*.[10–13] The skin is normally raised for only 2–3 cm anterior to the tragus, the SMAS is then

incised, and the rest of the dissection is done deep to the SMAS as far as the zygomaticus major muscle from which the SMAS is released. The skin and subcutaneous fat are left attached to the SMAS and the entire flap is then advanced and fixated as the surgeon desires. Advantages of this technique are the robustness and physical strength of the flap, and the requirement for only one plane of dissection. Ligaments are also thoroughly released. Certain variations of the technique also allow for repositioning of the malar fat pad.[10,13] Disadvantages include the inherent risk of dissecting under the SMAS with the potential for damage to the facial nerve. Also, these procedures are "monobloc" techniques where the skin, subcutaneous fat and SMAS are generally moved in one direction.

Subcutaneous facelift with separate SMAS flap (dual plane facelift)

Surgeons wishing to move the SMAS and subcutaneous fat in a different direction than the skin arrived at the concept of two separate flaps: the random pattern facelift skin flap and an SMAS flap carrying the superficial fat *(Fig. 11.2.7)*. Multiple variations of this popular concept have been developed with terminology introduced by different authors (extended SMAS: Stuzin; high SMAS: Connell and Marten; FAME: Aston).[14–22] As in plication, MACS and SMASectomy, proponents of this method feel that that moving the skin and subcutaneous soft

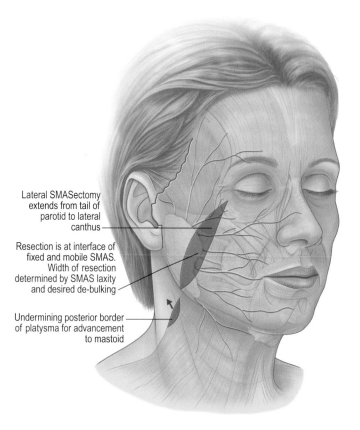

Lateral SMASectomy extends from tail of parotid to lateral canthus

Resection is at interface of fixed and mobile SMAS. Width of resection determined by SMAS laxity and desired de-bulking

Undermining posterior border of platysma for advancement to mastoid

Fig. 11.2.5 Subcutaneous flap with SMAS excision (SMASectomy).

Subperiosteal facelift

Paul Tessier, in 1979, first presented his concept for a subperiosteal approach using craniofacial principles to elevate facial tissue.[23,24] Variations were developed,[25,26] but it was not until the introduction of the endoscope that surgeons widely adopted this concept *(Fig. 11.2.8)*.

Approaching from the temple, the midface can be dissected in either the subperiosteal[27,28] or supra-periosteal plane.[29,30] Added exposure can be achieved with a lower eyelid or an intra-oral incision. The advantages are a dissection which is deep to all vital structures, a relatively short incision, and harmonious lifting of the midface and lateral brow. There is little or no tension on the skin thus eliminating problems from excess tension on the skin. Some surgeons feel this technique is uniquely advantageous for the patient requiring improvement in the infraorbital midface in conjunction with lateral browlifting. The younger patient who requires midface improvement without skin tightening has been proposed as a good candidate for this technique. Disadvantages of subperiosteal lifting include the additional technology and equipment involved, a limited effect in the lower face/neck region and limited effect on superficial structures, particularly loose skin. Furthermore, the early aging midface which seems suited to this technique may in fact be due to volume loss, a problem which can be correctable with less invasive procedures such as fat grafting.

Summary

Multiple techniques have been devised to elevate and reposition tissues in the aging face. In the following chapters, leading surgeons will address two issues: first, they describe how they handle the deep tissues of the face, and second, they explain the logic behind their own particular technique. This is a field where personal opinions are strong, and at the time of this writing, the greatest difference of opinion among facelift surgeons relates to the various methods used to manipulate deep facial tissue. All surgeons have been striving for the same objective: a procedure which will be effective, have a relatively a long-lasting result, and a high margin of safety. Over the years, a number of studies have been done to compare different facelift techniques.[31–40] In order to assess the available data, a systematic review of the world literature over a 60-year period was made in an attempt to locate reliable studies which could attest to the efficacy and safety of one method over another.[41] Despite this exhaustive review, no clear indication could be found that any one facelift technique was superior to the others. Therefore, surgeons must continue to use their own judgment for technique selection based on their patient's needs, balanced against their personal convictions about quality, longevity and safety.

tissues along different vectors will result in a more accurate reversal of the aging process. Typically, the deep tissue flap is shifted more vertically than the skin flap. A second advantage is the ability to reposition deep facial tissues by mobilizing and fixating the SMAS flap internally without the need to rely on skin tension for support. Theoretically, the disadvantages of excess skin tension are therefore avoided. Also, as in the deep plane technique, ligaments are surgically released, resulting in excellent mobilization and advancement for the SMAS and overlying fat. Disadvantages relate to a more time-consuming procedure because two different surgical planes are developed. In addition, these two planes introduce the inherent problems of each: potential damage to deep structure when doing the SMAS flap dissection, and potential problems with the skin flap if it is too thinly dissected or if it is placed on too much tension. In a thin patient, both layers can be quite thin, which increases the technical demands placed on the surgeon.

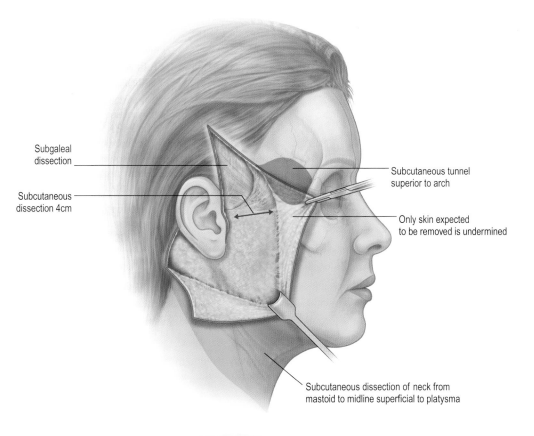

Subgaleal dissection

Subcutaneous dissection 4cm

Subcutaneous tunnel superior to arch

Only skin expected to be removed is undermined

Subcutaneous dissection of neck from mastoid to midline superficial to platysma

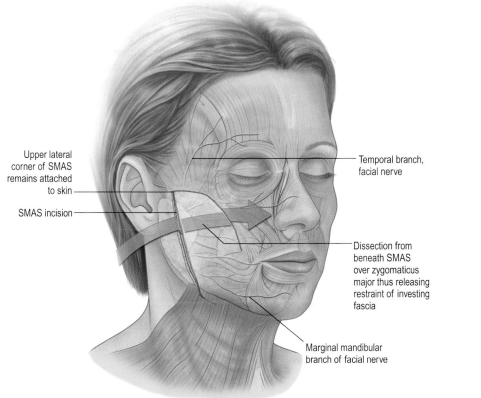

Upper lateral corner of SMAS remains attached to skin

SMAS incision

Temporal branch, facial nerve

Dissection from beneath SMAS over zygomaticus major thus releasing restraint of investing fascia

Marginal mandibular branch of facial nerve

Fig. 11.2.6 SMAS flap with skin attached (deep plane facelift).

11.3

Facelift: Platysma–SMAS plication

Dai M. Davies and Miles G. Berry

SYNOPSIS

- Allows multi-vector traction to individualise the facelift.
- Sutures placed closer to the point of lift have the best effect.
- Delivers a good malar auto-augmentation.
- Reduced downtime.
- Safe and ideal for thin, attenuated SMAS layers or repeat facelifts.

Introduction

As summarized in Chapter 11.2, facelifting has evolved appreciably from the simple, skin-only procedures of the early 20th century. Today, we have an almost bewildering array of techniques and tissue planes from which to choose. While each proponent may provide convincing support for their particular technique, most are in agreement about the central role of the superficial musculoaponeurotic system (SMAS), originally highlighted by Skoog in the 1970s[1] and detailed in Mitz and Peyronie's now classic treatise.[2] The question remains precisely what to do with the SMAS in order to balance invasiveness, and thus tissue trauma from which the patient must recover, in addition to potential complications, and its longevity.

The SMAS may be simply elevated and advanced,[3] dissected at various planes,[4,5] rolled upon itself with mesh to augment malar projection,[6] excised,[7] or plicated.[8] The multiplicity of techniques bears testament to the fact that a universal and standard procedure eludes us still. There is also some evidence that there may be little actual difference, in either the short[9] or the long term, between techniques of varying aggressiveness[10,11]; therefore, procedures with less inherent risk to important structures, such as the facial nerve may be safer. Problems noted include inconsistent results, a less-than-impressive effect on the nasolabial folds and jowls and long operating times, requiring extended periods of careful surgery, particularly with anterior SMAS dissection. Furthermore, the SMAS is relatively avascular,[12] behaving more as a graft in certain circumstances, and may be thin and attenuated, thus holding sutures poorly. During revision or secondary surgery, the poverty of vascular supply to the undermined SMAS may present the surgeon with a mass of scar tissue.

Given the recent paradigm shift towards minimally-invasive techniques, to limit facial nerve complications and reduce recovery time, the minimal access cranial suspension (MACS) lift was initially popularly accepted.[13] Since its description in 2002, the MACS has proven effective, particularly for younger patients concerned with early jowling, minimal neck ptosis and the desire for minimal downtime. Itself a derivation of Saylan's 'S-lift',[14] the MACS lift focussed on the anatomical basis, suture anchoring position and skin excision, but certain limitations have been shown by experience. One of these, the relative lack of malar augmentation was addressed by the addition of a third suture and quickly became commonly applied.[15] However, precise purse-string suture placement is not always easy and subcutaneous irregularities may not settle as well as described. Whilst good for younger patients, the authors feel it does not always have a sufficiently strong effect on the lateral neck of older patients, and is painful in the initial postoperative period, with a limitation of mouth-opening, acknowledged by the originators.[13] Finally, there are two areas of tissue excess, or dog-ears, in pure vertical-vector lifts, which may fail to settle satisfactorily. The first is infero-posterior to the lobule. The second, cutaneous bunching at the lateral canthus, is particularly pronounced with the powerful suture of the extended MACS[15] and may be addressed through a lower lid blepharoplasty incision, however, not all patients require this additional procedure. It has been demonstrated that by utilizing tension in the SMAS rather than the skin, both cutaneous dog-ears and scar stretch[3] are minimized.

Table 11.3.1 Comparison of chief features for the PSP and MACS facelifts

	PSP	MACS
Incision	Vertical temporal (± post-auricular extension)	Inverted L (anterior only)
Skin flap	As required	Limited to 5 cm oval
Dissection into neck	Yes	No
Platysmaplasty	Direct (infralobular excision)	Indirect
SMAS fixation	SMAS-SMAS	SMAS-DTF
Malar augmentation	Yes	No
Vector	Cephaloposterior	Predominantly vertical
Skin excision	Tailored, no tension	Tailored, high tension
Neck	Multiple procedures	Liposuction in >95%
Ancillary procedures	Yes	No

Experience with these limitations led the authors to the use of sutures to plicate the SMAS; a procedure termed the 'platysma-SMAS plication' (PSP) lift. Its advantages *(Table 11.3.1)* include the application of a postero-superior, as opposed to purely vertical, vector, which allows a lift tailored to each individual. The vertically-extended skin incision permits synchronous temporal lift and reduces sideburn elevation and a visible scar.[16,17] While concealing the scar within temporal hair risks alopecia, it allows greater flexibility with no risk of highly visible alopecia between the helical root and hairline. A post-auricular extension, not employed in all cases, is important to ameliorate the post-auricular skin dog-ear, which adds to down-time and has been reported as a problem with the MACS.[9]

With no sub-SMAS dissection, PSP is safer, particularly with respect to the facial nerve, and quicker. It is also beneficial where SMAS vascularity is poor. Large bites of SMAS allow greater security, and therefore potential longevity. A second layer of finer imbrication sutures is used, producing both a smooth finish and perhaps additional strength. It is, of course, not without sequelae and does produce two dog-ears in the subcutaneous layer. Fortunately, the first, overlying the malar prominence, has the effect of auto-augmentation and assists with the overall rejuvenation by reversion of the aged "square" to a youthful "triangular" face. The second, in the sub-lobule region is not so beneficial, but is simply excised; a manoeuvre common to both Baker's[7] and Waterhouse's modified SMASectomy procedures.[18]

Technique

The surgical procedure is as follows: patients are prepared as for a standard facelift with tumescent infiltration (20 mL 0.5% bupivacaine and 1 mL 1:1000 adrenaline in 200 mL normal saline) into the subcutaneous plane. The incision extends vertically in the temporal scalp, along the anterior helical sulcus then passes post-tragal, and on occasion into the post-auricular

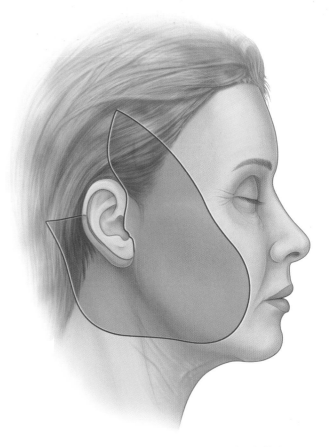

Fig. 11.3.1 Incision and area of subcutaneous dissection employed with the PSP-lift. Note that the posterior extension is not always required, but is useful where excess skin remains in the neck after SMAS plication.

sulcus *(Fig. 11.3.1)*. A post-auricular extension is used where required and subcutaneous dissection tailored to each patient. The anterior SMAS is grasped in a postero-superior direction to provide a satisfactory effect on the jowl *(Fig. 11.3.2)*. The key suture, using 2-0 PDS (Johnson & Johnson Medical Ltd), is then inserted to attach this SMAS to the relatively immobile pre-auricular parotid-masseteric fascia. Further sutures complete plication of the cervical platysma, below the mandibular angle, to the mastoid fascia *(Fig. 11.3.3)* and any surface irregularities are addressed by suture imbrication with 3-0 Vicryl (Johnson & Johnson). Excess SMAS in the infra-lobular region is excised, following hydrodissection, and closed with 3-0 Vicryl. Following meticulous haemostasis, excess skin, with low tension only, is trimmed and the wound closed over a small suction drain with 4-0 and 6-0 nylon. A light, compressive facelift dressing remains overnight and is removed with the drain the following morning. These can be similarly removed immediately prior to discharge in day-case patients. Sutures are removed at 4–6 days.

Evaluation

Patients and methods

In the authors' practice, the PSP-lift was initiated in 2004 and an initial evaluation was performed on a consecutive cohort

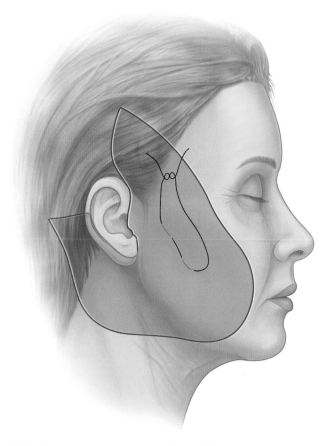

Fig. 11.3.2 Placement of the first and key suture, which takes a generous bite of anterior SMAS and tractions it postero-superiorly onto the parotido-masseteric fascia. It can be trialled and its effect easily measured externally by observing reduction of the jowl and effacement of the nasolabial fold as the SMAS is tractioned and the suture tied.

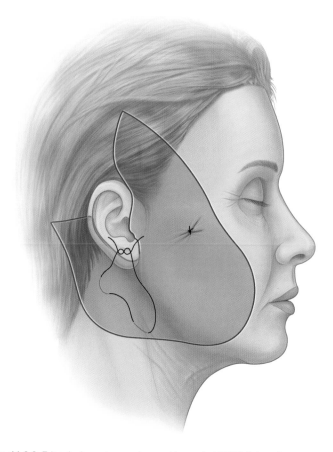

Fig. 11.3.3 Tying the key suture produces a 'dog-ear' of SMAS that produces a convenient malar autoaugmentation. A second suture passes between the posterior platysma and the mastoid fascia to complete the effect on the jowl and commence the necklift.

between August 2004 and May 2007. During this time, 122 patients were followed prospectively and specific assessment of outcome was performed. While specific, validated evaluation systems are available for surgical correction of the breast[19] and upper limb,[20] there is little available for evaluation of cosmetic facial surgery. Thus, a simple proforma *(Table 11.3.2)* was established allowing both patient and surgeon to contribute to the assessment employing a linear analogue scale (LAS), whereby poor and excellent results scored 1–5, respectively. Statistical analysis was performed with Kappa's correlation.

Results

Of the original cohort, five were lost to follow-up or had insufficient data for analysis. Of the remaining 117, all but eight were women (two male-female transgender patients were analyzed as biologically male). Mean age was 55 (range 29–79). General anesthesia was employed in the majority with three undergoing local anesthesia-sedation. Additional aesthetic procedures were performed in 104 patients *(Table 11.3.3)*. The neck was addressed with a variety of procedures in 92 (78.6%) patients *(Table 11.3.4)*.

Overall, there was a high correlation ($r = 0.76$) between the assessments of patient and surgeon. Mean scores of 4.45

Table 11.3.2 **Example of assessment proforma (blank)**

	Right	Left
Nerve damage		
Asymmetry		
Unevenness		
Scars		
Eye closure		
Subconjunctival		
Corneal symptoms		
Surgeon assessment		

5	4	3	2	1
Very happy	Happy	OK	Unhappy	Very unhappy

Patient assessment

5	4	3	2	1
Very happy	Happy	OK	Unhappy	Very unhappy

Table 11.3.3 Number of procedures synchronous with the PSP-lift

Procedure	n
Face alone	13
Face + 1 additional	40
Face + 2 additional	41
Face + 3 additional	12
Face + 4 additional	5
Face + non-face additional	6
Total	117

Table 11.3.4 Type and number of options employed in management of the neck

Management of the neck	n
Liposuction alone	54
Band division + platysmaplasty	11
Liposuction + band division + platysmaplasty	9
Lipectomy + band division + platysmaplasty	6
Liposuction + platysmaplasty	3
Liposuction + lipectomy + band division + platysmaplasty	2
Lipectomy + platysmaplasty	2
Band division alone	2
Liposuction + lipectomy	1
Liposuction + lipectomy + platysmaplasty	1
Liposuction + lipectomy + band division	1
Platysmaplasty alone	1
Total	92

(range 2–5) and 4.49 (3–5) were obtained for patients and surgeon, respectively initially and 4.43 (2–5) and 4.45 (3–5), finally. The same score was given at both stages in 42.9%, improved with time in 39.3%, and deteriorated in 17.8%.

Complications

The commonest complication was hematoma requiring a return to theatre which was required in four patients (3.4%); one following drain removal. All underwent evacuation under local anesthesia without apparent adverse effect on outcome (mean score 4.75). Some degree of nerve dysfunction was noted in five patients. Of the four with motor symptoms, only one lasted more than 6 weeks and was associated with ipsilateral infection. One with unilateral dysesthesia was followed-up at the chronic pain clinic after 3 months. The rate of temporary nerve injury overall was therefore 4.3%, motor 3.4%, and sensory 0.85%. Five patients experienced delayed wound healing, but all settled conservatively; oral antibiotics being required in one case, and the longest healed by 8 weeks. Two received intralesional steroid therapy for mild scar hypertrophy. One complained of a small area of alopecia, not

visible socially, in the temporal incision that improved spontaneously. A single patient underwent corrective fat transfer for a persistent surface irregularity. There was no statistically significant relationship between any complication and hypertension, smoking or secondary surgery.

Discussion

Facial rejuvenation is increasingly viewed by patients as a suitable recourse in a more ageist society that lives both longer and more healthily. Interestingly, studies directly comparing highly invasive with less aggressive procedures have shown no significant differences between the two[10,11] and more affluent, younger patients are requesting procedures with as little "down-time" as possible. The PSP facelift was designed to address these issues.

It must be remembered that SMAS advancement, whether composite or independent, exerts uniform traction, much like braces on trousers. Studies by Rohrich have elegantly demonstrated discrete facial partitions that go a long way to explaining why simple SMAS elevation-advancements often provide only partial correction.[21] PSP exploits the fact that the optimal effect from a suture derives from its proximity to the point of lift, and plication sutures can be placed wherever they are required. This answers one of the drawbacks of SMASectomies and conventional SMAS flaps where the excision is remote from both the jowl and nasolabial fold (NLF). With plication, the SMAS is sutured directly, rather than in a purse-string fashion used with the MACS lift, and has the potential for an infinite multiplicity of vectors, to obtain the precise effect tailored to the individual. This differs from Robbins' anterior plication, which employs a vertical row of SMAS sutures lateral to the NLF.[8] While addressing the NLF, this anterior only approach obliges antero-inferior traction on both lateral SMAS and malar fat thus counterbalancing malar augmentation.

Many have reported that the SMAS progressively thins anteriorly,[3,7,10] particularly in secondary surgery.[17] Saulis *et al.* demonstrated both the weakness and reduced suture-retention of the SMAS when raised alone,[22] as compared to an SMAS flap raised in continuity with the skin, a feature which has been cited by supporters of composite flaps. However, they also demonstrated less tissue creep and stress relaxation in the SMAS flap as compared to skin flaps, lending credence to SMAS tightening procedures such as plication, in the pursuit of surgical longevity. The degree of skin flap undermining is also much greater in the PSP than with procedures such as the MACS in observance of Baker's philosophy that SMAS vectoring to give maximal anatomic improvement is not adversely affected by employing a separate vector for skin redraping.[23]

Minimal access supporters stress the importance of vertical vectors in contemporary facelifts,[13] however, in our view, facial ageing occurs in multiple directions, according to gravity, the locations of retention ligaments, and local muscular forces,[16] and senescence is characterized by antero-inferior descent.[7] It seems counter-intuitive to disregard some vectors at the expense of others.[10]

Additionally, traditional SMAS techniques in which the malar fat is not specifically dissected, have a limited effect on both malar ptosis and the NLF.[3] As shown in *Figure 11.3.4,*

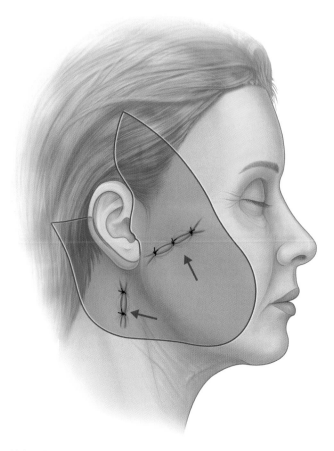

Fig. 11.3.4 Completion of the face and necklift, leaving the beneficial malar dog-ear and the undesirable infero-posterior lobule dog-ear.

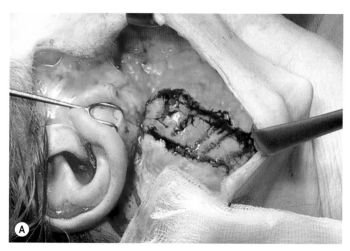

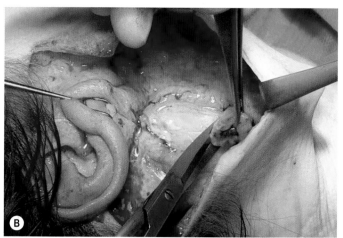

Fig. 11.3.5 Following the platysma-mastoid suture tying, the infero-posterior lobule excess is **(A)** marked and **(B)** excised. The cut SMAS edges are then sutured.

PSP can exert a powerful effect on the malar prominence and NLF due to individualized plication. Another advantage of the PSP lift is that after initial plication any residual SMAS irregularities are addressed with secondary imbrication to leave a smooth surface, this second layer further contributing to the integrity of the SMAS fixation. Personal experience has shown that the purse-string technique may lead to irregularities, which do not always resolve as claimed and can lead to patient dissatisfaction. Debate continues as to where the advanced SMAS should be fixed.[24] Deep fixation can also leave the patient with "marked pain and restricted mouth opening."[13] The success of SMASectomy procedures attests to the strength of SMAS-SMAS fixation.[7,18] Furthermore, there is the added benefit of autologous malar augmentation as proposed by Baker.[7] The infra-lobular platysma-SMAS excess is excised *(Fig. 11.3.5)*, and the defect closed, to remove the lateral swelling beneath the ear lobe, a feature typical of more minimal techniques.

Nerve dysfunction, particularly motor, remains the most feared complication of any facelift and in our series, none were permanently affected. Of note, half underwent synchronous endoscopic browlifts that more likely caused the frontal branch palsies. Interestingly, all nerve complications occurred in the first third of the study indicating a learning curve. That all motor function in this series recovered fully and rapidly indicates the inherent safety of PSP and assuages critics' fears that blind needle insertion into the pre-masseteric SMAS is dangerous.

The neck

The neck continues to be a problem area for several reasons: swelling and scarring always seem to mature slowly and correction of platysmal bands is often incomplete. In addition, aggressive submental lipectomy may leave irregularities and exacerbates the appearance of any residual jowling. Finally, seroma and excess skin are a frequent source of complaint and secondary surgery. The neck is a defining feature as small remnant anomalies can spoil an otherwise excellent result in the face. Management of the neck, therefore, remains controversial with supporters at both minimal and aggressive ends of the spectrum. That such a range and difference of opinion exists indicates the universal procedure remains elusive, although the pendulum appears to be swinging towards minimalism due to the limited margin for technical error and healing irregularities.[11,13] The viscoelastic properties of cervical flaps have been demonstrated to be inherently different from facial flaps with greater creep and stress-relaxation thereby allowing increased relapse, although the reason for this remains unclear.[22] The importance of the postero-superior region of the neck's anterior triangle has been highlighted in a recent publication, which demonstrated a gliding plane between the platysma and the sternocleidomastoid such that supero-lateral traction exerts a powerful effect on both lateral and anterior platysma.[25] Waterhouse emphasized a similar concept[18] for optimal results in the neck, which we fully endorse. It is worth reiterating the advantage of infra-lobular dissection, with or without a posterior incision, which allows SMAS anchoring to the mastoid fascia for a strong lateral platysmaplasty. A little over three-quarters of our patient cohort underwent some additional management of the neck, the majority (54 of 92) receiving liposuction alone. Following our assessment, nine (7.7%) were felt to have sub-optimal neck outcomes. Distribution was equal in the first and second halves of the study with no obvious features to assist in the preoperative selection of such patients.

Patient satisfaction was high with scores of 4.45. Inter-observer correlation was also high, lending some credence to what is effectively a subjective assessment. With respect to those who downgraded their scores, 75% had experienced a problem of some kind, including persistent dysesthesia, post-operative hematoma and skin flap telangiectasia; all were considered by the surgeon to have achieved at least a grade 4 surgical outcome.

Conclusion

The use of suture plication of the SMAS has been encouraging both for aesthetic outcome *(Figs 11.3.6–11.3.8)* and complication rate. The PSP-facelift seeks to combine the advantages of SMAS advancement with those of plication whilst minimizing complications and maximizing outcome. It has a sound anatomical basis, allowing individual, and differential, SMAS and skin vectoring that provides specific anatomical correction and ameliorates asymmetry. Moreover, the technique is safe to perform and easily acquired by trainees and less experienced aesthetic surgeons. The skin incision is standard and allows optimal access to the relevant anatomy. It is suitable for day-case surgery as a single procedure or with multiple concomitant aesthetic facial procedures and is particularly good for autologous malar augmentation. It works particularly well where the facial ptosis is concentrated primarily in the midface and at the jowl and has been noted by our patients to settle rapidly and thereby minimize "downtime".

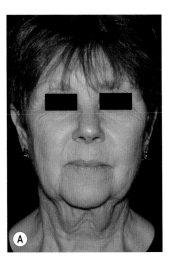 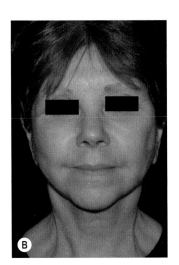 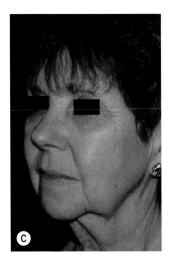 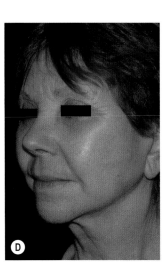

Fig. 11.3.6 A 67-year-old female shown 12 months following PSP-lift demonstrating its effect, particularly on jowl and cervical skin excess reduction. She also underwent synchronous bilateral upper and lower blepharoplasties and peri-oral CO_2 laser treatment. **(A,C)** preoperative; **(B,D)** postoperative.

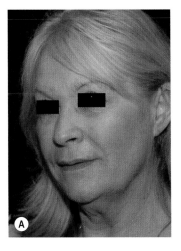 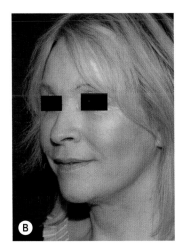 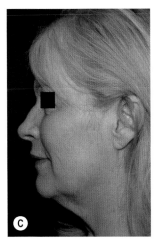 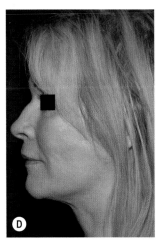

Fig. 11.3.7 Preoperative views **(A,C)** in a woman who underwent PSP-lift. Postoperative images **(B,D)** underline the malar autoaugmentation in addition to jowl diminishment and a good result in the cervical region.

Surgical foundation for the MACS-lift

The surgical foundation for facial rejuvenation should address the biomechanical effects of facial aging and volume loss for each patient, depending on their particular needs. Surgeons must be faulted in the past for not having a fundamental understanding of facial aging, volume loss, laminar anatomy, and biomechanical engineering. Our current understanding of the anatomy of facial aging is thoroughly reviewed in Chapter 10, giving insight into the complex biomechanics of facial aging. Aging involves the gravimetric effects on skin and SMAS, loss of elastic property of tissue, volume loss and descent within in fat compartments, and extrinsic effect of sun, genetics, weight loss/gain, and smoking.[11–13] Fat within the face does not exist as a confluent mass, but in discreet compartments separated by septae, formerly known as ligaments. Facial anatomy involves a laminar concept in which, movement between layers is possible without surgical delamination. Proponents of ligament release feel that such movement is inadequate for facial rejuvenation, but experience with the MACS-lift provides evidence that sufficient inter-layer movement is, indeed possible and surgically effective.

From the perspective of biomechanics, surgical approaches that rely on sheet tightening of attenuated facial structures (SMAS) may not produce a long-term effect due to the loosening of this layer over time (shear-yield). Suture line repairs such as linear plication or excision techniques (plication or SMASectomy) remain vulnerable to disruption (shear failure and "cheese wiring") by down-pulling the platysma whose fascia is contiguous with the SMAS facial rejuvenation, is therefore an exercise in biomechanical engineering in terms of how much force is required to vertically lift facial and neck structures and suspend them in place with approaches that are less prone to failure. Surgery is part of the solution for facial rejuvenation, but ancillary procedures found in cosmetic medicine such as medical skin care, fillers, neurotoxins, and light-based treatments work synergistically to produce a "wow effect" when used masterfully.

The MACS-lift concept involves the use of suture loops placed in a purse-string fashion in order to elevate deep facial tissue by anchoring to a fixed point. In the basic MACS-lift, there is one anchoring point on the deep temporal fascia, just above the lateral zygoma, and posterior to the passage of the temporal branch of the facial nerve. This is a very robust anchor point that will hold a 0-0 or 2-0 suture without a pull-out failure The "CS" part of the MACS-lift is "cranial suspension", which refers to the deep temporal fascia's attachment to the cranium along the temporal crest line. The MACS-lift does not utilize sheet tightening of the SMAS, SMAS plication, or SMASectomy, but relies purely on specialized suture suspension. The basic MACS-lift involves two suture loops, one vertical and one oblique, while the "extended MACS-lift" involves an additional suture to elevate the malar fat to a more anterior anchoring point (*Figs 11.4.1, 11.4.2*). Suture loops placed within facial tissues results in a gathering and suspension of tissue. Tonnard and Verpaele describe this as "micro-imbrication" (*Fig. 11.4.3*).

How the loops are designed and sequenced is crucial, as once the platysma is pulled upward, it is possible to rotate the layers of the face without a downward traction component of the platysma. By not dissecting skin off the platysma, there is

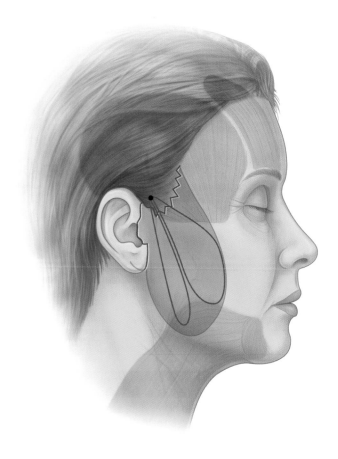

Fig. 11.4.1 The basic MACS-lift involves two suture loops placed into the SMAS in a purse-string fashion. The vertical loop captures the platysma muscle below the angle of the mandible, elevating soft tissues of the neck. The cheek loop captures and elevates soft tissue of the mid cheek and jowl.

tightening of the neck skin when the platysma is tightened.[7] The zone of adherence just anterior to the earlobe, called Lore's fascia, can be used as a fixed structure to pull against in order to achieve vertical tightening of the platysma as described by Labbé.[5]

The traditional skin incision for the MACS-lift utilizes a "short scar" anterior hairline approach with no retroauricular dissection. After deep tissue reposition, skin redraping is designed in a purely vertical direction (*Fig. 11.4.4*).

The amount of skin excision with the vertical approach of the MACS-lift is much less than seen with the classic SMAS-lift. Attention must be paid to a tension-free skin closure in order to promote excellent healing and avoid earlobe distortion. In a divergence of philosophy and practice from Tonnard and Verpaele, patients with greater facial and neck laxity will require extending the incision into the retroauricular area in order to manage lax skin (*Fig. 11.4.5*).

Therefore, the "MA" (minimal access) portion of the MACS terminology must be expanded to address situations where there is more tissue laxness necessitating a retroauricular incision. In optimal situations, with younger patients, the short scar approach is preferable, yet can be modified when the amount of loose tissues cannot be managed with a short scar approach. Extending the incisions into the post-auricular

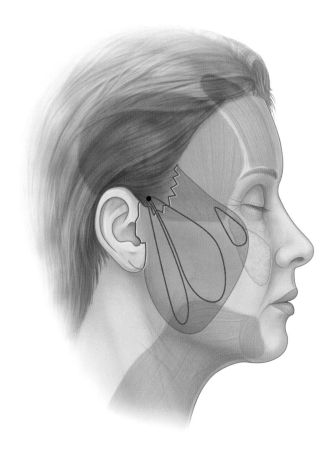

Fig. 11.4.2 The extended MACS-lift adds a third suture to elevate the malar fat pad.

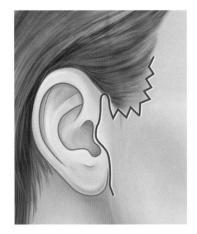

Fig. 11.4.4 The short scar incision used in the standard MACS-lift.

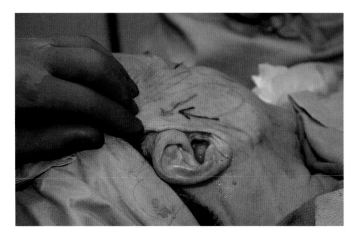

Fig. 11.4.5 Vertical skin advancement in the standard short scar approach for a MACS-lift.

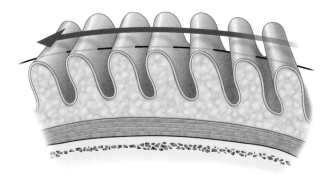

Fig. 11.4.3 MACS sutures result in a bunching up of soft tissue. This has been termed microimbrication.

region resolves bunching of loose skin at the level of the earlobe.

There are numerous advantages of the MACS-lift. Deep tissues are readily repositioned without deep plane dissection, which risks injury to the facial nerve. Less dissection is also likely to result in faster recovery. The short scar approach avoids dissection over the sternocleidomastoid muscle and therefore removes the potential for injury to the great auricular nerve. MACS sutures are anchored at fixed points which avoid the temporal branches of the facial nerve *(Fig. 11.4.6)*.

It has outcomes that are acceptable over time, and favorable biomechanics that address volume redistribution and facial tightening without deep layer work. This technique appears very adaptable to most patients seeking primary and secondary facial rejuvenation. It also has the advantage of being reversible during surgery, as suture loops can be changed or the entire technique be abandoned for a more traditional approach. The learning curve for successful adoption of the MACS-lift is something that can be mastered by most surgeons who are willing to invest the time required to learn a new approach to surgical facial rejuvenation.

Patient evaluation

Each patient is unique with respect to their particular needs for facial rejuvenation. It then is incumbent on the surgeon to formulate a strategy that will provide solutions for each patient. In the author's experience, a more holistic approach works best in his own patient population. This involves both cosmetic medicine and aesthetic plastic surgery, allowing for care to be ongoing and to advantage each patient with adjunctive services of medical skin care, fillers, neurotoxins, and light-based treatments.

The following components of a patient's face require evaluation and strategy.

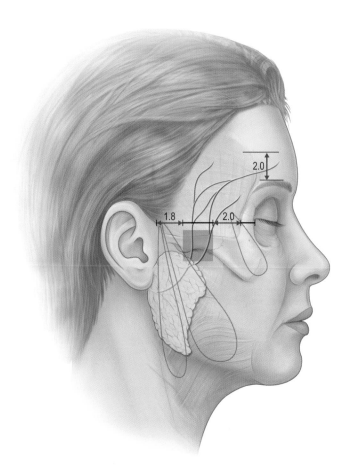

Fig. 11.4.6 The temporal branches of the facial nerve course over the middle third of the zygomatic arch. The MACS suture anchor points are designed to avoid damage to these nerve branches.

Facial skeletal structure and asymmetry

Structural needs such as cheek or chin deficiency must be addressed. Evaluate for facial nerve function, muscular function, any asymmetry.

Skin quality, character, and looseness

Photodamage and photoaging must be addressed and consideration given for medical skin care or light-based treatments. Rhytides and looseness in the perioral area cannot be resolved with rhytidectomy.

Forehead and glabellar rhytides

Forehead rejuvenation may involve the use of neurotoxins, or rejuvenation surgery through the endoscopic, or transpalpebral approach.

Facial volume

Assessment of the loss of facial volume is done. Volume enhancement in the submalar sulcus may be done with surgery, autologous fat grafts, or synthetic fillers. The recognition of volume loss that occurs due to attritional lipoatrophy is underestimated.

Ocular region

Dermatochalasis, brow position, brow ptosis, fat bags, lower eyelid looseness requiring lateral canthal work, lower eyelid skin, and malar bags should all be assessed. Given the substantive lift of the MACS-lift, a lower eyelid blepharoplasty is often an integral part of this approach.

Neck

Neck laxness and platysmal banding will influence the need to consider extended incisions and possibly a submental approach for direct work on platysma banding. The presence of submental fat may be addressed either through lipoplasty if superficial or direct excision if submuscular.

Jowls

The squareness of the jaw line is largely influenced by the downward descent of facial structures. Depending on the severity, dissection into the pre-masseteric space may be required.

Previous surgery

Patients seeking additional refinements or "maintenance" of facial rejuvenation from previous surgical procedure may present with distorted changes due to conflicting traction vectors or ineffectual outcomes. This type of patient requires thoughtful consideration of what can be safely addressed with reoperative surgery.

Medical history

Patients seeking facial rejuvenation may have medical conditions that can influence their safety during facial rejuvenation. Not everyone seeking facial rejuvenation surgery is a candidate for surgery, based on chronic medical disorders. Attention should be paid to a thorough review of systems with emphasis on cardiac and circulatory issues. Unique subsets of patients with surgical weight loss procedures may present with additional factors such as facial lipoatrophy, tissue wasting, and obstructive sleep apnea. DVT risk must be assessed and managed.

Patient expectations

The management of patient expectations becomes a major part of facial rejuvenation, whether surgical or medical. It is essential that patients see themselves for who they are before treatment and that realistic portrayal of outcomes be communicated. Occasionally, there is the need for revisionary surgery/procedures that must be addressed prior to treatment versus afterwards. Revision surgery may not be successful.

The better informed that patients are regarding their particular needs and your recommendations, both surgical and nonsurgical, they will be able to obtain the best outcome. If a patient does not appear to be capable of obtaining an outcome from treatments/procedures, it is better to communicate this up front and avoid the vexing problem of a dissatisfied patient who had unrealistic expectations.

Surgical strategy

The use of worksheets and templates has proven useful in many areas of aesthetic surgery and cosmetic medicine. A simple form based on your practice helps you develop your surgical strategy for each patient's care. It allows you to make notes, show specific details, and more importantly determine the tradeoffs involved. Such a form is a nice fit with your informed consent(s) for the surgical procedure or cosmetic treatments (fillers, neurotoxins, etc.).

How you choose to communicate your strategy with the patient is also important. Simple aids such as a 10×15 cm print from a digital camera on which you can draw, can be useful. Other approaches involve drawing on the patient with an eyeliner marker (easily removed) and taking a photograph. Both of these are good communication tools to make certain that your plans are in alignment with the patient's expectations and needs. Even something as simple as displaying a digital photograph on a large-screen LCD television works far better than using a hand mirror.

Anesthesia for the MACS-lift can be minimalistic: local anesthetic with conscious sedation; more complex with monitored anesthesia care – deep sedation (MAC) or general anesthesia (GA). If general anesthesia is contemplated, the author prefers an endotracheal tube (ET) over the laryngeal mask (LMA) device because of less neck distortion with the ET. Other important considerations would be DVT prophylaxis and a warming blanket for prevention of hypothermia. Although some surgeons consider chemoprophylaxis with fractionated heparin on long cases, there are reasonable concerns of increased risk of hematoma incidence. Some anesthesiologists prefer GA over MAC because of better airway management and the ability of a gas analyzer to measure end tidal CO_2 as an index of ventilation.

Care should be given during the procedure to installing protective eye ointment in order to prevent corneal exposure problems. Sterile tape strips may also be used to prevent eyelid opening. Individuals with a history of LASIK procedures are especially at risk for corneal problems due to diminished corneal sensory innervations that triggers tearing. When operating on a post-LASIK patient, consider an evaluation by an ophthalmologist for adequacy of tear production and tear film quality.

Surgical sequence

The patient is marked before the start of the procedure; key points are the planned incision, the degree of undermining, and the location of suture loops The degree of skin flap undermining typically extends inferiorly just past the mandibular angle and anteriorly 5–6 cm in front of the ear. If an extended MACS-lift is planned, undermining is marked over the malar prominence. The sequence of performing a MACS-lift is straightforward. If autologous fat grafting is considered, the author harvests and processes fat at the beginning, followed by injection prior to the incisions for the MACS-lift. It is preferred not to store AFT graft tissue at ambient temperature for long periods during the procedure. Any anterior neck surgery, such as lipoplasty is performed first. The cheek flap is then dissected and the loop sutures are placed. If a temporal lift or endobrowlift is contemplated, it is done next. A blepharoplasty, if planned, is done last.

Skin incision and undermining

Local anesthetic containing epinephrine is injected along the incision line. In the area of flap undermining, the author prefers lipoplasty wetting solution that contains epinephrine $1:500\,000$. The short scar incision extends from the earlobe below to the anterior hairline above. It follows the attachment of the earlobe from the retroauricular crease, around to the anterior attachment of the earlobe, following the tragal edge, the anterior helical attachment to the root of the helix, then across the lower portion of the sideburn and up the anterior hairline. Anteriorly, the incision is made in a zigzag pattern 1–2 mm within the hairline. The zigzag incision effectively increases the length of the temporal incision to better receive the elevated cheek flap. In the standard MACS-lift, the incision is carried up to the level of the lateral canthus, while in the extended MACS-lift, the incision extends up to a point opposite the tail of the eyebrow. Flap elevation is accomplished with scissor dissection. If an extended incision in the retroauricular zone is required, this is done early in the procedure as it generally facilitates suture loop placement and skin redraping when the neck is tightened vertically.

Anchor point

The deep temporal fascia anchor point is chosen to avoid the superficial temporal vessels and the temporal branch of the facial nerve. Small scissors are used to create a window in the subcutaneous tissue approximately 1 cm above the zygomatic arch and 1 cm in front of the helical rim in order to expose the deep temporal fascia *(Fig. 11.4.7)*.

When placing the suture into the temporalis fascia, the author sews away from the temporal vessel location. A single anchor point is used for both the neck loop and the cheek loop in order to diminish the amount of suture used and the palpability of knots. Absorbable monofilament sutures such as 0-polydiaxonone are preferred over nonabsorbable polypropylene or braided polyester suture.

The neck suture

The suture loop for the neck is placed first. Going inferiorly in the natural sulcus that is anterior to the tragus, firm bites between 1 cm and 1.5 cm long are taken into the SMAS. Progressing inferiorly past the angle of the mandible, two or three suture bites are taken into the platysma before the suturing is directed upward and back to the anchor point. A U-shape loop about 1 cm wide is created and the knot is then tied at the anchor point under tension. The suture loop is tied without any instrument that might be used to hold the first knot. This diminishes the possibility of suture damage

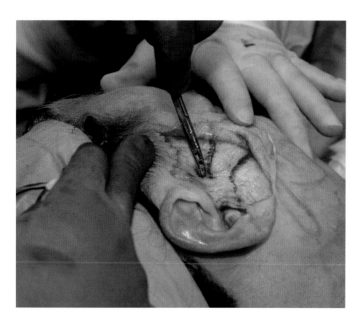

Fig. 11.4.7 The short scar incision has been made, and the skin flap raised. The zygomatic arch is marked in purple. Note the marks on the skin designating the location of the suture loops. The scissors are dissecting a window down to the deep temporal fascia which will be used as the anchor point for the vertical and cheek suture loops.

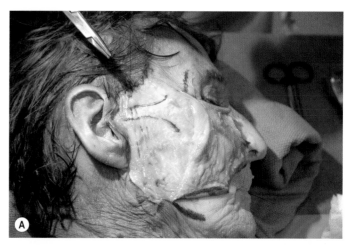

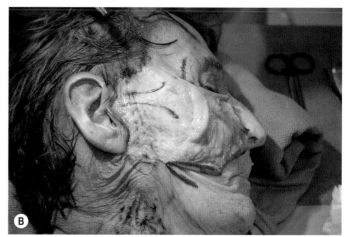

Fig. 11.4.8 (A,B) Cadaveric example demonstrating placement and the effect of the vertical neck suture. The orientation is vertical, and neck traction depends on achieving excellent suture purchase of the platysma muscle below the angle of the mandible.

and breakage. In my (the author) first few cases, I found that I did not have an adequate grip on the platysma fascia and that neck tightening was not optimal; for neck tightening to occur, adequate suture purchase of the platysma below the angle of the mandible is imperative. When performing the short scar variation, a fiberoptic retractor is helpful to visualize correct suture placement in the depth of the dissection. Should additional reinforcement of the neck be desired, 2-0 polydioxanone sutures can be placed from the platysma into the fascial zone of adherence just below the tragus (Lore's fascia) or from the platysma to the mastoid fascia. Suture knots in this area should be inverted to avoid knot palpability through the skin *(Fig. 11.4.8)*.

The cheek suture

The cheek loop is placed next. It originates at the same anchor point from the deep temporal fascia. Taking bites of the SMAS, suturing progresses inferiorly just anterior to the first loop and then curves more anteriorly, creating a wider loop above the jowl extending anteriorly as far as the skin flap has been raised. The author has found that the loop works best when it is in the configuration of a logarithmic spiral, like a Nautilus shell. This allows for upward rotation of facial structures and volume repositioning. The overall angle of the cheek loop is approximately 30° across the cheek, as compared to the vertical neck loop. The suture is then tied under tension. Novice MACS-lift surgeons tend to make too small of a cheek loop and are then faced with a situation of a peculiar wad of tissue when the loop is tied. Experience teaches that if a suture loop appears unsatisfactory, the best strategy is to take it out and replace it.

The malar suture

Once the cheek loop is tied, it is possible to add a third loop for elevation of the malar fat; this constitutes the "extended MACS-lift" variant. A different anchor point is used anterior to the temporal branch of the facial nerve. This point can either be the deep temporal fascia just lateral to the lateral orbital rim, or the periosteum of the zygoma, approximately 1.5 cm lateral to the lateral canthal area. Access to either of these anchor points requires a small window in the orbicularis muscle where the fibers run vertically. This purse-string suture travels obliquely toward the malar fat pad where at a point 2 cm below the lateral canthus, the direction is reversed, creating a narrow U-shaped loop that is tight under tension. In my experience, the direction of pull will be oblique, but ideally should be as vertical as possible. If the surgeon is dissatisfied with the placement of the loops, it is easy to cut and replace the loops until satisfied with their placement and tissue gathering.

Tissue bunching is an integral problem with the MACS suture loops. It is resolved with imbrications with 4-0 polyglactin braided suture. The author prefers the version of this suture that contains triclosan, an antibacterial agent in order to diminish risk of stitch abscess. Before leaving the deep tissue, it is necessary to place the skin flap over the tissue and observe for unresolved bunching and tissue tethering at the margins of the undermined area. Scissor removal of protruding fat may be needed in order to produce a smooth tissue surface inside the loops. Imbrication of tissue in the region just anterior to the tragus is important in order to preserve this normal sulcus.

Skin advancement and resection

The skin flap is then redraped along a vertical axis and the excess skin is resected. If there is excess skin at the level of the ear lobe, it must be resolved by incisions in the posterior ear region. My philosophy is to resolve this skin by extending my incisions in the posterior sulcus of the ear, instead of dealing with skin bunching post surgery. If necessary, the author uses a classic rhytidectomy incision in the post-auricular region, depending on the patient's neck laxity. The goal for skin

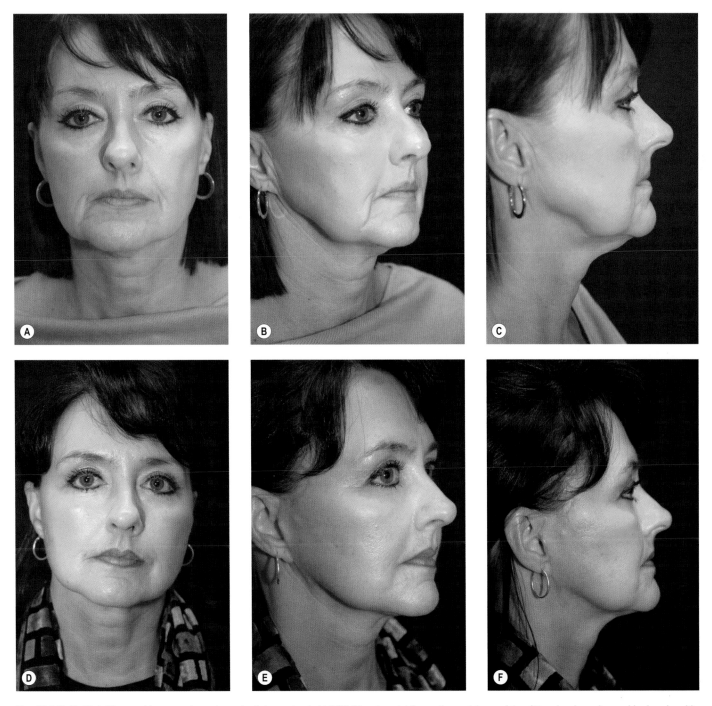

Fig. 11.4.9 (A–F) A 61-year-old woman who underwent a 3-loop extended MACS-lift, submental liposuction, autologous fat graft to submalar region, and hyaluronic acid fillers to the perioral area. The result shown is at 12 months.

excision is to have a tension free closure with wound margins coapted against each other.

The author's personal technique uses approximately 1 cc of fibrin glue (5 units/mL dilution) that is sprayed on the flaps and held for 3 min. I find that this diminishes ecchymosis formation and eliminates the requirement for drains. Care must be given to not apply excessive fibrin glue as it can interfere with revascularization of the flaps.

Wound closure is also straightforward with absorbable 5-0 monofilament in the deeper layers and 5-0 and 6-0 polypropylene skin sutures places as interrupted and continuous (horizontal mattress).

Dressings involve customary facelift dressings. The author personally prefers some silicone-backed foam for the anterior neck if lipoplasty has been performed. Otherwise, aftercare is similar to standard facelift procedures.

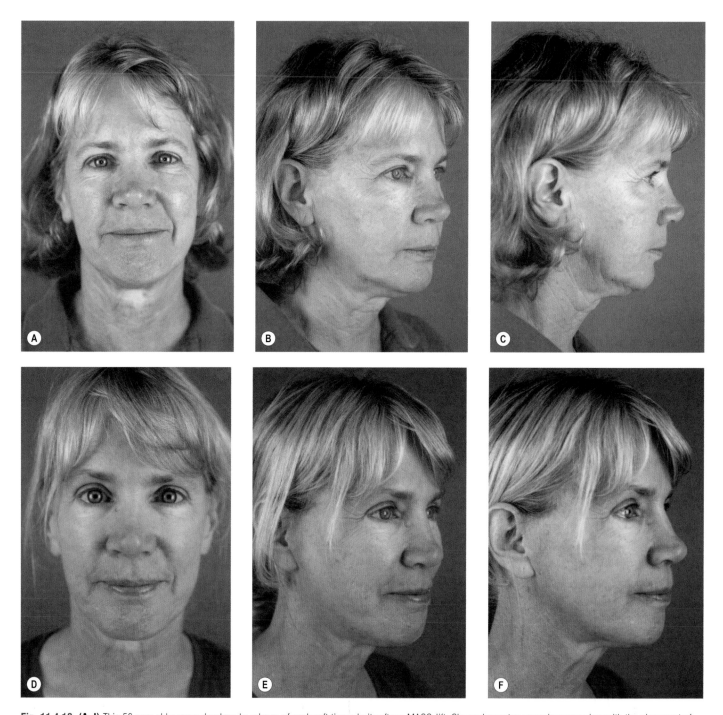

Fig. 11.4.10 (A–I) This 56-year-old woman developed a relapse of neck soft tissue laxity after a MACS-lift. She underwent a secondary procedure with the placement of both neck and cheek sutures. The result shown is at 12 months after the revision surgery.

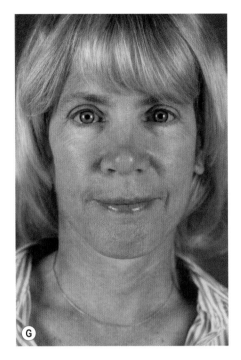 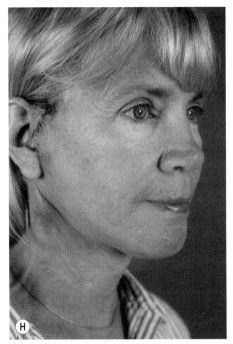 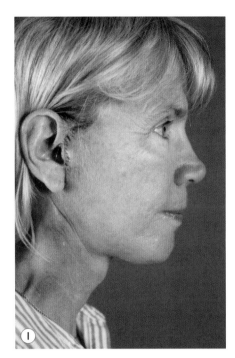

Fig. 11.4.10, cont'd

Three representative cases utilizing the MACS-lift concept are shown in *Figures 11.4.9 and 11.4.10*.

Summary

The MACS-lift is a facelift technique which is ideally suited for the lower and middle third of the face. By using strategically placed sutures, deep tissues are repositioned without the dangers of deeper dissection. The vertical vector ensures that many patients benefit from a short scar approach with a faster recovery. The technique is adaptable to a wide cross section of patients, and it can be mastered by most surgeons who are willing to learn a new technique.

References

1. Tonnard P, Verpaele A, Monstrey S, et al. Minimal access cranial suspension lift: a modified S-lift. *Plast Reconstr Surg*. 2002;109(6):2074–2086.

2. Tonnard P, Verpaele A. *The MACS-lift short-scar rhytidectomy*. St Louis: Quality Medical; 2004.

3. Tonnard P, Verpaele A, Gaia S. Optimising results from minimal access cranial suspension lifting (MACS-lift). *Aesthetic Plast Surg*. 2005;29:213.

4. Tonnard P, Verpaele A. *Short scar face lift, operative strategies and techniques*. St Louis: Quality Medical Publishing, 2007.

5. Aston S, Steinbrech, D, Walden J. MACS facelift. In: Tonnard P, ed. *Aesthetic plastic surgery*. Philadelphia: Saunders-Elsevier; 2009:137–149.

6. Labbé D, Franco R, Nicolas J. Platysma suspension and platysmaplasty during neck lift: anatomical study and analysis of 30 cases. *Plast Reconstr Surg*. 2006;117(6): 2001–2007.

7. Mendelson B, Muzaffar AR, Adams WP Jr. Surgical anatomy of the midcheek and malar mounds. *Plast Reconstr Surg*. 2002;110(3):885–896.

8. Besins T. The 'R.A.R.E.' technique (reverse and repositioning effect): the renaissance of the aging face and neck. *Aesthetic Plast Surg*. 2004;28(3): 127–142.

9. Rohrich RJ, Pessa, J E. The fat compartments of the face. *Plast Reconstr Surg*. 2007;119:2219–2227.

10. Gardetto A, Dabernig J, Rainer C, et al. Does a superficial musculoaponeurotic system exist in the face and neck? An anatomical study by the tissue plastination technique. *Plast Reconstr Surg*. 2003;111(2): 673–675

11. Mazza E, Papes O, Rubin MB, et al. Simulation of the aging face. *J Biomech Eng*. 2007;129(4):619–623.

12. Barbarino G, Jabareen M, Trzewik J, et al. *Biomedical Simulation: Physically based finite element model of the face*. Berlin: Springer-Verlag; 2008:1–10.

13. Barbarino G, Jabareen M, Trzewik J, et al. Development and validation of a three-dimensional finite element model of the face. *J Biomech Eng*. 2009;131:1–10.

11.5

Facelift: Lateral SMASectomy

Daniel C. Baker

SYNOPSIS

SMASectomy advantages
- Minimal SMAS dissection
- Greater tension can be put on SMAS re-approximation
- Malar fat pad can be elevated
- Reduces skin undermining
- Reduces tension of skin flap
- Simple and direct.

Avoiding SMASectomy pitfalls
- Keep parotid fascia intact
- Maintain correct plane from parotid edge to malar eminence
- Suture at proper level
- Feather all irregularities.

Introduction

Rhytidectomy is a procedure that continues to evolve as surgeons seek to offer patients natural rejuvenation with reduced morbidity. Over the years, we have witnessed an evolution of techniques ranging from basic skin lifts to superficial musculoaponeurotic system (SMAS) procedures to even more complex, deep-plane operations in search of an operation that reliably restores facial form with minimal morbidity.[1] More recently, the need for extensive incisions for rhytidectomy has also been questioned. It has become increasingly clear that not all patients require the full classic temporal preauricular and retroauricular incisions.[2] The incision, as well as the planes or levels of facial dissection, should be individualized for each patient, in-keeping with the physical changes related to aging and the desired result. As more patients seek facial rejuvenation at an earlier age, the need for surgical solutions that are less invasive and that involve less downtime is becoming increasingly important.[3]

When SMAS dissection first became popularized after the work of Mitz and Peyronie in 1976, many surgeons dissected the SMAS directly overlying the parotid gland developing a SMAS flap which was rotated to elevate the deeper tissue. I (the author) initially utilized this form of SMAS dissection beginning in the late 1970s and continued with it into the mid-1980s but overall, was disappointed with the effects of a simple elevation and tightening of the lateral superficial fascia. Specifically, there was little difference in overall facial contour whether I had performed a SMAS flap or plication.

As greater experience was gained with SMAS dissection, it became obvious that for the superficial fascia to produce any effective contour change in facelifting, it was necessary to elevate the SMAS anterior to the parotid gland. The problem of more extensive SMAS dissection is that facial nerve branches are placed in greater jeopardy.[4,5] It was also noted that the superficial fascia tends to thin out as it is dissected more anteriorly, making the SMAS easy to tear. A SMAS dissection that is not raised as a continuous fascial sheet but rather is raised with several tears in it is a poor substrate for holding the tension of contouring the face. For these reasons, the author felt that an extensive SMAS dissection was often not warranted in most patients and offered little long-term benefit when compared with SMAS plication.

In 1992, the author realized that an alternative to formal elevation of the SMAS was to perform a "lateral SMASectomy", removing a portion of the SMAS in the region directly overlying the anterior edge of the parotid gland at the interface of the fixed and mobile SMAS.[6] Excision of the superficial fascia in this region secures mobile anterior SMAS to the fixed portion of the superficial fascia overlying the parotid. The direction in which the SMASectomy is performed is oriented so that vectors of elevation following SMAS closure are perpendicular to the nasolabial fold or even more vertical, thereby producing improvement not only of the nasolabial fold but also of the jowl, jaw line, and midface.

The advantages of lateral SMASectomy are several when compared with formal SMAS elevation.[7] First, since the procedure does not require a formal SMAS flap elevation, there are fewer concerns about tearing of the superficial fascia. Second, the potential for facial nerve injury is less because the majority of the dissection is carried over the parotid gland. If the SMASectomy is performed anterior to the parotid, the deep fascia (parotid masseteric fascia) similarly will provide protection for the facial nerve branches as long as the resection of the superficial fascia is done precisely and the deep facial fascia is not violated. Third, because SMAS flaps have not been elevated, they tend to be more substantial in terms of holding suture fixation, and the problems of developing postoperative dehiscence and relapse contour are reduced.

Because of the design of the lateral SMASectomy along the anterior border of the parotid, the SMASectomy is performed at the interface of the superficial fascia fixed by the retaining ligaments and the more mobile anterior superficial facial fascia. On closure, this brings the mobile SMAS up to the junction of the fixed SMAS, producing a durable elevation of both superficial fascia and facial fat. In contrast, simple plication pulls on unreleased facial fascia (still bound by the retaining ligaments) such that proper vectors of elevation and obtaining long-lasting fixation can be problematic.

In the author's practice, utilizing the lateral SMASectomy technique, we are confident that we can obtain consistently good results with minimal risk, complications, and morbidity, and a speedy postoperative recovery. This method represents a rapid, safe, and reproducible operation, allowing the surgeon the versatility obtained with formal SMAS flap undermining while producing both the safety and rapidity of SMAS plication. However, we not apply this technique in every patient, and patients with a thin face, where fat needs to be preserved, get an excellent result with just a skin undermining, SMAS plication and redraping.

There are certainly other rhytidectomy techniques that produce excellent results.[8] Each surgeon must adopt a technique that serves his or her patients best. Ideally, the technique should be safe, consistent, easily reproducible, and applicable to a variety of anatomic problems. The surgeon must also have the versatility to adapt and modify his or her technique to the needs and desires of each patient. At present, the lateral SMASectomy provides this for many of my patients.

Operative technique

Anesthesia

Virtually all of the author's procedural facelifts are performed with the patient under monitored intravenous propofol sedation. Patients are given oral clonidine, 0.1–0.2 mg, 30 min before surgery to control their blood pressure. The face and neck are infiltrated with local anesthesia, 0.5% lidocaine with 1:200 000 epinephrine, through use of a 22-gauge spinal needle. The author injects the face before scrubbing to provide the requisite 10 min for vasoconstriction.

Incisions

When the temporal hairline shift is assessed as minimal, the preferred incision is well within the temporal hair. With this incision, it is often necessary to excise a triangle of skin below the temporal sideburn at the level of the superior root of the helix in order to prevent over elevation of the sideburn.

When a larger skin shift is anticipated or the distance between the lateral canthus and temporal hairline is >5 cm, the author prefers an incision a few millimeters within the temporal hairline. Although this is a compromise, the alternative of a receding temporal hairline is rarely acceptable to a female patient. When the incisions are executed properly, these scars heal well and are easy to revise or camouflage. The only exception might be in a patient who has deeply pigmented skin in whom the scar will contrast and appear as a white line. The temporal hairline incision should be made parallel to the hair follicles and no higher than the frontotemporal hairline.

The temporal hairline incision allows for more vertical elevation of the facial flap without changing the hairline. Other indications for this incision are a receding hairline from previous facelifts and a fine, fragile hairline.

The choice of preauricular incision is up to the surgeon. When executed properly, all of these incisions heal well and are imperceptible. I (the author) usually prefer a curved incision anterior to the helix and continue inferiorly anterior to the tragus in a natural skin fold. This practice preserves the thin, pale, hairless tragal skin and its demarcation from the usual coarser, thicker, darker cheek skin with its lanugo hairs. I perform intratragal incisions in patients in whom the cheek and tragal skin are similar and the tragal cartilage is not sharp or prominent. Closure must be without tension and the flap overlying the tragus should be defatted to dermis.

In short scar facelifting, efforts are made to end the incision at the base of the earlobe, but sometimes a short retroauricular incision is often necessary to correct a dog-ear after the facial flap rotation *(Fig. 11.5.1)*.

Skin flap elevation

All skin flap undermining is performed under direct vision (with scissors dissection) to minimize trauma to the subdermal plexus and preserve a significant layer of subcutaneous fat on the undersurface of the flap. Subcutaneous dissection in the temporal region is preferable, because the skin seems to redrape better. (I believe that hair loss results primarily from tension rather than superficial undermining.) Therefore, dissection in this area is done directly against superficial temporal fascia (temporoparietal fascia.) Subcutaneous dissection in the temporal region must be performed carefully to avoid penetrating the superficial temporal fascia that protects the frontal branch of the facial nerve. All dermal attachments between the orbicularis oculi muscle and the skin are separated up to the lateral canthus.

Dissection extends across the zygoma to release the zygomatic ligaments but stops several centimeters short of the nasolabial fold. I have never believed that further dissection provides significant benefits; on the contrary, the only result is increased bleeding. In the cheek, dissection releases the

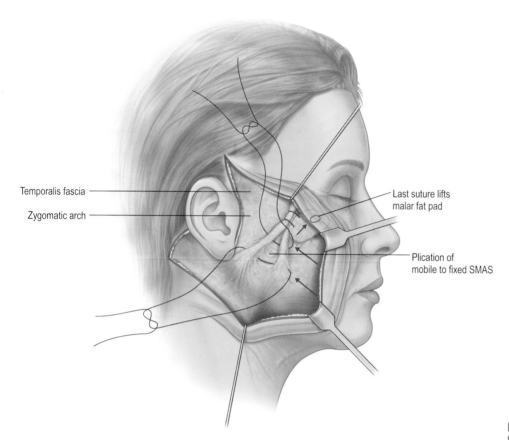

Temporalis fascia

Zygomatic arch

Last suture lifts
malar fat pad

Plication of
mobile to fixed SMAS

Fig. 11.5.4 Optional plication of SMAS, for thin
faces when debulking is not indicated.

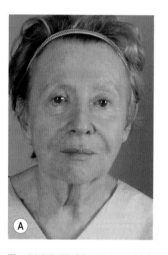

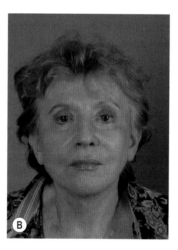

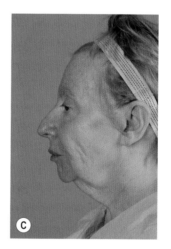

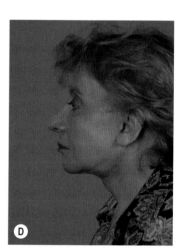

(A) (B) (C) (D)

Fig. 11.5.5 (A–D) A 79-year-old: face and neck, platysmaplasty, chin implant.

If firm monofilament sutures are used, such as PDA or
Maxon, the sutures should be buried and sharp ends on the
knot trimmed. Final contouring of any SMAS or fat irregularities along the suture line is completed with scissors. Fat can
also be trimmed at the sternomandibular trough, final contouring being accomplished with lipoplasty.

In the thin face where facial soft tissue should be preserved,
SMAS plication is a viable alternative. Instead of an incision
line into the SMAS, a row of plication sutures is placed, utilizing the same vectors, the same suture tension and the same
suture material as with the SMASectomy. Skin redraping completes the procedure *(Fig. 11.5.4)*.

Skin closure, temporal and earlobe dog-ears

After SMAS and platysma approximation, some tethering
of the skin might appear at the anterior and submandibular
skin. Suture fixation is at the level of the insertion of the superior helix. The author prefers to use a buried 3-0 PDS through
the temporal fascia with a generous bite of dermis on the
skin flap. Closure is under minimal to moderate tension.
Staples are used to close any incisions in the hair. A wedge
is usually removed at the level of the sideburn to preserve

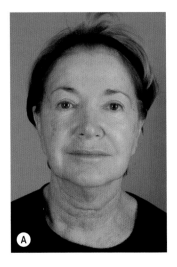
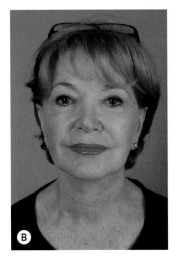
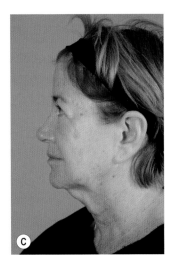
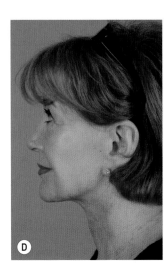

Fig. 11.5.6 (A–D) A 62-year-old: face and necklift-platysma, peel face.

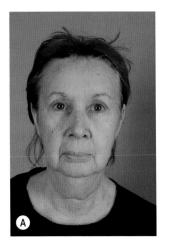
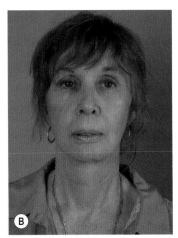
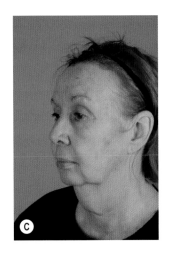
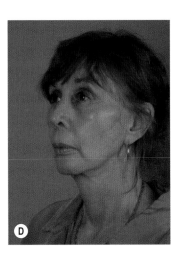

Fig. 11.5.7 (A–D) A 68-year-old: face and neck, platysmaplasty, chin implant, excise buccal fat.

the hairline. If an anterior hairline incision has been made, I like to close it with buried 5-0 Monocryl sutures (Ethicon, Inc.) and 5-0 nylon sutures. Extra time and attention must be sent on this closure to eliminate any dog-ears and obtain the finest scar.

Excess skin is then trimmed from the facial flap so that there is no tension on the preauricular closure. Wound edges should be "kissing" without sutures. Trimming at the earlobe must also be without tension, and the skin flap is tucked under the lobe with 4-0 PDS sutures, taking a bite of the earlobe dermis, cheek flap dermis, and conchal perichondrium to minimize any tension (if a short scar facelift is performed a small dog-ear might be present behind the earlobe; this is easily trimmed and tailored into a short incision in the retroauricular sulcus). A closed suction drain is usually brought out through a separate stab in the retroauricular sulcus *(Figs 11.5.5–11.5.7)*.

References

1. Baker DC. Deep dissection rhytidectomy: A plea for caution. *Plast Reconstr Surg*. 1994;93:1498–1499.

2. Baker DC. Lateral SMASectomy, placation and short scar facelifts: indications and techniques. *Clin Plast Surg*. 2008;35:533–550.

3. Baker DC. Short scar facelift. In: Aston SJ, Steinbrech D, Walden J, eds. *Advances in Aesthetic Surgery* London: Elsevier; 2009.

4. Baker DC, Conley J. Avoiding facial nerve injuries in rhytidectomy. Anatomical variations and pitfalls. *Plast Reconstr Surg*. 1979;64:781.

5. Baker DC. Complications of cervical rhytidectomy. *Clin Plast Surg*. 1983;10:543–562.

6. Baker DC. Lateral SMASectomy. *Plast Reconstr Surg*. 1997;100:509–513.

7. Baker DC. Lateral SMASectomy. *Semin Plast Surg*. 2002;16: 417–422.

8. Alpert BS, Baker DC, Hamra ST, et al. Identical twin face lifts with differing techniques: a 10-year follow-up. *Plast Reconstr Surg*. 2009;123:1025–1036.

11.6

Facelift: The extended SMAS technique in facial rejuvenation

James M. Stuzin

Introduction

Surgical rejuvenation of the aging face has evolved into one of the most frequently performed surgical procedures in the United States. Facelifting, initially performed as a skin tightening procedure since the early 1900s, has technically matured during the last quarter of a century. This evolution is directly related to the scientific investigation of facial soft tissue anatomy, resulting in a better understanding of the facial anatomic changes which occur with aging. Over the last 30 years, a plethora of procedures have evolved which utilize a variety of technical approaches, having as a common goal the reconstruction of aging-related anatomic changes.

Both the public's perception as well as the aesthetic concepts in facelifting have similarly evolved over time. Initially, both patients and surgeons focused solely on the laxity which occurs with facial aging, attempting to tighten what was loose rather than shape the face. Hence the term "facelift" (as opposed to "facialplasty"), a mechanical term implying a procedure, the goal of which is to lift what has fallen. Unfortunately, this mechanical approach to facial rejuvenation often produced a tight-appearing, operated look, the stigma of the "wind-tunnel appearance" so often associated with surgical rejuvenation of the aging face. Nonetheless, based on a better understanding of facial soft tissue anatomy and the anatomic changes which occur in aging, facelifting has developed into both a reconstructive procedure (whose goal is to reconstruct the anatomic changes which occur in aging) as well as a more artistically defined technique, which attempts to enhance facial appearance while minimizing signs that a surgical procedure, has been performed.

There are many treatment goals in facelifting besides simply correcting the hallmarks of the aging face, including improvement of the nasolabial folds, facial jowling and correction of obliquity of cervical contour. As important as the mechanical aspects of tightening a loose, aged face, are the aesthetic concepts of improving facial shape and bringing out the beauty in the face which existed during youth. To these goals, the surgeon attempting facial rejuvenation must have a thorough understanding of facial soft tissue anatomy, comprehend the anatomic changes which occur in aging which produce a change in facial shape, and understand the ideal facial shape which can be obtained for a particular patient. Artistic design of surgical access incisions to minimize scar perceptibility, as well as prevent hairline distortion, is also key in preventing surgical stigmata.

The evolution of aging in the human face is complex and multifactorial. Problems that the plastic surgeon confronts in midface rejuvenation include: (1) the dermal component of aging related to intrinsic and extrinsic skin changes (dermal elastosis); (2) facial fat descent; (3) facial deflation, which tends to be regionally specific; (4) radial expansion as facial fat becomes situated centrifugally away from the facial skeleton; and (5) the degree of skeletal support of the soft tissue which influences both loss of volumetric highlights, as well as the descent of facial fat.[1-4] All of these factors influence facial shape changes with aging. Individual patients will exhibit various degrees of these problems at the time they request surgery, and each component of the aging face should be addressed according to individual patient needs.

Evaluation of patient photographs taken during youth and middle age are helpful in determining how a specific patient has aged. Young photographs will usually demonstrate the location of the volumetric highlights present in youth, or serve to document areas which have deflated over time, delineating both the position and vector of facial fat descent. These factors illustrate patient-specific changes in facial shape from youth to middle age, as well as clarifying the possibilities of methods which facial fat repositioning can improve and restore shape. From my perspective, the restoration of facial shape is a more worthy aesthetic goal than attempting to tighten a loose face.

Anatomic considerations

The anatomic basis that allows rhytidectomy to be performed safely is that the facial soft tissue is arranged as a series of concentric layers. This concentric arrangement allows dissection within one anatomic plane to proceed completely separate from structures lying within another anatomic plane. The layers of the face are the: (1) skin; (2) subcutaneous fat; (3) SMAS (superficial facial fascia); (4) mimetic muscles; (5) parotidomasseteric fascia (deep facial fascia); and (6) plane of the facial nerve, parotid duct, buccal fat pad, and facial artery and vein. (This information is thoroughly reviewed in Chapter 6.)

In an overview of the architectural arrangement of the facial soft tissue, the essential point is that there is a superficial component of the facial soft tissue which is defined by the superficial facial fascia and includes the SMAS and those anatomic components which move facial skin (including superficially situated mimetic muscle invested by SMAS, the subcutaneous fat, and skin). This is in contrast to the deeper component of the facial soft tissue, which is defined by the deep facial fascia and those structures related to the deep fascia (including the relatively fixed structures of the face, such as the parotid gland, masseter muscle, periosteum of the facial bones, and facial nerve branches). As the human face ages, many of the stigmata which are typically seen in aging relate to a change in the anatomic relationship which occurs between the superficial and deep facial fascia. With aging, facial fat descends in the plane between superficial and deep facial fascia, and the radial expansion of the superficial soft tissue away from the facial skeleton occurs within this plane. In the author's opinion, these anatomic changes justify repositioning facial fat through subSMAS dissection to restore facial shape.[5,6]

Retaining ligaments

The communication between the superficial and deep facial fascia occurs at the level of the retaining ligaments which are discussed in Chapter 11.1. These structures fixate facial soft tissue in normal anatomic position, resisting gravitational forces.[1,7] In the evolution of midface aging, the zygomatic and masseteric cutaneous ligaments bear particular attention. The zygomatic ligaments originate from the periosteum of the malar region. Their function is to fixate the malar pad to the underlying zygomatic eminence in the youthful face.

Support of the soft tissues of the medial cheek is provided from a series of fibrous bands that extend along the entire anterior border of the masseter muscle. These are the "masseteric cutaneous ligaments", and are identified superiorly in the malar area where they mingle with the zygomatic ligaments and extend along the anterior border of the masseter as far inferiorly as the mandibular border. These fibers represent a coalescence between the superficial and deep fascia, extending from the masseter muscle vertically to insert into the overlying dermis. These masseteric ligaments support the soft tissues of the medial cheek superiorly above the mandibular border in youth.

The surgical significance of the retaining ligaments is that they represent the anatomic communication between superficial and deep facial fascia. As this support system becomes

attenuated, facial shape changes. The position of the retaining ligaments also dictates the degree of dissection required in a facelift. To adequately mobilize the skin flap, the dissection needs to be carried at least to the peripheral extent of the retaining ligament system, specifically dissecting the skin flap into the malar region, as well as past the anterior border of the masseter. Similarly, the location and restrictiveness of the retaining ligaments dictates the degree of SMAS elevation required to adequately release the superficial fascia. In general, this requires the surgeon to extend the SMAS dissection into the malar region, releasing the superficial fascia from the restraint of the zygomatic ligaments, the upper masseteric ligaments, as well as medial to the anterior border of the parotid.

Aesthetic analysis and treatment planning

As the human face ages, facial shape changes, morphologic facial changes are multifactorial. Some of these changes are straightforward to address, while others remain difficult technical challenges. A paradox has always been that facial anatomy (in terms of basic soft tissue architecture) is essentially unchanged from youth to middle-age, but facial appearance changes greatly over time and is patient specific. Although each face ages differently, there are common themes noted in all aging faces.

Descent of facial fat

As the human face ages, facial fat descends and with it facial shape changes. Typically, the youthful face is full of well-supported fat. Volumetric highlights are located within facial aesthetic subunits, which have a high density of retaining ligaments (zygomatic eminence and zygomatic arch, preparotid, orbital rim) and serve to fixate this volume of fat to underlying structures. Juxtaposed to the volumetric fullness (or convexity) of the malar and preparotid region is commonly a concavity within the submalar region, overlying the buccinator muscle and buccal recess. The combination of fullness in the malar region and lateral cheek, associated with submalar concavity and a well-defined mandibular border, accounts for the angular, tapered appearance of the youthful face.

With aging, facial fat can descend and produce significant changes in facial shape. In middle-age, as ligamentous support becomes attenuated, facial fat volumetrically becomes situated anteriorly and inferiorly in the cheek, producing a contour that is square and bottom heavy with little differential between malar highlights and submalar fat. As facial fat is situated more inferiorly in the face, middle-aged faces appear vertically longer than young faces *(Fig. 11.1.4)*.[3,4]

Volume loss and facial deflation

Youthful faces are full of well supported facial fat. Over time, deflation occurs, and tends to be most apparent in regions of the face with a high density of retaining ligaments. For this reason, the areas which are noted to be volumetrically full in

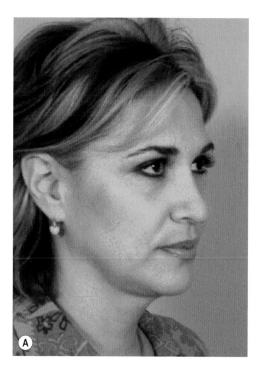
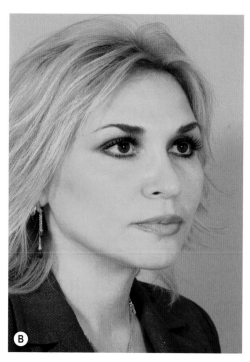

Fig. 11.6.1 (A) Preoperative appearance of a 42-year-old patient with early facial aging resulting primarily from deflation. Note the hollowing effect within the lateral cheek and preparotid region. Deflation in this young patient has occurred in the fat compartments lateral to the zygomaticus major muscle. **(B)** Postoperative result following face and necklift. Note, as anteriorly situated fat is brought into the upper lateral midface, it fills the areas of deflation, thereby blunting the lines of demarcation between aesthetic subunits which develop with age. Notice also the change in facial shape, which now appears more structured and supported following facial fat repositioning.

youth (malar, preparotid, lateral and infraorbital rim, lateral chin) become volumetrically deflated over time. With deflation, soft tissue becomes less supported and therefore appears lax. Youthful faces have a smooth blending of contour between the aesthetic subunits of the face. Middle-aged faces, secondary to both deflation and facial fat descent, develop lines of demarcation between one region of the face and another, which is intuitively identified as old. An accurate aesthetic treatment plan to improve facial shape requires repositioning descended soft tissue into areas of facial deflation to improve shape, not only by restoring volume to the position noted in youth, but also serving to blunt the lines of demarcation between aesthetic subunits. Volumetric augmentation through autologous fat injection or other injectable soft tissue fillers are ancillary agents, which can be useful in augmenting areas of deflation.

Deflation in the aging face is a complex process which tends to be regional and age-specific. Key elements in understanding how deflation occurs have been enlightened following an elucidation of the compartmentalization of subcutaneous fat within the cheek as defined by Rohrich and Pessa.[8] What these investigators realized was that the cheek subcutaneous fat, rather than being homogeneous, is compartmentalized, with each facial fat compartment surrounded by specific septal membranes and with each compartment having an independent perforator blood supply. Aesthetically, the significance of compartmentalization of facial fat is that deflation tends to occur within a specific region of the cheek, explaining why the entire cheek does not deflate homogeneously *(Fig. 11.6.1)*.

At the risk of over-simplification, one key to understanding facial deflation is the recognition of the location of zygomaticus major muscle, which traverses from the malar eminence to the oral commissure. Deflation of the cheek lateral to the zygomaticus major muscle tends to occur independently from deflation in the malar region, medial to the zygomaticus major. For many patients, lateral cheek deflation develops at an earlier age than malar pad deflation, and is often noted in patients in their forties. Medial cheek and malar pad deflation tend to occur later in life and is responsible not only for the loss of volumetric support within the anterior cheek, but also leads to the development of what has been termed the infraorbital V-deformity. Deflation in this region results in an apparent increase in the vertical length of the lower lid, as the lid–cheek junction visually descends inferiorly into the poorly supported anterior cheek *(Fig. 11.6.2)*.

An interesting region of deflation develops in some patients in the submalar region lateral to the oral commissure. In these patients, deflation can result in accentuation of the submalar concavity, which can become more obvious following the vertical soft tissue shifts associated with facelifting procedures. An accentuation of submalar depression lateral to the oral commissure can result in the development of what has been termed "joker lines" or cross-cheek depressions, which are a typical stigmata that a patient has undergone a facelift. Avoidance of vertical soft tissue repositioning in conjunction with volume addition in the submalar recess lateral to the oral commissure is useful in preventing the accentuation of postoperative cross-cheek depressions *(Fig. 11.6.3)*.[9]

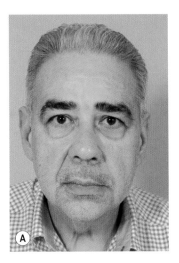
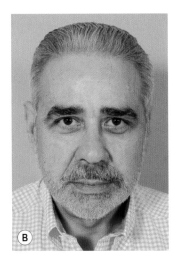
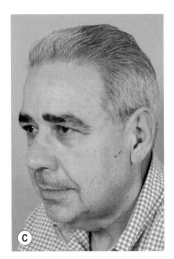
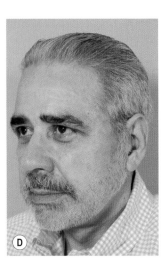

Fig. 11.6.2 (A,B) Preoperative appearance of a 59-year-old male following a 90 pound weight loss from a gastric bypass procedure. Notice the significant areas of facial deflation along the infraorbital rim, lateral orbital rim and malar region. Also note the apparent length of the lower lid as the infraorbital V-deformity develops in association with malar pad deflation. Note also the radial expansion of skin and fat lateral to the nasolabial fold, most marked on the right side. Not only does malar fat deflate and descend, but attenuation of the retinacular connections between skin, fat and deep facial fascia lateral to the nasolabial line allows centrifugal prolapse of soft tissue which accentuates nasolabial prominence. **(C,D)** Postoperative result. The areas of deflation along the infraorbital rim, lateral orbital rim, and malar region are improved as facial fat has been repositioned into these regions. The nasolabial folds are somewhat improved following malar pad repositioning, but correction is incomplete, especially on the right. Malar pad elevation helps to flatten the prominent nasolabial fold, and improve the infraorbital V-deformity, but does little to correct radial expansion, with the skin lateral to the nasolabial line remaining prolapsed from its attachments to the facial skeleton. (From Stuzin JM. Restoring facial shape in facelifting: The role of skeletal support in facial analysis and midface soft-tissue repositioning. Plast Reconstr Surg 2007;119:362.)

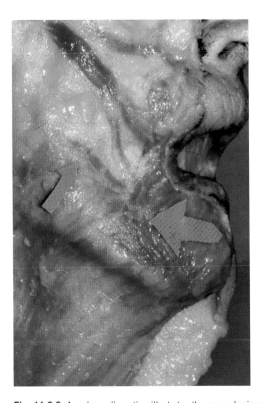

Fig. 11.6.3 A cadaver dissection illustrates the muscular insertions into the oral commissure and modiolus. The small arrow overlies the facial portion of the platysma, and points to the risorius muscle. The large arrow points to the depressor anguli oris in the region where it merges with the platysma. Superiorly, note the insertion of the zygomaticus major into the lateral commissure with a slip of muscle inserting inferiorly into the modiolus. Following deflation in this area, the medial component of the cross cheek depression develops in the watershed between the elevator and the depressors of the lip. (From Lambros V, Stuzin JM. The cross-cheek depression: surgical cause and effect in the development of the "Joker Line" and its treatment. Plast Reconstr Surg 2008;122:1543.)

Radial expansion

Not all facial aging is vertical and a major challenge in facial rejuvenation is the radial expansion of facial soft tissue which occurs along specific areas of the midface. In youth, the skin and underlying subcutaneous fat are densely attached to the deep facial fascia by retinacular fibers which transverse between skin, subcutaneous fat, superficial fascia and insert into the deep fascia and facial musculature. Over time, with prolonged animation such as smiling, the skin along the nasolabial line is forced deep to the subcutaneous fat, positioned lateral to the nasolabial fold, attenuating these retinacular attachments. Prolonged animation therefore forces the skin and fat lateral to the nasolabial fold to expand radially and prolapse outward from the facial skeleton, accounting for much of the nasolabial fold prominence in the aging face. Radial expansion lateral to the oral commissure and marionette line similarly accounts for the prominence of the jowl in many middle-aged patients, making the older face appear square in shape and bottom heavy.[4,10]

Radial expansion is technically difficult to correct, as there are few surgical solutions to re-establish the retinacular attachments between skin, subcutaneous fat and deep fascia. Nonetheless, repositioning of facial fat through some form of support to the superficial fascia will not only reposition fat vertically, but will also provide some degree of internal repositioning such that the superficial facial soft tissues lie closer to the facial skeleton. As the soft tissues become situated closer to the underlying deeper structures of the face, facial morphology tends to be restored to a more youthful configuration. Because of the technical difficulty to completely treat radial expansion in many faces, incomplete correction of both the jowl and nasolabial fold resulting in under-correction can be noted postoperatively despite heroic efforts at repositioning descended facial fat.

Role of skeletal support in formulating a surgical treatment plan

Facial shape and contour is intuitively evaluated when analyzing a patient for facial rejuvenation. Often the two-dimensional considerations seen in photographs are the easiest aspects of aging to identify, and such factors as nasolabial fold depth, jowl prominence, and cervical contour become the primary objectives to improve appearance in the middle-aged face. While these factors are certainly important considerations in treatment planning, the more subtle three-dimensional qualities of facial shape are equally important to evaluate, and are greatly influenced by underlying skeletal support.

In evaluating facial shape during preoperative analysis, there follow some of the major factors which are helpful to consider.[4]

Facial width, bizygomatic diameter, and malar volume

The emphasis in facelifting over the last 30 years has focused on malar pad elevation.[2,11–19] While malar pad elevation and restoration of malar highlights is an important factor in improving facial shape, it needs to be patient-specific. Many patients present preoperatively with wide faces, strong malar eminences and large malar volume, with little evidence of malar fat descent. In these individuals it is necessary to evaluate preoperatively the degree of malar pad elevation required to improve facial shape. While limited degrees of malar pad elevation can be helpful in patients who present with wide bizygomatic diameters, in general, if the malar volume is significantly enhanced in these types of individuals, the aesthetic effect is to make a wide face appear even wider on the front view postoperatively. In patients with adequate facial width, the author tends to limit both SMAS release and malar pad elevation to the lateral aspect of the zygomatic eminence such that bizygomatic diameter is not increased postoperatively *(Fig. 11.6.4)*.

Facial length and the relative vertical heights of the lower and middle-third of the face

Compared with wide faces, patients who present with vertical maxillary excess often have long, thin faces on front view. As facial fat descends in middle age, it becomes situated anteriorly and inferiorly in the face, and the face appears even longer with age. Malar pad elevation and enhancing malar volume in these types of patients is usually beneficial. As malar volume is enhanced and bizygomatic diameter is increased, the face appears wider on the front view, detracting from relatively excessive facial length *(Fig. 11.6.5)*.

Convexity of the malar region juxtaposed to the concavity of the submalar region

In youth, facial fat is situated overlying the malar and preparotid region. This malar fullness is juxtaposed to a concavity

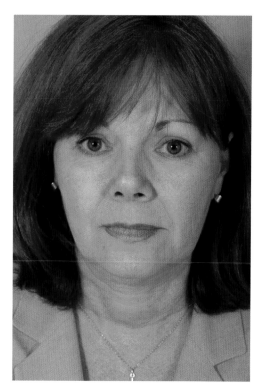

Fig. 11.6.4 Facial width and bizygomatic diameter reflect the underlying degree of skeletal support. Patients who exhibit strong malar eminences and wide bizygomatic diameter often benefit from having malar highlights restored, but usually do not require significantly enhancing malar volume (which will cause a wide face to appear wider postoperatively). Shaping considerations in these types of faces usually focus on improving the appearance of the lower two-thirds of the cheek, specifically addressing jowl fat repositioning, as well as creating submalar hollowing which improves the aesthetic relationship between malar and submalar regions. (From Stuzin JM. Restoring facial shape in facelifting: The role of skeletal support in facial analysis and midface soft-tissue repositioning. Plast Reconstr Surg 2007;119:362.)

within the submalar region overlying the buccinator. As patients age, the relationship between the malar and submalar regions changes and with it, facial shape changes. As facial fat descends and facial deflation occurs, there is less volume overlying the malar eminence and an associated increase in fullness resulting from radial expansion within the submalar region. As the aesthetic relationship between the malar and submalar region becomes modified with time, there is a loss of the angular, tapered configuration in shape noted in youth, and middle-aged faces often appear oval. With greater facial fat descent, and an increase in submalar fullness, older faces appear square.

Preoperatively, an evaluation of the relationship between the malar and submalar region on front view is an essential component of aesthetic treatment planning. For many patients, a restoration in this relationship by increasing malar highlights and malar volume, in association with a restoration of concavity in the submalar region through repositioning fat internally overlying the buccinator muscle becomes a central component in improving facial shape *(Figs 11.6.6, 11.6.7)*.

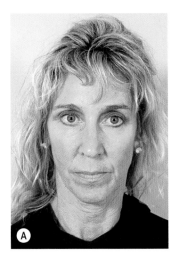
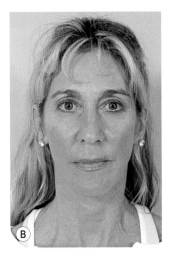
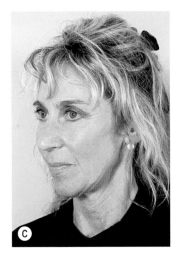
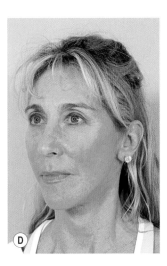

Fig. 11.6.5 Long, thin faces often benefit from an enhancement of malar volume. SMAS dissection and facial fat repositioning carried anteriorly over the zygomatic eminence allows the surgeon to restore malar volume, thereby increasing bizygomatic diameter. When malar volume is enhanced, the face appears wider, detracting from the relatively excessive facial length. (From Stuzin JM. Restoring facial shape in facelifting: The role of skeletal support in facial analysis and midface soft-tissue repositioning. Plast Reconstr Surg 2007;119:362.)

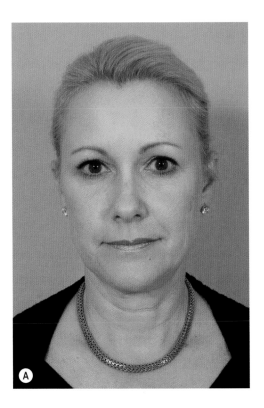
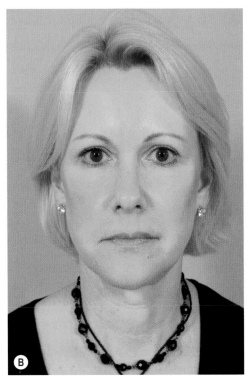

Fig. 11.6.6 (A) Preoperative appearance. Note that facial shape is oval, secondary to malar deflation associated with an increase in submalar fullness. **(B)** Postoperatively, following malar pad elevation, malar volume is enhanced in association with a restoration of submalar concavity, producing a more angular appearance to facial shape. (From Stuzin JM. Restoring facial shape in facelifting: The role of skeletal support in facial analysis and midface soft-tissue repositioning. Plast Reconstr Surg 2007;119:362.)

The vertical height of the mandibular ramus and the horizontal length of the mandibular body

The vertical height of the mandibular ramus and the horizontal length of the mandibular body provide skeletal support for the lower two-thirds of the face. Patients who present with a normal mandibular ramus height, as well as adequate horizontal length of the mandibular body, usually have excellent skeletal support for soft tissue repositioning and are, therefore, less of a surgical challenge. In contradistinction, patients with a short mandibular ramus, an open mandibular plane angle and a short length of the mandibular body typically have poor skeletal support for midface and perioral soft tissue repositioning. These patients are a greater surgical challenge in restoring facial shape, and often benefit from volumetric augmentation, either alloplastic or autogenous, to enhance skeletal support.

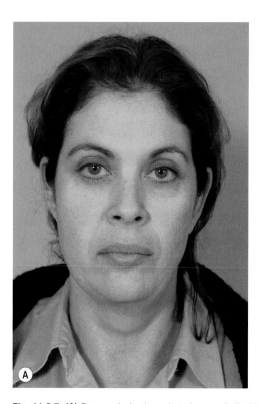
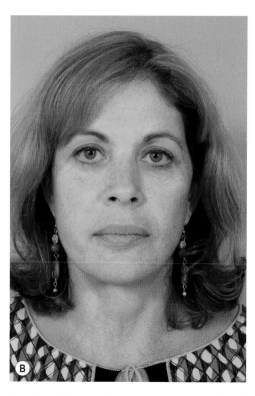

Fig. 11.6.7 **(A)** Preoperatively, the patient shows a similar blunting of the relationship between the malar and submalar regions. **(B)** Postoperative appearance. Enhancing malar volume (and bizygomatic diameter) and restoring the concavity within the submalar region make the face appear more angular, as well as vertically shorter. (From Stuzin JM. Restoring facial shape in facelifting: The role of skeletal support in facial analysis and midface soft-tissue repositioning. Plast Reconstr Surg 2007;119:362.)

The aesthetic advantages of formal SMAS elevation in a two-layer dual plane SMAS facelift

All modern techniques share a commonality in that postoperative contour is largely dependent on facial fat repositioning through some form of SMAS manipulation. The advantage of formal SMAS flap elevation lies in its aesthetic versatility. Once the superficial fascia has been freed from the restraint of the retaining ligaments, it offers the surgeon several advantages, including: (1) vector versatility; (2) greater control in terms of long-term vertical facial fat repositioning; and (3) greater control in terms of long-term internal facial fat repositioning.

Regarding vector versatility, dermal elastosis and skin laxity in the aging face often does not occur in the same direction nor at the same rate as aging related to the descent of fat. The main advantages of performing skin dissection separate from SMAS dissection is that it allows these two layers to be draped along vectors which are independent of one another *(Fig. 11.6.8)*.[2,19–21] Another advantage of a two-layer SMAS facelift is that the tension of contouring is placed on the superficial fascia, thereby allowing the surgeon to use less tension for skin closure. This improves control regarding scar perceptibility.[20,21] In terms of vectors, in the author's experience, facial fat is commonly repositioned in a more vertical vector than skin flap redraping. Strong vertical shifting of the cervicofacial flap is a maneuver that has traditionally been utilized in many facelift techniques. While skin tightening can produce a dramatic effect in terms of improvement of facial laxity, the

aesthetic effects of vertical skin vectoring unfortunately have been poorly delineated. Specifically, when skin is shifted in a cephalad direction, the effect of skin tension commonly produces an accentuation of flatness in the preparotid region, an area that typically deflates with aging. In my opinion, vertical skin shifting can produce an unnatural tightness to facial shape, producing some of the typical stigmata associated with rhytidectomy. If the surgeon has been successful in repositioning descended facial fat, the use of strong vertical skin tension is neither desirable nor required to enhance the postoperative result *(Fig. 11.6.9)*.

Surgical technique: extended SMAS dissection

Restoration of support to the underlying deeper facial soft tissues has become the key ingredient to the approach to improve facial aging. If the SMAS is thin, plication is an alternative method. Nonetheless, better contouring and longer lasting results are obtained following a formal dissection of the superficial fascia. In the author's experience, after the superficial fascia is freed from the restraint of the retaining ligament, it slides freely, allowing greater control in vertically repositioning of facial fat. Full release of the SMAS also allows the superficial fascia to better conform internally to the underlying deeper facial soft tissue and facial skeleton. Greater control of internal fat repositioning provides for more complete correction of radial expansion.

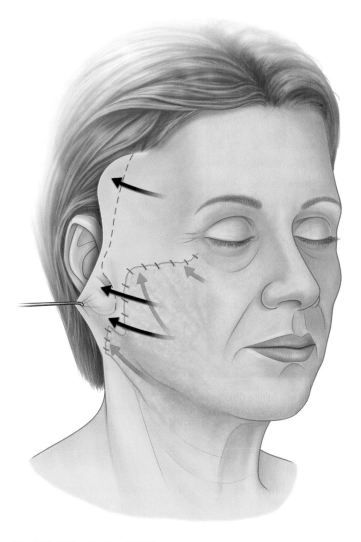

Fig. 11.6.8 The direction of SMAS redraping in the face tends to be cephalad in its orientation as opposed to skin flap redraping, which is oriented along a more horizontal vector. The aesthetic versatility of vectoring the SMAS in a direction independent of skin flap redraping is a major advantage of a two-layer SMAS-type facelift.

The key to performing successful dissection of an extended SMAS flap is precise dissection of the skin flaps during subcutaneous undermining, with care to leave a moderate amount of fat intact on the superficial surface of the SMAS, especially in the regions where the SMAS is to be dissected. If the skin flaps are dissected so that little fat is left along the superficial surface of the SMAS, the SMAS becomes more difficult to raise, appearing thin, tenuous and prone to tearing. In a SMAS-type facelift, much of the contouring that is obtained is due to elevation and fixation of the SMAS layer. The more substantial the SMAS flap, often the better long-term results that can be obtained in terms of facial contouring. The use of contralateral transillumination is helpful in providing a clearer definition of the interface between subcutaneous fat and superficial fascia, allowing for greater precision in skin flap elevation.

Preoperatively, I (the author) decide the extent of subcutaneous skin flap undermining based on the most medial aspect of where I want to end the SMAS dissection, which typically is situated just medial to the retaining ligaments. I prefer to limit the skin undermining several centimeters lateral to the nasolabial fold rather than undermining the skin to this facial landmark. The reason is that if one limits the dissection of the skin flap in the medial aspect of the cheek, this will preserve some of the attachments that go from the deep fascia through the SMAS to facial skin. The preservation of these attachments, followed by adequate undermining of the superficial facial fascia (SMAS), will allow the surgeon to re-elevate anteriorly displaced fat and skin through SMAS rotation rather than to redrape the superficial fascia completely independent of skin flap redraping. The ability to re-elevate and resuspend facial soft tissue through SMAS rotation produces a more pleasing aesthetic result and a greater degree of correction of radial expansion within the cheek, as the facial fat is brought internally to conform to the underlying buccinator muscle (*Fig. 11.6.10*).

SMAS elevation

The dissection of the superficial fascia allows the surgeon to re-elevate jowl and descended malar fat back upwards into the face toward their previous, normal anatomic location.[2,5] In patients with prominent nasolabial folds and significant infraorbital hollowing, it is my feeling that the SMAS dissection should extend into the malar region in an effort to re-elevate the malar fat pad back upward overlying the zygomatic eminence. An added benefit of performing a more extensive anterior dissection of the SMAS is that it frees this layer from the restraint of both the zygomatic and masseteric ligaments, and this anterior release provides for a more complete elevation of the facial fat below the oral commissure and along the anterior portion of the jowl.

The incisions (*Fig. 11.6.11*) for extended SMAS dissection begin approximately 1 cm inferior to the zygomatic arch to ensure frontal branch preservation. This horizontal incision is continued several centimeters forward to the region where the zygomatic arch joins the body of the zygoma. At this point, the malar extension of the SMAS dissection begins with the incision angling superiorly over the malar eminence toward the lateral canthus for a distance of 3–4 cm. On reaching the edge of the subcutaneous skin flap in the region of the lateral orbit, the incision is carried inferiorly at a 90° angle toward the superior aspect of the nasolabial fold. A vertical incision is designed along the preauricular region, extending along the posterior border of the platysma to a point 5–6 cm below the mandibular border. In essence, the malar extension of the SMAS dissection simply represents an extension of a standard SMAS dissection into the malar region in an attempt to obtain a more complete form of deep layer support.

The SMAS in the malar region is then elevated in continuity with the SMAS of the cheek. When elevating this flap, the fibers of the orbicularis oculi, as well as the zygomaticus major and minor, are usually evident and the flap is elevated directly along the superficial surface of these muscles. It is important to carry the dissection directly external to these muscle fibers, where a natural plane exists, remembering that the facial nerve branches lie deep to these muscular bellies. The malar SMAS is then elevated until the flap is freed from the underlying zygomatic prominence. Freeing of the SMAS completely from the zygomatic attachments is

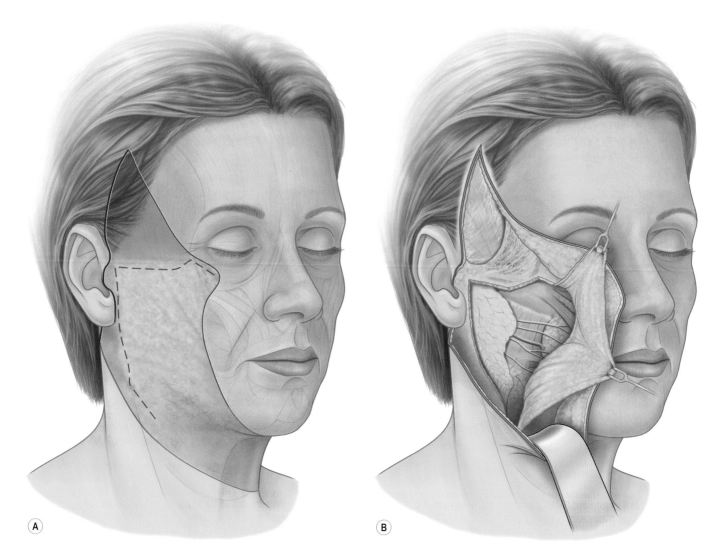

(A)   (B)

Fig. 11.6.11 (A) In patients with malar deflation or malar pad descent, the author typically performs what is termed an extended SMAS dissection. By this, I mean I extend the SMAS dissection into the malar region in an attempt to re-elevate ptotic malar fat back upward over the zygomatic prominence. The incisions begin at the junction where the zygomatic arch joins the body of the zygoma. From this point, the incision in the SMAS is angled superiorly toward the lateral canthus and along the lateral orbital rim. The incision in the SMAS is then carried medially and inferiorly toward the peripheral extent of skin flap undermining, angling toward the uppermost portion of the nasolabial fold (the amount of subcutaneous undermining is shaded in pink, whereas the amount of SMAS undermining is shaded in yellow.) **(B)** The malar-SMAS dissection is then performed in continuity with the cheek-SMAS dissection. Dissecting in the malar region carries the dissection directly along the superficial surface of the zygomaticus major and usually exposes the lateral aspects of the zygomaticus minor as well. To obtain adequate mobility in terms of SMAS dissection, it is necessary to elevate the malar portion of the dissection completely from the zygomatic eminence and free it from the zygomatic ligaments. To obtain mobility in terms of SMAS movement affecting the jowl contour, the uppermost portions of the masseteric cutaneous ligament commonly are divided, especially where they merge with the zygomatic ligaments of the malar area. If these fibers are not divided, they will restrict the upward redraping of jowl fat. On division of the upper portion of the masseteric cutaneous ligaments, the buccal fat pad becomes evident, and commonly the zygomatic nerve branches traversing toward the undersurface of the zygomaticus major muscle are visualized. This diagram illustrates the typical degree of mobilization performed in our extended SMAS dissection.

Variations in extended SMAS technique to affect a restoration in facial shape

The biomechanics of SMAS repositioning have been previously described and are influenced by the degree of release, vector of fat repositioning and how the superficial fascia is fixated.[22] As postoperative contour is dependent on each of these factors, preoperative planning needs to be patient-specific in terms of the degree of SMAS release required, the vectors in which facial fat is repositioned, and the location and method for SMAS fixation.

Release

The incision design of an extended SMAS dissection allows for complete release of the SMAS from its underlying retaining ligamentous attachment in the lateral midface. As surgeons, there is a tendency to believe that a greater degree of SMAS dissection equates with a better result, but this

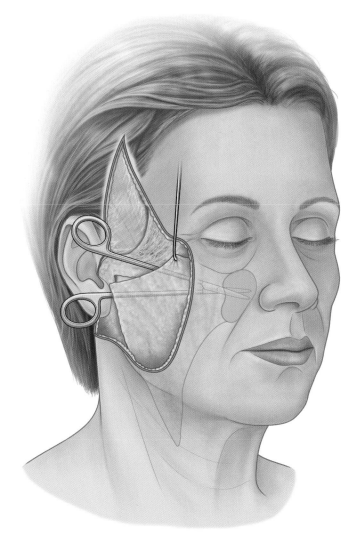

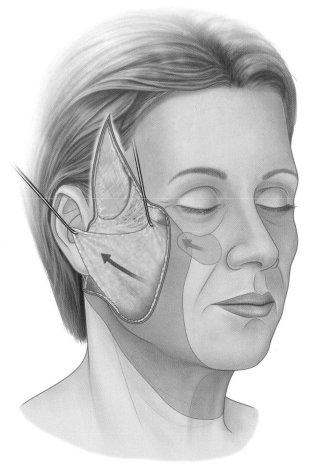

Fig. 11.6.13 The vectors of redraping of the extended SMAS flap are determined according to the preoperative evaluation of the patient and are generally more cephalad than skin flap redraping.

Fig. 11.6.12 It is commonly necessary to extend the malar SMAS dissection more peripherally than the subcutaneous dissection to obtain adequate flap mobility of the soft tissues lateral to the nasolabial fold. This portion of the dissection is easily performed by simply inserting the scissors in the plane between the superficial surface of the elevators of the upper lip and the overlying subcutaneous fat. Once the scissors are inserted in the proper plane, the surgeon bluntly dissects in a series of passes past the nasolabial fold (area marked in green). As long as the scissors remain superficial to the elevators of the upper lip, motor nerve injury will be prevented. Usually three or four passes are required to obtain adequate flap mobility.

has not been my experience. Rather, precision in the degree of SMAS dissection and its release from the retaining ligaments as dictated by the aesthetic needs of a patient increases surgical control and consistency in while minimizing morbidity.[3]

How much to release the SMAS, and how high and anterior to carry the SMAS dissection, needs to be decided preoperatively. As discussed previously, in patients who present with adequate malar volume, wide bizygomatic diameter and little evidence of malar pad descent, it is usually unnecessary to carry the SMAS dissection medial to the lateral orbital rim (although the author usually carries the dissection high within the malar eminence to allow fat repositioning along the

infraorbital and lateral orbital rims). Most commonly, these types of patients require only a restoration of malar highlight and not significant anterior malar volume enhancement. Limiting the SMAS dissection to the lateral aspect of the malar eminence will not increase facial width on the front view.[4] Typically, the shaping considerations for these patients is focused on reducing fullness in the submalar region (*Fig. 11.6.14*).

Vertically long faces often benefit from carrying the malar portion of the extended SMAS dissection anteriorly, medial to the lateral orbital rim so that malar volume restoration is performed along the anterior aspect of the zygomatic eminence. Carrying the SMAS dissection more medially allows the surgeon to enhance malar volume and restore malar highlights anteriorly over the zygomatic eminence, thereby increasing facial width on the front view (*Fig. 11.6.15*).

Vectors of fat elevation: facial asymmetry

All patients exhibit some degree of facial asymmetry. Commonly, one side of the face is vertically longer and the

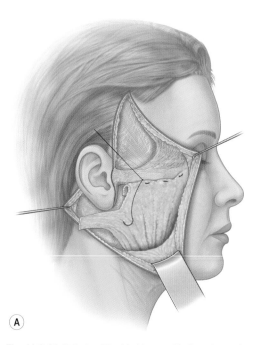

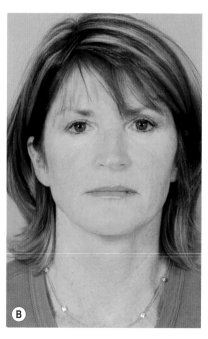

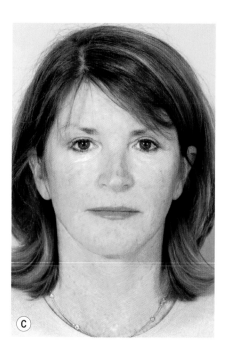

Fig. 11.6.14 Patients with wide bizygomatic diameters and good underlying skeletal support typically do not require a significant anterior malar dissection to improve facial shape. Most commonly, the SMAS dissection in these patients (while kept high), is extended only as medial as the lateral orbital rim, so that malar volume restoration is limited to the lateral aspect of the zygomatic eminence. The shaping considerations for these types of faces usually emphasize reducing fullness within the submalar area, as well as jowl fat elevation. Notice that postoperatively the patient's face appears more tapered and thinner in morphology through facial fat repositioning without removal of facial fat. (From Stuzin JM. Restoring facial shape in facelifting: The role of skeletal support in facial analysis and midface soft-tissue repositioning. Plast Reconstr Surg 2007;119:362.)

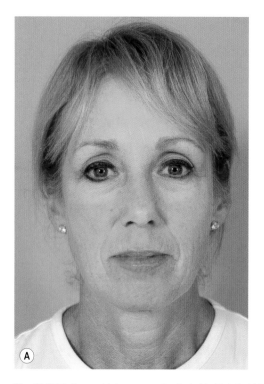

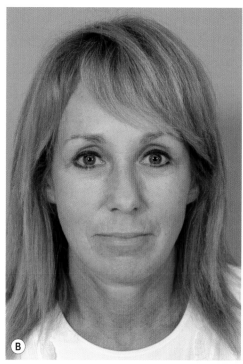

Fig. 11.6.15 Faces which are more dominated by their facial length (especially the lower third of the face) usually benefit from malar volume restoration. To enhance malar volume requires the SMAS dissection be carried toward the anterior aspect of the zygomatic eminence, such that malar volume is increased in this region. (From Stuzin JM. Restoring facial shape in facelifting: The role of skeletal support in facial analysis and midface soft-tissue repositioning. Plast Reconstr Surg 2007;119:362.)

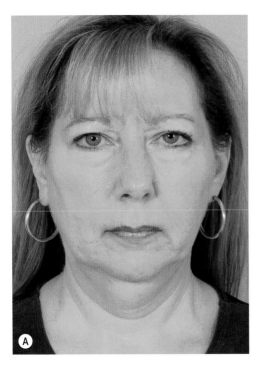 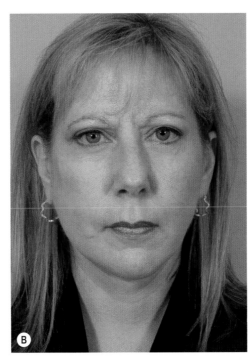

Fig. 11.6.16 Vectors of SMAS elevation have a significant impact on facial shape. Vertical repositioning of the SMAS allows the surgeon to enhance malar volume and reduce fullness within the submalar region, as fat is forced up along the concavity of the buccinator. Restoration of submalar hollowing through SMAS vectoring is useful in contouring full faces, making them appear thinner postoperatively. In this patient, a small amount of jowl defatting through needle aspiration was also performed. (From Stuzin JM. Restoring facial shape in facelifting: The role of skeletal support in facial analysis and midface soft-tissue repositioning. Plast Reconstr Surg 2007;119:362.)

short side of the face is usually wider than the long side. Malar highlights are typically more superiorly located on the long side of the face and, with age, facial fat tends to descend in a more vertical direction on the long side. As facial asymmetry and facial skeletal configuration are asymmetric in most individuals, it follows that the vectors of fat elevation (SMAS repositioning) should be specific for the right and the left side of the face.

The vector in which the SMAS is repositioned has a significant impact on the location and volume of elevated facial fat, thereby influencing facial shape. Decisions regarding the direction of SMAS vectoring for the right and left side of the face are best determined preoperatively, as it is very difficult to make aesthetic vector judgments intraoperatively with the patient recumbent.

SMAS vectors influence postoperative facial shape. Vertical SMAS repositioning typically provides a larger amount of fat for malar eminence enhancement, as well as allowing for a reduction in fullness within the sub-malar region as fat is forced internally along the concavity of the buccinator. For this reason, vertical SMAS vectors are often indicated to reshape round, full faces, allowing them to appear more tapered and thinner postoperatively *(Fig. 11.6.16)*. If the SMAS is vectored more obliquely, there is less volume of fat brought into the malar region and a greater volume of fat repositioned into the submalar region. Oblique SMAS repositioning is therefore helpful in elderly patients who appear gaunt over the buccal recess, as it allows the surgeon to volumetrically enhance the submalar region *(Fig. 11.6.17)*.

SMAS fixation

In a two-layer SMAS-type facelift, the tension of contouring is placed on the superficial fascia rather than the skin envelope. For this reason, the fascial quality and tensile strength of the superficial fascia has an influence on both the longevity of result, as well as the volume of fat which can be repositioned intraoperatively and maintained postoperatively. In other words, soft tissue quality influences long term contour, and is the primary reason why facelifts in young patients are more predictable.

In an effort to improve fascial quality in a SMAS facelift, for over a decade I incorporated Vicryl mesh into the SMAS fixation.[3] It was my initial observation that incorporating Vicryl mesh into fixation improved not only longevity of result, but greater aesthetic control. Nonetheless, I have stopped using Vicryl mesh, as I have come to realize that what was the predominant factor in improving fixation is the method in which the superficial fascia was secured. Obtaining a secure fixation utilizing multiple sutures placed deeply within the superficial fascia allows the surgeon greater control in postoperative shape. Suturing the SMAS securely under moderate tension affects facial shape in two ways: (1) adding more sutures allows the surgeon to stack volume in specific areas of the midface, which is useful in augmenting areas of deflation, as well as augmenting volume along the malar eminence; (2) as the superficial fascia is sutured under tension, facial fat is not only repositioned vertically, but also

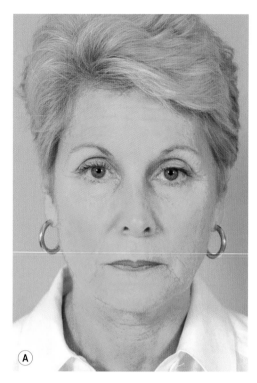
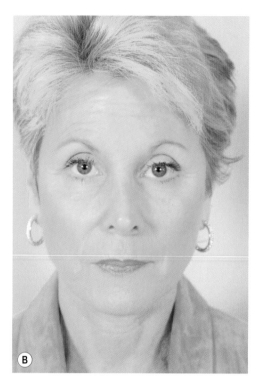

Fig. 11.6.17 This patient exhibits asymmetry in the submalar region preoperatively. Notice that she appears hollow and concave on the right, while she is fuller on the left side. For this reason, the SMAS was vectored obliquely on the right to volumetrically enhance the submalar region, while it was vertically vectored on the left side to restore submalar hollowing and balance the two sides of her face. (From Stuzin JM. Restoring facial shape in facelifting: The role of skeletal support in facial analysis and midface soft-tissue repositioning. Plast Reconstr Surg 2007;119:362.)

repositioned internally, forcing the soft tissue to conform to the underlying deep facial structures. This gives the surgeon greater control in improving radial expansion *(Fig. 11.6.18)*.

Correction of platysma bands and cervical obliquity

Correction of the neck is thoroughly reviewed in Chapter 13. In the author's hands, the best approach to the anterior platysma is via a submental incision, placed just caudal to the submental skin crease.[5,23–26] If this crease is very deep, the skin cephalad is elevated toward the base of the chin pad and along the caudal mandibular border to free any retaining mandibular ligaments, which tend to accentuate the crease. Following this, the cervical skin is carefully elevated. The cervical skin is usually undermined at least to the level of the cricoid.

Upon exposing the platysma muscle anteriorly, most patients exhibit a decussation of platysmal fibers across the midline, at least for a few centimeters below the mentum. When platysma band surgery is contemplated, these decussating fibers must be sharply divided with scissor dissection directly in the midline. Following this, the medial edge of the platysma is mobilized from the mentum inferiorly at least to the hyoid and commonly as caudal as the cricoid cartilage. Mobilization, usually performed using a combination of sharp and blunt dissection, separates the platysma from the

underlying subplatysmal fat, the anterior belly of the digastric muscle, and the strap muscles overlying the thyroid cartilage. At times, numerous small venules are encountered within the subplatysmal fat and careful hemostasis must be obtained. Following mobilization of the medial edges of the platysma, the subplatysmal fat is conservatively contoured according to preoperative planning.

Following mobilization, the medial edge of the platysma muscle is grasped on either side and overlapped in the midline in order to estimate the amount of excess muscle present. Muscle excess will vary from patient to patient. A portion of the medial edge can be excised to remove redundancy within the platysma. A conservative resection is performed so that undue tension is not present at the time of suture plication.

Muscular plication consists of edge-to-edge approximation using multiple interrupted sutures at the mentum and extending at least to the level of the hyoid. Suture placement back from the leading edge of the muscle, in areas of intact muscular fascia, is an important technical point in preventing suture pull-through postoperatively.

In most patients, the edge-to-edge suturing below the hyoid is continued inferiorly toward the cricoid cartilage. The goal of muscular plication is to produce an even, smooth contouring of the platysma that is tightly adherent to the underlying floor of the mouth and thyroid cartilage, providing a flat framework for redraping of cervical skin. A low plication joining a widely separated platysma over a prominent thyroid cartilage also tends to blunt a prominent larynx and produce a rounder, more feminine appearance to the neck.

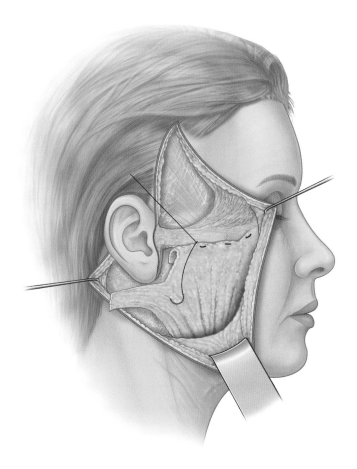

Fig. 11.6.18 This diagram illustrates how the excess SMAS, rather than being excised, is rolled onto itself to form a double layer of SMAS thickness. Once the SMAS has been rolled, it is fixated to the periosteum of the zygomatic eminence. An added benefit of preserving the excess SMAS rather than excising it is that, as the thickened SMAS layer is secured to the zygomatic eminence, it highlights the malar region, serving as an autogenous malar augmentation. Highlighting the malar area tends to enhance angularity in facial contour. (From Stuzin JM. Restoring facial shape in facelifting: The role of skeletal support in facial analysis and midface soft-tissue repositioning. Plast Reconstr Surg 2007;119:362.)

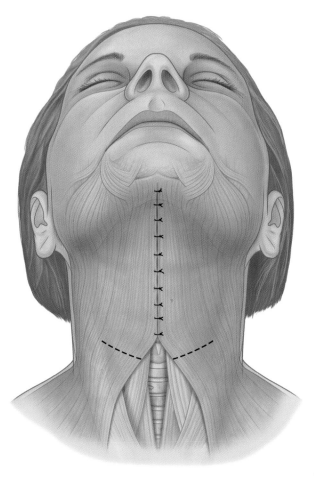

Fig. 11.6.19 After edge-edge approximation of the platysma from the mentum to the cricoid cartilage, some form of muscular release is performed. This usually consists of a horizontal cut extending from the midline to the anterior border of the sternocleidomastoid muscle.

Following edge-to-edge approximation of the platysma, some form of muscular release is performed. This muscular release commonly involves a partial transection of the platysma muscle with the myotomy performed inferiorly within the neck.

Platysma transection is an effective technique in the treatment of platysma bands and in obtaining the desired cervical contour. This procedure must be performed meticulously because the early experience with transection was fraught with complications. Specifically, if the transection is performed at a high level, it can be associated with unveiling of the submaxillary glands and denervation of the platysma associated with lower lip dysfunction. Also, obvious contour depressions associated with divided muscular edges can be noted in the overly thin neck *(Fig. 11.6.19)*.

The key to platysma transection is that the transection of the muscle be performed lower in the neck, often as inferior as the level of the cricoid cartilage. The disadvantage of horizontal transection at this level is that a depression in the neck can develop if preplatysmal fat has been removed at the level

where the transection is performed. Preservation of preplatysmal fat lower in the neck where the transection is to be performed is obviously an important factor in preventing this problem.

In most patients, only partial division is required. The myotomy is performed from the midline laterally until the tension is completely released from the platysmaplasty closure (approximately the anterior border of the sternocleidomastoid muscle in most patients).

The muscular release seen following platysma transection serves many purposes:

1. It alleviates tension along the medial portion of the platysma transection following plication.

2. It allows the platysma to shift superiorly, producing a deeper cervicomental angle.

3. It prevents the conversion of two platysmal bands to a single band following edge-to-edge approximation, which can be visible when the neck is extended.

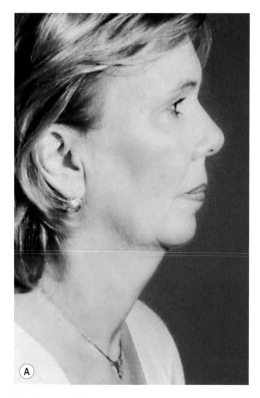
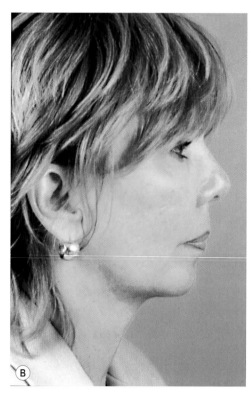

Fig. 11.6.20 **(A)** Preoperative appearance. Note the hollowed contour in the lateral cheek, which represents the region from which the facial fat has descended and deflated, as well as the marked cervical obliquity. **(B)** Postoperative result following extended SMAS dissection. If the surgeon can re-elevate descended facial fat back to its previous anatomic location and secure it there postoperatively, this will help to enhance the mandibular border, providing for predictable cervical contouring through platysmaplasty. This lessens the need for preplatysmal fat removal. In general, necks look softer if cervical fat is preserved. (From Stuzin JM, Baker TJ, Baker TM. Refinements in facelifting: Enhanced facial contour using Vicryl mesh incorporated into SMAS fixation. Plast Reconstr Surg 2000;105:290.)

In most patients in whom I perform a platysmaplasty, small drains are placed and left in place until drainage is minimal and the skin flaps are adherent. In my experience, the use of drains has lessened postoperative edema, ecchymosis and seroma formation *(Fig. 11.6.20)*.

Sequence of SMAS fixation versus platysmaplasty

Because the SMAS and the platysma represent the same anatomic layer, if platysmaplasty is performed before the SMAS dissection, it can adversely affect facial contour.[3,20,21] Contouring the neck before the midface can also be problematic. When the platysmaplasty is performed first, the descended jowl fat is locked down into the neck, and movement of the superficial fascia diminishes following elevation of the SMAS. This diminished movement tends to lessen surgical ability to modify facial shape; it also produces a loss of aesthetic contour. If the SMAS dissection is performed before platysmaplasty, descended jowl fat is brought cephalad to the mandibular border and easily repositioned. After the SMAS has been securely sutured bilaterally, the mandibular border appears more distinct, making cervical contouring less demanding. When performing platysmaplasty subsequent to SMAS

fixation, the surgeon will notice less redundancy along the medial borders of the platysma; there is also less need to resect muscle at the time of platysmaplasty. The enhanced contour effects of extended SMAS dissection, associated with precise platysmaplasty, tend to diminish the need to remove cervical fat. In general, the neck and jaw lines appear softer if preplatysmal fat is preserved when contouring the neck *(Fig. 11.6.21)*.

Incisions

Incisions have been reviewed in Chapter 11.1. The importance of incision quality cannot be over-emphasized in diminishing signs that the patient has undergone a surgical procedure. One of the major advantages of a two-layer facelift is that the tension of contouring is along the superficial fascia and thus there is less need to redrape the skin flap with great force. Decreased tension on the key sutures in both the preauricular and postauricular region provides greater control for scar perceptibility. If the incisions are artistically designed, patients can typically wear their hair up off their ears without obvious stigma that a facelift has been performed.[21]

Whereas many authors have described the salient factors regarding incision design, we would delineate the main points:

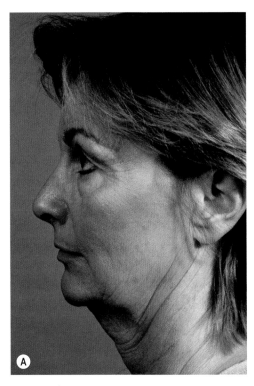 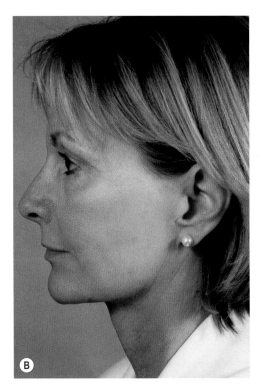

Fig. 11.6.21 (A) Preoperative appearance. **(B)** Postoperative appearance. Another example of how facial fat re-elevation influences cervical appearance. Sequencing errors can lead to loss in contour; it is my preference to perform SMAS elevation and fixation before performing platysmaplasty. As the facial fat and skin is re-elevated back into the midface through SMAS rotation, the mandibular border becomes more distinct, making cervical contouring more predictable.

1. The author prefers tragal incisions, performed at the margin of the tragus, rather than preauricular incisions, because the color difference between the pale skin of the ear and the blush skin of the cheek is usually better camouflaged when the incision is brought internally into the ear.

2. Tragal incisions are more demanding than preauricular incisions, requiring precise design and insert so that the tragus is not distorted. The aesthetic unit of the tragus is rectangular as opposed to semilunar. If the surgeon designs the tragal incision properly, respecting the incisura of the tragus, the tragus will appear normal in its shape postoperatively, exhibiting both a visual beginning at its junction with the helix and a visual ending along the preserved incisura.

3. Detached earlobes tend to appear more natural than attached earlobes. If a small cuff of cheek skin is left attached to the earlobe, it will allow surgical rotation of the skin up under the earlobe during skin flap redraping, suturing the earlobe distinctly from the cheek flap. The earlobe should be inset in an axis posterior to the axis of the pinna, thereby avoiding a pixie deformity.

There is increasing public demand for natural appearing results in facial rejuvenation. This places the onus on the surgeon to create incisions that are imperceptible if these procedures are to be justified. No matter how well deep-layer support is obtained, and facial contour improved by SMAS elevation and platysmaplasty, if the incision is obvious, scar quality poor, the hairline disturbed, or the earlobe deformed, the overall result remains disappointing

Summary

From a personal perspective, after two decades of striving to improve techniques in facial rejuvenation, it is my firm conviction that improving technical control when contouring the superficial facial fascia and platysma provides for a more consistent, aesthetically pleasing result, which is non-surgical in appearance. The difficulty in performing a two-layer SMAS-type facelift is that it requires a commitment on the part of the surgeon, not only to understand facial soft tissue anatomy, but also to perform a procedure which demands technical precision. A two-layer SMAS-type facelift is a time consuming operation, with both the skin flap elevation, as well as the dissection of the SMAS, requiring meticulous and accurate dissection. Obtaining consistency with this procedure is challenging because of the variability in thickness of subcutaneous fat and the SMAS which exists among individual patients. Following precise dissection, secure fixation of both SMAS and platysma is mandated to maintain the shaping desired in postoperative contour. Meticulous hemostasis followed by careful skin flap inset are required to minimize postoperative scar perceptibility and ensure a rapid postoperative recovery.

Despite these demands, this author has found the extended SMAS technique to be personally rewarding, with a high degree of patient satisfaction. All techniques have advantages and disadvantages. For me, the biggest advantage of the extended SMAS technique remains its aesthetic versatility, allowing the surgeon to vary the contouring aspects of the procedure according to the aesthetic needs of the patient.

Access the complete references list online at **http://www.expertconsult.com**

1. Stuzin JM, Baker TJ, Gordon HL, et al. Extended SMAS dissection as an approach to midface rejuvenation. *Clin Plast Surg.* 1995;22:295.

2. Stuzin JM, Baker TJ, Gordon HL. The relationship of the superficial and deep facial fascias: Relevance to rhytidectomy and aging. *Plast Reconstr Surg.* 1992;89:441.

   Facial anatomy is characterized as a series of concentric layers based on cadaveric and intraoperative dissection. These findings inform a discussion of the anatomic basis of facial aging.

4. Stuzin JM. Restoring facial shape in facelifting: The role of skeletal support in facial analysis and midface soft-tissue repositioning. *Plast Reconstr Surg.* 2007;119: 362.

   The authors emphasize the importance of establishing patient-specific aesthetic goals in planning a facelift. Skeletal anatomy is a key component of this analysis.

7. Furnas DW. The retaining ligaments of the cheek. *Plast Reconstr Surg.* 1989;83:11.

   The anatomy of the facial retaining ligaments is reviewed. The importance of addressing these structures in facelift procedures is addressed.

8. Rohrich RJ, Pessa JE. The fat compartments of the face: Anatomy and clinical implications for cosmetic surgery. *Plast Reconstr Surg.* 2007;119:2219.

   Cadaveric dissection demonstrated multiple discrete compartments of subcutaneous fat in the human face. The clinical significance of this finding is addressed.

10. Lambros V. Fat contouring in the face and neck. *Clin Plast Surg.* 1992;19:401.

11. Lemmon ML, Hamra ST. Skoog rhytidectomy: a five-year experience with 577 patients. *Plast Reconstr Surg.* 1980;65:283.

14. Barton Jr FE. Rhytidectomy and the nasolabial fold. *Plast Reconstr Surg.* 1992;90:601.

    The Skoog facelift was modified to free the SMAS from the underlying mimetic muscles of the face. A sizeable clinical series demonstrated improvement in nasolabial fold aesthetics.

15. Owsley Jr JQ. Lifting the malar fat pad for correction of prominent nasolabial folds. *Plast Reconstr Surg.* 1993;91:463.

22. Mendelson BC. Surgery of the superficial musculoaponeurotic system: Principles of release, vectors, and fixation. *Plast Reconstr Surg.* 2001;107:1545.

11.7

Facelift: SMAS with skin attached – the "high SMAS" technique

Fritz E. Barton Jr.

SYNOPSIS

- The patient consultation considers both the potential for anatomic improvement as well as the patient's expectations.
- Maintenance of facial "harmony" is paramount.
- A "high SMAS" facelift vertically repositions the skin and the subcutaneous tissues as a single unit.

 Access the Historical Perspective section online at
http://www.expertconsult.com

Patient consultation

The patient consultation is divided into three portions: (1) evaluation of the patient's health; (2) evaluation of the facial anatomic features; and (3) evaluation of the patient's appropriateness.

First and foremost, cosmetic surgery is only appropriate for healthy patients. As physicians, our overriding responsibility is to do no harm. A patient's life should never be placed at significant risk for improvement of appearance. Intercurrent illnesses such as cardiac disease, cerebrovascular disease, major organ dysfunction, and potential healing impairment may preclude safe surgery.

Assuming the patient is healthy, the evaluation turns to the anatomic analysis. From my perspective, maintaining facial harmony is paramount. The worst of all outcomes is to look "operated". The are a number of causes of an "operated" look, and these will be addressed in more detail later in the chapter. But surgical disharmony – that is, correcting one aging feature while leaving other aged areas uncorrected – is disharmony by design. Regardless of the effectiveness of the surgical technique, segmental disharmony compromises the result.

Young patients may have only segmental aging. Most commonly, early aging involves the forehead and orbit before the lower face and neck. If the only disharmony is brow ptosis, a forehead procedure alone may suffice. The same may be true regarding the eyelids in young patients. In such a situation, correcting a single aged feature, so as to match the remaining youthful features, actually restores facial harmony.

However after the age of 40, most patients have aging changes throughout multiple areas. They may look slightly aged, but they look natural, since all areas match. If natural facial harmony is to be maintained, all aged areas need simultaneous correction.

Such an approach is often met with resistance by patients, particularly young patients. They are used to the traditional approach of sequential segmental surgery – an approach that most of us were trained to do. Adding to the confusion is the patient's faulty logic that, by doing less at a single stage, they are less likely to look operated.

While debate remains regarding the relative roles of *deflation* (loss of fat) and *descent*, there are several inescapable truths.

The practical fact is that aging patients have lax facial tissues. And when standing erect (as most people judge their appearance), gravity causes the facial tissues to descend. The second fact is that aged people have excess facial skin. Re-inflating the skin envelope to the point of eliminating laxity would create an unattractively puffy face. Third, the descended tissues look better when repositioned superiorly. Finally, a method of maintaining the tissues in their upward position has to be found, even if the repair is non-anatomic.

While the "high SMAS" approach to the cheek is the assigned focus of this chapter, the need to maintain facial harmony necessitates a brief description of pan-facial analysis.

Starting at the top, forehead analysis begins at the hairline. The determination of hairline height is assessed from mid-pupil to hairline – not brow to hairline. While forehead rejuvenation is colloquially referred to as a "browlift", the brow is actually only one element of forehead improvement. Lateral brow hooding, corrugator lines, and procerus creases also

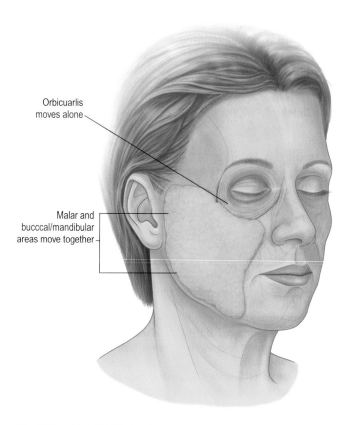

Orbicuarlis moves alone

Malar and bucccal/mandibular areas move together

Fig. 11.7.3 "High SMAS" elevation of the subcutaneous fatty mass with orbicularis suspension separately.

added. Otherwise, I have remained consistent with the "high SMAS" technique for over 25 years *(Fig. 11.7.3)*.[24,33,34]

Surgical planning

Surgical planning involves both the surgical sequence as well as patient preparation. As previously mentioned, in the patient who has not had previous surgery, I believe a pan-facial approach is usually necessary. The actual components of the procedures of the forehead, orbit and neck vary with the patient's anatomy and aging deformity. (Those planning details are beyond the scope of this chapter, however.)

Preoperative patient preparation means stabilizing any intercurrent medical problems or medications not serious enough to preclude surgery. The most common intercurrent illness to stabilize is hypertension.

Preparation of the healthy facelift patient involves mainly avoidance of any interference with wound healing. It has been my observation that the body will heal well if not interfered with. Avoidance focusses on nicotine products and medications that interfere with clotting (e.g., Aspirin, NSAIDs, etc.).

Surgical technique

The initial incision location in the temporal area depends upon what is to be done with the forehead. If a bicoronal or hairline incision is to be utilized for the forehead, then that extension is used for the cheek dissection. If only an endoscopic approach or no forehead surgery is planned, then only a horizontal sideburn incision is done. With use of the sideburn incision, it is critical to limit the upward extent. The fine, posterior-directed upper temple hair will not hide an incision.

A post-tragal auricular incision is used routinely in both males and females. The only exception is dark skinned males with very dark, heavy beards. In most males, skin displaced to the tragus can have the hair follicles excised from beneath the dermis. Any remaining hair can be controlled with an Alexandrite laser. The location and extent of the mastoid incision depends upon the amount of neck skin laxity.

Sequencing of the facial units is the next consideration. The author usually starts at the midline of the neck and works in an upward sequence. This moves the redundancy upward through the cheek and eyelid, then out the top. One criticism of this sequence is that the anterior platysmal closure in the neck might restrict the upward motion of the platysma (SMAS) in the cheek. This restriction can be avoided by merely connecting the medial platysmal borders loosely to each other in the midline, so as to allow later upward motion in the cheek.

The cheek dissection is begun by elevating the skin in the pre-auricular area sharply. Above the level of the tragus, a subcutaneous tunnel is formed to the lateral border of the orbicularis oculi muscle. This tunnel will facilitate later horizontal division of the upper SMAS. From the tragus down, the skin flap is thinly dissected only to the extent of estimated skin excision *(Fig. 11.7.4)*. Care is taken not to overly separate the skin from the SMAS, especially at the upper corner where the previous tunnel was made. The lower extent of the subcutaneous cheek dissection extends below the mandibular border. If no previous neck skin dissection has been done, the submandibular skin dissection is carried approximately one-half way down the neck and one-half way to the midline. This release is necessary to allow partial division of the lateral platysma, and its investing fascia, to facilitate upward displacement of the cheek composite tissues.

With the skin dissection complete, attention is turned to the SMAS. The safest place to penetrate the SMAS is between the top of the tragus and the bottom of the ear lobule. Here, the SMAS is the thickest, and the facial nerve lies deep within the parotid gland. In this location, the SMAS is a multilayer fibro-fatty structure laminated to the parotid capsule. The proper dissection plane leaves a thin translucent fibrous layer over the visible parotid acini. As this dissection plane is extended anteriorly and inferiorly an areolar plane on the underside of identifiable platysma fibers can be visualized. Once in this areolar plane, dissection is carried to the anterior border of the parotid gland, and down the anterior border of the sternocleidomastoid muscle.

At the anterior border of the parotid gland, the dissection method changes from sharp to blunt spreading in the anterior areolar plane. Over the parotid gland, the SMAS is fixed to the gland capsule – the so-called "fixed SMAS". Anterior to the parotid gland, in the buccal area, there is an areolar gliding plane which can be separated bluntly, to avoid any risk to the underlying facial nerve branches. It is imperative to maintain the filmy, near-transparent deep fascia over the masseter muscle, since the facial nerve branches lie just beneath.

Inferiorly, the dissection continues down the fascial fusion plane at the anterior border of the sternocleidomastoid muscle.

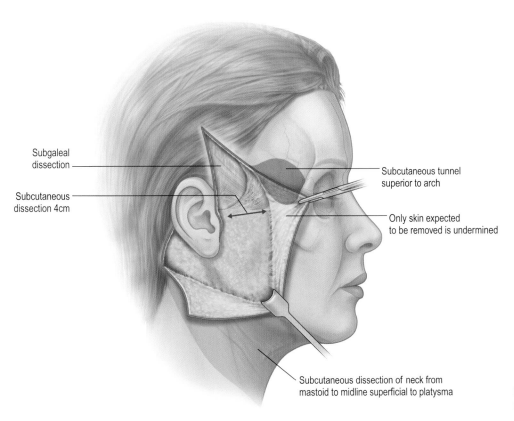

Subgaleal dissection

Subcutaneous dissection 4cm

Subcutaneous tunnel superior to arch

Only skin expected to be removed is undermined

Subcutaneous dissection of neck from mastoid to midline superficial to platysma

Fig. 11.7.4 The skin flap is thinly dissected only to the extent of estimated skin excision.

Here the cervical investing fascia of the platysma continues to invest the sternocleidomastoid muscle. Without a "back cut" in this fascia, upward motion of the platysma (SMAS) can be restricted. Thus, a short 2–3 cm "back cut" in the investing fascia and platysma is made about 4 cm below the mandibular border. The "back cut" is made at this level to avoid any aberrant branches of the marginal mandibular facial nerve.

At this point in the dissection, the buccal-mandibular portion of the cheek will mobilize well, but the upper (malar) portion of the cheek mass is little affected.

Completion of cheek mobilization is achieved by release of the anterior ligament and fascial restrictions. The SMAS is divided horizontally above the zygomatic arch over to the lateral orbicularis. Using the visible edge of the orbicularis as a depth marker, the dissection is carried over the malar area to release the zygomatic retaining ligaments. Again, using the inferior-lateral border of the orbicularis oculi muscle as a depth gauge, the dissection is carried over the lateral border of the zygomaticus major muscle into the subcutaneous plane. Since the anterior SMAS is attached to the zygomaticus major as its investing fascia, the muscle attachment will restrict upward cheek mass mobilization unless released. By making a transition in the cheek dissection plane from a subSMAS plane to over the surface of the zygomaticus major muscle, the investing fascia is released. Dissection is then carried down the lateral border of the zygomaticus major muscle to the level of the modiolus *(Fig. 11.7.5)*. The extent of anterior subcutaneous dissection depends upon the characteristics of the nasolabial fold.

In patients with minimal nasolabial fold depth, dissection stops short of the fold to preserve attachment of the fat to the cheek flap *(Fig. 11.7.6)*. This allows elevation of the cheek to spread the medial fat away from the fold. The limited

dissection also minimized swelling by preserving the anterior facial venous and lymphatic supply.

In patients with moderately deep nasolabial folds, the same limited cheek dissection is done, but a fibro-fatty SMAS graft,[35,36] trimmed from the lateral dissection, is tunneled beneath the nasolabial fold *(Fig. 11.7.7)*. I find this graft to survive most of the time, such that, accurate placement is critical.

In patients with deep nasolabial folds, usually associated with a thin face, complete dissection across the nasolabial fold into the lip is done *(Fig. 11.7.8)*.

In the rare patient, the upper one-third of the nasolabial fold may be quite deep. In such a case, more anterior cheek elevation is needed. In this situation, the author combines the "high SMAS" cheek lift with a subperiosteal "malar lift".[38,39] With the cheek supporting its own weight, rather than being suspended from the lid, the risk of secondary ectropion is greatly reduced.

With completion of this release, the entire subcutaneous cheek mass, from mandible to orbit, will freely move superiorly. *It is paramount to mobilize the cheek in a pure vertical – not horizontal or oblique – direction. The primary vector is vertical along the lateral orbital rim (Fig. 11.7.9).*

Key sutures are placed in the deep temporal fascia and in the mastoid fascia. The periauricular SMAS is then completely closed with a continuous suture to disperse the tension from the key sutures.

Redundant skin is trimmed in place – with no additional tension. *It is paramount to the "high SMAS" concept that all suspension load is placed on the fascia (SMAS) – the skin is never placed under greater than normal tension.*

This upward cheek mobilization, however, does not elevate or redrape the ptotic orbicularis oculi. Care is taken not to undermine the lower orbicularis with the cheek dissection,

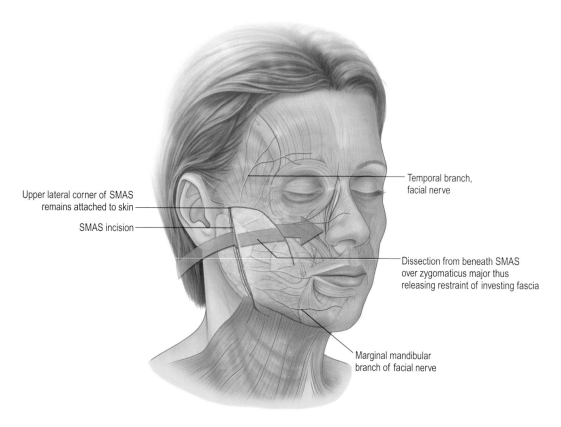

Upper lateral corner of SMAS remains attached to skin

SMAS incision

Temporal branch, facial nerve

Dissection from beneath SMAS over zygomaticus major thus releasing restraint of investing fascia

Marginal mandibular branch of facial nerve

Fig. 11.7.5 Complete release of the SMAS.

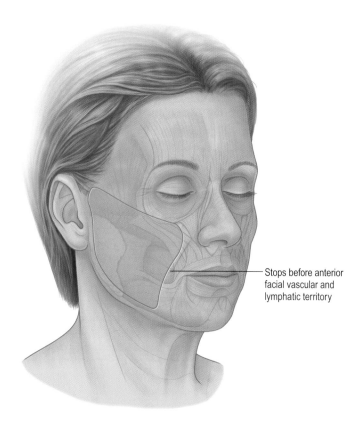

Stops before anterior facial vascular and lymphatic territory

Fig. 11.7.6 Cheek dissection I stops short of the nasolabial fold.

in order to avoid denervation. But by leaving the ptotic orbicularis in place, upward cheek movement accentuates the shelving of the lower orbicularis. It is therefore necessary to add orbicularis suspension, with or without correction of other lower lid malformations, to the routine "high SMAS" cheek lift.

While the cheek mass, including anterior cheek skin, moves in a vertical direction, correction of neck redundancy necessitates posterior (horizontal) redraping. This is accomplished by lateral suspension of the SMAS to the mastoid fascia, accompanied by lateral skin redraping and excision. As opposed to the cheek, where the skin and subcutaneous fat are mobilized as a composite, the neck dissection separates the skin from the underlying platysma. Thus, the redundant cervical skin can be mobilized horizontally, while the cheek mass moves vertically.

Ancillary procedures

Defatting the face presents a different challenge when using the "high SMAS" facelift. The dissection plane is deep to the platysma at the jowl, while the jowl fat lies superficial to the platysma. The author finds liposuction, through a nasal vestibule incision, to be most expeditious. A 2.4 mm cannula works quite well. It should be cautioned, however, that liposuction the buccal area should be avoided. Secondary grooving is too likely.

Two areas respond well to fat grafting. There is often a small redundant strip of excess in the SMAS mobilized to the

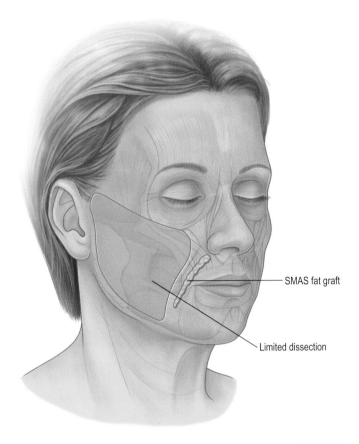

Fig. 11.7.7 Cheek dissection II stops short of nasolabial fold with tunneled SMAS graft.

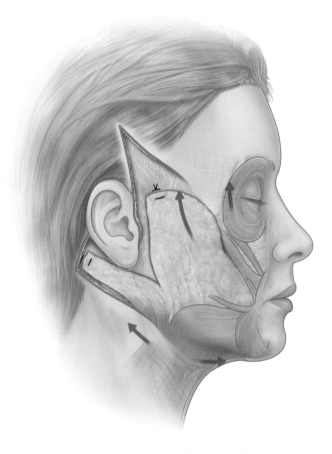

Fig. 11.7.9 The cheek mass is suspended vertically (shown with key sutures), and the entire SMAS flap is closed with a continuous suture to disperse the tension from the key sutures. An orbicularis flap is then done to suspend the orbicularis.

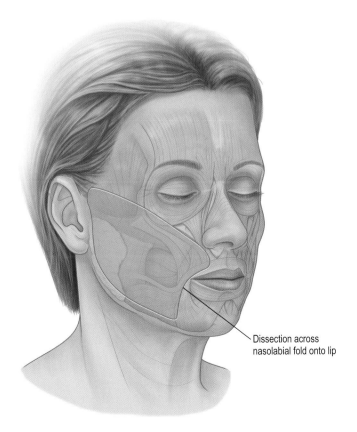

Fig. 11.7.8 Cheek dissection III across the nasolabial fold into the lip.

mastoid. This fibrofatty strip can be used to tunnel beneath the nasolabial fold or to provide lip fullness.[35–37] As previously mentioned, the graft takes reliably in the nasolabial area, but survives only about 50% of the time in the lips.

Vertical upper lip lengthening is present in some patients. In the properly selected individual, a "gull wing" excision at the nostril sill[40,41] will provide subtle improvement.

Perioral lines, either from actinic damage or recurrent orbicularis contraction, are very common in aging patients. While a number of corrective methods exist, all have limited benefit. The dilemma is that in order to completely remove deep wrinkles, you often remove pigment and skin appendages. This can leave the patient with a smooth, but white, waxy appearance. Lighter peels and fractionated lasers have fewer side-effects, but less complete correction *(Fig. 11.7.10)*.

Postoperative care

Immediate postoperative care consists of basic post-anesthesia recovery and avoidance of hematoma. Due to the depth and precision of dissection, most patients are under general anesthesia.

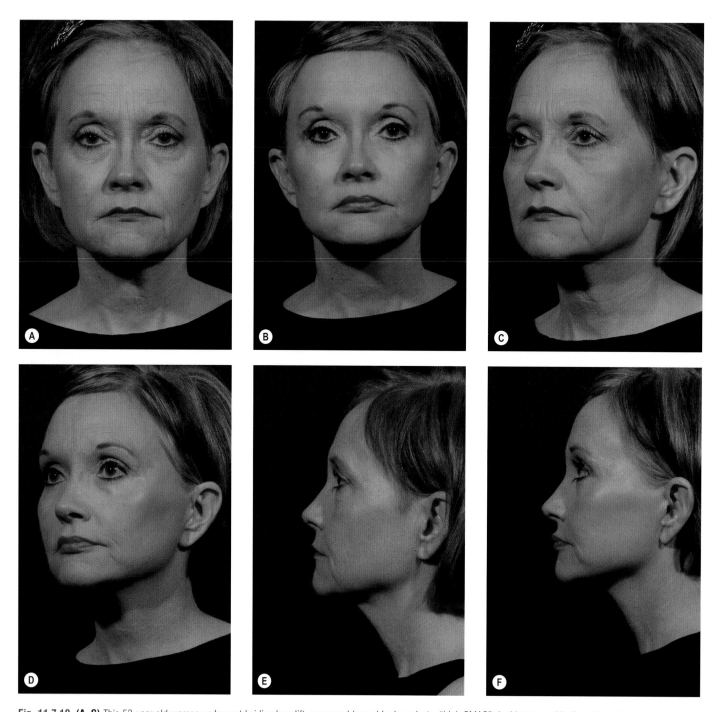

Fig. 11.7.10 (A–C) This 53-year-old woman underwent hairline browlift, upper and lower blepharoplasty, "high SMAS" rhytidectomy with dissection short of the nasolabial fold, submental plication and SMAS grafts to the lips. **(D–F)** The result is shown at 6 months postoperatively.

Intraoperatively, a 0.2 mg clonidine dermal patch is placed. The maximal onset of action coincides nicely with maximum absorption peak of the adrenalin in the local anesthetic solution, 4–6 h postoperatively. The patch is usually left in place until the first postoperative morning, unless the patient demonstrates hypotension.

Xylocaine 0.5% with 1:400000 adrenalin is used for local anesthesia and hemostasis. The 1:400000 adrenalin strength seems to provide adequate tissue hemostasis, and results in less postoperative rebound hypertension than the stronger dilutions.

The other major element to control in the postoperative period, is swelling. Any facial dissection, whether subcutaneous or sub-SMAS, temporarily interrupts part of the lymphatic drainage. While the lymphatics reconstitute over 3–6 months,[42] during that interval, swelling can compromise the result. Even young skin, maintained under stretch, undergoes stress relaxation. But young patients' skin can recoil back to normal dimension. Older patients, however, do not have skin recoil. If skin is held under stretch from prolonged edema, the initial surgical improvement can be compromised.

judged by digitally elevating the brow to an aesthetically pleasing position. This will give an estimate of the needed skin excision. If there is any doubt it is better to postpone the blepharoplasty for a second stage when the brow and forehead has settled. The combination browlift and blepharoplasty allows the surgeon to be conservative for both procedures: brow positioning and the extent of upper eyelid excision. The combined procedure prevents over-resection of eyelid skin that may occur by trying to correct upper eyelid fullness and excess skin with a blepharoplasty only. Consequently, the combined procedure will make the upper blepharoplasty resultant scar shorter and more confined to the inner orbit. Conversely, if an attempt is made to correct fullness and excess skin with a browlift only, a surprised look by hyper-elevation of the brow position may be the result.

Dissection in the frontal area is done entirely in the subperiosteal plane and in the temporal area between the superficial temporal fascia and the temporal fascia proper in the upper temporal area and over the intermediate temporal fascia in the lower temporal area. Both areas of dissection (temporal and frontal) are connected across the temporal line of fusion with the undermining coming from temporal to frontal orientation (four incision technique, see below). The lower limit of the temporal dissection is about 1 cm above the zygomatic arch.

My endoforehead can be done with 2, 3, or 4 incisions, depending on the complexity of the surgery and the difficulty imposed by the patient's anatomy. If two incisions are used, these are located about 3 cm from the midline. If three incisions are used, one is made centrally and the other two are paramedian, 4 cm from the midline. If four incisions are used, two are paramedian at 2.5 cm from the midline and the other two, one on each temporal area, are located 2 cm inside the temporal scalp in a line tangential to a line extending from the nasal alae and external canthus.

The more lateral incisions (paramedian or temporal) are used to do the periosteal release of the lateral brow in cases of hooding of the brow. The paramedian incisions in general are used to do corrugator and procerus ablation. The multiple incisions are utilized for the introduction of two separated instruments for the standard triangulation technique used in endoscopic surgery. After the muscle manipulation and periosteal release are done, one "butterfly" drain of 2 mm diameter is introduced to the glabellar area. The drain is introduced through a separate mini stab wound incision in the scalp posterior to the entrance ports for dissection. Fixation in the majority of cases is done with two percutaneous self-retaining self-stabilizing screws (Synthes®). These are applied at the superior projection of the tails of the brows in the frontal scalp with the vector of traction in the superomedial direction *(Fig. 11.8.4)*. Upper blepharoplasty, if indicated, is done at the end of the endoforehead procedure. In the majority of cases the lateral extent of the blepharoplasty excision does not extend beyond the lateral orbit.

Another important functional interrelation is the function of the frontalis muscle and the levator muscle. It is important to understand this critical connection because this will affect not only function of the eyelid and brow but also will have very important aesthetic consequences. The basic functional fact is that the frontalis and levator muscles are agonist muscles. The frontalis will usually contract forcefully every time an individual wants to look up or at a distance. Similarly,

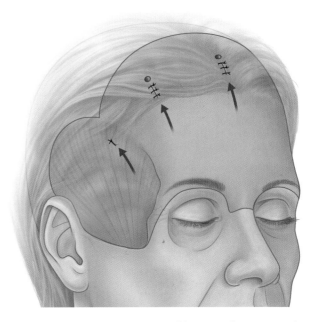

Fig. 11.8.4 The forehead and the upper eyelids are treated as one cosmetic unit. The forehead is usually approached through four small endoscopic ports. Fixation is obtained via a suspension of the superficial temporal fascia to the temporal fascia proper and by percutaneous screws in the frontal area. Direction of traction is superomedially.

when eyes are being closed, the frontalis muscle will usually relax. In patients with congenital unilateral or bilateral weakness of the levator system, the individual will use the frontalis muscle to compensate for this function. This will create forehead lines and creases. This is more frankly seen in the severe eyelid ptosis. The same situation is seen in cases of acquired eyelid ptosis. However, there is a condition of gradual development with aging that at an early stage may not be quite apparent. In this scenario, there is a gradual weakening of the aponeurosis insertion into the tarsal plate. This may eventually progress to a frank disinsertion of the levator aponeurosis. To compensate for this weakness, the patient will contract the frontalis muscle. At an early stage, this will produce a tonic contraction of the frontalis without the development of significant lines and creases. As the process continues, the collagen composition of the skin deteriorates and the additive effect of the brow ptosis occurs, the patient will develop severe lines and creases in the forehead. During this stage, the patient will develop a condition that I have coined "spastic frontalis syndrome".[5] This is characterized by the severe contraction of the frontalis muscle, elevated brows, severe forehead wrinkles and inability of the patient to relax the forehead, Even when the brow is pushed down digitally this immediately moves upwards like a rubber band. When the patient is asked to relax the forehead they are unable to do it voluntarily. Even when they are asked to close the eyes the frontalis remains spastic. In the early stages however, the diagnosis can be difficult and ptosis surgery may be a proposition to the patient that he/she did not expected. The treatment for this is usually carried out in two stages. Ptosis repair is done first under local anesthesia. The frontalis muscle is allowed to relax and the brow will subsequently drop. This may take weeks or months. After the final position of the brow is determined, a decision can be made about how much brow elevation is required. In this situation, performing both operations

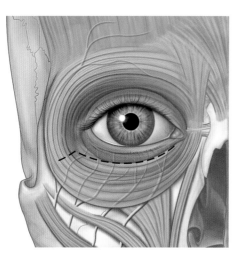

Fig. 11.8.5 During lower eyelid blepharoplasty, the author avoids transecting the orbicularis oculi muscle when entering the preseptal-suborbicular plane, because this will denervate its pretarsal portion. The motor nerves travel perpendicular to the orientation of the muscle incision.

simultaneously becomes a guessing game in determining the most appropriate brow position.

Video
1

Midface and lower eyelid

The lower eyelid is a structure in which the functional and aesthetic effect of aging is more critical than in any other structure in the face. This makes its surgical approach equally critical.

Although some controversies have arisen in relation to its innervations, I stand by the original conclusions of my original research in which we showed that the innervations of the lower orbicularis muscle fibers comes in a perpendicular direction to its fibers *(Fig. 11.8.5)*.[6] If these fibers come from the zygomaticus branch or the buccal branch or from both, it is irrelevant as far as the planned incision is made. If the classic skin-muscle flap is used (the original McIndoe operation), the pretarsal portion of the lower orbicularis oculi muscle will at its best be temporarily denervated and at worst will be totally denervated. The degree of denervation will depend of the extent of the original muscle transection. The recovery process will also depend of the degree of neurotization of the pretarsal orbicularis. A better chance of neurotization will occur when more contact between the preseptal and pretarsal segments of the muscle exist at the end of the operation. This is accomplished by preseptal orbicularis suspension methods, such as the orbicularis "hitch". Canthopexy methods will also prevent the flabby tarsal orbicularis to heal in a relaxed position and will make innervations functionally more effective. Some of the secondary effects of incomplete innervations in order of severity are: tilting of the ciliary border with anterior exposure of the white line of the lower eyelid, sclera show, bowing of the lateral third of the lower eyelid and frank ectropion. Lesser degrees of the problem still will affect how the tear film is distributed across the cornea and from the aesthetic point of view will show an eye that looks "funny" even if the patient or the surgeon can not pinpoint the exact cosmetic defect.

The midfacelift combined with my functional blepharoplasty is an excellent tool to rejuvenate the lower eyelid while preserving its function. Additional improvements will be seen with better lower eyelid position, improvement of laxity and correction of the V deformity of the lower orbit/upper cheek.

The midfacelift begins with Xylocaine 0.5% mixed with epinephrine at 1/200000 dilution, which is infiltrated in the temporal and midface areas.

The midface is approached from above through a temporal incision, and from below through an intraoral buccal mucosal incision. The length of the incision in the temporal area will depend on the technique used. In the open approach the incision is either a coronal incision if the forehead lift is also done concomitantly or a limited temporal-frontal incision. Dissection in the temporal area separates the superficial temporal fascia from the temporal fascia proper in the upper temporal area and the superficial temporal fascia from the intermediate temporal fascia in the lower temporal area. In the endoscopic technique, dissection continues in this plane until the superior border of the zygomaticus arch is reached. With upward traction of the temporal flap, the periosteum of the zygomaticus arch is elevated with a sharp periosteum elevator. In the open approach the intermediate temporal fascia with its attached intermediate fat pad is elevated 2–3 cm above the zygomaticus arch and the periosteum is dissected in continuity.[1] This fascial flap will be used as an anchor suspension of the midface. Alternatively, in the open technique this fascial flap elevation can be avoided and rely on the suspension points of the midface used in the endoscopic approach. In either of the alternatives the temporal nerve branch of the facial nerve is protected in the elevated flap. It is important although not critical to save the temporal vein #2 (sentinel vein) and the zygomaticus-temporal nerve(s). This will minimize ecchymosis, swelling, and hypoesthesias.

Next, the intraoral buccal incision is made. This is located at the level of the first premolar and done either vertically or slightly obliquely. The initial incision is done through the mucosa only, then the buccinator muscle is spread with the periosteal elevator and a subperiosteal dissection is carried out on the maxilla and malar bones. Medially, this extends to the pyriformis area and laterally underneath the fascia of the masseter muscle. This lateral extension goes about 2.5 cm over the masseter tendon. Dissection superiorly is done to separate the orbicularis muscle attachments to the inferior orbital rim, thus releasing the arcus marginalis. The attachments around the infraorbital nerve are freed after the fixation points on the midface are applied and just before their fixation in the temporal fascia proper. That will avoid traction neuropathy by excessive manipulation. The zygomaticofacial nerve is also preserved to avoid the occasional painful neuropathy and/or localized anesthesia. Subperiosteal dissection of the midface is connected with the temporal optical cavity over the anterior two-thirds of the zygomatic arch *(Fig. 11.8.6)*. Dissection includes elevation of the soft tissues from the external lateral orbital rim.

The sutures applied to the midface have the following effects: suspension, volumetric remodeling and lifting. I routinely use four sutures per side, although in some particular cases it may be three or two depending on the aesthetic objectives *(Fig. 11.8.7)*. The first one to be applied is to the anterior central SOOF (suborbicularis oculi fat), which is anchored to the most anterior portion of the temporal fascia proper near the lateral orbital rim. This is a 4-0 polydioxanone (PDS) suture that prior to its passing to the temporal area can be

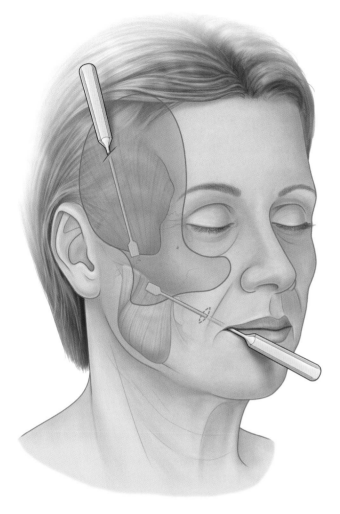

Fig. 11.8.6 The "endo-midface" is approached by a single temporal and an intraoral incision. For this reason, it is better called an endotemporo-midface procedure. The midface and temporal cavities are connected across the zygomatic arch. The subperiosteal dissection here is critical to avoid injuring the frontal branch of the facial nerve. The midface dissection extends under the masseteric fascia for 2–3 cm.

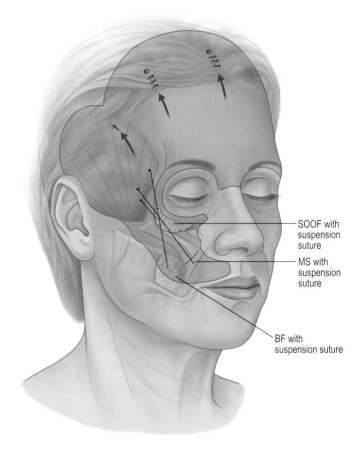

SOOF with suspension suture

MS with suspension suture

BF with suspension suture

Fig. 11.8.7 An endoscopic browlift is shown in conjunction with an endoscopic midfacelift. For the midfacelift, four sutures are used to obtain the maximal remodeling and beneficial effect of the subperiosteal dissection. The anterior SOOF (suborbicularis oculi fat) effaces the infraorbital V deformity. The lateral SOOF lifts the midface. The MS (modiolus suspension) lifts the corner of the mouth. These three sutures also produce imbrication, thus increasing the anterior projection of the cheek. The last suture suspension is the buccal (Bichat's) fat pad (BF). This is the structure that helps more than any other to create the Ogee line of the midface.

anchored to the immediately superior arcus marginalis which will act as a pulley to direct the anterior SOOF towards the orbital rim area helping to efface the tear trough area. This is anchored before passing the rest of the sutures to the temporal area because this does not restrict with the placement of the rest of the sutures and it may become entangled with the rest of the other sutures if left for later. The next suture is the lateral SOOF that is applied to the compound periosteum/ SOOF tissue 3 cm inferior and vertical to the lateral canthal tendon insertion. This is done with a 3-0 PDS suture. The next suture is the modiolus suspension. This is applied to the fibroadipose tissue just inferior to the most anterior portion of the intraoral incision. This is done with 4-0 PDS suture. These two sutures are tunneled to the temporal area end exited through the temporal port. The last suture is applied to the Bichat's fat pad. This is perhaps the most difficult and the one that has the steepest learning curve among the different sutures applied to the midface. Once this technique is mastered, there is nothing to replace it in the finesse and beautifying effect of its mobilization.[7] The Bichat's or buccal fat pad is located in

the so-called buccal space *(Fig. 11.8.8)*. To enter here, you need to open the periosteum/buccinator that forms its anteromedial wall. This is just medial to the masseter tendon. This is best done with a blunt and long scissor. The blades of the scissors are opened and the fat pad will extrude from its encased buccal space. The fat pad is then gently pulled with two blunt scissors. Simultaneously, the surgical assistant will push with his finger from the external lower cheek/jowl area encouraging the most inferior portion of the fat pad to migrate toward the oral cavity. During this process, the fascia that forms the wall of the buccal space is gently teased. The buccal fat pad has a very thin fascial layer that protects the fat pad and carries the nourishing vessels. This has to be maintained to maintain the integrity of the pad. Separating the buccal wall fascia from the fat pad itself is similar to the maneuver used to reduce an inguinal hernia. Once the fat pad has been delivered, it is still attached to buccal fat remaining inside the buccal space and to the deeper structures of the modiolus. A 4-0 PDS suture with an RB1 needle is weaved into the fat pad utilizing two or three passes. The next step is to anchor these sutures. The first one to be anchored is the Bichat's fat pad suture, which is done to the loop of SOOF suture applied beforehand. We call this technique "piggy backing" the SOOF

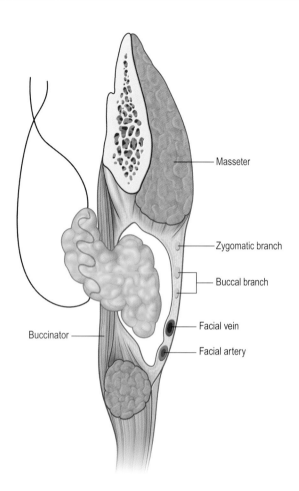

Fig. 11.8.8 The Bichat's (buccal) fat pad has its own facial covering and its own blood supply. It is located inside the buccal space. This space has a gliding surface that allows the buccal fat pad to work as a syssarcosis but also makes it prone to pseudo-herniation towards the para commissural/jowl area. This fat pad can be mobilized towards the malar area after opening the periosteum/buccinator layer.

Labels in figure: Masseter; Zygomatic branch; Buccal branch; Facial vein; Facial artery; Buccinator

anterior SOOF area and the localization of this deformity. If the deformity is mostly in the area medial to the location of the infraorbital nerve then the improvement will be minimal. This technique improves mostly the laterally and centrally located defect. A different procedure such as fat grafting or orbital rim implant will be required to obtain a significant improvement of the centrally located defect. Another effect is the volumetric augmentation of the midface. This is created by the combination of the lateral SOOF lift and Bichat's fat pad repositioning. During aging or in chubby faces, Bichat's fat pad will usually migrate towards the lower anterior cheek area just above the area of the jowl. In the oblique view, this contributes to the flat, linear configuration of the upper cheek and convex shape in the lower cheek. Changing the anatomical position of the buccal fat pad will simultaneously, with one maneuver, augment the upper cheek and change the lower cheek from a convexity to either a flat surface or to a concavity. This helps create the "Ogee line", which is a feature of beauty and youth. Bichat's fat pad, the imbrication by the lateral SOOF suspension and the direction of traction of the modiolus suture all will converge at the so-called "zygomaxillary point".[9] This is the point that will get the maximal augmentation. This is also the point that has the maximal convexity in the outline of the Ogee in the young and beautiful individual. Therefore, this technique allows creating or recovering this line of beauty.

- The midface cavity is irrigated with antibiotic solution and closure of the intraoral incision is done with interrupted 4-0 chromic catgut sutures.
- After the blepharoplasty is done, the forehead and midface are tapped with brown colored micropore tape for additional support and temporary splinting effect.
- The lower blepharoplasty is then done in a totally different fashion to the traditional technique.

There are two fundamental differences here, compared with traditional methods. First, I usually do not remove any fat from the lower eyelids/orbits. In the few cases that I have done, it was done in an extremely conservative manner and using muscular or transconjunctival tunnels. Second, I do not detach the pretarsal muscle from the preseptal portion. The continuity of the orbicularis oculi is maintained. The preservation of fat prevents the sunken eye appearance with postsurgical enophthalmos that eventually leads to small beady eye look, seen in many post-blepharoplasty patients. The preservation of muscle integrity will maintain its innervation and its function. The eye after this type of blepharoplasty will look healthy, vibrant, and fuller, with a slight pretarsal roll typical of a youthful eye. The ciliary margin will be in an excellent position, facilitating good lacrimal tear film distribution and normal pumping of tears by the good muscle function.

Lower eyelid blepharoplasty is done after the midfacelift is completed. A skin incision 2 mm below the ciliary border is extended directly into the crow's foot area without making any sharp curves as traditionally we were taught. The full thickness lower eyelid skin is "peeled" off the orbicularis muscle layer for an average of 1.5–2 cm inferiorly, creating a pure skin flap. The exposed lateral extension of the preseptal portion is anchored to the most anterior portion of the temporal fascia proper with a 5-0 or 6-0 Prolene suture. For this maneuver, a window in the lateral orbital portion of the

suture. The objective is to limit the upward mobilization of the buccal fat pad and its potential accidental tearing off of this structure. The next maneuver is to anchor the modiolus stitch to the anterior part of the temporal fascia proper just behind the anchor point of the anterior SOOF. Last is the fixation of the lateral SOOF to the most posterior portion of the temporal fascia proper. All the sutures anchored to the temporal area are done using the endoscopic sliding Peruvian fisherman's knot.[8] This suture technique allows control of the tension applied to each structure. It is also reversible up to some point, therefore it can be made a bit looser if needed. A 2 mm "butterfly" drain is introduced via a mini stab incision. The last suspension suture is applied to the superficial temporal fascia at the inferior lip of the temporal entrance port and anchored to the temporal fascia proper above and anterior to it. During this process, the temporal scalp is pulled in a superomedial direction. This prevents posterior shifting of the sideburn and encourages a more vertical lift of the upper cheek temple areas. The scalp is closed with staples.

One effect of this multiple and independent suture suspension is that the lower eyelid will be elevated in relation to the orbital rim, and the V deformity of the lower orbit will be totally or partially effaced *(Fig. 11.8.9)*. The degree of this effacement will depend on the amount of soft tissue in the

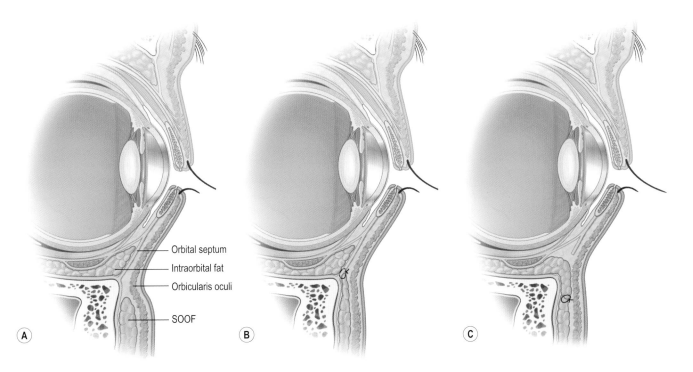

Fig. 11.8.9 The medial suborbicularis oculi fat (SOOF) located below the inferior orbital rim can be elevated to efface the V deformity. This can be sutured to the arcus marginalis or to the post-septal fat pads which are advanced over the infraorbital rim. OOM, orbicularis oculi muscle.

orbicularis muscle is created with a blunt dissection. This maneuver will lift the entire lower orbicularis and apply tension on the post-septal fat pushing the fat inside the eye orbit. The skin will also be brought up by the orbicularis elevation and thick soft tissue will be positioned over the inferior orbital rim giving additional support to the intraorbital fat and improving the infraorbital V deformity. The upward lifting of the orbicularis will also roll up muscle fibers from preseptal to pretarsal areas, providing to this area the natural fullness seen in younger individuals.

Methods to enhance midface rejuvenation

The methods described above will work in the majority of patients, particularly in the younger group (up to age 50), However those patients with thin faces, those with poor skeletal support and the much older individuals will require other ancillary procedures to improve the results of the midface rejuvenation and provide three-dimensional rejuvenation. As indicated in one of my previous articles, there are several methods to enhance the tri-dimensional or volumetric rejuvenation of the entire face.[10] In relation to the midface these include implants (cheek, periorbital, paranasal) and fat grafting.

Fat grafting techniques can be easily incorporated into the operation because fat can be injected anywhere from the dermis down to the periosteum. Fat is usually obtained from the periumbilical area and after it is spun in a centrifuge the fluid elements are separated. Using a 1 cc Luer Lock type of syringe with mini-cannulas the fat is injected to correct any residual asymmetries, to improve the nasolabial folds and into the brow and glabellar areas as needed. I use an average of 30 cc of fat for the entire face as an adjunctive technique.

However, I do not rely on fat grafting for the volumetric augmentation of the cheek unless the patient is too thin and emaciated and does not have enough soft tissues to create volume with the imbrications techniques and advancement of Bichat's fat pad.

Facial implants to the paranasal areas, to the lower periorbita and to the cheek are used as a way to enhance the aesthetic results but in cases of atrophy of those areas by the aging process as a way to restore the facial skeleton volume and provide long term support to the tissues that has been lifted. Since the dissection has been done at the subperiosteal plane, the field is ready for the use of this implant. Those implants are customized to the facial contour with the use of physical facial skeletal model obtained from a reformatted facial CT scan. This is an advanced methodology to obtain the most precise fitting of those implants to the facial skeleton. Implants are fixed in place with titanium miniscrews.

Lower face and neck

The lower face and neck is another facial aesthetic unit that traditionally has been treated with various methods of cervicofacial lift that are covered elsewhere in this text. I rarely do isolated cervicofacial lifts because that will create a disharmony with rest of the face. Furthermore, the horizontal/oblique pull that is done with these techniques will create tension bands in a horizontal or oblique direction. These tension bands may not be visible on photographs taken in neutral expression but are much more evident during facial animation. These are, in my observation, more prevalent in those patients who have had SMAS facelifts because the SMAS is attached to the facial mimetic muscles and is pulled

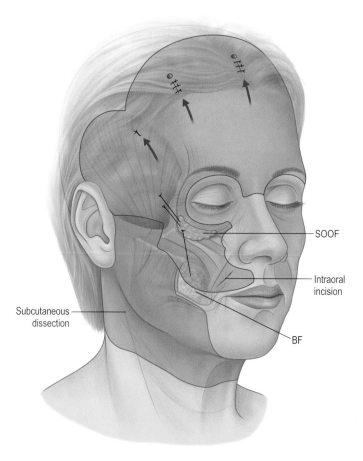

Fig. 11.8.10 An endoscopic browlift is shown in conjunction with a midfacelift and a subcutaneous facelift. This creates a biplanar facelift in which the central oval of the face (forehead, midface, and chin) is addressed at the subperiosteal level and the peripheral hemicircle is dissected at the subcutaneous plane. The vectors of traction are different in both regions. There is some overlap between both planes of dissection but the intermediate lamella of the face is preserved.

laterally, affecting those muscles. Consequently, on muscle contraction during facial animation tension bands become evident.

I include the cervicofacial lift during facial rejuvenation of patients with significant laxity or excessive fat accumulation of those areas. This is usually in patients above the age of 50 years *(Fig. 11.8.10)*. After the midface rejuvenation has been done, the lower face is approached at the same surgical stage or as a second stage through a periauricular incision extending posteriorly into the occipital scalp. The anterior auricular incision extends up to the sideburn. No temporal scalp incision is done. I prefer the marginal tragal incision as opposed to the pretragal one in both female and male patients. In males, I trim the root of the hair follicles on the periauricular flaps.

My retroauricular incision in done at the crease itself and not against the conchae, as is sometimes taught. I make the incision high in the anterior mastoid area at the level of the superior insertion of the ear. From here, the incision angles sharply (about 45° angle), initially for 1–2 cm at the hairline and gradually into the occipital scalp in an oblique direction. That way, I avoid a visible scar and a sharp contrast of skin color and texture in the mastoid area. It also avoids distortion of the ear due to pull in the conchae. The dissection is done at the subcutaneous plane. I make a thick subcutaneous dissection initially with the scissors and after the very adherent areas are separated using a sharp periosteal elevator. This separates the subcutaneous plane from the SMAS in an anatomical plane and does not make perforations of the subcutaneous plane that often occur with the scissors. Dissection is usually extended as far as an oblique line from the sideburn to the jowl area. The neck dissection is through-and-through across the midline. If needed, a submental incision is done to defat the area, do a platysmaplasty or do a subplatysmal dissection. After the appropriate amount of skin is removed, the flaps are inset and closed in two layers using 5-0 and 4-0 Prolene. To create a natural parotid area-ear interface, a

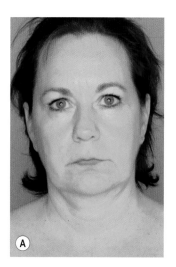
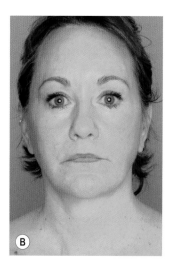
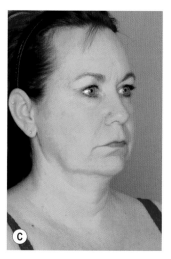
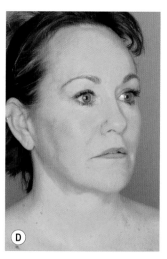

Fig. 11.8.11 **(A)** Preoperative front view of a 55-year-old woman without history of previous facial surgery requesting total facial rejuvenation. Observe the heavy face and neck and the poor chin bone support. **(B)** Postoperative front view 2 years after. She underwent endo-forehead, endo-midface, functional lower blepharoplasty, cervicofacial component with short preauricular incision, deep neck defatting, 5 mm Medpor RZ geniomandibular custom carved chin implant and liplift, with the bull's horn incision. No upper blepharoplasty was done. **(C)** Preoperative three-quarters view. More evident is the heaviness of her face, particularly around the jaw line and neck. Also, observe the "witch's chin". **(D)** Postoperative three-quarters view. Observe the brow elevation, improvement of the lower orbital V deformity, and the creation of the "double Ogee line" on the oblique outline. Also, observe the improvement of the perioral aesthetics and dynamics due to the combined effect of the midfacelift, liplift and chin implant. Make particular note of the reversal of the suprajowl convexity to a slight concavity and the increase of the zygomaxillary point.

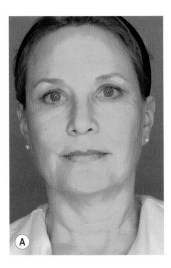
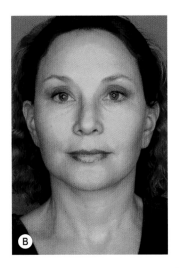
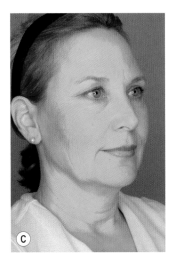
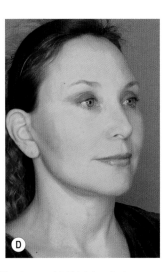

Fig. 11.8.12 (A) Preoperative front view of a 48-year-old woman with generalized aging of the face. Observe the periocular aging with a lower orbital V deformity, brow ptosis, nasolabial fold, jowls. **(B)** Postoperative front view 18 months after. She had the author's biplanar version of facial rejuvenation: endo-forehead, endo-midface, lower blepharoplasty, cervicofacial lift and a small amount of fat grafting. There was no upper blepharoplasty done. Observe the generalized rejuvenation without the typical stigmata of a "facelift". **(C)** Preoperative three-quarters view. Observe corrugator hyperactivity, sagging of brows, V deformity on the lower orbits, sagging cheeks, jowls and laxity of neck. **(D)** Postoperative three-quarters view. Patient has not changed her features but looks significantly younger and more beautiful. Observe the double Ogee line of the oblique outline, her beautiful cheeks and excellent jawline. There is no windswept appearance.

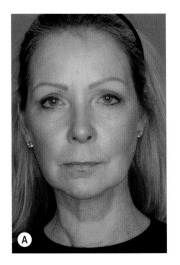
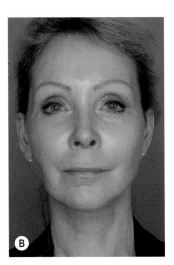
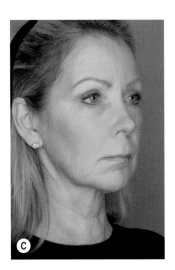
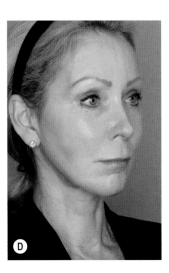

Fig. 11.8.13 (A) Preoperative front view. Observe the depressed and tired look typical of the aging face. Notice the hooding of the upper eyelids and the V deformity of the lower orbit. The woman's corrugator hyperactivity gives her a tense and angry look. Her cheeks are sagging and the lower face presents jowls and jaw line laxity. Her neck is loose and presents platysma bands and horizontal creases. She had previous neck surgery via a submental incision, performed somewhere else. **(B)** Postoperative front view at 36 month's follow-up. She underwent endo-forehead, endo-midface, lower blepharoplasty, cervicofacial lift and small amount of fat grafting. **(C)** Preoperative three-quarters view. Hyperactivity of the frontalis is more evident in this view. **(D)** Postoperative three-quarters view. Observe the more sophisticated outline of the Ogee line and a natural and beautiful look. There is no windswept appearance.

pretragal depression is created with the technique previously published.[11]

The role of subperiosteal dissection

Subperiosteal dissection of the chin and anterior mandible is done to insert the different shapes of implant designed to enhance the rejuvenation of the lower face. Subperiosteal mentopexy is another procedure used to lift the ptotic chin. Dissection of the gonial area and lateral mandible is done to insert mandibular ramus or gonial angle implants. These implants give support and enhance the lower face. The upward lifting of the midface also helps to lift the detached soft tissues of the jaw line area. Also, once subperiosteal detachment of the soft tissues is done, the flaps of the cervicofacial lift helps to remodel these areas.

Results

Well over 800 patients have had subperiosteal facial rejuvenation of the midface. The complication rate has been minimal and of no long-term duration or significance. It is a safe operation and the surgical results speak for themselves, as is shown in the random sample of patients included in this chapter *(Figs 11.8.11–11.8.13)*.

References

1. Ramirez OM, Maillard GF, Musolas A. The extended subperiosteal facelift: a definitive soft tissue remodeling for facial rejuvenation. *Plast Reconstr Surg.* 1991;88: 237–238.

   The authors report favorable results with their technique for deep plane rhytidectomy. Salient operative details are discussed.

2. Ramirez OM. Endoscopic full facelift. *Aesthetic Plast Surg.* 1994;18:363–371.

3. Ramirez OM, Volpe CR. Double ogee facial rejuvenation. In: Panfilov DE, ed. *Aesthetic surgery of the facial mosaic.* New York: Springer Verlag; 2007:288–299.

4. Ramirez OM. Transblepharoplasty forehead and upper face rejuvenation. *Ann Plast Surg.* 1996;37:577–584.

   A technique for facelifting through blepharoplasty incisions is detailed. Indications, procedural details, and outcomes are reviewed.

5. Ramirez OM. Spastic frontalis: a description of a new syndrome. Presented at the Annual Meeting of the American Society of Aesthetic Plastic Surgery, Dallas, Texas; 1994:April.

6. Ramirez OM, Santamarina R. Spatial orientation of motor innervation to the lower orbicularis oculi muscle. *Aesthetic Surg J.* 2000;20:107–113.

   Cadaveric dissections were performed to detail the course of the facial nerve as it supplies the lower portion of orbicularis oculi. Implications for blepharoplasty and midface access are addressed.

7. Ramirez OM. Three-dimensional endoscopic midface enhancement. A personal quest for the ideal cheek rejuvenation. *Plast Reconstr Surg.* 2002;109:329–340.

   Midface rejuvenation is achieved by a combined open/ endoscopic approach through a temporal slit and upper oral sulcus incisions. Complications were minimized and results compared favorably with those achieved by the author with other midface rejuvenation techniques.

8. Ramirez OM, Tezel E, Ersoy B. The Peruvian fisherman's knot: a new, simple, and versatile self-locking sliding knot. *Ann Plast Surg.* 2009;62:114–117.

9. Nahai F. *The art of aesthetic surgery: principles and techniques.* St Louis: Quality Medical; 2005.

10. Ramirez OM, Heller L. The anchor tragal flap: A method of preserving the natural pretragal depression during rhytidectomy. *Plast Reconstr Surg.* 2005;116: 1115–1121.

    The tragus and pre-tragus depression are facial landmarks often sacrificed during rhytidectomy. A technique to preserve these structures is described.

11. Ramirez OM. Full face rejuvenation in three dimensions: a "face-lifting" for the new millennium. *Aesthetic Plast Surg.* 2001;25:152–164.

12

Secondary deformities and the secondary facelift

Timothy J. Marten and Dino Elyassnia

SYNOPSIS

- Although many aspects of planning and performing secondary facelift surgery are similar to those of the primary procedure, one must identify and treat not only new problems that are the product of age, but those that have resulted from any prior procedure as well. Often it is these secondary deformities that present the biggest challenge in terms of creativity, planning, preparation, and technique.

- Recognizing the problems in the secondary facelift patient and appreciating their underlying anatomical abnormalities is fundamental to planning and performance of any repair. Although not all problems can always be completely corrected, any surgeon able to recognize their anatomic basis can, through the application of logic and careful planning, select techniques that are safe, effective, and rational.

- Secondary deformities are worth every surgeon's consideration, even if he or she performs only the occasional secondary procedure, as they exist as compelling reminders of mistakes to avoid in the planning and performance of any primary procedure.

- Hairline displacement and disruption remain predictable outcomes of many currently used facelift plans and are a source of disappointment and frustration for patients and surgeons alike. These problems are the result of poor analysis and planning and failure to use an incision along the hairline when indicated.

- The placement of an incision and thus of the resultant scar along a hairline at secondary surgery represents a choice between two imperfect alternatives but the best overall artistic and aesthetic compromise in many patients.

- Using the SMAS to lift sagging facial tissues and restore facial contour circumvents the problems associated with skin-only facelifts, as it is an inelastic structural layer capable of providing meaningful and sustained support. Although skin must be excised in SMAS procedures, only redundant tissue is sacrificed and closure can be made under normal skin tension.

- "Lamellar" dissections, in which the skin and SMAS are dissected as two separate layers, offer the important advantage that skin and SMAS can be advanced different amounts, along separate vectors,

and suspended under differential tension. This allows each layer to be addressed individually as indicated and, in turn, results in a more comprehensive and natural appearing improvement.

- It is not enough in most secondary facelift procedures to limit treatment of the neck to pre-platysmal lipectomy and post-auricular skin excision in secondary facelift patients. For many patients, subplatysmal fat accumulation, submandibular salivary gland "ptosis", and digastric muscle hypertrophy will contribute significantly to their neck deformity and necessitate additional treatment.

- As experience is gained in evaluation of patients presenting for secondary surgery, prominent submandibular glands will increasingly be recognized as a frequent part of the secondary neck deformity and the underlying cause of objectionable residual bulges in the lateral triangle of the lateral submental region. In most instances, the secondary facelift will provide an opportunity for proper diagnosis and appropriate treatment, when present.

- The secondary facelift will generally require a comparatively small resection of skin and an increased focus on correcting deep layer problems and secondary deformities, depending upon the skill of the surgeon performing the primary procedure and the type of technique used.

- Secondary facelifts are often time consuming and technically demanding when compared to primary procedures and are likely to test the patience and composure of most surgeons.

- Many patients requesting secondary facelifts are chronologically elderly, but deceptively young in appearance. A careful medical history must be taken because they often have medical problems consistent for their age group.

- The opportunity to perform a facelift is a unique artistic privilege granted to us by our patients that carries a significant responsibility. It deserves nothing less than our best effort, and a few extra hours of our time in the operating room benefits them for the rest of their lives.

- Performing a secondary facelift if frequently a considerable undertaking and its difficulty should not be underestimated.

The procedure must be carefully planned, meticulously carried out, and the patient's safety and wellbeing unfailingly insured.

- Performance of the procedure itself only fulfills part of our obligation to the patient and the care they receive perioperatively is arguably as important as the surgery itself. Diligent perioperative care will ensure the best result and reduce the likelihood that problems and complications will occur.

Introduction

The increased number of patients seeking facelifts at a younger age, coupled with the continued good health of an older group of patients who have already undergone one or more procedures, has resulted in a significant increase in requests for secondary and tertiary procedures. Although many aspects of planning and performing secondary surgery are similar to those of the primary procedure, additional considerations must be taken into account in the evaluation and treatment of the patient presenting for secondary facelift, as one must identify and treat not only new problems that are the product of age, but those that have resulted from any prior procedure as well. Often, it is these *secondary deformities* that present the biggest challenge to the surgeon in terms of creativity, planning, preparation, and technique.

Consideration must also be given to possible underlying anatomical damage that may have resulted from previous procedures but is not evident as a visible deformity. This includes possible damage to skin, fat, SMAS and deeper layer structures. Injury to these tissues at the time of the primary procedure can preclude certain maneuvers and limit the overall amount of improvement possible at the time secondary surgery is performed. "Red flag" procedures in this regard include radiofrequency and ultrasonic "skin tightening" treatments, prior "suture lifts", and prolonged large volume use of facial fillers ("filler fibrosis").

As in primary procedures, recognizing the problems in the secondary facelift patient and appreciating their underlying anatomical abnormalities is fundamental to planning and performance of any repair. Although not all problems can always be completely corrected, any surgeon able to recognize their anatomic basis can, through the application of logic and careful planning, select techniques that are safe, effective and rational.

Identification and analysis of secondary aging deformity

Surgery does not halt the aging process and patients requesting secondary or tertiary facelifts usually present with many of the same problems seen when they presented for their primary procedures. This is particularly true if the primary facelift was limited and consisted of skin excision and skin tightening only. In such instances, a tight or pulled appearance will typically be present, but problems of deep layer origin will still be evident and will likely have worsened over time. These include nasolabial folds, labiomental folds, cheek ptosis, infraorbital hollowing, malar flattening, jowl laxity,

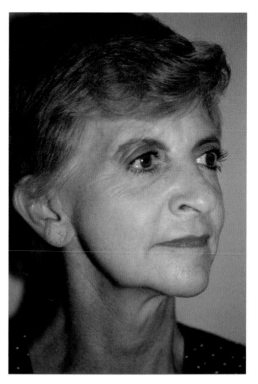

Fig. 12.1 Identification of secondary aging deformities. Surgery does not arrest the aging process, and patients requesting secondary facelifts usually present with many of the same problems seen when they presented for their primary procedures. This is particularly true if the primary facelift was limited and consisted of skin excision and skin tightening only, as with this patient. Problems typically seen include nasolabial folds, labiomental folds, cheek ptosis, infraorbital hollowing, malar flattening, jowl laxity, submental fat accumulation, and platysma band formation. Note that although some wrinkling and atrophy are present, the patient's predominant problem is deep layer tissue ptosis. Additional skin excision and tightening under these circumstances will be of little benefit to the patient. (Previous procedure performed by an unknown surgeon.)

subplatysmal fat accumulation, submandibular gland hypertrophy, and cervical band formation *(Fig. 12.1)*.

Regrettably, many surgeons have been traditionally taught to perform a limited "tuck" or "touch-up" in secondary procedures consisting of additional skin excision and skin tightening. This does not address the true underlying problems however, and compounds the secondary deformities present in many patients.

Identification and analysis of secondary surgical deformities

The number and degree of secondary deformities present will determine the difficulty of any additional surgery and the overall potential for improvement possible. Typical problems seen in the patient presenting for secondary facelift include hairline displacement, hair loss, poorly situated scars, thick scars, wide scars, scleral show, eyelid dysfunction, tragal distortion, earlobe distortion, over-excision of cervicofacial fat, distortion and abnormal appearances due to inappropriate tissue shifts, and abnormal appearance when emoting. Less commonly, problems related to nerve injury, skin slough, or other surgical complications may be present. These problems are worth every surgeon's consideration, even if he or she

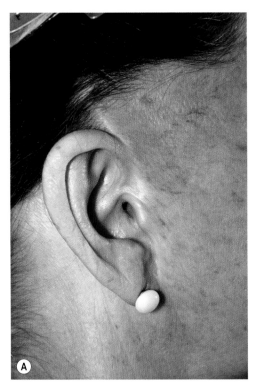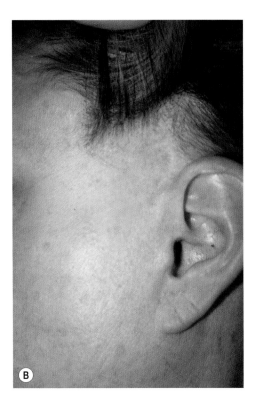

Fig. 12.2 (A,B) Displacement of the sideburn and temple hair due to poor incision planning. The temporal portion of the facelift incision was made in the temporal scalp in a well-intended effort to hide the resulting scar. Because cheek flap redundancy was large and skin elasticity poor, advancement of the cheek skin flap has resulted in objectionable hairline displacement. An incision along the hairline would have prevented this deformity. (Procedures performed by an unknown surgeon.)

performs only the occasional secondary procedure, as they exist as compelling reminders of mistakes to avoid in the planning and performance of any primary procedure.

Hairline displacement and disruption

Hairline displacement and disruption remain predictable outcomes of many currently used facelift plans and are a source of disappointment and frustration for patients and surgeons alike. These problems are the result of poor analysis and planning at the time of the primary procedure and failure to use an incision along the hairline when indicated. Although hairline displacement may be acceptable after some primary facelifts in which incisions were made in the traditional location within hair bearing scalp, it will almost always be intolerable after a secondary facelift if such an incision plan is used again. For this reason, thoughtful planning of secondary and tertiary facelifts frequently requires the use of incisions placed along hairlines, rather than behind them.

The placement of an incision and thus of resultant scar along a hairline at secondary surgery represents a choice between two imperfect alternatives but the best overall artistic and aesthetic compromise in many patients. Although incisions upon the scalp produce concealed scars within the hair, they will result in tell-tale and objectionable hairline displacement in many patients that is usually readily apparent upon casual glance and at some distance. These deformities are often not subtle and frequently result in an unnatural or even grotesque appearance *(Fig. 12.2)*. In addition, they are uniformly difficult for the patient to disguise and a challenge for the surgeon to correct.

Placing the incision along a hairline, however, usually results in a fine scar only visible on close inspection when correctly planned and proper technique is used. And unlike displaced hair, a scar along the hairline can usually be easily concealed with make-up or tattooed if necessary, but generally go unnoticed in most social situations and casual encounters. Often, they are difficult to detect even on close inspection (see *Fig. 12.5*). Attempts to disguise displaced hair by combing adjacent hair over these areas is no more effective than the "comb-over" hairstyles worn by many balding men. Although this is perhaps preferable to the patient to having bald spots and missing hair showing, it is immediately evident that the problem is still present in most cases.

The temporal portion of the facelift incision traditionally placed within the temporal scalp will frequently result in a tell-tale and unnatural-appearing superior elevation and posterior displacement of the temporal hairline. Secondary or tertiary facelifts using the same incision plan will compound this problem and often result in a bizarre appearing and objectionable absence of temple hair *(Fig. 12.3)*.

This can best be minimized or avoided at secondary facelift by the use of an incision along the hairline *(Fig. 12.4)*.

If it is appropriately planned and carefully executed, an acceptable scar will result that is artistically and aesthetically superior to additional hairline displacement *(Fig. 12.5)*.

In choosing the location of the temporal portion of the facelift incision, it is important to note the degree of existing temple "skin show" *(Fig. 12.6)* and consider it in conjunction with skin redundancy present over the cheek *(Fig. 12.7)*.

This allows an estimate to be made of the degree of elevation and/or displacement of the sideburn and temporal hair

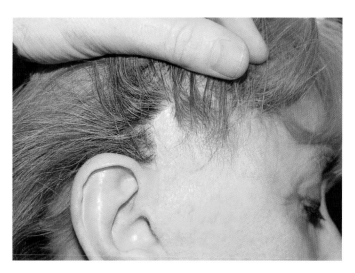

Fig. 12.3 Sideburn elevation and displacement of the temporal scalp after multiple facelifts. A secondary facelift using the same incision plan as at the primary procedure has resulted in the telltale displacement of temple hair and elevation of the sideburn (procedure performed by an unknown surgeon).

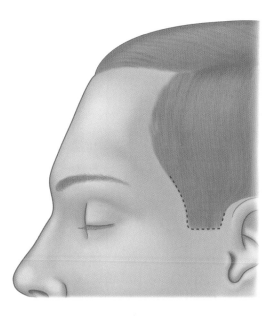

Fig. 12.4 Plan for incision along the temporal hairline. An incision along the temporal hairline should be considered whenever objectionable displacement of the sideburn and temple hair is predicted. Although a fine scar is present in these patients, it is not evident upon casual inspection. Note the preservation of lush temple hair and a full, youthful appearing sideburn.

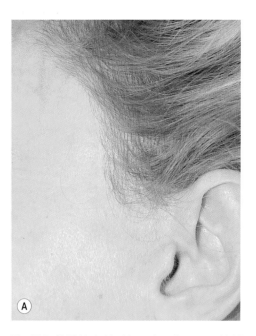

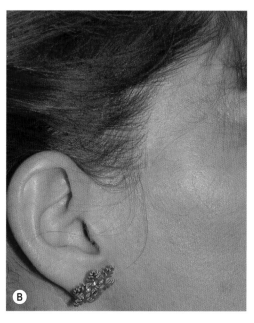

Fig. 12.5 (A,B) Healed incisions along the temporal hairline. The use of an incision along the hairline, when indicated, can prevent hairline and sideburn displacement without compromising the end result. Although a fine scar is present in these patients, it is not evident upon casual inspection. Note the preservation of lush temple hair and a full, youthful appearing sideburn (compare with Figs 12.2 and 12.3). (Procedures performed by Timothy J Marten, MD, FACS.)

that will occur when facelift flaps are shifted, and thus facilitates rational planning of incision placement. In certain instances, a sub-sideburn incision used in conjunction with a traditional incision on the temporal scalp will be adequate in preventing objectionable sideburn elevation and/or hairline displacement. In other situations, however, the incision must extend more superiorly along the temple hairline. Such an incision will accommodate large posterior-superior skin shifts and prevents tell-tale hairline displacement.

The occipital portion of the facelift incision is traditionally placed high upon the occipital scalp, in a well intended, but almost always counter-productive effort to hide the resulting scar. Unfortunately, any such a plan embodies an inherent defect in design that will preclude optimal improvement in the neck and frequently result in a tell-tale and unnatural appearing displacement of the occipital hairline (*Fig. 12.8*).

A high transverse post-auricular incision plan presumes that the resultant vector of skin redundancy is directed mostly superiorly and that the majority of skin redundancy is present over the lateral neck. Both careful consideration and direct observation will reveal the proper direction of post auricular flap shift to be in a mostly *posterior*, slightly superior direction that roughly parallels the mandibular border if an optimal result is to be achieved in the cervicosubmental area. This is because it is along this vector that the majority of neck skin redundancy is present. As the flap is shifted along a more superiorly directed vector, as it must be with any high transverse occipital incision plan, tension will rise across the cervicomental angle, but a diminished effect will be seen over the anterior neck and submental regions. In addition, transverse cervical rhytides, if present, will be unnaturally shifted

superiorly over the upper lateral neck and sometimes onto the pre-lobular and post auricular area. It must also be kept in mind that neck contour should be the result of deep layer repair, and not skin tightening. Thus, neck skin should be shifted and excised along a vector that allows maximum elimination of redundancy, and not one that appears to produce the most neck tightness.

Although occipital hairline displacement may sometimes be acceptable to patients after their primary procedure, secondary or tertiary facelifts using the same incision will compound this problem and usually result in an unnatural and intolerable absence of occipital hair and notching of the occipital hairline *(Fig. 12.9)*.

If an attempt is made to reconstitute the hairline by superior shifting of the post- auricular flap, a wide scar will usually result as the tissue discarded in any such maneuver is necessary for side-to-side head tilt and shoulder drop when the patient is in an upright position. These problems can best be minimized at the time of secondary facelift by the use of an incision along the occipital hairline *(Fig. 12.10)*.

If the incision is appropriately planned and carefully executed, an acceptable scar will result that is artistically and aesthetically superior to additional hairline displacement. In addition, this plan will sometimes allow scalp displaced at the primary procedure to be partially advanced back towards its proper position *(Fig. 12.11)*.

When and incision is used along the occipital hairline it should be planned in such a way that the inferior portion of the incision and thus the resulting scar is turned back into the scalp and at the junction of thick and fine hair on the nape of the neck (see *Figs 12.10, 12.11*). It should not be carried more inferiorly because it will be incompletely concealed and is likely to be visible to others *(Fig. 12.12)*.

Fundamental to obtaining an inconspicuous, well-healed scar when incisions are placed along the temporal or occipital hairline is the diversion of tension to deeper tissue layers and precise flap trimming so that wound edges abut each another under little if any tension before sutures are placed. The incision is then closed using a combination of half buried vertical

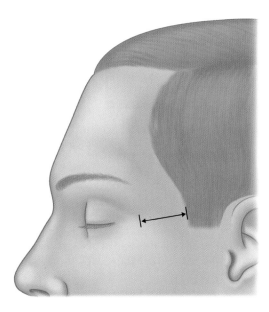

Fig. 12.6 Temporal skin show. The distance between the lateral orbit and the temple hairline and how it will change with flap shift must be considered when planning the temple portion of the facelift incision.

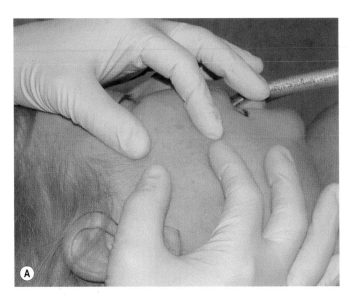

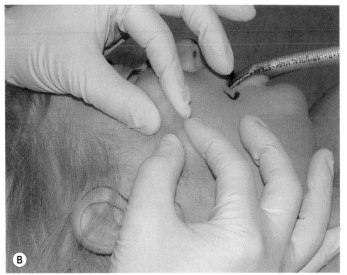

Fig. 12.7 (A,B) Estimating skin redundancy over the upper cheek. Gauging the skin redundancy over the cheek assists in predicting the degree of temporal hairline displacement that will occur when the facelift flap is shifted.

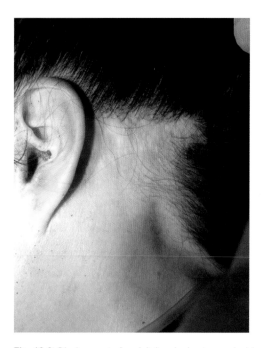

Fig. 12.8 Displacement of occipital scalp due to poor incision planning. The occipital portion of the facelift incision was made high within the occipital scalp in a well-intended effort to hide the resulting scar. Because cervical redundancy was large and skin elasticity poor, advancement of the neck skin flap has resulted in objectionable hairline displacement. An incision along the hairline would have prevented this deformity (procedure performed by an unknown surgeon).

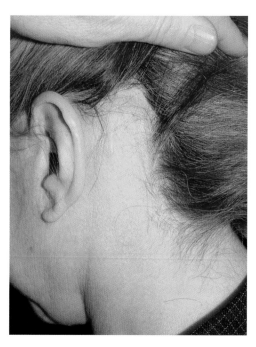

Fig. 12.9 Elevation and displacement of the occipital scalp after multiple facelifts. A secondary facelift using the same incision plan as at the primary procedure has resulted in the objectionable displacement of the hairline (procedure performed by an unknown surgeon).

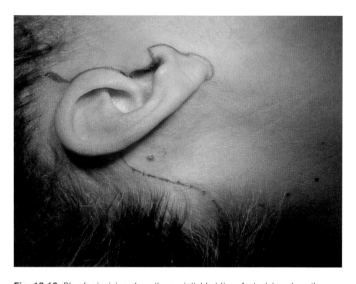

Fig. 12.10 Plan for incision along the occipital hairline. An incision along the occipital hairline should be considered whenever objectionable displacement of the occipital hairline is predicted. This incision plan protects the hairline and prevents hairline displacement.

mattress sutures of 4-0 nylon with the knots tied on the scalp side and multiple simple interrupted sutures of 6-0 nylon. The 6-0 sutures provide precise wound alignment and are removed in 5 days. The half buried vertical mattress sutures of 4-0 nylon provide wound support, while simultaneously avoiding cross-hatched marks. These sutures are removed 7–10 days after surgery.

Although incisions placed along the frontal, temporal, and occipital hairlines will prevent additional hairline

displacement at a secondary procedure, they do not provide for correction of large and severe problems sometime seen (see *Figs 12.2, 12.3, 12.8, 12.9*). In these situations, consideration must be given to the use of hair flaps, hair transplantation, and scalp expansion.

Hair loss

Hair loss is an all too common and avoidable stigmata of facelift surgery seen in many patients presenting for secondary procedures. Hair loss is generally the result of technical errors, including improperly made incisions that damage hair follicles, placement of overly tight sutures, or the closure of inadequately mobilized scalp flaps under too much tension. It may occur, however, in smokers, certain individuals with scalp disease (alopecia areata), eating disorders, or patients with a variety of systemic illness in the absence of any wrong doing on the part of the surgeon. Consideration should be given to an origin of this sort before hair loss experienced by the patient at the primary procedure is attributed to technical error. Hair loss is also frequently the result of the ill-conceived shifting of scalp flaps along the wrong vector. This is commonly seen on the temporal scalp after erroneous attempts to smooth the forehead and glabella by applying lateral traction on the forehead flap *(Fig. 12.13)*.

The use of cautery near or within the plane of hair follicles can also result in hair loss, as can rough flap handling and pinching or prolonged folding of scalp flaps beneath retractors.

Small areas of hair loss resulting from tight suture placement or attempts at spot suspension of the scalp can often be corrected at the time of secondary facelift by direct excision after adequate mobilization of surrounding tissue or by incor-

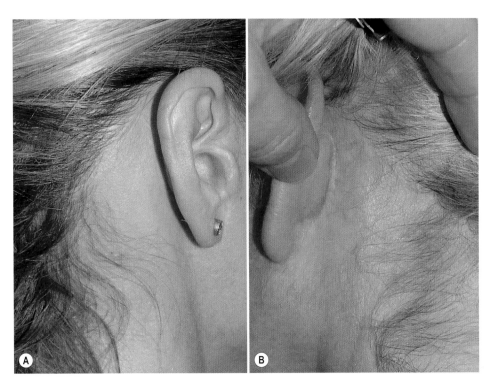

Fig. 12.11 Healed incision along the occipital hairline. The use of an incision along the occipital hairline will prevent hairline displacement without compromising the end result. Although a fine scar is present in these patients, it is not evident upon casual inspection and they are free to wear their hair up off their neck in any manner they choose. (Procedures performed by Timothy J Marten, MD, FACS.)

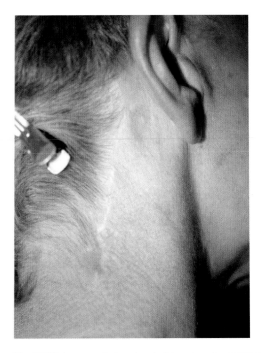

Fig. 12.12 Improper design of an incision along the occipital hairline. The incision has been made too low and carried too far inferiorly in front of the fine hair on the nape of the neck. It would have been better concealed if it had been made more superiorly and turned posteriorly into scalp hair more superiorly. (Procedure performed by an unknown surgeon.)

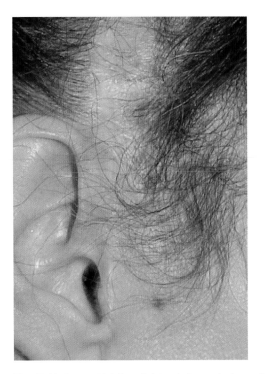

Fig. 12.13 Temporal hair loss. Hair loss is frequently the result of improper shifting of scalp flaps along the wrong vector. This is commonly seen on the temporal scalp after well intended but misguided attempts to smooth the forehead and glabella by excising temporal scalp and applying lateral traction on the forehead flap (procedure performed by an unknown surgeon).

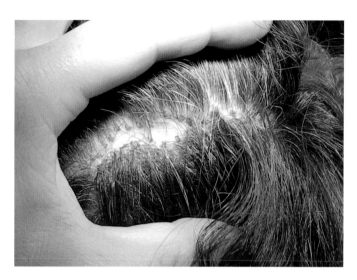

Fig. 12.14 Hair loss resulting from tight suture placement or attempts at spot suspension of the scalp. These problems can often be corrected at the time of secondary facelift by direct excision after adequate mobilization of surrounding tissue or by incorporation of the hairless area into a more comprehensive incision plan (procedure performed by an unknown surgeon).

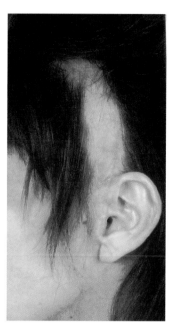

Fig. 12.15 Large areas of hair loss. Large areas of hair loss are usually difficult to correct, especially if scalp excision was aggressive at the primary procedure and little residual redundancy is present. In such cases, complete correction may not be possible at the time of secondary facelift and that hair transplantation, scalp flaps and scalp expansion may be required (procedure performed by an unknown surgeon).

poration of the hairless area into a more comprehensive incision plan *(Fig. 12.14)*.

Larger areas of hair loss resulting from excessive flap tension, an overly tight closure or ill-conceived scalp flap shifting are usually much more difficult to correct, especially if scalp excision was aggressive at the primary procedure and little residual redundancy is present *(Fig. 12.15)*. In such instances, the patient and surgeon must accept that complete correction may not be possible at the time of secondary facelift and that hair transplantation, scalp flaps and even scalp expansion may be necessary at a later date. The goal at any secondary procedures in these patients is to select a surgical plan that does not further compound the problem.

Poorly situated scars

Poorly situated scars are a common problem after primary facelift and the result of artistic insensitivity, poor planning, and tension-based surgical techniques. In many patients, secondary facelift will provide the opportunity to relocate these to a more appropriate, less conspicuous location, but in others it must be recognized and accepted that complete correction is not possible if additional problems are to be avoided.

Poorly situated scars are typically seen in the pre-auricular, peri-lobular, and post-auricular areas. They can also be found in the submental region in many patients. Proper placement of incisions is important, particularly in the pre-auricular area, because even a thin, well-healed scar will ultimately be visible and noticed by others in most cases as a result of the gradient of skin color and texture typically present on each side of it. Although differences in skin color can sometimes be concealed with make-up, differences in texture usually cannot. Scars placed along natural anatomic interfaces tend to be overlooked by the eye however, where a gradient of color and texture is expected to be seen and where the scar appears to be a natural crease on the face. Make-up becomes less necessary as the scar is lost in shadow, appears to be a natural

part of the face, or is mistaken to be a reflected highlight *(Fig. 12.16)*.

The pre-auricular region is a common point of reference for those seeking to identify the facelift patient, and, as such, it is of concern to patients and worthy of careful consideration by the surgeon. The pre-helical portion of the pre-auricular scar is often situated too far anteriorly in the patient presenting for secondary surgery and the illusion of the scar as an anatomical feature is lost. Moving this scar so that it rests in the helical-facial sulcus will result in a less conspicuous scar and a more natural appearance. This is generally possible in most secondary and tertiary cases if skin resection has not been overly excessive at prior procedures *(Fig. 12.17)*.

Although it is not possible to move a pre-tragal scar to a "retro-tragal" position along the margin of the tragus in every patient presenting for secondary surgery, this is preferred when possible, for the reasons outlined above *(Fig. 12.18)*. The feasibility of relocating a pre-tragal scar to a retrotragal position will depend on the amount of cheek skin redundancy that remains after the primary procedure. Because preoperative assessment of residual cheek skin redundancy can be difficult and exceedingly deceptive at the tragus, it is sometimes best to make the initial incision along the existing pre-tragal scar, when present. The decision to sacrifice the remaining skin over the tragus and move the scar to the tragal margin can then be delayed until after cheek flaps have been mobilized, SMAS advanced, and the actual amount of cheek skin recruited through these maneuvers, if any, determined. Often, skin recruited is needed to recreate an absent pre-tragal sulcus and to correct a "buried tragus" deformity. In such instances, relocation of a pre-tragal scar to the margin of the tragus will not be possible and the existing pre-tragal location of the scar

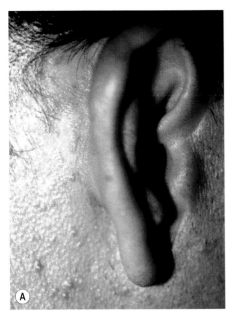 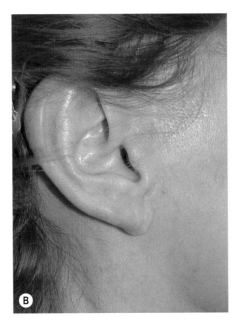 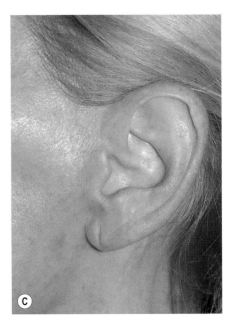

Fig. 12.16 Retrotragal scar. **(A)** The scar resulting from a properly situated retrotragal incision will usually be inconspicuous, even if it is suboptimally healed, as the eye will mistake it for a reflected highlight. Note the well-concealed scar on this darkly complexioned patient. A scar of the same type would be more obvious if the incision had been placed in a pretragal position. **(B)** A healed retrotragal face lift incision in another patient with fair skin. Transitions of color and texture are hidden along natural interfaces. **(C)** A healed retrotragal incision in another patient. If the incision is closed carefully, a natural appearance without anatomic distortion should result.

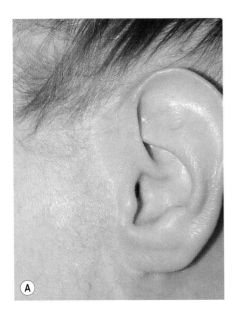 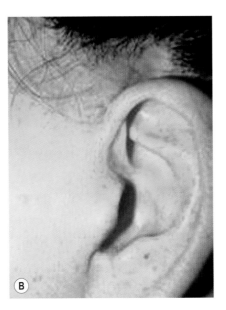 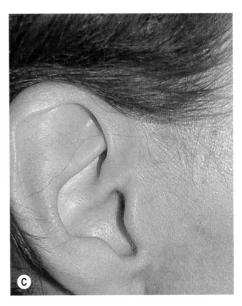

Fig. 12.17 Improper and proper placement of pre-helical scar. The pre-helical portion of the pre-auricular scar is often poorly situated **(A,B)** and the illusion of it as an anatomical feature is lost. **(A)** The pre-helical incision has been made too far anteriorly and the illusion of the scar as an anatomical feature is lost. (Procedure performed by unknown surgeon.) **(B)** The pre-helical incision has been made too far posteriorly and has obliterated the helical facial sulcus and part of the helix itself. The illusion of the scar as an anatomical feature is lost. (Procedure performed by unknown surgeon.) **(C)** A patient with a properly placed pre-helical incision. The scar has been placed directly in the helical facial sulcus. In this location a transition of color and texture is expected and the scar appears to be a natural anatomical feature. (Procedure performed by Timothy J. Marten, MD, FACS.)

must be accepted. If the secondary facelift incision is initially made along the margin of the tragus when a pre-tragal scar is present but before intraoperative assessment of skin redundancy can be made, needed skin may be erroneously excised. This will force an inappropriately tight closure and result in tragal distortion, tragal retraction, and obliteration of the pre-tragal sulcus.

The peri-lobular area is a common location for poorly situated facelift scar in secondary and tertiary facelift patients. Typically, it is low lying due to poor planning and the skin settling that occurs after "skin only", non-SMAS facelift techniques *(Fig. 12.19)*.

Unlike the pre-helical and post-auricular portions of the facelift scar, however, which should be placed directly in their

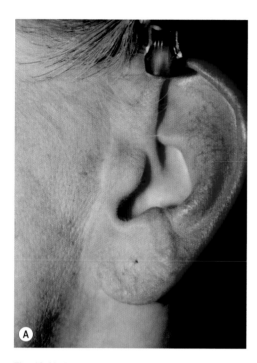
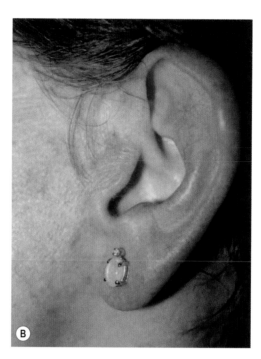

Fig. 12.18 Pre-tragal and retrotragal incisions compared. **(A)** Pre-tragal incision in a patient presenting for secondary facelift. The scar has healed satisfactorily but attention is drawn to it due to differences in color and texture on each side of it. (Procedure performed by an unknown surgeon.) **(B)** Same patient after secondary facelift in which incision was moved to a retrotragal position. Color and texture differences, and the scar itself, are hidden along natural anatomic interfaces. (Procedure performed by Timothy J. Marten, MD, FACS.)

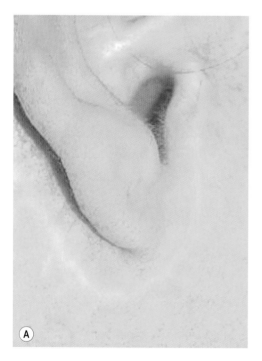
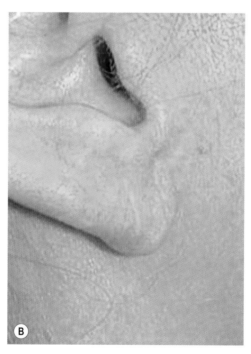

Fig. 12.19 Improper and proper placement of the peri-lobular incision. **(A)** The peri-lobular incision has been made too far inferiorly and is evident even on casual inspection. (Procedure performed by an unknown surgeon.) **(B)** A different patient seen after facelift. The peri-lobular scar has been placed more superiorly and in such a manner that it is hidden by the lobule itself. In this location it cannot be seen. (Procedure performed by Timothy J. Marten, MD, FACS.)

respective anatomic creases the peri-lobular scar should not lie directly in the lobular-facial crease because the crease itself constitutes a delicate, aesthetically significant anatomical subunit that cannot be reconstructed and should not be disrupted. Other factors being equal, a superior result will be obtained if the scar is situated a few millimeters inferior to this junction and an attempt is not made to join thin, soft earlobe skin directly with course, thick cheek skin. As is the situation with the relocation of other scars about the ear, relocation of the peri-lobular portion of the facelift scar at the time

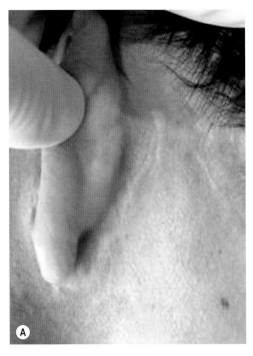 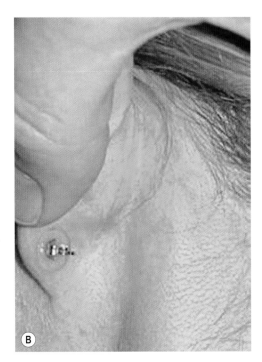

Fig. 12.20 Improper and proper placement of the post-auricular incision. **(A)** The post-auricular incision has been made too far posteriorly. The scar lies outside the auriculomastoid sulcus and is evident if hair is worn short or up off the neck (Procedure performed by an unknown surgeon.) **(B)** A different patient seen after facelift. The post-auricular scar has been placed in the auriculomastoid sulcus. In this location it mimics a natural anatomic feature and is overlooked on even close inspection. (Procedure performed by Timothy J Marten, MD, FACS.)

of secondary or tertiary facelift will depend on the amount of cheek skin that remains after the primary procedure. If cheek skin excision has been excessive at the primary procedure, or if a "pixy" earlobe is present, relocation may not be possible. For these patients, it must be accepted that only partial correction can be accomplished.

A poorly situated post-auricular scar, although not as readily apparent and easier to disguise in most social situations than a poorly situated scar in the pre-auricular region, is nonetheless an objectionable deformity that should be corrected when possible. Typically, the poorly situated post-auricular scar will be seen to lie outside the auriculo-mastoid sulcus, and too low over the mastoid to be concealed by the pinna. Such a deformity is the result of poor planning and inferior–posterior migration of the post-auricular flap due to excessive tension placed upon it at the primary procedure *(Fig. 12.20)*.

Moving the post-auricular scar so that it rests directly in the auriculo-mastoid sulcus is sometimes possible in secondary and tertiary patients, if tissue sacrifice has not been excessive or along an improper vector at the primary procedure. Moving the scar more superiorly, although seemingly straight forward, is often not possible because of the common practice of inappropriately excising tissue from the superior tip of the post-auricular flap at the primary procedure. Attempts to do so will often result in a forced closure under excessive tension and eventual inferior migration and widening of the scar due to inferior traction on the post-auricular flap. Although an apparent redundancy will be present in the supine patient on the operating table due to a high lying position of the shoulders, this will be seen to vanish in the upright position when the shoulders fall to a normal position. As a result, little if any

redundant skin is available along the needed superior vector of shift.

The submental incision will frequently be seen to have been erroneously placed directly along the submental crease in a well-intended effort to hide the resulting scar *(Fig. 12.21)*. Regrettably, this serves only to reinforce the submental retaining ligaments and accentuate a "double chin" or "witch's chin" appearance. In such situations, consideration should be given to moving the submental incision 1–2 cm posterior to the crease so that the existing scar car be undermined and released. Although this results in a new scar, it will be inconspicuously hidden in the shadow of the mandible in all but the unusual case *(Fig. 12.22)*. This is preferable and a worthwhile trade-off for correction of the more obvious and objectionable contour deformity that would result if the incision were made again in the same place upon the existing scar. If limited work in the neck only is needed and minimal or no double chin deformity is present, it may be possible and appropriate to use an existing scar in the submental crease as the site for secondary incision. If more extensive maneuvers are required and a marked double chin deformity is present however, a new more posteriorly situated submental incision is indicated *(Fig. 12.23)*.

If skin excision has been aggressive and excessive at the primary procedure, relocation of poorly situated scars may not be possible at the time of request for secondary facelift, regardless of how much the patient and surgeon would wish otherwise. These patients have typically undergone aggressive skin-only, non-SMAS procedures and have overly tight faces with wide and/or hypertrophic scars *(Fig. 12.24)*. Often earlobes have been pulled or placed too far inferiorly into the cheek as well, compounding the problem. In such cases, it is

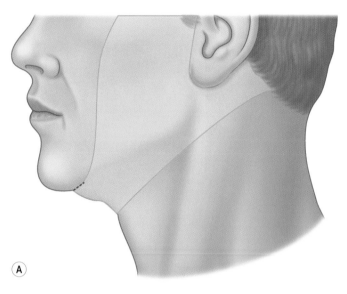

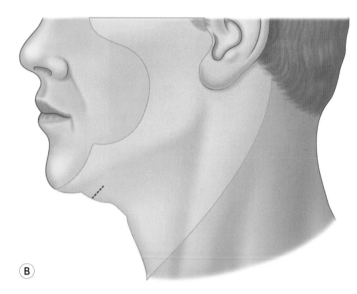

(A)

(B)

Fig. 12.21 Incorrect and correct plan for the submental incision. **(A)** Incorrect position for the submental incision. The incision should not be placed directly along the submental crease because this will accentuate it and reinforce the double chin appearance. Note that the traditional plan of skin undermining (shaded area) also promotes a double chin. **(B)** Correct position for the submental incision. Placement of the submental incision posterior to the submental crease prevents accentuation of the double chin and witch's chin deformities and provides for easier dissection and suturing in the anterior neck. Note that this incision plan allows the submental crease to be undermined (shaded area) and released and the fat of the chin pad and neck to be blended.

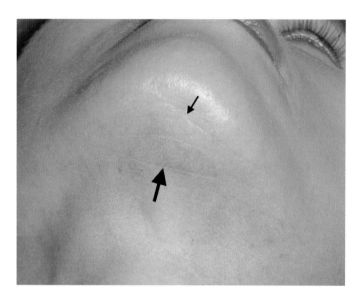

Fig. 12.22 Placement of the submental incision. Close-up view of the submental region of a patient after secondary face lift. A previous incision had been made directly in the submental crease (small arrow). The incision used at the secondary procedure was made posterior to the prior incision (large arrow), and the scar and crease were released. Smooth submental contours are present, and both scars are inconspicuous.

usually best to defer surgery until scars are mature, skin has relaxed, and adequate tissue is available to make proper repair. In most cases, this will mean waiting until 2–3 cm or more of skin can be pinched up along each jaw line along a line extending from the chin to the lobule. Re-operation in the absence of adequate skin to make proper repair will be a frustrating act of futility in which little if any benefit will be gained.

Wide scars

Wide, thick, hypertrophic, and keloid scars, often attributed to be the result of the patient's own poor healing, are more often due to the over excision of skin along improper vectors in procedures in which the surgeon has employed skin tension as a vehicle to lift sagging deeper layer tissue, rather than the SMAS and platysma. In fact, it is noteworthy that scar widening and hypertrophic healing have rarely seen after a primary facelift in patients of all skin types, providing a technique of no skin tension has been employed.

Because the factors underlying suboptimal healing leading to wide or hypertrophic scars are still present to some extent in the patient requesting secondary surgery, each must be approached with caution. Like the patient with a skin shortage and poorly situated scars, the patient with wide or hypertrophic scars may be impossible to effectively treat if skin excision has been excessive at the primary procedure (*Fig. 12.25*). This is true, regardless of how much the patient and surgeon wish otherwise. Re-operation in the absence of adequate skin to make proper repair will be a frustrating act of futility in which little, if any, benefit will be gained.

Cross-hatched scars

Cross-hatched scars are a completely avoidable deformity commonly seen in patients presenting for secondary facelift. Like most secondary facelift deformities, they are the product of errors in both planning and technique. The underlying cause of most cross-hatched scars can be traced directly to skin tension and tension-based facelift techniques. When incisions are closed under tension, larger sutures must be used, and these must be tied tighter and left in longer. Inevitably, varying degrees of necrosis occur beneath each, and these

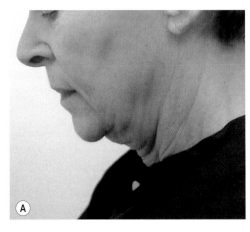
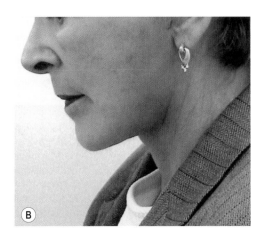

Fig. 12.23 Correction of the double chin and witch's chin deformities. If the submental incision is placed posterior to the submental crease, the submental retaining ligaments can be released and the fat of the chin and the neck blended. **(A)** Patient with double chin before secondary facelift. (Procedure performed by an unknown surgeon.) **(B)** Patient after secondary facelift. The submental incision was made 1 cm posterior to the submental crease, the submental restraining ligaments released, and the subcutaneous fat of the chin and the submental areas sculpted and blended to achieve optimal contour. Platysmaplasty, transverse platysma myotomy, and submandibular gland reduction were also performed. (Procedure performed by Timothy J Marten, MD, FACS.)

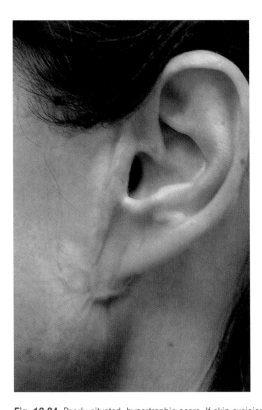

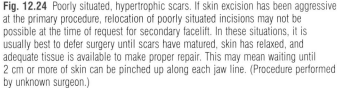

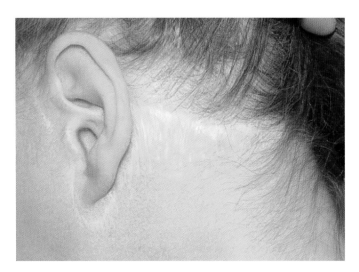

Fig. 12.25 Wide scars. Wide, thick, hypertrophic and keloid scars, often attributed to be the result of the patient's own poor healing, are usually due to the over excision of skin along improper superiorly directed vector in procedures in which the surgeon has employed skin tension as a vehicle to lift sagging deeper layer tissue. As is the case in the patient with poorly situated scars, the patient with wide or hypertrophic scars may be impossible to effectively treat if skin excision has been excessive at the primary procedure. (Procedure performed by unknown surgeon.)

Fig. 12.24 Poorly situated, hypertrophic scars. If skin excision has been aggressive at the primary procedure, relocation of poorly situated incisions may not be possible at the time of request for secondary facelift. In these situations, it is usually best to defer surgery until scars have matured, skin has relaxed, and adequate tissue is available to make proper repair. This may mean waiting until 2 cm or more of skin can be pinched up along each jaw line. (Procedure performed by unknown surgeon.)

spots go on to heal as scars. As skin relaxation occurs over time the hatch marks and suture hole scars stretch and migrate away from the incision scar, giving the appearance that the wound was closed in a crude fashion with large, widely placed sutures. Almost always cross-hatched scars are accompanied by other signs of over reliance on skin tension including hairline displacement, hypertrophy, and wide scars *(Fig. 12.26)*.

Cross-hatched scars can simply and easily be avoided by employing a facelift technique that does not rely on skin tension. Diverting tension to the SMAS allows skin incisions to be closed under little if any tension with loosely tied, fine sutures that can safely be removed in 4–5 days after surgery.

Diverting tension to the SMAS and platysma will not, in and of itself, prevent cross-hatched scars. If skin is closed under tension, or shifted along an improper vector after SMAS and platysma fixation, the opportunity to avoid tension-based secondary deformities will be lost and one of the major benefits of the utilization of the SMAS and other deep layer tissue will be subverted.

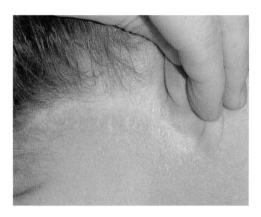

Fig. 12.26 Cross-hatched scars. The underlying cause of most cross-hatched scars can be traced directly to skin tension and tension based facelift techniques. When incisions are closed under tension, necrosis occurs beneath sutures and these spots go on to heal as scars. As skin relaxation occurs over time the hatch marks and suture hole scars stretch and migrate away from the incision scar, giving the appearance that the wound was closed with large, widely placed sutures. (Procedure performed by unknown surgeon.)

Accepting that skin need not be tight is difficult for most surgeons trained in classical facelift technique. For many, it seems not only counter-intuitive, but also at cross-purposes with traditional goals and objectives. Dismissing this idea, and failing to accept related concepts, however, are major stumbling blocks to achieving high quality scars and a "non-surgical" and natural postoperative appearance.

The correction of cross-hatched scars is often difficult because the factors leading to the problem are still present to some extent in the patient requesting secondary surgery, and each must be approached with caution. As is the situation in the patient with hairline displacement and wide or poorly situated scars, for the patient with cross-hatched scars, it may be impossible to effectively treat the patient with cross-hatched scars if skin excision has been excessive at the primary procedure or if enough residual skin redundancy is not present to allow simultaneous excision of scars, skin flap advancement along an appropriate vector, and closure without tension.

It is a common error to think that scars can simply be excised and the skin needed for closure can be recruited by wide undermining of overly tight adjacent areas. Experience will show that re-operation in the absence of adequate skin to allow excision along a proper vector along with a tension free closure will result in a recurrence of the problem and other associated tension-based deformities. In most patients, it is best to accept partial correction of the problem, rather than create new or worse problems by attempting complete elimination. Make-up, tattooing or restyling of hair may be necessary to conceal the residual scars.

Distortion of tragal anatomy

Distortion of tragal anatomy is a common problem in patients presenting for secondary facelifts. Like many other problems associated with secondary surgery, it is the result of artistic insensitivity, poor planning, and errors in technique. In many patients, the secondary facelift will provide an opportunity to improve or correct tragal distortion, but in others complete correction may not be possible if additional problems are to be avoided.

Common types of tragal distortion seen after primary facelift include changes in tragal shape, changes in tragal contour, tragal retraction, and obliteration of the pre-tragal sulcus. Less commonly, more severe degrees of distortion can also be present. In rare cases, the tragal cartilage has been excised and the tragus is absent.

The most commonly observed forms of tragal distortion seen in patients presenting for secondary facelift are loss of tragal contour and obliteration of the pre-tragal sulcus. These are frequently seen concurrently, although they have somewhat different underlying causes. Loss of tragal contour is usually the result of improper incision planning, superior overshifting of cheek skin, and imprecise trimming of the tragal skin flap. The tragus is seen to have no distinct beginning or end and no posterior projection. A tell-tale "chopped-off" appearance results (*Fig. 12.27A*). This is generally correctable if tension is diverted to the SMAS, skin can be recruited from secondary advancement of the cheek skin flap, and the skin flap is properly trimmed and fit over the tragal cartilage.

Loss of the pre-tragal sulcus results from failure to leave enough skin to fill the pre-tragal depression when the tragal flap is trimmed and is almost unavoidable in any technique in which tension is placed on the cheek skin flap. The over-trimmed skin flap bridges the pre-tragal sulcus which in turn is gradually filled with fibrotic tissue and scar over time. The tragus appears "buried" and indistinct from the cheek anterior to it. It can also be seen to have a flat, two-dimensional contour (*Fig. 12.27B*).

Correction of the buried tragus deformity requires recruitment of sufficient skin from the cheek at the secondary procedure to fill the three dimensional contours of the pre-tragal area. Pre-tragal subcutaneous scar filling the pre-tragal sulcus must also be excised, and the tragal skin flap must be redraped under no tension. Skin must then be trimmed to a precise fit while the flap is depressed and held in the pre-tragal sulcus. No deep suture is necessary to hold the skin flap in the pre-tragal hollow if the above steps are properly carried out.

The "retracted tragus" represents an extreme case of the "buried tragus" deformity. It too, is the result of technical error and has its origin in an overly tight and excessively trimmed cheek skin flap. The retracted tragus deformity differs from the buried tragus deformity, however, in that not only is the pre-tragal sulcus obliterated by subcutaneous scar, but the tragal cartilage itself is pulled anteriorly by the over-trimmed skin flap. This results in an open auditory canal and a tell-tale and unnatural appearance (*Fig. 12.27C*). Simple recruitment of skin from the cheek and excision of pre-tragal subcutaneous scar is not sufficient to correct the retracted tragus deformity because the retracted tragal cartilage is usually stiff, fibrotic, and unable to return to its natural position and configuration on its own. Correction usually requires that the cartilage be scored on its anterior surface and then secured with a mattress suture once in its proper anatomic position (*Fig. 12.28*).

Distortion of earlobe anatomy

There is perhaps nothing as tell-tale and objectionable in the patient who has undergone a prior facelift as distortion or

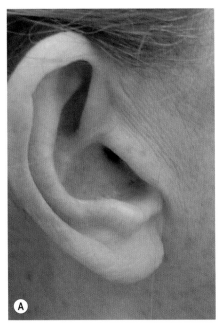 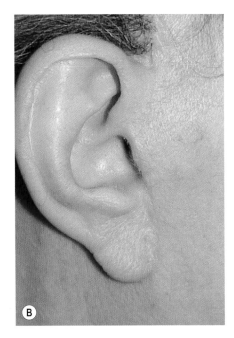 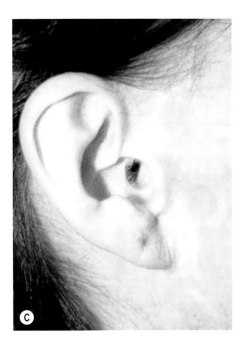

Fig. 12.27 "Chopped-off", "buried" and "retracted" tragal deformities. **(A)** In the "chopped-off" tragus deformity the tragus is seen to have no distinct beginning or end and no posterior projection. It is usually the result of improper incision planning, superiorly overshifting of the cheek skin and imprecise trimming of the tragal flap. **(B)** In the "buried" tragus deformity the tragus appears indistinct from the cheek anterior to it and the pre-tragal depression is absent. This deformity results from failure to leave enough skin to fill the pre-tragal sulcus and is commonly seen when tension is placed on the cheek skin flap. **(C)** The "retracted tragus" represents an extreme case of the "buried tragus" deformity and is the result of an over trimmed cheek skin flap. The retracted tragus deformity differs from the buried tragus deformity, however, in that not only is the pre-tragal sulcus obliterated, but the tragal cartilage itself is pulled anteriorly. This results in an open auditory canal and a tell-tale and unnatural appearance. (All procedures performed by unknown surgeons.)

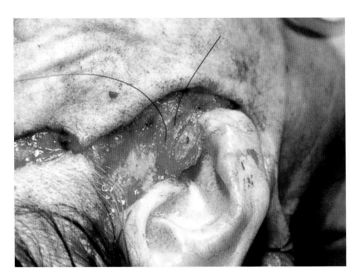

Fig. 12.28 Correction of the "retracted tragus" deformity. To correct the retracted tragus deformity cheek skin is undermined and subcutaneous scar in the pretragal sulcus be excised. The anterior surface of the tragal cartilage then incised to allow it to bend posteriorly to its proper anatomical position. The cartilage is secured in this configuration with a mattress suture of 4-0 nylon. Skin is then recruited by facelift flap advancement and the tragal flap is carefully trimmed to ensure that adequate skin is preserved to fill the pre-tragal sulcus. (Procedure performed by Timothy J. Marten, MD, FACS.)

mal-position of the earlobe. Like most other problems associated with secondary surgery, it is the result of artistic insensitivity, poor planning and errors in technique. Common types of earlobe distortion seen after primary facelift include the "pixy ear" and the "loving cup" ear.

"Pixy ear" is a pejorative term used by some to describe the unnatural, impish, or elf-like appearance the ear assumes when the lobule is attached directly to the cheek and pulled anteriorly and inferiorly *(Fig. 12.29A)*.

It is often the result of inartistic, improper, or careless resetting of the earlobe into the cheek after the cheek flap has been suspended. It can also result as a delayed effect after artistically appropriate resetting of the lobule at the time of surgery in a skin only – non-SMAS facelift. The lack of deep layer support in such cases will inevitably lead to some inferior migration and settling of the cheek skin flap and eventual traction on the lobule. "Loving cup" ear is used to describe the situation in which the ear resembles the handles commonly seen on vase-like trophy cups. In this deformity, the earlobes are joined to the cheek in a less extreme fashion, but also have been inset or pulled too far inferiorly *(Fig. 12.29B)*.

This problem is often made worse by inferior migration of the cheek skin flap over time when a skin-only, traction-based facelift technique is used.

A full understanding of the origin of lobular deformity requires that the surgeon understands and appreciates normal lobular anatomy. This sets the stage for appropriate and natural resetting of the lobule into the cheek at the time of the primary procedure and the avoidance of unnatural secondary deformities. Young patients presenting for other procedures and friends and family members who have not undergone plastic surgery serve as useful subjects for study in this regard. Photographs of actors, models, and celebrities are less valuable however, as many have secondary lobular deformities that may not be immediately recognized due to concealment of scars by photo-retouching or make-up.

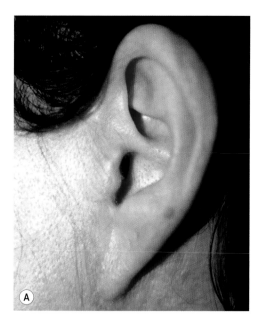
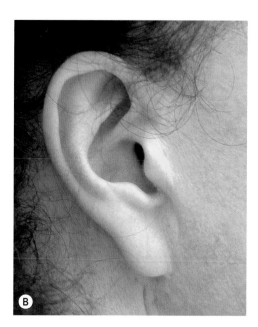

Fig. 12.29 The "pixy ear" and "loving cup ear" deformities. **(A)** "Pixy ear" describes the unnatural, impish or elf-like appearance the ear assumes when the lobule is attached directly to the cheek. It is the result of inartistic resetting of the earlobe into the cheek after the cheek flap has been suspended. It can also result as a delayed effect after artistically appropriate resetting of the lobule at the time of surgery in a "skin only" facelift. **(B)** "Loving cup ear" describes the state in which the ear resembles the handles commonly seen on vase like trophy cups. In this deformity, the earlobes are not only attached to the cheek, but have been inset or pulled too far inferiorly. (Procedures performed by unknown surgeons.)

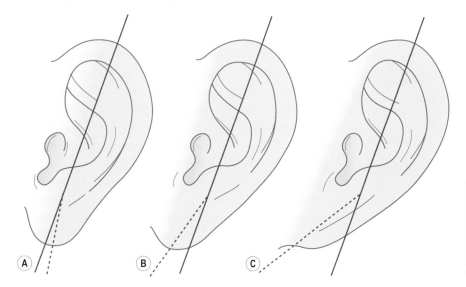

Fig. 12.30 Earlobe aesthetics. **(A)** In the youthful appearing attractive ear, the long axis of the lobule (dotted line) will be seen to rest 15° posterior to the long axis of the pinna (solid line). **(B)** As the long axis of the lobule is shifted anterior to the long axis of the pinna a less natural "surgical" appearance is produced. **(C)** If the long axis of the lobule is shifted further anteriorly and/or inferiorly an objectionable deformity will result.

A careful examination of the youthful lobule will show that it is distinct from the cheek and that its long axis lies approximately 15° posterior to the long axis of the pinna *(Fig. 12.30A)*. As the axis of the lobule is moved anteriorly to rest anterior to the long axis of the pinna, a tell-tale "surgical" appearance is produced *(Fig. 12.30B)*. If the long axis of the lobule is shifted well anterior to the long axis of the pinna and/or is drawn inferiorly, an objectionable and grotesque appearance can result *(Fig. 12.30C)*.

On occasion a patient presenting for primary facelift will be encountered, in whom the lobule naturally sits in an anterior–inferior position. In these patients, it is best to reset the lobule in an attractive, artistically appropriate, more posterior position, rather than where it was originally found. If the lobule is reset in its original position, a "surgical" appearance is likely to result. This will not only raise suspicion that

the patient has had a facelift, but also will make appropriate positioning of the lobular difficult at a secondary procedure.

Correction of the pixy and loving cup ear deformities requires that sufficient skin can be recruited along the jaw line at the secondary procedure to allow the lobule and cheek flap to be elevated to a natural position under no tension. As is the case in the patient with a skin shortage and poorly situated, cross-hatched, or wide scars, the patient with a pixy or loving cup earlobe may be impossible to effectively treat if skin excision has been aggressive and excessive at the primary procedure or if the ear lobe has been reset too far inferiorly into the cheek. In addition, if deep layer support is not provided, it is likely that skin elevated at a secondary procedure will migrate inferiorly over time and the deformity will recur. This is true, regardless of how much the patient and surgeon wish otherwise, and re-operation in the absence of adequate skin to

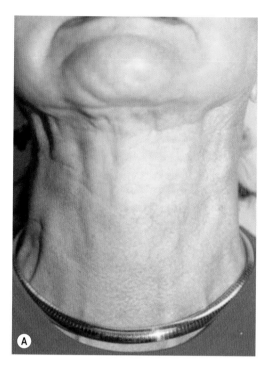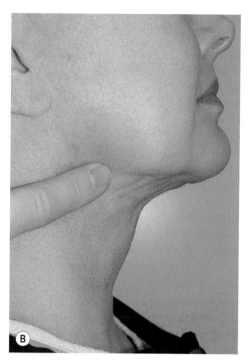

Fig. 12.31 Over-excision of subcutaneous fat. **(A)** The patient has undergone a "weekend" facelift in which aggressive liposuction was performed and too much fat was removed. The neck and submental region are irregular and unattractive. **(B)** A different patient who has had a previous facelift. Submental "microliposculpture" was performed as part of the procedure. Inappropriate over-resection of fat has resulted in harsh and unnatural contours. Note the contrast with the soft contours of the cheek and neck. (Procedures performed by unknown surgeons.)

make proper repair will be a frustrating act of futility in which little, if any, benefit will be gained.

Redundant skin available over the jaw line and in the upper neck can be assessed by pinching it up and measuring it. In general, if <2–3 cm is present, it is best to advise the patient that complete correction will most likely not be possible. The extent to which correction can be made will depend, of course, on the degree of deformity present. Although commonly practiced, anchoring the lobule to auricular cartilage or adjacent deep tissue with buried sutures will not be effective if enough skin is not present to allow closure to be made under minimal skin tension. Over time, the lobule will migrate inferiorly.

In all but the unusual case, there will not be enough skin present to correct loving cup earlobes by undermining and elevating the cheek skin. It will also be an artistic error to simply place the lobule back in an inappropriate position. In such instances, it may be best to move the lobule into a normal position and carefully close the defect into which it was originally inset using meticulous technique. The resulting scar will go unnoticed because the eye will not be drawn to the area as it once was by the abnormal appearing lobule. In addition, the scar itself will often heal well following this maneuver, as the incision can be closed under minimal tension under these circumstances. A small amount of make-up or a cosmetic tattoo is often usually sufficient to conceal it. If the healed scar is raised or irregular and is incompletely concealed with make-up dermabrasion can be performed as a subsequent step. For most patients, a scar on the cheek will be less noticeable than a displaced lobule, and an acceptable trade-off for obtaining proper lobular position.

Over-excision of subcutaneous fat

The introduction of liposuction, along with ill-conceived procedures in which subcutaneous fat of the face and neck is aggressively curetted, excised or even subjected to laser and ultrasound treatment, has resulted in a group of patients with excessively defatted necks and concomitant deformities *(Fig. 12.31)*.

These patients with "cadaver necks" have little fat between their cervical skin and the underlying platysma and present a difficult problem when they request secondary procedures. Often, they require platysma surgery, although they have little superficial fat to disguise any irregularities that may arise from these procedures. In addition, if isolated surgery on the neck was performed as the primary procedure, pseudoptotic jowl fat and fat lying along the mandibular border has usually been erroneously excised. This can result in harsh or irregular contours when the SMAS is subsequently elevated and defatted areas are unavoidably advanced superiorly onto the face *(Fig. 12.32)*.

In these situations, care must be taken in any secondary procedure to preserve as much fat as possible and to carefully contour fat at the interface between face and neck.

It should be the aim of every surgeon who endeavors to rejuvenate the face to create an attractive neck and not one simply devoid of fat. Excessive fat excision does not produce attractive or youthful contours, and often exposes and accentuates other neck problems. These problems include platysma bands, prominent submandibular glands and large digastric muscles. Each of these neck problems generally requires that wide cervical skin undermining be performed if appropriate

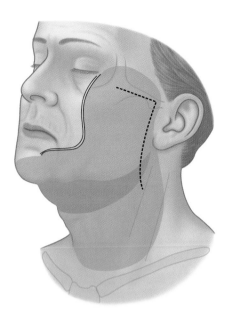 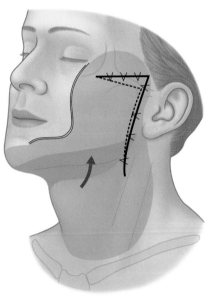

Fig. 12.32 Erroneous excision of submental and pseudoptotic jowl fat. Aggressive liposuction is performed as a primary procedure over the neck and jowl (shaded area) in a misguided attempt to rejuvenate the face. When the patient returns for formal facelift and ptotic deep layer tissues are properly repositioned, denuded areas are advanced up onto visible areas of the face. This can result in harsh and irregular contours.

correction is to be made. This is often difficult when little fat is present. Any such dissection must be carried out with great care to avoid any injury to residual subdermal fat, the platysma, and regional motor nerves. Excessive fat excision can also result in troublesome dermomuscular adhesions. These frequently result in tethering and abnormal appearances in animation and generally require careful division if an open dissection of the neck is planned. If no modification of the platysma or other deep layer structures is needed, dermomuscular adhesions can be treated transcutaneously with a "V" tipped needle dissector and carefully placed fat injections.

Although judicious excision of cervical fat is often necessary as part of rejuvenation of the aging neck, the excision of *facial* fat will usually produce an aged and haggard look, inconsistent with the intended goal of producing an improved appearance. This haggard appearance is evident in many patients presenting for secondary surgery who have undergone "minilifts", "weekend" facelifts, "microliposculpture", and other procedures in which facial liposuction is often performed. In these cases, remaining fat must be carefully tailored to produce the best contours possible. These patients will also often benefit from facial fat injections.

Over-excision of subplatysmal fat

Although not all surgeons routinely explore the subplatysmal space and excise subplatysmal fat, patients with an unappealing "dug out neck" deformity are increasingly presenting for secondary procedures. The dug out neck deformity is a term used by some to describe situations in which subplatysmal and/or deep cervical fat has been erroneously over-excised resulting in an objectionable depression in the submental region *(Fig. 12.33)*. Typically, this depression is more evident when the neck is flexed somewhat or when the patient swallows.

Correction of the dug out neck deformity is best made using fat injections if it is the only problem present. If large digastric muscles and/or large submandibular glands are

present, reducing these as part of the procedure may be sufficient to hide the deformity. If secondary surgery is planned and adequate platysma is present, an anterior invagination (rather than excision) of the redundant portion of the medial platysma borders can also produce some improvement.

Over-excision of buccal fat

Although the judicious excision of buccal fat will occasionally benefit certain patients seeking primary or secondary facelift, it will usually result in an ill or haggard look inconsistent with the intended goal of producing an improved appearance *(Fig. 12.34A)*. This is evident in many patients presenting for secondary surgery who have undergone "minilifts", "weekend facelifts", and limited incision procedures in which buccal fat excision is often performed. In these patients, SMAS advancement or midfacelifts can exacerbate this situation by elevating the over-reduced buccal pad. These patients will often benefit from less aggressive SMAS surgery and avoidance of midfacelifting.

Correction of the over-resection of buccal fat is most easily made using fat injections and these can generally be performed as part of the secondary facelift procedure *(Fig. 12.34B)*. Injections should be made meticulously in small amounts and in multiple passes in multiple planes with a small blunt infiltration cannula. In general, 3–7 cc of centrifuged fat is needed for each cheek. Alternatively, free fat grafts, or dermis fat grafts can be used. Facial fat injections can also be performed as a separate procedure after secondary facelift is performed. This allows the patient and surgeon to examine what was accomplished during the secondary procedure, and adjust the fat injection procedure accordingly.

Prominent submandibular glands

As experience is gained in evaluation of patients presenting for secondary surgery, prominent submandibular glands will increasingly be recognized as a frequent part of the secondary neck deformity and the underlying cause of objectionable

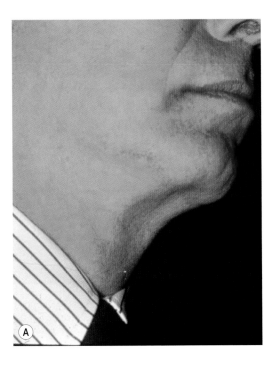

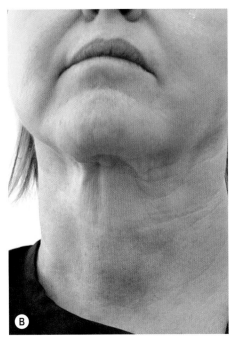

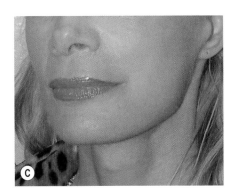

Fig. 12.33 **(A,B)** The "dug out neck" deformity. The "dug out neck" deformity is a term used to describe situations in which subplatysmal and/or deep cervical fat has been erroneously over excised resulting in an objectionable depression in the submental region. (Procedures performed by unknown surgeons.)

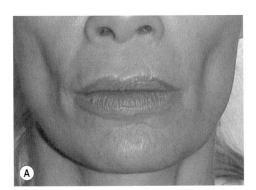

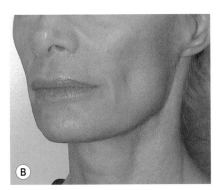

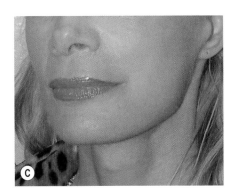

Fig. 12.34 **(A)** Inappropriate excision of buccal fat. Excision of buccal fat as part of a "mini" face lift has resulted in an ill or haggard look. This problem is most easily corrected by fat injections, and these can generally be performed as part of the secondary face lift procedure. (Procedure performed by unknown surgeon.) **(B,C)** Correction of the overresected buccal fat pad. **(B)** Secondary face lift patient who had buccal fat removed as part of her primary procedure. An unattractive, ill appearance has resulted. (Procedure performed by unknown surgeon.) **(C)** Same patient after secondary face lift that included fat injections. The lower face has been filled and lost buccal volume restored. A healthy, youthful, and attractive appearance results. (Procedure performed by Timothy J. Marten, MD, FACS.)

residual bulges in the lateral triangle of the lateral submental region *(Fig. 12.35)*. Often, these bulges go unnoticed at the time of the primary procedure owing to the fact that they are obscured by neck fat and lax platysma muscle. In most instances, the secondary facelift will provide an opportunity for proper diagnosis and appropriate treatment, when present.

If a large or ptotic sub-mandibular gland is present, it can usually be seen and/or palpated lateral to the ipsilateral anterior belly of the digastric muscle within its respective submandibular triangle.

Large glands can be incrementally resected through the sub-mental incision after raising the ipsilateral platysma but before submental platysmaplasty is performed, if indicated. Submandibular glands are usually firm and have a distinctive lobulated appearance. Reduction is begun by incising the glandular capsule inferomedially and grasping the inferior most portion of the gland. The gland can then easily

be separated from its capsule and adjacent tissue using a combination of gentle blunt and sharp scissors technique. Care should be taken when mobilizing the superior-lateral portion of the gland as both the retromandibular vein and the marginal mandibular branch of the facial nerve are in proximity in this area.

An examination of the dissected submandibular gland will show it to be large, and not "ptotic", and careful consideration of this fact will reveal that attempts to reposition it more superiorly with sutures or by tightening the platysma are misguided and will ultimately be fruitless. This observation forms the basis of the recommendation that partial resection be performed in these patients.

After the protruding portion of the gland has been exposed and freed from adjacent tissue, the redundant portion of the submandibular gland is excised using a long tipped cautery and a long pair of shielded forceps. Adequate exposure is

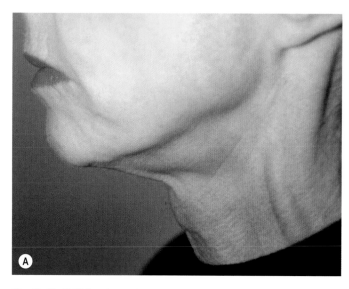

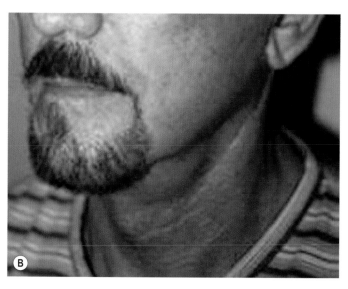

Fig. 12.35 **(A,B)** Prominent submandibular glands. Prominent submandibular glands are commonly seen in patients presenting for secondary facelifts. They are typically evident as objectionable residual bulges in the lateral triangle of the lateral submental region. Prominent glands often go unnoticed at the primary procedure because they are obscured by neck fat and lax platysma muscle. (Procedures performed by unknown surgeons.)

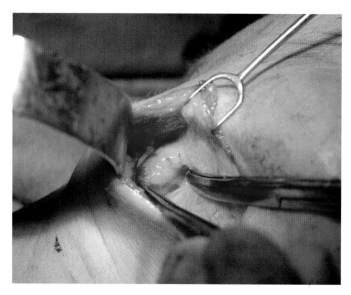

Fig. 12.36 Overview of the technique for reduction of prominent submandibular gland. A submental incision has been made approximately 1 cm posterior to the submental crease and the neck subcutaneously undermined. The right platysma muscle has been elevated and is retracted with a double pronged skin hook and a malleable retractor. The gland will be seen as a distinct bulge just lateral to the ipsilateral anterior belly of the digastric (scissors tips rest on digastric). The capsule has been incised inferiorly and medially and the submandibular gland isolated using blunt dissection. The gland, once isolated, is gently pulled inferiorly (forceps). The protruding portion is then excised incrementally with electrocautery. (Courtesy of Timothy J. Marten, MD, FACS.)

This corresponds to a plane tangent with the ipsilateral inferior mandibular border and anterior belly of the digastric muscle. Intraglandular vessels are often encountered and these must be carefully divided and immediately cauterized in a controlled fashion. Any bleeding points on the raw surface of the gland are then further cauterized once the redundant portion has been excised. Platysmaplasty (suturing the medial borders of the right and left platysma muscles together in the midline) and platysmamyotomy (transverse division of the platysma at the level of the cricoid cartilage) are then performed as indicated. A 10F closed suction drain is placed in both the pre-platysmal and subplatysmal spaces when submandibular gland reduction is performed. It is not necessary to remove the entire gland to create an attractive cervical contour. Complete submandibular gland excision risks injury to the marginal mandibular branch of the facial nerve and is likely result in a depression or other contour abnormality. Subtotal submandibular gland excision to date has resulted in no cases of nerve injury, hematoma, seroma formation, salivary fistula, or gustatory sweating.

Large digastric muscles

As experience is gained in evaluation of patients presenting for secondary surgery, large, low lying anterior bellies of the digastric muscles will increasingly be recognized as a frequent part of the secondary neck deformity and the underlying cause of objectionable linear paramedian fullness in the submental region. These bulges often go unnoticed at the primary procedure because they are often obscured by neck fat and lax platysma muscle. In most cases, the secondary facelift will provide an opportunity for proper diagnosis and appropriate treatment *(Fig. 12.37)*.

Prominent anterior bellies of the digastric muscles can be treated by superficial subtotal myectomy. Superficial, *subtotal anterior digastric myectomy* is performed under direct vision, working through the submental incision after the subplatysmal space has been opened and the medial

necessary, as is good light, an attentive assistant, and a good source of suction. It should be noted that all vital structures are situated lateral to the dissection and lie outside the glandular capsule. Excision is begun by grasping the inferior portion of the gland and gently pulling it inferiorly and medially out of its fossa and away from adjacent structures. The redundant portion is subsequently incised incrementally along the planned line of resection *(Fig. 12.36)*.

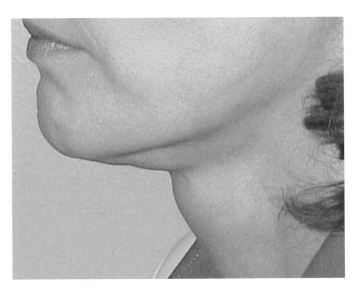

Fig. 12.37 Prominent anterior belly of the digastric muscle. The patient has had prior face and necklift. The anterior belly of the digastric muscle can be seen as objectionable linear paramedian fullness in the submental region that spoils and otherwise good result. Prominent digastric muscles often go unnoticed at the time of the primary procedure due to the fact that they are frequently hidden by cervical fat and lax platysma muscle. (Procedure performed by unknown surgeon.)

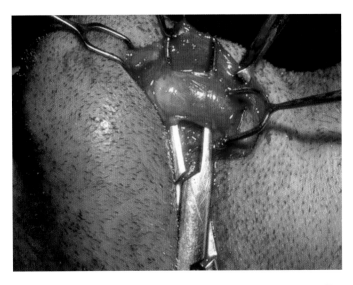

Fig. 12.38 Isolation of the protruding portion of the anterior digastric muscle. The tips of curved hemostatic forceps are bluntly pushed through the midbody of the muscle belly. (View from patient's right of right digastric muscle through submental incision. Patient's chin is on the left and neck on right.)

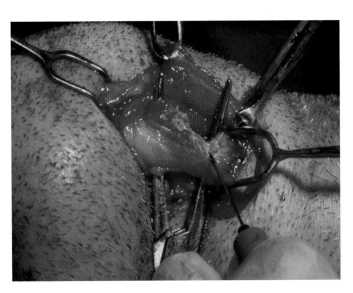

Fig. 12.39 Excision of protruding portion of anterior digastric muscle. The muscle has been isolated on a hemostat. The isolated muscle segment is then divided near the hyoid and mandible using electrocautery. (Courtesy of Timothy J Marten, MD, FACS.)

platysma muscle borders mobilized. Partial digastric myectomy is usually best performed after subplatysmal fat excision and submandibular gland reduction have been performed, if indicated, as it is easiest to assess the muscles at that time. Two basic techniques can be used: incremental tangential shave excision and muscle splitting myectomy. In the former the protruding portion of the muscle is shaved tangentially in an incremental fashion using a DeBakey forceps and medium Metzenbaum scissors until appropriate contour is obtained. The neck is re-examined and the maneuver repeated until an improved contour is obtained. Usually this entails the excision of 25–50% of the superficial most part of the anterior muscle belly, but occasionally 50–90% of the muscle must be removed. In the muscle-splitting partial myectomy technique the protruding portion of the muscle is isolated on a tonsil forceps, or similar instrument, by pushing the instruments tips transversely through the muscle belly *(Fig. 12.38)*. The isolated segment is then excised with scissors or electrocautery by dividing the muscle near the mandible and the hyoid *(Fig. 12.39)*. Contours are checked and the maneuver repeated as indicated. Platysmaplasty (suturing the medial borders of the right and left platysma muscles together in the midline) and platysmamyotomy (transverse division of the platysma at the level of the cricoid cartilage) are then performed as indicated.

A 10F closed suction drain is usually placed in the subplatysmal space when digastric myectomy is performed, and almost always if subplatysmal fat excision or submandibular gland reduction is concomitantly carried out. Digastric myotomy has not resulted in dysphagia, dysphonia, or other functional problem.

Residual platysma bands

The introduction of liposuction has resulted in many surgeons adopting a closed plan of treatment for the neck, consisting

of suction excision of preplatysmal fat with and without postauricular skin excision. Although this occasionally yields a good result in a younger patient with modest deep layer problems, more often it accomplishes little more than exposing underlying platysma bands, resulting in an objectionable and elderly appearance.

Primary and secondary platysma bands are best treated by *transverse platysma myotomy* (transverse division of the platysma at the level of the cricoid cartilage), as the underlying problem is one of platysma hyperfunction, not horizontal platysmal laxity. Dividing the muscle defunctionalizes the muscle similar to the way in which the gastrocnemius muscle is defunctionalized when the Achilles tendon is ruptured. Platysmaplasty alone (suturing the right and left platysma

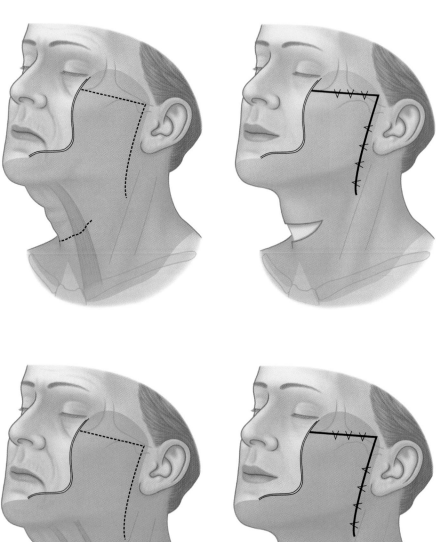

Fig. 12.40 Treatment of residual anterior platysma bands. Schematic showing anterior band and plan for platysma myotomy. After myotomy and SMAS flap advancement.

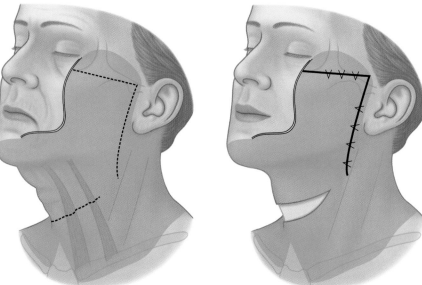

Fig. 12.41 Treatment of residual anterior and lateral platysma bands. Schematic showing anterior and lateral bands and plan for platysma myotomy. After myotomy and SMAS flap advancement.

muscles together in the midline) is usually insufficient as it does not address the underlying cause of the problem.

Transverse platysma myotomy generally requires complete subcutaneous undermining of the neck because myotomy must be preformed at or near the level of the cricoid cartilage where the platysma muscle is thin if visible irregularities are to be avoided. Bleeding will also be minimal when myotomy is performed at this location, and there is minimal chance that lower lip dysfunction will be produced. If platysma transection is performed higher where the muscle is thicker, bleeding from cut muscle edges is more common, and contour irregularities are likely to be evident once swelling is gone and healing is complete. A high division of the platysma can also precipitate lower lip dysfunction. If wedge resection of the platysma is made near the hyoid as is often traditionally taught, muscle and low lip dysfunction is common and an unattractive overly sharp cervicomental angle is likely to result.

Anterior bands require transection of the platysma to a point lateral to the band to the midpoint of the muscle *(Fig. 12.40)*. If lateral bands are present, transection is extended further laterally to a more lateral point in the muscle to include them as well *(Fig. 12.41)*.

Platysma bands are the result of platysma muscle hyperfunction they are not logically or effectively treated in most cases by suspension sutures or direct excision. Suspension sutures and straps, especially those extending from mastoid to mastoid, often result in an overly rigid noose that is disturbing and uncomfortable to patients, especially when they look down. Sutures extending partially across the neck are better tolerated and may be helpful for minor muscular irregularities. Neither, however, addresses directly the anatomical basis of the problem.

Excision of platysma bands, although recommended and practiced for some time, can result in nerve injury and muscle dysfunction, and typically results in visible irregularity, and recurrent deformity. Excision does not address the anatomic basis of the problem and often results in new bands on each side of the excised muscle.

Uncorrected and under-corrected midface deformities

A careful examination of the typical patient presenting for secondary surgery is commonly remarkable for an uncorrected or under corrected midface evident as infraorbital hollowing, malar flattening, and nasolabial fold formation. These changes often appear more obvious and more objectionable after the patient's primary procedure as they typically stand in contrast to an overly tight jaw line and against a background of aggressive rejuvenation of other adjacent areas.

Treatment of midface problems remains controversial and a consensus of opinion as to the best way to correct them has yet to arise. A major short-coming of "skin lifts" and the typical "low" SMAS flap elevated below the zygomatic arch, is that neither is able to produce significant improvement in the midface area. Skin lifts fail because skin provides little in the way of support of the malar fat pad. "Low" SMAS flaps are ineffective, as they are unable by design to exert a significant vector of pull over the midface and infraorbital region. Incising and elevating the SMAS flap "higher", along the mid-body of the zygomatic arch, and extending the dissection medially to release and mobilize midface tissue, however, enables problems in these areas to be addressed (*Figs 12.42, 12.43*). This high SMAS plan, as such, provides a means for both elevating ptotic infraorbital and malar tissue, and increasing lower lid support.

It is common at the time of secondary facelift surgery to find that the SMAS has been dissected timidly at the primary procedure and that the high, extended dissection described above can easily be performed in a virgin plane. Fortunately, a secondary SMAS dissection is also still possible after a more extensive primary SMAS procedure, and the subSMAS plane usually offers little in terms of scar, adhesions, or other encumbrances.

Advancing the cheek SMAS flap superiorly and suspending it without excising its superior margin or folding it superior edge upon itself at the primary procedure, provides the ideal setting for secondary SMAS surgery. The overlapping tissue segments are easily dissected at some future date and minimal subSMAS cicatrix is produced. A high SMAS plan also precludes dimpling and irregular contours over the upper cheek when the patient smiles ("smile block") due to impingement of the cheek pad at suture sites and tethering of tissue there. This can occur, however, if attempts are made to suspend midface or malar pad over the superior aspect of the zygoma or to the periosteum along the infraorbital rim.

It should be recognized that the nasolabial fold and crease are a product of the patient's individual anatomical make-up and in many cases a specific familial trait. In such cases, elevation of the midface as described should not be expected to eliminate or obliterate these features. Indeed, in such cases there is little artistic imperative to do so.

Most midfacelifts are generally conceptually flawed and of limited utility in the secondary facelift patient in that they erroneously assume the problem seen in the anterior upper cheek to be solely one of tissue sagging. Failure to acknowledge the fact that atrophy is present to a significant degree in most cases has led to general disappointment following many procedures for both patients and surgeons, and has resulted in the addition of dermis fat grafts, orbital fat transposition and "septal resets" to "midfacelift" procedures. It is questionable and remains to be answered however, whether these procedures can produce a restoration of lost volume as simply, naturally, and effectively as can be obtained with fat

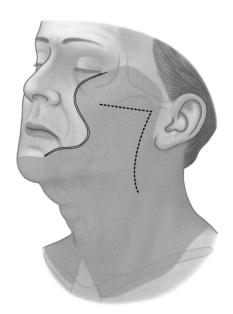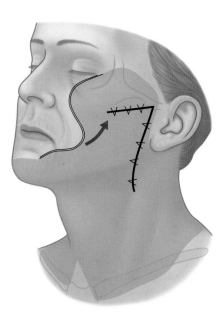

Fig. 12.42 "Low" SMAS flap. The traditional "low" plan for the cheek SMAS flap is by design only able to apply a vector to the lower cheek and jowl, but not the midface. Plan for low SMAS flap. Low SMAS flap after advancement and fixation. Arrow indicates that flap elevation results in improvement in the lower cheek and jowl only.

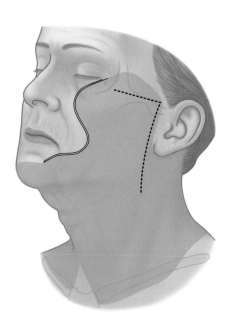
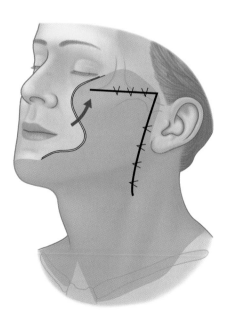

Fig. 12.43 "High" SMAS flap. The "high" plan for the cheek SMAS flap allows a vector to be applied to not only the lower cheek and jowl, but not the midface and infraorbital region as well. Plan for High SMAS flap. High SMAS flap after advancement and fixation. Arrow indicates that flap elevation results in not only improvement in the lower cheek and jowl, but in the midface and infraorbital region as well (compare with *Fig. 12.42A,B*).

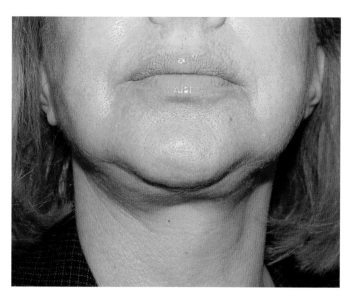

Fig. 12.44 Residual jowl and jaw line laxity. Incomplete elevation of the jowl is commonly seen in patients presenting for secondary facelifts and represents incomplete or under utilization of the cheek SMAS. Although liposuction and direct excision of jowl fat may straighten mandibular contours, this fat more appropriately belongs higher on the face and should not be arbitrarily sacrificed. (Procedure performed by unknown surgeon.)

injections. The current trend seems to strongly favor a "filling" rather than a "lifting" approach.

Residual jowl

Incomplete elevation of the jowl, or recurrent jowl ptosis, is a common problem seen in patients presenting for secondary facelifts that in all but the unusual case, represents incomplete mobilization, improper shift, inadequate fixation or other improper or under utilization of the cheek SMAS *(Fig. 12.44)*.

In most patients, the secondary facelift will provide an opportunity to reposition sagging jowl tissues and to restore attractive mandibular contour. Although liposuction and direct excision of jowl fat can be used to improve mandibular contours in some instances, this fat more appropriately belongs higher on the face and should not be arbitrarily sacrificed (see *Fig. 12.33*). In addition, in most instances liposuction and/or direct jowl fat excision was performed aggressively at the primary procedure, and little residual superficial fat is typically present in secondary cases. Almost all patients with residual jowls presenting for secondary surgery will be better served by formal SMAS dissection and suspension, than by fat excision. Occasionally, patients with very heavy jowls will require the combination of repositioning of jowl fat via SMAS elevation and conservative jowl fat removal via direct excision or liposuction. In a minority of instances however, residual large jowls present after a primary facelift represent a combination of residual excess fat, jowl tissue ptosis, and atrophy at the geniomandibular groove, and a combination of SMAS elevation, judicious fat excision, and geniomandibular groove fat grafting may be indicated.

Distortion and abnormal appearances due to inappropriate skin shifts

Many patients presenting for secondary facelift will have abnormal appearances due to inappropriate shifts of skin flaps. This problem is particularly common in the older patient with deep rhytides and poor skin elasticity and will typically be evident as superiorly over-shifted cervicofacial rhytides in the lower lateral cheek, perilobular area, and upper lateral neck sometimes referred to as a "wrinkle shift deformity" *(Fig. 12.45)*.

Superior over-shifting of cervicofacial rhytides is commonly seen in skin-only facelifts and "composite" type procedures, and in MACS (minimal access cranial suspension) lifts, and other "short-scar" procedures in which a short postauricular incision is used and skin is obligatorily shifted along

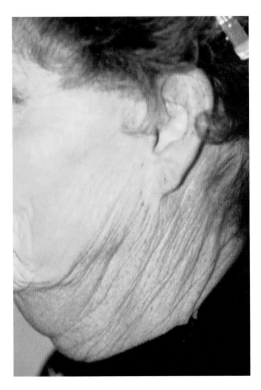

Fig. 12.45 Abnormal appearance due to inappropriate skin shifts. Wrinkles originally present on the neck have been moved up over the jaw line and in front of the lobule. This occurs in "skin lift" procedures when the skin is advanced along a superiorly directed vector in a mistaken attempt to improve neck contour. It can also occur in Skoog and "composite" procedures as skin and SMAS must obligatorily be advanced in the same direction. (Procedure performed by unknown surgeon.)

superiorly directed vector. This deformity is commonly accompanied by temporal hairline displacement, unless an incision along the temporal hairline has been used. The fundamental problem with these procedures is that they fail to address the fact that skin and SMAS age at different rates and along different vectors. *In general, skin needs to be advanced along a vector perpendicular to the nasolabial fold whereas the SMAS and deep layer tissue needs to be advanced along a more superiorly directed vector roughly parallel to the long axis of the zygomaticus major muscle.* In skin-only lifts, skin is typically over-shifted along a superiorly directed vector in a misguided attempt to correct problems of deep layer origin seen in the lower face and along the jowl. In deep plane and composite procedures, skin is obligatorily advanced as a composite with underlying SMAS and skin must be over-shifted superiorly to obtain the best SMAS effect. The "wrinkle shift deformity" is most problematic in MACS lifts and short scar procedures, and any similar procedure in which an attempt is made to shorten or eliminate the post-auricular scar. These procedures, by design, require that cervicofacial skin flaps be shifted along a purely vertical vector, and do not provide a means for wrinkled cervical skin to be partially excised, shifted more posteriorly, and kept on the cervical area.

Separating the skin and SMAS from one another into separate lamella and advancing each along independent vectors allows each layer to be treated most appropriately and as indicated. When this is done, wrinkled cervical skin can be shifted posteriorly and partially excised, and kept off the face. This minimizes cervical wrinkle shift onto the face and other secondary irregularities resulting from improper skin shifts. This treatment of the skin and SMAS as separate layers is referred to as a "lamellar" or "bi-directional" facelift.

Neck to face wrinkle shift is difficult to correct, especially in the patient with little residual skin redundancy. Although skin flap elevation and re-advancement along a more posteriorly directed vector can produce some improvement, the degree to which the flap can be shifted back into a normal position will be limited by the severity of the previous skin over-shifting, the previous cut-out made for the lobule at the primary procedure, and the amount of recurrent redundant skin present at the time that secondary surgery is requested *(Fig. 12.46)*.

Compression of the temporal face

Although advancement of the SMAS along a mostly superiorly directed vector will produce the most comprehensive improvement in the midface, cheek, jowl, and infraorbital areas, it will also inevitably produce compression of the temporal face and lateral orbital region if tissue shifts have been meaningful and temple lift or foreheadplasty is not performed. This compression and wrinkling not only contribute to a "young face–old forehead" deformity, but also will be worse after a secondary facelift if temple and lateral upper facial tissue are not correspondingly repositioned.

Patients are often aware that a problem exists in the temple area after their primary facelift but often mistakenly assume it to be a problem of skin wrinkling and residual "crow's feet". Many rightly observe that tissue compression is worse upon smiling. These patients will benefit from repositioning of temporal tissues or formal foreheadplasty if not performed as part of the primary procedure.

Skin deficiencies and "tight look"

Whenever prospective patients and the lay public discuss facelift surgery they inevitably express the most concern and dismay over the tight faces of various celebrities and their friends and acquaintances who have undergone the procedure. Many unhesitatingly demonstrate what they see to be the problem by pulling forcefully on their cheeks, eyes, and eyebrows asking either not to look that way after their surgery, or stating they will never undergo surgery for fear of ending up with a similar appearance. This concern is reinforced by the numerous jokes and references in the popular press to "masks", "wind tunnels", and "faces so tight they will crack" if their wearer smiles. Despite these expressed concerns and the frequent popular ridicule of the typical outcome of multiple skin-only facelifts, procedures based predominantly on skin excision that produce a tight look continue to be widely performed.

The fundamental problem with a "skin-only" facelift, especially if multiple such procedures are performed, is that skin is meant to serve a covering function and not a supporting one. Most of the changes seen in the aging face, however, are the result of an attenuation of support and subsequent descent of deep layer facial tissues, and not sagging of skin. Any attempt to lift significant sagging of deep facial tissue with

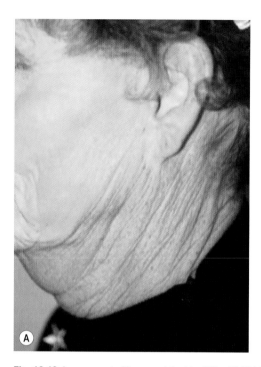
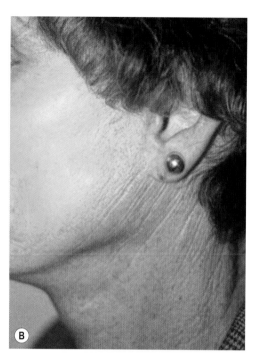

Fig. 12.46 Improvement of inappropriate skin shifts. **(A)** Wrinkles originally present on the neck have been moved up over the jaw line and in front of the lobule at the patient's primary procedure. (Procedure performed by unknown surgeon.) **(B)** After secondary facelift. Contour has been created using the SMAS and platysma and cheek skin has been shifted inferiorly to the extent possible. (Procedure performed by Timothy J. Marten, MD, FACS.)

skin will be short-lived, destined to produce an overly tight appearance, and doomed to result in secondary deformities.

As the elastic limits of skin are exceeded in a skin-only facelift, a tight or pulled appearance develops and facial contour is flattened. Tightness and flattening will be most pronounced in the pre-auricular region where tension is highest and the threshold of elasticity exceeded the most. More inferiorly, in the jowl and peri-oral region, skin will be under less tension and below its threshold of inelasticity. Less tightness will thus be present in these areas, where it is needed most. Further tightening of the skin usually results in more pre-auricular flattening but little improvement in jowl and peri-oral contour. Over time, "tight lines" *(Fig. 12.47)* will appear across the lower cheek and upper lateral neck upon neck flexion and "drapery lines" *(Fig. 12.48)*, or "lateral sweep" will develop over the lower cheek and jowl. Drapery lines and lateral sweep develop because skin is fixed and tethered in the pre-auricular and peri-stomal regions, but has no support in between where deep layer tissue sagging is greatest. Wrinkling and tightness extending from the lobule to the jowl and submental area when the patient looks down ("tight lines") also occurs after well-intended attempts to contour the face by skin excision because the elastic limits of cheek skin is exceeded when the neck is flexed and its normal covering function is corrupted *(Fig. 12.47)*. This tell-tale deformity is typically evident when the patient is looking down and the neck is markedly flexed (e.g., when looking at a menu, book, or theater program).

The patient presenting for secondary facelift who had skin excision only at their primary procedure is the quintessential patient in need of deep layer support. Additional skin

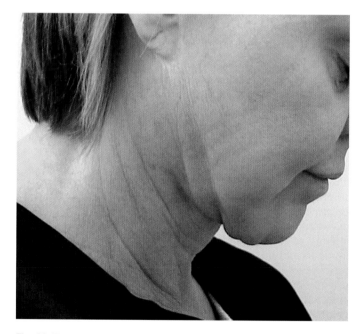

Fig. 12.47 "Tight lines". Wrinkling and tightness extending from the lobule to the jowl and submental area when the patient looks down ("tight lines") occurs after well-intended attempts to contour the face by skin excision because the elastic limits of cheek skin is exceeded and its normal covering function is corrupted. (Note other tension artifacts including retracted lobule and wide, cross-hatched peri-lobular scar.) (Procedure performed by unknown surgeon.)

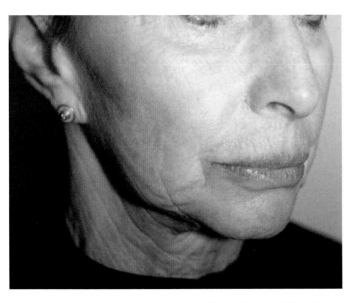

Fig. 12.48 "Drapery lines" and "lateral sweep". "Drapery lines" and "lateral sweep" are common problems following a "skin-only" facelift. In these procedures skin tightness is most pronounced in the pre-auricular region where it is least needed. More inferiorly, in the jowl and peri-oral region, skin will be under less tension where it is needed most. "Drapery lines" develop because skin is fixed and tethered in the pre-auricular and peri-stomal regions, but has little no support in between where deep layer tissue sagging is greatest. (Procedure performed by unknown surgeon.)

excision will result in an accentuation of their deformities, and little improvement in facial contour.

Skin slough

The continued popularity of procedures in which the skin of the face and neck is extensively undermined and then suspended under abnormal tension in an attempt to create youthful contour has resulted in the continued occurrence of potentially avoidable secondary deformities resulting from skin slough. Skin slough is also frequently the result of inappropriately aggressive surgery on smokers and arguably risky procedures in which a facelift is performed concomitantly with aggressive laser resurfacing of undermined skin.

Small areas of scarring resulting from skin slough in patients presenting for secondary surgery can sometimes be corrected at the time of the secondary procedure by direct excision after adequate mobilization of surrounding tissue or by incorporation of the scarred area into a more comprehensive incision plan. Larger areas of skin loss resulting from excessive flap undermining, excessive flap tension, rough tissue handling, or overly tight facial bandages are usually much more difficult to correct, especially if skin excision was aggressive at the primary procedure and little residual redundancy is present. Regrettably, this is all too frequently the case. In such situations, the patient and surgeon must accept that complete correction is not possible at the time of the secondary procedure no matter how much they wish it were so.

It is a common error to assume that scarred areas can simply be excised and that the skin needed for closure can be recruited by wide undermining of adjacent cheek or neck tissue. Even the surgeon who knows better will often set good judgment aside when subjected to the persistent pleading of a patient desperate for some kind of improvement. Experience has shown however, that simple scar excision and adjacent tissue undermining in these patients will result in inadequate skin for a tension free repair and a forced, excessively tight closure. This tight closure, in turn, will inevitably result in wound dehiscence, scar widening, and associated tension-related deformities including scar hypertrophy, cross hatched suture marks, facial distortion, tragal irregularities, and lobular malposition. In these patients it is best to accept partial correction of the problem, rather than creating a new one, or injuring remaining normal tissue. Make-up, camouflage tattooing, or restyling of hair are better alternatives to conceal the residual scars in these circumstances.

If make-up is ineffective in concealing scars due to ridges and step-offs where they abut normal tissue, dermabrasion may be helpful in reducing the discrepancy in tissue height and smoothing the transition between the two areas. Even if discrepancies in tissue height can be reduced in this manner, there is usually a marked difference in tissue texture that prevents the scar from being completely concealed. Patients wishing further improvement may benefit from scar excision and full thickness skin grafting as this technique can provide cover with more natural appearing skin texture. Several follow-up dermabrasion procedures may be necessary to smooth the interface between the skin and skin grafts and these patients are likely to benefit from the use of a silastic gel sheet and/or facial compression garments during the healing process. In some circumstances, it may be better to excise some normal skin along with scarred areas and graft a large anatomical sub-unit, rather than creating a patch quilt of smaller grafts. In extreme situations, consideration may have to be given to cheek or neck skin expansion.

Skin slough can be minimized or avoided by exercising caution, using common sense, and adhering to basic plastic surgery principles. All patients who smoke or have a history of smoking should be identified and their surgery planned in a way that recognizes their increased risk for compromised healing skin necrosis. Consideration should be given to not performing a facelift on heavy smokers with a long history of tobacco use, or employing a facelift technique that does not involve wide skin flap undermining and skin flap tension. Many of these patients will be satisfied with a combination of limited lower risk procedures including closed forehead-plasty, eyelid surgery, conservative submental liposuction, fat injections, and laser resurfacing. Smokers should always be approached with caution however, and every surgeon should recognize these patients have a higher risk of experiencing healing problems after surgery.

Flap necrosis is dependent upon a variety of factors under the surgeon's control and can be minimized by procedure design. These factors include tissue trauma, the extent of skin undermining, and skin tension. Because deep layer techniques limit skin undermining, preserve important cheek perforators, and avoid excessive tension on cervicofacial skin flaps, a careful surgeon employing a gentle, atraumatic, technique in carefully selected patients should infrequently encounter skin slough. And when the procedure is performed in this manner, skin slough, should it occur, should be limited and easily managed.

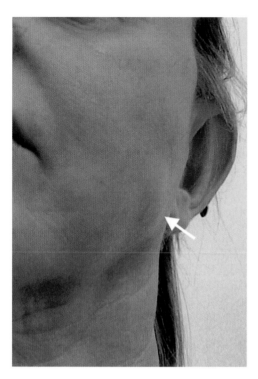

Fig. 12.49 Contour irregularity (arrow) due to prior SMAS injury. A common type of SMAS injury resulting in secondary deformity occurs when the SMAS is knowingly or unknowingly "button-holed" at the primary procedure. This can result in bulges or contour irregularities when the patient animates or clenches her teeth. (Note the bulge in the lower cheek in this patient when clenching her teeth.) (Procedure performed by unknown surgeon.)

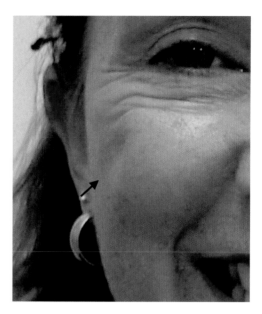

Fig. 12.50 "Smile block". If the SMAS is suspended too low, too far medially over the zygoma, or too rigidly directly to the periosteum, tissue tethering can result in dimpling and other irregularities when the patient smiles (arrow). This problem can also be seen when attempts are made to directly suspend the malar pad or when the malar midface or other mobile area of the face is suspended to the infraorbital rim or other part of the bony skeleton. (Procedure performed by unknown surgeon.)

Distortion and abnormal appearances due to inappropriate SMAS shifts or SMAS injury

Many patients presenting for secondary facelift will have had skin only, non-SMAS procedures and as such, will be potentially free from deformities related to inappropriate SMAS maneuvers. SMAS injury during non-SMAS surgery can, however, result in distortion and irregularities of SMAS origin, even though no actual SMAS surgery was performed. The typical SMAS injury resulting in secondary deformity occurs when the SMAS is knowingly or unknowingly "button-holed". This will result in asymmetries and contour irregularities, especially when the patient is in animation or clenches their teeth *(Fig. 12.49)*. Identification and repair of these SMAS defects at secondary surgery will eliminate many of these types of problems. Larger rents or defects in the SMAS, resulting from larger areas of SMAS injury, SMAS excisions, and failed plications present a bigger challenge and can be difficult to fully correct.

Patients who have had prior SMAS lifts may have other secondary SMAS deformities that must be recognized and addressed as well. These deformities include ridges from SMAS plication or SMAS excision, irregularities from an uneven or overly tight SMAS suspension, and distortion and unnatural appearances from advancement of the SMAS along an improper vector.

Ridges and irregularities from prior plication or SMAS excision may limit the potential for improvement in secondary procedures, and secondary correction techniques must be individualized according to the specific problems present. Some correction is usually possible if tissues are carefully examined and the origins of the problem can be ascertained.

SMAS advancement along an improper vector can result in distortions in animation and at rest. These typically occur when the cheek SMAS flap has been erroneously advanced and suspended under tension along a predominantly *posterior*, rather than mostly superior vector and are typically evident as a "clown mouth" or "pulled mouth" appearance and bizarre and unusual facial movements in animation.

The proper vector of advancement of the SMAS is along a vector parallel to the long axis of the zygomaticus major muscle. If the SMAS is advanced along another vector, the zygomaticus major muscle will be bowed off its axis of normal function and its action corrupted. Posterior traction also exaggerates risorius action and results in an objectionable change in the resting posture of peri-oral tissues. Secondary deformities related to an improper advancement of the SMAS flap are often markedly improved during secondary surgery when the SMAS is re-elevated and re-advanced along a proper vector.

"Smile block"

Attempts to directly suspend the midface or malar fat pad with sutures, or low rigid suspension of the SMAS to the facial skeleton, will prevent natural gliding of cheek and midface tissue during animation. This will be clinically apparent postoperatively, when the patient emotes as dimpling and contour irregularities often referred to as "smile block" *(Fig. 12.50)*.

Smile block can usually be improved at a secondary procedure by a thorough release of the tethered area and re-suspension of ptotic tissues using a technique that allows unrestrained and natural gliding of malar pad and midface.

This is usually best accomplished by high suspension of the cheek and midface using a high SMAS flap *(Fig. 12.43)*, or by employing a subperiosteal midfacelift technique. Techniques that require suture fixation of more superficially situated tissue, or "low" fixation on the face, should be avoided. Smile block can also often be corrected percutaneously by release of tethered areas with a small "V" tipped lipo-infiltration needle and concomitant fat injection.

Unaesthetic facial implants

It is not uncommon to find patients presenting for secondary facelift who have inappropriate or unaesthetic facial implants that detract from their appearance and limit the potential for improvement at any secondary procedure. Frequently, these implants were placed in an attempt to offset the deficiencies and shortcomings of a "minilift", "laser facelift", "infomercial lift", "franchise facelift", or "weekend" procedure, or placed in an isolated procedure in a patient who would have arguably been better served by formal facelift surgery. These can include under and over-sized malar implants, submalar implants, chin implants, and mandibular angle implants. Often even more troublesome are PTFE (Gore-Tex®) strips and similar implants placed in the lips and nasolabial folds. These can be seen to result in visible surface irregularities and buckle and fold upon facial animation.

Although facial implants collectively comprise a significant advance in aesthetic surgery and have helped many patients, they were devised primarily to be used in individuals with skeletal deficiencies. Patients troubled by age-associated soft tissue ptosis are more logically, appropriately, and effectively treated by procedures that reposition and redistribute ptotic tissue, rather than those designed to augment the facial skeleton. Patients troubled predominantly by soft tissue atrophy are likewise more appropriately treated by fat injections than with facial implants.

Many patients with unaesthetic facial implants are aware that all is not right with their appearance and are more than willing to consent to implant exchange or removal. These patients are typically seen to have small button-like chin or cheek implants, oversized malar implants, or submalar implants placed in a failed attempt to improve their nasolabial folds.

A more difficult situation exists when the patient does not see the problem and is unwilling to consider implant exchange or removal. In these patients, one must decide whether it is possible to work around this, or if it is preferable to let the patient enlist the services of another surgeon.

In general, the removal or exchange of facial implants at the time of secondary facelift is not difficult and results in a few untoward occurrences. If implants were originally placed subcutaneously, a more natural appearance can usually be obtained when they are moved to a subperiosteal position. Submalar implants often can be removed at secondary procedures, as cheek and midface repositioning will often result in abnormal appearances if these are left in place. Alternatively, they can be left in place and removed in a subsequent procedure, if necessary, if the patient desires.

PTFE ("Gore-Tex") implants placed in the lips and nasolabial folds present a particular problem in that they can be exceedingly difficult to remove. In addition, removal can often result in troublesome and difficult to correct secondary deformities. It is often best to encourage the patient to return to the surgeon who originally placed these implants before secondary surgery is performed if he or she wishes them to be removed. This allows problems associated with implant removal to be clearly defined prior to the secondary surgery, and an appropriate plan for correction to be made. If implant removal is made as part of the secondary facelift, problems may be erroneously attributed to that procedure or the technique used.

The un-rejuvenated forehead

Rarely does isolated aging occur in the cheek and neck. Nonetheless, most attempts to rejuvenate the face are targeted at these areas and many patients presenting for secondary facelift will have a distinct and tell-tale "young face–old forehead" deformity. This results from a failure to recognize and treat forehead aging at the primary procedure *(Fig. 12.51)*.

A careful consideration of the typical patient presenting for secondary facelift frequently reveals that isolated tightening of the neck and cheeks is often an artistically inappropriate undertaking. This is due, at least in part, to the fact that changes in the forehead are more likely to be mistakenly assigned emotional significance than those in the lower face and neck, and as such, play a greater role in how we interact with and are regarded by others. In addition, rejuvenating the lower face and neck only will typically result in facial disharmony and an unnatural, unbalanced, and "surgical" appearance.

Recognizing the "young face–old forehead" deformity is necessary for it to be corrected and a pre-requisite to communicating the need for forehead surgery to the patient. To appreciate the "problem", the surgeon must examine the patient's face in its entirety and consider the way in which his or her appearance might make others *feel*. This is often best accomplished by viewing the patient's face at a distance and momentarily deferring to one's intuition.

Because a patient's hairstyle can conceal important signs of forehead aging, and compensatory frontalis spasm can give the false impression that the eyebrows are in an appropriate position, *it is imperative that the face of the patient presenting for secondary facelift be examined with the patient's hair pushed well back off their forehead.* In addition, because patients who wear forehead concealing hairstyles often do not see the full extent of these problems, it is helpful, as it is during the rest of their evaluation, for the patient to hold a hand mirror during this part of the examination. They can then be shown these important findings and counseled as to how they are actually the product of forehead ptosis.

The erroneous assumption that forehead ptosis is not present because the eyebrow appears to be in a normal position is the single biggest stumbling block in evaluating the forehead for patients and surgeons alike. Patients are accustomed to optimizing the appearance of their face when looking at their reflection by unconsciously raising their eyebrows. This is often further compounded by the fact that many women aggressively pluck the inferior-lateral portion of their eyebrow to give the allusion that it is higher and more arched. In many cases, the entire outer third of the eyebrow will be seen to be missing and has been drawn on in a higher position with an eyebrow

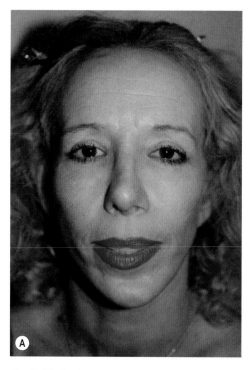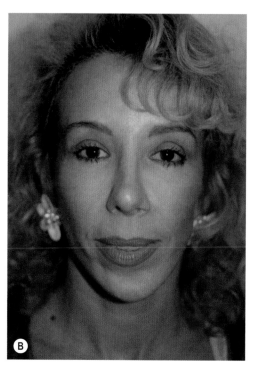

Fig. 12.51 The "young face–old forehead" deformity. **(A)** Patient seen after face lift, neck lift, genioplasty, and eyelid surgery performed elsewhere. Her forehead appears older than the rest of her face, and her overall appearance is disharmonious and unnatural. (Procedure performed by unknown surgeon.) **(B)** Same patient seen after hairline lowering foreheadplasty. No eyelid surgery or other procedures have been performed. Her face appears more natural, harmonious, and balanced, and all areas appear to be the same age. (Procedure performed by Timothy J. Marten, MD, FACS.)

pencil. The all too commonly observed circumstance is one in which the patient with a marked frontalis spasm and marked transverse forehead wrinkling holds a hand mirror during his or her consultation and sees only that his or her eyebrows appear in a normal position.

Because many patients presenting for secondary facelift will have un-rejuvenated foreheads, foreheadplasty will usually be an important component of the planned facelift procedure. (Forehead rejuvenation is discussed in Chapter 7.)

Un-rejuvenated peri-oral region

Although advanced peri-oral aging is usually appreciated at the time of primary facelift, more subtle deformities often go unnoticed, especially when viewed against a background of advanced aging elsewhere on the face. As a result, peri-oral deformities often go untreated at the primary procedure and usually appear more apparent after rejuvenation of adjacent areas is done. This can result in a tell-tale "young face–old mouth" deformity.

Recognizing the "young face–old mouth" deformity is necessary if improvement is to be made and a pre-requisite to communicating the need for the procedure to the patient. Because many patients presenting for secondary facelift will have an un-rejuvenated peri-oral area, peri-oral rejuvenation will often be an important component of the planned secondary "facelift" procedure. This will usually require some form of skin resurfacing to improve skin quality and reduce skin wrinkling, and fat or filler injections to counteract peri-oral atrophy. Other treatments such as upper liplifts and corner lifts of the mouth are also very useful in secondary facelift patients.

Facial atrophy

Traditionally, the aging face has been thought of and defined in terms of tissue relaxation and surface wrinkling, but more recently surgeons have come to appreciate atrophy and lipodystrophy as integral parts of the aging process. A careful examination of patients presenting for secondary facelift will reinforce this assertion and reveal that *simply smoothing wrinkles and lifting sagging tissues will fall short of truly rejuvenating the face in most cases.* This is particularly true if the patient is thin, buccal fat was removed as part of the primary procedure, or facial liposuction was performed *(Fig. 12.52).*

Atrophy is usually most profound and most easily observed around the orbits, upper midface, and infraorbital and peri-oral areas but can be seen on close inspection of many patients in the forehead, brow, temple, cheek, jaw line, chin and neck. Atrophy is not corrected by traditional "facelift" procedures, and is usually incompletely or poorly corrected by traditionally used facial implants. These procedures may even exacerbate the problem, and result in an arguably more unnatural, hard and objectionable appearance.

Correction of facial atrophy requires the addition of volume to the face, not a subtraction, lifting, or tightening, and a rethinking of the traditionally taught approach to rejuvenation of the face. Unlike problems corrected by a "lift" of the face, correction of atrophy requires the surgeon to employ techniques that "fill" and *"sculpt"* the face, and to think in three, instead of just two, dimensions *(Fig. 12.52).*

Currently, the most effective and natural correction of facial atrophy is best achieved through the use of fat injections. Fat injections, when properly performed produce soft and natural

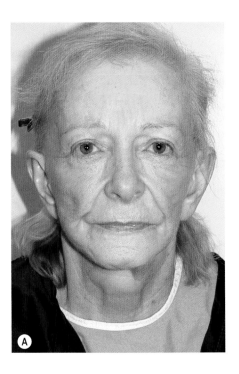

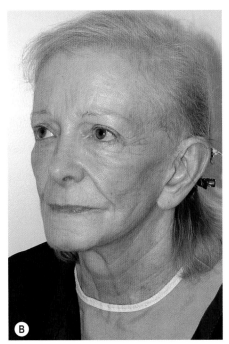

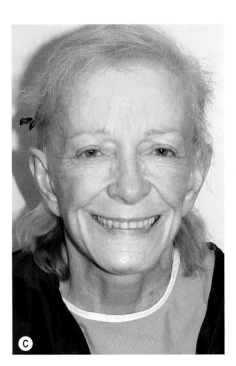

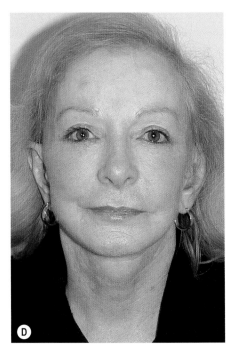

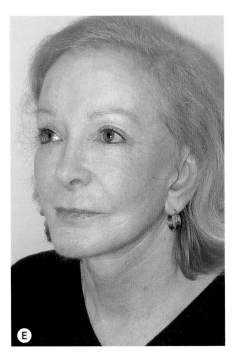

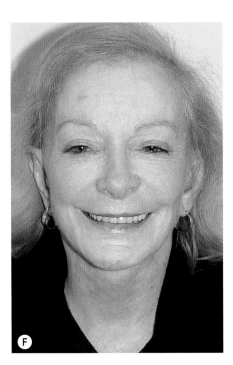

Fig. 12.52 Facelift and fat injection example. **(A–C)** Before surgery view of a woman, aged 75, who has had multiple prior facelifts and related procedures, including laser resurfacing, performed by unknown plastic surgeons. Note marked, uncorrected panfacial atrophy and, despite her multiple traditional lifts, a frail, ill, and elderly appearance. **(D–F)** Same patient, 1 year 4 months after secondary facelift, necklift, foreheadlift, upper and lower blepharoplasties, canthopexy, and aggressive fat transfer to the forehead, temples, cheeks, upper and lower orbits, lips, peri-oral area, buccal recess, chin, and jaw line. A total of 90 cc of fat was injected. No skin resurfacing, facial implants, or ancillary procedures were performed. Note that the patient has soft, natural facial contours and absence of a tight or pulled appearance. Atrophy in all treated areas has been markedly improved with fat injections to create a softer, more youthful, fit, healthy, athletic, and energetic appearance. Such an improvement cannot be obtained with traditional lifting and tightening. It can only be achieved by volume replacement. As was the case in this patient, for many secondary facelift patients, volume replacement is more important than the facelift itself.

contours and afford one the opportunity to correct problems traditional surgery cannot (*Fig. 12.53*). ⊛ FIG **12.53** APPEARS ONLINE ONLY

As a practical matter, fat injections are most effectively performed in areas where tissue planes have not been opened. As a result, they are less applicable and less commonly performed concurrently with a facelift in some areas. These areas include the pre-auricular cheek and the neck. Other areas, however, including the temples, forehead, brows, glabella, radix, orbits, cheeks, midface, "tear troughs", buccal recess, lips, nasolabial folds, nasal base, stomal angles, geniomandibular grooves, chin, and jaw line lend themselves to concurrent treatment, when indicated.

Eyelid skin deficiencies and eyelid malposition

Many patients presenting for secondary facelift have undergone aggressive excision of eyelid skin at their primary procedure and are secondarily troubled functionally by nocturnal lagophthalmos, lid retraction, canthal laxity, scleral show, and dry eye problems, and aesthetically by orbital hollowing, change in eye shape, and unnatural ocular appearance. (These problems and deformities and their treatment are discussed in Chapter 9.)

Over reliance on laser resurfacing

Motivated by largely unscientific claims of laser manufacturers and enticing, but deceptive, early postoperative photographs of patients shown at meetings and included in commercial advertisements, many plastic surgeons and physicians in other specialties embraced laser resurfacing as a substitute for traditional surgical maneuvers in which ptotic deep layer tissue was repositioned and redundant tissue excised. Indeed, laser resurfacing was often referred to as a "laser facelift" and numerous claims were made regarding the lasers ability to incite skin contraction and "tighten" the facial skin. Although laser resurfacing has proven to have clinical utility, experience has shown that it does not produce the skin tightening once hoped for. In addition, "wrinkle relapse" is common once patients are fully healed and all traces of swelling are gone.

Many patients who have undergone laser resurfacing are now presenting for formal facelifts, disappointed in the lack of "lift" gained from their "laser facelift" and concerned over associated secondary deformities including hypopigmentation, skin sensitivity, abnormal skin texture, lower lid malposition, and an unnatural "smooth face-wrinkled neck" appearance. Radiofrequency and ultrasound-based technologies suffer the additional drawback that they often result in a loss of subcutaneous facial fat.

Artistically, the fundamental problem with laser resurfacing is that its primary effect is to smooth skin, and that it does little, if anything, to reposition ptotic tissue, to reduce skin redundancy, or to correct facial atrophy. Its misapplication to the patient with ptotic deep layer tissue and redundant skin typically produces an unnatural, incongruent and "smooth skin-sagging face" appearance. Because this combination appears rarely in nature, the patient is left with a tell-tale "surgical" appearance, often easily recognized by even the untrained eye at a considerable distance.

In all but the unusual instance, *facial contour takes artistic precedent over smooth skin*. Indeed, a few surface wrinkles will be overlooked by the eye if youthful facial contour is successfully re-established. A more balanced, harmonious and natural appearance will result, and a less "surgical look" will be present.

If the patient presenting for secondary facelift has had good repositioning of ptotic tissue at the primary procedure, and little recurrent ptosis is present, skin resurfacing may be worthwhile and appropriate if residual surface textural wrinkling is present. It must be kept in mind, however, that *skin resurfacing will do little to permanently reduce wrinkles that are the product of muscle hyperactivity*. These include glabellar frown lines, transverse forehead wrinkles, and lateral periorbital lines. Correction of these "expression lines" will require reduction or resection of hyperactive muscles, repositioning of ptotic tissue, or removal of excess tissue stimulating muscle contraction. Although skin resurfacing will temporarily disguise forehead wrinkles by inciting swelling, it is no substitute for formal foreheadplasty.

Patients who have undergone prior skin resurfacing can present a number of technical problems at the time of secondary facelift as well. The most vexing of these is the inevitable shift of the line of demarcation between resurfaced and un-resurfaced areas below the jaw line onto the lower face. This "demarcation line shift" usually requires that a second resurfacing procedure be performed to lower this line back into the shadow of the submental area.

Although many surgeons now assert concomitant facelift and laser skin resurfacing to be safe (and cheek skin has arguably been "delayed" at the primary procedure) this combination of procedures still carries significant risk in any case in which skin has been undermined. For this reason it is preferable to defer resurfacing until three months or more after the facelift procedure, at which time the face can be safely, comprehensively, and aggressively treated, if necessary.

The patient who has had a previous combined facelift and skin resurfacing procedure is often an excellent candidate for secondary facelift. This is because the previous surgeon, fearing complications might result from aggressive surgical undermining or relying heavily on resurfacing to make up for shortcomings of the chosen surgical procedure, has been conservative in his or her surgical approach and timid during dissection. Indeed, examination usually shows that these patients have residual uncorrected or under corrected deep layer ptosis and residual forehead deformities.

A new generation of "skin shrinking" technologies has now been introduced that have been widely embraced and said by some to eventually supplant the traditional facelift. In its current form this certainly is not the case, and for the time being at least, facelifts and secondary facelifts offer improvements unobtainable by other means.

Patient considerations

Many patients requesting secondary or tertiary facelifts are chronologically elderly, but deceptively young in appearance. A careful medical history must be taken because they often have concomitant medical problems consistent for their age group that were not present at the time of their primary procedure. It is also wise to obtain independent medical clearance prior to surgery as this group of patients will commonly minimize existing problems and deny important symptoms of age related illness.

A careful documentation of all existing secondary problems and deformities must also be made in patients undergoing secondary facelift procedures, including, but not limited to, facial muscle weakness, dyskinesias, numbness, paresthesias, eye dryness, visual disturbances, and chronic pain. These problems do not show up in a photograph and are not always recognized or volunteered by the patient. If not documented preoperatively, they will inevitably be attributed to be the result of the secondary procedure.

Technical considerations in secondary facelift

The secondary or tertiary facelift will present technical problems and certain risks not seen in primary procedures. In addition, the general approach to secondary procedures is somewhat different depending upon the type of secondary deformities present.

The secondary or tertiary facelift will generally require a comparatively small resection of skin and an increased focus on correcting deep layer problems and secondary deformities, depending upon the skill of the surgeon performing the primary procedure and the type of technique used. This is because the focus of most primary procedures is usually on skin resection and this is more easily and quickly performed than deep layer maneuvers. In addition, skin resection and skin tightening are the underlying cause of many secondary problems. Very often, the skin elevated and recruited by deep layer maneuvers at the secondary or tertiary procedure is needed to correct these problems and will not be excised.

It should also be recognized that secondary facelifts are often time consuming and technically demanding when compared with primary procedures and are likely to test the patience and composure of most surgeons. It is highly recommended that additional operating room time be allotted for the procedure and that the services of an anesthesiologist or competent nurse anesthetist be enlisted. This is particularly true if the procedure is being performed on a patient who is overly apprehensive or has a history of anesthetic difficulties, hypertension or other medical problems.

Although less bleeding is often encountered in elevation of the skin flap in secondary surgery, skin flap undermining is often more taxing because of subcutaneous scar and adhesions resulting from the previous dissection. Scissors pushing techniques should not be used and it is wise that dissection be made carefully, under direct vision, in good light, with an experienced assistant.

Patients undergoing secondary procedures have at least some areas of their face or neck that have been aggressively stripped of fat and these areas must be carefully dissected when skin flaps are elevated. Not uncommonly, dermomuscular adhesions are present in the upper lateral neck over the superficial most portion of the great auricular nerve. Similar caution must be taken when subcutaneous dissection is made secondarily in the temple. It is also very common for the anterior neck and submental regions to have been aggressively defatted at the primary procedure by aggressive small cannula liposuction, ultrasonic lipectomy, excessive direct excision, or by other means. In such patients, it is very easy to perforate, get under the platysma or damage it while attempting to re-elevate the cervicosubmental skin. Entry under the platysma can result in nerve injury and platysma dysfunction, and can render the SMAS or platysma useless in the planned repair. For these reasons, all skin flap dissection must be made with great care in secondary procedures and it is not advisable to use aggressively patterned "super-sharp" or serrated scissors for flap elevation. These scissors tend to pick up and cut delicate structures and are more likely to result in the inadvertent fenestration of the platysma, or unintended excision of subdermal fat.

Subcutaneous fat is generally precious in the secondary facelift patient and as much of it as possible should be preserved until the surgeon is certain that its sacrifice is artistically appropriate and of benefit to the patient. Care must be taken however, not to injure the SMAS and platysma, while elevating skin flaps as these will serve as the workhorse tissue layers in restoring more youthful facial contours. The margin for error is thus very small, and often critically so. The careful infiltration of dilute local anesthetic solutions is often helpful in these situations in pre-establishing the proper plane by hydrodissection. This beneficial effect will be lost if infiltration is made carelessly or in the wrong plane.

A satisfactory and uncomplicated SMAS dissection can usually be performed in most secondary procedures particularly if the primary surgeon previously elevated the SMAS in a skilled manner. Occasionally, the SMAS will be found to have been damaged or thinned however, or compromised by previous plication or suture lifts, making elevation difficult and putting facial nerve branches at risk. Use of a nerve stimulator or raising the flap with cautery on a low setting can be helpful in such instances to differentiate retaining ligaments from nerve branches. Ultimately, however, no amount of aesthetic improvement is worth a facial nerve injury and dissection should not be continued if overly difficult and motor nerve branches are put at unacceptable risk. In such cases, a formal SMAS elevation may have to be abandoned and replaced by an arguably safer alternative treatment such as SMAS plication.

Not all deformities resulting from the primary procedure can necessarily be corrected and the patient needs to have their expectations set in this regard. In addition, the secondary facelift patient will often need ancillary procedures in addition to secondary facelift surgery if maximum improvement is to be obtained *(Figs 12.53–12.55)*. FIGS **12.54**, **12.55** APPEAR ONLINE ONLY

Bonus images for this chapter can be found online at **http://www.expertconsult.com**

Fig. 12.53 Case study 1. Multiple views of a 57-year-old woman before and 12 months after secondary cervicofacial rejuvenation. The primary facelift was performed by an unknown surgeon using conventional techniques and included aggressive upper and lower blepharoplasty but no forehead surgery. The secondary procedure consisted of a high cheek SMAS advancement with post-auricular transposition flaps, preplatysmal and subplatysmal cervical lipectomy, anterior platysmaplasty, and platysma myotomy. Incisions along the hairline were used in the temporal and occipital areas and the preauricular incision was moved from a pretragal position to the margin of the tragus. Foreheadplasty, lower blepharocanthoplasty, bilateral ptosis correction, and perioral dermabrasion were also performed. Full thickness skin grafts taken from the postauricular areas were applied to the upper lids to allow foreheadplasty to be performed and the eyebrows elevated to an appropriate position. No resurfacing or other ancillary procedures were performed. (A) Patient, aged 57, several years after primary conventional facelift, necklift and upper and lower blepharoplasty were performed elsewhere. Note residual and secondary deformities including unrejuvenated forehead, bilateral senile ptosis, midface ptosis, and residual jowl laxity. (B) Same patient, 12 months after secondary facial rejuvenation. Note improvement in forehead, cheeks, periorbital area, and along jaw line that has been achieved without a tight or pulled appearance. (C) Aged 57, several years after conventional facelift was performed elsewhere. Note residual and secondary deformities including obvious preauricular scar. (D) Same patient, 12 months after a secondary facial rejuvenation. (Secondary facelift and related procedures performed by Timothy J. Marten, MD, FACS.) (E) Aged 57, several years after conventional facelift was performed by an unknown surgeon. Note residual and secondary deformities midface ptosis, malar flattening, residual jowl, residual cervical obliquity and "witch's chin" deformity. (F) Same patient, 12 months after a secondary facial rejuvenation. Cheek and midface tissue has been elevated, the pretragal scar has been moved to the margin of the tragus, and cervical contour improved. The witch's chin deformity has also been corrected. (G) Aged 57, several years after conventional facelift and upper and lower blepharoplasty was performed elsewhere. Note severe, untreated residual brow ptosis. When the patient's eyebrows were held up in an appropriate position, she was unable to close her eyelids. (H) Same patient, 12 months after a secondary facial rejuvenation. Full thickness postauricular skin grafts were applied to the upper eyelids so that foreheadplasty could be performed without compromising lid function. Canthopexy and bilateral ptosis correction was also performed. (I,J) Improved periorbital appearance is evident..

Fig. 12.54 Case study 2. Multiple views of a 64-year-old woman before and 13 months after tertiary cervicofacial rejuvenation. The primary facelift and secondary necklift were performed by an unknown surgeon using conventional techniques. The secondary procedure consisted of trifurcated cheek SMAS advancement with temporal and postauricular transposition flaps, preplatysmal and subplatysmal cervical lipectomy, anterior platysmaplasty, platysma myotomy and correction of "loving cup" ear. Incisions along the hairline were used in the temporal and occipital areas and the preauricular incision was moved from a pretragal position to the margin of the tragus. Foreheadplasty, lower blepharoplasty, bilateral ptosis correction and crow's feet reduction were also performed. No resurfacing or other ancillary procedures were performed. (A) Patient, aged 64, 8 years after primary conventional facelift was performed by an unknown surgeon. A secondary necklift had also been performed by the same surgeon at a later date. Note residual and secondary deformities including unrejuvenated forehead, bilateral senile ptosis, midface ptosis, and residual jowl laxity. (B) Same patient aged 65, 13 months after tertiary facial rejuvenation. Note improvement in forehead, cheeks, periorbital area, and along jaw line that has been achieved without a tight or pulled appearance. Note also residual aging in perioral area ("young face–old mouth" deformity). Regrettably, the patient declined recommended perioral rejuvenation. (C) Patient age 64, 8 years after primary conventional facelift was performed elsewhere. A secondary necklift had been performed by the same surgeon at a later date as well. (D) 13 months after tertiary facial rejuvenation. Note that SMAS and platysma surgery has not resulted in abnormalities during expression. (E) Patient aged 64, 8 years after conventional facelift was performed by an unknown surgeon. Note residual and secondary deformities. (F) 13 months after a secondary facial rejuvenation. Note improvement in jowl contour has achieved made without the creation of skin tightness or flattening of facial contour. (G) Patient aged 64, 8 years after conventional facelift was performed elsewhere. Note residual and secondary deformities midface ptosis, malar flattening, shift of cervical wrinkles onto lower face, loving-cup ear, residual jowl and residual cervical obliquity. (H) 13 months after a secondary facial rejuvenation. Cheek and midface tissue has been elevated, the pretragal scar has been moved to the margin of the tragus, the lobular-facial junction has been improved, overshifted wrinkles have been partially moved back onto neck, and cervical contour improved. (I) Patient aged 64, 8 years after conventional facelift was performed by an unknown surgeon. Note shift of cervical wrinkles onto lower face, loving-cup ear, and residual cervical obliquity. (J) 13 months after a secondary facial rejuvenation. The pretragal scar has been moved to the

margin of the tragus, the lobular-facial junction has been improved, overshifted wrinkles have been partially moved back onto neck, and cervical contour improved. (K) An incision along the temporal hairline was used to prevent objectionable hairline displacement. Although the scar can be seen on close inspection, it is not evident on casual glance and in social situations.

Fig. 12.55 Case study 3. Secondary cervicofacial rejuvenation. Multiple views of a 68-year-old woman seen before, and 1 year and 8 months after secondary facelift and related procedures. The primary procedure was performed by an unknown surgeon. The secondary procedure consisted of a high SMAS facelift, neck lift, small incision closed forehead lift, upper and lower blepharoplasties with reinsertion of the levator aponeurosis and canthopexy, facial fat injections, peri-oral dermabrasion, scalp scar revisions, and nevus excision. The neck procedures included excision of residual subplatysmal fat, submandibular gland reduction, superficial digastric myectomy, anterior platysmaplasty with post-auricular transposition flaps, and full width platysmamyotomy. No subcutaneous cervical fat was removed. Fat injections were performed in the temples, upper and lower orbits, the upper nasal dorsum, the cheeks, midface, piriform, nasolabial, stomal angle, peri-oral, lips, chin, GMG (geniomandibular groove), and jaw line areas. No resurfacing or other ancillary procedures were performed. (A) Preoperative AP view. The patient can be seen to have suboptimal eyebrow position and configuration with over-elevation of the medial brow, residual cheek and jowl ptosis, and poor posture of the peri-oral tissues. The peri-ocular appearance suggests aggressive upper and lower blepharoplasty had been previously performed. Marked atrophy can be seen in the temples, orbits, cheeks, oral and peri-oral, and peri-mental areas. Marked facial asymmetry, mild peri-oral wrinkling, and bilateral senile ptosis, worse on the left, are also present. Overall, the face has an ill, tired, and aged appearance. (B) Postoperative AP view. The patient has a soft, natural nonsurgical appearance. The lateral portion of each eyebrow has been raised and eyebrow position and configuration have been improved creating a more alert and engaged appearance. The cheek mass and jowls have been raised and the posture of tissues around the mouth improved. The temples and the upper and lower orbits have been filled using fat injections. A slight under correction of upper orbital atrophy on the left can be seen. Atrophy present in the oral, peri-oral, chin, geniomandibular groove and upper nasal dorsum areas has been nicely improved using fat injections as well. The lips have been subtly filled with fat and the lip border enhanced without a "stung by a bee" or "filler lip" appearance. The combination of fat injections and peri-oral dermabrasion has produced natural appearing correction of peri-oral wrinkling. Overall improved facial symmetry can also be seen. The patient's ptosis has been improved. (C) Preoperative smiling view. Smiling reveals mandibular asymmetry and a poor transition from the lower eyelid to the cheek. (D) Postoperative smiling view. The patient appears natural when smiling. The transition from the lower eyelid to the cheek is improved. The chin is integrated with the jaw line and the two together form one continuous and desirable aesthetic line. The lips are fuller but the shape of the mouth is unchanged. (E) Preoperative oblique view. The patient has a sad, forlorn appearance and the orbital area looks sunken and hollow. The lower face lacks strength and aesthetic appeal and appears elderly. Suboptimal eyebrow position and configuration is evident and residual cheek and jowl ptosis can be seen. Atrophy can be seen in the temples, orbits, upper cheek, oral and peri-oral, and peri-mental areas. The chin is frail and narrow appearing and is poorly integrated with the jaw line. The posterior jaw line is weak and the mandible has a diminutive appearance. The lips are thin and have an elderly retruded appearance. (F) Postoperative oblique view. Overall, the patient has a soft, natural, nonsurgical look and a youthful, athletic, aesthetic, and healthy appearance. The lateral eyebrow has been raised and the eyebrow position and configuration have been improved. The cheek mass and jowls have been re-positioned and the temples and the upper and lower orbits have been filled. An improved transition from the lower eyelids to the cheeks is present. Atrophy present in the oral, peri-oral, chin, and geniomandibular groove areas has been

nicely improved and the posterior jaw line has been strengthened with fat injections. This has resulted in a broader more aesthetic and youthful appearing chin that is integrated with a stronger, more photogenic jaw line. The lips have been subtly filled and the lip border enhanced, and the entire peri-oral area can be seen to have been filled and strengthened. Fat injections to the upper nasal dorsum have also resulted in a more aesthetic and attractive nasal line. A better overall aesthetic balance between facial features is present and the patient has a more attractive and feminine appearance. (G) Preoperative lateral view. The patient can be seen to have a poor transition from the lower eyelid to the cheek, cheek and jowl ptosis, residual cervicosubmental fullness and platysmal bands, a large submandibular gland, suboptimal jaw line contour, a retracted tragus, and a mild "loving-cup" earlobe. Marked atrophy can also be seen in the upper and lower orbits, cheeks, oral and peri-oral, and peri-mental (geniomandibular) areas. (H) Postoperative lateral view. Overall, the patient has a soft, natural, nonsurgical look. Improved balance between facial features can be seen and the patient has an attractive, photogenic appearance. Scars are well concealed and the retracted tragus and loving cup earlobe have been corrected. The cheek mass and jowl have been raised resulting in improvement in "drool lines" and nasolabial folds. Atrophy present in the oral and peri-oral areas has been improved with fat injections and the lips have been subtly filled and the lip border enhanced creating a more youthful and attractive mouth. The geniomandibular groove ("pre-jowl sulcus") has been filled

integrating the chin and the jowl into a strong, aesthetically desirable, continuous line. The posterior jaw line has also been strengthened with fat injections adding to the effect. The protruding portion of the enlarged submandibular gland has been reduced, the cervicomental angle improved, and platysma bands corrected. The improved cervicosubmental configuration provides a youthful, fit, decisive, and attractive appearance. (I) Preoperative lateral flexed view. The patient can be seen to have a poor transition from the lower eyelid to the cheek, cheek and jowl ptosis, residual cervicosubmental fullness, an indistinct jaw line, and a "double chin". Residual poor neck contour results an overweight, indecisive, and unattractive appearance. The lips are flat and the peri-oral area is retruded resulting in an elderly appearance. (J) Postoperative lateral flexed view. The patient now has a fit, athletic look and an attractive, photogenic appearance. A strong mandibular contour is present with the chin and the jowl integrated into a distinct, aesthetically desirable, continuous line. Residual subplatysmal fat and protruding portions of the submandibular glands have been removed, and platysma laxity corrected. The posterior jaw line has also been strengthened with fat injections adding to the effect. The double chin deformity has been eliminated by dissecting subcutaneously in a retrograde fashion onto the chin to release the submental retaining ligaments, and blending the fat of the chin and submental regions. The orbits have been filled using fat injections, and the lips and peri-oral are project to produce a more aesthetic and youthful appearance.

Conclusion

The increased number of patients seeking early facelifts at a younger age, coupled with the continued good health of an older group of patients who have already undergone one or more procedures, has resulted in an increase in requests for secondary facelift procedures. Although many aspects of planning and performing secondary surgery are similar to those of the primary procedure, additional considerations must be taken into account in the evaluation and treatment of the patient presenting for secondary facelift as one must identify and treat not only new problems that are the product of age, but those that have resulted from the prior procedure as well. Often, it is these secondary deformities that present the biggest challenge to the surgeon in terms of creativity, planning, preparation and technique. The secondary facelift patient is also usually short on skin and will typically present with problems of deep layer origin. Additional excision of large amounts of skin is likely to be counterproductive, result in unnatural appearances and compound existing deformities. Many of the problems seen in the secondary facelift

patient are worth careful consideration, even for the surgeon who performs only the occasional secondary procedure, as they exist as compelling reminders of mistakes to avoid in the planning and performance of any primary procedure.

References

1. Guyuron B, Eriksson E, Persing JA, et al., eds. *Facelift in plastic surgery: indications and practice*. Philadelphia: Saunders; 2009.

2. Marten TJ. High SMAS facelift: combined single flap lifting of the jaw line, cheek, and midface. *Clin Plast Surg*. 2008;35(4):569–603.

3. Marten TJ. Lamellar high SMAS face and midfacelift: a comprehensive technique for natural-appearing rejuvenation of the face. In: Nahai F, ed. *The art of aesthetic surgery: principles and techniques*. 2nd ed. St Louis: Quality Medical; 2010:1525.

4. Marten TJ, ed. Facelift – state of the art. *Seminars in plastic surgery*. New York: Thieme Medical; 2002.

5. Marten TJ, ed. Maintenance facelift: early facelift for younger patients. In: *Facelift: state of the art. Seminars in plastic surgery.* New York: Thieme Medical; 2002.

6. Marten TJ. Facelift: planning and technique. *Clin Plast Surg.* 1997;24:269.

7. Connell BF, Marten TJ. Deep layer techniques in cervicofacial rejuvenation. In: Psillakis J, ed. *Deep face-lifting techniques.* New York: Thieme Medical; 1994.

8. Connell BF, Marten TJ. Facelift. In: Cohen M, ed. *Mastery of plastic and reconstructive surgery.* Boston: Little Brown; 1994:1873–1902.

9. Connell BF, Marten TJ. Orbicularis oculi myoplasty: surgical treatment of the crow's feet deformity. In: Jurkiewicz MJ, Culbertson JH, eds. *Operative techniques in plastic and reconstructive surgery.* Philadelphia: WB Saunders; 1995.

13

Neck rejuvenation

James E. Zins, Colin Myles Morrison, and Claude-Jean Langevin

SYNOPSIS

- Aging affects the face globally. Therefore, the neck is an important component of any facelift procedure.
- Improvement in neck contour is predicated upon skin release from retaining ligaments, appropriate removal of fat from the subcutaneous and subplatysmal plane and alteration of the medial platysma.
- In selected instances, the neck can be treated as an isolated entity including submental approach only (anterior lipectomy and platysmaplasty) and direct excision of neck skin.
- For best results, skeletal developmental abnormalities are treated at the time of face/necklift.

Access the Historical Perspective section online at
http://www.expertconsult.com

Introduction

Neck laxity is one of the earliest signs of facial aging and is, therefore, most often present when the patient presents with other signs of facial aging. It is best integrated into a global approach to cervicofacial rejuvenation. However, under appropriate circumstances as detailed in this chapter, it can be treated as an isolated entity.

Improvement in the neck contour is predicated upon: (1) skin release from retaining ligaments and septae; (2) appropriate fat removal from the subcutaneous (superficial) and subplatysmal (deep) plane; (3) alteration of the platysma and on occasion the digastric muscles; and (4) submandibular gland alteration.

Skin tension should generally be avoided in facelift/necklift procedures, as it results in poor scar quality at best and skin slough at worst. Skin tension adds little to further neck improvement.

When corrected by skin and platysmaplasty techniques, neck surgery results are long-lasting. In fact, neck correction when performed as described, is generally the longest-lasting component of the face/necklift procedure.

Anatomy and the effect of aging

The critical anatomical areas in the neck are the cervicomental angle, the submental/submandibular triangles and the gonial angles. The paired anterior bellies of the digastric muscles extend from the lesser cornu of the hyoid bone to the posterior surface of the mandible on each side of the symphysis. The motor innervation of the anterior belly of the digastric muscle is the mandibular division of the trigeminal nerve. The muscles act as weak depressors of the mandible. Excision produces no noticeable functional deficit but does cause retropositioning of the hyoid bone and, therefore, a favorable deepening of the cervicomental angle.[1]

The borders of the submandibular triangles are formed by the digastric muscles and the inferior border of the body of the mandible. These bilateral triangles each contain the submandibular salivary gland, facial artery and vein, lingual nerve and the marginal mandibular branch of the facial nerve. The submandibular gland may produce a bulge in the submandibular triangle if it is hypertrophied and/or ptotic.

In the lower face, the marginal mandibular nerve exits from under the anterior-inferior portion of the parotid gland. In this location the course is deep to the parotid masseteric fascia. It runs horizontally along the lower border of the mandible passing from deep to the parotid masseteric fascia into the subSMAS cleavage plane and continuing superficial to the facial vessels to innervate the depressor anguli oris and mentalis muscles.[2] This is the area most prone to marginal mandibular nerve injury during facelift surgery (*Fig. 13.1*). Both the lingual and hypoglossal nerves lie deep to the submandibular gland. Therefore, intracapsular resection of the gland minimizes the risk of bleeding and nerve injury.

Three important planes exist in the neck: the superficial plane between the skin and the platysma; the intermediate plane composed of the platysma and the interplatysmal fat; and the deep plane containing the subplatysmal fat, the anterior belly of the digastric muscles and the submandibular glands.[3]

The platysma muscles are thin, bilateral structures that are continuous with the SMAS in the face.[4,5] The platysma is vertically oriented in the neck extending from the clavicles inferiorly and predominantly horizontal in the lower face (*Fig. 13.2*). The platysma has osseous connections to the mandible as it ascends over the mandibular border. And while separate, the platysma is intimately related to the mandibular septum, both structures sending fibers to the mandibular border.[6] Reece *et al.* recently described the mandibular septum. They suggest that the septum may act as a sling impeding fat descent below the mandible and hence lead to jowl formation.[6] Because the platysma is continuous with the SMAS and has minimal bone contact, laxity in the SMAS is transmitted to the neck.[2,4,5,7] There are three variations of platysmal anatomy in the submental region:

Type I (75%)

Interdigitation of the platysmal muscles 1–2 cm posterior to the mandibular symphysis.

Type II (15%)

Interdigitation of the platysma muscles from the mandibular symphysis to the thyroid cartilage.

Type III (10%)

No interdigitation of the platysma muscles (*Fig. 13.3*).[8]

With age, the retaining ligaments attenuate from the free medial edges of the platysma muscle to the deep cervical fascia. The platysmal edges then pull away from the underlying structures, shorten and form visible bands.

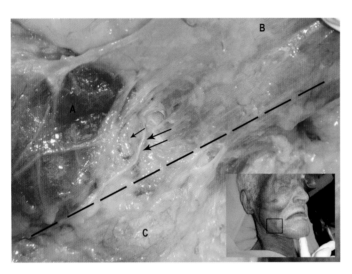
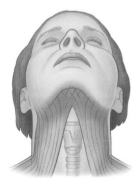

Fig. 13.1 Fresh cadaver dissection demonstrating the marginal mandibular nerve (large arrows) coursing superficial to the facial vessels (small arrow) but deep to the SMAS. It is here where the marginal mandibular nerve passes from deep to the parotid masseteric fascia into the subSMAS cleavage plane and superficial to the facial vessels that it is most prone to injury during facelift surgery. The dotted line represents lower mandibular border. (A) Represents the masseter muscle; (B) represents platysma muscle reflected anteriorly; (C) represents the submandibular gland. Rectangle seen at the lower mandibular border of the full face fresh cadaver orients the reader to close-up view of cadaver dissection.

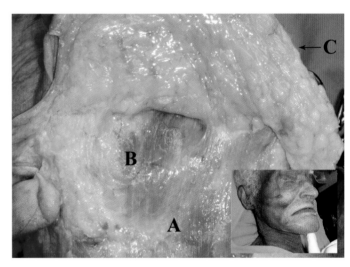
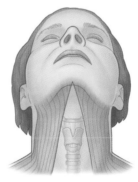

Fig. 13.2 The platysma muscle is vertically oriented in the neck (A) but becomes predominantly horizontally oriented in the lower face (B). (C) Represents superiorly-based skin flap turned upward.

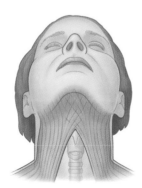

Type I
Occurs in 75% of cases (most common). Demonstrates a limited decussation of platysma muscles, extending 1 to 2 cm below the mandibular symphysis.

Type II
Occurs in 15% of cases. Demonstrates decussation of the platysma from the mandibular symphysis to the thyroid cartilage.

Type III
Occurs in 10% of cases. Demonstrates no decussation or interdigitations.

Fig. 13.3 Variations in platysma anatomy in the submental region. Type I: interdigitation of the platysma muscle 1–2 cm posterior to the mandibular symphysis. Type II: interdigitation of the platysma muscles from mandibular symphysis to the thyroid cartilage. Type III: no interdigitation of the platysma muscles.

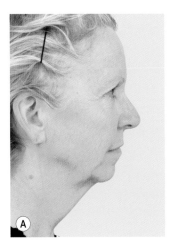
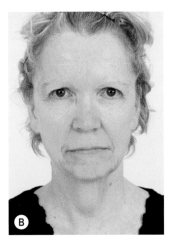
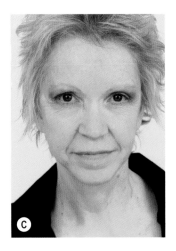
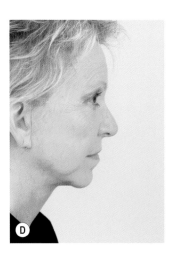

Fig. 13.4 **(A)** Preoperative photograph of a 58-year-old female with sagittal microgenia and facial aging. **(B)** Postoperative photograph of a patient 15 months following a facelift, with extended SMAS and anatomic silicone chin implant. **(C)** Front view. **(D)** Profile view.

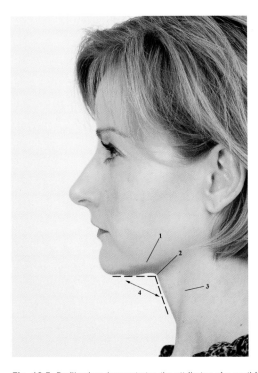

Fig. 13.5 Profile view demonstrates the attributes of a youthful neck including: **(1)** a cervicomental angle of approximately 105°; **(2)** a distinct inferior mandibular border; **(3)** a slightly visible thyroid cartilage; and **(4)** a visible anterior border of the sternocleidomastoid muscle.

In addition to skin quality, soft tissue laxity and fat maldistribution, developmental variations of the bony anatomy, will have a decided effect on the aging process. Specifically, sagittal and vertical microgenia and/or a skeletal Class II appearance will have a negative impact on support of the lower face and neck. Similarly an obtuse gonial angle or mandibular plane will negatively affect lower facial aging. Conversely, correction of these skeletal deformities will have a decidedly positive effect on the facial aging process *(Fig. 13.4)*.

The hallmark of a youthful face is a well-contoured neck.[9–12] Several criteria of a youthful neck have been defined

including a curving or blunt cervicomental angle of 105–120°, a distinct inferior mandibular border, a slightly visible thyroid cartilage and a visible anterior sternocleidomastoid border *(Fig. 13.5)*.[13,14] Knize grades the degree of neck deformity on a I–IV scale. Grade I represents an ideal neck angle and increasing numbers indicate increasing deformity. Using this system, he documented consistent and significant long-term neck correction following anterior lipectomy and platysmaplasty.[15,16] It is important to note, however, that an isolated necklift in the presence of significant jowling and descent of the neck–face junction will generally not produce a pleasing aesthetic result.[3]

Effects of aging/disease process

In patients with facial aging the neck and face are ideally treated simultaneously. Therefore, a necklift is an important component of virtually any facelift procedure. Similarly, it is the rare patient who will be best treated by neck surgery alone. While this chapter is devoted to the aging neck, the maneuvers described should be considered as part of the facelift technique. Virtually all techniques used for neck correction can be performed through the submental incision.

Aging in the lower face is due to varying degrees of laxity which develops in the skin, retinaculum cutis and cutaneous ligaments of the face. Which component is most responsible for facial aging dictates the type of face/necklift procedure chosen. The importance of laxity in the lower masseteric cutaneous ligaments as a major factor in the development of the jowl has been established for some time.[17] More recently, this anatomy and its implications for aging have been further clarified by Mendelson.[2] This information is thoroughly reviewed in Chapter 6. Mendelson's "premasseteric space" overlies the lower one-half of the masseteric muscle. The roof of the space is the platysma, the posterior border of the masseter represents its posterior border, the inferior border of the mandible and mandibular septum its inferior border, the anterior border of the masseter and the lower masseteric-cutaneous ligaments its anterior border. Superiorly are the stout upper masseteric-cutaneous ligaments. This is a potential space in

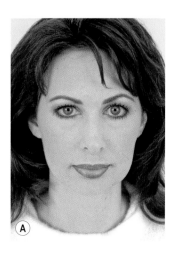
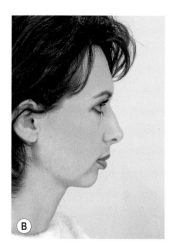
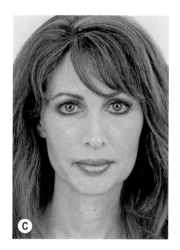
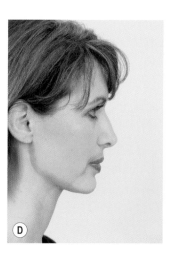

Fig. 13.6 Preoperative photograph of a 30-year-old female with sagittal and vertical microgenia. **(A)** Front view. **(B)** Profile view. One year following horizontal advancement genioplasty. **(C)** Front view. **(D)** Profile view.

youth, but becomes a true space with facial aging, expanding and bulging onto the masseteric ligaments. This results in stretching and jowl formation.

In Chapter 11, facelift techniques are reviewed and authors present their preferred method to manipulate the deeper soft tissues of the face. Conceptually, techniques which involve the SMAS are based on the premise that a major component of facial aging is due to laxity in the SMAS and the cutaneous ligaments. Not only do the SMAS procedures correct this laxity, but the SMAS also acts as a vehicle for repositioning lower face and submental fat. Whether SMAS plication,[18] SMAS excision and closure (lateral SMASectomy)[19] or ligament release, SMAS advancement and reattachment (extended SMAS procedures)[9–12,20–23] is superior, is open to question. Furthermore, certain techniques favor a vertical advancement of the SMAS,[9–11,20–26] while others utilize an oblique vector.[18,19]

Laxity in the lower face is transmitted to the neck because the SMAS and the platysma are located in the same plane with minimal bony attachments. Therefore, tightening of the SMAS has a decided effect on the platysma. In sequencing SMAS manipulation in the face and platysmaplasty in the neck, SMAS procedures should be performed first. Theoretically, if the platysmaplasty is done first, this locks the platysma in place and prevents repositioning of jowl and neck fat into the face by SMAS elevation (J. Stuzin, pers. comm.).

In Chapter 11, the MACS lift principle, originally described by Tonnard, was reviewed. In that technique, platysma tightening is accomplished along a mostly vertical vector utilizing purse-string sutures in the cheek. Fogli borrows on and extends this concept by relying on posterior-superior traction on the neck platysma rather than anterior (medial) platysma tightening. He believes that it is counterproductive to separate skin from platysma. He addresses the platysma with a vertically oblique vector, to Lore's fascia (platysma auricular fascia, or parotid cutaneous ligaments). Higher in the cheek, he utilizes oblique vectors, suturing submalar fat to the malar bone and a running suture continues as an oblique vector ending at the anterior parotid fascia. His technique is predicated on the concept of addressing laxity where the laxity is greatest. Lax SMAS is sutured to immobile areas such as the malar bone and parotid fascia.[7]

While soft tissue changes associated with facial aging have received widespread attention, the effect of facial aging on the bony skeleton has not. Aside from the clear adverse effect of tooth loss on the lower vertical facial height on the maxilla and mandible, bony changes associated with facial aging have been limited to the correction of developmental abnormalities of the cheek and chin and infraorbital rim.[27–30] However, certain dicta described in the orthognathic surgery literature should be applied to the aging lower face and neck.[27,31–34] Rosen has demonstrated that just as expansion of the soft tissue envelope is desirable in the patient with facial aging, expansion of the bony envelope with augmentation techniques should be favored over reduction procedures in the aging face even when taken beyond normal cephalometric bounds.[35,36]

Horizontal advancement genioplasty tightens suprahyoid musculature, expands the skin envelope and improves the profile *(Fig. 13.6)*, while chin reduction procedures lead to a relative excess of the skin envelope, chin ptosis and an adverse effect on the profile with aging.

Preoperative assessment

An analysis of facial proportions on the patient with facial aging is a good starting point for patient assessment from both a diagnostic and treatment standpoint. This can be done rapidly during the patient examination in the office, as well as from patient photographs after the initial interview. There are a number of good methods of both frontal and profile assessment. The analysis in *Figure 13.7* depicts ideal frontal facial proportions, *Figure 13.8*, the ideal transverse and, *Figure 13.9*, the ideal proportions in profile. Facial aging is exacerbated by deficiencies in lower vertical facial height *(Fig. 13.10)* and by lower face sagittal deficiencies *(Fig. 13.4)*. Vertical deficiency in the frontal plane is corrected at the time of facelift/necklift surgery by vertical lengthening genioplasty. Sagittal microgenia is corrected by horizontal genioplasty or alloplastic chin augmentation *(Figs 13.4 and 13.6, respectively)*.

Midface weakness in the pyriform aperture area or the submalar area results in premature aging, deepening of the nasolabial folds and a relative excess of the soft tissue

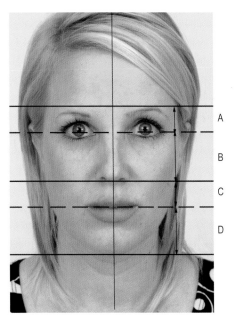

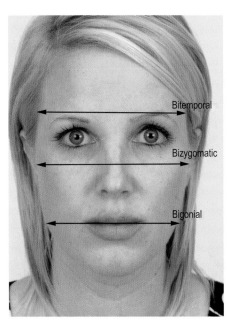

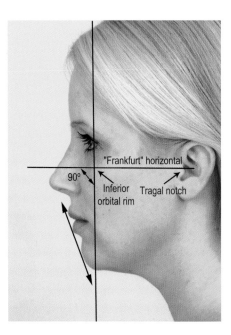

Fig. 13.7 Ideal facial proportion in frontal view. Distance from medial canthus to top of the brow **(A)** is roughly equal to the vertical distance of the upper lip **(C)** medial canthus to alar base **(B)** is roughly equal to the vertical distance from commissure to Menton **(D)**.

Fig. 13.8 Transverse dimensions. The bitemporal distance is equal to the bizygomatic distance, which is equal to the bigonial distance.

Fig. 13.9 Ideal profile dimensions: Reidel's line. A tangent is drawn from upper lip to lower lip. Ideal chin position should fall on this line.

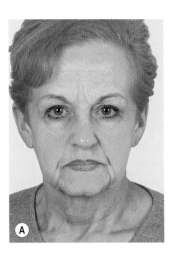

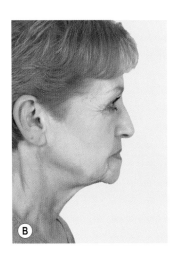

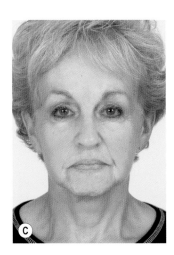

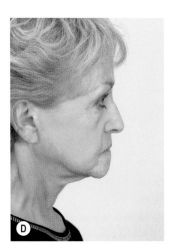

Fig. 13.10 (A) Preoperative frontal view demonstrates less than ideal facial proportions with eyebrow height significantly less than the vertical height of the upper lip (see Fig. 13.6). **(B)** The patient also demonstrates ptosis of the chin in preoperative profile view. **(C)** A 6-year postoperative frontal view demonstrates maintenance of corrected brow position following endoscopic browlift and extended SMAS facelift surgery. **(D)** A 6-year postoperative profile view demonstrates maintenance of soft tissue chin correction.

envelope. Expansion of the soft tissue envelope by soft tissue augmentation with fat injection or with a submalar implant has a beneficial effect on facial aging *(Fig. 13.11)*.

An attractive gonial angle may be masked by the fatty neck. Conversely defatting just posterior to the ramus of the mandible and inferior to the gonial angle will define and enhance the lower face. When defatting is combined with SMAS tightening the surgical result is significantly enhanced *(Fig. 13.12)*.

In evaluating the neck proper, aging in the neck may be due to skin excess, fat accumulation, platysma laxity,

digastric, submandibular gland abnormalities or anatomic variants such as a low hyoid bone (i.e., abnormalities in the superficial, intermediate or deep planes).[3] Evaluation of the skin is relatively straightforward. Marked laxity or excess skin dictates the need for a pre and postauricular incision for proper skin redraping. Mild to moderate skin laxity may be treated by a short-scar facelift approach or submental incision and skin undermining through the submental approach. Numerous authors have stated that skin often need not be removed from the neck during face/neck

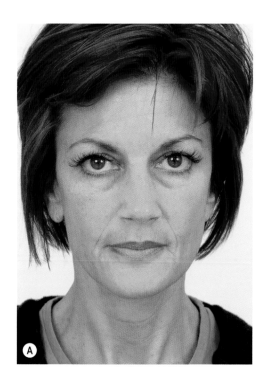
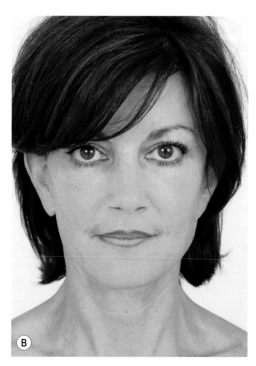

Fig. 13.11 **(A)** Preoperative photograph of a 38-year-old female with facial aging, submalar hollow and deep nasolabial folds. **(B)** At 1 year following facelift with extended SMAS and submalar implants.

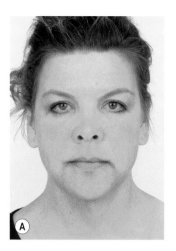
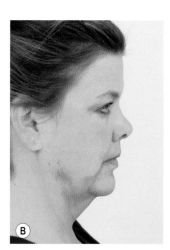
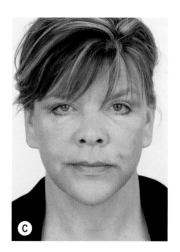
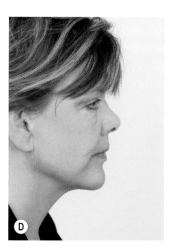

Fig. 13.12 A 45-year-old female with facial aging, obtuse cervicomental angle and loss of gonial angle. **(A)** Front view. **(B)** Profile view. At 1 year following extended SMAS facelift, submental lipectomy and platysmaplasty and defatting of the gonial angle. **(C)** Front view. **(D)** Profile view.

rejuvenation.[13–16,27,28,37–46] This is due to: (1) the unique ability of neck skin to contract once released from the platysma and (2) more, not less skin, is needed once the obtuse angle of the neck becomes more acute, i.e., the hypotenuse of a triangle is less than its two sides *(Fig. 13.13)*.

The degree of platysmal banding should be assessed and, when present, where the platysma is most lax, i.e., medially. Skin tightening and necklift without platysmaplasty will lead to early platysmal band correction. However, if present and not addressed platysmal bands will invariably recur shortly after surgery.

In evaluating neck fat, assessment should be made both above and below the platysma. While fat above the platysma is generally readily apparent, the amount of fat deep to the platysma is more difficult to gauge. The proper estimate of subplatysmal fat often requires platysma opening for accurate assessment. A reasonable maneuver at the time of the patient exam is to ask the patient to grimace. Fat above the platysma should remain within the examining fingers while subplatysmal fat will be less apparent.

In general, if there is a question as to the presence of subplatysmal fat, the platysma should be opened because of the inaccuracy of preoperative assessment. With regard to neck defatting, the trend is towards conservatism. The majority of defatting is done centrally, over the jowl and posterior to the gonial angle. Skin flaps should be left relatively thick in order to avoid irregularities and an over-resected unnatural appearance of the neck.

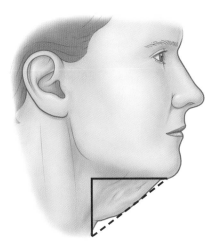

Fig. 13.13 More, not less skin is needed in the neck once the obtuse cervicomental angle is converted to a pleasing neckline, i.e., the hypotonuse of a triangle is a shorter distance than the sum of its limbs.

Nonsurgical options

Some nonsurgical treatments have been advocated for neck rejuvenation. These include botulinum toxin,[47] injectable fillers,[48,49] lasers[50] and intense pulse light.[51] Although these alternatives have a role in the treatment of facial aging either as ancillary or stand-alone procedures, they do not exert the same impact on facial aging that is seen with face/necklift surgery.

Minimally invasive options

Threadlift in facial rejuvenation

A variety of internal sutures, anchored barbed sutures and threadlift techniques have been introduced as minimally invasive alternatives to traditional facelift surgery. These varieties include the Contour Threads (Surgical Specialties Corp., Reading, PA), the APTOS Threads (APTOS, Moscow, Russia) and the Isse Endo Progressive Facelift suture.[52–54] Outcomes using these barbed sutures are few and the follow-up is short. In one of the best outcomes studies using the Contour Threads, complication rates were high. Of 72 patients, 46 (64.8%) developed at least one complication. Revision surgery was also high with some type of revision performed on an average of 8.4 months post Contour Thread placement. Further, in this series, 11% of the patients ultimately required removal of their threads. Initial claims of short recovery were also not found with ecchymoses and "chevron" contour irregularities or contour irregularities frequently present for weeks following surgery.[55] Others have reported a complication rate of 20%. In a group of 20 patients with an average of 11.5 months follow-up, barbed sutures were said to meet their patients' expectations with satisfaction ratings of 6.9 on a scale of 1–10. Higher scores were noted in the midface and lower scores in the neck region.[54,56] Contour threads produced by Quill are no longer available for the correction of soft tissue ptosis; Quill

sutures are now available for wound closure only. The APTOS and ISSE Endo Progressive Facelift suture remain available for facial suspension. Based on the above experience, initial enthusiasm for the barbed sutures has been muted.

Surgical options

The most effective approach to the aging face and neck is through the facelift approach, either using a short scar technique for patients with minor neck laxity[3,19,57,58] or using a standard pre- and postauricular incision for those with significant laxity in the neck. These techniques are reviewed in Chapter 11. As mentioned earlier, when the SMAS is tightened through a facelift approach, there is a decided benefit on the neck platysma because there is minimal bony attachment of the platysma to the mandible. Hence, SMAS tightening above the mandible leads to platysma tightening below the mandible. That being said, all other maneuvers used to address the aging neck may be performed through the submental approach except for skin excision and horizontal genioplasty. Direct neck procedures include the following:

1. Defatting superficial to the platysma
2. Subplatysmal and interplatysmal defatting
3. Medial platysmaplasty/platysma tightening
4. Platysma plication over the submandibular gland
5. Submandibular gland resection
6. Alloplastic anatomic chin implant placement when indicated.

Open surgical rejuvenation of the aging neck usually includes some form of platysma modification. The platysma is approached in the midline, opened, interplatysmal and subplatysmal fat removed and the platysma is tightened by closing it vertically. In addition, the muscle may be partially divided in the horizontal direction low in the neck. This is performed to allow the platysma to ride up superiorly further defining the cervicomental angle.

A wide variety of platysmaplasties have been described including lateral plication,[59] varying degrees of low, horizontal, partial transaction either medially or laterally,[9] simple midline suturing,[60,61] the corset platysmaplasty[37] and the pants over vest platysma plication in the midline.[62]

Suspension sutures designed to improve the jawline and neck-jaw angle were first described by Guerrerosantos[63] and then popularized by Giampapa.[64] The principle is to create a permanent artificial "ligament" under the mandible to correct the deformities of the aging neck. However, the long-term efficacy of suture suspension techniques in improving and masking abnormalities deep to the platysma has been questioned by a number of authors.[46,65] These authors prefer muscle modification to suture suspension.

The submental approach to the neck can, therefore, be considered either as an integral step to facial rejuvenation or as a standalone procedure in selected individuals. In Giampapa's submental approach, liposuction was used to defat the neck and for skin release. Medial platysmal bands were resected when necessary and two interlocking sutures from one digastric muscle to the opposite mastoid region were placed.[64,66,67] Since his description, a number of authors have described a variety of submental approaches combining platysmaplasty with skin undermining.[15,16,27,38–46,68–70] While each of these

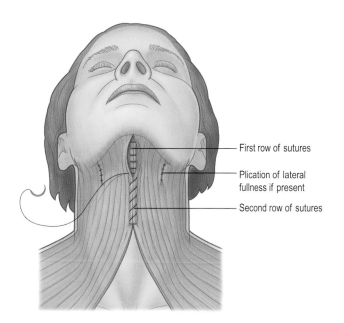

First row of sutures

Plication of lateral fullness if present

Second row of sutures

Fig. 13.14 The Corset (Feldman[37]) Platysmaplasty. The platysma is opened in the midline and subplatysmal modifications performed including defatting, digastric shave or submandibular gland partial resection as indicated. The corset consists of a running suture from chin to thyroid cartilage, reapproximating and tightening medial platysma edges. The suture is then run back up to the chin outside the first suture line and halfway down again, progressively tightening the platysma corset. Plication over the ptotic gland may also be performed.

techniques varies to some degree, conceptually they owe a good deal of their efficacy to lessons learned from neck liposuction.[71,72] We learned a number of years ago that neck skin, unlike many other areas, has the unique ability to contract when released from fibrous septae and cutaneous ligaments. Knize's[15,16] anterior lipectomy and platysmaplasty which he practiced beginning in the early 1980s utilizes a submental approach, medial platysmal plication and submental undermining with excellent, long-term results. Feldman has presented his technique[37–44] since the early 1990s and published his textbook in 2006, detailing his technique.[73] His approach includes a submental incision, defatting, a corset platysmaplasty and varying degrees of undermining through the submental and minimal access postauricular approach. Zins and Fardo's description is similar to that described by Feldman *(Fig. 13.14)*.[45]

Ramirez has also described his anterior approach. Most recently, he has added a horizontal plicating, submandibular suture to his technique.[74]

Feldman has taken this concept yet further, stating that he rarely resects postauricular neck skin even during facelift surgery. He merely uses the postauricular approach for access and redraping the neck skin at the completion of the procedure.[73] Whether this concept of no skin resection in the postauricular area during standard facelift gains widespread acceptance is not clear, but it does emphasize the importance of placing minimal tension on the postauricular closure. This maximizes scar quality and minimizes postauricular healing problems.

The authors of the anterior approach to neck rejuvenation are also in agreement on where to most effectively address platysma tightening. They address it medially where it

demonstrates the most laxity. This is in direct contrast to Tonnard and Fogli who depend on a posterior vertical vector to effect neck rejuvenation. Early on, Tonnard and Verpaele[57] avoided the anterior approach, although more recently, they and their colleagues appear to be moving toward more medial platysmal plications in older individuals.[7,58,75]

Surgical approaches to neck rejuvenation include:

1. Liposuction
2. Anterior (submental) incision
3. Direct skin excision and Z-plasty.

Liposuction

Liposuction exerts its affect via a combination of subcutaneous fat removal and release of skin-muscle attachments. Release of the skin from underlying platysma muscle allows for avid skin contraction in young and middle aged patients.

The ideal patient for neck liposuction is the relatively young patient with good skin elasticity who has localized submental and submandibular fat. In such patients, the technique is straightforward and uniformly excellent results should be obtained. The result can be further enhanced in patients with sagittal microgenia with the addition of a genioplasty. Correction of the skeletal deficiency combined with submental liposuction can yield a dramatic result *(Fig. 13.15)*.

The operation can be extended to treat patients with markedly fat necks or patients with mild or moderate skin excess. In such patients submental and postauricular approaches are used to minimize skin contour abnormalities. Wider skin undermining should also be practiced to maximize skin contraction *(Fig. 13.16)*. While not ideal patients, this group will demonstrate significant improvement.

Liposuction of the neck can either be undertaken with suction-assisted lipectomy (SAL) or ultrasound-assisted liposuction (UAL).

Ultrasound-assisted liposuction (UAL) emulsifies the supraplatysmal fat which is then evacuated. Ultrasonic energy causes an inflammatory reaction which some believe causes enhanced skin contraction.[3] However, the use of UAL carries the potential risk of thermal injury, dysesthesias and marginal mandibular nerve palsy.[76] Ultrasound-assisted lipoplasty (UAL) has therefore not been widely adopted in the submental region because of its increased potential for complications, complex and bulky instrumentation and additional cost.

Newer technologies include VASER (vibration amplification of sound energy at resonance) and SmartLipo (Cynosure, Westford, MA). VASER is a fat pre-treatment device based on the emission of pulsed or continuous ultrasound energy to emulsify fat before its aspiration. With thinner cannulas and decreased use of ultrasonic energy, it is theoretically a safer and more efficient process than standard ultrasonic liposuction.[77,78]

SmartLipo® uses an internal neodymium:yttrium-aluminum-garnet laser (1064 nm) to rupture fat cells. The laser energy also interacts with the dermis theoretically resulting in collagen shrinkage, improving skin tightness and smoothness on the neck.[79] However, higher concentrations of free-fatty acids after laser-assisted lipoplasty may cause possible hepatic and renal toxicity.[80]

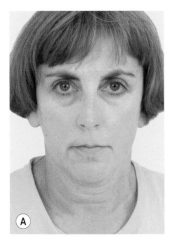
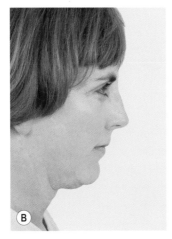
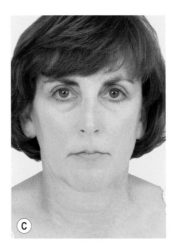
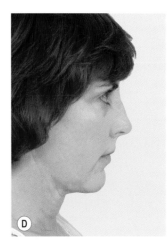

Fig. 13.15 A 40-year-old female with an obtuse cervicomental angle and submental fat. **(A,B)** Preoperatively. **(C,D)** At 13 months following liposuction using a submental approach only.

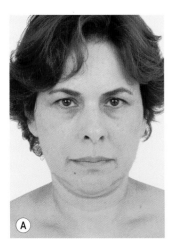
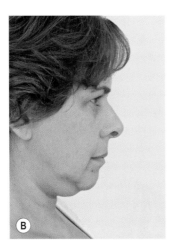
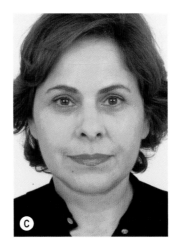
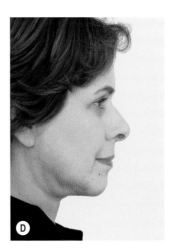

Fig. 13.16 A 62-year-old female with submental fullness, moderate neck skin laxity. **(A)** Front view. **(B)** Profile view. Same patient 1 year postoperatively following submental lipectomy, subplatysmal defatting and platysmaplasty without a preauricular incision. **(C)** Front view. **(D)** Profile view.

Technique for liposuction of the neck

Liposuction of the neck can be performed readily under local or general anesthesia. The patient is marked in the sitting position prior to surgery noting the location of submental and/or submandibular fat and the extent of tunneling to be performed. A large volume (50 cc) of 0.5% lidocaine (Xylocaine; AstraZeneca, Wilmington, DE) and 1:2 000 000 epinephrine is injected through the submental and postauricular approach. For maximum vasoconstriction effect, 15 min is allowed to elapse.

A small caliber (2.4 mm) suction cannula with single or multiple holes is used. Holes are directed toward the soft tissue, liposuction is begun through the submental incision using wall suction fanning out from the submental incision. Additional postauricular stab incisions can be utilized to cross liposuction. Relatively little fat is generally removed and overly aggressive liposuction is to be avoided to minimize postoperative adverse sequelae such as contour irregularities, banding and skeletonization of the neck. Less is generally more with this procedure. Normally, little change is seen on the operating table. No drains are used. An elastic garment is worn for 5 days postoperatively and for 2 weeks at night only.[45]

Anterior (submental) incision

The anterior approach to neck rejuvenation (anterior lipectomy and platysmaplasty, necklift without a preauricular incision) improves upon the results of previous neck liposuction techniques. In addition to skin contraction, neck contour is further improved by: (1) subplatysmal and interplatysmal fat removal; (2) the options of digastric muscle shave or plication; and (3) platysmaplasty and the resultant muscle tightening *(Fig. 13.17)*.[1,3]

Proper patient selection is critical to surgical success. This procedure is not an alternative to facelift, since no changes will be noted above the lower mandibular border. Many patients assume that the anterior approach will also correct jowl formation, which it generally does not. In fact, there is little change in the frontal view. Significant change will be seen in profile only. To assure patient satisfaction, careful explanation of the benefits and limitations of the procedure are to be emphasized.

Patient selection is best guided by the degree of skin laxity.[74] We, therefore, arbitrarily divide our patients into four groups depending on their laxity of skin: grade I (no laxity); grade II (mild); grade III (moderate); and grade IV (severe).[46]

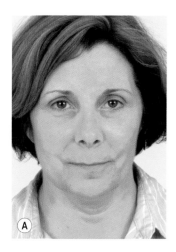
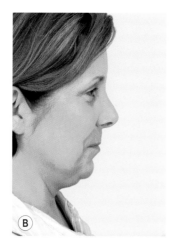
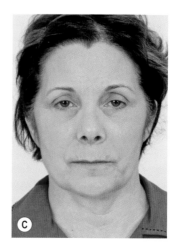
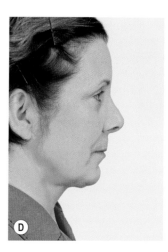

Fig. 13.17 A 55-year-old female with mild skin laxity and an obtuse cervical angle secondary to fat. **(A)** Front view. **(B)** Profile view. Same patient 1 year following submental lipectomy and medial platysmaplasty and subplatysmal fat removal. **(C)** Front view. **(D)** Profile view.

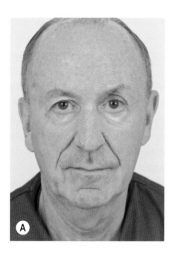
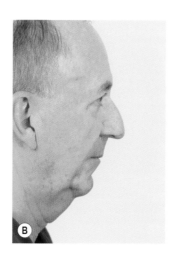
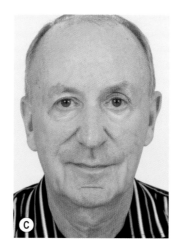
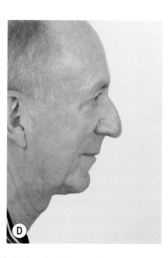

Fig. 13.18 A 67-year-old male with deep nasolabial folds and neck laxity due to skin excess and platysmal laxity. **(A)** Front view. **(B)** Profile view. Same patient 1 year following direct excision of neck skin, Z-plasty and direct excision of nasolabial folds. **(C)** Front view. **(D)** Profile view.

These four patient grades fall relatively neatly into our treatment paradigm: grade I patients (no skin laxity) may be treated by liposuction alone through single or multiple incisions. If, however, subplatysmal fat is suspected, at the completion of liposuction, the submental incision is opened and subplatysmal and interplatysmal fat is sought out. Since it is often difficult to determine whether subplatysmal fat is present without opening the platysma, the platysma is opened if there is any question. Grade II patients (mild skin laxity) with an obtuse cervicomental angle are good candidates for the anterior approach. Fat above the platysma, interplatysmal fat and subplatysmal fat are all readily treated through the submental incision. The degree of skin undermining is dictated by the degree of skin laxity. A good rule of thumb is that the amount of undermining should be similar to the amount one would do for that given patient if a standard facelift were being performed. These patients with mild laxity will need undermining to the anterior border of the sternocleidomastoid, while those with moderate laxity (grade III) will require more extensive undermining over the sternocleidomastoid muscle for adequate skin redraping *(Figs 13.16, 13.17)*. Patients with marked skin excess (grade IV) are not candidates for the anterior approach and will need standard

facelift techniques or a direct excision of neck skin and Z-plasty for correction of facial aging *(Fig. 13.18)*.[45,81–84]

While skin laxity is the most important factor in patient selection, others come into play. Patients with diffusely fat necks tend to be more difficult patients. Smooth contours are more difficult to obtain and irregularities are more common. Men tend to have less impressive results, presumably because of thicker more sebaceous skin and less avid skin contraction.[46]

Technique for anterior lipectomy and platysmaplasty

As described for the patient undergoing neck liposuction, the patient is marked preoperatively in the sitting position marking the submental fullness, the location of submandibular fat, the extent of planned undermining and the submental and posterior sulcus incisions. Infiltration with 50 cc of 0.5% Xylocaine with 1:400 000 epinephrine, is similar to that described for neck liposuction. A 3.5 cm submental incision is made and superficial subcutaneous undermining is performed. The extent of undermining is dictated by the degree of skin laxity and excess. Once superficial undermining and superficial defatting have been completed, the platysma is opened in the midline, interplatysmal and subplatysmal fat is removed. Fat is removed flush with the anterior belly of the digastric muscles. Defatting using the Colorado Needle (Stryker, Portage, MI) is continued inferiorly. Fat distribution in the subplatysmal and interplatysmal location is in the shape of an inverted "T" extending laterally as dissection extends inferiorly. Lymph nodes and anterior jugular branches are routinely encountered. Nodes are removed and vessels cauterized. Once defatting has extended down to the thyroid cartilage, dissection is complete and the platysmaplasty of choice is performed.

A postauricular sulcus incision is made on each side and through this incision, the posterior dissection is completed. If moderate laxity exists, the dissection extends over the sterno-cleidomastoid. If not, a posterior sulcus incision is made merely for ease of drain placement. The neck is drained with a 7 mm J-Vac drain (Ethicon Inc., Somerville, NJ) in all cases.

Direct excision of neck skin and Z-plasty

Although frowned upon by many, the direct excision of neck skin and Z-plasty is a reasonable alternative in the elderly. This generally applies to men in their mid- to late 70s or older with significant submental skin excess, but on occasion can be used in males or females as an adjunct to facelift surgery in patients with massive weight loss. This procedure will appeal to those elderly males who are unwilling to undergo a more involved facelift procedure with its associated longer recovery, added risk and cost. However, the patient must understand the location and extent of the neck scar before proceeding. Photographs are particularly helpful in this regard *(Fig. 13.19)*.

The procedure has the added benefit of being readily performed under local anesthesia with or without sedation. Skin excision tends to produce perhaps even a better neckline than a standard facelift in this patient population, once again, because skin excision is performed where laxity is greatest *(Fig. 13.18)*.

Ideal candidates are non-obese elderly males with significant skin excess. Diffusely fatty necks can be problematic as smooth contour can be difficult to obtain.

Postoperatively, occasional mild hypertrophic scarring can occur at 3 months, which readily resolves with dilute triamcinolone injections.

Technique for direct excision necklift

Although numerous techniques have been described in the literature,[82–86] we prefer the Gradinger technique.[87]

With the patient in the sitting position, the ultimate central limb of the Z-plasty is chosen by placing a measuring tape from gonial angle to gonial angle *(Fig. 13.20)*. The central limb is then marked making certain to extend the horizontal line beyond the central ellipse. Once this horizontal limb has been decided on, a vertical ellipse is chosen by conservatively

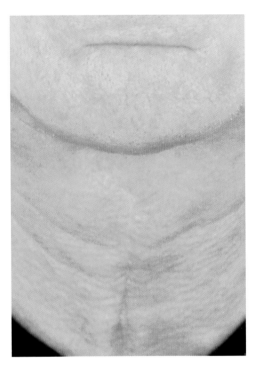

Fig. 13.19 Well-healed neck scar 1 year following direct excision of neck skin and Z-plasty.

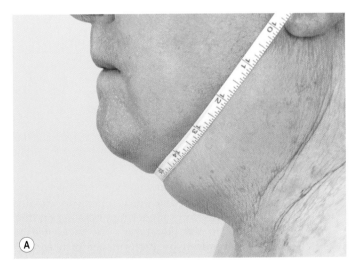

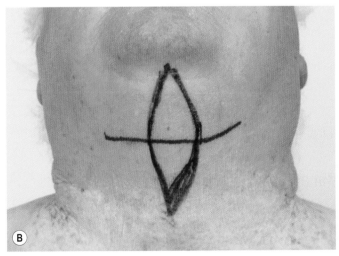

Fig. 13.20 **(A)** The ideal location for the new cervicomental angle is determined using a measuring tape running from ear to ear. **(B)** A horizontal line then marks this location. A vertical ellipse is drawn estimating the amount of skin to be excised.

pinching skin excess in the vertical dimension and drawing the ellipse *(Fig. 13.19)*. This should be taken the entire extent of the skin excess. An elliptical excision is completed according to preoperative markings and the skin is undermined for 3–5 cm in either direction to allow adequate draping postoperatively. The platysma is then undermined on its deep surfaces and a Z-plasty with its long axis in the vertical direction and limbs of approximately 2 cm and 60° angles are designed. The completed Z-plasty lies on the original horizontal line drawn preoperatively. The "Zs" are transposed and the platysma closure is completed. The skin is then temporarily closed in the vertical direction. Again, a Z-plasty identical to the one completed on the platysma is then drawn with the central limb in the vertical direction and limb lengths and angles also identical. The Z-plasty is incised, transposed and inset. An additional Z-plasty can be added inferiorly if the vertical skin scar is still of significant length.

Postoperative care

Minimizing postoperative problems begins in the operating room. Control of bleeding should be meticulous. The anesthesiologist should raise the blood pressure to the preoperative blood pressure level as hemostasis is being gained. Relative hypotension will mask bleeding. Raising the pressure toward the end of the procedure will conversely minimize postoperative hematoma. The recovery from anesthesia should be smooth without coughing or retching. With the exception of liposuction, patients are seen the morning following surgery. At that time, the operative dressing and drain are removed. Drains are used in all cases when there is significant neck dissection. However, if drainage is significant, i.e., >30 cc in 24 h, the drain remains in place until the drainage has subsided. Drainage is likely to be significant in fat necks or if electrocautery is used to raise flaps. Therefore, scissor dissection is favored for skin flap elevation.

A chinstrap is worn continuously for 5 days and at night for 2 weeks for those undergoing platysmaplasty and fat resection. Patients are instructed to sleep with their heads elevated and necks gently extended. A single pillow positioned behind the head should be avoided. Cervical flexion can increase edema through venous obstruction, place excess tension on mastoid region closures and diminish adherence of the skin to underlying structures.

There should be no heavy lifting or bending in the immediate postoperative period. NSAIDs and anticoagulants are best avoided for at least 1 week after neck rejuvenation. Finally, good communication between the surgeon and patient increases cooperation and helps achieve a better surgical outcome.

Management of the submandibular glands

Ptotic submandibular glands should be noted preoperatively as they will detract from the surgical result. Platysmaplasty, direct plication over the gland and submandibular gland suspension will improve but not eliminate their visibility. Indirectly re-establishing fascial support by SMAS plication or platysmal suspension has also not proven to be effective in the long term. Numerous authors have described suspension or cable sutures from the submental or digastric muscle to the mastoid process with reported success,[64,68,69] while others question these long-term results.[65]

While these authors do not remove submandibular glands due to the possibility of significant complications, others do.[3,19,74,88,89]

Technique for submandibular gland suspension

This technique is well described by Sullivan *et al.*[90] The position of the submandibular gland is marked preoperatively, the neck is approached through a submental incision and the platysma is opened. The capsule of the gland is found by dissection underneath the platysma and lateral to the digastric muscle. A 1.5 cm incision along the anterior surface of the capsule parallel to the body of the mandible allows access to the gland. Gentle dissection releases adhesions allowing complete mobilization.

A hemostat is then used to create a subperiosteal tunnel around the gland and along the lingual aspect of the mandibular body. A stab incision over the tip of the hemostat establishes intraoral access. The end of a 2-0 suture is then brought out through the neck incision.

A second pass lateral to the gland is performed. The periosteal tunnel created for this suture is parallel but 3 cm anterior to the initial one. The opposite end of the suture is grasped and again pulled down into the neck. This creates a suspension arc. The submandibular gland is then elevated with gentle digital pressure and the knot secured. Finally, the incised capsule is imbricated with a permanent suture and the intraoral incision closed with chromic.[90]

Complications

Complications following neck rejuvenation surgery are similar to those seen with standard facelift surgery.

Early complications

- Hematoma
- Seroma
- Sialoma
- Injury to the marginal mandibular branch of the facial nerve
- Injury to the frontal branch of the facial nerve.

Late complications

- Contour irregularities
- Asymmetrical fat removal
- Inadequate reduction
- Overcorrection.

The incidence of hematoma following facelift or the variety of necklift procedures described in this chapter vary greatly to as low as 1% to significantly higher numbers depending upon the study cited in the literature.[91] The incidence of hematoma can be minimized by performance of a careful history, making certain that anticoagulants and antiplatelet medications are avoided for 1–2 weeks preoperatively and careful attention to detail is carried out intraoperatively.

Other time-honored means of reducing incidence of hematoma include the avoidance of postoperative hypertension, nausea and vomiting. As mentioned earlier, attention to blood pressure at the time of flap closure has been helpful in our experience. Other adjuncts such as platelet-rich plasma,[92] and fibrin glue have been cited as effective in some hands while others have found these ancillary-type techniques ineffective.[93–95]

There is no crime in getting a hematoma but there certainly is a crime in not recognizing one. Clearly, early evacuation of both small and large hematomas minimize postoperative morbidity. An expanding hematoma is a surgical emergency due to the potential for airway compromise and skin flap necrosis. Small hematomas, however, can also be troublesome postoperatively. They are frequently missed because of facial swelling and lead to long-term irregularities and patient concerns. Large hematomas obviously need to evacuated in the operating room. However, small hematomas can often be aspirated, milked out through the drains or evacuated with a suction cannula. If a small hematoma goes unrecognized in the early postoperative period, they can be drained 7–14 days following surgery when the clot lysis and the hematoma drained percutaneously.

Seromas are most frequent in the neck area and can also be troublesome postoperatively. Unrecognized seromas lead to neck contour irregularities which are difficult or impossible to correct. While it is not universally performed, most surgeons drain the neck postoperatively. Our preference is to use suction drains to obliterate dead space and minimize seroma fluid collections. Drains are removed when output is minimal. This may require drainage for 24 h or more. Should a seroma occur in the neck following drain removal, repeat aspiration is indicated until the seroma subsides.

Sialoma is a rare but not unheard of face/necklift complication. This may occur following subSMAS surgery or submandibular gland resection. It should be suspected when clear fluid is found in the drain or by aspiration. The diagnosis of parotid fistula is confirmed by measuring the amylase level in the aspiration fluid. In the case of parotid fistulas, the amylase level will be quite high. Suction drains which obliterate dead space rather than repeated aspiration appears to be the most effective means of resolving the fistula. In the absence of distal obstruction, the fistula will close.

Facial nerve injury is also rare, most commonly involving the marginal mandibular branch of the facial nerve, or the frontal branch, if a facelift approach is used. Most injuries are relatively distal and resolve. However, marginal mandibular nerve injury is more likely than frontal branch injury to be permanent due to its peculiar anatomy. Re-exploration for facial nerve injury is generally not indicated since injury is most likely distal. The use of botulinum toxin A to weaken the contralateral muscles is a reasonable temporizing approach while waiting for the nerve injury to resolve.

Late complications of face and neck rejuvenation are generally aesthetic and include contour abnormalities due to the irregular resection of fat, the unmasking of ptotic submandibular glands, pixie ears and abnormalities of scar formation. Neck banding due to overresection of fat, unrecognized seromas or irregularities caused by platysma plication are notoriously difficult to treat. Conservative defatting is the best prevention.

 Access the complete references list online at **http://www.expertconsult.com**

2. Mendelson BC, Freeman ME, Wu W, et al. Surgical anatomy of the lower face: the premasseter space, the jowl, and the labiomandibular fold. *Aesthetic Plast Surg.* 2008;32:185–195.

   The areolar cleavage plane overlying the lower masseter has specific boundaries and is a true space named the "premasseter space." This space is rhomboidal in shape lined by membrane and reinforced by retaining ligaments. The masseter fascia lines the floor and branches of the facial nerve pass under its deep surface. The roof, lined by a thin transparent and adherent membrane on the underside of the platysma, has a less dense collagen network and contains more elastin. With aging, there is a significant reduction in the collagen density of the roof. Expansion of the space with aging, secondary to weakness of the anterior and inferior boundaries, results in formation of the jowl. Medial to the premasseter space is the buccal fat in the masticator space which descends with aging and contributes to the labiomandibular fold and jowl. The premasseter space should be considered as the preferred dissection plane for lower (cervicofacial) facelifts because the space is a naturally occurring cleavage plane and dissection is bloodless and safe as all the facial nerve branches are outside of it.

3. Nahai F, ed. Neck lift. In: The art of aesthetic surgery: principles and techniques, Vol. 2. St. Louis: Quality Medical; 2005:1239–1284.

7. Fogli AL. Skin and platysma muscle anchoring. *Aesthetic Plast Surg.* 2008;32:531–541.

13. Ellenbogen R, Karlin JV. Visual criteria for success in restoring the youthful neck. *Plast Reconstr Surg.* 1980;66: 826–837.

    Five visual criteria for achieving and assessing success in aesthetic neck surgery are suggested: (1) A distinct inferior mandibular border from mentum to angle with no jowl overhang. (2) Subhyoid depression. (3) Visible thyroid cartilage bulge. (4) Visible anterior border of the sternocleidomastoid muscle. (5) Cervicomental angle between 105 and 120°.

17. Furnas DW. The retaining ligaments of the cheek. *Plast Reconstr Surg.* 1989;83:11–16.

19. Baker DC. Lateral SMASectomy. *Plast Reconstr Surg.* 1997;100:509–513.

    With the advent of liposuction in the 1980s, the author found that he could obtain excellent neck contouring in many patients utilizing liposuction combined with strong, lateral platysmal suturing. In a lateral SMASectomy, a portion of the SMAS in the region directly overlying the anterior edge of the parotid gland is removed. Because of this design the SMASectomy is performed at the interface of the superficial fascia fixed by the retaining ligaments and the more mobile anterior superficial facial fascia. On closure, this brings the mobile SMAS up to the junction of the fixed SMAS producing a durable elevation of both superficial fascia and facial fat. The direction in which the SMASectomy is performed is oriented so that the vectors of elevation following SMAS closure lie perpendicular to the nasolabial fold, thereby producing improvement not only of the nasolabial fold but also of the jowl and jawline.

26. Little JW. Three-dimensional rejuvenation of the midface: volumetric resculpture by malar imbrication. *Plast Reconstr Surg.* 2000;105:267–269.

37. Feldman JJ. Corset platysmaplasty. *Plast Reconstr Surg.* 1990;85:333–343.

   The corset platysmaplasty was developed to avoid producing necks that display persistent or recurrent paramedian muscle bands, visible submandibular gland bulges and various contour irregularities. The two medial edges of the platysma are joined together with a continuous suture that runs down almost the full height of the neck to create a smooth, flat, multilayered seam, leaving no free muscle edges. Progressive side-to-side tightening along the midline defines the "waistline" of the neck. Additional submandibular suturing may then be done to create strong, flat, vertical muscle pleats that correct submandibular gland bulging and refine the jawline and anterolateral neck contours.

46. Zins JE, Menon N. Anterior approach to neck rejuvenation. *Aesthet Surg J.* 2010;30:477–484.

   The anterior (submental) approach to neck rejuvenation is one of the minimally invasive procedures with clear documentation of long-term efficacy. The procedure improves upon previous neck liposuction because in addition to skin contraction, the results are enhanced by the removal of subplatysmal and interplatysmal fat, the options of digastric muscle alterations and platysmal muscle tightening. The technique is described in detail, potential complications noted and technical limitations of the procedure described.

57. Tonnard P, Verpaele A. The MACS-lift short scar rhytidectomy. *Aesthet Surg J.* 2007;27:188–198.

58. Tonnard P, Verpaele A, Morrison C. MACS facelift. In: Aston SJ, Steinbrech DS, Walden JL, eds. *Aesthetic plastic surgery.* New York: Saunders Elsevier; 2009:137–148.

14

Structural fat grafting

Sydney R. Coleman and Alesia P. Saboeiro

SYNOPSIS

- The concepts of aging are changing, placing more emphasis on volume loss and volume restoration.
- Fat grafting provides a long-lasting, minimally invasive means to restore volume and rejuvenate the face, hands, or body.
- Proper harvesting, refinement, and placement of the fat is essential for consistent results.
- The most forgiving area to learn structural fat grafting is the dorsum of the hand and the least forgiving area is the eyelid.
- Fat grafting can be used to replace tissue lost due to aging, trauma, and/or disease, as well as to rejuvenate and dramatically alter the contours of the face, hands, and/or body.
- The future use of adipose-derived stem cells in regenerative medicine and tissue engineering is promising.
- Numerous aesthetic and reconstructive problems can be addressed with structural fat grafting, but patient selection is very important.
- Fat must be harvested gently to preserve its natural architecture.
- Predictable volume changes are possible when fat is refined and condensed by centrifugation and decanting.
- Centrifugation at 1286 g is considered optimal (Yoshimura) and may enhance fat graft take and prevent long-term atrophy of the transplanted tissue.
- Oil present after centrifugation can indicate adipocyte destruction as well as the desired separation of oil from fatty components.
- Growth factors and stem cells have been isolated and appear to be concentrated in the densest portions of centrifuged fat.
- Frozen or stored fat is not considered viable and should not be used.
- Fat should be grafted in very small aliquots using multiple passes of the cannula and should not be molded after placement.
- While technically considered minimally invasive, significant bruising and tissue edema generally result from fat grafting.
- Continued research on the applications of adipose-derived stem cells is of utmost importance.

 Access the Historical Perspective section online at
http://www.expertconsult.com

Introduction

Basic science/disease process

Since the 1890s when fat grafting first began, there has been controversy regarding the predictability and consistency of results that may be obtained with fat grafting. With some studies reporting up to a 70% rate of reabsorption, this is not surprising, especially with the dramatic variations in technique which have been used to transplant and study fat.[15] Initially, a reasonable explanation for this was based on Lyndon Peer's cell survival theory,[16] whereby the number of viable adipocytes transplanted correlates with the volume of grafted fat that survives. Pu and colleagues have looked at a number of different laboratory assays that determine the viability of fat grafts, including viable adipocyte counts, colorimetric assays, adipocyte-specific enzyme assays, and routine histologic examinations.[17,18] Their *in vitro* studies have looked at fat grafts obtained by direct excision, conventional liposuction, a fat graft harvest and transfer device, and the Coleman technique.[19] The results favored the Coleman method, as it yields a greater number of viable adipocytes and maintains a more optimal level of cellular function.

The future

An exciting new potential of fat grafts is in reparative and regenerative medicine. Fatty tissue has been found to not only contain adipocytes, but also a subpopulation of cells consisting of adipose-derived stem cells (ADSCs), MSCs, endothelial cells and their progenitor cell lines, smooth muscle cells and smooth muscle progenitor cell lines, and numerous other stem cells that are multipotent and have the potential to aid in tissue regeneration.[20] ADSCs serve a number of functions and may be induced to differentiate into many different cell types in culture, including ectodermal, mesodermal and endodermal lineages. Additionally, ADSCs have been shown to induce blood vessel formation, mitigate fibrosis and promote bone formation and wound healing. It is now believed that this particular population of cells within a fat graft may be a major contributor to the therapeutic potential of the graft.[21]

Rigotti *et al.* have used fat grafting in the irradiated breast and consistently showed an improvement or complete healing of the damaged tissues.[22] As our understanding of fat and its constituent cells improves, so will our ability to positively affect other areas of medicine.

Aging and atrophy

What is the process by which we age?[23] Our concepts of how the face and body change with time are evolving, and the traditional ways of thinking about the problems and their solutions are being modified. We have been taught that over time, there is loss of elasticity of the tissues which results in descent and sagging of the skin. In the face, our traditional response to the descent has been to resuspend the tissues and to remove the excess skin. What we have ignored is the reason for the descent in the first place. While there are obvious environmental and genetic components to aging, one of the main reasons that the tissue starts to sag is lack of support, or lack of volume beneath it. One component of this volume is fat, but there are also components including collagen, elastin, hyaluronic acid, etc. that are involved. The goal then should be to replace the missing fullness, which will support and reposition the skin. In most cases, the body supplies us with a significant source of filling material to restore the volume lost with aging in the form of fat. There are, of course, limitations as to the ability of volume to support the overlying tissues. If there is a tremendous amount of sagging or excess skin, then manual resuspension and trimming may be necessary.

The easiest way to analyze a face to determine how it has changed is to study photographs of patients when they were younger compared to their current state. Depending on the degree of aging, one can often easily see that as the face ages, typical patterns emerge. The model shown in *Figure 14.1* exemplifies the changes that occur, from left to right, going from age 20 to 50 to 70 years.

The 20-year-old model *(Fig. 20.1A,D)* has a full, smooth face. Her temples are flat and her brow and glabella are unfurrowed. Her upper eyelids are full beneath the brow and there is a short distance between the ciliary margin and the lid crease. The lower eyelids are smooth and there is minimal hollowing medially. Her cheeks are round with the zygomatic arches well covered with soft tissue. There is a slight hollowing in the buccal cheek, but she does not look gaunt. She has mild nasolabial folds compared with her full cheeks, but she does not have deep folds or creases within the folds. The lips are full, pouty and everted and the lower lip is slightly larger than the upper lip. Her jaw line and chin are well-defined and smooth.

As we move from left to right in this model of aging, we have a 20-year-old followed by a 50-year-old and finally a 70-year-old. As we go across, we see hollowing of the temples with skeletonization of the area. Wrinkles become more and more obvious in the forehead and glabella secondary to loss of youthful fullness over areas of muscular activity, especially in the glabella. The fullness that was previously present beneath the brow is now diminished and the upper eyelids appear to either collapse and fold anteriorly or collapse posteriorly to reveal the hollow orbit. There may be a real excess of skin, but there may also be merely the illusion of excess skin that disappears when the volume is restored. The lower eyelids begin to deflate, making the orbital rim more apparent and elongating the lid-cheek junction. The tear trough extends diagonally into the anterior cheek, breaking up the continuous line of cheek fullness and accentuating the nasolabial folds.

The zygomatic arches lose their soft tissue covering to reveal the bony outlines beneath and hollow buccal cheeks. The vermillion of the lips becomes thinner and thinner with time and the lips begin to invert, which accentuates the length of the cutaneous upper lip. The anterior chin becomes less well-defined and more rounded like one button instead of two defined mounds with a central cleft. As volume and support is lost along the posterior aspect of the jaw line, the mandibular border becomes less well-defined and wavy, and the lower face slides forward to accentuate the jowls and perimental hollows/pre-jowl sulci.

Diagnosis, patient presentation, indications

Patients who desire fat grafting to the face will present for numerous different reasons. One of the most common reasons is aging. These patients are generally over 40 years of age and present with loss of facial fullness, resulting in skin laxity, wrinkles, or a gaunt, skeletal appearance. As volume is restored to their face, their appearance will begin to resemble their younger photographs.

The younger patient who presents for facial fat grafting is generally one who is unhappy with a facial feature such as the cheeks, chin, or jaw line. These patients can benefit from fat grafting to augment these deficient structures in a manner similar to bone grafts or solid implants. The facial proportions can be significantly altered to create a more aesthetically pleasing balance.

Patients may also present for facial fat grafting for corrective purposes. This includes patients with congenital deformities such as hemifacial microsomia and Treacher Collins syndrome. In addition, patients who have sustained previous trauma resulting in significant scarring or tissue loss can often benefit from fat grafting.[24] Patients who have undergone previous facial cosmetic surgery often present with iatrogenic deformities such as hollow upper and/or lower eyelids and flattening of the posterior jaw line. These areas can be restored to a more youthful and natural appearance with fat grafting.

Facial atrophy from etiologies other than aging[25,26] have been increasing over the last few decades, especially drug-related lipodystrophy seen in patients taking antiretroviral and protease inhibitor therapies. These patients often present with a maldistribution of not only facial fat but also body fat. While an excess of fat may appear as a dorsal hump on the

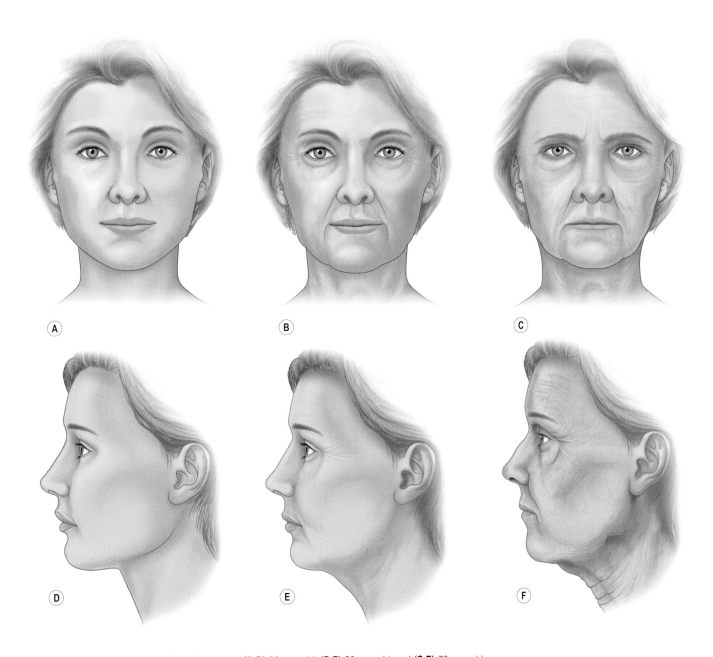

Fig. 14.1 Model of aging. From left to right in each row: **(A,D)** 20-year-old, **(B,E)** 50-year-old, and **(C,F)** 70-year-old.

upper back/lower neck, the face usually appears hollow in the temples and buccal cheeks, creating an appearance pathognomonic for the drug-related lipoatrophy. Fat can be removed from the dorsal hump by suctioning, but should probably not be used for grafting purposes, as it could have an unusual growth pattern.

What happens to the hands over time that will give away the age of the patient if the face does not? Again, there is a loss of volume, or soft tissue coverage over the veins and tendons of the dorsal hand. The hands of a 20-year-old are generally smooth and full, with the extensor tendons and dorsal veins barely visible. There is naturally little fat over the dorsum of the hands, but with thinning of the skin and loss of interosseous muscle fullness, the hands can take on a wasted appearance that can be reversed with fat grafting. Fat

grafting not only restores a subtle fullness to the dorsal hand, but appears to thicken the skin as well, which partially obscures the tendons and veins so obvious in aging skin.[27]

As liposuction has become a more common procedure, and with an increasing number of practitioners performing the procedure, there are more deformities being created as a result of liposuction and variations of liposuction. These liposuction deformities range from very slight irregularities that are barely perceptible, to large indentations and even full thickness skin loss. The large and complex tissue deficiencies often require several operative procedures, with the occasional release of adhesions, to restore the necessary volume and smoothness. In addition to large defects, there can also be significant disturbances of body proportion, such as making the feminine shape more boxy and masculine or creating an unusually deep buttock crease that makes the buttock appear droopy.

A new use of fat appears to come from its apparent healing properties. Rigotti has grafted fat beneath tissue ulcerations in the breast that occurred after radiation therapy, and has noted remarkable restoration and healing of the involved tissues.[22] Radiated tissue that is stiff and noncompliant can be restored to a more normal consistency and texture and allows filling of contour deformities. In addition, anecdotal reports have been made regarding the improvement of the appearance of scars and skin quality after fat grafting.[21,24]

Patient selection

There are few contraindications to fat grafting to the face and body. The first contraindication is true for all procedures, which is poor patient health prohibiting anesthesia. Small areas of fat grafting can often be performed under local anesthesia, but anything involving more than a few milliliters of fat usually requires sedation. In addition, patients with unrealistic expectations are not good candidates for this or any other procedure. A contraindication specific for fat grafting is the extremely thin patient who does not have sufficient fat for transfer. Since large volumes of fat are generally not needed for the face, enough fat can usually be harvested in all but the most anorexic patient or muscle-bound body builder. For fat grafting to the hands, breasts or body, significantly more fat is usually needed; and often there is a limit as to the correction that can be made given the paucity of fat in some patients. Asking the patient to gain weight prior to the procedure only makes sense if the patient is willing and able to maintain that weight afterwards.

In aging patients with a tremendous amount of loose, excess skin, fat grafting can be disappointing. These patients are either left with residual skin excess or if completely filled, may have an unusual appearance to their face. In these cases,

it is usually advisable to first tighten the skin with a more traditional facelift and then to add volume with fat. The aging patient in *Figure 14.2* represents a typical patient that might present for a facelift. She is instead an excellent candidate for fat grafting to the face, particularly along the jaw line and chin, where there is an apparent slight excess of skin secondary to deflation. The jowls and irregular jaw line that are present and this degree of laxity in the neck can be improved significantly with fat grafting without any cutting or suspension techniques. By adding volume back into the face the contours are improved and the skin is effectively tightened and lifted by radial expansion.

Younger patients usually do not have as much facial atrophy and subsequent sagging of the skin, but the overall appearance of the face can be changed drastically with a shift in facial proportions. The patient in *Figure 14.3* is an example of how a more balanced upper and lower lip and more defined chin can make the face look more balanced and attractive. The patient in *Figure 14.4* is an example of a chin augmentation in a younger patient to improve the overall facial proportions. The patient in *Figure 14.5* is an example of an upper and lower lip augmentation. Filling the lips gives her a much softer appearance.

Patients with more severe deformities such as those seen in Treacher Collins syndrome are excellent candidates for fat grafting. This is true despite the fact that the problem is complex, with both bony and soft tissue abnormalities. The unusual facial contours present in *Figure 14.6* would be very difficult to address with anything other than fat, as different volumes can be tailored to the specific defects to create a more norm.

Patients with facial lipoatrophy are also excellent candidates for fat grafting, regardless of the cause of their disease process. Like Treacher Collins syndrome patients *(Fig. 14.6)*, these patients have specific soft tissue defects, making fat an ideal long-lasting filler. A temporary filler could theoretically be used in a patient such as this, but the volume of product that would be needed on a regular basis would likely be cost-prohibitive *(Fig. 14.7)*.

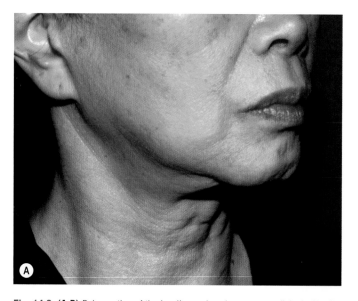 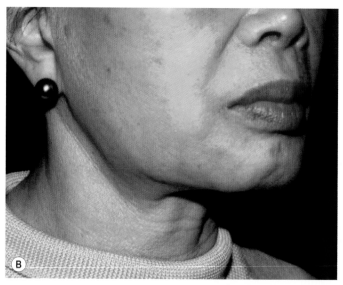

Fig. 14.2 (A,B) Rejuvenation of the jaw line and neck was accomplished with placement of structural fat along the border of the mandible back to the angle of the mandible and forward into the chin. Significant augmentation of the lower lip also adds to her improved proportion and rejuvenation.

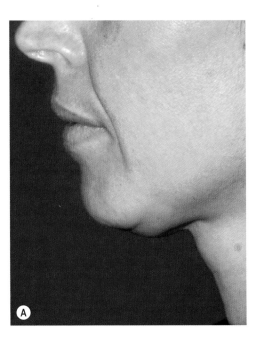

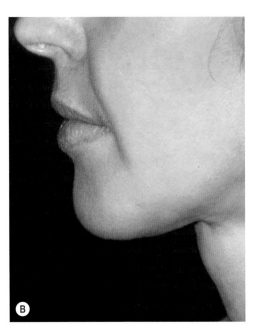

Fig. 14.3 (A,B) Patient 6 years after fat grafting to the lower face: 17 cc to chin; 12.5 cc to the left border of the mandible, and 8.0 cc to the lower lip. Please note that no fat was placed into the upper lip, so that the size of the upper lip can be used as a meter to evaluate the degree of change present.

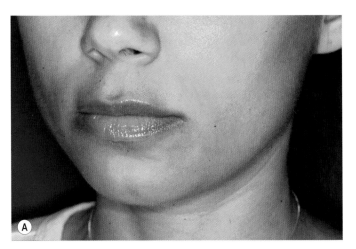

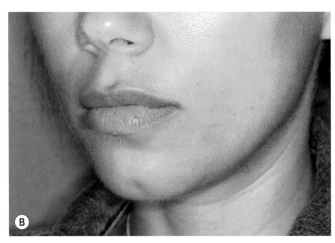

Fig. 14.4 (A,B) This young woman presented for improved balance of her lower face; 5 cc of fat was placed into her anterior and inferior chin to elongate it. Note that the natural dimple was preserved.

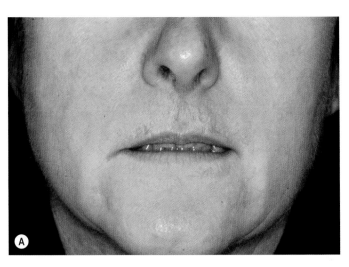

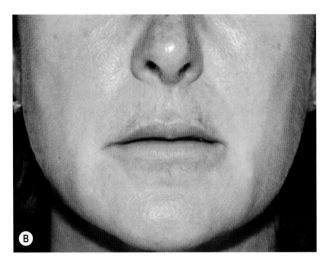

Fig. 14.5 (A,B) This 50-year-old woman had fat grafting to her upper and lower lips in three stages to minimize the postoperative swelling. She is seen here 15 months after her last fat grafting procedure.

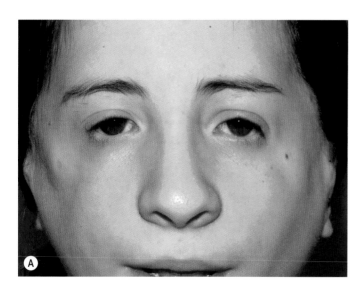
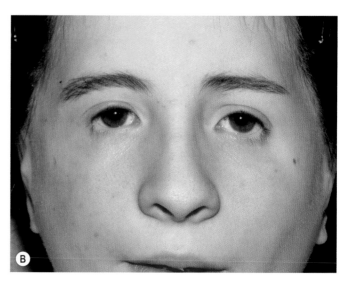

Fig. 14.6 (A,B) This 22-year-old woman presented after multiple reconstructive attempts at treating her Treacher Collins syndrome. She presented with not only malproportion of her face, but also impending extrusion of hardware in her zygoma. Diffuse fat grafting from the lateral lower eyelids extending out to the zygomatic arch not only reinforced the thin lateral eyelid skin, but also covered the obvious hardware visible through the thin cheek skin.

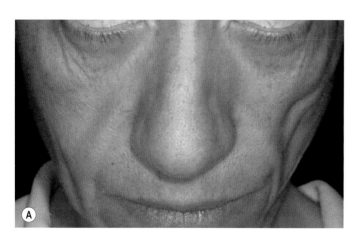
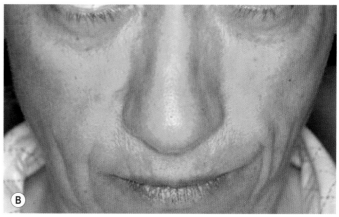

Fig. 14.7 (A,B) This patient presented with idiopathic facial atrophy with the primary involvement on the left side of the face. At her first procedure, 13 cc was placed into the left cheek and 4 cc into the right. At the second procedure, an additional 12.2 cc was placed diffusely over the left cheek and nothing further was done on the right. The photograph below shows her 15 months after the second procedure.

There are very few options to rejuvenate the aging hand. If there is a problem of pigmentation, lasers can be helpful in removing the spots. Topical treatments can also be of some help, however it is impossible to lessen the prominence of obvious tendons and veins without the addition of some volume. The patient in *Figure 14.8* demonstrates the loss of volume in the dorsum of the hand due to aging. The hand has a somewhat wasted appearance, with poor quality skin. After fat grafting to the dorsum of the hand, the veins and tendons are less visible and the quality of the skin appears improved.

Patients presenting with post-liposuction deformities are excellent candidates for fat grafting. The patient in *Figure 14.9* has irregularities created by liposuction. Grafted fat is really the only option to correct areas of significant deficiency, whereas small depressions can occasionally be corrected with temporary fillers.

The patient in *Figure 14.10* is an example of atrophy that has occurred in the temple secondary to radiation therapy.

After grafting fat to the region, the area is not only filled in but it is also of a more normal texture and consistency.

Treatment/surgical technique

The Coleman method of fat grafting is essentially unchanged since the original inception more than two decades ago.[11] The process involves harvesting the fat gently to preserve the delicate architecture, refining the fat with centrifugation to remove nonviable components and provide a predictable volume,[28] and placement of the fat in small aliquots to increase the surface area and ensure a blood supply to the grafted tissue.[29] When these principles are adhered to, structural fat grafting can be a relatively predictable and safe procedure. Recent histologic studies have shown that this method of harvesting and refinement with centrifugation yields fat with a high

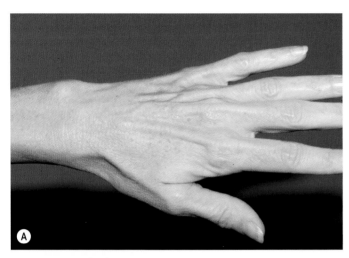

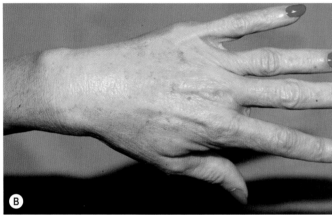

Fig. 14.8 (A,B) This 46-year-old woman presented complaining of visible tendons and ropey veins on her hand and wrist (above). She had 40 cc of fat diffusely infiltrated over the dorsal surface from the distal forearm to the PIP joints.

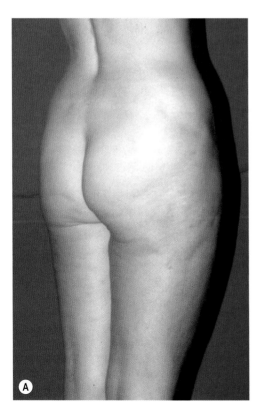

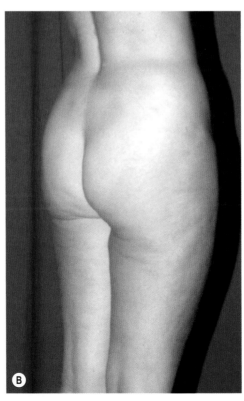

Fig. 14.9 (A,B) This 50-year-old woman presented after liposuction to her thighs and lateral buttock, followed by an attempted fat grafting (left). 69 cc was grafted to the hip and 156 cc to the lateral buttock and thigh. Ten months later, an additional 20 cc was grafted to the lateral thigh. She returned 1 year after the second procedure (right).

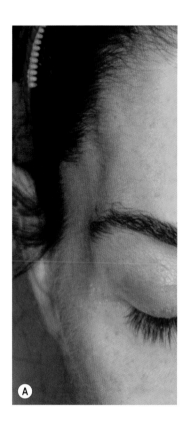
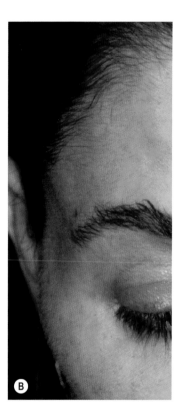

Fig. 14.10 This patient presented after resection of a nonsecreting pituitary adenoma through a craniotomy incision, followed by a 6-week course of radiation. The craniotomy left her with a significant depression in her temple, which extended into her temporal-parietal scalp. **(A)** Cranioplasty was attempted 5 years after the radiation, but it "fell in", making the condition worse than before the procedure. She presented with the above depression extending from her temple and into her scalp, which also had some alopecia. **(B)** Her appearance 26 months after 9 cc was placed into the visible temple depression and another 17 cc into the scalp behind her hairline. Not only was the contour deformity completely corrected, but the patient felt that the quality of her skin was improved, as well as her alopecia (although it was difficult to photograph the improved hair growth).

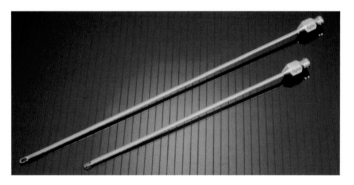

Fig. 14.11 Harvesting cannulas.

percentage of survival and near-normal adipose cellular enzyme activity.[19]

Harvesting

The choice of donor site for fat grafting is dependent on the desires of the patient and accessibility of the fat, as no conclusive differences in viability or "graft take" have been demonstrated from one site to another in scientific studies. In general, the love handle, posterior hip, back, and lateral thighs are more forgiving and do not have as much potential to wrinkle as the abdomen and medial thighs. Incisions are hidden in creases, scars, stretch marks, or hair-bearing areas, if possible. Through these incisions, local anesthetic solution is infiltrated using a blunt Lamis infiltration cannula. For straight local cases, the local anesthetic solution consists of 0.5% lidocaine with 1:200000 epinephrine, however for general anesthesia cases, where larger volumes of fat are harvested, a solution containing 0.2% lidocaine with 1:400000 epinephrine is used. The amount of solution infiltrated is essentially equal to the amount of fat removed.

Fat is then harvested using a two-hole Coleman harvesting cannula attached to a 10 cc syringe. This harvesting cannula is designed to harvest intact fatty tissue parcels that are large enough to survive, but small enough to pass through the standard infiltration cannula (17 gauge). The plunger of the 10 cc syringe is pulled back only a few milliliters during suctioning, so as not to create too much negative pressure and rupture the fat cells. Incisions are closed with interrupted nylon sutures *(Figs 14.11, 14.12)*.

Refinement

As fat is harvested, the first few syringes occasionally have more local anesthetic present than later. As the suctioning continues, many of the later syringes contain less infiltrate and more blood. After the 10 cc syringe is full, the cannula is disconnected from the syringe and a Luer-Lok plug is used to cap the syringe. The plunger is then removed, and the syringe is placed into the centrifuge. To maintain sterility during the centrifugation process, a centrifuge with a sterilizable central rotor and sleeves that are sterilizable, is essential. Centrifugation at 1286 g for 2 min concentrates the fat so that the aqueous components (the local anesthetic and blood) can be removed and discarded by releasing the Luer-Lok plug. In addition, any ruptured fat cells that release their oil can be decanted off the top and/or wicked away with Telfa pads *(Fig. 14.13)*.

The fat is then transferred to a 1 cc syringe for placement into the face and hands or a 3 cc syringe for placement into the breasts or body. This process yields relatively pure fat for grafting, providing a much more predictable volume of tissue

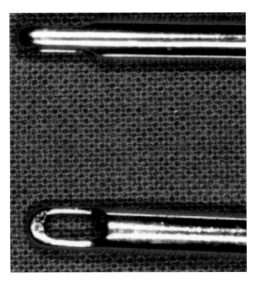

Fig. 14.12 "Bucket handle" tip of harvesting cannulas.

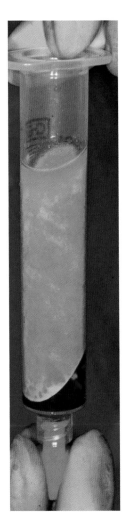

Fig. 14.13 Appearance of a syringe after centrifugation. Note the small oil layer at the top; the large volume of fat in the mid-portion, and the small layer of local anesthetic/blood at the bottom.

than a sample with excess liquid and/or oil might. Allowing the syringe of harvested fat to sit on end and sediment will separate the fat from the oil and aqueous component to some extent, but it is more time consuming and has less of a concentrating effect than centrifugation. The uncentrifuged sample will initially appear to provide the proper correction, but in a short period of time, much of it will be reabsorbed and the procedure will have been considered a failure *(Fig. 14.14)*.

Placement

Planned incision sites are anesthetized with 0.5% lidocaine with 1:200000 epinephrine and small stab incisions are made for the placement of fat through one of three Coleman cannulas *(Figs 14.15, 14.16)*.

Small amounts of 0.5% lidocaine with 1:200000 epinephrine are usually infiltrated into the face for vasoconstriction of the vessels prior to placement of the fat. This not only helps to reduce bruising, but also decreases the chance of accidental intravascular embolization of the fat. The success of the fat grafting procedure depends not only on the harvesting and refinement, but also on the placement of the fat in a manner that increases its chance for survival and graft "take". This means maximizing the contact surface area of the fatty parcel with the surrounding tissue, such that a blood supply can be conferred to the newly grafted fat *(Fig. 14.17)*.

Transferring large globules of fat can result in central necrosis of the mass with subsequent resorption and loss of volume, or possibly even cyst formation *(Fig. 14.18)*.

The fat is placed gently during the withdrawal of a blunt Coleman infiltration cannula. Fat can be placed at different levels to accomplish different effects. For instance, grafting fat immediately beneath the dermis can improve the quality of the skin, decreasing wrinkles, decreasing pore size and even reducing scarring. Special care must be taken, however, when placing fat superficially, as irregularities are more apt to be apparent in this plane. This is especially true in areas that have thin skin, such as the lower eyelid. To make changes in the shape of the face or body that relate to the underlying bony skeleton, fat can be placed above the periosteum. The structure should be purposefully built up with tiny aliquots of fat rather than attempting to insert larger aliquots and then mold the tissue after it is placed. Molding may displace the fat or cause necrosis of some or all of the fat in an area, resulting in uneven contours. The only time molding should be considered is if an irregularity is noted at the time of placement, as the surface must be smooth before you leave the operating room. The stab incisions used to place the fat are closed with single interrupted nylon sutures.

Postoperative care

Care of the patient after fat grafting has evolved over time. Initially, all areas of the face, except the upper eyelids, were covered with Microfoam® tape, forming a sort of mask. Now occasionally, we will use Tegaderm®, which is more flexible, tolerable, and socially acceptable. Around the eyes, dressings must be applied carefully so as not to pull the lower eyelids down. In areas of the face that were suctioned,

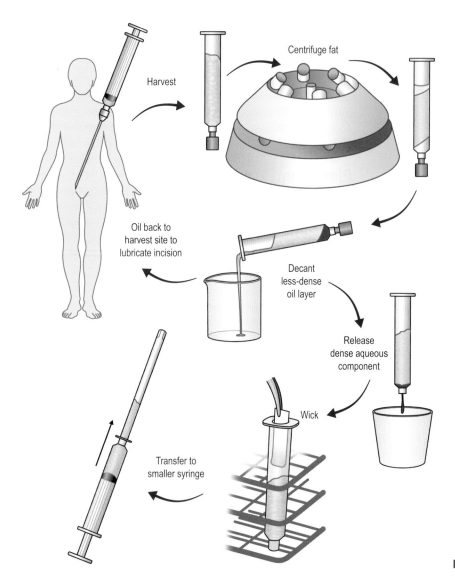

Harvest

Centrifuge fat

Oil back to harvest site to lubricate incision

Decant less-dense oil layer

Release dense aqueous component

Wick

Transfer to smaller syringe

Fig. 14.14 The Coleman refinement and transfer process.

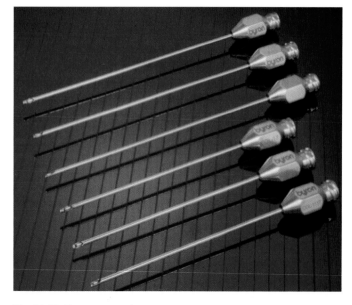

Fig. 14.15 Placement cannulas.

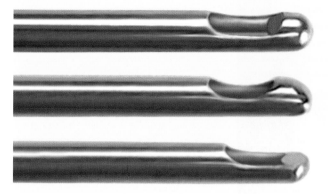

Fig. 14.16 Various placement cannula tips, from the most blunt to the least blunt.

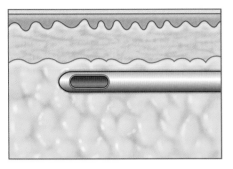

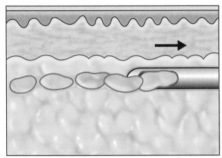

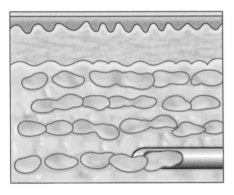

Fig. 14.17 Placement of fat into the recipient site. Note that placement is performed during the withdrawal of the cannula and is placed in different layers to build up the structure.

½" Reston foam is usually applied, followed by Tegaderm or Microfoam tape to compress the foam. In addition, cold therapy is usually recommended for up to 72 h postoperatively.

The hands are generally still dressed with Microfoam tape, and the donor sites are dressed with a compression garment or abdominal binder. The dressings are usually left in place for 3–4 days, at which time the patient is seen in the office, the dressings are removed, and the facial sutures are removed. Body sutures at the donor sites and on the hands are usually removed at 5–7 days. Lymphatic drainage techniques using a very light touch can be performed on the face and/or body, but deep massage is to be avoided during the first month.

Outcomes, prognosis, complications

In addition to the obvious volumetric changes that can occur with fat grafting, it has been noted by many to also improve the quality of the overlying skin. Rigotti has grafted fat

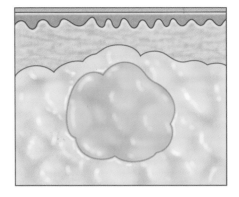

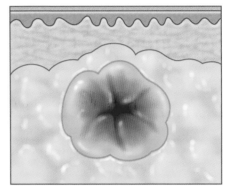

Fig. 14.18 Injection of a large mass of fat and the central necrosis that can occur when this is done.

beneath irradiated, ulcerated breast skin and has noted healing and normalization of the affected skin. Mojallal *et al.* have also demonstrated improvement in adherent scars, skin texture, skin suppleness, skin color and scar quality in their patients.[24] This group has demonstrated similar findings histologically in the nude mouse.

The most common complications, or side-effects, of fat grafting to the face, hands, or body are aesthetic. There is generally considerable swelling and bruising that occurs with the multiple passes of the cannula used to place the fat. Bruising generally resolves in 2–3 weeks, but there have been a few cases of prolonged subcutaneous pigmentation that is easily visible through the thin skin of the lower eyelids. This has the appearance of "tea staining" and can take many months to resolve.

More problematic is the potential for subcutaneous irregularities visible through the skin, which can occur in both the recipient and donor sites. In the recipient sites, excess grafted fat will appear as a lump beneath the skin. This can be the result of placement of a volume that was too large just beneath thin skin, particularly in the periorbital region. These bits of unwanted fat can be difficult to remove, therefore caution should be employed when grafting into this area (*Fig. 14.19*).

Potential remedies for irregularities caused by excess fat include suctioning of the fat using the same cannula used for infiltration,[30] direct excision of the fat under visualization,[31] and Lipodissolve,[32] which is not approved by the FDA in the United States. Irregularities in the donor sites can also be problematic, particularly if too much fat is removed.

The most catastrophic potential complication is an intravascular embolization, which fortunately, is extremely rare.

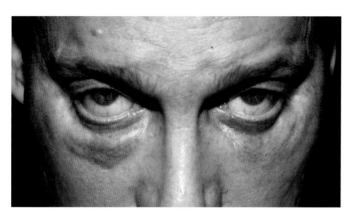

Fig. 14.19 This 48-year-old man presented with large protuberant masses on his lower eyelids after fat grafting to the lower eyelids and cheeks. The surgeon had attempted to correct the problem with the injection of catabolic steroids into the transplanted fat. According to the patient, the steroids made his irregularities more visible as the skin appeared thinner.

Such an event can occur when fat is inadvertently injected under pressure into a small artery, with retrograde filling of the vessel. With the next pump of the heart, this intra-arterial fat can embolize to an end arteriole resulting in tissue ischemia. This has never been reported when using a blunt cannula, therefore sharp needles are discouraged except when placing fat directly into the dermis. For similar reasons, the injection of large boluses of fat and injection guns are not recommended.[33]

Infections in the recipient or donor site are also extremely rare, but if they do occur, they can result in resorption of the grafted fat and loss of the desired correction. Strict sterile technique should be employed during fat grafting and cannulas that penetrate the oral mucosa should be considered contaminated. Lip augmentation, therefore, should be performed last if fat grafting is performed elsewhere on the face.

Significant changes in weight can result in concomitant changes in the size of the area grafted, therefore patients are encouraged to have the procedure performed when they are at their ideal body weight and to maintain that weight, if possible.

Secondary procedures

With fat grafting, secondary procedures, or touch up procedures, are possible if the correct volume of fat was not placed initially. Due to the difficulty in the lower eyelid of removing fat, it is far better to under correct the area and return to the operating room for a second stage, if necessary, at a later date. In complicated liposuction deformity cases, a second stage is often part of the original plan, as it can be very difficult to make an area smooth enough in one procedure. Generally, the goal of the first procedure is to fill in large deficits with significant amounts of fat and later to come back and refine the area.

Access the complete references list online at **http://www.expertconsult.com**

11. Coleman SR. The technique of periorbital lipoinfiltration. *Oper Tech Plast Reconstr Surg.* 1994;1:20–26.
    This article was the first published on the Coleman technique of fat grafting.
13. Coleman SR. *Structural fat grafting.* 1st ed. St. Louis, MO: Quality Medical; 2004.
    This is a comprehensive text on fat grafting.
19. Pu LL, Coleman SR, Cui X, et al. Autologous fat grafts harvested and refined by the Coleman technique: a comparative study. *Plast Reconstr Surg.* 2008;122(3):932–937.
20. Zuk PA, Zhu M, Mizuno H, et al. Multilineage cells from human adipose tissue: implications for cell-based therapies. *Tissue Eng.* 2001;7(2):211–228.
    This is the first clear description of the presence of stem cells in fat grafts. This article had four plastic surgeons among the authors.
21. Coleman SR. Structural fat grafting: more than a permanent filler. *Plast Reconstr Surg.* 2006;118(3 Suppl):108S–120S.

This article is the first article to clearly spell out the healing effect of fat grafting on the surrounding tissues.
22. Rigotti G, Marchi A, Galie M, et al. Clinical treatment of radiotherapy tissue damage by lipoaspirate transplant: a healing process mediated by adipose-derived adult stem cells. *Plast Reconstr Surg.* 2007;119(5):1409–1424.
23. Coleman SR, Grover R. The anatomy of the aging face: volume loss and changes in 3-dimensional topography. *Aesthet Surg J.* 2006;26(1):S4–S9.
24. Mojallal A, Lequeux C, Shipkov C, et al. Improvement of skin quality after fat grafting: clinical observation and an animal study. *Plast Reconstr Surg.* 2009;124(3):765–774.
27. Coleman SR. Hand rejuvenation with structural fat grafting. *Plast Reconstr Surg.* 2002;110(7):1731–1743.
33. Coleman SR. Avoidance of arterial occlusion from injection of soft tissue fillers. *Aesthet Surg J.* 2002;22(6):555–557.
    The avoidance of intravascular embolization should be always on the mind of anyone injecting fat.

15

Skeletal augmentation

Michael J. Yaremchuk

SYNOPSIS

- Facial skeletal augmentation can add angularity, definition, or balance to a face of normal dimensions.
- Given acceptable occlusion, implant surgery can be an alternative or an adjunct to orthognathic surgery in disproportioned faces.
- Most skeletal augmentation is done with alloplastic implants.
- Solid silicone and porous polyethylene are the materials most commonly used for facial skeletal augmentation.
- Incisions should be placed remote from implant placement.
- The subperiosteal plane is preferred for implant placement.
- Gaps between the implant and the skeleton result in unanticipated increases in augmentation.
- Screw fixation of the implant prevents gaps between the implant and the skeleton.
- Screw fixation of the implant prevents implant movement.
- All faces are asymmetric. Facial asymmetries should be discussed with patients preoperatively.

 Access the Historical Perspective section online at
http://www.expertconsult.com

Introduction

- The size and shape of the facial skeleton are fundamental determinants of facial appearance.
- Small asymmetries in skeletal morphology can be noticeable.
- Small changes through surgical intervention can be powerful.
- Augmentation is the predominant means of aesthetic contouring of the facial skeleton in non-Asian populations.
- The use of autogenous bone as an onlay graft is conceptually appealing, but limited by the morbidity associated with its harvest and the unpredictability of the result.
- Most facial skeletal augmentation is performed with alloplastic implants.

Basic science/disease process

Most often, facial skeletal deficiencies are perceived in disease-free individuals whose dimensions fall within the normal range. These patients desire more definition, angularity, or balance to their facial dimensions.

Craniofacial deformities which are disfiguring and of functional consequence usually require skeletal osteotomy and rearrangement as primary treatment. Alloplastic augmentation of the skeleton is often adjunctive in the treatment of the aesthetic sequelae of these diseases.

In less severe deformities, for example, midface or mandibular hypoplasia with normal or compensated occlusion, alloplastic augmentation may be a preferable alternative to osteotomy.

Recently, senescent changes in the facial skeleton have been investigated. Studies revealed retrusion of the midface and mandibular skeleton over time. This supports the concept of alloplastic augmentation of the facial skeleton as part of the algorithm for facial rejuvenation and enhancement.[1]

Diagnosis/patient presentation

For patients presenting with reconstructive problems, implant surgery is performed to return the involved area to its original appearance, or, if that is not possible, to create a face that is symmetric and accepted as normal. For patients presenting for aesthetic enhancement, the surgical goal is more arbitrary. Because implant augmentation of the facial skeleton results in measurable changes in facial dimensions and proportions, it is intuitively advisable and appropriate to use facial measurement and proportion to evaluate the face and to help guide surgery.

Physical examination

Physical examination is the most important element of preoperative assessment and planning. Reviewing life-size photographs with the patient can be helpful when discussing aesthetic concerns and goals as well as demonstrating the asymmetries common to all faces. The recognition of facial asymmetries is important to the surgeon in planning and to the patient in anticipating the postoperative result. As asymmetries become more obvious, it is important to recognize that they are more complex than relative skeletal deficiencies or excess. Rather, they reflect three-dimensional differences that are most easily conceptualized as twists of the facial skeleton that can only be partially compensated for with surgery.

Neoclassical canons and facial anthropometries

For the purposes of painting and sculpture, Renaissance scholars and artists formulated ideal proportions and relations of the head and face. These were largely based on classical Greek canons. Although usually referenced in texts discussing facial skeletal augmentation, neoclassical canons have a limited role in surgical evaluation and planning, because they are based on idealizations. When the dimensions of normal males and females were evaluated and compared to these artistic ideals, it was found that some theoretic proportions are never found, and others are one of many variations found in healthy normal people, or those determined more attractive than normal.[2] The neoclassical canons do not allow for the facial dimensions that are known to differ with sex and age. Most of these canons of proportion (e.g., the width of the upper face is equal to five eye-widths) are interesting but hold for few individuals and cannot be obtained surgically or, if obtainable, only with extremely sophisticated craniofacial procedures. For these reasons, we have found it more useful to use the anthropometric measurements of normal individuals to guide our gestalt in the selection of implants for facial skeletal augmentation (see Ch. 16). Normal-dimensioned faces are intrinsically balanced. That is, the relations between the various areas of the face relate to one another in a way that is not distracting to the observer. By comparing a patient's dimensions to the average, the surgeon has some objective basis as to what anatomic area may be amenable to augmentation, and by how much.

Radiology

Most aesthetic procedures are done without preoperative radiology assessment. In general, the size and position of the implant are largely aesthetic judgments. Cephalometric X-rays are most often used for planning chin and mandible augmentation surgery. These studies define skeletal dimensions and asymmetries as well as the thickness of the chin pad. Computed tomographic (CT) scans provide the ability to view the skeleton in different planes and, through computer manipulation, in three dimensions. CT imaging provides digitized information that can be transferred to design software. This can be used to create life-sized models and custom implants, and these are particularly helpful when augmenting facial skeletons with significant asymmetries.

Patient selection

Patients with normal, deficient, and surgically altered or traumatically deformed anatomy may all benefit from implant augmentation of their craniofacial skeleton.

Skeletal enhancement

Most often, facial skeletal augmentation is done to enhance facial appearance in patients whose skeletal relationships are considered within the normal range. They want more definition and angularity to their appearance. Other patients desire to "balance" their facial dimensions.

Alternative to orthognathic surgery

Midface and mandibular hypoplasia are common facial skeletal variants. In patients with these morphologies, occlusion is normal or has been compensated by orthodontics. These patients have neither respiratory nor ocular compromise. In skeletally deficient patients whose occlusion is normal or has been previously normalized by orthodontics, skeletal repositioning would necessitate additional orthodontic tooth movement. Such a treatment plan is time-consuming, costly, and potentially morbid. It is, therefore, appealing to few patients. In these patients, the appearance of skeletal osteotomies and rearrangements can be simulated through the use of facial implants. Diagrammatic representations of how implant surgery can mimic the appearance of skeletal osteotomies are shown in *Figures 15.1* and *15.2*.

Adjunct to orthognathic surgery

Alloplastic implants can enhance the results of certain orthognathic surgery procedures, including the LeFort I maxillary advancement, the sagittal split mandibular osteotomy, and the sliding genioplasty.

The LeFort I advancement may fulfill its functional role by creating appropriate occlusal relations but inadequately treats midface hypoplasia since only the lower half of the midface is advanced. This may result in a convexity confined to the lower half of the midface. Alloplastic augmentation of the infraorbital rim with or without malar implants can create a truly convex midface. Posterior mandible implants can camouflage osteotomy-induced irregularities along the mandibular border as well as malpositions of the mandibular angles. Chin implants can correct mandible border contour irregularities after sliding genioplasty *(Fig. 15.3)*.

Rejuvenation

Traditional concepts of periorbital and midface aging and rejuvenation focus on the soft tissues. Recently, senescent changes in the supporting facial skeleton have been investigated. Findings in these studies revealed retrusion of the

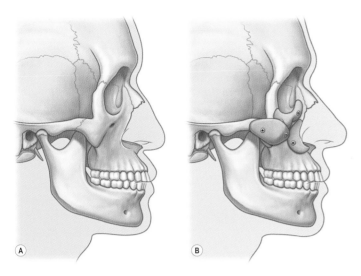

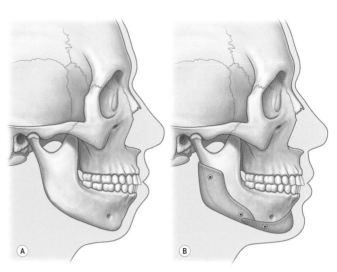

Fig. 15.1 **(A)** Illustration of midface concavity and compensated occlusion. **(B)** Multiple midface implants provide visual effect of LeFort III osteotomy and advancement but do not alter occlusion.

Fig. 15.2 **(A)** Mandibular deficiency with compensated occlusion. **(B)** The visual effect of sagittal split osteotomy and horizontal osteotomy of the chin with advancement has been simulated with mandible and chin implants. Note that the class I occlusion is unchanged. Notice also that the border regularities inherent with skeletal osteotomies are avoided when implants are used.

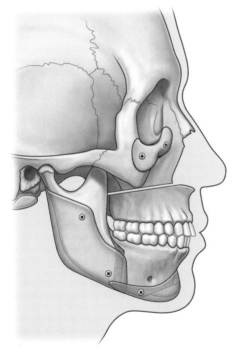

Fig. 15.3 Infraorbital rim implants create upper midface convexity to compensate for lower midface advancement. Posterior mandible implants can camouflage osteotomy-induced irregularities along the mandibular border as well as malpositions of the mandibular angles. Chin implants can correct mandible border contour irregularities after sliding genioplasty.

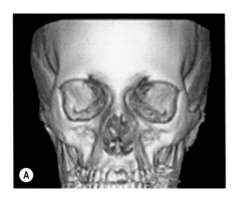
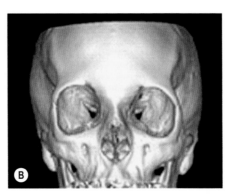
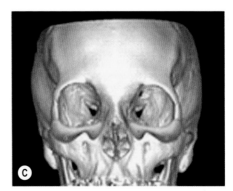

Fig. 15.4 Illustration showing how the placement of infraorbital rim implant on an aged orbit creates contours that mimic a youthful orbit. **(A)** CT scan of a youthful face and orbit. **(B)** CT scan of an aged orbit. **(C)** Implant augmentation of the infraorbital rim restores a youthful orbital contour.

midface skeleton and mandible *(Fig. 15.4)*. This diminution in projection would hasten the gravitational-induced descent of their overlying and now, less supported soft-tissue envelope.[3] Alloplastic skeletal augmentation can both restore skeletal contours and support the overlying soft-tissue envelope.[1]

Provision of these functions supports the concept of selective alloplastic augmentation of the facial skeleton as part of the algorithm for facial rejuvenation and enhancement.

Selective augmentation of the infraorbital rim, malar and pyriform aperture of the old midface skeleton can mimic the contours of its youthful counterpart. Selective augmentation of the chin and mandible can restore youthful contours of the lower jaw.

Skeletal versus soft-tissue augmentation

Both the soft tissues and the skeleton contribute to facial contour and both components are impacted by the aging process. Hence, both soft-tissue and skeletal augmentation can be appropriate to restore youthful facial contours. However, these modalities are not equivalent in their impact on facial appearance. Free fat grafting and the injection of various fillers are intuitive for the restoration of soft-tissue volume loss due to senile atrophy. They have a limited role in simulating the effect of an increase in skeletal projection. Whereas augmenting the facial skeleton results in an increase in the projection of the skeleton, augmenting the soft-tissue volume results in an inflation of the soft-tissue envelope and blunting of the contours of the skeleton. Overaugmentation of either component brings home the point. If overly large implants were placed on the skeleton, the appearance would be too defined and, ultimately, skeletal. If too much fat were placed in the soft-tissue envelope, an increasingly spherical and otherwise undefined shape would result.

Treatment/surgical technique

Anesthesia and preparation

Facial skeletal augmentation can be performed under either local anesthesia supplemented with sedation or general anesthesia. When implants are placed through intraoral approaches, general anesthesia with nasotracheal or endotracheal intubation assures protection of the airway and the best possible antiseptic preparation of the oral cavity. Patient positioning and exposure for implant placement are also optimized when the airway is controlled. Prior to preparation and draping, a dilute solution of Marcaine with epinephrine is infiltrated into the operative site for postoperative pain control and intraoperative hemostasis. Cephalosporins are administered perioperatively. 0.12% chlorhexidine gluconate oral rinse is prescribed for daily use beginning 3 days before and including the day before surgery.

Facial implant surgery is routinely performed on an outpatient basis.

Incisions

Incisions for skeletal access and implant placement are borrowed from craniofacial and aesthetic surgery.

Transconjunctival retroseptal incisions are routinely used to access the infraorbital rim and internal orbit. The lateral extent of the lower lid blepharoplasty incision provides access to the lateral orbit and zygomatic arch. This small cutaneous incision leaves an inconspicuous scar. Skin or skin muscle flap lower lid incisions provide alternative approaches to the periorbital area. Intraoral sulcus incisions are used to augment the midface as well as the mandibular body and ramus. These incisions are made with a generous labial cuff to allow watertight mucosal closure. Chin area augmentation is performed through submental or intraoral incisions. Placement of incisions directly over implants is avoided.

Implant materials

Implant materials used for facial skeletal augmentation are biocompatible – that is, there is an acceptable reaction between the material and the host. In general, the host has little or no enzymatic ability to degrade the implant with the result that the implant tends to maintain its volume and shape. Likewise, the implant has a small and predictable effect on the host tissues that surround it. This type of relationship is an advantage over the use of autogenous bone or cartilage which, when revascularized, will be remodeled to varying degrees, thereby changing volume and shape. The alloplastic implants presently used for facial reconstruction have not been shown to have any toxic effects on the host.[4] The host responds to these materials by forming a fibrous capsule around the implant, which is the body's way of isolating the implant from the host. The most important implant characteristic that determines the nature of the encapsulation is the implant's surface characteristics. Smooth implants result in the formation of smooth-walled capsules. Porous implants allow varying degrees of soft-tissue ingrowth that result in a less dense and less defined capsule. It is a clinical impression that porous implants, as a result of fibrous incorporation rather than encapsulation, have a lower tendency to erode underlying bone or migrate due to soft-tissue mechanical forces and, perhaps, are less susceptible to infection when challenged with an inoculum of bacteria. The most commonly used, commercially available materials today for facial skeletal augmentation are solid silicone, which has a smooth surface, and porous polyethylene.

Silicone

Solid silicone or the silicone rubber used for facial implants is a vulcanized form of polysiloxane. Polysiloxane is a polymer created from interlinking silicone and oxygen with methyl side groups.

Silicone implants have the following advantages: they are easily sterilized by steam or irradiation; they can be carved with either scissors or scalpel; and they can be stabilized with a screw or suture. There are no known clinical or allergic reactions to silicone implants. Because they have a smooth surface, there is no soft-tissue ingrowth, allowing them to be easily removed. Disadvantages to silicone implants include: the tendency to cause resorption of underlying bone; the potential to migrate if not fixed to the underlying skeleton; and the likelihood of its fibrous capsule to be visible when placed under a thin soft-tissue envelope.

Polyethylene

Polyethylene is a simple carbon chain of ethylene monomer. Polyethylene used for facial implants is porous with intra-material porosity between 125 and 250 µm. The porosity allows fibrous tissue growth into the surface of the implant. The porosity of this implant has both advantages and disadvantages. Soft-tissue growth into the implant lessens the tendency to migrate and to erode underlying bone. Porosity also allows some flexibility and adaptability of the implant. However, its porosity causes its soft tissue to adhere to it, making placement more difficult and requiring a larger pocket to be made than with smoother implants. The soft-tissue ingrowth also makes implant removal more difficult.

The firm consistency of porous polyethylene allows it to be easily fixed with screws and contoured with a scalpel or power equipment without fragmenting.

Requisites of implant shape, positioning, and immobilization

Shape

The external shape of the implant should mimic the desired shape of the bone it is augmenting. Its posterior surface should be one that molds to the bone to which it is applied. The implant margins must taper imperceptibly into the native skeleton so that they are neither visible nor palpable.

Positioning

Although some surgeons prefer to place implants in a soft-tissue pocket, clinical experience has led this surgeon to adopt a policy of strict subperiosteal placement. Placement in a subperiosteal pocket involves a dissection that is safe to peripheral nerves and relatively bloodless. It allows visualization and, therefore, more precise augmentation of the skeletal contour desired for augmentation. The size of the pocket will be determined by the type of implant used and its method of immobilization. The long-standing teaching using smooth silicone implants is to make a pocket just large enough to accommodate the implant and, therefore, guarantee its position. Porous implants require a larger pocket, because they adhere to the soft tissues during their placement. This author, whether using smooth or porous implants, dissects widely enough to have a perspective of the skeletal anatomy being augmented, which allows more precise, symmetric implant positioning. Wide subperiosteal exposure of the area to be augmented optimizes accuracy of implant placement.

Immobilization

Facial implants should be immobilized. Many surgeons stabilize the position of the implant by suturing it to surrounding soft tissues or by using temporary transcutaneous pull-out sutures. Screw fixation of the implant to the skeleton is preferred. Screw fixation prevents any movement of the implant and also assures application of the implant to the surface of the bone. Because each facial skeleton has a unique and varying surface topography, a nonconforming implant will leave gaps between the implants and the skeleton. These gaps between the implant and the skeleton are problematic for two reasons. The space between the implant and the skeleton is equivalent to an additional augmentation. This can lead to overaugmentation and asymmetries. Gaps are also potential spaces for hematoma and seroma formation. Finally, screw fixation allows for final contouring with the implant in position. This final contouring is particularly important where the implant interfaces with the skeleton. Any step-off between the implant and the skeleton will be palpable and possibly visible in patients with thin soft-tissue cover.

> **Hints and tips**
>
> Screw fixation of implants not only prevents implant movement but also obliterates gaps between the implant and the native skeleton. Gaps result in unanticipated increase in augmentation.

Preventing hematoma

The adequacy of hemostasis shortens convalescence, and minimizes morbidity. My impression is that hematomas are associated with most postoperative infections. To optimize hemostasis, the soft tissues are infiltrated with epinephrine-containing solution, the operative field is packed with epinephrine-soaked neuropaddies until the wound is closed, suction drains are routine, and mildly compressive tape dressings are placed at the completion of each procedure.

> **Hints and tips**
>
> A suction drain placed at the site of augmentation minimizes hematoma formation.

Midface implants

Video 1

Virtually all aesthetic augmentation is performed on the middle and lower thirds of the facial skeleton. The midface is best conceptualized as having three zones, alone, or in combination, amenable to augmentation. Implants are designed to augment these three areas, which include the infraorbital rim, the malar, and the pyriform aperture.

Infraorbital rim

Because the infraorbital rim and upper midface skeleton support the lower eyelids and the cheek soft tissues, their projection impacts on lid and cheek position. Patients with retrusive skeletons are more likely to undergo premature lower lid and cheek descent with aging. This lack of skeletal support predisposes to lower lid malposition after blepharoplasty and limits the efficacy and longevity of midfacelifting procedures.

Jelks and Jelks[5] categorized globe–orbital rim relationships and the tendency for the development of lower lid malposition after blepharoplasty. On sagittal view, they placed a line or vector between the most anterior projection of the globe and the malar eminence and lid margin. A positive vector

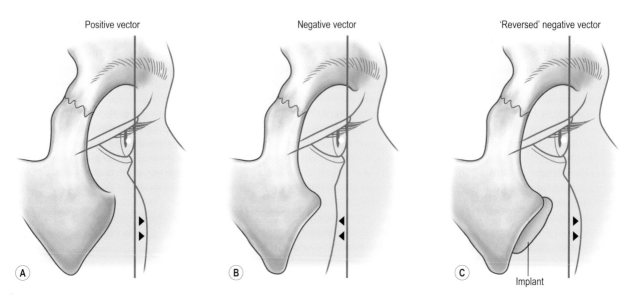

Positive vector   Negative vector   'Reversed' negative vector

(A)   (B)   (C)
Implant

Fig. 15.5 Jelks and Jelks[5] categorized globe–orbital rim relationships by placing a line or "vector" between the most anterior projection of the globe and the malar eminence and lid margin. **(A)** Positive vector relationship. In the youthful face with normal globe-to-skeletal rim relations, the cheek mass supported by the infraorbital rim lies anterior to the surface of the cornea. The position of the cheek prominence beyond the anterior surface of the cornea is termed a positive vector. **(B)** Negative vector relationship: In patients with maxillary hypoplasia, the cheek mass lies posterior to the surface of the cornea. The position of the cheek prominence beyond the anterior surface of the cornea is termed a negative vector. **(C)** "Reversed" negative vector relationship: Alloplastic augmentation of the infraorbital rim can reverse the negative vector. (Redrawn after Yaremchuk, M.J. Restoring palpebral fissure shape after previous lower blepharoplasty. Plast. Reconst. Surg. 111:441–450. © 2003, with permission of Lippincott Williams and Wilkins.)

relationship exists when the most anterior projection of the globe is posterior to the lid margin and the malar eminence. A negative vector relationship exists when the most anterior projection of the globe lies anterior to the lower lid and the malar eminence. They warned that patients whose midface skeletal morphology has a negative vector relationship are prone to lid malposition after lower blepharoplasty. Augmentation of the infraorbital rim in patients with a retruded infraorbital rim can bring it into a better relationship with the globe, thereby "reversing the negative vector"[6,7] *(Fig. 15.5)*. Infraorbital rim augmentation is part of the strategy for normalizing the appearance in patients who are "morphologically prone." It can be adapted for morphologically prone patients who are first seeking improvement in their periorbital appearance or for those whose lid malposition and round-eye appearance have been exaggerated by previous lower blepharoplasty.[6]

Surgical technique

The infraorbital rim and adjacent anatomy must be exposed sufficiently to assure ideal implant placement, smooth implant facial skeleton transitions, and screw fixation. Direct, subciliary skin or skin muscle flap incisions can provide this exposure. A transconjunctival retroseptal incision may require lengthening with a lateral canthotomy. I prefer to use a transconjunctival incision along with an intraoral sulcus incision to free the entire midface skeleton in the subperiosteal plane.

It is important to identify the infraorbital nerve as it exits from the infraorbital foramen. The foramen is located about 1 cm below the margin of the orbit in the midpupillary line. The arcus marginalis, the orbicularis oculi and the origins of the lip elevators are separated from the underlying skeleton in a subperiosteal plane to expose the infraorbital rim.

Implants are designed to increase the sagittal projection of the infraorbital rim. The implants are then carved to fit the specific needs of the patient. Since, inevitably, there is a varying discrepancy between the contours of the posterior surface of the implant and the anterior surface of the facial skeleton, segmenting the implant may allow better adaptation of the implant to the skeleton. It may also facilitate placement of the implant through limited skeletal access. The implant is fixed to the skeleton with titanium screws. Most often, the cheek soft-tissue mass is resuspended by sutures tied to the rim implant (subperiosteal midfacelift). This technique is summarized in *Figure 15.6*. A clinical example is shown in *Figure 15.7*.

Pyriform aperture

The average Caucasian face is convex. A relative deficiency in lower midface projection may be congenital or acquired, particularly after cleft surgery and trauma. Patients with satisfactory occlusion and lower midface concavity can have their aesthetic desires satisfied with skeletal augmentation. Implantation of alloplastic material in the paranasal area can simulate the visual effect of LeFort I advancement and other skeletal manipulations. Pyriform aperture augmentation increases the projection of the nasal base and, therefore, opens the nasolabial angle.[8]

It also tends to lessen the depth of the nasolabial fold.by effacing it from below *(Fig. 15.8)*.

Surgical technique

Paranasal augmentation is done through an intraoral incision made approximately 1 cm above the sulcus. The medial extent of the incision is made just lateral to the piriform aperture to avoid placing incisions directly over the implant. Subperiosteal

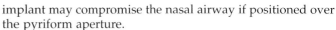

dissection exposes the area to be augmented. The infraorbital nerve is identified and preserved. The patient's anatomy will determine whether the entire crescent, or just the horizontal or vertical limb of the crescent, will be utilized. The root of the canine usually lies in the field to be augmented and should be avoided if the implant is immobilized with screws. The implant may compromise the nasal airway if positioned over the pyriform aperture.

The technique is illustrated in *Figure 15.9*.

A patient who underwent aesthetic rhinoplasty and augmentation of the pyriform aperture area is shown in *Figure 15.10*.

Malar

Prominent malar bones are considered attractive. Hence, the malar area is frequently augmented with implants. The lack of anthropometric and cephalometric landmarks precludes the availability of normative data, making analysis and augmentation of the malar area largely subjective. Malar deficiency is often part of a generalized midface deficiency for which malar augmentation alone may be inadequate or even inappropriate. Clinical experience has shown that when malar projection is deemed inadequate, malar augmentation is most effective when it recreates the contours of a normal skeleton with prominent anterior projection. Malar skeletal augmentation is not a substitute for soft-tissue augmentation or repositioning.

Since full cheeks are associated with youth, malar augmentation is often performed to provide a youthful appearance. This may provide an aesthetic benefit if there is a relative malar hypoplasia or if the implants are of modest size and projection. This skeletal augmentation is not equivalent to a soft-tissue augmentation or resuspension. Similarly, malar implants are often advocated as a means to obliterate lower-eyelid wrinkles or secondary bags. Malar augmentation impacts poorly on these surface irregularities. More often, they may detract from periorbital aesthetics by contributing to lower lid malposition, particularly when placed through an eyelid approach.[9]

Surgical technique

Malar augmentation can be performed through intraoral, coronal, or eyelid incisions. It is the author's preference to access the malar midface through an intraoral approach. An upper sulcus incision is made far enough from the apex of the sulcus so that sufficient labial tissue is available on either

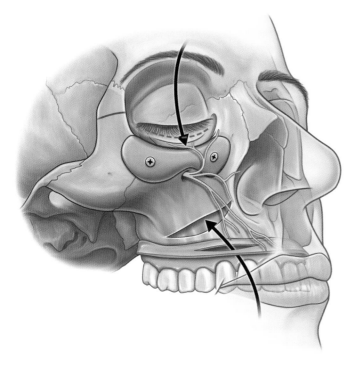

Fig. 15.6 Overview of operation to increase projection of infraorbital rim and "reverse the negative vector" in patients with upper midface skeletal deficiency. I prefer a transconjunctival retroseptal incision (broken line) and, if necessary, the lateral extent of a lower lid blepharoplasty incision (solid line) to expose the infraorbital rim. This approach preserves the integrity of the lateral canthus, and hence, the palpebral fissure. Transcutaneous blepharoplasty or transconjunctival with lateral canthotomy incisions are alternative approaches which provide greater exposure but are accompanied by a greater risk of palpebral fissure distortion. An intraoral incision is used to access the lower midface skeleton and to identify and protect the infraorbital nerve. The lower lid and midface soft tissues are freed by subperiosteal dissection. The implant is immobilized with titanium screws.

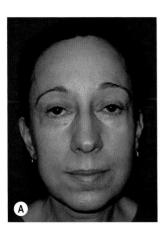 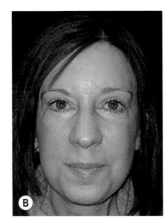 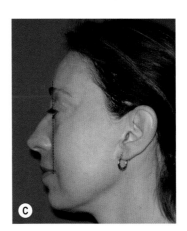 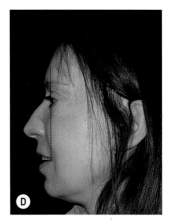

Fig. 15.7 A 52-year-old woman had undergone previous browlift, rhytidectomy, and upper and lower lid blepharoplasty. Lower lid retraction was treated by multiple canthopexies, spacer grafts, and full-thickness skin grafts. Dry-eye symptoms persisted. Infraorbital rim augmentation, midfacelift, and lateral canthopexy resolved her symptoms. Her brows and hairline were repositioned. **(A),** Preoperative frontal view; **(B)** postoperative frontal view; **(C)** preoperative lateral view; **(D)** postoperative lateral view. Note the vertical line defining globe–rim relations. The procedure transformed the preoperative negative vector to a positive vector globe–rim relationship.

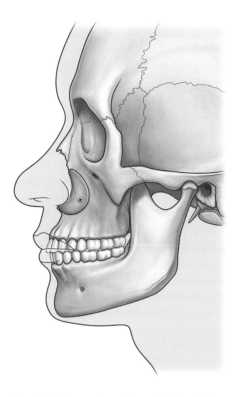

Fig. 15.8 Diagram shows impact of implant relative to profile and nasolabial angle.

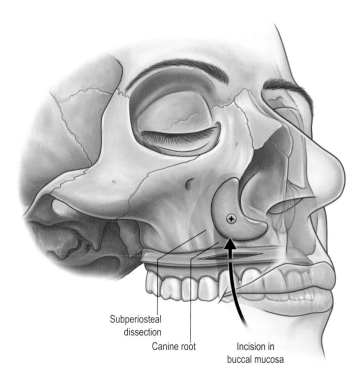

Fig. 15.9 Diagrammatic overview of paranasal implant surgery. The green area indicates the area of subperiosteal dissection. Note proximity of infraorbital nerve. Note that the root of the canine tooth lies below the area to be augmented. It must be avoided during screw immobilization of the implant.

Subperiosteal dissection

Canine root   Incision in buccal mucosa

side for secure incision closure. Taking care to identify the infraorbital nerve, subperiosteal dissection is carried over the malar eminence and on to the zygomatic arch almost up to the zygomaticotemporal suture. The pocket size should allow precise insertion of the implant to the area of the skeleton desired for augmentation. Extending a malar implant onto the zygomatic arch has a profound impact on midfacial width. Although implants with greater projection are available, I rarely provide more than 3 mm of augmentation at the point of maximum projection. Larger implants may become obvious with time as the overlying soft tissues atrophy and sag. The capsule formation that accompanies smooth-surfaced implants further exaggerates the tendency towards implant visibility. In my experience, implants with large surface areas do not mimic natural skeletal topography and cause unnatural implant-dictated contours. The intraoperative position of both smooth and porous implants can be guaranteed with screw fixation of the implant to the skeleton (*Fig. 15.11*).

A clinical example is shown in *Figure 15.12*.

Mandible implants

Each of the anatomic areas of the mandible – chin, body, angle, and ramus – may be deficient and is amenable to augmentation with alloplastic materials.

Chin

There is consensus that the ideal profile relation portrays a convex face with the upper lip projecting approximately

2 mm beyond the lower lip and the lower lip projecting approximately 2 mm beyond the chin.[9] Note that, on the average, men tend to have larger, more projecting chins than women.[10]

Early implant designs augmented the mentum only and, if prominent, often created a stuck-on appearance due to failure of the lateral aspect of the implant to merge with the anterior aspect of the mandibular body (*Fig. 15.13*). "Extended" chin implants with tapered lateral extensions were later designed to allow the chin implant to merge better with more lateral mandibular contours.[11] However, as implants become larger with more complex three-dimensional configurations, they often are less likely to fit the needs of a given patient. A one-piece chin implant with lateral extensions is unlikely to have an arc, projection, and inclination appropriate for every mandible. Furthermore, with one-piece implants, asymmetry in horizontal positioning increases as one proceeds laterally. It is not uncommon to find one end of an extended silicone implant impinging on the mental nerve, while the other end extends beyond the edge of the mandibular border (*Fig. 15.14*). A two-piece chin implant design allows adaptation of each of these parameters for a given mandible (*Fig. 15.15*).[12]

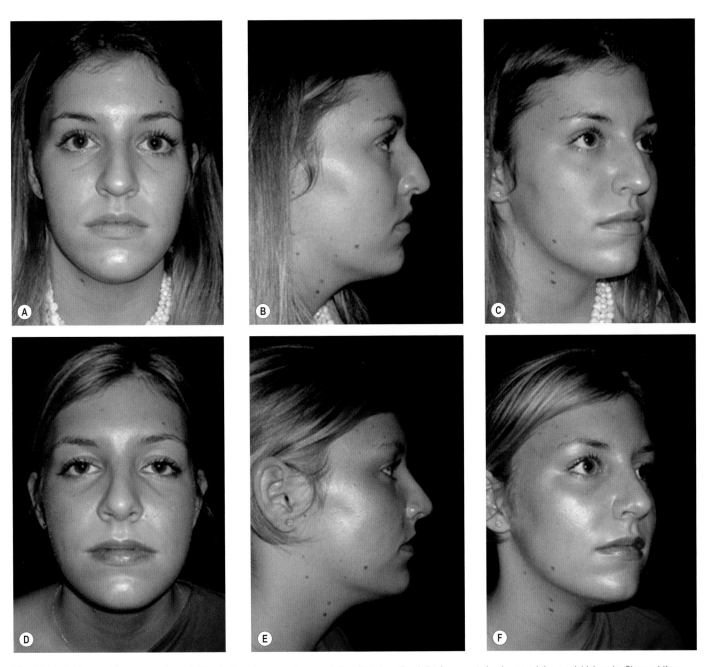

Fig. 15.10 A 20-year-old woman underwent rhinoplasty and paranasal augmentation. Note how the skeletal augmentation increased the nasolabial angle. Since midface concavity tends to increase the relative projection of the nose, creating midface convexity tends to lessen the relative projection of the nose. **A–C,** Preoperative frontal, lateral, and oblique views. **D–F,** Postoperative frontal, lateral, and oblique views.

Technique

The midline of the chin is marked as a reference point. The chin is accessed through either a submental or intraoral incision. An intraoral incision should be placed 1 cm above the sulcus to provide adequate tissue inferiorly for ease and security of closure. This incision also avoids pooling of saliva over the suture line, which risks implant contamination if the closure is not secure. The technique of intraoral placement of chin implants avoids a cutaneous scar but provides limited exposure to the menton while compromising the mentalis muscle. As a result, the intraoral approach can be associated with superior malposition of implants and lower lip dysfunction resulting from mentalis muscle division or detachment.[13]

After reviewing his series of more than 100 cases of postoperative chin problems, Zide[14] noted that almost all chin implant problems that he had seen were caused by implants that were placed through intraoral incisions.

The submental approach and extended dissection avoid damage to the mentalis muscle and allow better visualization of the mental nerve.

Subperiosteal dissection should extend approximately 1 cm beyond the area of augmentation to provide a panoramic view of the complex and varying contours of the mandible, thereby allowing precise implant placement.

The implant is immobilized with titanium screws *(Fig. 15.16)*.

Clinical examples of alloplastic augmentation of the chin are shown in *Figure 15.17*.

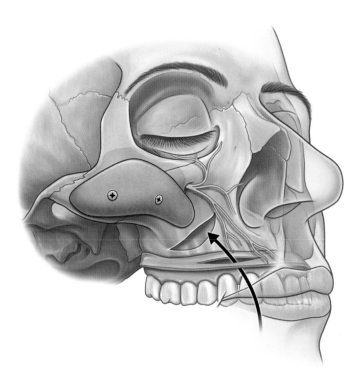

Fig. 15.11 Overview of the operative technique for malar augmentation. The upper sulcus incision is at least 1 cm above the apex so that sufficient tissue is available for closure. Taking care to identify the infraorbital nerve, the subperiosteal dissection is carried over the malar eminence and on to the zygomatic arch just beyond the zygomaticotemporal suture. It is useful to identify or create landmarks (for example, scoring the zygoma relative to the infraorbital foramen) to allow symmetric placement of the implants. Implants are fixed with titanium screws for immobilization, and for the obliteration of dead space between the posterior surface of the implant and the anterior surface of the facial skeleton. The implants are contoured so that they are identical in size and shape, are appropriate for the area to be augmented, and merge imperceptibly with the native skeleton. A trochar-attached suction drain is placed. It exits through temporal hair-bearing scalp or the postauricular area. The colored area denotes the area of subperiosteal dissection. The implant usually extends from the temperozygomatic suture on the zygomatic arch to just below the foramen of the infraorbital nerve.

Hints and tips

Many chin implant problems are caused by transoral placement.

Implant augmentation versus sliding genioplasty

In most clinical situations, I prefer to augment the sagittal projection of the chin with alloplastic implants rather than with horizontal osteotomy and advancement. Chin point advancement after osteotomy has the advantage of stretching the attached suprahyoid muscles, thereby decreasing submental fullness and improving submental contour. The major disadvantage intrinsic to sliding genioplasty is the unnatural bony and border contours that accompany the selective movement of the chin point. The contour result is one that has a poor transition, resulting in the stuck-on appearance of the chin, much like a large button chin implant. There are also step-offs at the osteotomy sites along the mandibular body.

The notchings or indentations are particularly detrimental to those who have an existing prejowl sulcus. Extending the osteotomy to the second molar can minimize both of these deformities but may exaggerate mandible asymmetry after advancement.

Horizontal osteotomy of the chin with inferior repositioning of the chin point is a key procedure to increase the vertical height of the severely deficient chin. Horizontal osteotomy with chin lengthening may also efface the deep labiomental sulcus, affecting some patients. Implants placed on the inferior border of the chin can effect small increases in chin height.

Ramus, angle, and body

Aside from chin augmentation, there are three patient populations who may benefit from other mandibular augmentation procedures. One group has mandibular dimensions that relate poorly to the upper and middle thirds of the face which are within the normal range. These patients perceive a wider lower face as an enhancement to their appearance. Patients in this treatment group often present with a desire to emulate the appearance of models, actors, and actresses who have a defined, angular lower face. This patient group benefits from implants designed to augment the ramus and posterior body of the mandible and, in so doing, increase the bigonial distance.

Patients with mandibular deficiency who have had their malocclusion treated with orthodontics may benefit from mandible implants. Implants are designed to correct the obtuse mandibular angle with steep mandibular plane, as well as the decreased vertical and transverse ramus dimensions *(Fig. 15.18)*. The addition of an extended chin implant will camouflage the poorly projecting chin.

Patients who have had orthognathic surgery often have contour irregularities after skeletal osteotomy and rearrangement. Posterior mandible implants can camouflage osteotomy-induced irregularities along the mandibular border as well as malposition irregularities after sliding genioplasty.

Technique

An intraoral incision is made to expose the ramus and body of the mandible. It is made at least 1 cm above the sulcus on its labial side. The anterior ramus and body of the mandible are freed in the subperiosteal plane from their overlying soft tissues *(Fig. 15.19)*. If the mental area is also being augmented, a submental incision is made for access and exposure of the anterior mandible. The mental nerve is visualized as it exits its foramen to avoid its injury. It is important to free both the inferior and posterior borders of the mandible of soft-tissue attachments to allow implant placement.

To assure the desired placement of the implant and its application to the surface of the mandible, the implant is fixed to the mandible with titanium screws. With vigorous retraction, this is performed intraorally. It can also be done transcutaneously by making small incisions in the neck skin to allow passage of a trochar and a protective sleeve for drilling. Screws are placed to avoid the anticipated path of the inferior alveolar nerve prior to its exit from the mental foramen.

It is crucial to soften any transitions between the implant and the mandible, particularly where the implant extends

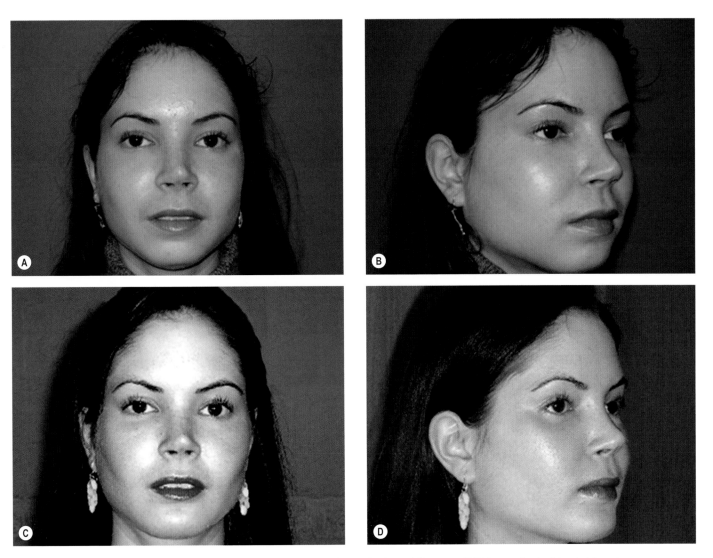

Fig. 15.12 A 24-year-old woman underwent malar augmentation, chin augmentation, and submental lipectomy. **(A,B)** Preoperative frontal and oblique views; **(C,D)** postoperative frontal and oblique views.

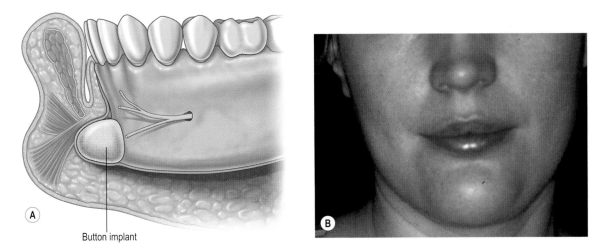

Button implant

Fig. 15.13 (A,B) Illustration and clinical example of a large button chin implant resulting in a poor implant mandible transition with a stuck-on appearance.

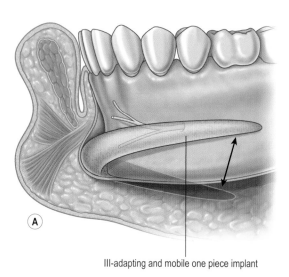

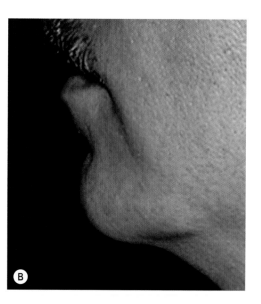

Fig. 15.14 Malpositioned one-piece extended implant. **(A)** When placed through an intraoral approach it is common for one end to extend beyond the mandibular border while the other end impinges upon the mental nerve. **(B)** Clinical example: extended one-piece implant protruding beyond the mandibular border.

Ill-adapting and mobile one piece implant

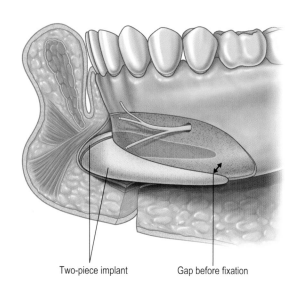

Two-piece implant   Gap before fixation

Fig. 15.15 Illustration of a two-piece chin implant placed in a subperiosteal pocket. Note two-piece design, which allows the lateral extension of the implant to follow the inclination of the mandibular border. Because the contour of the posterior surface of the implant does not mimic the contour of the anterior surface of the mandible, there is a gap between the mandible and the implant.

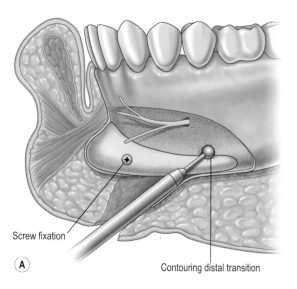

Screw fixation

Contouring distal transition

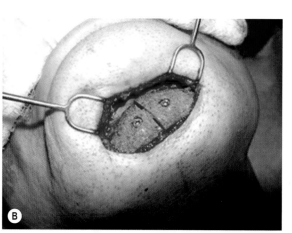

Fig. 15.16 Screw fixation of the implant to the mandible prevents implant movement and obliterates gaps between the implant and anterior surface of the mandible. Screw fixation also allows in-place contouring of the implant to ensure desired contour and an imperceptible implant–skeleton transition. **(A)** Illustration showing "in-place" contouring of the implant fixed to the mandible with titanium screws. **(B)** Clinical example of screw-fixed two-piece porous polyethylene chin implant exposed through a submental incision.

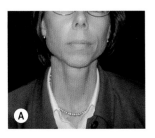
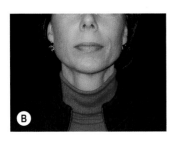
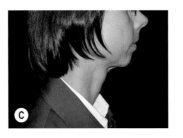
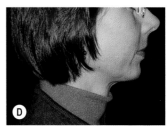

Fig. 15.17 A 35-year-old woman with microgenia underwent chin augmentation with an alloplastic implant. **(A)** pre- and **(B)** 1 year postoperative frontal views; **(C)** pre- and **(D)** 1 year postoperative lateral views.

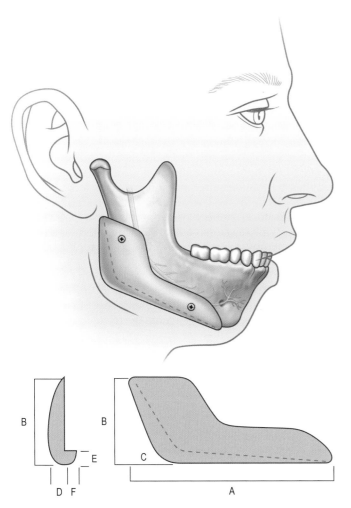

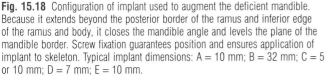

Fig. 15.18 Configuration of implant used to augment the deficient mandible. Because it extends beyond the posterior border of the ramus and inferior edge of the ramus and body, it closes the mandible angle and levels the plane of the mandible border. Screw fixation guarantees position and ensures application of implant to skeleton. Typical implant dimensions: A = 10 mm; B = 32 mm; C = 5 or 10 mm; D = 7 mm; E = 10 mm.

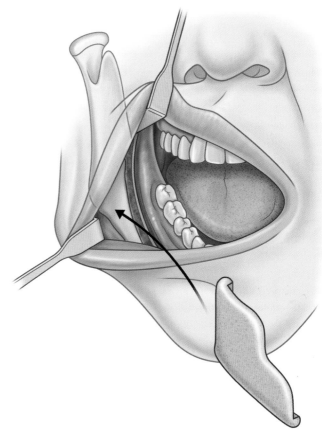

Fig. 15.19 An intraoral mucosal incision is made along the ramus and posterior body of mandible. It is made approximately 1 cm above the sulcus on its labial side. A subperiosteal pocket is created for placement of the mandible implant.

> ### Hints and tips
>
> Make the intraoral incision at least 1 cm above the sulcus on the labial side to provide adequate soft tissue for two-layer closure and to avoid saliva pooling over the suture line in the early postoperative period.

beyond the anterior mandibular border's inferior edge. Any step-offs between the implant and the mandible in this area may be visible in thin patients. Screw fixation of the implants allows scalpel or mechanical burr final contouring with the implants in place. A small suction drain is placed at the operative site and exits through the skin behind the ear. The incision is closed in two layers with absorbable sutures.[15]

A clinical example is shown in *Figure 15.20*.

Postoperative care

A suction drain is routinely placed at the operative site. After midface and chin procedures, the drain is routinely removed the morning after surgery. Drains usually remain in place for 72 hours after placement of mandible implants. A supportive

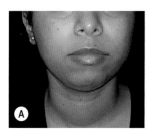
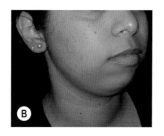
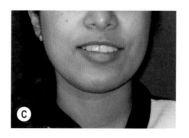
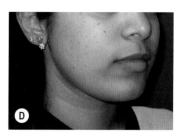

Fig. 15.20 A 28-year-old woman with micrognathia underwent horizontal osteotomy of the chin with lengthening as well as placement of chin and mandible implants. **(A,B)** Preoperative frontal and oblique views. **(C,D)** Postoperative frontal and oblique views.

tape dressing placed after the completion of surgery is usually removed the morning after surgery. Oral antibiotics are prescribed for 7 days after surgery.

When intraoral incisions are used, patients are asked to eat a soft diet for the first 72 hours after surgery. Patients are instructed to refrain from strenuous exercise for 2–3 weeks after surgery.

Outcomes, prognosis, and complications

The best available data support the biocompatibility of the currently used implant materials.[4] No cases of cancer have been reported in association with a polymer craniofacial implant. True hypersensitivity reactions to prefabricated polymer implants are extremely rare. There are no truly scientific data to document the surgical complication rate related to facial skeletal augmentation. Prospective studies that control for surgical technique, implant site, patient selection, and follow-up time do not exist. We reviewed almost 200 reports in the literature that provided sufficient data to compare complication rates related to both implant material and implant site. The accumulation of these clinical data can provide some useful information about factors that can contribute to morbidity with implants. For example, the quality of the soft-tissue coverage is clearly related to morbidity. Complication rates are lowest in the chin and malar region, where the soft-tissue cover is relatively thick, and highest in the nose and ear, where the soft-tissue cover is thin and often under tension from the underlying device. The surface characteristic of an implant may also be important.

Porous implants allow a certain ingrowth of tissue which may allow the presence of host defenses within the implant to decrease the risk of infection. Given that several biomaterials are well tolerated in the human body, the actual chemical structure of an implant is important only to the degree that it influences the consistency and surface characteristics of the device.

In 2003, I reported my personal experience with porous implants used for facial skeletal reconstruction.[16] This report was based on experiences with 162 patients who were operated on over an 11-year period (1990–2001). In this series no implants migrated or were extruded, formed clinically apparent capsules, or caused symptoms attributable to bioincompatibility. The overall reoperation was 10%, which included operations to remove implants because of acute infection (2%) or late infection (1%), or to remove or adjust implants causing displeasing contours. The rate of complications has not changed in facial implant procedures in the subsequent 250 patients.

The low incidence of infection after facial implant surgery precludes a strict formulation for the treatment of postoperative infections. The presence of a foreign body decreases the minimal infecting dose of *Staphylococcus aureus* in an animal model due to impaired bacterial clearance. If microorganisms are not eliminated rapidly from an implant surface they will adhere to the implant initially by nonspecific physical forces and then by the formation of biofilms characterized by clustering together in an extracellular matrix attached to the implant. Biofilms protect bacteria from host defenses and antibiotics. Only aggressive debridement and long-term suppressive therapy have been effective in treating orthopedic implant-related infections.[17] This approach is usually not appropriate in facial implant patients since both debridement and chronic infection may be deforming in this appearance-conscious population. Since antibiotic treatment alone is usually not successful, facial implant-related infections are usually treated by implant removal, antibiotics, and appropriate wound care. Implants may be replaced in 6–12 months.

Common causes for patient dissatisfaction after facial implant surgery include malposition, asymmetry, and sensory nerve dysfunction. Although bone resorption beneath facial implants is often cited as a complication of implant surgery, the process is rarely clinically significant unless a chin implant that overrides the lower incisor tooth roots creates symptoms. Wide subperiosteal exposure of the area to be augmented optimizes implant placement, screw fixation prevents implant movement, and visualization of the infraorbital and mental nerves before and after implant placement avoids problems with nerve compression.

Secondary procedures

The most common indication for secondary surgery is to treat the visibility of facial implants. Since it is inevitable that the volumes of soft tissues change with time and that of alloplastic implants does not, large implants placed under a thin soft-tissue cover will become visible in time. This phenomenon is exaggerated when smooth-walled implants which elicit a vigorous capsule response are used. Patients with thin soft tissue are advised preoperatively that soft-tissue augmentation with fillers or fat injections may later be appropriate.

Access the complete references list online at **http://www.expertconsult.com**

1. Yaremchuk MJ, Kahn DM. Periorbital Skeletal Augmentation to Improve Blepharoplasty and Midfacial Results. *Plast Reconstr Surg*. 2009;124:2151–2160.

   Describes the impact of the projection of the skeleton on the soft-tissue envelope and periorbital appearance.

5. Jelks GW, Jelks EB. The influence of orbital and eyelid anatomy on the palpebral aperture. *Clin Plast Surg*. 1991;18:193.

   Emphasizes the importance of globe rim relations and morbidity in lower lid blepharoplasty

7. Yaremchuk MJ. Restoring palpebral fissure shape after previous lower blepharoplasty. *Plast Reconst Surg*. 2003;111:441.

   Introduces the concept of negative-vector reversal with implants.

9. Yaremchuk MJ. Secondary malar implant surgery. *Plast Reconstr Surg*. 2008;121:620.

   Avoidance and correction of malar implant-related problems

14. Zide BM. The mentalis muscle: An essential component of chin and lower lip position. *Plast Reconst Surg*. 1989;83:413.

    Warns of potential damage to the mentalis muscle with the intraoral approach to chin augmentation and presents techniques for repair.

16. Yaremchuk MJ. Facial skeletal reconstruction using porous polyethylene implants. *Plast Reconst Surg*. 2003;111:1818.

    Reports one surgeon's clinical experience.

16

Anthropometry, cephalometry, and orthognathic surgery

Daniel I. Taub, Jordan M.S. Jacobs, and Jonathan S. Jacobs

SYNOPSIS

- Anthropometry is the study of the human body in relation to size and proportion. The division of the face into proportions is a convenient way for surgeons to analyze facial esthetics.
- Presurgical analysis of soft tissue points, photographs, cephalometrics and prediction tracings are critical for diagnosis and surgical planning.
- The most successful orthognathic surgical outcome is one in which a team approach is used. The primary objective is to correct facial skeletal discrepancies and achieve optimal aesthetics and dental occlusion.
- Presurgical orthodontics positions the teeth within the alveolar bone and permit successful surgical repositioning of the maxilla and/or mandible in three dimensions.
- Modern anthropometrics allows comparison of many soft tissue and skeletal data points to a database of normative values based on age, sex, and ethnicity.
- A detailed facial analysis remains one of the most important elements during evaluation of the orthognathic surgical candidate, and has been greatly enhanced with the development of three-dimensional imaging systems.

Introduction

Perhaps the most important responsibility in the treatment of a patient with an aesthetic problem is the ability to critically study their facial morphology and recognize deviations from normative values. The contours of an individual's face represent a complex interaction between skeletal and soft tissue anatomy as well as static and dynamic forces. This chapter will focus on the various tools used to diagnose aberrations in a patient's skeletal proportions and the surgical correction of these abnormalities. The relationship between the facial skeleton and the overlying soft tissue will also be examined so that predictions of the final surgical result can be made preoperatively. Specifically, this chapter will emphasize treatment of the lower two-thirds of the face. Treatment of the nose, eyes, and forehead will be covered elsewhere.

Anthropometrics

Anthropometry involves the study of the human body in relation to its variations in size and proportions. The use of well-established aesthetic standards allows facial, craniofacial, and maxillofacial surgical techniques to achieve cosmetic results.[1] Throughout history, there has been a fascination with the human form. While the ancient Egyptians are reported to have been the first to divide the human body into equal parts, the Greek sculptor Polycleitus is credited with the development of canons as exemplified in his statue of Doryphorus (Fig. 16.1).[2] During the Renaissance, artists such as da Vinci, Dürer, Pacioli, and Alberti developed the Neoclassical Canons, which divided the face into symmetric ideal proportions. The 18th and 19th centuries brought the concept of physical anthropology, in which the majority of measurements were performed directly on skulls with less attention given to soft tissue points. Camper introduced the concept of the facial angle and used this measurement to challenge the hypothesis of an evolutionary basis to racial inequality.[3] Later anatomists, however, such as De Gobineau, Broca, Topinard, and Lombroso, accepted variations in skull proportions as evidence of inferiority of all non-white individuals.[4–6] The 20th century was highlighted by the development of radiographic techniques to indirectly measure the facial skeleton. Broadbent's concept of cephalometrics[7] allowed the initial compilation of normative facial data in 5400 children over 36 years as part of the Bolton study.[8,9]

The idea of the "golden proportion" having application to facial analysis, although introduced by Seghers et al.,[10] was popularized by Ricketts.[11–14] The aesthetically attractive 1:1.618 ratio, indicated by the Greek letter phi (Φ), was first recorded in the 3rd century BC by the Pythagoreans and has

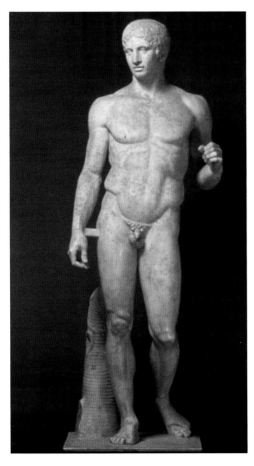

Fig. 16.1 The Greek sculptor Polycleitus' Doryphorus.

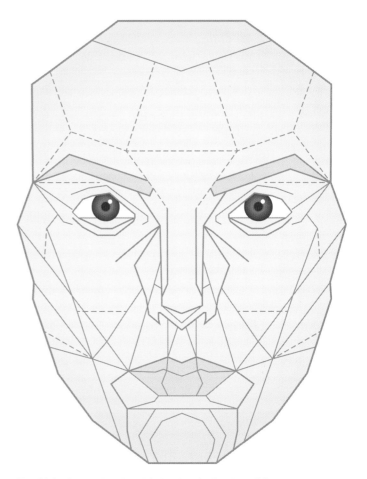

Fig. 16.2 Marquardt's phi mask is based on the "golden ratio".

applications dating back to the architecture of the Egyptians.[1] Ricketts' use of the golden divider caliper to demonstrate, e.g., the relationship between the width of the nose to mouth or the height of pupils to nasal alae and alae to chin has allowed application of the golden proportion to preoperative planning.[15] Marquardt has attempted to further objectify the concept of an aesthetic face with his development of the golden ratio phi mask *(Fig. 16.2)*. Although the validity of this concept has been supported by superimposing the mask on young, white individuals of European descent,[16] there are many limitations, as Guyuron points out,[17] in the use of two-dimensional photographs to define an attractive face.

Modern-day anthropometrics has been perhaps led by the work of Leslie Farkas. He has defined and measured countless soft tissue points and dimensions in hundreds of people of varying ethnicities and ages.[18,19] His extensive work has allowed the development of a database of normative values to which subsequent facial analyses may be compared. Perhaps of equal importance, Farkas has realized the limited application of the neoclassical canons and the golden ratio to only a select group of patients.[20,21]

With the development of three-dimensional scanning systems, a new layer of complexity has been added to facial analysis. Data points can be obtained from a variety of different technologies, including computed tomography (CT); magnetic resonance imaging (MRI); ultrasonography;[22] facial morphometry;[23] 3-D video imaging system;[24] moiré-stripe photography;[25] liquid crystal range finder system;[26] surface

scanner system, and stereophotogrammetry. The accuracy of these techniques has been tested and appears to correlate well with direct measurements. The clinical application of these systems allows not only a detailed facial analysis by the physician, but also a more realistic and conceptually tangible postoperative result for the patient.

Facial analysis

The standardization of soft tissue facial analysis and the application of the neoclassical canons relies on consistent facial landmarks *(Table 16.1, Box 16.1)*. By use of the classic two-dimensional photograph, facial proportions can be examined both vertically and horizontally.

The initial proportional analysis of the face begins with the division into halves, with the height of the vertex to endocanthion being equal to the endocanthion to gnathion height *(Fig. 16.3)*. Perhaps one of the most utilized canons is the division into thirds *(Fig. 16.4)*. The distance from the trichion to the glabella equals the distance from the glabella to subnasale, which equals the subnasale to gnathion distance. Obviously, a limitation of this technique is the position of the hairline which may change with age, most notably in the male patient. When examining the lower third, it can be further divided into thirds such that the distance from the subnasale to the stomion is one-third and the distance from the stomion to gnathion is two-thirds *(Fig. 16.5)*. The four section canon

Table 16.1 Soft tissue landmarks

Vertex (v)	The highest seen point on the head with the head in Frankfort horizontal
Trichion (tr)	The junction of the hairline and the forehead in the midline
Glabella (g)	The most prominent point of the forehead in the midline between the eyebrows
Nasion (n)	The midline point of the junction of the frontonasal suture and the superior nasal bones. Externally, nasion often corresponds to the point of greatest concavity of the nasal dorsum near a line level with the upper lid lash line
Orbitale (or)	The palpable point of the lowest margin of the inferior orbital rim
Porion (po)	The most superior point of the external auditory meatus
Frankfort horizontal (FH)	The line connecting porion and orbitale. This line is parallel to the floor for anthropometric measurements. It is an approximation of neutral head position in straight gaze
Endocanthion (en)	The point of the medial canthus where the upper and lower lids join
Pronasale (prn)	The most prominent point of the nasal tip
Subnasale (sn)	The deepest point at the junction of the base of the columella and the upper lip in the midline
Stomion (sto)	The midline point where the upper lip touches the lower lip
Sublabial (sl)	The midline point at the junction of the lower border of the cutaneous lower lip and the superior border of the chin. It is the deepest point of the labiomental groove
Pogonion (pg)	The most prominent point of the chin in the midline
Gnathion (gn)	The most inferior point of the lower border of the mandible; also called menton (me). In cephalometric analysis, gnathion and menton are two different points on the mandible

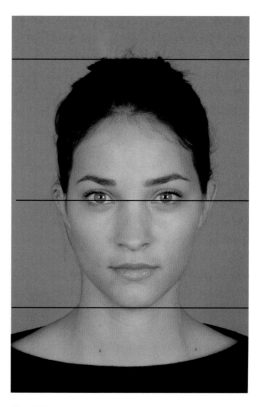

Fig. 16.3 The division of the face into halves. The height from the vertex to endocanthion is equal to the endocanthion to gnathion height.

states that the distances from vertex to trichion, trichion to glabella, glabella to subnasale, and subnasale to gnathion are all equal *(Fig. 16.6)*. Farkas examined the reliability of these relationships and found that a majority of patients deviate from these proportions.[20] The upper half of the face, especially in women is actually greater than the lower half, and the height of the nose is typically less than the upper and lower thirds. Men typically have a larger lower third due to a more prominent mandible while women tend to have more equal lower and middle thirds. Further consideration must be given to proportional variations due to ethnicity, and these differences must be respected when considering surgical changes. Further division of the face into five major aesthetic masses[27] (forehead, eyes, nose, lips, and chin) allows a more detailed analysis.

Forehead

The aesthetic forehead has a slight convexity to it, with the apex lying just above the nasion. The nasofrontal angle is formed between the inferior forehead and the nasal dorsum *(Fig. 16.7)*. In an aesthetic profile, this angle is between 125° and 135°. The forehead is the most stable unit of the face and small changes in its prominence at the supraorbital ridges can have dramatic effects on nasal length and projection. The

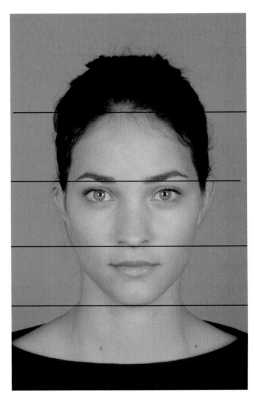

Fig. 16.4 The division of the face into thirds. The distance from the trichion to glabella equals the glabella to subnasale distance, which equals the subnasale to gnathion distance.

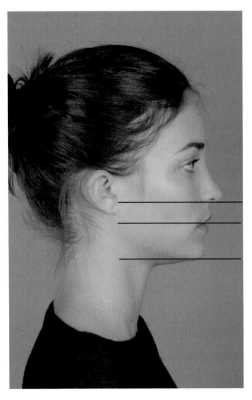

Fig. 16.5 The lower third of the face can be divided into thirds, with subnasale to stomion equal to one-third and stomion to gnathion equal to two-thirds.

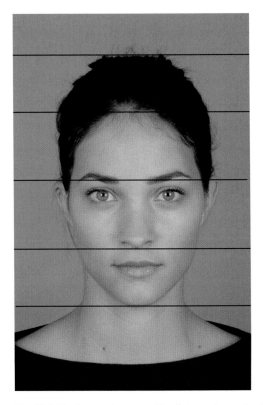

Fig. 16.6 The four section canon. The distances from vertex to trichion, trichion to glabella, glabella to subnasale, and subnasale to gnathion are equal.

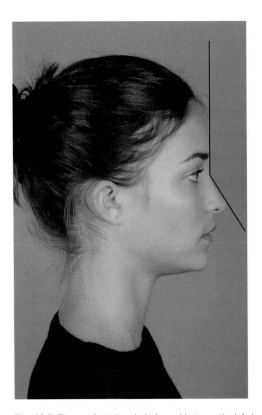

Fig. 16.7 The nasofrontal angle is formed between the inferior forehead and the nasal dorsum. This angle is between 125° and 135°.

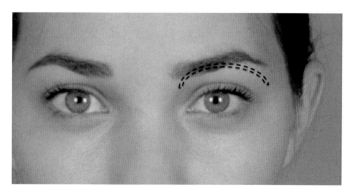

Fig. 16.8 The aesthetic eyebrow in women lies just above the supraorbital rim and the lateral brow is more elevated than the medial brow.

nasal radix depth should be tangent to the fronto-subnasal line.[28] The eyebrows should lie just above the supraorbital rim in women and have the apex of their arch above the lateral limbus. An important aesthetic feature is the lateral brow in women, which should be more elevated *(Figs 16.8, 16.9)*. In men, the eyebrows are less arched and should lie at the level of the supraorbital rim. (Eyebrow aesthetics are thoroughly reviewed in Chapter 7.)

Eyes

The shape, color, and cant of the eyes, as well as the quality of the eyelids are very important components of facial aesthetics (aesthetic issues are reviewed in Chapter 6). The width of the eye from medial to lateral canthus should equal the distance between the medial canthi. This distance is typically one-fifth of the width of the face with the most lateral fifths lying between the lateral canthus and helix *(Fig. 16.10)*. The distance from the lid margin to the supratarsal crease, which changes with ethnicity, varies between 7 and 15 mm. The upper lid should cover 1–2 mm of the superior limbus, while the lower eyelid should be at the level of the inferior limbus. A vertical line through the medial limbus should intersect with the oral commissure.

Nose

As the central and most prominent unit of the face, the nose plays a major role in facial aesthetics. Although nasal anatomy and nasal aesthetics are reviewed in Chapter 17, a few basic relationships will be discussed here. The nasofacial angle is formed by the nasal dorsum and the facial plane (defined by a line drawn from the glabella to pogonion), and ranges from 35° to 40° *(Fig. 16.11)*. The nasolabial angle formed between the columella and upper lip is between 100–103° in men and 105–108° in women *(Fig. 16.12)*. This angle is a very important component of nasal aesthetics and may be affected dramatically with changes in tip rotation or projection.

Tip projection is closely related to the nasofacial angle and can be measured in many ways. In Chapter 17, tip projection is defined as the distance from the alar base to the nasal tip; ideally 50–60% of the projection will lie anterior to a vertical line drawn over the most projecting part of the upper lip. The Byrd method suggests that tip projection should be 0.67 of nasal length. In the Goode method, a vertical line is drawn

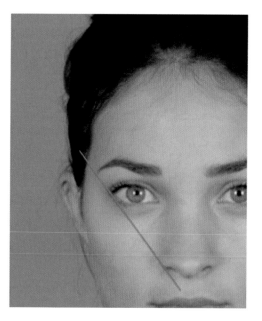

Fig. 16.9 An oblique line drawn from the alar margin through the lateral canthus should cross the lateral extent of the eyebrow.

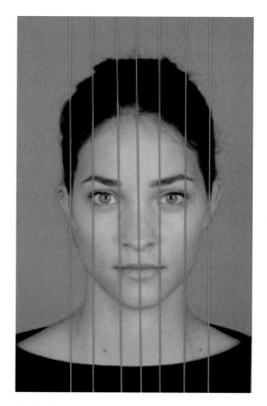

Fig. 16.10 The width of the face can be divided into fifths. The distance from the helix to lateral canthus equals the distance from the lateral canthus to medial canthus, which equals the distance between the medial canthi.

from nasion to the alar groove. The horizontal distance from ala to tip is then measured and a ratio of ala-tip:nasion-tip is typically 0.55–0.60, corresponding with a nasofacial angle of approximately 36°. The Baum method uses the nasofrontal angle as the vertical axis. A line is drawn from the nasofrontal angle vertex to the subnasale. A perpendicular horizontal line drawn to the tip should give a ratio of dorsum:tip of 2:1,

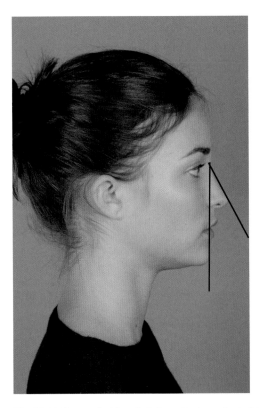

Fig. 16.11 The nasofacial angle is formed between the facial plane and the nasal dorsum. This angle is between 35° and 40°.

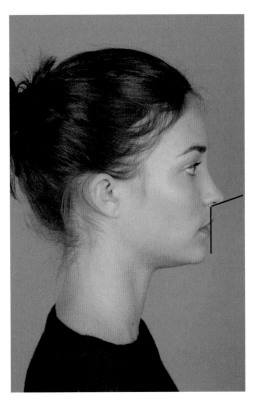

Fig. 16.12 The nasolabial angle is formed between the columella and the upper lip. This angle is between 100° and 103° in men and between 105° and 108° in women.

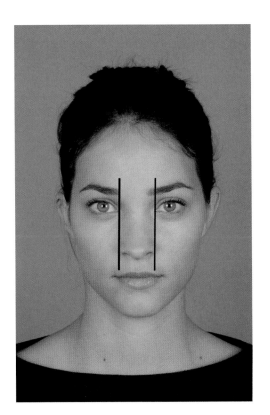

Fig. 16.13 The intercanthal distance should equal the width of the nose from ala to ala.

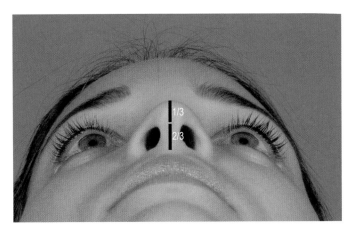

Fig. 16.14 On basilar view, the nostrils comprise two-thirds the length of the columella. The tip occupies the remaining one-third.

which corresponds to a nasofacial angle of 42°. Powell[27] suggests modifying this ratio to 2.8:1 to produce a nasofacial angle of 36°. The Simons method relates tip projection to upper lip length. The distance from the skin-vermilion junction to the base of the columella should equal the distance from the subnasale to the tip.

The ideal width of the nose at base from ala to ala should equal the intercanthal distance *(Fig. 16.13)*.[29] The nasal width:length ratio (from nasion to tip) should be approximately 0.7.[30] On basilar view, the nostrils comprise two-thirds the length of the columella and the tip occupies the remaining one-third *(Fig. 16.14)*.

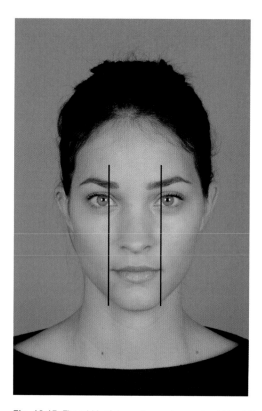

Fig. 16.15 The width of the oral commissure should be defined by a vertical line drawn from the medial limbus.

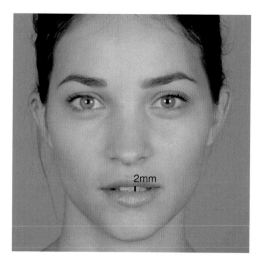

Fig. 16.16 In repose, the amount of maxillary incisal show should be 2 mm.

Lips

The upper lip extends from subnasale to stomion, while the lower lip and chin are measured from stomion to gnathion. The ratio of these distances should be 1:2. The ideal width of the oral commissure should be defined by a vertical line drawn from the medial limbus *(Fig. 16.15)*. On lateral view, the lip protrusion can be measured as the perpendicular horizontal distance from a vertical line drawn from subnasale to pogonion. The upper lip typically lies 3.5 mm from this line and should protrude over the lower lip, which typically lies 2.2 mm anterior to the line.[31] The underlying dentition has a profound impact on the fullness of the lips. In repose, the amount of maxillary incisal show should be 2 mm *(Fig. 16.16)*. In a full smile, approximately two-thirds of the crown should show. This relationship is obviously impacted significantly by surgical changes in maxillary vertical position, which will be discussed later in this chapter.

Chin

The chin is defined superiorly by the labiomental sulcus and inferiorly by the gnathion. Changes in both the vertical and horizontal positions of the chin have a significant impact on not only the appearance of the lower lip and the labiomental sulcus, but also the contour of the neck. The vertical height of the chin, as previously stated, is included with the measurement of the lower lip (stomion to gnathion), and should be twice the length of the upper lip (subnasale to stomion). It is important also to consider the horizontal dimension of the chin while analyzing the face. Chin projection can be measured by drawing a line from glabella through subnasale and another line from glabella to pogonion. This angle should be approximately 11°. Additionally, a perpendicular line drawn from Frankfort horizontal through subnasale should lie approximately 3 mm posterior to pogonion. The depth of the labiomental sulcus should be approximately 4 mm and is measured from a vertical line drawn from the inferior lip margin to the pogonion.

The mentocervical angle *(Fig. 16.17)* is measured by a vertical line drawn from the glabella to the pogonion and a horizontal line drawn from the gnathion to the cervical point (intersection of the neck and submental areas). This value ranges from 80–95° and is affected by both the position of the chin and the overlying soft tissue of the chin and neck. A more acute mentocervical angle gives a more pronounced, aesthetic jaw line *(Table 16.1, Box 16.1)*.

Cephalometrics

The planned and precisely executed surgical procedures that permit the re-arrangement of the maxillomandibular complex and tooth-bearing segments in horizontal, transverse and vertical spatial dimensions are collectively termed orthognathic surgery.

Historically, the primary purpose of these procedures was to correct the skeletal mandibular and/or maxillary jaw relationship that orthodontic movement of teeth alone could not accomplish to produce "normal" functional dental occlusion. Concomitantly, it was recognized that the surgical procedures on the underlying facial skeleton will produce nuanced as well as profound esthetic facial changes.

Abnormalities of the maxillomandibular complex may be secondary to genetic malformations, developmental malformations or acquired deformities. This chapter will focus on the more common developmental abnormalities that involve one or both jaws.

A broad classification permits recognition of the location of the facial abnormality as maxillary or mandibular (occasionally in both jaws). Those commonly occurring are maxillary hypoplasia or maxillary hyperplasia and mandibular hypoplasia (retrognathia) and mandibular hyperplasia (prognathia). In addition, growth disturbances may occur in any

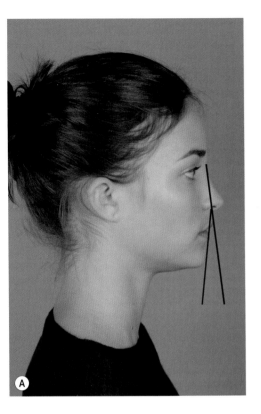

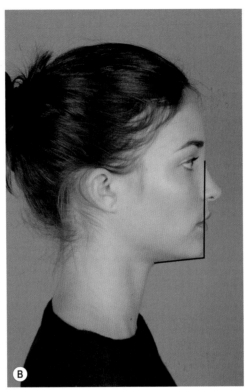

Fig. 16.17 (A) Chin projection can be measured by the angle between a line through glabella and subnasale and a line from subnasale through pogonion. This angle should equal 11°. **(B)** The mentocervical angle ranges from 80° to 95° and is formed between a line from glabella to pogonion and a line from gnathion to the cervical point.

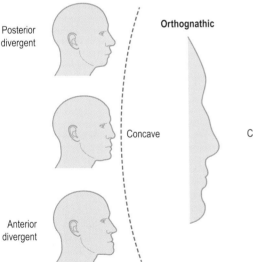

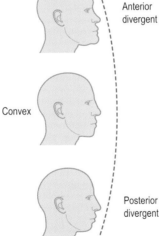

Fig. 16.18 A facial profile may be classified as convex or concave, based on the facial outline created by two lines. One line extends from the nasal bridge to the base of the upper lip, and the second line extends from that point downward to the chin. A convex facial profile denotes a skeletal class II jaw relationship and a concave facial profile denotes a class III relationship. (From Graber T, Swain B: Current Orthodontic Concepts and Techniques, 2nd ed. Philadelphia, WB Saunders, 1975.)

spatial plane (i.e., anterior posterior, horizontal, vertical, transverse).

A convex facial profile can result from an over-projecting maxilla or a mandible positioned too far posteriorly. A concave facial profile can result from a maxilla being too far posterior or a mandible that protrudes forward *(Fig. 16.18)*.

The relationship between the maxillary and mandibular dentition and occlusion was classically defined by Angle in 1899.[32] He described the position of the maxillary and mandibular first molar teeth to each other as follows:

- Class I: normal relationship of the mesial buccal cusp of the maxillary first molar fits the buccal groove of the first mandibular molar (orthognathic)

- Class II: mandibular molar posteriorly positioned relative to the upper first molar (retrognathic)
- Class III: mandibular molar anteriorly positioned relative to the upper first molar (prognathic).

The correction of the first molar position is an important guide to achieve class I jaw and dentition relationships *(Fig. 16.19)*.

Additionally, vertical jaw abnormalities may produce "open-bites" and "over-bites" and transverse abnormalities may produce buccal and lingual "cross-bites" that need to be evaluated for correction *(Fig. 16.20)*.

Although aesthetic beauty is a subjective concept, surgeons primarily use objective aids to establish a treatment plan.

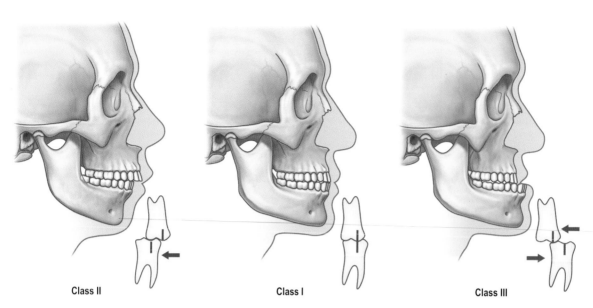

Fig. 16.19 Angle's classification may be used to describe the anterior–posterior relationship of the maxillary and mandibular dental arches. In a class I relationship, the mesial buccal cusp of the upper first molar articulates in the buccal groove of the mandibular molar. In a class II relationship, the mesial buccal cusp of the upper first molar articulates between the mandibular first molar and second premolar. In a class III relationship, the mesial buccal cusp of the upper first molar articulates between the first and second mandibular molar teeth. In a class III relationship, the mandible is said to be prognathic-more anterior when compared with the maxilla.

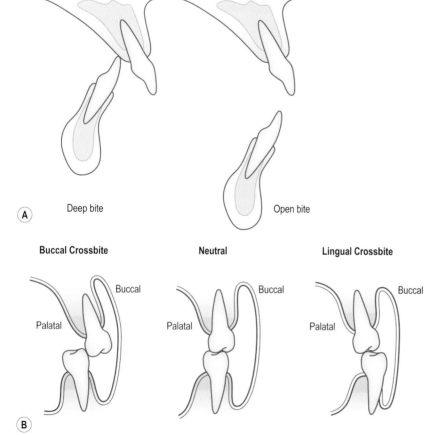

Fig. 16.20 (A) Malocclusions in the vertical plane are measured from the incisal edge of the upper central incisor to the incisal edge of the lower central incisor while the teeth are in occlusion. An anterior open bite is present when the molars are in occlusion and there is an anterior open space between upper and lower incisors. The opposite relationship is termed a deep bite. Anterior open bites usually are present in patients with excessive vertical dimension of the lower face. **(B)** Buccal and lingual crossbites. Malocclusions are classified in the transverse dimension by the position of the maxillary posterior molar cusp relationship to the mandibular molar central fossa. These relationships are either buccal, lingual, or neutral. A buccal crossbite exists when the maxillary posterior teeth are lateral to the mandibular molar teeth without contact. A lingual crossbite exists when the buccal cusps of the maxillary posterior teeth occlude with the central fossa of the mandibular posterior teeth.

Cephalometrics is one technique that helps to provide surgeons with normative values. The cephalometric concept was first introduced by Broadbent in the United States in 1934.[33,34] His research provided normative data that was applicable in the diagnosis of skeletal abnormalities. Cephalometrics requires the patient to be properly positioned with the jaws in centric relation and lips in repose. It is important to have the head parallel to the floor so Frankford Horizontal is oriented correctly. A PA cephalometric radiograph is generally only useful in assessing transverse discrepancies and/ or asymmetries; the normal cephalometric view is a lateral. By the geometric measurement of established points and

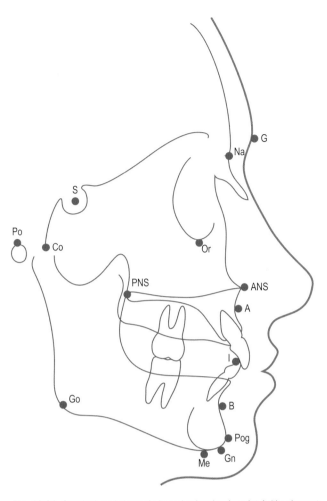

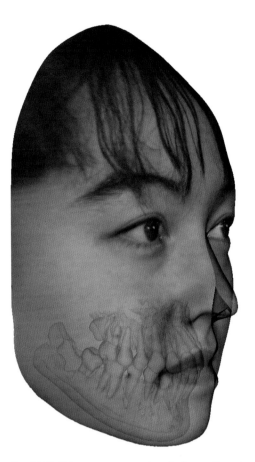

Fig. 16.22 Software programs such as Anatomage™ can be used to predict facial soft tissue outcomes in response to skeletal movement.

Fig. 16.21 Standard cephalometric bone landmarks. A, point A (the deepest midpoint on the maxillary alveolar process); ANS, anterior nasal spine; B, point B (the deepest midpoint on the mandibular alveolar process); Co, condylion; G, glabella; Gn, gnathion; Go, gonion; I, incision superius; Me, menton; Na, nasion; O, orbitale; Pog, pogonion; PNS, posterior nasal spine; Po, porion; S, sella.

landmarks, reliable analysis of the vertical and horizontal components of the facial and cranial skeleton may be made *(Fig. 16.21)*.

Efforts to correlate dental and skeletal relationships by the use of cephalometrics have resulted in different analyses by several researchers.[35,36] The Ricketts analysis[37] attempted to establish the positional relationship of the functional components of the face and jaws, taking into consideration future growth predictors. McNamara in 1983,[38] produced an analysis that combined elements of the previous works with more precise jaw and teeth relationships. However, a number of limitations of the two-dimensional cephalometrics are recognized such as:

1. Head position errors

2. Facial asymmetry may make analysis and identification of key landmarks inaccurate

3. An inability to visualize internal structures of the skull with inadequate soft tissue visualization

4. Magnification produced by the imaging

5. Inter-observer differences.[39]

Precise three-dimensional technology is available now for orthognathic surgical treatment planning. It's use in orthognathic surgery was discussed by Cutting et al in 1986,[40] and by Ono *et al*. in 1992,[41] and Cavalcanti *et al*. in 2004.[42] Several studies have also compared the accuracy of three-dimensional CT analysis with two-dimensional cephalometry.[43,44] Cone-beam CT (CBCT) makes it possible to capture the patients head in "one-pass" instead of multi-planar cytometry (MSCT). The reduction in radiation exposure with CBCT compared with MSCT is desirable.[45]

The combination of CBCT with specific application software (such as Anatomage™ and Dolphin Imaging™) allows surgeons to use visual treatment objectives (VTOs) as an aid to plan and predict surgical outcomes. VTOs are based on cephalometric radiographs independent of the analysis. This prediction tracing along with the facial analysis permits the surgeon to view the surgical plan *(Fig. 16.22)*.

Orthodontic considerations

The most successful orthognathic surgical outcomes are those in which a team approach is utilized. In most circumstances, patients have been treated by an orthodontist prior to surgical evaluation. If not, it is necessary to compare pretreatment records with the patient's existing condition. Prior to performing any surgical treatment objectives (STO) or prediction tracings, orthodontic treatment goals must be established by way of physical examination, study models, and cephalometrics.

The majority of tooth movement should occur in the pre-operative phase. The main goal is to eliminate all dental compensations so dental arches can be leveled and aligned. The following cephalometric goals should be used as ideal references:

• Position long axis of the maxillary central incisor so its final position will be 22±2° to the NA line. In the Steiner analysis, the NA line is drawn from Nasion to point A.
• The incisal tip of the maxillary central incisor should be 4 mm anterior to the NA line
• Position the long axis of the mandibular incisor so its final position will be 20±2° to the NB line. This is the same line as above except drawn from Nasion to B point.
• The mandibular incisor tip of the mandibular incisors should be 4 mm anterior to the NB line.
• Satisfy all arch length requirements.

These fundamental concepts will position the teeth within the alveolar bone and allow for ideal repositioning of the jaws. With the occlusion properly leveled and aligned, the surgeon should be able to obtain maximum intercuspation of teeth. The classical dental compensations include proclined (flared) maxillary incisors uprighting in the class II patient and excessive uprighting of the mandibular incisors in the class III patient. Apertognathia or "open-bite" occurs if these compensations occur in the vertical dimension. It is important to advise patients that their dental deformity may worsen during the orthodontic phase of treatment due to such decompensation.

Temporomandibular joint

The temporomandibular joint (TMJ), its musculature and function occupies an important consideration in the correction of jaw deformity. While most agree that orthognathic surgery has significant aesthetic implications for patients, it serves no benefit to effect aesthetic changes, only to find that the function of the joint as well as the subsequent dental occlusion has been affected adversely. It is necessary therefore, that the planning and operative correction of jaw deformities be predicated on continued normal function of the temporomandibular joint. To that end, a brief discussion of TMJ anatomy and function are appropriate.

The temporomandibular joint is a ginglymoarthrodial joint that is subtended by the action of a series of muscles about the proximal portions of the face. The muscles are in relation to both closing and opening, creating a sling that surrounds the ramus of the mandible. The masseter muscle originates in two parts from the zygomatic process of the maxilla and the lower border of the zygomatic arch and inserts on the lateral side of the ramus and angle of the mandible, coincident with the medial portion of the sling, the medial pterygoid muscle. The medial pterygoid arises from the medial surface of the lateral pterygoid plate, and inserts similarly on the angle and ramus of the mandible on its medial side. These two powerful muscles form a sling at the mandible angle that supports the mandible. During function, the mandible is elevated and the teeth are brought into occlusion.

At the same time, the fan-shaped temporalis muscle originates in the temporal fossa and inserts via tendinous attachment to the coronoid process of the mandible under the arch of the zygoma, completing the group of muscles that allow for the powerful action of closing.

It is estimated that 300 psi of force can be generated by the combined actions of these three groups of muscles acting on both sides of the face during closure. The muscles are innervated by branches of the third division of the fifth cranial nerve and function in a coordinated fashion to allow a hinge closing motion. Muscles that work to open the jaw exist in two groups, the first of which is the suprahyoid group. The anterior belly of the digastric and geniohyoid muscles originates from the hyoid bone and insert into the symphysis of the mandible. The anterior belly of the digastric originates at the hyoid bone around its tendinous insertion and inserts into the more proximal inferomedial border of the mandible. Each of these, in contraction, cause rotatory movement at the chin point with opening. Concomitantly, contraction of the lateral pterygoid muscle originating on the lateral pterygoid plate and inserting on the anterior portion of the mandibular condyle as well as the articular disc of the joint causes anterior positioning of the condylar head. This allows both hinge opening and anterior translation of the mandibular condyle.

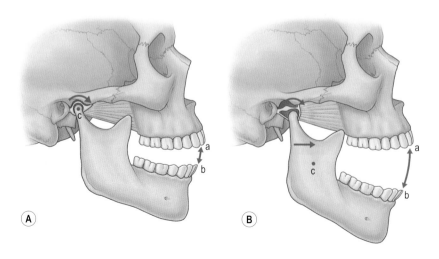

Fig. 16.23 (A) Lower joint space allows rotation. Isolated function of 2 cm (a–b). Center of rotation is center of condyle (c). **(B)** Combined translation under disk of lower joint space allows 4–5 cm opening a–b with center of rotation in the mid-ramus.

The temporomandibular joint is therefore also described as a hinge joint in a movable socket. With anterior positioning, the condylar head finds itself in a position slightly anterior to the articular eminence of the temporal bone and with closure it must reposition itself back under the eminence.

The function of the articular disc, a fibrocartilaginous cushion between the condylar head and the glenoid fossa, is an important component of the temporomandibular joint.

The disc is positioned firmly over the mandibular condylar head and lies loosely in the glenoid fossa. Its posterior attachment is fibroelastic allowing for anterior positioning with each movement. The disc's function is coordinated with the movement of the condylar head such that in opening, contraction of the lateral pterygoid, which inserts on the disc as well as the anterior portion of the condyle allows for the disc to move anteriorly with the translation of the condyle. Rotation takes place in the inferior joint space and translation in the superior joint space. This complicated mechanism can be affected in two ways: by the uncoordinated function of the muscles and by the position of the disc *(Fig. 16.23)*.

The dental opposition of the teeth (occlusion) in the maxilla and mandible has significant effect on the position of the condyle. It is obvious that any alteration in occlusal position will effect the condylar position each time the teeth are interdigitated. This usually occurs in a rather limited portion of our waking hours and other than clenching, the mandible finds itself free floating in its position, determined by the rest position of the muscles of mastication and the positioning of the condyle within the glenoid fossa under the articular disc.

Orthognathic surgical procedures

A detailed description of surgical techniques or a complete historical reiteration of the development of these procedures, will not be given here. However, for the sake of clarity, a limited exposition is necessary to appreciate how orthognathic surgical procedures developed and how they can be used to obtain aesthetics and normal jaw function. It is also necessary to emphasize that the relationship between soft tissue and hard tissue changes are carefully considered in planning, the most important of which are the maxillary lip-to-tooth relationship, the position and depth of the labiomental fold, the relationship of the anterior nasal spine to changes in the position of the nasal tip and the width of the alar base, and the effect of chin positioning on the hyoid angle. In all instances, these soft tissue parameters must be considered in planning for desirable cosmetic results.

The technique for immobilization of segments in orthognathic surgery changed remarkably with the development of rigid fixation.[46,47] Previously, when simple wire fixation was used, procedures to reposition the jaws were troubled by problems of an immediate tendency to relapse. The development of rigid fixation with the use of position plates and screws has allowed for immediate stability and quick return to function.[48] The original techniques of plate and screw fixation emphasized dynamic compression and primary bone healing; however, it is more common in orthognathic surgery to use plate positioning and position screws rather than compression screws.[49] This permits some "leeway" in segment positioning and also permits the ability to bend plates without

the precision which is required for long bone fixation. The use of plate and screw fixators has been revolutionary in orthognathic surgery; however, the clinical application of techniques has been modified so that the practical aspects of segment positioning are emphasized.

The philosophy of the authors in their general plan for correction of congenital jaw deformities, is to first correct the occlusal deformity on dental casts and then to adjust to that occlusion in the most cosmetic position for the patient. Preoperative surgery on dental models allows the surgeon to plan the osteotomies *ex-vivo*. It is necessary to accurately mount the patient's dental cast on a semi-adjustable articulator utilizing a face bow and bite registration. Model surgery allows the surgeon to fabricate an acrylic intermediate splint and final surgical splint. It is not the author's intent to outline this entire process, however, the importance of precision and accuracy during this step cannot be over-stressed. It is appropriate also to review the expected changes with the patient, and their families if underage, preoperatively. It is not the intent, necessarily, to correct to a cephalometric norm, but it is the intent to correct to a maximum aesthetic and functional position of the jaws. In general that means filling the soft tissue facial envelope to an increased volume rather than decreased volume. It has become more and more evident that increasing the hard tissue projection of the face leads to a more aesthetic facial appearance.[50,51] This is tempered by the patient's ethnicity and desires. Prediction tracings and visual treatment objectives (VTOs) are necessary aids in treatment planning *(Fig. 16.22)*. To reiterate, the position of the nasolabial angle, the proportions of the maxilla and the mandible, the labiomental fold, and the need for maintaining lip competence are of greatest importance. The aforementioned relationship of the maxillary lip to tooth and the amount of "show" of the maxillary teeth in both repose and in animation is the cardinal yardstick for success in surgery.

Orthognathic surgery is made possible because of the excellent vascular supply to the upper and lower jaws and to the teeth. It is important to note that the maxilla has a widespread vascular network from the labiobuccal mucoperiosteum and the palatal mucoperiosteum. The ability to surgically move the maxilla based on either of these blood supplies has been established with good documentation *(Fig. 16.24)*.[52,53] However, it is necessary to maintain at least one of the two vascular networks intact or a surgical disaster may occur. It should be clear that the maxillary blood supply through the palatal mucosa or through the labiobuccal mucosa is adequate for the healing of moved bone segments. This rule is especially important in the cleft lip/palate patient, who may require orthognathic manipulation of the jaws and in whom the palatal blood supply may be compromised having been previously disrupted. Special care should be taken to maintain a labiobuccal vascular curtain where compromised segments may be anticipated in this special group.[54,55]

The blood supply to the teeth is similarly found within the labiobuccal blood supply or the palatal blood supply *(Fig. 16.25)*. There are significant anastomosing vessels that enter the alveolus through the periosteum that will supply the apical vessels to the teeth and maintain their integrity. It is possible, especially with significant movement of the jaws, that sensation to the teeth and gingiva may be lost, at least temporarily, by these procedures, this may be annoying but not disastrous. It may also be emphasized that when plate and

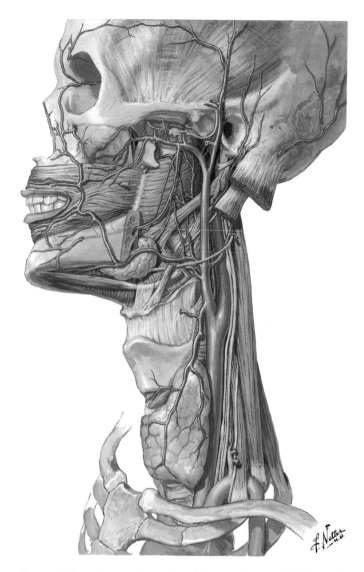

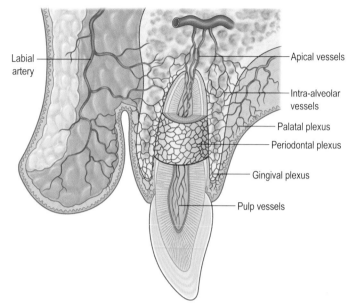

Fig. 16.25 Cross-section of a maxillary incisor associated with osseous and soft tissue. A rich plexus of vessels anastomose from the labial, apical, alveolar, periodontal and gingival which maintain the integrity of teeth.

Great care should be taken to assure appropriate long-term stability of the orthognathic result. Frequently, long-term use of orthodontic retention devices is required to assure dental stability.[48,56,57]

Mandibular osteotomies

It is appropriate to begin a discussion of orthognathic surgery with a synopsis of the types of mandibular osteotomies that are currently popular, the most useful of which, and the most frequently performed, is the sagittal split osteotomy *(Fig. 16.26)*. Historically, this procedure is advantageous to the patient because of its stability and to the surgeon because of its adaptability to clinical requirements.

The sagittal split osteotomy was developed in the mid-1950s by Trauner and Obwegeser,[58] as an intraoral procedure to divide the mandibular ramus by splitting the lateral cortical bone plate from the medial cortical bone plate. The original procedure was modified by Dal Pont[59] to bring the vertical corticotomy forward to the position of the second molar teeth. This allowed for a wider bone-on-bone contact in advancement procedures.

A secondary modification was made by Hunsuck[60] in the 1960s who proposed that the horizontal portion of the lingual osteotomy should be completed to a position only behind the mandibular lingula, because the mandible frequently becomes unicortical proximal to the lingula and splits behind that area were difficult, if not impossible, to achieve.

The resultant design of the sagittal split osteotomy as presently performed, is demonstrated in *Figure 16.26*. The procedure, done intraorally, allows separation of the lateral cortical plate of the ramus extending from the medial cortical plate of the ramus extending to the area of the second molar tooth anteriorly, from the area just superior to the lingula

screw fixators are used, the condylar position is extremely important since the fixation is "non-forgiving." If fixation is instituted when the mandibular condyle is out of position, the long term function will be adversely affected. For this reason, techniques to assure proper condylar position have been proposed. However, most techniques depend upon the operator's ability to achieve the appropriate position of the condyle prior to the fixation.

Relapse tendencies may occur as a result of the following:

1. Type of fixation
2. Condylar displacement
3. Direction of movement (clockwise vs counterclockwise)
4. Functional pull of the suprahyoid musculature
5. The inappropriate positioning of the posterior facial height.
6. Improper or insufficient presurgical orthodontic treatment also may lead to relapse.

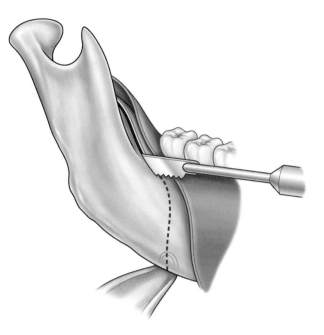

Fig. 16.26 The initial osteotomy cut can be made with a fissure bur or reciprocating saw along the medial surface of the ramus just above the mandibular foramen (lingula) extending to the posterior ascending ramus. The cut is then extending down the anterior ramus onto the superior aspect of the body of the mandible, and finally curving inferiorly along the external oblique line through the lateral cortical plate. This vertical cut is made at a 45° angle from the sagittal plane cutting only the lateral cortex and then inferior border.

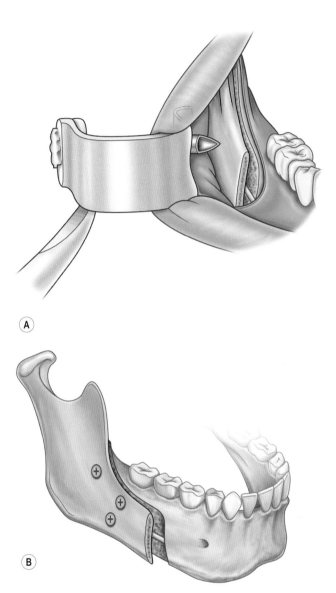

Fig. 16.27 (A) Trocar insertion to place. **(B)** Positioning screws. These screws are used to fixate the proximal and distal segments without torquing the condyle.

proximally while protecting the entrance of the inferior alveolar nerve and artery at the mandibular foramen.

Although the inferior alveolar nerve usually remains intact with the tooth-bearing segment (distal segment), it is frequently visualized and often stretched during the procedure. The primary disadvantage of the sagittal split osteotomy is that paresthesias do occur. This technically difficult procedure, however, allows for anterior positioning of the mandible to a significant degree and also permits all posterior positioning, especially if sections of the lateral cortical plate are excised.

The sagittal split technique lends itself to positional fixation with lateral screws *(Fig. 16.27)*; thus favoring immediate stability and quick return to function. Another disadvantage, beside the potential paresthesia, is the long-term instability of an elongated ramus. This is true of all procedures. Elongation of the ramus against the strong muscle memory of mastication is one of the frequently described reasons for relapse of orthognathic procedures, especially in the effort to solve an open bite. It is appropriate to mention here that removal of third molars should be 6–9 months prior to the planned sagittal split to avoid unfavorable osteotomy patterns.[61]

The vertical subcondylar osteotomy for the correction of class III malocclusion (prognathia) was developed as an extraoral procedure in the 20th century; which was later modified by Caldwell and Letterman[62] as an intraoral operation. However, relatively small proximal mandibular movements are permissible with this simple osteotomy of the mandibular ramus (from sigmoid notch to gonion). Although initially popular, the posterior movement causes displacement of the temporalis muscle insertion on the coronoid process, does not allow easy fixation of the cut bone segments with plate and screw techniques, and induces displacement of the condylar position. For these reasons the intraoral vertical subcondylar osteotomy finds less suitability in modern orthognathic surgery. Yet, it is applicable for the modest correction of prognathism in a patient willing to accept intermaxillary fixation for 4–6 weeks. A primary advantage of the technique is the ability to protect the inferior alveolar nerve. Larger retropositioning of the mandible can also be accomplished by L-osteotomy in an inverted fashion to leave the coronoid position intact. This osteotomy occasionally becomes necessary if one anticipates large posterior movements, in order to preserve the inferior alveolar nerve.

Genioplasty

Genioplasty or horizontal osteotomy of the mandible was a procedure first described by Larré in 1896. It had been modified by multiple authors since that time. The modern genioplasty, generally, is attributed to Hofer.[63] This procedure was described in the 1950s and designed as an advancement of the chin point for correction of retrogenia. The original procedure has been modified by many authors to demonstrate its usefulness in regard to both macrogenia and asymmetries. Because of advancements in bone replacement materials and bone grafting, correction of the short chin is possible. Modifications that were permitted by bone plate and screw fixation are significant *(Fig. 16.28)*. In general, the simplest genioplasty is a horizontal advancement, and the simplest technique allows wire fixators placed from the lingual cortical plate of the advanced segment to the buccal cortical plate of the proximal segment. In instances in which height is required, bone plate fixation will allow inferior positioning of the advanced distal segment. In addition, if further advancements are required, and bone contact is to be maintained, double steps for the advancement can be developed. In the correction of mandibular anterior asymmetries, sections of bone from the elongated side of the mandible can be removed allowing for a return of the chin point to the midline while the excised removed bone is used as a free graft for the short

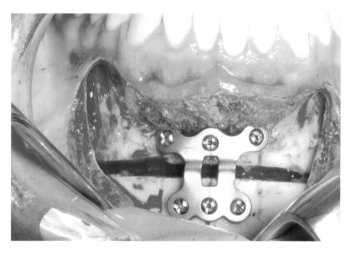

Fig. 16.28 Miniplates are used to achieve segment stability and optimum bony union.

side. Genioplasty has become the most popular of the mandibular procedures for esthetic correction of mandibular deformity. Studies indicate that these procedures may aid tongue positioning and help relieve symptoms of sleep apnea.[64] The origin of the genioglossus and geniohyoid may be advanced with the segment. However, functional results are secondary to cosmetic goals for genioplasty. Case examples are provided for illustrative purposes *(Fig. 16.29)*.

Maxillary osteotomy

The historical evolution of maxillary osteotomy *(Fig. 16.30)* was developed to allow segmental movements of the maxillary arch. However, the current maxillary osteotomy primarily involves the LeFort I procedure. It is useful to trace the development of procedures that are used to reposition the upper dental arch.

The anterior segment of the maxilla was first described as a separate osteotomy in 1921 by Cohn-Stock.[65] This procedure produced a greenstick fracture with little mobility. It was not until 1927 that Wassmund[66] described the procedure as a bipedicled repositioning of the anterior six teeth leaving both the palatal and labial blood supply intact. Later a six-tooth segment divided in the midline based on palatal blood supply was described by Cupar[67] in 1954. The procedure was further modified as a labially-based flap of anterior labial mucosa musculature and dental segments by Wünderer[68] in 1962. It is most important to understand the variety of vascular pedicles to this anterior segment, especially in consideration of patients with the cleft-lip palate deformity who may not be candidates for repositioning of anterior segments based on palatal blood supply alone. The anterior segment's mobility, and the ability to widen the arch between the canines allows for greater flexibility in the repositioning of the anterior maxilla in order to develop normal occlusal patterns. The maxilla and its posterior segments, usually taken as tooth segments from proximal of the canine to the second molar, was first proposed and done by Wassmund[66] in 1927. This procedure was described as a bipedicled-flap, one designed to close an anterior open bite,

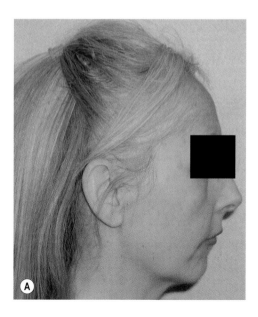

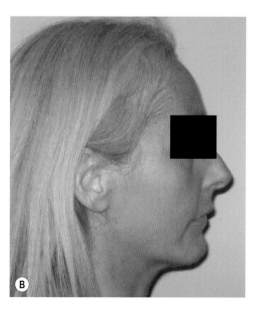

Fig. 16.29 (A,B) Profile photographs of a patient who underwent advancement genioplasty.

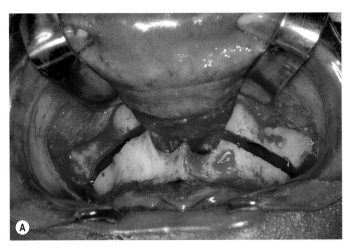

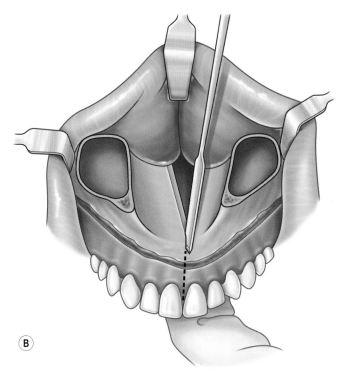

Fig. 16.30 (A) LeFort I osteotomy cut begins along the piriform aperture superior to canine root and then tapers inferiorly below the zygomatic buttress ending at the junction of the maxillary tuberosity and pterygoid plates. **(B)** Once the maxilla is mobilized it can be moved in all directions or segmentalized into multiple pieces.

The LeFort I osteotomy has become the most commonly preferred maxillary procedure *(Fig. 16.30)*.

It finds wide applicability to both advancement and intrusion of the dental arch to allow shortening of a long face, but also allows the elongation of the mid face, to correct a short face. In such instances interpositional grafting may be necessary.

The modern LeFort I osteotomy was investigated experimentally and initiated by Bell[52] in 1969 who described the palatal blood supply as being adequate in regard to the support of the entire segment. The ability to downfracture the entire maxilla was followed by the demonstration that segmental procedures on the maxilla could also be accomplished after initial downfracture. Once again, admonition must be given in regard to the care of the cleft and/or the trauma patients who may have compromised the palatal blood supply because of previous surgery. The total maxillary osteotomy reported as a combined anterior segmental and posterior segmental procedure has been largely abandoned because it was necessary to strip the palatal mucosa to accommodate the intrusion.

The maxillary osteotomy has been effective in the treatment of dysmorphia of the face with disparity between the soft tissues and the bony skeleton *(Box 16.2)*.

The "long face syndrome" is a common dentofacial abnormality. There are cardinal signs, which lead to the diagnosis and should result in a subsequent treatment plan.

The long face syndrome is characterized in radiographs by increased bone height found over the apices of the maxillary teeth *(Fig. 16.31)*.

The palatal vault is found to be high on physical examination. There is generally increased exposure of the maxillary incisors, especially in animation with significant amounts of gingiva visible. The lips are often incompetent in closure; therefore requiring excessive mentalis and circumoral muscle strain necessary for competence. There is a relative backward rotation of the mandible and a secondary retrogenia in occlusion. The cephalometric analysis will demonstrate an increased mandibular plane to SN angle, and the overall length of the face will be long in the lower face and long in the total face. There is considerable disparity between the bony skeleton and the ability of the facial soft tissues to cover that skeleton the vertical dimension.

The short face syndrome is characterized by many opposite findings. There is generally intrusion of the maxillary incisor teeth with little incisal "show", and a decreased dimension of the upper facial height and decreased total facial height on

seeking to obviate the issue of autorotation of the mandible. As we will demonstrate, this will become more important in regard to the treatment of the long face syndrome. In 1942, the procedure was described in two stages by Schuchardt,[69] and modified in 1965 by Obwegeser[70] to demonstrate that a palatal pedicle was adequate for blood supply for the posterior segment along with an anterior labial pedicle. In 1967, Hogeman and Wilmer[71] described the palatal pedicle alone, and in 1975, the procedure was further modified as a segmental portion of the LeFort I downfracture. To reiterate, the repositioning of the posterior segment allowed flattening of the dental arch to achieve a more normal occlusion, and permitted either widening of the arch or autorotation of the mandible.

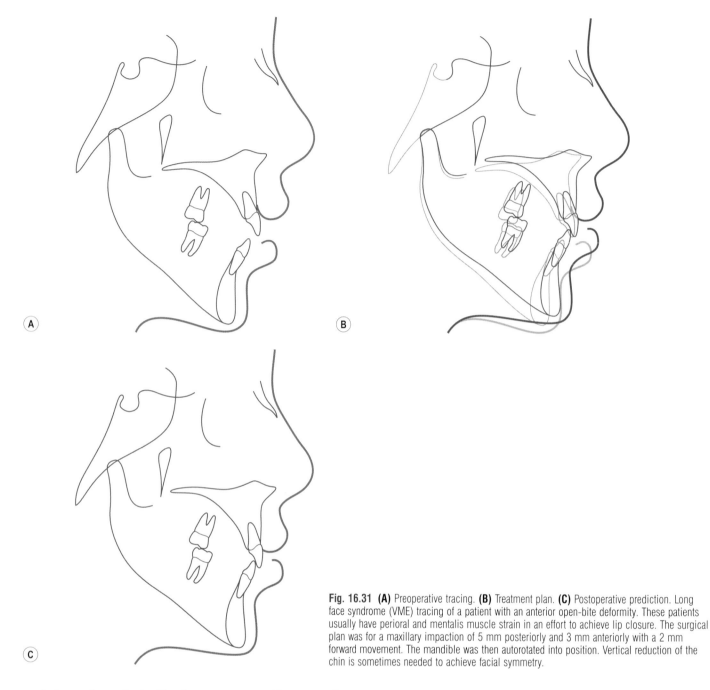

Fig. 16.31 (A) Preoperative tracing. **(B)** Treatment plan. **(C)** Postoperative prediction. Long face syndrome (VME) tracing of a patient with an anterior open-bite deformity. These patients usually have perioral and mentalis muscle strain in an effort to achieve lip closure. The surgical plan was for a maxillary impaction of 5 mm posteriorly and 3 mm anteriorly with a 2 mm forward movement. The mandible was then autorotated into position. Vertical reduction of the chin is sometimes needed to achieve facial symmetry.

cephalometric analysis. The free-way space, if measured, is found to be increased and the palatal arch is flattened. The classic short-faced patient is illustrated by the repaired cleft lip palate with limited maxillary growth, both in the horizontal and vertical dimension, causing overclosure of the mandible and pseudoprognathism. In general, corrections are designed to recreate an adequate facial profile and fill the facial soft tissue dimensions to their appropriate position Combined osteotomies show versatility for the correction of almost any dentofacial deformity.

Postoperative care

Following surgery, patients frequently experience pain, nausea and swelling. Peak swelling usually occurs between the 3rd and 4th days after surgery and resolves by the fourth postoperative week. During surgery and the first postoperative day, the patient should receive intravenous steroids to help decrease swelling. NG tube suction prior to extubation is recommended as well as antiemetics to help reduce postoperative nausea and vomiting. Immediately after surgery, the patient's head position should be in the semi-Fowler position with ice packs placed to both sides to further limit swelling for 48–72 h. Preoperative antibiotics are frequently administered prior to incision and then continued for two hospital days. After discharge, oral antibiotics may be used for 5–7 days. Patients should be instructed to use a mouth rinse and soft toothbrush. This is especially important if the patient is wearing a surgical splint. Mouth rinses can be started immediately postoperatively. The patients should be instructed to avoid heavy brushing against the incision areas for the first week. A liquid diet for the first 48 h followed by a soft diet may be beneficial for the first 2 weeks. Initial bone healing in young patients who are in rigid fixation is usually completed within four weeks. During this time period, patients should not participate in contact sports or strenuous physical activity. Other factors may also affect healing, e.g., medical conditions, smoking, poor nutrition or clenching. Outpatient follow-up should be routinely performed on week 1, 3, and 6. The resumption of active orthodontic movement should not begin until the 6th postoperative week. Follow-up care should continue at 3 months, 6 months, and 1 year intervals. A lateral cephalometric film and panographic radiograph should be used to evaluate skeletal stability. Clinical photographs should be taken during all visits and then final photographs after orthodontic bands are removed.

Complications

Neurosensory loss

Neurosensory loss is the most common complication following orthognathic surgery. It may occur when either maxillary or mandibular procedures are performed. In mandibular procedures the third division of the trigeminal nerve may be injured during soft tissue retraction, transected during BSSRO osteotomies, stretched or torn during fixation of bone segments, or impaled by fixation screws. Clinical evaluations of patients postoperatively have revealed sensory disturbances in more than 80% of the patients undergoing BSSRO.[72] The lower lip is most frequently affected and sensory loss may persist for more than a year in 4–20% of patients.[73] If the inferior alveolar nerve is transected, it should be mobilized and repaired immediately to increase the chance for nerve regeneration. Special care should be taken when performing osteotomy cuts, and drilling should be accompanied copious irrigation to prevent heat injury. Documentation of anticipated neurosensory deficits at the time of injury should be carefully noted.

During maxillary osteotomies, injuries can occur to the infraorbital division. Traction injuries to the infraorbital nerve at the foramen are possible and symptoms are usually transient. Temporary palatal anesthesia should be anticipated at the time of maxillary procedures. Paresthesia or anesthesia generally recovers spontaneously but may be permanent depending upon the extent of the osteotomy and the nature of the bone cuts.

Unfavorable aesthetic outcomes

Repositioning and reattachment of the tissues of the upper lip and nose during closure of LeFort I osteotomy notoriously is associated with widening of the alar base. In order to maintain nasal aesthetics, the alar base is sutured in conjunction with a V-Y closure and is used to prevent flaring and thinning of the upper lip. Changes in the skeleton are reflected favorably or unfavorably by the overlying soft tissues; thus orthognathic surgery is a basic form of aesthetic surgery.[74] Careful preoperative facial analysis of both hard and soft tissues will

maximize favorable aesthetic outcomes. As previously stated, "relapse" tendencies may occur because of the type of fixation, the position of the condyle, the direction of movement (clockwise or counter clockwise), the strength of the pull of the suprahyoid musculature and inappropriate elongation of the posterior facial height exceeding the resting length of the muscles of mastication. If relapse occurs, it should be documented on both cephalograms and by postoperative models. Follow-up is recommended to evaluate patient's long-term occlusal relationships.

Hemorrhage

The incidence of major intraoperative hemorrhage has decreased over the years principally because of advances in surgical technique and use of the hypotensive anesthetic protocols (mean systolic blood pressures of 65 mmHg). Hypotensive anesthesia coupled with injection of local anesthetic with vasoconstrictor minimizes blood loss and increases visualization of the operative field. In a LeFort I procedure, properly positioning the osteotome in an anterior and inferior direction when separating the pterygomaxillary junction should decrease the risk of injury to the descending palatine vessel. It is important to inform patients that they may experience periodic nasal bleeding, which can usually be controlled by direct pressure or packing. It is also highly important to explain preoperatively, that blood transfusion may be required, and that if autotransfusion is desirable the blood should be drawn and banked.

Dental complications

Dental and periodontal complications may usually be avoided with proper incision design, accurate osteotomies and an in-depth understanding of dental anatomy. The risks of such complications escalate when segmental interdental osteotomies are performed. If an injury should occur to a tooth or tooth apex, endodontic therapy may be necessary. Good preoperative orthodontic preparation helps limit these risks.

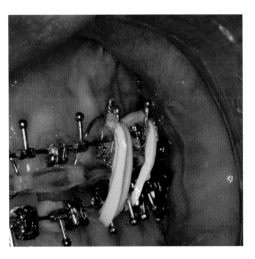

Fig. 16.32 Avascular necrosis of the left posterior maxilla after segmental LeFort I surgery in three pieces with interdental osteotomies.

Avascular necrosis

Avascular necrosis of the condyle is a known potential complication. The cause is thought to be secondary to either trauma or disruption of the blood supply when multiple osteotomies or combined temporomandibular joint surgery is performed. Therefore, caution should be taken to avoid compromise of blood supply to this area. This is an iatrogenic problem and caused by excessive stripping of mucosa from osteotomized segments. These technical difficulties can be limited with careful preoperative planning and execution *(Fig. 16.32)*. Infection is rare in orthognathic procedures and usually is associated with poor vascular supply to segments.

 Access the complete references list online at **http://www.expertconsult.com**

8. Broadbent BH. The face of the normal child. *Angle Orthod.* 1937;7:183.

9. Broadbent BH, Broadbent BH, Golden WH. *Bolton standards of dentofacial developmental growth.* St Louis: Mosby; 1975.

11. Ricketts RM. Esthetics, environment, and the law of lip relation. *Am J Orthod.* 1968;54:272.

16. Bashour M. An objective system for measuring facial attractiveness. *Plast Reconstr Surg.* 2006;118:757.

    The "phi mask" is presented as a mathematical model to assess facial attractiveness. Validating this approach may lead to standardized assessment of facial aesthetic harmony.

20. Farkas LG, Hreczko TA, Kolar JC, et al. Vertical and horizontal proportions of the face in young adult North American Caucasians: Revision of neoclassical canons. *Plast Reconstr Surg.* 1985;75:328.

    Conventional ideals of facial proportion were assessed with reference to 153 North American Caucasians 6, 12, or 18 years of age. These standards were not found to be consistent with average facial proportions in this cohort.

38. McNamara JA Jr. A method of cephalometric analysis. In: *Clinical alteration of the growing face. Monograph 12, Craniofacial growth series.* Ann Arbor: University of Michigan, Center for Human Growth and Development; 1983.

50. Rosen HM. Facial skeletal expansion: treatment strategies and rationale. *Plast Reconstr Surg.* 1992;89:798.

    This report stresses the importance of considering patient-specific aesthetic assessment in planning facial reconstruction.

54. Posnick JC, Thompson B. Modification of the maxillary LeFort 1 osteotomy in cleft – orthognathic surgery: the bilateral cleft lip and palate deformity. *J Oral Maxillofac Surg.* 1993;51:2.

    Techniques to improve outcomes of LeFort I osteotomies in patients with bilateral cleft lip and palate are presented. Outcomes ranging from relapse to persistent fistulas are addressed.

70. Obwegeser HL. Surgical correction of small or retrodisplaced maxillae: the "dish-face" deformity. *Plast Reconstr Surg.* 1969;43:351.

72. Bagheri SC, Meyer RA, Khan HA, et al. Microsurgical repair of the peripheral trigeminal nerve after mandibular sagittal split ramus osteotomy. *J Oral Maxillofac Surg.* 2010;68(11):2770–2782.

    An algorithm for the management of inferior alveolar nerve and lingual nerve injury during sagittal split ramus osteotomy is presented, and clinical outcomes are assessed.

17

Nasal analysis and anatomy

Joel E. Pessa and Rod J. Rohrich

SYNOPSIS

- Surgery begins with a careful preoperative analysis utilizing standardized measurements.
- All tissues including bone, cartilage and soft tissue may contribute to any one measurement, e.g., nasal length.
- Nasal anatomy is considered within the context of facial shape, facial proportions, and the size and shape of adjacent structures.
- Knowledge of nasal anatomy facilitates the use of an algorithmic approach to surgery that increases the predictability of surgery.
- A knowledge of blood supply increases the safety of the open approach to rhinoplasty.
- Any rhinoplastic problem can be analyzed by the component structures and their relationship to one another.

Introduction

A thorough understanding of nasal anatomy enables the practitioner to accurately perform reconstructive and aesthetic rhinoplasty.[1] Nasal surgery is recognized as one of the most difficult procedures in plastic surgery, and accomplishing predicable results is a challenging task for the surgeon. Rhinoplastic surgery can be approached with these points in mind.

A discussion of nasal anatomy begins with a description of the terms commonly used. These terms are the language that describes nasal anatomy, shape, and form.

Surgery begins with a careful preoperative analysis utilizing standardized measurements. One must accurately describe the deformity in order to establish an operative goal. Less than hoped for results often occur as a direct result of failure to recognize one or more features prior to surgery.[2]

All tissues including bone, cartilage and soft tissue may contribute to any one measurement, e.g., nasal length. This is the main reason that understanding nasal anatomy is so critical to the performance of successful rhinoplasty surgery. Any rhinoplastic problem can be analyzed by individual components and their relationship to one another.[3]

Nasal anatomy is considered within the context of facial shape, facial proportions, and the size and shape of adjacent structures.[4] The size and position of the chin, facial width, and facial height, are examples of factors that may influence the operative goal.

A basic knowledge of blood supply increases the safety of the open approach to rhinoplasty. This information is also important to avoid injury to the angular artery during external percutaneous osteotomy, and to avoid inadvertent intravascular injections.[5]

Knowledge of nasal anatomy combined with the ability to preoperatively analyze the nose facilitates the use of an algorithmic approach to surgery that increases the predictability of surgery.

The nose is described employing a standardized terminology (*Fig. 17.1*). These terms allow standardized measurements to be defined (*Fig. 17.2*).

The nasolabial angle gives an approximation of tip rotation relative to the Frankfort Horizontal plane, drawn through the external auditory canal to the orbital rim. The nasofrontal angle is defined from the glabella to radix to nasal tip. Normative values exist for these measurements and vary according to gender (*Fig. 17.3*).

The normative values for tip projection, the distance from the alar crease to the nasal tip, is calculated in three ways, and described later in the text. The tip defining points seen on anterior view are located where the lateral crurae begin to diverge.

The crurae themselves consist of three sections or parts, each with its own curvature. The pyriform aperture, best visualized on basal view, corresponds with the bony aperture of the maxilla along the inferior nasal passage (*Fig. 17.4*).

The algorithm for preoperative assessment follows that previously described.[1] The relationship of the nose to the face is first analyzed. The nose is thus considered in the context of overall facial proportions for precise analysis. A simple technique for understanding facial proportions is using the fractal

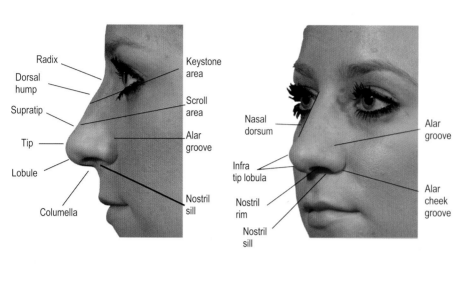

Radix
Dorsal hump
Supratip
Tip
Lobule
Columella

Keystone area
Scroll area
Alar groove
Nostril sill

Nasal dorsum
Infra tip lobula
Nostril rim
Nostril sill

Alar groove
Alar cheek groove

Fig. 17.1 Standardized terminology of external nasal landmarks exists that facilitates a discussion of proportionate and disproportionate nasal aesthetics. These landmarks, essentially reference points of nasal topography, often relate directly to the shape and relationship of underlying structures.

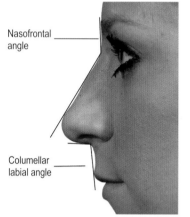

Nasofrontal angle
Columellar labial angle

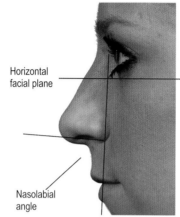

Horizontal facial plane
Nasolabial angle

Fig. 17.2 Angular measurements assess multiple factors such as nasal length, alar base position, and lip aesthetics.

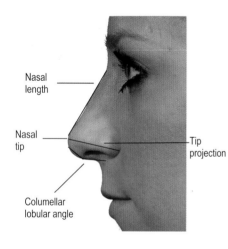

Nasal length
Nasal tip
Columellar lobular angle

Tip projection

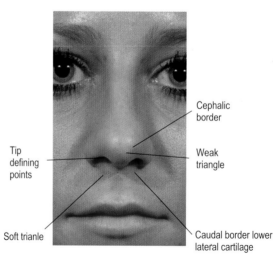

Tip defining points
Soft trianle

Cephalic border
Weak triangle
Caudal border lower lateral cartilage

Fig. 17.3 Tip projection, a critical measurement in preoperative analysis, is defined as the maximal distance from alar base to the nasal tip.

technique of thirds: the upper, middle, and lower face vertical heights are considered to be equal thirds. The lower face is the distance from the alar base to the chin (menton). This is further divided into thirds with the distance from the alar base to lip crease (stomion) being one-third of this height.

Frontal view allows nasal length to be analyzed relative to lower facial proportions. One measurement suggests that the

distance from radix to tip defining points is equal to the distance from stomion to menton. *(Fig. 17.5)*

The nose is viewed from the frontal view *(Fig. 17.6)*. A line drawn from the glabella, radix through the middle lip and chin helps to assess nasal deviation. The vertical line drawn from the radix to the midline lip and chin analyzes several structures. It helps to determine septal deviation, the position

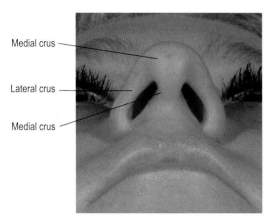

Medial crus

Lateral crus

Medial crus

Fig. 17.4 The lower lateral cartilages, comprising the lower third nasal vault, have three defined segments. These segments are determined by where the lower lateral cartilages display marked changes in curvature.

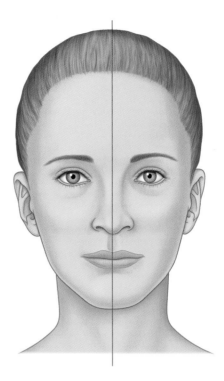

Fig. 17.6 A line drawn from midline glabella to menton helps to assess nasal symmetry. This simple method is one of the best means to analyze septal deviation and the position of the nasal bones. It also emphasizes asymmetries of the maxilla or mandible.

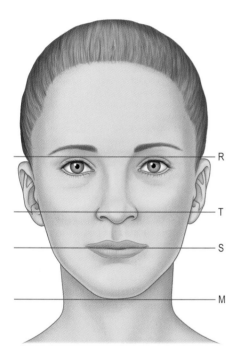

R

T

S

M

Fig. 17.5 General guidelines exist to assess nasal aesthetics in relation to the rest of the face. One guideline suggests that nasal length is equal to lower facial height. M, menton; R, radix; S, stomium; T, tip.

of the nasal bones and upper vault, and points out asymmetries of the lower lateral cartilages.[6]

The dorsal aesthetic lines are determined by a line drawn from the medial brow to the tip defining points, and should be two gently diverging curves. These can be judged relative to vertical lines drawn from the medial brows through the lateral nostril *(Fig. 17.7)*.

The distance between the alar bases is approximately equal to intercanthal width. Alar shape is analyzed on frontal view and has a gull wing shaped curve, defined by the curvature of the lateral and middle crurae *(Figs 17.8, 17.9)*.

The lateral view is then reviewed. As with the frontal view, the nose is analyzed in the context of position and facial proportions *(Fig. 17.10)*.

On lateral view, the alar base should lie slightly anterior to the medial canthus. The upper lip is slightly anterior to the lower lip; the lower lip slightly anterior to the chin. This analysis can reveal micro or macrogenia, as well as skeletal disharmonies including maxillary retrusion with a retro displaced alar base.

The nose itself is analyzed in lateral view beginning with the position and depth of the nasal root at the nasofrontal angle (radix). The radix lies at a point between the lash line and supratarsal crease with the eyes in horizontal gaze. The depth of the radix, or the nasion-medial canthal distance is approximately 15 mm.

Radix is an important point that helps to define the nasofrontal angle defined as the angle formed by the frontal bone, and a line drawn parallel to the nasal bone. If the nasofrontal angle is positioned more anteriorly or superiorly than normal, the nose appears elongated, and the tip projection will appear less, while if the nasofrontal angle is more posterior and inferior than normal, the nose will look shorter, and the tip will appear to project more. The radix forms the cephalic end for the measurement of nasal length, which is the distance from the radix to the nasal tip. Normally, nasal length is equal to the distance from stomion to menton *(Fig. 17.11)*.

The nasal dorsum is then analyzed. The nasal dorsum lies slightly behind a line drawn from the radix to the nasal tip, more so in females than in males. The supratip break occurs cephalad to the tip defining points, and 2–3 mm behind the

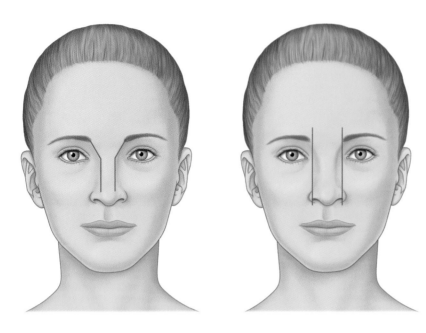

Fig. 17.7 The dorsal aesthetic lines should be a gentle curve from brow to tip.

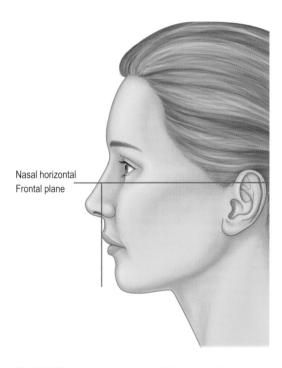

Nasal horizontal
Frontal plane

Fig. 17.8 For measurements, especially angular values to be reproducible, head position is standardized. Here the Frankfort horizontal is shown: the line from the external auditory canal to the orbital rim is parallel to the horizon.

line from radix to nasal tip in women *(Fig. 17.12)*. A slightly lower value is more desirable in males.

The nasolabial is then assessed. It is formed by a line drawn through the anterior and posterior ends of the nostril and the vertical facial plane. The nasolabial angle is usually 95–100° in females, and 90–95° in males *(Fig. 17.13)*. This is slightly different than the columellar-labial angle which is formed by the columella and the upper lip, an angle which is often influenced by a prominent caudal septum which gives the impression of increased tip rotation despite a normal nasolabial angle.

Another determinant of tip rotation is the columellar-lobular angle, formed at the junction of the columella and the infratip lobule and represents the junction between the middle and medial crura. The ideal columellar lobular angle is 30–45° in females.

The relationship between the ala and columella is assessed. A line drawn through the long axis of the nostril should bisect the oval formed by the nostril in lateral view *(Fig. 17.14)*. A greater distance below the long axis may indicate a hanging columella, and a greater distance above the long axis may indicate retracted ala. This issue is reviewed more thoroughly in Chapter 18.

Tip projection is then assessed. Tip projection is defined as the distance from alar base to the nasal tip *(Fig. 17.13)*. If 50–60% of the tip lies anterior to the vertical line adjacent to the most projecting part of the upper lip, tip projection is considered normal. If it is >60%, the tip may be overprojecting. Inadequate tip projection is suggested by a value <50%.

Similar to the rule of thirds used to evaluate the nasal proportions relative to the overall face, tip projection is 0.67 of total nasal length as measured from radix to tip defining points. If the ratio is <0.67 there is inadequate tip projection.

Basal view provides information regarding alar shape, tip projection, and alar width. The base of the columella and alar

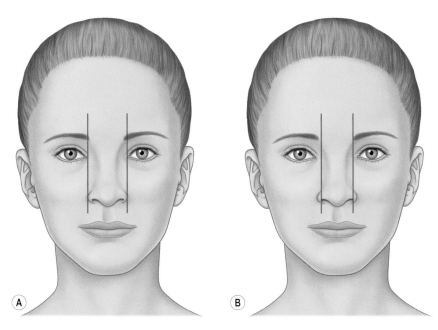

Fig. 17.9 The width of the bony base relative to the alar base is then assessed. **(A)** The bony base width should be 80% of the normal alar base width. **(B)** A normal alar base width is equal to the intercanthal distance or the width of one eye.

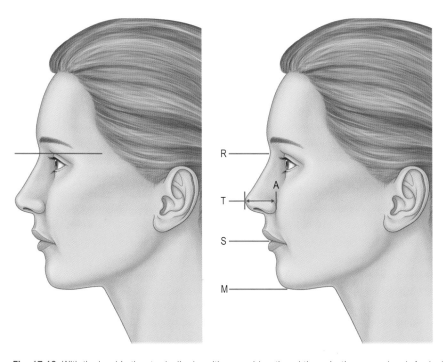

Fig. 17.10 With the head in the standardized position, nasal length and tip projection are analyzed. A, alar base; M, menton; R, radix; S, stomium; T, tip.

rims should form an equilateral triangle *(Fig. 17.14)*. The infratip lobule is one-third of the distance from alar base to tip. The alar base view also visualizes alar base width and flaring. The alar rims on basal view should have a flare of 2 mm. Any asymmetries in alar shape are noted. This analysis provides the information necessary to formulate a detailed operative plan including the techniques required to meet the surgical goals.

The technical maneuvers of open rhinoplasty are facilitated by an understanding of the details of nasal anatomy. Blood supply to the nasal tip is the one anatomical point of overwhelming significance that has contributed most to the safety of open rhinoplasty. Understanding the vascular supply of the nose, and how to preserve its intricate network, enhances the safety of the open approach in not only primary rhinoplasties, but secondary and tertiary procedures as well.

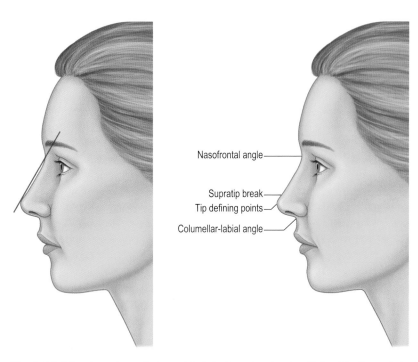

Fig. 17.11 A line drawn from radix to nasal tip helps to analyze dorsal aesthetics. The dorsum is located behind this line, and the steepest curve occurs just cephalad to the nasal tip. This supratip break is determined by the relationship between tip projection and septal and upper lateral (middle vault) height.

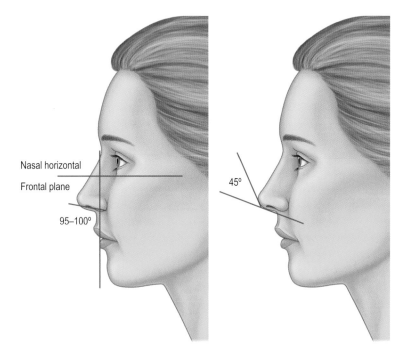

Fig. 17.12 The nasolabial angle is shown on the left and the columellar lobular angle is shown on the right. While less discussed, it is important to remember that the nasolabial angle is determined by alar base position as well as tip projection and nasal length. Maxillary deficiency has a tremendous effect in determining the nasolabial angle. The columellar lobular angle is determined by fewer variables: it simply represents the transition from medial to middle crura.

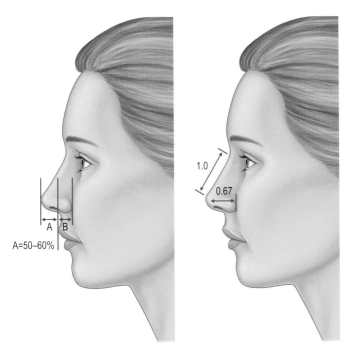

Fig. 17.13 Tip projection can be analyzed by three techniques, either relative to the nostril or relative to nasal length. Here, two methods are shown.

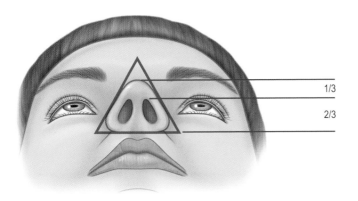

Fig. 17.14 Tip projection is determined here relative to nostril position. In addition, basal view should reveal the nose as an equilateral triangle.

Blood supply

The extensive collateral blood supply of the nose makes the open approach a safe procedure. Local flaps and wide undermining are possible because the multiple vessels supplying the nasal tip. Latex injection gives some indication of the degree of collateralization encountered during rhinoplasty. Both a branch of the internal carotid, the supratrochlear, and a branch from the external carotid, the facial artery, give rise to branches that cross the midline. These form a vascular network that crosses the dorsum.

The supratrochlear branch gives rise to lateral nasal, descending external nasal, and angular vessels *(Fig. 17.15)*. The supratrochlear artery gives rise to the angular vessel, and the lateral nasal and external nasal arteries *(Fig. 17.16)*. These course directly below the dermis, superficial to the intrinsic nasal muscles.

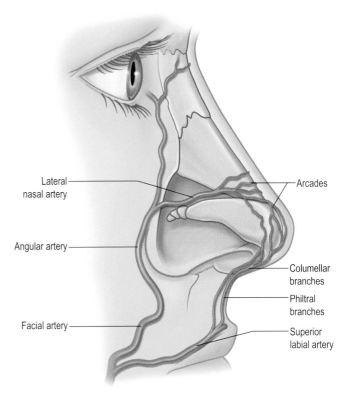

Fig. 17.15 Vascular supply to the nose. This is derived from branches of the ophthalmic and facial arteries.

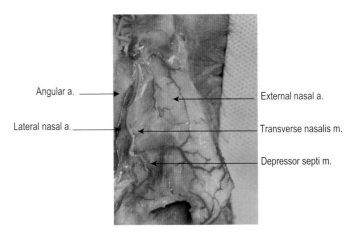

Fig. 17.16 The blood supply to the nose arises from both the internal and external carotid arteries. a., artery; m., muscle.

The facial artery travels superiorly to connect with the angular vessel. Along the way, inferior to the nose, it gives rise to the superior labial artery.

The sill artery is a small branch that arises from the superior labial artery *(Fig. 17.17)*. The superior labial also gives rise to the philtral arteries, these providing the main contribution to the ascending columellar arteries.

The columellar artery is transected during the external nasal approach, but this has little effect because of the multiple branches that perfuse the region of the nasal dome. There likewise exist multiple arcades, which arise from both the supratrochlear as well as the facial arteries. The arcades are transected during surgery that removes any part of the ala.

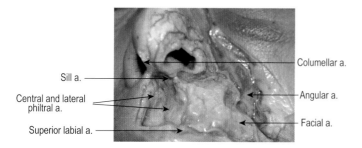

Fig. 17.17 All major nasal arterial branches lie above the muscles and nasal fascia. Dissection deep to this plane spares collateral blood supply during the open rhinoplasty technique. a., artery.

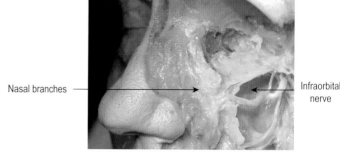

Fig. 17.18 The infraorbital nerve travels through its canal and exits through the foramen to supply much of the lateral nose and tip. Supratrochlear and ethmoidal branches supply the superior nasal skin.

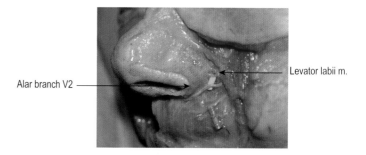

Fig. 17.19 Clinically, nerve block at the alar base leads to anesthesia of the nasal alae, side walls and tip. A dense confluence of branches from V2 is found at this location. m., muscle.

Again, extensive collateralization protects the remaining medial and lateral areas of the nose.

Two points are suggested by this anatomy. The first is that dissection in the correct plane preserves the blood supply, even in compromised nasal tips. The safety of the external approach in secondary procedures is increased by dissection directly above perichondrium. This way, the delicate subdermal plexus is spared further trauma that could compromise blood supply. The second point is that the arteries of the nasal vasculature are significant and should be cauterized if cut. This must be done with care because imprecise cauterization can injure adjacent vessels. One can draw an analogy of the blood supply of the nose to that of any other aperture on the face. The eye, nose, and mouth are each protected by a dual blood supply that travels circumferentially around each aperture. In the case of the eyelid, the facial and supratrochlear give rise to the marginal arteries; the facial and angular contribute to the superior and inferior labial vessels, and the supratrochlear and facial arteries provide blood supply to the skin around each nostril. In each instance, these blood vessels are directly beneath dermis.

It is during subdermal dissection, as may occur during excessive defatting of a nasal tip, that the delicate blood supply is at risk and may result in skin necrosis. The lateral nasal artery is one of the main sources of blood supply to the nose; this vessel is at risk during wide lateral skin undermining.

The venous drainage of the nose consists mainly of vessels anastomosing with the facial vein, either through veins traveling from the dorsum and lateral nasal wall, or via vessels accompanying the philtral and superior labial vessels.

Nerve supply

The main sensory nerves to the nose are branches of the infraorbital nerve and the external nasal nerve, both of which are terminal branches of the trigeminal nerve.

The infraorbital nerve, exiting the foramen rotundum and coursing through the maxillary sinus in its own canal, exits the maxilla through the infraorbital foramen (*Fig. 17.18*). This foramen generally lies 10–12 mm below the orbital rim, although there is significant variation depending on factors including the age of the individual. There are multiple branches of this nerve, and these provide sensation to the alar base, upper lip, and lateral nasal wall. The dense confluence of sensory branches of V2 at the alar base makes local

anesthesia possible with subdermal infiltration. Infiltration at the alar base is an ideal point with which to anesthetize the nasal tip (*Fig. 17.19*).

An important consideration is that the alar and sill arteries are located in direct contact with the sensory branches of the infraorbital nerve at this location, and requires care during infiltration to prevent bleeding or intra-arterial injection. Another approach to local block of the infraorbital nerve includes direct infiltration at or within the foramen.

The second main sensory nerve supply to the nose is via the external nasal branch of the V1. This arises from the anterior ethmoidal branch of the frontal nerve, and exits through a small foramen in the mid-portion of the nasal bone. The placement of local anesthetic at this location and at the alar base will result in near complete anesthesia of the nasal skin.

Intrinsic and extrinsic nasal musculature

The intrinsic muscles of the nose are the nasalis and its lower portion, which is known as the dilator naris or as the levator alae. The external muscles of the nose are the procerus, the orbiculars, the depressor septi and the levator labii alaeque nasi. The importance of the nasal muscles if frequently understated. They are important for animation, but intrinsic muscles are also important to maintain a patent nasal airway.

The transverse part of the nasalis muscle inserts into the edge of the upper lateral cartilage (*Fig. 17.20*). Contraction

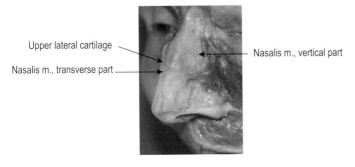

Upper lateral cartilage

Nasalis m., transverse part

Nasalis m., vertical part

Fig. 17.20 Nasal muscles can be intrinsic or extrinsic. Both are important as a dynamic means of providing nasal airway patency. Airflow can be diminished by inadvertent injury to these muscles, especially the transverse nasalis; middle vault disturbances are common in Bell's palsy. m., muscle.

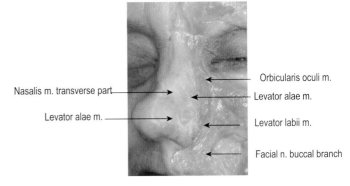

Nasalis m. transverse part

Levator alae m.

Orbicularis oculi m.

Levator alae m.

Levator labii m.

Facial n. buccal branch

Fig. 17.21 As seen in this dissection, nasal muscles may run together and intertwine. This is important physiologically, as contraction of groups of muscles usually occurs rather than contraction of one isolated muscle. Flaring of the nostrils to increase nasal airflow is accomplished by contraction of the levator alae, transverse nasalis, and orbicularis oris muscles. m., muscle; n., nerve.

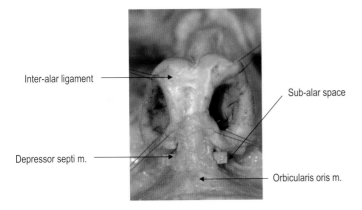

Inter-alar ligament

Sub-alar space

Depressor septi m.

Orbicularis oris m.

Fig. 17.22 The depressor septi muscle, beneath orbicularis oris muscle, may cause the transverse upper lip crease. This muscle insert into the caudal septum. m., muscle.

of this muscle splays the upper lateral cartilage, increasing nasal airflow. A front view emphasizes the relationship of the transverse part of the nasalis muscle to the upper lateral cartilage.

Two muscles control the position of the alar rim. The small levator alae and the levator labii muscles flare the nostril rim with contraction. Moreover, tonic contraction of these muscles contributes to patency of the external nasal valve. One sees a loss of function of these muscles with facial nerve paralysis that results in collapse of the external nasal valve. Similarly, the internal nasal valve is compromised by loss of function of the transverse part of the nasalis muscle. The origin and insertion of each of these muscles determines their contribution to nasal airflow. Another situation that may result in diminished nasal airflow is ablation of the alar rim, with loss of the elevator alae muscle.

Both the thickness of alar skin and tonic contraction of this small, fine muscle are important in maintaining alar rim shape and position. Cartilage grafts provide static support to substitute for loss of these muscles from any cause.

There is some debate whether the levator labii is separate from the levator alae; hence the frequent name levator labii alaeque nasi. However, careful dissection shows that these muscles are distinct *(Fig. 17.21)*. The levator alae muscle originates at the upper maxilla along the nasal bone. The levator labii muscle (m.) arises from along the orbital rim, and lies beneath orbicularis oris muscle.

The levator alae m. elevates the ala and increases the area of the external valve, as well as serving as a muscle of expression. The levator labii muscle primarily elevates the lip during smiling and increases oral aperture size. The levator anguli m. described in the section on facial muscles, is termed the caninus: however, this is a misnomer, at least from a functional point of view. It is the levator labii m. that exposes the canine, whereas the levator anguli m. controls vertical commissure position.

The depressor septi has its origin at the caudal septum. Its insertion is the orbicularis muscle of the upper lip, and is part of the lip elevator complex *(Fig. 17.22)*. The presence of the depressor septi muscle is occasionally accompanied by a transverse upper lip crease in some individuals. Denervation of this muscle will diminish this crease, albeit at the expense of increasing central upper lip height.

The intrinsic and extrinsic nasal muscles are interrelated such that they usually contract as units of two or more muscles. Therefore, the term "muscle of expression" is not entirely accurate, since one muscle may be expressive and functional as is the case of the levator alae muscle. Muscles are also part of static support nasal position; such is the case with the alar rim and alar base. Inadvertent injury to an intrinsic muscle, such as the transverse part of the nasalis, may de-stabilize the upper lateral cartilages and contribute to decreased nasal airflow.

Nasal ligaments

Ligaments are another part of static support.[7] There are fibrous connections between the upper portion of the lateral crura and the lower portion of the upper lateral cartilage. Fibrous connections also stabilize the medial crura to the distal septum. Dorsally, the alar domes are interconnected by a superficial ligament in the superficial fascia and by the inter-alar ligament proper, often referred to as Pitanguy's ligament *(Figs 17.23, 17.24)*. The inter-alar ligament stabilizes the lower lateral cartilages at the level of the medial–middle crura junction. Its disruption can lead to widening and distortion of the nasal tip. For this reason, one can see why interdomal sutures are necessary after open rhinoplasty, where there these structures are frequently divided.

While muscles and ligaments are important for nasal support, dissections demonstrate that the alar base position is stable with all soft tissue removed (sub-alar space). Usually, sub-muscular fat lies in this space. However, with all the adipose tissue and muscles removed, the alae are still stable in their anterior posterior position. This one point stresses the importance of the nasal septum in providing support for the entire nose.

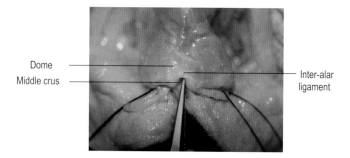

Fig. 17.23 Ligaments, as condensations of deep fascia, exist throughout the nose. These ligaments are released during rhinoplasty, highlighting the importance of knowing their anatomic location as well as the importance of reconstructing them with the various suturing techniques.

Nasal bones, cartilages and septum

The upper third of the nose is a bony pyramid formed by the nasal bones and the frontal process of the maxilla. This constitutes the upper nasal vault *(Fig. 17.25)*.

The paired upper lateral cartilages form the middle third of the nose. They are triangular in shape and attach to the nasal bones cranially and to the nasal septum dorsally. At their most superior extent, they are overlapped by the nasal bones for 4–5 mm in the so-called "keystone area", normally the widest part of the nasal dorsum *(Fig. 17.26)*.

The importance of the relationship of the upper lateral cartilages to the nasal septum is that an "I-beam" structure is formed *(Fig. 17.27)*. This provides stability for the middle third of the nose, so that collapse and subsequent airway constriction does not occur.[8] At the same time, lateral motion of the upper lateral cartilages can occur, with contraction of the transverse part of the nasalis muscle. Functionally, this attachment of the upper lateral cartilages to the nasal dorsum is the framework of the internal nasal valve *(Fig. 17.28)*.

The anatomical relationship between the septum and upper lateral cartilages *(Fig. 17.29)* explains why removing upper lateral cartilage, or over zealous septal trimming, can result in airway collapse.[9] If this occurs, recreating the "I-beam" construction with a spreader graft restores patency of the internal nasal valve. This will be covered in Chapters 18, 19 and 20.

The upper lateral cartilages are not in contact with the maxillary bone. However, at the pyriform rim, these cartilages are held in place by a membrane that encompasses them as well as the edge of the nasal bone and lower lateral cartilage.

The lower third of the nose is defined by the lower lateral cartilages, which have three components: a medial, middle, and lateral crura *(Fig. 17.30)*. The upper portion of the lateral crura interconnect with the upper lateral cartilages at the so-called "scroll area".

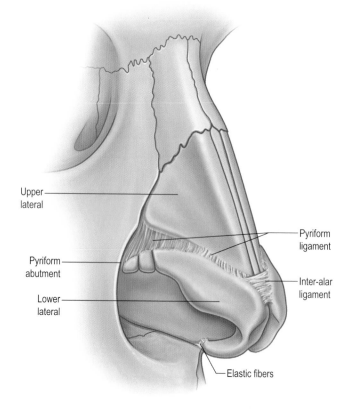

Fig. 17.24 Cartilaginous framework. The cartilages are connected to each other, the upper lateral cartilages and the septum by fibrous tissue and ligaments.

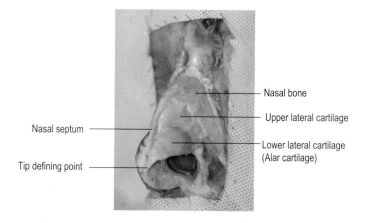

Fig. 17.25 The three nasal vaults: upper, middle, and lower, are shown with their corresponding anatomical structures. The upper vault is formed by the nasal bones, the middle vault by the upper lateral cartilages, and the lower vault by the lower lateral cartilages. Upper lateral cartilage lies deep to both the nasal bone and lower lateral cartilage.

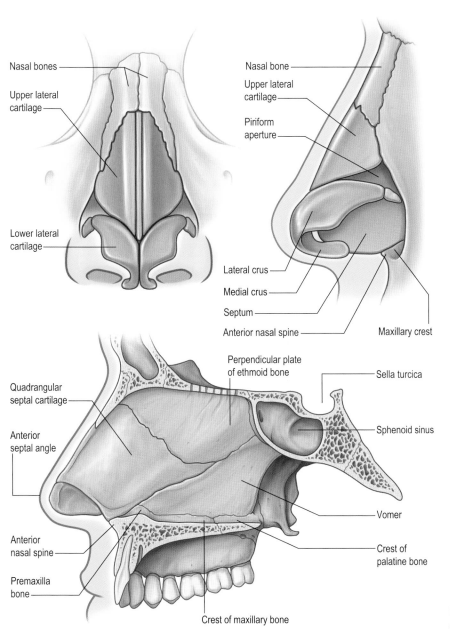

Fig. 17.26 Diagrams of the cartilaginous and bony nose and septum.

The lower lateral cartilages lie in a more prominent position than the upper lateral cartilages. Consequently, they have a greater impact on surface anatomy, with their upper border defining the nasal dome and the most anterior portion determining the tip defining points *(Fig. 17.25)*. Functionally, the lower lateral cartilages support the external nasal valve *(Fig. 17.28)*.

The edges of the lower lateral cartilages are visible when there is little subcutaneous tissue, enabling one to assess the anatomy before surgery. The lower lateral cartilages do not lie parallel to the alar rim, but rather angle along an oblique path towards the maxillary bone. The amount of angulation contributes significantly to subtle differences in the external shape of the nasal tip angulation along an axis toward the lateral canthus of the eye is considered normal, whereas a more cephalic orientation with angulation toward the medial canthus contributes to the so-called "parentheses deformity".

The pyriform ligament is a fibrous membrane that encases the nasal cartilages *(Fig. 17.31)*. As such, the cartilages can function as a unit, each adding stability to the other.[10] In this way, the inferior (caudal) border of the upper lateral cartilage stabilizes the lower lateral cartilage.

The nasal septum is the principle support structure for the nose. It is comprised of hyaline cartilage and bone; a cross-section reveals the varying thickness and translucency of these regions. The junction of the anterior septum with the caudal border is defined as the septal angle *(Figs 17.32, 17.33)*.

The mucosa overlying the perichondrium of the septum is highly vascularized, and receives its blood supply from primarily from the labial, sphenopalatine and ethmoidal arteries

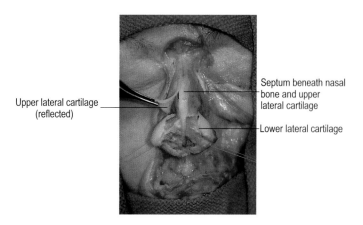

Fig. 17.27 Upper lateral cartilage constitutes the middle nasal vault. Transverse nasalis inserts onto the edge of upper lateral cartilage such that muscular contraction enables increased nasal airflow. Either disruption of the relationship of the upper lateral cartilage to the septum, or paralysis of the nasal musculature, can lead to diminished middle vault patency.

(Fig. 17.34). The dense area of vascularity in the anterior septum is referred to as Kiesselbach's area, and is a likely area of epistaxis.

If one stays in the subperichondrial plane during septal dissection, there is less chance of significant bleeding.

The principle intranasal structures are the superior, middle and inferior turbinates, which are essentially bony structures covered by thickened mucosa. The mucosa removes particulate matter, warms and humidifies the incoming air, and regulates airflow by undergoing a normal cycle of expansion and contraction *(Fig. 17.35).*

The turbinates are likewise highly vascular. The inferior turbinate has the greatest impact on airway resistance and therefore, it is commonly reduced in size in order to improve nasal airflow. It is important clinically to understand that vessel diameter increases in the posterior turbinate, and that posterior resection can therefore risk significant bleeding. Submucosal dissection, and removal of bone alone, is another

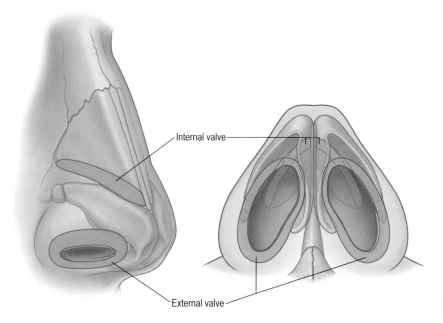

Fig. 17.28 Cartilaginous framework showing the location of internal and external valves.

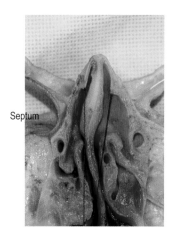

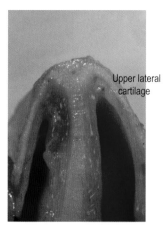

Fig. 17.29 The critical relationship of septum to the upper lateral cartilage can not be stressed enough. This "T" configuration of cartilage to septum prevents middle vault collapse. The narrowed middle vault after rhinoplasty is pathognomic of disruption of this critical anatomy.

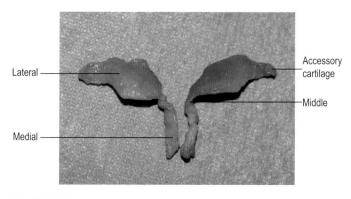

Fig. 17.30 The lower lateral cartilages, along with skin, subcutaneous tissue, and the diminutive elevator alae muscle constitute the external nasal valve. Their height, width, shape, and contour determine the aesthetics of the nasal tip.

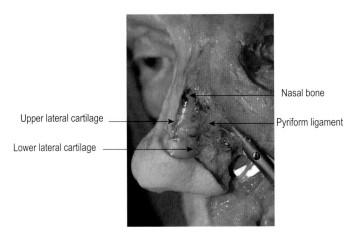

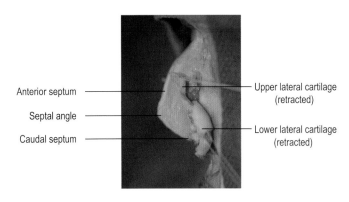

Fig. 17.31 Cartilages are attached to bone, nasal and maxillary, to increase their stability. The pyriform membrane is one mechanism that exists to stabilize these cartilages to the pyriform rim.

Fig. 17.32 The dorsal and caudal septum is noted, their junction occurring at the septal angle.

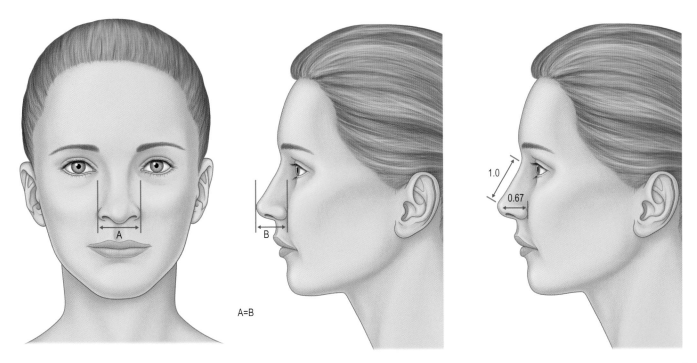

Fig. 17.33 Other methods for assessing tip projection. **(A)** A second method the authors use to help access tip projection is by comparing it to the alar base width – they should be equal. **(B)** When comparing the ratio of the nasal length (radix-to-tip, RT) to the tip projection (alar base-to-tip), the ideal tip projection is 0.67 × RT.

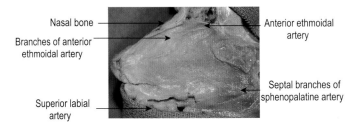

Fig. 17.34 The nasal septum consists of cartilage, attached to nasal bone, maxilla, vomer, and ethmoid. It is highly vascularized, having multiple blood supplies. Septum is the key support structure of the nose, with cartilages and ligaments attached and suspended from it. This cross-section also shows the proximity of the sphenoid sinus, and superiorly located cribriform plate, to the posterior ethmoid bone. Removing ethmoid bone with a twisting motion can inadvertently damage either of these structures.

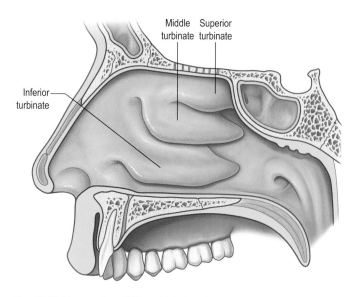

Inferior turbinate

Middle turbinate

Superior turbinate

Fig. 17.35 The superior, middle and inferior turbinates.

practical method of avoiding bleeding during turbinate resection.

The nose is thus created by a number of structures built upon the scaffold of maxillary and frontal bone. Its three-dimensional structure is able to be analyzed with knowledge of these structures, and their relationship to one another.

References

1. Menick FJ. Nasal reconstruction. *Plast Reconstr Surg.* 2010;125:138e–150e.

   An excellent overall review article of nasal anatomy and physiology.

2. Courtiss EH, Goldwyn RM. The effects of nasal surgery on airflow. *Plast Reconstr Surg.* 1983;72:9–21.

   This clinical paper describes the four anatomical structures that determine nasal airflow, important for approaching any patient who presents with the complaint of nasal obstruction.

3. Han SK, Lee DG, Kim JB, et al. An anatomic study of the nasal tip supporting structures. *Ann Plast Surg.* 2004;52:134–139.

   The authors describe the micro and macroscopic anatomy of the supporting structures of the nasal tip and the relevance of this anatomy to nasal tip surgery.

4. Sheen JH. Spreader graft: a method of reconstructing the roof of the mid nasal vault following rhinoplasty. *Plast Reconstr Surg.* 1984;73:230–239.

   The classic paper that details the anatomy of the middle nasal vault, crucial for prevention of mid-vault collapse after rhinoplasty.

5. Rohrich RJ, Muzaffar AR, Gunter JP. Nasal tip blood supply: confirming the safety of the transcolumellar incision in rhinoplasty. *Plast Reconstr Surg.* 2000;106: 1640–1641.

   The arterial blood supply to the nasal tip is discussed. This anatomical study is important with the emergence of open rhinoplasty technique as a preferred method for rhinoplastic surgery.

6. Constantian MB. The boxy nasal tip, the ball tip, the alar cartilage malposition variations on a theme – a study in 200 consecutive primary and secondary rhinoplasty patients. *Plast Reconstr Surg.* 2005;116: 268–281.

7. Rohrich RJ, Hoxworth RE, Thornton JF, et al. The pyriform ligament. *Plast Reconstr Surg.* 2008;121: 277–281.

8. Byrd HS, Salomon J, Flood J. Correction of the crooked nose. *Plast Reconstr Surg.* 1998;102:2148–2157.

9. Rohrich RJ, Muzaffar AR, Janis JE. Component dorsal hump reduction: the importance of maintaining dorsal aesthetic lines in rhinoplasty. *Plast Reconstr Surg.* 2004; 114:1298–1308.

10. Pitanguy I. Surgical importance of a dermatocartilaginous ligament in bulbous noses. *Plast Reconstr Surg.* 1965;36:247–253.

18

Open technique rhinoplasty

Rod J. Rohrich and Jamil Ahmad

SYNOPSIS

- Accurate preoperative analysis and clinical diagnosis set the foundation for successful primary open rhinoplasty.
- Open rhinoplasty allows anatomic exposure, identification, and correction of nasal deformities.
- Component dorsal hump reduction allows accurate and incremental reduction of the nasal dorsum while preventing problems with internal valve collapse or dorsal irregularities.
- Nasal tip suturing techniques allow control of definition without damaging the osseocartilaginous framework and compromising support.
- Knowledge of the normal course of recovery and potential complications is key to managing patient expectations in the postoperative period.

Access the Historical Perspective section online at
http://www.expertconsult.com

Introduction

Rhinoplasty remains one of the most commonly performed aesthetic surgical procedures in plastic surgery, with over 279 000 performed in 2008.[1] The trend over the past 20 years in modern rhinoplasty has shifted away from ablative techniques involving reduction of the osseocartilaginous framework to conserving the native anatomy with cartilage sparing, augmentation of deficient areas, and suture techniques to correct contour deformities and restore structural support.[2] Emphasis on preoperative analysis and clinical diagnosis, refinements in techniques, and the popularization of the open approach in rhinoplasty *(Table 18.1)*[3] have advanced the understanding of nasal anatomy and nasal surgery, leading to more predictable and consistent aesthetic and functional outcomes.

Success in primary rhinoplasty is predicated on comprehensive perioperative care of the rhinoplasty patient. Accurate preoperative analysis and clinical diagnosis, identification of both the patient's expectations and the surgeon's goals, and a thorough review of the plan of care and expected postoperative recovery will form the foundation for a successful experience for both patient and surgeon. Intraoperatively, adequate anatomic exposure of the nasal deformity, preservation and restoration of the normal anatomy, correction of the deformity using incremental control, maintenance and restoration of the nasal airway, and recognition of the dynamic interplays between the composite of maneuvers lead to excellence in execution. Finally, care and reassurance during postoperative recovery will lead to increased patient satisfaction.

Basic science/disease process

A thorough knowledge of nasal anatomy and understanding of nasal airflow and physiology are the foundations for successful aesthetic and functional rhinoplasty. Nasal anatomy is covered in detail in Chapter 17 and nasal airflow and physiology are covered in depth in Chapter 20. Deformities of the external and internal nose can be congenital or acquired, and may be secondary to soft-tissue and/or osseocartilaginous abnormalities, leading to aesthetic and/or functional consequences.

Diagnosis/patient presentation

Consultation

The initial consultation for rhinoplasty serves as an opportunity for the surgeon to obtain the patient's nasal history and perform an anatomic examination. In addition, the surgeon should solicit the expectations of the patient. If the patient is a suitable candidate for rhinoplasty, informed consent should

Table 18.1 Advantages and disadvantages of the open approach

Advantages	Disadvantages
Binocular visualization	External nasal incision (transcolumellar scar)
Evaluation of complete deformity without distortion	Prolonged operative time
Precise diagnosis and correction of deformities	Protracted nasal tip edema
Allows use of both hands	Columellar incision separation
More options with original tissues and cartilage grafts	Delayed wound healing
Direct control of bleeding with electrocautery	
Suture stabilization of grafts (invisible and visible)	

Table 18.2 External nasal analysis

Frontal view	
Facial proportions	
Skin type/quality	Fitzpatrick type, thin or thick, sebaceous
Symmetry and nasal deviation	Midline, C-, reverse C-, S- or S-shaped deviation
Bony vault	Narrow or wide, asymmetrical, short or long nasal bones
Midvault	Narrow or wide, collapse, inverted-V deformity
Dorsal aesthetic lines	Straight, symmetrical or asymmetrical, well or ill defined, narrow or wide
Nasal tip	Ideal/bulbous/boxy/pinched, supratip, tip defining points, infratip lobule
Alar rims	Gull-shaped, facets, notching, retraction
Alar base	Width
Upper lip	Long or short, dynamic depressor septi muscles, upper lip crease
Lateral view	
Nasofrontal angle	Acute or obtuse, high or low radix
Nasal length	Long or short
Dorsum	Smooth, hump, scooped out
Supratip	Break, fullness, pollybeak
Tip projection	Over- or underprojected
Tip rotation	Over- or underrotated
Alar–columellar relationship	Hanging or retracted alae, hanging or retracted columella
Periapical hypoplasia	Maxillary or soft-tissue deficiency
Lip–chin relationship	Normal, deficient
Basal view	
Nasal projection	Over- or underprojected, columellar–lobular ratio
Nostril	Symmetrical or asymmetrical, long or short
Columella	Septal tilt, flaring of medial crura
Alar base	Width
Alar flaring	

be obtained and preoperative instructions are given along with a general overview of postoperative care. Each patient should receive an information sheet containing the information shown in *Figure 18.1*. ✍ FIG 18.1 APPEARS ONLINE ONLY

Nasal history

During the nasal history, the surgeon should obtain information on the patient's medical and emotional suitability to undergo rhinoplasty. In addition to reviewing the patient's past medical history, the patient should be asked specifically about a history of allergic disorders, including hayfever and asthma, and other problems, including vasomotor rhinitis and sinusitis.[16] These conditions should be well controlled prior to rhinoplasty. However, exacerbations of these conditions may occur in the postoperative period and may persist for several weeks to months; the patient should be informed about this before surgery. Nasal obstruction is usually found in patients with a long history of allergic rhinitis secondary to inferior turbinate hypertrophy.[17] Engorgement of the inferior turbinates causes these symptoms to be worse at night. The patient may also complain of headache because of the inadequacy of the inferior turbinate to warm inspired air. Prior nasal trauma and surgeries, including rhinoplasty, septal reconstruction/septoplasty and sinus surgery, should be noted. Smoking, alcohol consumption, and use of illicit drugs, in particular cocaine, can compromise outcomes. Medications including acetylsalicylic acid, nonsteroidal anti-inflammatory drugs, fish oil, and certain herbal supplements may cause increased risk of bleeding[18] and postoperative ecchymosis.

As with other aesthetic procedures, assessment of the emotional stability of the patient is critical when evaluating the patient seeking rhinoplasty.[19–21] Motivating factors should be identified and the surgeon must differentiate between healthy and unhealthy reasons for seeking rhinoplasty. Feelings of inadequacy, immaturity, family conflicts, divorce, and other major life changes may be unhealthy motivating factors behind the patient seeking aesthetic surgery. Poor postoperative patient satisfaction is often based on emotional dissatisfaction as opposed to technical failure, and this can be avoided by the preoperative identification of these unhealthy motivating factors.[18]

Anatomic examination

Anatomic examination includes both external nasal analysis *(Table 18.2)* and internal nasal exam *(Table 18.3)*. In addition, facial analysis plays a key role in achieving facial harmony after rhinoplasty.[22] External nasal examination provides information about the underlying osseocartilaginous framework. Nasal skin is typically thinner and more mobile superiorly and thicker around the nasal tip.[23,24] Skin is thinnest over the osseocartilaginous junction and thickest over the nasion and supratip area. Nasal skin characteristics such as thick

Table 18.3 Internal nasal exam

External valve	Collapse
Internal valve	Narrowing, collapse
Mucosa	Edema, irritation
Inferior turbinates	Hypertrophy
Septum	Deviation, tilt, spurs, perforation, cartilage
Masses	Polyps, tumors

sebaceous or thin skin will influence the outcome and recovery following rhinoplasty. Patients with thick nasal skin are prone to prolonged postoperative edema and scar formation requiring a longer recovery. More dramatic intraoperative manipulation of the osseocartilaginous framework is required in patients with thick nasal skin while subtle changes will be visible in patients with thin skin. Systematic nasal analysis is important to identify deformities, evaluate anatomical relationships, and establish goals for surgery. This is covered in depth in Chapter 17.

Prior to performing internal nasal examination, external evaluation of the nasal airway should be performed. In particular, collapse of the external nasal valve on deep inspiration and a Cottle test should be performed. Internal nasal examination is aided with the use of a nasal speculum. If mucosal edema is present, the use of oxymetazoline nasal spray facilitates mucosal constriction. Internal valve narrowing or collapse with inspiration should be noted. Inferior turbinate hypertrophy, which typically occurs on the side opposite septal deviation, should be noted. Septal deformities including deviation, tilt, spurs and perforations are identified. The quality and the quantity of available septal cartilage are assessed as this is the primary source of autogenous graft material. To assess for the presence of septal cartilage, a cotton-tipped applicator is inserted into one nostril and pressed against the septal mucosa. A nasal speculum is inserted into the opposite nostril and if the cotton tip applicator is visible through the translucent septal mucosa, then the septal cartilage is absent. The presence of nasal polyps or tumors may require further investigation and treatment.

Imaging

Standardized photography is obtained for every patient presenting for rhinoplasty and includes frontal, lateral, oblique, and basal views of the patient.[25] These are a critical component of the medical record for preoperative planning and evaluation of postoperative results. It is useful to review photographs with the patient to identify areas of concern that can be addressed with surgery and deformities that may persist after surgery, including notches, grooves, and irregularities. In addition, facial disproportions and asymmetries should be pointed out to the patient as these may require orthognathic surgery to address.

Expectations

Identifying the patient's expectations preoperatively is a key component to postoperative patient satisfaction and successful rhinoplasty. The patient should list specific concerns about his or her nasal appearance and/or function. Common concerns include asymmetry, tip deformities, dorsum irregularities, and nasal airway obstruction. The patient should attempt to rank these concerns in order of importance. Taking all of this into account, the surgeon has to determine if the patient's expectations are realistic and can be met adequately. Most patients have realistic expectations for surgery and can understand the limitations of rhinoplasty with adequate discussion and review of photographs with the surgeon. Reviewing photographs with the patient allows patients to appreciate different views of their face and nose which can help them identify specific areas of concern for the surgeon to address. A patient who focuses on minor or uncorrectable problems or who has unrealistic expectations despite extensive discussion will likely be disappointed following surgery regardless of the aesthetic improvement; it is better to avoid operating on these patients.

Informed consent

Prior to surgery, informed consent should be obtained following discussion about the surgery, alternative treatments, and disclosure of risks. The patient should be made aware of the possibility of additional surgery in the event of a complication or the need for revisionary surgery and his or her financial responsibilities if this situation were to arise.[18]

Patient selection

After completion of a detailed nasal history and anatomic examination, and the patient's concerns and expectations have been discussed, the surgeon can decide if the patient is a good candidate for rhinoplasty. In general, the ideal candidate for surgery has legitimate concerns and realistic expectations, and is secure, well informed and understands the limitations of surgery. The acronym SYLVIA has been used to describe the ideal patient: secure, young, listens, verbal, intelligent, and attractive. The poor candidate for surgery has excessive concerns about minimal deformities and unrealistic expectations, and is insecure, poorly informed, and fails to recognize the limitations of surgery. The acronym SIMON has been used to describe this patient: single, immature, male, overly expectant, and narcissistic traits.[19,26] These patients are likely to be unsatisfied following surgery regardless of the aesthetic improvement. They should be approached with caution and in most cases should not be operated on.

Treatment surgical technique

Video 1

Anesthesia and preoperative management

It is our preference to perform primary open rhinoplasty under general endotracheal anesthesia. Following induction and intubation with a Mallinkrodt endotracheal tube, a moist throat pack is placed to prevent intragastric blood leading to postoperative nausea and vomiting. The patient is positioned so that his or her head is slightly past the head of the operating room table, allowing moderate hyperextension of the neck and improving visualization for the surgeon.

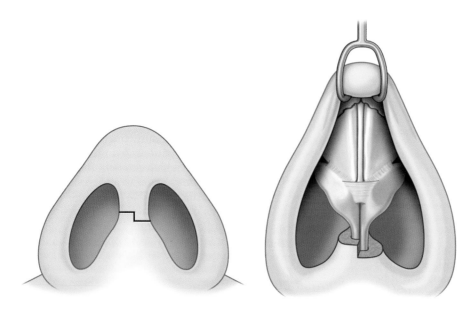

Fig. 18.2 Transcolumellar stair-step incision.

Prior to sterile prep, the nose and septum are infiltrated with a total of 10 mL 1% lidocaine with 1:100 000 epinephrine. Injection in the submucoperichondrial plane of the nasal septum is performed followed by infiltration of the soft-tissue envelope. Injection of the highly vascular areas of the nose, including the columella, tip, dorsum, lateral side walls, alar base, and along the caudal margin of the lower lateral cartilages, is important for hemostasis. If inferior turbinoplasty is anticipated, the anterior head of the inferior turbinates is also injected. Oxymetazoline-soaked cottonoid pledgets are inserted into the nasal cavities. One drop of methylene blue is instilled in the oxymetazoline to differentiate this from the local anesthesia and prevent inadvertent injection. Typically, two or three cottonoid pledgets are placed in each nasal cavity. Comparable hemostasis can be obtained using lidocaine with oxymetazoline while avoiding the use of a controlled substance with potential cardiac effects, as seen with cocaine.[27,28]

A headlight is worn to assist in visualization of the internal nasal structures. The entire face and neck are prepped sterilely, which allows for intraoperative assessment of the nose in relation to the rest of the face.

Incisions and approach

Adequate exposure during primary open rhinoplasty is best obtained using a transcolumellar incision with infracartilaginous extensions. Several transcolumellar incisions are commonly used, including stair-step, inverted-V, and transverse. Blood supply to the nasal tip is preserved with the transcolumellar incision provided that extensive defatting of the nasal tip or extensive alar base resections above the alar grooves are not performed.[29,30] We prefer to use a stair-step incision which camouflages the scar, provides landmarks for accurate closure, and prevents linear scar contracture. Broken-line transcolumellar incisions may lead to better scar formation and less notching.[31]

The stair-step transcolumellar incision is made at the narrowest part of the columella, which is typically at its

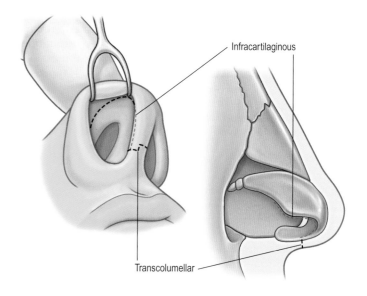

Fig. 18.3 Transcolumellar stair-step incision with infracartilaginous extensions.

midportion *(Fig. 18.2)*. A 15-blade scalpel is used to incise the skin superficially, avoiding damage to the underlying medial crura. The incision is carried into the nasal vestibule and then continued along the caudal border of the medial crus towards the middle crus of the lower lateral cartilage. After everting the ala using external digital pressure against a double hook placed within the alar rim, a separate incision is started at the caudal border of the lateral crura and connected with the medial incision, caudal to the middle crus *(Fig. 18.3)*. The lower edge of the lateral crus can be palpated after the ala has been everted to assure precise infracartilaginous incision placement. Fine dissecting scissors are used to elevate the nasal skin in a supraperichondrial plane starting from the columellar incision in a superior direction to the nasal tip. Next, dissection is started over the lateral crus and continued in a medial direction connecting the supraperichondrial dissection planes over the middle crus. Dissection to elevate the nasal skin in the supraperichondrial plane is carried superiorly to 2 mm above the keystone area. A Joseph elevator is then used to elevate nasal skin in a subperiosteal plane off nasal bones to radix. This dissection over the nasal bones is only performed in the central area to allow for bony dorsal hump reduction while the lateral periosteal attachments of the bony side wall should not be disrupted as they provide necessary stability to the bony vault after percutaneous osteotomies have been performed.[32]

Component dorsal hump reduction

An aesthetically pleasing nasal dorsum is critical to a successful result after rhinoplasty. Dorsal hump reduction without careful attention to the anatomic and physiologic functions of the nasal dorsum and internal nasal valve can lead to irregularities of the nasal dorsum, excessive narrowing of the midvault, the inverted-V deformity, and underresection or overresection of the osseocartilaginous hump.[33] We prefer a graduated approach using component dorsal hump reduction *(Box 18.1)* over earlier techniques of composite dorsal hump reduction.[33,34] This incremental reduction of the osseocartilaginous structures of the nasal dorsum offers increased control and reproducibility over composite dorsal hump reduction performed with an osteotome.

The nasal dorsum is initially modified prior to addressing the nasal tip, which establishes balance between the dorsum

---

Box 18.1 Component dorsal hump reduction

- Separation of the upper lateral cartilage from the septum
- Incremental reduction of the septum proper
- Incremental dorsal bony reduction (using a rasp)
- Verification by palpation
- Final modifications, if indicated (spreader grafts, suturing techniques, osteotomies)

---

and tip essential to achieving the optimal aesthetic result.[34] Component dorsal hump reduction is performed using five essential steps: (1) separation of the upper lateral cartilage from the septum; (2) incremental reduction of the septum proper; (3) incremental dorsal bony reduction (using a rasp); (4) verification by palpation; and (5) final modifications, if indicated (spreader grafts, suturing techniques, osteotomies).[33,34]

After dorsal undermining of the nasal soft tissues has been carried over the central aspect of the bony vault, the lower lateral cartilages are separated from each other and the septum by taking down the interdomal suspensory ligament. The creation of bilateral submucoperichondrial tunnels along the dorsal septum is essential prior to component dorsal hump reduction. This allows extramucosal resection of the osseocartilaginous components of the dorsal hump preventing late cicatricial narrowing of the internal nasal valve and webbing of the vestibule causing potential nasal airway obstruction. The perichondrium is scored at the nasal septal angle with a 15-blade scalpel and then, using a Cottle elevator, dissection in a submucoperichondrial plane is performed from caudal to cephalad along the dorsal septum until the nasal bones are reached. Once in the correct plane, there should be little resistance elevating the mucoperichondrium off the septal cartilage. The upper lateral cartilages are separated from the septum sharply using a 15-blade scalpel. By incising along the surface of the septal cartilage to separate the upper lateral cartilages, the transverse projections of the T-shaped dorsal septum are kept attached to the upper lateral cartilages *(Fig. 18.4)*. This helps to minimize the need for spreader grafts to maintain the internal valve. Following this, angled septal scissors are used to reduce the septal cartilage incrementally. This cartilage is saved and can be used later for grafts, including as a columellar strut graft if large enough.[35] Preservation of the upper lateral cartilages during dorsal reduction of the cartilaginous septum is important in achieving smooth dorsal aesthetic lines while equal resection of the septum and upper

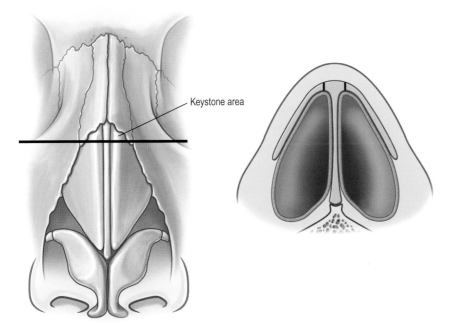

Keystone area

Fig. 18.4 Nasal dorsum.

lateral cartilages results in rounding of the dorsum and excessive resection of the upper lateral cartilages results in the inverted-V deformity. For dorsal reduction of the bony hump less than 3 mm, a down-biting diamond rasp is used to reduce the bony dorsum incrementally. Rasping should proceed along left and right dorsal aesthetic lines and then centrally, employing short excursions of the rasp for maximal control. Care is taken to avoid avulsing the attachments of the upper lateral cartilages from the undersurface of the nasal bones. If a larger reduction of the bony dorsum is required, a guarded 8-mm osteotome can be used. The osteotomy should start at the caudal aspect of the nasal bones and is directed towards the radix. A rasp is used for final adjustments. Only in limited circumstances is reduction of the upper lateral cartilages indicated. Overresection must be avoided to prevent internal valve collapse or long-term dorsal irregularities. Patients with short nasal bones and high and narrow osseocartilaginous framework are at higher risk for these problems.[35] Most importantly, after each incremental modification of the dorsum, the nasal skin is replaced and the contour of the nasal dorsum is assessed using the three-point dorsal palpation test in order to avoid overresection of the dorsum.[33,34]

When the transverse projections of the T-shaped dorsal septum are kept attached to the upper lateral cartilages, they act as autospreader grafts, maintaining the patency of the internal valves and contour of the dorsal aesthetic lines. In thicker-skinned patients, upper lateral cartilage-septal sutures are used to reapproximate the upper lateral cartilages to the septum to re-establish the integrity of the nasal dorsum. They can be reapproximated into their anatomic position, or rolled inward as cartilaginous spreader flaps. Spreader grafts may be added, and are indicated in primary rhinoplasty to recreate the dorsal aesthetic lines, widen the midvault, or correct the deviated nose *(Fig. 18.5)*.[36] They may be fashioned from harvested septal cartilage and are typically 5–6 mm in height and 30–32 mm in length. They can be placed either unilaterally or bilaterally parallel to the dorsal septum. If indicated for improvement of the dorsal aesthetic lines they can be visible, placed above the plane of the dorsal septum, and if indicated to improve function of the internal nasal valve they can be invisible, placed below the plane of the dorsal septum. Additionally, an extended spreader graft with its caudal extent projecting below the caudal septum can be used to lengthen the short nose.[37] Spreader grafts are secured to the septum using 5-0 PDS horizontal mattress sutures. Overuse of spreader grafts in primary rhinoplasty can lead to excessive width of the midvault.[33,34]

Following re-establishment of the cartilaginous midvault, percutaneous osteotomies are performed to correct widened or asymmetrical nasal bones, or close the open-roof deformity if present after dorsal reduction.[33,34] Osteotomies will be discussed later in this chapter.

The nasal airway

Proper identification of causative factors of nasal airway obstruction is key to successful treatment. Nasal airway obstruction can have both medically and surgically correctable causes. Common surgically correctable causes include nasoseptal deviation, internal or external valve dysfunction, and inferior turbinate hypertrophy.[17] Management of issues related to the nasal airway is covered in detail in Chapter 20. However, septal reconstruction and inferior turbinoplasty/submucous resection are discussed here as they are commonly performed during primary open rhinoplasty in the patient with nasal airway obstruction secondary to septal deviation or inferior turbinate hypertrophy, respectively.

Septal reconstruction

Septal deviation can involve deviation of the septal cartilage, perpendicular plate of the ethmoid bone, or vomer away from the midline and can cause obstruction of one or both of the nasal airways, along with external deviation of the nose. In our experience, nasal deviations can be classified into three basic types: (1) caudal septal deviations; (2) concave dorsal deformities; and (3) concave/convex dorsal deformities *(Box 18.2)*.[38,39] Septal tilt is the most common type where the quadrangular cartilage and perpendicular plate of the ethmoid are straight but the quadrangular cartilage is tilted to one side

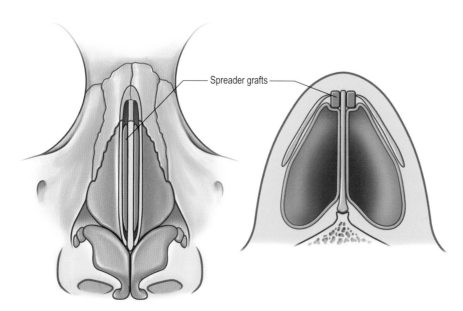

Spreader grafts

Fig. 18.5 Dorsal spreader grafts.

internally and to the opposite side externally. Hypertrophy of the inferior turbinate contralateral to the side of internal deviation is usually present. Correction of septal deviation is key to improving nasal airflow and correcting the deviated nose and is executed using the following principles: (1) exposure of all deviated structures through the open approach; (2) release of all mucoperichondrial attachments to the septum, especially the deviated part; (3) straightening of the septum, and if necessary septal reconstruction, while maintaining an 8–10-mm caudal and dorsal L-strut; (4) restoration of long-term support with buttressing caudal septal batten or dorsal nasal spreader grafts; (5) if necessary, submucous resection of hypertrophied inferior turbinates; and (6) precisely planned and executed external percutaneous osteotomies.[38]

As opposed to septoplasty, where the septal cartilage is scored in an attempt to straighten it, or submucosal resection, where the entire septum is removed other than the L-strut, septal reconstruction differs in that only the portion of the septum causing airway obstruction is removed, with the idea that native cartilage is preserved. It is of critical importance to preserve an L-strut of septal cartilage for structural integrity. The technique for septal reconstruction is similar to that for septal cartilage harvest and is discussed later in this chapter.

Inferior turbinoplasty/outfracture/ submucous resection

The turbinates exist as three or four bilateral extensions from the lateral nasal cavity. The inferior turbinate consists of highly vascular mucoperiosteum covering a thin semicircular conchal bone.[40] It is involved in regulation of filtration and humidification of inspired air. In combination with the internal nasal valve, the anterior extent of the inferior turbinate can be responsible for up to two-thirds of the upper airway resistance.[17,41] Posteriorly, the inferior turbinate diverges away from the nasal septum, allowing for reduced upper-airway resistance in this area.[17,42]

Inferior turbinoplasty is performed in patients with nasal airway obstruction secondary to inferior turbinate hypertrophy refractory to medical management. We prefer a more conservative surgical approach to correct inferior turbinate hypertrophy as we have found it to be effective with low morbidity. Overly aggressive surgical management may be complicated by bleeding, mucosal crusting and desiccation, ciliary dysfunction, chronic infection, malodorous nasal drainage, or atrophic rhinitis.[17] In most cases, inferior turbinoplasty with outfracture of the inferior turbinate or submucous resection is adequate to achieve significant improvement *(Fig. 18.6)*.

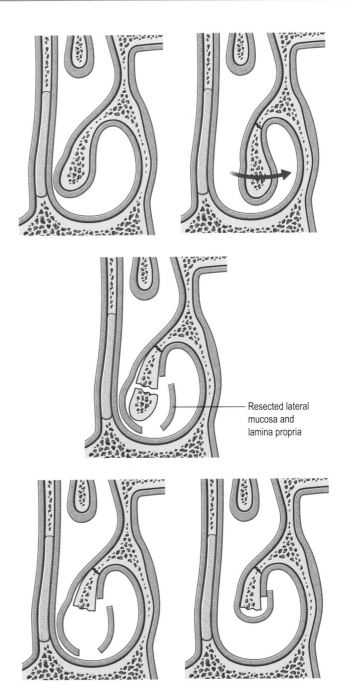

Resected lateral mucosa and lamina propria

Fig. 18.6 Inferior turbinate outfracture and submucous resection.

After removal of the previously placed oxymetazoline-soaked cottonoid pledgets, the inferior turbinates are inspected after vasoconstriction of the overlying mucosa has occurred. In cases of mild to moderate inferior turbinate hypertrophy, a long Vienna speculum is used to outfracture the inferior turbinates. In cases of severe inferior turbinate hypertrophy, submucous resection of the inferior turbinate is indicated. Outfracture is performed so that the entire inferior turbinate is visible. Needle point electrocautery is used to incise the inferior border of the anterior 1.5–2 cm of the inferior turbinate down to the conchal bone. A Cottle elevator is used to develop a medially based submucoperichondrial flap to expose the portion of the conchal bone to be resected.

Takahashi forceps are used to resect the bone sharply from the anterior third of the turbinate. The mucoperichondrial flap is replaced down over the cut edge of the conchal bone; no suturing is necessary as this will adhere to the raw surface. Replacement of the flap will avoid postoperative hemorrhage or crusting.

Harvesting autologous cartilage

The trend over the past two decades in rhinoplasty has shifted away from ablative techniques involving reducing the osseo-cartilaginous framework to conserving the native anatomy and augmentation of deficient areas to correct contour deformities and restore structural support. As such, certain situations require harvest of autologous cartilage for graft material. Autologous grafts are preferential to homografts and alloplastic implants because of their high biocompatibility and low risk of infection and extrusion.[43] Their disadvantages include donor site morbidity, graft resorption, and unavailability of sufficient quantities for graft material.[43] Autologous cartilage grafts are most commonly obtained from septal, ear, and costal cartilage. Other donor sites for autologous grafts include calvarial and nasal bone, and the olecranon process of the ulna.[43] Concerns regarding donor site morbidity, graft availability, and graft resorption will necessitate the use of homologous or alloplastic implants.[44]

Septal cartilage

Septal cartilage is the primary choice for autogenous grafts in rhinoplasty. It can be used in all areas including tip grafts, dorsal onlay grafts, columellar strut grafts, and nasal spreader grafts. It is easily harvested, leaves minimal donor site morbidity, and is available in the operative field. Septal cartilage harvest is performed as previously described for septal reconstruction.

Open rhinoplasty allows for ease of septal cartilage harvest with improved exposure and visualization. Septal cartilage harvest is performed only after component dorsal hump reduction is complete as it is essential to preserve an 8–10-mm L-strut for nasal support. Dorsal reduction of the septum after septal cartilage harvest may leave an L-strut that is too narrow to provide adequate nasal support. Septal cartilage harvest is performed after the lower and upper lateral cartilages have been separated from the quadrangular cartilage. A 15-blade scalpel is used to score the mucoperichondrium of the septal angle and then a Cottle elevator is used to develop the sub-mucoperichondrial pocket on one side of the septum (*Fig. 18.7*). Once in the correct plane, the denuded septal cartilage has a gray-blue hue, the septal cartilage has a gritty texture, and there should be little resistance elevating the mucoperichondrium off the septal cartilage until the dissection reaches the osseocartilaginous junction between the quadrangular cartilage and the vomer.

Dissection of the submucoperichondrial pocket is done towards the floor of the nasal cavity to the maxillary crest and posteriorly to the vomer (*Fig. 18.8*). The contralateral mucoperichondrium may be left attached to the septum and only the portion of the septal cartilage to be harvested is released. This method leaves contralateral mucoperichondrium attached to the L-strut for more support and decreases the amount of dissection and dead space with the potential for hematoma formation. Alternatively, development of these submucoperichondrial pockets can be performed bilaterally, allowing for improved visualization. During development of the submucoperichondrial pockets, care is taken to avoid perforations of the mucosa. Anterior perforations should be repaired with 5-0 chromic gut sutures while posterior perforations can be left as they allow for drainage of any blood. An 8–10-mm wide dorsal and caudal L-strut is created using a 15-blade scalpel to incise the septal cartilage parallel to the dorsal edge of the septum from the perpendicular plate of

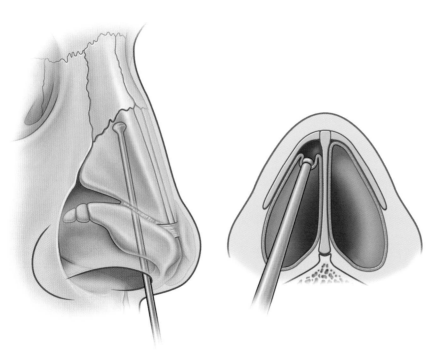

Fig. 18.7 Submucoperichondrial dissection.

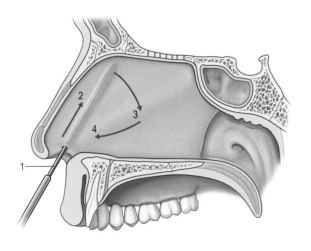

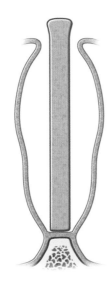

Fig. 18.8 Submucoperichondrial flaps.

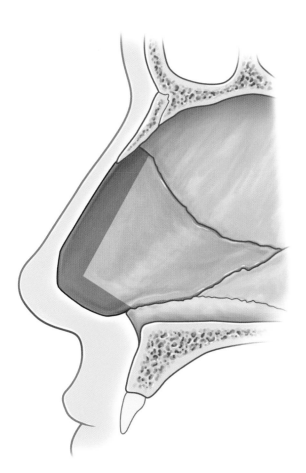

Fig. 18.9 Septal L-strut.

the ethmoid to a point 8–10 mm from the caudal edge of the septum *(Fig. 18.9)*. This incision is then continued posteriorly and parallel to the caudal edge of the septum until the crest of the maxilla. Straight Mayo scissors are used to continue the dorsal incision across the osseocartilaginous junction of the quadrangular cartilage and the perpendicular plate of the ethmoid. A Cottle elevator is then used to elevate the septal cartilage from the maxillary crest and vomer and then to fracture the perpendicular plate between the dorsal incision

and the vomer, liberating the septal cartilage. This septal cartilage is placed in a saline-moistened gauze until it is needed. During septal cartilage harvest, pressure on the L-strut must be avoided to prevent its fracture. If this occurs, it should be repaired to restore nasal support.[45] Once the septal cartilage has been removed, any remaining septal spurs or deviations of the perpendicular plate of the ethmoid or vomer can be osteotomized or rongeured to remove these potential sites for nasal airflow interference. After cartilage grafts have been fashioned, any excess material should be replaced between the mucoperichondrial flaps in case it is required in subsequent procedures. The mucoperichondrial flaps can be sutured together using a 5-0 chromic gut quilting suture and are bolstered by placement of Doyle splints to support the mucoperichondrial flaps and minimize dead space.

Ear cartilage

The ear can provide a significant amount of cartilage for rhinoplasty when septal cartilage has been depleted. It can be used for tip grafts, dorsal onlay grafts, alar contour grafts, and reconstruction of the lower lateral cartilages.[46–48] However, its flaccidity does not allow it to be used where structural support is necessary. Donor site morbidity and scarring are minimal.[49]

An anterior approach is used if autogenous graft material is required for tip grafts or lower lateral cartilage reconstruction *(Fig. 18.10)*. For hemostasis and hydrodissection of the subperichondrial plane overlying the conchal cartilage 3 mL of 1% lidocaine with 1:100 000 epinephrine is injected. An incision is made through the anterior auricular skin 3 mm inside the rim of the conchal bowl using a 15-blade scalpel. Fine dissecting scissors are used to dissect the anterior auricular skin off the conchal cartilage in the subperichondrial plane. A 15-blade scalpel is used to incise through the conchal cartilage, again 3 mm inside and parallel to the rim of the conchal bowl; this rim maintains the structural integrity of the remaining ear cartilage. Fine dissecting scissors are again used to dissect the posterior skin off the posterior aspect of the conchal cartilage in the subperichondrial plane. Once the desired amount of cartilage has been dissected away from the overlying anterior and posterior auricular skin, it can be excised with a 15-blade scalpel. Hemostasis is obtained and the

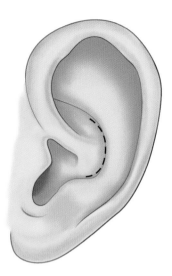
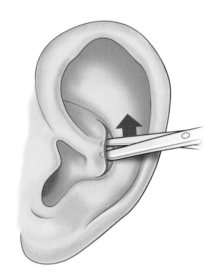
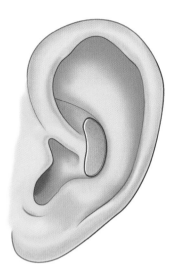

Fig. 18.10 Harvesting ear cartilage.

incision is closed with a 5-0 plain gut running suture. A tie-over Xeroform-cotton bolster held in place with a 3-0 nylon suture through the anterior and posterior auricular skin is used to obliterate dead space and prevent hematoma formation. This is removed on postoperative day 3.

A posterior approach is used if a longer, more malleable piece of cartilage is required. Prior to harvest, injection of 3 mL of 1% lidocaine with 1:100 000 epinephrine aids in hydrodissection of the subperichondrial plane overlying the ear cartilage to be harvested. A 3-cm posterior auricular skin incision is made with a 15-blade scalpel over the conchal bowl. Fine dissecting scissors are used to dissect the posterior auricular skin off the conchal cartilage in the subperichondrial plane up to the postauricular sulcus. The amount of cartilage required is marked by passing a 25-gauge needle dipped in methylene blue from anterior to posterior to tattoo the ear cartilage. A 3-mm rim of conchal bowl is preserved along with a small buttress of cartilage superiorly at the root of the antihelix and inferiorly at the incisura intertragica, preventing donor site deformity. The outlined ear cartilage is then incised using a 15-blade scalpel and fine dissecting scissors are again used to dissect the anterior auricular skin off the anterior aspect of the conchal cartilage in the subperichondrial plane. Once the desired amount of cartilage has been dissected away from the anterior and posterior auricular skin, it is excised with a 15-blade scalpel. Hemostasis is obtained and the incision is closed with a 5-0 plain gut running suture, followed by placement of a tie-over Xeroform-cotton bolster as previously described.

Costal cartilage

Costal cartilage provides abundant autogenous graft material. It can be used for tip grafts, columellar strut grafts, nasal spreader grafts, alar cartilage grafts, and dorsal onlay grafts. Given the size, amount, and intrinsic qualities, costal cartilage lends itself well to use as a dorsal onlay graft and where structural support is required. It can be carved into any shape. However, allowing at least 30 minutes to pass prior to carving allows initial warping to occur, minimizing late deformity.[50]

In addition, utilizing centrally over peripherally located cartilage may help to minimize late deformity.[50,51] Some authors advocate the use of internal stabilization of costal cartilage grafts with Kirschner wire to prevent warping.[52]

Various authors[53–56] have described harvesting costal cartilage from different ribs but it is our preference to harvest the ninth rib because it is straight medially and provides 4–5 cm of autogenous graft material (*Fig. 18.11*). The ninth rib is a floating rib and can be located by palpation. A 2-cm incision is made on the anterolateral aspect of the chest wall. Since the skin overlying the rib is mobile in this area, a long segment of rib can be harvested through this relatively small incision. The external oblique muscle is split in the direction of its fibers, exposing the underlying rib. The perichondrium is lightly scored and is dissected away from the underlying rib cartilage using both a dental elevator and a Joseph elevator. When freeing the cartilage away from the deep perichondrium, care is taken to avoid damaging the parietal pleura and creating a pneumothorax. After the amount of cartilage needed is determined, it is harvested by incising through the rib using a 15-blade scalpel. Slightly more cartilage should be harvested than needed because cartilage is lost secondary to carving. Hemostasis is obtained and the perichondrium is closed using 3-0 Vicryl. The wound is closed in layers using 4-0 Vicryl followed by a 5-0 PDS intradermal suture. Injection of 0.25% bupivacaine into the donor site for postoperative pain control is followed by application of SteriStrips.

If there is concern about pneumothorax during costal cartilage harvest, the wound is filled with saline and positive-pressure ventilation can be performed by the anesthesia provider to ensure that there are no gas bubbles escaping from the chest cavity. If the parietal pleura has been violated, the tip of a red rubber catheter is inserted into the defect and a 3-0 Vicryl purse-string suture is performed around the catheter. The anesthesia provider performs a Valsalva maneuver while suction is applied to the red rubber catheter. As the catheter is withdrawn, the purse-string suture is tied to seal the parietal pleural defect followed by wound closure. An upright chest X-ray should be performed postoperatively to confirm resolution of the pneumothorax.

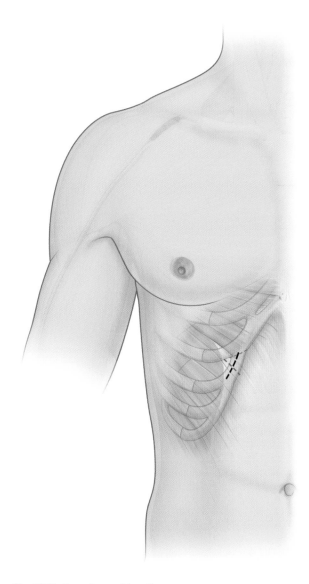

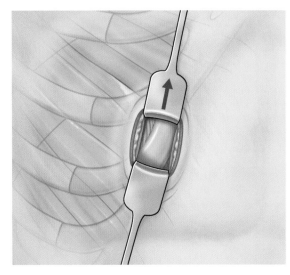

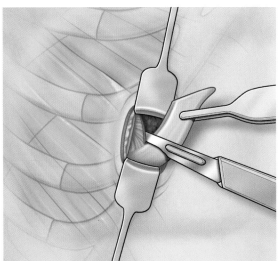

Fig. 18.11 Harvesting costal cartilage.

The nasal tip

A graduated approach to nasal tip surgery requires a combination of techniques including the cephalic trim, the use of a columellar strut graft, nasal tip suturing, and nasal tip grafting. Application of these techniques will help to correct tip deformities and improve tip shape while minimizing deformities secondary to loss of support. In addition, compared with the closed approach, the open approach may cause mild loss of tip projection due to disruption of ligamentous support and increased skin undermining.[57] As such, we commonly employ columellar strut graft and nasal tip suturing techniques to maintain nasal tip support during open rhinoplasty.

Cephalic trim

Cephalic trim should be performed with the bulbous or boxy tip *(Fig. 18.12)*.[58] Paradomal fullness is secondary to prominence of the cephalic border of the middle and lateral crura of the lower lateral cartilages. Cephalic trim of this area reduces paradomal fullness and helps to define the tip and narrow the distance between the tip defining points. A rim strip of at least 5 mm is preserved for adequate support of the external valve. Calipers should be used to measure the rim strip accurately. The excised cartilage can also be used as a source of autogenous grafts.

A lower lateral crural turnover flap is another useful technique to address paradomal fullness while providing additional support to the lower lateral cartilages.[59] It is beneficial for deformities, weakness, and collapse of the lower lateral crura and can also be used to improve lower lateral crural strength during tip reshaping. However, there must be sufficient lower lateral crura to leave a 5-mm rim strip. It can be used in combination with other external valve and alar arch supporting techniques.

Columellar strut graft

An intercrural columellar strut graft is used to maintain or increase nasal tip projection, and aids in unifying the nasal tip. It can be either floating or fixed *(Fig. 18.13)*. A floating columellar strut graft is used more commonly to maintain tip

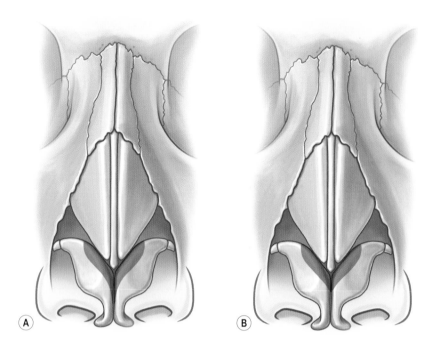

Fig. 18.12 Cephalic trim. **(A)** Lateral and middle crura; **(B)** lateral crus.

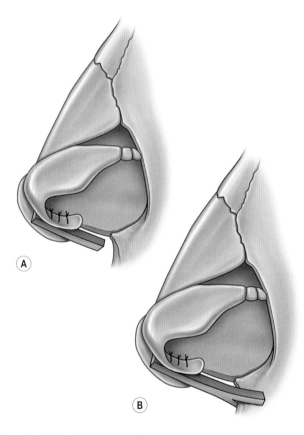

Fig. 18.13 (A) Floating and **(B)** fixed columellar strut grafts.

Box 18.3 **Tip suturing techniques**

- Medial crural suture
- Interdomal suture
- Transdomal suture
- Joined transdomal suture
- Intercrural septal suture
- Lateral crural mattress suture

is placed with a hook in the vestibular apex of each lower lateral cartilage. Upward traction is placed and scissors are used to dissect a pocket between the medial crura down towards the nasal spine. A 2–3-mm pad of soft tissue is preserved over the nasal spine to keep the graft from moving back and forth over the nasal spine with lip movements.[60] The columellar strut graft is placed in the pocket. With the tip defining points held at the same level, a 25-gauge needle is placed through the medial crura and columellar strut graft to stabilize the complex for suturing. A 5-0 PDS suture is used to stabilize the medial crura to the columellar strut graft, followed by two additional 5-0 PDS sutures to unify the nasal tip complex. The columellar strut graft is then trimmed to alter or refine the infratip lobule.

Nasal tip suturing techniques

Tip suturing techniques *(Box 18.3)* are used to refine the tip by controlling the subtle contours of the lower lateral cartilages. Various authors have described their approaches to nasal tip suturing techniques.[61–66] We commonly use four primary suture techniques *(Fig. 18.14)*.[32,67,68] Medial crural sutures are the first sutures placed and can be used to correct medial crural asymmetries, to reduce flaring, and to control the overall width of the columella.[68] In addition, medial crural suture techniques stabilize the columellar strut and have been previously described. Interdomal sutures can increase infratip columellar projection and definition or further increase tip

projection and is positioned between the medial crura and rests in the soft tissues 2–3 mm anterior to the nasal spine. A fixed columellar strut graft is used to increase tip projection and is positioned between the medial crura and rests on the nasal spine. The columellar strut graft is typically fashioned from septal cartilage, to measure 3×25 mm. A double hook

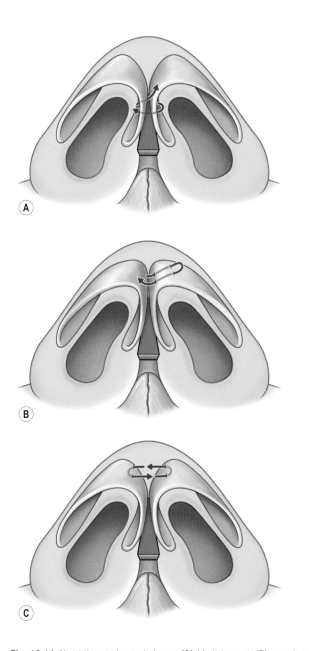

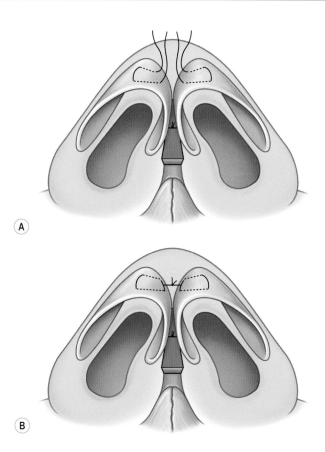

Fig. 18.15 (A, B) Joined transdomal sutures.

Fig. 18.14 Nasal tip suturing techniques. **(A)** Medial crural; **(B)** transdomal; **(C)** interdomal.

projection. A 5-0 PDS suture is placed through the medial walls of the domes and tied to narrow the interdomal distance. Transdomal sutures control dome asymmetry. A 5-0 PDS horizontal mattress suture is placed from the medial surface of the dome through to the lateral surface, staying deep to the vestibular skin, and then back from lateral to medial. A double surgeon's knot is placed in the suture and tightened until the desired angulation of the dome is achieved. If narrowing of the distance between the tip defining points is required, one end of the suture is cut short and the other left approximately 2 cm long *(Fig. 18.15)*. Another transdomal suture is performed on the opposite side, leaving one end of the suture long. The long end is tied to the long suture end on the opposite side. The knot is tightened until the desired distance between the tip defining points is achieved and then tied. Intercrural septal sutures are used to alter tip rotation

(Fig. 18.16) and for this, 5-0 clear nylon is used for permanency. Additionally, the lateral crural mattress suture has been described to reduce the convexity and straighten the lateral crus *(Fig. 18.17)*.[66] The area of maximal convexity of the lateral crus is grasped with a forceps. A 5-0 PDS suture is placed beginning at the caudal aspect of the lateral crus and passed perpendicular to the length of the lateral crus on one side of the forceps and then on the other side of the forceps forming a mattress suture. The usual width of the mattress suture is approximately 6–8 mm. The knot is tightened until the convexity of the lateral crus disappears. The suture should not penetrate the vestibular lining on the deep surface of the lateral crus.

Nasal tip grafting techniques

Nasal tip grafts are used in primary rhinoplasty only if adequate tip projection, definition, or symmetry cannot be obtained by the use of the previously discussed techniques. Visible nasal tip grafts are used infrequently in primary rhinoplasty because of the potential for long-term resorption leading to asymmetries or sharp angulations requiring revision. When nasal tip grafts are used, it is important that they have smooth, tapered edges. Nasal tip grafts of all shapes and sizes have been described *(Fig. 18.18)*.[60] A shield graft is placed adjacent to the caudal edges of the anterior middle crura and extends into the tip. It is used to increase tip projection, and improve definition of the tip and the infratip lobule.[34,69,70] A shield graft is approximately 8 mm wide and 10–12 mm long. The width of the base of the graft is the same as the distance

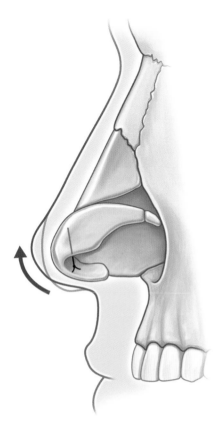

Fig. 18.16 Intercrural septal suture.

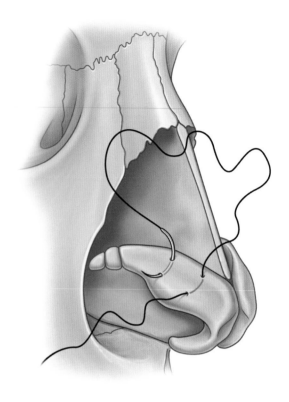

Fig. 18.17 Lateral crural mattress suture.

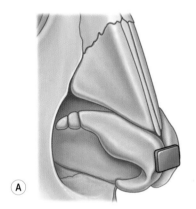

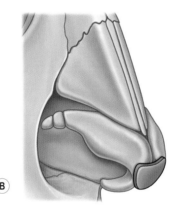

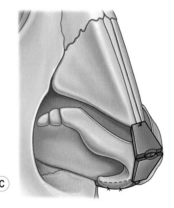

Fig. 18.18 Nasal tip cartilage grafts. **(A)** Supratip; **(B)** infratip; **(C)** anatomic.

between the caudal margins of the medial crura. It is placed so that it extends 2–3 mm past the tip defining points and should be sutured with at least two 5-0 PDS sutures to the caudal margins of the dome and medial crura. An onlay graft is placed horizontally over the alar domes and is used to camouflage tip irregularities and can provide increased tip projection.[71,72] Cartilage removed from the lower lateral cartilages after cephalic trim is usually sufficient for use as an onlay graft.[73] A 6 × 8 mm onlay graft is sutured to the tip defining points with two 5-0 PDS horizontal mattress sutures with the knots tied on the underside of the domes. An anatomic tip graft is a combination of the shield and onlay grafts and reflects the surface anatomy of the ideal tip.[74] The upper part of the graft represents the area between the domes and the lower part represents the area between the middle crura. In primary rhinoplasty, the anatomic tip graft is reserved for the patient with inadequate tip projection or thick skin.

The alar rims

The presence of deformities of the alar rims such as alar notching or retraction, facets of the soft-tissue triangles, malposition of the lateral crura, or functional problems including external valve collapse may require the use of lateral crural horizontal mattress sutures, lower lateral crural turnover flaps, alar contour or lateral crural strut grafts to correct.

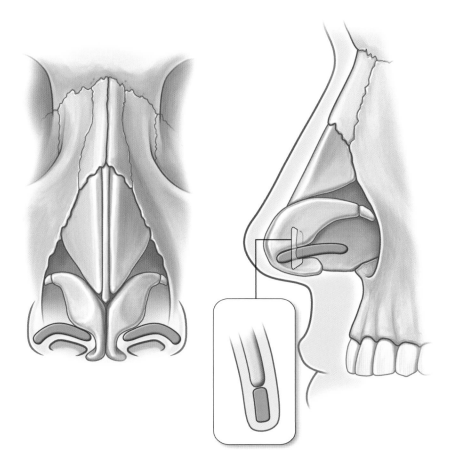

Fig. 18.19 Alar contour grafts.

Alar contour grafts

Alar contour grafts are used as a simple and effective method to correct and prevent alar notching or retraction, and facets of the soft-tissue triangles, after correcting the tip deformity *(Fig. 18.19)*.[75] Sharp dissection scissors are used to dissect a subcutaneous pocket below the infracartilaginous incision and parallel to the alar rim. The pocket should span the length of the deformity and extend 3 mm to each side of it. An alar contour graft is typically 4 × 10 mm but it may be need to be larger depending on the size of the deformity.

Lateral crural strut grafts

Lateral crural strut grafts are used to support weak lateral crura, prevent collapse of the external nasal valve, address malposition of the lateral crura, or increase tip projection *(Fig. 18.20)*.[76] The vestibular skin is dissected from the deep surface of the posterior two-thirds of the lateral crus. The lateral crus is separated from the accessory cartilages. Sharp dissection scissors are used to dissect a subcutaneous pocket below adjacent to the accessory cartilages posteriorly to the pyriform aperture. To correct malposition of the lateral crura, the pocket is dissected below the infracartilaginous incision and parallel to the alar rim. A 4 × 25 mm lateral crural strut graft is placed in the pocket and rests on the pyriform aperture posteriorly. The anterior aspect of the graft is placed deep to the lateral crus and secured with two or three 5-0 PDS simple interrupted sutures.

The alar–columellar relationship

The alar–columellar relationship demonstrated on the lateral view is dictated by the relative positions of the alar rim and the columella to a line drawn through the long axis of the nostril *(Fig. 18.21)*. The ideal distance from the long axis to both the alar rim superiorly and the columella inferiorly is 1–2 mm.

Six classes of alar–columellar relationship have been described.[77] A class I relationship, in which the distance from the long axis to the columella is greater than 2 mm while the distance from the long axis to the alar rim is 1–2 mm, is known as a hanging columella. Correction involves resection and reapproximation of the membranous septum to reposition the columella superiorly. It may also be necessary to resect part of the caudal septum or medial crura if they contribute to the hanging columella. A class II relationship, where the distance from the long axis to the columella is 1–2 mm while the distance from the long axis to the alar rim is greater than 2 mm, is secondary to alar retraction. Correction may involve caudal repositioning of the lateral crus, the use of alar contour or lateral crural strut grafts, or composite grafts from the septum or concha. A class III relationship is a combination of both classes I and II and requires the use of techniques described for both classes. A class IV relationship, in which the distance from the long axis to the columella is 1–2 mm while the distance from the long axis to the alar rim is less than 1 mm, is known as a hanging ala. Correction involves resection of a horizontal ellipse of vestibular skin no more

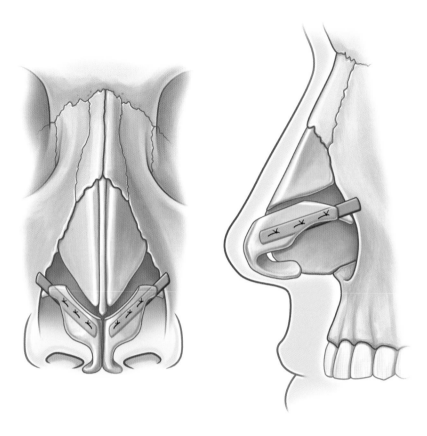

Fig. 18.20 Lateral crural strut grafts.

than 3 mm in width to raise the hanging ala. A class V relationship, in which the distance from the long axis to the columella is less than 1 mm while the distance from the long axis to the alar rim is 1–2 mm, is secondary to columellar retraction. Correction involves placing a contoured columellar strut graft between the medial crura to push the columellar skin inferiorly. A class VI relationship is a combination of both classes IV and V and requires the use of techniques described for both classes.

Percutaneous lateral nasal osteotomies

Nasal osteotomies are a key component to shape the bony vault in rhinoplasty. Osteotomies are used to narrow a wide bony vault, close an open-roof deformity, or straighten deviated nasal bones.[78,79] The goals of nasal osteotomies are maintenance or creation of smooth dorsal aesthetic lines and obtaining a desirable width of the bony vault.[80] Osteotomies can be classified by approach (external or internal), type (lateral, medial, transverse, or a combination), and level (low-to-high, low-to-low, or double-level) *(Fig. 18.22)*. A transition zone of decreased bony thickness exists along the frontal processes of the maxilla near its junction with the nasal bone, from the pyriform aperture to the radix. This area of relatively thin bone allows for consistent osteotomies and predictable fracture patterns. Relative contraindications to the use of osteotomies during rhinoplasty include patients with short nasal bones, elderly patients with excessively thin nasal bones, those with relatively thick nasal skin, and some noncaucasian patients with extremely low and broad noses.[34,79–84]

Various authors have described their experience using different approaches, including intranasal, intraoral, and percutaneous techniques.[78,85–104] We prefer percutaneous lateral discontinuous osteotomies because this technique results in a more controlled fracture with less intranasal trauma while minimizing morbidity, including bleeding, ecchymosis, and edema *(Fig. 18.23)*.[81–84] Although osteotomies can be performed at any point during rhinoplasty, we typically perform lateral osteotomies during the final stages of the operation. A 2-mm incision is made in the nasofacial groove at the level of the inferior orbital rim. A sharp 2-mm straight osteotome is inserted through the incision and parallel to the surface of the maxilla, down through the periosteum. A lateral subperiosteal sweep to the bony nasofacial groove is performed to displace the angular artery laterally and prevent its injury. The osteotome is oriented so that only one edge is in direct contact with the bone for improved accuracy. The discontinuous osteotomy is performed from inferiorly, preserving the caudal aspect of the frontal process of the maxilla at the pyriform aperture to prevent collapse of the internal nasal valve, to the level of the medial canthus superiorly and then continued into a superior oblique osteotomy medially. The osteotomy should not be continued superior to the medial canthus to avoid injury to the lacrimal system. A mallet is used to strike the osteotome, with the endpoints being loss of resistance and change in sound. After the osteotomies have been completed, the thumb and index finger are used to exert gentle pressure to perform a greenstick fracture of the nasal bones to reposition them in the desired location. If more than gentle pressure is required, the osteotome should be reinserted to ensure that there are no significant

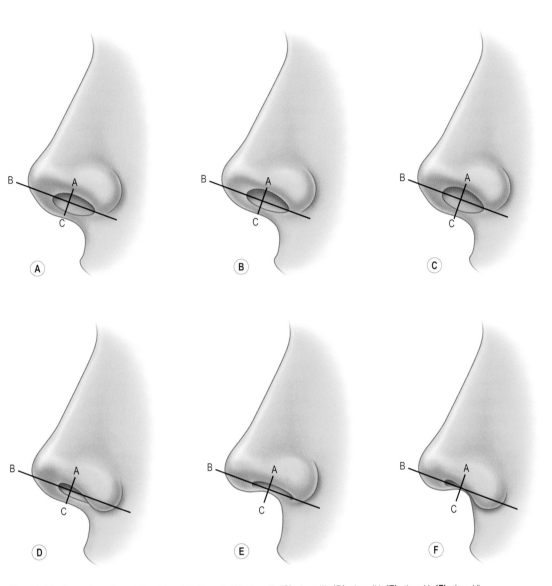

Fig. 18.21 Alar–columellar relationships. **(A)** Class I; **(B)** class II; **(C)** class III; **(D)** class IV; **(E)** class V; **(F)** class VI.

areas of nonosteotomized bone between the discontinuous perforations.

Closure

Prior to closure, the wound is irrigated with warm sterile saline to remove debris that can cause deformity. Closure of the incisions is begun by lining up the transcolumellar stair-step incision in the midline and at the junction of the columellar skin and nasal vestibule bilaterally. This incision is closed with simple interrupted sutures using 6-0 black nylon on a PC-3 needle. This closure must be meticulously performed to prevent notching leading to a noticeable columellar scar. The bilateral infracartilaginous incisions are closed next with simple interrupted sutures using 5-0 chromic gut on a PC-3 needle. The mucosa should be exactly reapproximated, particularly around the middle crura, to prevent distortion of the soft triangle or webbing at the nasal vestibule.

Depressor septi muscle translocation

The depressor septi muscles are small, paired muscles attached to the medial crural footplates and interdigitating with the orbicularis oris muscle fibers (type I) or originating on the periosteum of the maxilla (type II).[105] In some patients, these muscles are diminutive or nonexistent (type III). The action of the depressor septi muscles creates or accentuates the deformity characterized by descent of the nasal tip, shortening of the upper lip, and a transverse crease in the mid philtral area.[103] If the patient has a tension tip that with animation causes a foreshortened upper lip and decrease in tip projection, the depressor septi muscles are released through an upper gingivolabial sulcus approach **(Fig. 18.24)**. A horizontal incision between 8 and 10 mm centered on the frenulum is made in the upper gingivolabial sulcus using needle tip electrocautery. The depressor septi muscles are dissected using needle tip electrocautery and then released near their origin with the orbicularis oris muscle or maxillary periosteum. The

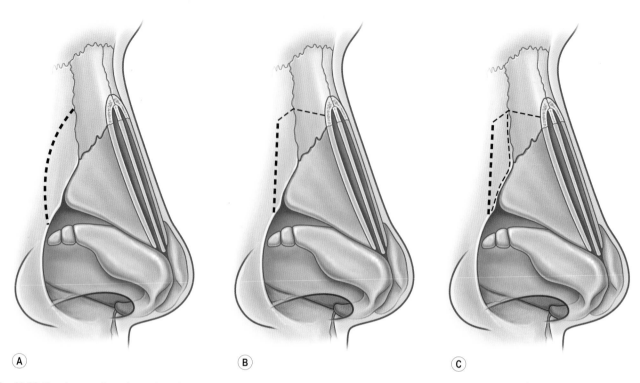

Fig. 18.22 Percutaneous discontinuous lateral nasal osteotomies. **(A)** Low-to-high; **(B)** low-to-low; **(C)** double-level.

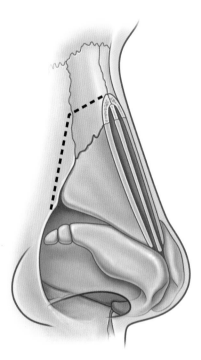

Fig. 18.23 Percutaneous discontinuous lateral nasal osteotomies.

depressor septi muscles are then transposed and their cut ends are sutured with 4-0 chromic gut suture, providing fullness to the central upper lip. The upper gingivolabial sulcus incision is closed vertically to elongate and enhance fullness to the central upper lip.

Alar base surgery

Alar base surgery is indicated for abnormalities including alar flaring, nostril asymmetry, excessively large nostrils, elongated alar side walls, widened alar base, large alae, and alar asymmetry *(Fig. 18.25).*[30] Alar flaring is the most common problem requiring modification of the alar base. The relationship between the alar and basal planes, alar base width, and the nostril shape and size should be taken into consideration when choosing the appropriate surgical technique. The ideal configuration for alar base modification is when the alar plane diverges laterally, forming an acute angle of less than 90° with the basal plane. When the alar and basal planes form a perpendicular or obtuse angle, alar base resections will cause a disproportionately narrow alar base width, resulting in a "bowling pin" appearance.[106] With open rhinoplasty, alar base resections should be kept inferior to the alar groove to avoid damage to the lateral nasal arteries.[29,30,107]

Alar flaring

Alar flaring in the presence of normal nostril shape and symmetry is corrected by limiting excision to the alar lobule; the incision is not continued into the vestibule.[31,108] The incision is not made directly in the alar-cheek groove but within 1 mm of the groove, allowing for an everted closure with improved scarring. In addition, 1–2 mm of the alar base is preserved, preventing alar base notching. The wound is closed with 6-0 black nylon suture on a PC-3 needle using the "halving principle" since the incision adjacent to the alar-cheek groove is longer than the incision on the alar surface.

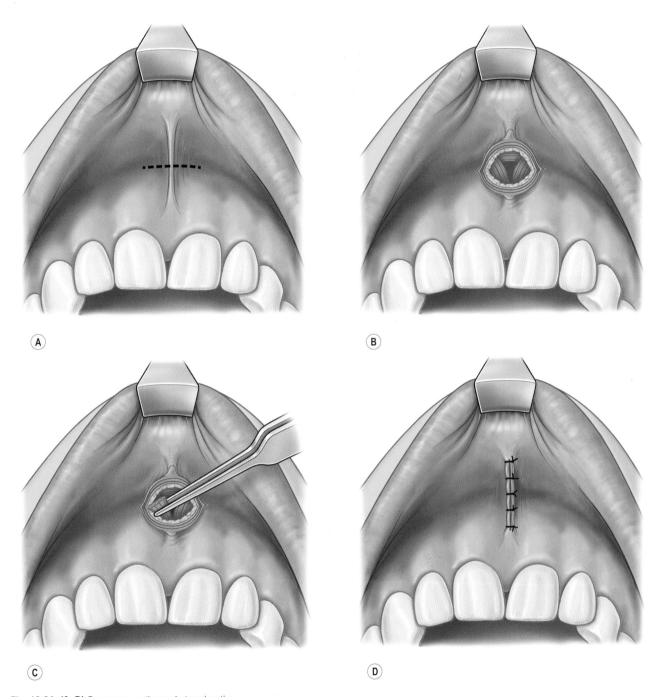

Fig. 18.24 (A–D) Depressor septi muscle translocation.

Alar flaring with modification of nostril shape

Alar flaring with nostril asymmetry or excessively large nostrils requires a wedge excision of the alar lobule and vestibule.[32] The alar lobule incision is continued into the vestibule 2 mm above the alar groove. The medial incision is made using an 11-blade scalpel angled 30° laterally, resulting in a small medially based flap. Straight-line closure is avoided to prevent distortion of the nostril or notching of the nostril sill. The wound is closed with 6-0 black nylon suture on a PC-3 needle using the "halving principle" and careful eversion to avoid a depressed scar across the nostril sill.

Correction of specific deformities

Deviated nose with dorsal hump

Systematic analysis

The patient illustrated in this example had the following complaints: (1) a dorsal hump; (2) a bulbous nasal tip; and (3) deviation of the nose to the left *(Fig. 18.26)*. On frontal view, she has Fitzpatrick type IV thick skin and good facial proportions. She has a reverse C-shaped dorsal septal deformity,

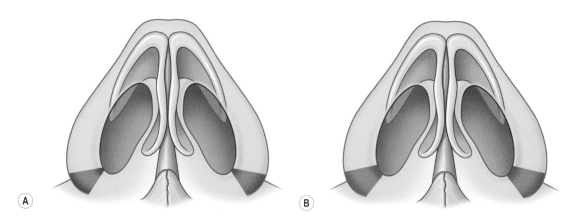

Fig. 18.25 Alar base surgery. **(A)** Alar flaring; **(B)** alar flaring with modification of nostril shape.

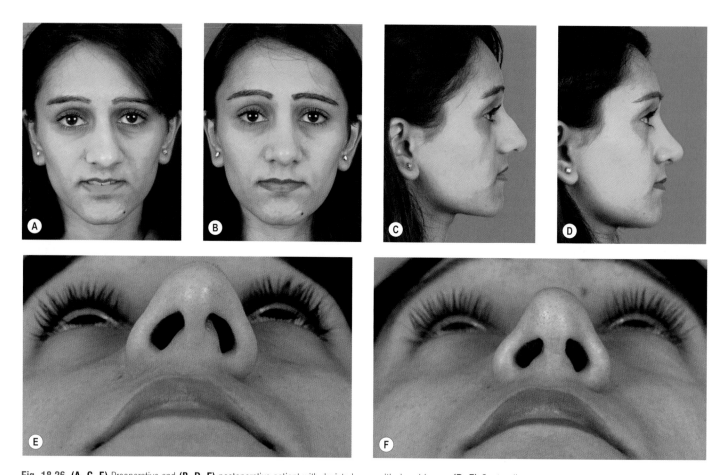

Fig. 18.26 **(A, C, E)** Preoperative and **(B, D, F)** postoperative patient with deviated nose with dorsal hump. **(D, E)** Gunter diagrams.

nasal deviation to left, the nasal base is wide, and the nasal tip is bulbous with slight alar flaring (greater on the left). On lateral and oblique views, the radix position is good, there is a moderate dorsal hump about 4 mm, but tip projection and nasal length are adequate. She has a short upper lip. On basal view, there is a left caudal septal deviation, and a bulbous tip and slight alar flaring are again demonstrated. Internal nasal examination reveals pink mucosa with septal deflection to the left.

Operative goals

1. Correct the nasal airway obstruction.
2. Reduce the dorsal hump.
3. Correct the nasal deviation.
4. Correct and refine the bulbous nasal tip.
5. Narrow the wide nasal base.
6. Lengthen the short upper lip.

Surgical plan

1. Open approach with transcolumellar and infracartilaginous incisions to expose nasal framework.

2. Carry out component dorsal hump reduction to reduce cartilaginous and bony dorsum by 4 mm.[34]

3. Expose nasal septum and perform septal reconstruction with septal cartilage harvest to correct nasal airway obstruction and provide material for cartilage grafts.

4. Perform 50% full-thickness inferior cuts into the deviated L-strut and place figure-of-eight suture to contralateral periosteum of anterior nasal spine with 5-0 PDS suture to correct septal deviation.[38]

5. Place right nasal spreader graft to prevent deviation of L-strut and strengthen dorsal aesthetic lines.

6. Perform cephalic trim of bilateral lower lateral cartilages, retaining 5-mm rim strip to correct and refine bulbous nasal tip.

7. Secure floating columellar strut graft with 5-0 PDS intercrural sutures to support and unify nasal tip.

8. Perform graduated approach to nasal tip suturing with medial crural and interdomal sutures and place cap graft from cephalic trim to refine nasal tip.[68]

9. Perform percutaneous low to low lateral osteotomies to reposition the bony nasal base.

10. Release and transpose depressor septi muscles through upper lip gingivolabial incision.[103]

Outcome

The patient is shown at 2-year follow-up. Frontal view reveals a straight nose, improved dorsal aesthetic lines, and a refined nasal tip. Lateral view shows a normal radix position, a smooth, straight dorsum, a slight supratip break, and improved nasal length. Tip projection is good. There is a subtle increase in the upper lip length that enhances the tip–lip relationship. Basal view again demonstrates an aesthetic triangular nasal tip with an improved alar–columellar relationship.

Long, wide nose with a drooping tip and nasal airway obstruction

Systematic analysis

The patient illustrated in this example had the following complaints: (1) nasal airway obstruction; (2) a long, drooping nose; and (3) a poorly defined nasal tip (*Fig. 18.27*). On frontal

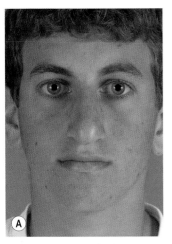
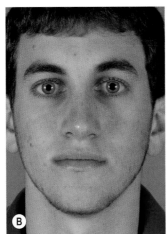
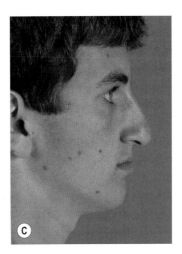
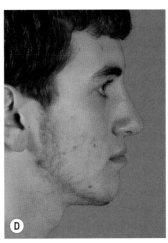

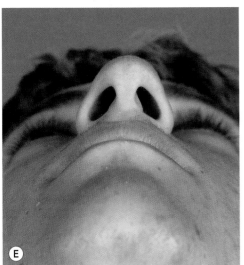
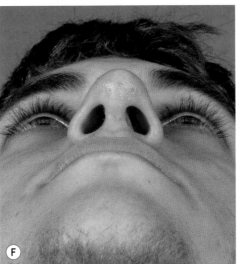

Fig. 18.27 (A, C, E) Preoperative and **(B, D, F)** postoperative patient with long, wide nose with a drooping tip and nasal airway obstruction.

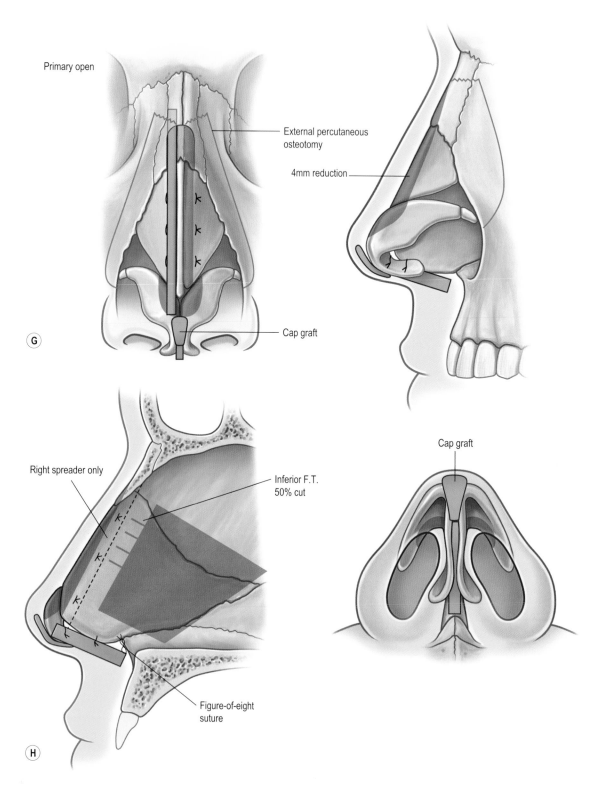

Primary open

External percutaneous osteotomy

4mm reduction

Cap graft

G

Right spreader only

Inferior F.T. 50% cut

Cap graft

Figure-of-eight suture

H

Fig. 18.27, cont'd (G, H) Gunter diagrams.

view, the patient has Fitzpatrick type II moderately thick skin and good facial proportions. He has deviation of the nose to the right, the nasal base is wide, and the nasal tip is poorly defined with a wide angle of divergence and domal arch. On lateral and oblique views, he has a moderate dorsal hump, and a dependent nasal tip with infratip lobule excess giving the appearance of poor tip projection. On basal view, the poorly defined nasal tip is again apparent with a wide angle of divergence. Internal nasal examination reveals a septal deflection to the right.

Operative goals

1. Correct the nasal airway obstruction.
2. Reduce the dorsal hump.
3. Correct the nasal deviation.
4. Decrease nasal length by correcting infralobular excess.
5. Narrow the wide nasal base.
6. Correct and refine the nasal tip.

Surgical plan

1. Open approach with transcolumellar and infracartilaginous incisions to expose nasal framework.
2. Carry out component dorsal hump reduction to reduce cartilaginous and bony dorsum 4 mm.[34]
3. Expose nasal septum and perform septal reconstruction with septal cartilage harvest to correct nasal airway obstruction and provide material for cartilage grafts.
4. Perform cephalic trim of bilateral lower lateral cartilages, retaining 5-mm rim strip to correct and refine bulbous nasal tip.
5. Secure floating columellar strut graft with 5-0 PDS intercrural sutures to support and unify nasal tip.
6. Perform graduated approach to nasal tip suturing with medial crural, transdomal, and interdomal sutures to refine nasal tip.[68]
7. Perform columellar-septal suture to increase tip projection and derotate nasal tip.
8. Carry out infralobular onlay graft to improve nasal tip balance.
9. Perform percutaneous low to low lateral osteotomies to narrow the bony nasal base.

Outcome

The patient is shown at 1-year follow-up. Frontal view reveals a straight, narrower nose, improved dorsal aesthetic lines, and a refined nasal tip. Lateral view shows a smooth, straight dorsum, improved tip rotation and projection, and improved balance between the nasal tip and dorsum. Basal view again demonstrates improved nasal tip definition and an aesthetic triangular nasal tip.

Postoperative care

Postoperative care begins preoperatively with a thorough review of the plan of care and expected postoperative recovery. The patient is provided with both oral and written detailed postoperative instructions at the initial visit, establishing the foundation for successful postoperative care. At each subsequent visit, including the day of surgery, postoperative instructions are reviewed with the patient to reinforce and clarify these details. This helps to improve patient understanding, involve the patient in his/her own care, and minimize patient anxiety. Dressings and wound care, medications, activity restrictions, general instructions, and management of complications are the core elements in postoperative care of the rhinoplasty patient.[109]

Dressings and wound care

At the end of the procedure, edema is gently compressed from soft tissues of the lobule, the nasal skin is cleansed with an alcohol prep pad, Skin-Prep protective barrier wipe (Smith & Nephew, St. Petersburg, FL) is applied, followed by ¼-inch (0.6-cm) Steri-Strips (3M, St. Paul, MN). SteriStrips are applied starting at the supratip break, carefully contouring the soft tissue to the underlying osseocartilaginous skeleton and then continuing superiorly along the dorsum with SteriStrips of progressively shorter length.

A Denver dorsal splint (Shippert Medical Technologies, Centennial, CO) is shaped over a cylindrical object with a diameter similar to the width of the osseous base of the nose. This splint is applied over the superior two-thirds of the dorsum and the edges are compressed medially to support the osteotomized nasal bones. The inferior edge of this splint should be superior to the supratip area. If septal reconstruction and/or inferior turbinoplasty was performed, Doyle septal splints (Micromedics, St. Paul, MN) are applied to avoid hematoma formation deep to the mucoperichondrial flaps, support and stabilize the structures, protect the septal mucosa, and prevent synechiae formation between adjacent mucosal surfaces. These splints are covered with antistaphylococcal antibiotic ointment, inserted into each of the nasal cavities and secured using a 3-0 nylon horizontal mattress suture through the membranous septum, loosely tied to prevent ischemia of this delicate tissue. Both Denver and Doyle splints are removed, typically on postoperative day 7, along with the columellar sutures. If the patient has undergone extensive septal reconstruction, the splints are left in place for approximately 10 days. Alar base sutures are also removed on postoperative day 10.

A nasal drip pad is fashioned using 2 × 2 gauze and held in place under the nose with paper tape secured to tape on the cheeks. The tape on the cheeks helps to prevent skin maceration secondary to frequent removal and reapplication of the tape. The patient will gently clean the incisions with half-strength hydrogen peroxide and apply antistaphylococcal antibiotic ointment twice daily for 7 days.

Generally, most of the nasal swelling and ecchymosis will resolve within 3–4 weeks of following surgery; however soft-tissue edema, both external and internal, may take 6–12 months to resolve and external subtle nasal definition and internal nasal airflow will continue to improve over this period.

Medications

First- or second-generation cephalosporins are generally used for antibiotic prophylaxis. The patient receives preoperative prophylactic intravenous antibiotics in the holding area 30 minutes prior to surgery. Several studies[110–112] have shown no difference in infection rate with the use of postoperative prophylactic antibiotics. We do not prescribe any postoperative oral antibiotic prophylaxis.

A short course of high-dose corticosteroids is started intraoperatively and continued in the early postoperative period to minimize edema and ecchymosis. Intraoperatively, 8 mg intravenous dexamethasone is given and continued postoperatively in the form of oral methylprednisolone (Medrol Dose Pack) for 6 days. Although the efficacy of high-dose corticosteroids remains debatable, newer data suggest their utility in open rhinoplasty.[113,114]

Postoperative pain and discomfort are highly variable. In general, oral narcotic analgesia is used for several days, after which nonsteroidal anti-inflammatory drugs are adequate. While using narcotics, the patient should also receive stool softeners to prevent constipation as straining may precipitate postoperative bleeding.

Activity restrictions

During the initial 48 hours following rhinoplasty, the patient should keep his/her head elevated greater than 30° degrees and gently apply cold compresses to help decrease postoperative edema and ecchymosis. Head elevation should be continued until there is no longer edema in the morning. This is typically 7–10 days. The patient should avoid any straining, including strenuous activity or heavy lifting, for 3 weeks. Trauma and pressure on the nose, including wearing glasses, should be avoided for 6 weeks.

General instructions

In addition to the previous postoperative instructions, the patient is instructed to call the physician if he/she experiences fever (temperature greater than 38.5°C or 101.5°F), pain not controlled with medication, or persistent nasal bleeding with bright red blood or changing the nasal drip pad more frequently than every 30 minutes.

Follow-up

The first follow-up appointment is at 1 week postoperative where sutures and splints are typically removed. Typically, the patient is seen again at 3 months, 6 months, 1 year, and then every 1–2 years following surgery. Postoperative photographs are taken at the 6-month follow-up appointment and then yearly thereafter.

Outcomes, prognosis, and complications

Outcomes

At this time, there are no standardized measures for assessing the aesthetic or functional outcomes following rhinoplasty. Various authors have proposed different methods, including image analysis, measurement tools and computer programs, to assess these outcomes.[115–122]

Following rhinoplasty, most patient dissatisfaction is seen in the lower third of the nose, including the nasal tip, followed by the middle and upper thirds. Poor results in the lower third typically arise from nasal tip asymmetries, notching of the alae, and inadequate tip rotation. Common problems in the middle third include supratip fullness or a pinched supratip. Complaints in the upper third include excessive reduction of the dorsum, asymmetrical or ill-defined dorsal aesthetic lines, and other dorsal irregularities.

Box 18.4 Complications following rhinoplasty

- Anosmia
- Arteriovenous fistula
- Bleeding (ecchymosis, epistaxis, hematoma)
- Deformities and deviation
- Epiphora
- Infection (cellulitis, abscess, granulomas, toxic shock syndrome)
- Intracranial injury
- Nasal airway obstruction (external valve collapse, internal valve collapse, septal deviation, synechiae, vestibular stenosis)
- Nasal cyst formation
- Nasolacrimal apparatus injury
- Prolonged edema
- Scarring
- Septal perforation

Prognosis

Several studies have attempted to assess the impact of rhinoplasty on the patient's quality of life.[123] Rhinoplasty has been reported to improve the quality of life significantly for patients following this procedure regardless of whether the indication was cosmetic or posttraumatic.[124]

Complications

The reported incidence of significant complications following rhinoplasty ranges from 1.7 to 18%.[125–129] Common complications following rhinoplasty include bleeding, infection, prolonged edema, deformities and deviation, and nasal airway obstruction *(Box 18.4)*.[109]

Bleeding

Patients who are at risk for bleeding complications include those with hypertension, a family history of bleeding diatheses, and those taking aspirin and other nonsteroidal anti-inflammatories. Hypertension should be well controlled perioperatively. Patients should be instructed about which antihypertensive medications to take on the morning of surgery. There should be good communication with the anesthesia provider regarding intraoperative blood pressure control. Patients with intraoperative hypertension may benefit from placement of a Catapress-TTS-2 (0.2 mg clonidine transdermal therapeutic system) (Boehringer Ingelheim Pharmaceuticals, Ridgefield, CT) for prevention of transient postoperative hypertension. Patients with a family history of bleeding diatheses should have preoperative laboratory investigations that may include prothrombin time, partial thromboplastin time, and platelet count. Aspirin and other nonsteroidal anti-inflammatories should be stopped 10 days prior to surgery and avoided for 2 weeks after.

Epistaxis is one of the most common complications following rhinoplasty.[130] It is usually mild and originates from the incisions or areas of mucosal trauma. Head elevation greater than 60°, oxymetazoline nasal spray into the affected nostril, and gentle pressure for 15 minutes are usually enough to stop any mild epistaxis. These measures may be attempted twice by the patient; however if bleeding persists, the patient should be seen immediately. Oxymetazoline nasal spray may be used again and anterior nasal packing with saline-moistened ribbon gauze or Surgicel (Ethicon, San Angelo, TX) lubricated with antistaphylococcal antibiotic ointment should be gently placed in the affected nostril. If bleeding continues, the Doyle splints should be removed and the nasal cavity should be irrigated with saline and suctioned to remove blood clots and crusting to allow identification of the origin of the bleeding. Silver nitrate can be used to cauterize the offending area, followed by anterior nasal packing. If bleeding remains refractory, posterior nasal packing should be considered along with hospital admission for observation. In less than 1% of patients, major epistaxis occurs and should be addressed in the operating room with exploration and cauterization. Inferior turbinate resection is usually the source. If all of the above measures fail, consultation for angiographic embolization should be obtained.

Hematoma is another common bleeding complication following rhinoplasty. Regardless of the location, all hematomas should be drained following rhinoplasty. Hematomas deep to the skin will cause fibrosis leading to scarring and contour deformities affecting the final nasal appearance. Septal hematomas can create septal perforations or necrosis of septal cartilage leading to a saddle-nose deformitiy. A septal hematoma appears as an ecchymotic septal mass that resembles a "blackberry" on physical examination. Hematomas can usually be drained in the office with appropriate lighting. Following drainage, the area should be packed with ¼-inch (0.6-cm) ribbon gauze to prevent recurrence. This should be removed the following day and the area should be reinspected.

Infection

Although infections are rare following rhinoplasty, diligent physical examination to identify early signs of infection allows early initiation of treatment to prevent serious complications such as tissue necrosis, toxic shock syndrome, and cavernous sinus thrombosis. In the event of an infection, internal nasal splints or packing may need to be removed.

Mild cellulitis usually responds to cephalosporins. If infection has developed where a course of postoperative prophylactic antibiotics has been prescribed, treatment with a different antibiotic such as a fluoroquinolone should be started. In the event that cellulitis is refractory to these antibiotics, consideration of methicillin-resistant *Staphylococcus aureus* should be given and empirical antibiotic treatment with levofloxacin, sulfamethoxazole/trimethoprim, or minocycline should be started based on local antibiotic resistance patterns. In cases of severe cellulitis, the patient may need to be admitted for intravenous antibiotics. Abscesses are usually found at the nasal dorsum, nasal tip, and the septum. Any abscess identified should be drained and irrigated, and purulent material should be cultured to guide antibiotic therapy.

Toxic shock syndrome has been described after rhinoplasty with the use of both nasal packing[131,132] and internal nasal splints.[133] It is an acute, multisystem disease caused by release of exotoxins from *Staphylococcus aureus* or *Streptococcus pyogenes* causing excessive activation of inflammatory cells and release of inflammatory cytokines, often resulting in tissue damage and organ dysfunction.[134] Patients can present with fever, a diffuse macular erythroderma rash, desquamation, nausea, vomiting, diarrhea, tachycardia, and hypotension.[134] Removal of nasal packing or internal nasal splints, administration of intravenous antibiotics, supportive care, and intensive care unit monitoring are indicated in this rare event.

Prolonged edema

Soft-tissue edema in the early postoperative period is largely prevented by preoperative patient education about postoperative care and recovery, perioperative corticosteroid use, head elevation, taping, and application of cold compresses. Most edema will resolve within 4 weeks.

Late soft-tissue edema persists several months to more than a year postoperatively and represents scar remodeling. It can be seen in situations such as secondary rhinoplasty or patients with thick skin. Patients should be reassured that it will resolve on its own. In certain circumstances where excessive scarring threatens to cause loss of definition, such as in the supratip area or radix, corticosteroid injection may be indicated to decrease the production of scar tissue.[109] Triamcinolone acetate 3–5 mg (10 mg/mL) mixed with 2% lidocaine in a 1:1 ratio is injected into the supratip area with a 27-gauge needle. Care is taken to avoid superficial injection that can lead to dermal atrophy resulting in contour deformities and visibility of the underlying osseocartilaginous framework or hypopigmentation. Depending on the clinical scenario, injections may be administered as early as 1 week postoperatively and repeated at 4- and 8-week intervals.

Deformities and deviation

Deformities may be identified in the postoperative period. Mild deformities should be observed. If they persist beyond 1 year, surgical treatment is required. Significant deformities should be corrected as soon as they are identified to avoid patient dissatisfaction.

Deviations are managed similarly to deformities. Mild deviation may be corrected using nasal molding techniques.[130] The patient is instructed to apply controlled pressure using his/her thumb along the nasal side wall 3–4 times per day for 4–6 weeks postoperatively. If the deviation is significant or persistent beyond 1 year, surgical treatment is required.

Nasal airway obstruction

Following rhinoplasty, most patients experience transient nasal airway obstruction secondary to edema. This typically resolves over 2–3 weeks as edema subsides. When nasal airway obstruction persists after 3 weeks, internal nasal examination using a topical vasoconstrictor should be performed to identify the cause. If it is secondary to edema, nasal decongestants can be used but topical vasoconstrictors should not be used for more than 7 days because of rebound congestion following cessation of these medications. If an anatomical cause of obstruction is identified, such as internal nasal valve collapse or synechiae, surgical treatment will be required but should be delayed for at least 1 year to allow for complete resolution of edema and maturation of scar tissue.

Secondary procedures

Although it is difficult to determine an exact revision rate following primary open rhinoplasty, a recent survey of plastic surgeons and otolaryngologists revealed that 58% of those surveyed cited their revision rate less than 5% while another 33% reported their revision rate between 6 and 10%.[135] This survey also revealed that the open approach was preferred by 73%, compared with 20% preferring the closed approach for revision rhinoplasty. Revision or secondary rhinoplasty poses a significant challenge due to the complex nature of the problems causing the anatomical deformity or functional abnormality, alteration of native nasal anatomy, presence of scarring, and depletion of autogenous cartilage needed for grafting. Secondary rhinoplasty is covered in detail in Chapter 21.

 Bonus images for this chapter can be found online at **http://www.expertconsult.com**

Fig. 18.1 Patient information sheet and informed consent for rhinoplasty.

Access the complete references list online at **http://www.expertconsult.com**

2. Rohrich RJ, Ahmad J. Rhinoplasty. *Plast Reconstr Surg.* 2011;128:49e–73e.

16. Howard BK, Rohrich RJ. Understanding the nasal airway: principles and practice. *Plast Reconstr Surg.* 2002;109:1128–1146.

19. Rohrich RJ, Janis JE, Kenkel JM. Male rhinoplasty. *Plast Reconstr Surg.* 2003;112:1071–1085.

34. Rohrich RJ, Muzaffar AR, Janis JE. Component dorsal hump reduction: the importance of maintaining dorsal aesthetic lines in rhinoplasty. *Plast Reconstr Surg.* 2004;114:1298–1308.

   Dorsal hump reduction may result in dorsal irregularities caused by uneven resection, overresection or underresection of the osseocartilaginous hump, the inverted-V deformity, excessive narrowing of the midvault, and collapse of the internal valve. The authors present a technique for component dorsal hump reduction that allows a graduated approach to the correction of the nasal dorsum by emphasizing the integrity of the upper lateral cartilages when performing dorsal reduction.

38. Rohrich RJ, Gunter JP, Deuber MA, et al. The deviated nose: optimizing results using a simplified classification and algorithmic approach. *Plast Reconstr Surg.* 2002;110:1509–1523.

   The deviated nose frequently causes both functional and aesthetic problems. The authors present a classification and approach to the deviated nose that relies on accurate preoperative planning and precise intraoperative execution of corrective measures to return the nasal dorsum to midline, restore dorsal aesthetic lines, and maintain airway patency. An operative algorithm is described that emphasizes simplicity and reproducibility.

39. Gunter JP, Rohrich RJ. Management of the deviated nose: the importance of septal reconstruction. *Clin Plast Surg.* 1988;15:43–55.

60. Gunter JP, Landecker A, Cochran CS. Frequently used grafts in rhinoplasty: nomenclature and analysis. *Plast Reconstr Surg.* 2006;118:14e–29e.

68. Ghavami A, Janis JE, Acikel C, et al. Tip shaping in primary rhinoplasty: an algorithmic approach. *Plast Reconstr Surg.* 2008;122:1229–1241.

   Underprojection and lack of tip definition often coexist. Techniques that improve both nasal tip refinement and projection are closely interrelated. The authors present a simplified algorithmic approach to creating aesthetic nasal tip shape and projection in primary rhinoplasty to aid the rhinoplasty surgeon in reducing the inherent unpredictability of combined techniques and improving long-term aesthetic outcomes.

75. Rohrich RJ, Raniere J Jr, Ha RY. The alar contour graft: correction and prevention of alar rim deformities in rhinoplasty. *Plast Reconstr Surg.* 2002;109:2495–2505.

   Deformity of the alar rim is a common problem after primary and secondary rhinoplasty. It is caused by congenital malposition, hypoplasia, or surgical weakening of the lateral crura, with the potential for both functional and aesthetic consequences. The authors describe the use of the alar contour graft to provide the foundation for the re-establishment of a normally functioning external nasal valve and an aesthetically pleasing alar contour.

83. Rohrich RJ, Krueger JK, Adams WP Jr, et al. Achieving consistency in the lateral nasal osteotomy during rhinoplasty: an external perforated technique. *Plast Reconstr Surg.* 2001;108:2122–2130.

   The lateral nasal osteotomy is an integral element in rhinoplasty. The authors present a reproducible and predictable technique for the lateral nasal osteotomy and discuss the role of the external perforated osteotomy technique in reproducing consistent results in rhinoplasty with minimal postoperative complications.

108. Rohrich RJ, Muzaffar AR. Rhinoplasty in the African-American patient. *Plast Reconstr Surg.* 2003;111: 1322–1339.

Closed technique rhinoplasty

Mark B. Constantian

SYNOPSIS

The author's system of thinking about and performing rhinoplasty can be summarized by the following principles:

- Nature is predictable – therefore nasal phenomenology can be understood.
- Rhinoplasty has consistent "behavioral" rules, like all surgery – therefore the surgeon can control the result.
- Nasal deformities are not limitless or lawless but follow patterns – therefore their solutions follow patterns.
- Sequential intraoperative photography teaches nasal behavior and structural interactions.
- Follow the technical rules that apply to all other surgery: limit dissection, morbidity, and tension on closure.
- Reconstruct anatomically.
- Never forget function.
- Never forget the patient's own aesthetic.
- Remember that most problems are under the surgeon's control.
- Always follow your patients closely.

Introduction

Rhinoplasty is uniquely difficult and uniquely rewarding surgery. The very fact that surgeons calculate and publish their nasal surgery revision rates (a practice uncommon in other aesthetic procedures) distinguishes the diminutive "nose job" as an operation that can accomplish harm as well as good, producing favorable or highly unfavorable results. Some excellent surgeons stop performing rhinoplasty, with great relief; others abandon it early in their careers after unsuccessful attempts to produce the desired results. This need not be the case. The goal of this chapter is to outline a system of understanding and treating nasal deformities that is based on functional analysis, knowledge of critical anatomical variants, soft tissue and skeletal behavior, and careful, logical surgical technique.

The anatomy and science necessary for surgical success

Why rhinoplasty is difficult

The advocates of the open approach argue that rhinoplasty (especially endonasal rhinoplasty) is difficult because the surgeon does not have good binocular vision through small incisions, the dissection is blind, the anatomy is complex, and the operation is technically difficult.

There is a small amount of truth in each of those statements – but the same can be said of many plastic surgical operations. Actually, rhinoplasty is primarily difficult because the nasal soft tissues have limited contractility; the nasal regions are structurally and functionally interrelated, not independent; the operation is dynamic and interactive; and because rhinoplasty is a right brain operation.

Modern rhinoplasty is not simply the reduction rhinoplasty model to which grafts have been added; viewed only in that way, current techniques will seem unnecessarily convoluted. Instead, a new rhinoplasty paradigm has emerged in which nasal skin is recognized to be more fixed than variable; in which aesthetics, proportion, and function depend on structural interdependencies and skeletal balance; and in which rhinoplasty therefore becomes an operation of reduction, augmentation, and equilibration. In turn, the new paradigm has widened the spectrum of surgical problems that may be solved. Rhinoplasty remains difficult, but becomes easier when viewed in the context of a model that considers both function and aesthetics and prescribes techniques that effectively modify them together.

Rhinoplasty as a right brain operation

Rhinoplasty is probably the most right-brain operation that plastic surgeons perform.[1] Unfortunately, our educational system cultivates the verbal, rational, analytical, and numerical left side of the brain, tending to ignore the right side. This is one of the reasons that most adults draw with the same level of sophistication that they possessed as a 10-year-old child, which is, not coincidentally, the age at which the left brain becomes dominant. The ease with which surgeons can perform rhinoplasty correlates directly with the facility with which they can deliberately involve right-brain function.

The most attractive noses in nature do not look assembled but unified as a whole, in which every part seems to belong. This principle should also apply to rhinoplasty results. The beauty of the assembled result, the finished surgical product, depends on the ability to see the preoperative excesses and deficiencies in shape and proportion as they really are, with no preconceptions; balance them against the patient's surgical goals; and from those accurate observations create an effective surgical plan. The most direct means to this kind of analysis involves significant right-brain contributions. Right brain function can be cultivated[2] by analytic exercises and by studying silhouettes of patient profiles.[1]

Equilibrium and balance

The fact that many post-rhinoplasty nasal configurations, and all "end-stage" noses, look the same, is not a coincidence. The response of any nasal skeleton and its investing soft tissues to reduction is not idiosyncratic but consistent and therefore predictable.[3,4] These forces collapse the upper nose caudally and medially over the pyramidal bony and upper cartilaginous vaults, cephalad at the columella, posteriorly over the maxillary arch, and posteriorly and concentrically around the tip lobule (*Fig. 19.1*). Whether the nasal skeleton has been reduced by surgery, trauma, congenital anomalies, or Wegener's granulomatosis, the essential external appearance remains the same. Variations occur because of disequilibrium between skeletal and soft tissue volumes or differences in soft tissue thickness and elasticity, not because biologic forces differ from patient to patient.

If the reaction of the nose to reduction rhinoplasty is not idiosyncratic but predictable, it follows that the surgeon who

can predict the nasal response to certain interventions can control the result. Useful here is the concept of a dynamic equilibrium,[3] in which preoperative nasal shape represents not a static structure but rather a dynamic equilibrium, the sum of balanced, opposing forces between the nasal soft tissues and their underlying support. At the start of a rhinoplasty, the nose is equilibrated. Skeletal reduction during rhinoplasty disrupts this preoperative skeletal and soft tissue equilibrium; the nose in disequilibrium at the conclusion of a rhinoplasty cannot remain the same. Soft tissue and skeletal contraction occurs until the nose re-establishes its internal equilibrium or until contraction can no longer occur. The degree of disequilibrium at the end of the procedure thus determines the amount of redraping and contraction that will occur postoperatively: the bigger the disequilibrium, the bigger the postoperative surprise. The surgeon therefore ideally controls the postoperative equilibrium by permitting soft tissue contraction only where it is most predictable (e.g., over the bony and cartilaginous dorsa) and by minimizing contraction where it is less predictable (e.g., the lower nasal third). In doing so, the surgeon immediately gains a powerful tool for influencing postoperative nasal contour.

The structural nasal layers

In understanding structural nasal interrelationships, it is helpful to conceptualize the nose as a system of two interrelated layers (*Fig. 19.2*). The outer layer, like a soft, elastic sleeve, slides over the inner semi-rigid layer and contains the entire investing nasal soft tissues plus the alar cartilages and their associated lining. The inner layer contains everything else (the bony and upper cartilaginous vaults, the nasal septum, and their associated linings). This two-layer concept associates those structures that behave together anatomically and functionally, and provides an explanation for the "global" manifestations of some surgical changes (e.g., the effect of dorsal reduction or augmentation on nasal length).[5]

Upper cartilaginous vaults

The width and stability of the upper cartilaginous vault (formed by the upper lateral cartilages and the anterior septal edge), the critical area of the internal nasal valves, depend not only on the width of the bony vault but also on the height and width of the middle vault roof.[6] Resection of the middle vault roof during hump reduction removes this most critical anterior stabilizing force on the upper lateral cartilages, which will fall medially and produce a characteristic "inverted V" deformity and consequent narrowing at the internal valves.[7] Middle vault collapse virtually always occurs when the cartilaginous roof has been resected, whether or not osteotomy has been performed, but may not be visible if the overlying soft tissues are sufficiently thick; when the nasal skin is thin, the deformity can be impressive (*Fig. 19.3*). To avoid middle vault collapse and internal valvular incompetence, the surgeon should plan to reconstruct the normal distracting forces by a substantial dorsal graft or by spreader grafts,[8,9] which provide the same degree of functional mean nasal airflow improvement (see below).

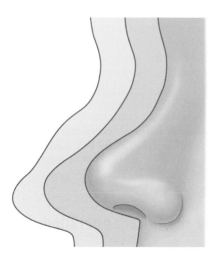

Fig. 19.1 The pattern of soft tissue contraction after skeletal reduction, the end stage of which is supratip deformity.

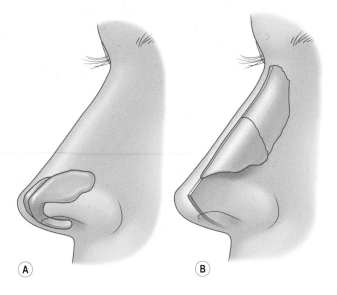

Fig. 19.2 The structural layers of the nose, which separate those anatomical units that move together. The investing soft tissues and alar cartilages glide over the inner, fixed, semirigid layer, which contains the bony vault, the upper cartilaginous vault, and the nasal septum.

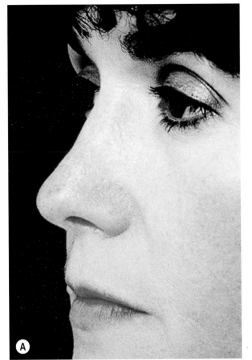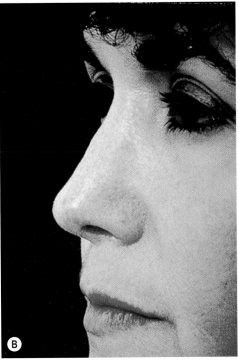

Fig. 19.3 The characteristic appearance caused by resection of the roof of the middle vault, which produces the so-called inverted V deformity and internal valvular incompetence. The most effective corrections are spreader or dorsal grafts. (From Constantian MB. The middorsal notch: an intraoperative guide to overresection in secondary rhinoplasty. Plast Reconstr Surg. 1993; 91:477.)

Middle and lower cartilaginous vaults

The upper lateral cartilages are supported caudally by their relationship to the cephalic margins of the lateral crura in the region of the so-called 'scroll'; radical alar cartilage resection can compromise middle vault support and may leave an external deformity typified by deepening and lengthening of the alar creases. Resect the upper lateral cartilages submucosally only when failure to do so would allow them to prolapse into the airway or when necessary to shorten the nose.

The point of intersection of the upper and lower lateral cartilages creates the "watershed" area between the internal and external nasal valves, and aggressive surgery in this area also affects external valvular competence, particularly in patients whose alar cartilage lateral crura are cephalically rotated.[9,10] Compared with caudal support of the upper lateral cartilages, however, anterior support provided by the intact cartilaginous roof is more profound and more critical to airway function.

Dorsum and tip

Tip projection, that is, the intrinsic ability of the alar cartilages to support the tip lobule independent of dorsal height,

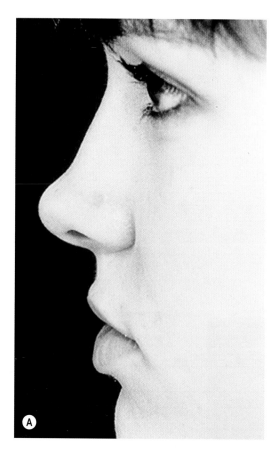
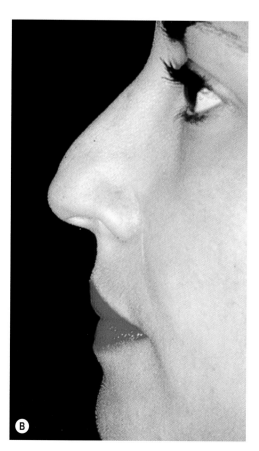

Fig. 19.4 Examples of adequate **(A)** and inadequate **(B)** tip projection, which can be defined by the relationship of the alar cartilages to the septal angle. (B from Constantian MB. Distant effects of dorsal and tip grafting in rhinoplasty. Plast Reconstr Surg. 1992; 90:405.)

depends on alar cartilage middle crural size, shape, and substance *(Fig. 19.4)*. Tip projection extremes are the easiest to identify. The nasal tip in *Figure 19.4A* depends not on bridge height but on intrinsic alar cartilage strength and projection. Conversely, the nasal tip in *Figure 19.4B* is partially dependent on bridge height; therefore, tip projection will decrease when the dorsum is resected. It is important to identify inadequate tip projection preoperatively so that its correction can be incorporated in the surgical plan; inadequate tip projection cannot be rendered adequate by bridge resection alone. The tip, the lower nasal skin, and in many patients nearly the lower half of the profile line depend on suspension of the skin sleeve by the alar cartilages, which, like a "cap" anterior to the remaining skeleton, maintain lower nasal tension. The alar cartilages carry a larger responsibility for caudal nasal support than may at first be evident.

Four common anatomic variants that predispose to unfavorable results

A great deal can be learned about primary rhinoplasty by observing the deformities of secondary rhinoplasty patients seen in consultation and by examining one's own unsatisfactory results. A retrospective study of 150 consecutive secondary rhinoplasty and 50 primary rhinoplasty patients suggests that only four anatomic variants in the primary nose

particularly predispose to unfavorable rhinoplasty results: low radix/low dorsum, narrow middle vault, inadequate tip projection, and alar cartilage malposition.[11]

Low radix or low dorsum

Low radix or low dorsum begins caudal to the level of the upper lash margin with the patient's eyes in primary gaze; this variant was present in 93% of the secondary patients and 32% of the primary patients in the series.[11] First described by Sheen, the low radix is one of several primary causes of nasal imbalance: an upper nose that seems too small for its lower nasal component.[12] When the radix begins lower than the upper lash margin, dorsal length is therefore shorter and so nasal base size appears larger. The classic imbalance may take the form of the depression or notch in the upper nasal third, or a low, straight dorsum may accompany a large nasal base. Whether or not the patient has a dorsal convexity, the surgeon often hears the same complaint: "The tip of my nose sticks out too far." The surgical dilemma is as follows: If the surgeon reduces the nasal dorsum, the patient's preoperative skeletal and skin sleeve maldistribution will worsen: the lower nose will appear even larger. The surgeon fortunately has two other choices: either limit tip reduction or raise the dorsum segmentally or entirely to balance the nasal base. Variations of the latter option are generally safer because they require less contraction of the thicker nasal base tissues.

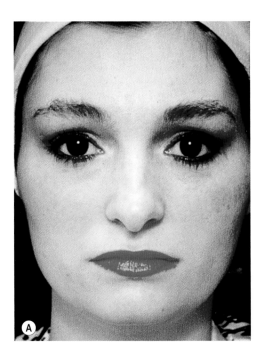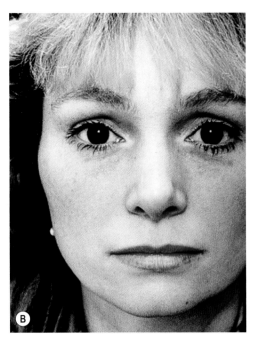

Fig. 19.5 Narrow middle vault treated with spreader grafts. Many of these patients have preoperative internal valvular incompetence and will develop increased airway obstruction after resection of the cartilaginous roof. (From Constantian MB. Experience with a three-point method for planning rhinoplasty. Ann Plast Surg. 1993; 30:1.)

Narrow middle vault

A narrow middle vault *(Fig. 19.5)* is arbitrarily defined as any upper cartilaginous vault that is at least 25% narrower than the upper or lower nasal third (present in 87% of the secondary patients and 38% of the primary patients in this series). This variant was described by Sheen in conjunction with short nasal bones[13] but has been discussed subsequently by that author and others[11,14–16] as a trait that places the patient at special risk for internal valvular obstruction, which can exist preoperatively or may be produced by dorsal resection. Descriptions of valvular collapse had appeared earlier in the rhinoplasty literature[17–19] but the missing puzzle piece had been the link between resection of the cartilaginous roof and postoperative internal valvular collapse, a phenomenon previously attributed to traumatic or surgical avulsion of the upper lateral cartilages from the nasal bones. Resection of even 2 mm of the cartilaginous roof during hump removal ablates the stabilizing confluence that braces the middle vault, 80 which can now collapse toward the anterior septal edge, restricting airflow at the internal valves and producing a characteristic inverted "V deformity". Rhinomanometric studies indicate that valvular obstruction is 4 times more common than pure septal obstruction in primary rhinoplasty patients and 12 times more common in secondary patients; reconstruction of incompetent, internal valves by dorsal or spreader graft doubles nasal airflow in most patients.[8,20]

Inadequate tip projection

A tip with inadequate projection is defined as any tip that does not project to the level of the anterior septal angle. Inadequate tip projection was present in 80% of the secondary patients and 31% of the primary patients in the reported series.[11] Despite its common use and importance, the term "tip projection" has been used to connote different things by different authors. Some surgeons assess tip projection by measuring the distance of the most projecting point of the tip from a facial parameter,[21,22] and others by the relative proportion of the nasal base segments anterior and posterior to the upper lip[23,24] or the relative lengths of the nasal base and upper lip.[25] Although these definitions apply in some cases, there are patients whose nasal bases are large but whose tip cartilages are nevertheless poorly projecting (i.e., reflecting a disproportionate amount of lower nasal skin, rather than excessive cartilage size). In these individuals, tip projection may be inaccurately assessed as "adequate" or even "excessive", even though the alar cartilages still lack the substance required to create a straight bridge line.

An alternative functional definition of tip projection is the relationship of the tip lobule to the anterior septal angle. Alar cartilages sufficiently strong to support the tip to the level of the septal angle are "adequately projecting" *(Fig. 19.4A)*; alar cartilages too weak to do so are "inadequately projecting" *(Fig. 19.4B)*. The practical value of this definition lies in its ability to define treatment: adequately projecting tips do not need increased support, whereas inadequately projecting tips do. Further, by defining tip projection relative to the septal angle, the surgeon can distinguish between two associated but distinct entities: (1) intrinsic anterior supporting strength supplied by the alar cartilages and (2) skin sleeve volume and distribution in the lower nasal third. Inadequately projecting nasal tips often appear to "hang" from the septal angle *(Fig. 19.4B)*. Because an inadequately projecting tip owes its position to dorsal height and not only to tip cartilage support, the surgeon must employ some tip-strengthening method (sutures, struts, or grafts) to create that support. A straight dorsum requires the nasal tip to support itself independent of bridge height; that is, to be adequately projecting. Interestingly, rhinoplasty pioneer Jacques Joseph instinctively solved the problem of inadequate tip resection in his patients by limiting bridge resection and deliberately leaving a dorsal convexity.[26]

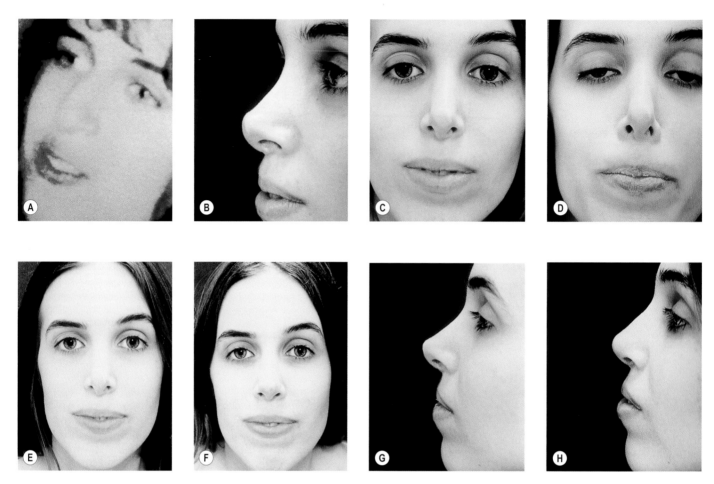

Fig. 19.6 Patient with alar cartilage malposition (as well as low radix, narrow middle vault, and inadequate tip projection) **(A)** preoperatively and **(B)** after primary rhinoplasty. **(C)** Quiet and **(D)** forced inspiration demonstrate incompetence of the internal and external nasal valves. **(E–H)** After dorsal, spreader, tip, and alar wall grafts. Postoperative airflow typically triples or quadruples in such patients.

Alar cartilage malposition

"Alar cartilage malposition" describes cephalically-rotated lateral crura whose long axes run on an axis toward the medial canthi instead of toward the lateral canthi, the position of orthotopic lateral crura *(Fig. 19.6)*. This anatomic variation was first recognized by Sheen[27] as an aesthetic deformity that produced a round or boxy tip lobule with characteristic "parentheses" on frontal view. Initially believed to be a rare variant, malposition is present in approximately 50% of primary patients and 80% of secondary patients.[28] Malposition also has two additional ramifications that are not aesthetic. First, the abnormal cephalic position of the lateral crura places them at special risk if an intercartilaginous incision is made at its normal intranasal location.[10] This maneuver could transect the entire rotated lateral crus instead of only splitting the intended cephalic portion: the entire lateral crus may thus be inadvertently removed. Resected or whole, most malpositioned lateral crura do not provide adequate external valvular support, and so malposition is not only associated with boxy or ball tips but also the leading cause of external valvular incompetence.[20] The secondary deformity is characteristic.

The adequate treatment of cephalic rotation of the lateral crura requires resection and replacement of these structures, relocation of the lateral crura to support the external valves, or supporting the areas of external valvular collapse with autogenous grafts.[29] Prior reports have indicated that approximately 50% of patients presenting with external valvular obstruction have alar cartilage malposition. Correction of external valvular incompetence doubles mean nasal airflow in most patients (2.5 times for primary patients; 4.0 times for secondary patients).[8]

None of these four anatomical variants (low radix or low dorsum, narrow middle vault, inadequate tip projection, and alar cartilage malposition) always requires treatment. For example, the low radix must always be assessed relative to nasal base size: if the base is small, a low radix may create the best balance. But they do supply cautionary notes. At least one of these four anatomic traits was present in each of the 150 secondary patients in the reported series.[11] Some 78% of the secondary patients and 58% of the primary patients had three or all four of the traits. The most common grouping in both primary and secondary patients was the triad of low radix, narrow middle vault, and inadequate tip projection (40% and 28%, respectively) *(Fig. 19.7)*. The second most common grouping was the association of all four anatomic traits (27% of secondary and 28% of primary patients). None

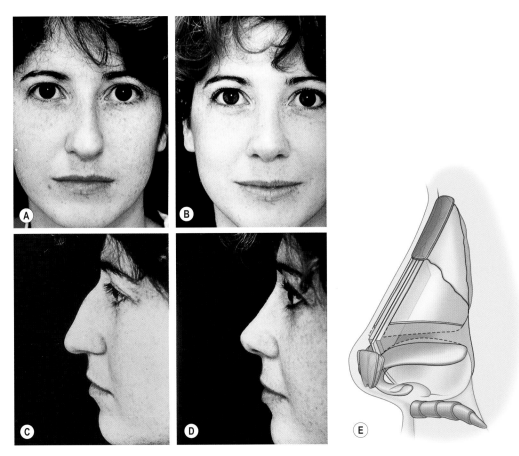

Fig. 19.7 The most common grouping of the four anatomic variants that predispose to unfavourable results; low radix, narrow middle vault, and inadequate tip projection. **(A)** Preoperative view. **(B)** 1 year postoperative frontal. **(C)** Preoperative view and **(D)** 1 year postoperative oblique view (now symmetric). **(E)** Schematic of the surgical correction, involving dorsal reduction; conservative reductions of the lateral crura and caudal upper lateral cartilages; maxillary augmentation; and radix, spreader, and tip grafts with left unilateral osteotomy. (From Constantian MB. Elaboration of an alternative, segmental, cartilage sparing tip graft technique: experience in 405 cases. Plast Reconstr Surg. 1999; 103:237.)

of these anatomic variants is adequately treated by classic reduction rhinoplasty, emphasizing the importance of careful preoperative diagnosis.

The effect of rhinoplasty on the airway

Traditional concepts and clinical observations

For many years, the following concepts provided the basis for analysis of the obstructed nose:

1. The bony and cartilaginous septal partition, deformed by congenital or traumatic causes, may obstruct the nasal airway.

2. Compensatory hypertrophy of the contralateral inferior turbinate frequently occurs, so that both airways eventually become obstructed.

Although many patients with obstructed nasal airways undoubtedly improve after septoplasty or submucous septal resection with or without inferior turbinectomy, not all do. Adding to the frustration of patient and surgeon are three other common observations: that there is often a poor correlation between a patient's symptoms and the apparent site of clinical septal or turbinate obstruction; [18–21] that patients frequently breathe better (preoperatively and even

postoperatively) on the "narrower" side (ipsilateral to the septal deviation); and that many patients who have undergone prior successful septoplasty and turbinectomy or who have straight, unoperated nasal septa still complain of airway obstruction.

These apparently inconsistent observations are more understandable if the reader considers airway size to be the product of at least four factors: (1) mucosal sensitivity to the environment or hereditary factors; (2) inferior turbinate hypertrophy from many causes; (3) septal deviation; and (4) position and stability of the lateral nasal wall during the dynamic process of ventilation.[8,9,20] Thus, any congenital or acquired weakness or instability of the upper or lower lateral cartilages or their investing soft tissues (which compose the internal and external nasal valves, respectively), along with septal and inferior turbinate size and position, becomes a factor that may profoundly influence the ability to draw adequate volumes of air through the nose.

The internal nasal valve is formed by the articulation of the caudal and anterior (or dorsal) edges of the upper lateral cartilages with the anterior septal edge *(Fig. 19.8)*; the external nasal valve is composed of the cutaneous and skeletal support of the mobile alar wall (the alar cartilage lateral crura with their associated external and vestibular skin coverings). The watershed area between the valves occurs at the transverse portion of the alar crease and at the articulation of the caudal

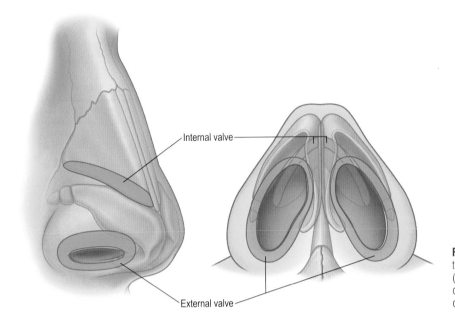

Fig. 19.8 The nasal valves. The internal valves are formed by the articulation of the upper lateral cartilages with the anterior (dorsal) septal edge; the external valves are formed by the alar cartilage lateral crura and their associated investing soft tissue cover.

edge of the upper lateral cartilages with the alar cartilage lateral crura.

Until recently, efforts to correlate nasal airflow with clinical symptoms had yielded equivocal conclusions. There was argument on both clinical and rhinomanometric grounds that septoplasty either did or did not improve nasal airflow.[30–34] For such a commonly and easily diagnosed clinical problem as septal deviation, one would expect to find more unanimity in clinical series. These observations were clouded further by the fact that some 80% of nasal septa in the population at large are "deviated", and by imprecision in distinguishing internal from external valvular incompetence. Nevertheless, mounting clinical evidence indicates that obstruction at either set of valves may profoundly obstruct the airway, even in the absence of septal deviation.[35–58]

Adding to the confusion, is the absence of consensus in the literature about whether rhinoplasty itself impairs airflow, which is surprising in view of the number of patients who have postoperative airway obstruction. In fact, the second most common cause for malpractice litigation after rhinoplasty is unrelieved or new nasal airway obstruction (M. Gorney, pers comm, March 2000).

Results of an airway outcome study in 600 patients

To help resolve some of these conflicting clinical observations and to provide quantitative measurements of the relative increases in nasal airflow after functional septal or valvular surgery, an ongoing study of 600 consecutive patients undergoing surgery for airway obstruction was undertaken between 1991 and 2008.[8,59] Patients with septal perforation, atopic patients, and patients requiring turbinectomy were excluded. The diagnosis of septal obstruction or valvular incompetence was made by observation of the nasal airway and nasal sidewall movement with and without a nasal speculum during quiet and forced inspiration *(Fig. 19.9)*. When a flaccid or collapsible valve was supported during inspiration by a cotton-tipped applicator, the patient could usually appreciate an

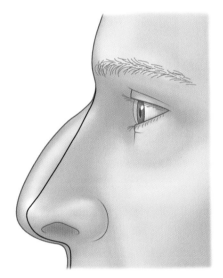

Fig. 19.9 The common "straight line" strategy used to plan rhinoplasty. The assumptions implicit here are that the skin sleeve will contract infinitely and uniformly to any skeletal size and shape, and that dorsal and tip resections will affect only those structures. The ideas are all very logical; they are just not true.

immediate improvement in nasal airflow, thus directing the surgeon toward appropriate operative treatment. Septoplasty and valvular reconstruction by cartilage or bone grafts were performed as indicated. Anterior, active, mask rhinomanometry was performed according to the method of Mertz *et al.*[42,60–62]

That study comprised 600 patients: 78% women and 22% men; 36% primary rhinoplasties and 64% secondary rhinoplasties (median follow-up 14.3 months, mean 27 months). The longer-term data of 362 patients observed for a minimum of 12 months (median 29 months) supported the numbers in the entire group.

The data may be summarized as follows:

1. Overall, septal and valvular surgery corrected the airway obstruction in more than 95% of patients in a single operation.

2. Although septoplasty improved airflow ipsilateral to the obstruction, there was no significant improvement in total (geometric mean) nasal airflow after septoplasty alone.

3. Internal valvular reconstruction by dorsal or spreader grafts doubled nasal airflow.

4. Spreader grafts and dorsal grafts were equally effective in supporting the internal nasal valves.

5. External valvular reconstruction doubled mean nasal airflow.

6. The largest postoperative improvement was seen in patients after correction of both internal and external valvular incompetence (more than four times preoperative values).

7. Septoplasty in addition to valvular reconstruction did not significantly improve nasal airflow over the results obtained by valvular reconstruction alone, even in patients observed more than 100 months postoperatively.

8. These results were produced without performing inferior turbinectomy in any of the patients.

9. In those patients with lateralized symptoms, the septum was contralateral to the more obstructed side in 45% of cases.

10. Of the 384 secondary rhinoplasty patients, 94% had previously undergone an adequate septoplasty but were still symptomatically obstructed. Within this group, valvular reconstruction alone corrected the airway in 97% after one operative procedure.

11. When primary and secondary rhinoplasty patients were stratified, the improvement in primary patients equaled or exceeded the improvement achieved in secondary rhinoplasty patients in six of the eight obstructed sites examined.

12. Valvular obstruction was 4 times more common than pure septal obstruction in primary rhinoplasty patients and 12 times more common than pure septal obstruction in secondary rhinoplasty patients.

13. When the entire 600-patient group was stratified, the greatest improvement was observed in those patients observed more than 12 months, supporting the view that the airway continues to enlarge as edema resolves.

14. By measuring airflow during quiet and forced inspiration, sidewall stiffness could be quantified and shown to increase following valvular reconstruction.

15. A decrease in nasal airflow was not obligatory, even in patients with preoperative airway obstruction.

In conclusion, current rhinomanometric data support the concept that lateral nasal wall movement caudal to the bony arch (containing both the internal and external valves) constitutes a cause of airway obstruction equal to or greater than septal deviation in many rhinoplasty patients. By visualizing the airway as a structure in which the septal partition forms one side and the mobile lateral nasal wall forms the other, and in which the turbinates and mucosa function as additional dynamic structures, the inconsistencies in prior clinical observations become easier to explain. Inspired airflow passes through the nose at 15–65 km/h, the latter equivalent to gale force winds.[63] The size of any nasal airway thus depends not only on the position and configuration of the septum and turbinates but also on the stability and competence of the nasal valves under significant transmural pressures. The observation that patients often breathe worse on the side contralateral to the septal obstruction (45% of our patients with lateralized obstructions) can therefore be explained through valvular incompetence. In patients with septal deviation and valvular incompetence, the side with the greater airflow and greater transmural pressure (i.e., the side contralateral to the septal deviation) will collapse first and therefore become more symptomatic.

This study did not answer the question of where turbinates fit into the hierarchy of nasal obstructions. In atopic individuals with gross turbinate hypertrophy or polyps, turbinectomy is unquestionably valuable.[64] However, the mean nasal airflow improvements listed above were achieved without turbinectomy, even in a population of patients with secondary deformities, valvular incompetence, prior intranasal scars, webs, or vestibular atresia, suggesting that turbinate obstruction in many patients may be largely reactive or secondary and that radical turbinectomy may not often be necessary if septal and valvular factors have been addressed properly.

Resection of nasal lining, alar cartilage malposition, excessive alar wedge resection, and inadequate or excessive nasal shortening may also obstruct the airway.

Patient selection

Fallacies of planning: two false assumptions that lead to unsatisfactory results

Two principles underlie the logic of reduction rhinoplasty, neither of which is always valid:

- FALSE ASSUMPTION NUMBER ONE: *The nasal soft tissue cover has the infinite ability to contract to the shape of any underlying skeleton.*

If the nose is being reduced, the entire surgical result depends on the validity of this assumption. The nasal skin sleeve does contract according to its quality, thickness, and preoperative distribution, but not necessarily to the shape of the surgically reduced skeleton. The vectors of skin sleeve contraction are related to, but independent of, the volume and contour of the underlying skeleton; the end stage of these vectors is the classic shape of supratip deformity *(Fig. 19.1)*. If this assumption was always true, supratip deformity would never occur and augmentation would not correct it.[65]

- FALSE ASSUMPTION NUMBER TWO: *Alterations in the nasal skeleton produce purely regional changes.*

The classic application of this assumption is a preoperative plan in which the surgeon plans to resect all nasal dorsum anterior to a straight line drawn from the nasal radix to the point of the tip *(Fig. 19.9)*. Underlying this strategy is the assumption that dorsal reduction affects bridge height alone.

Changes in the nasal skeleton are not independent, however, but rather have global effects outside their areas. Resection of the nasal bridge affects nasal width and length, apparent nasal base size, middle vault support, alar rim contour, and columellar position. Similarly, alar cartilage reduction can affect tip support and projection, nasal length, alar rim contour, and external valvular support. These structural interdependencies are not just regional. Recognizing them is necessary to preoperative planning, interpretation of intraoperative nasal appearance, postoperative success, and the correction of secondary deformities.

The interview

Although rhinoplasty presents unique difficulties for the surgeon, it is difficult for the patients as well. Those surgeons who have seen secondary rhinoplasty candidates devastated by the results of one or more prior operations should immediately recognize the importance of a safe and biologically sound surgical plan and of an accurate understanding between patient and surgeon of the aesthetic goals and the realities of the surgical problem – that is, what is possible and what is not.

Making the interview more difficult is the prevalent misconception that many patients hold about their nasal deformities and therefore about the corrective plan. Many patients do not recognize that a simple nasal reduction may not achieve their goals. Patients without airway obstruction do not appreciate the importance of maintaining nasal function, and most do not realize that an improperly performed rhinoplasty can jeopardize the airway.

The patient must therefore be guided to understand that every rhinoplasty is a compromise between the patient's preferred aesthetic goals and the limitations that a predetermined preoperative skeletal and soft tissue configuration imposes. Donor materials vary in quantity, character, and composition, determining their usefulness.[66] Finally, many preoperative noses already have some desirable features; patient and surgeon should be careful not to destroy them.

It is important to elicit the patient's goals in the greatest possible detail and to prioritize them. Is the major issue bridge height, tip projection, nasal length, asymmetry, or airway? How long has the sense of deformity existed? This latter question is more critical in older than in younger patients: the 60-year-old patient who has disliked her nasal shape for 40 years may tolerate a larger change than will one who has been troubled for only 5 years and who may be noticing only signs of recent aging.

For any patient older than 14 years, the author prefers to interview and examine the patient alone (in minors after parental permission), before involving the family, spouse, or others of significance in the discussion. Although some protective family members or spouses initially object to this policy, it is important to establish an individual relationship with the patient and to hear his or her concerns and complaints free of outside influences. Not surprisingly, it is usually the family members who object most strongly who should most be excluded from the initial consultation, when their presence invariably distracts the patient, and questions to the patient (like some odd ventriloquist act) elicit responses from the family member instead. If, after an adequate explanation, the patient's family will not accept an initial interview with the patient alone (which occasionally happens), their response is a significant sign that should not be overlooked.

When the patient has had prior surgery, it is important to obtain a careful chronology and, if possible, photographs that reflect the preoperative appearance. Such pictures provide information about the prior surgeon's goal and how the current deformities may have occurred and place the patient's original objectives in current perspective. For the younger surgeon, a comparison of preoperative photographs to outcomes is invaluable and teaches an enormous amount about the consistencies and variabilities of nasal skeletal and soft tissue responses to surgery.

Inquire about the airway first to avoid becoming distracted by the patient's aesthetic considerations, which always seem more pressing. Ask about periodic or cyclic airway obstruction; which airway is worse; any history of nasal trauma; seasonal allergies that obstruct the airway; clear rhinitis; episodes of suppurative sinusitis requiring antibiotics; snoring, epistaxis, and sinus headache; and what nonsurgical remedies the patient has previously tried, successfully or unsuccessfully. Not infrequently, secondary rhinoplasty patients with poor airways chronically self-medicate with steroid or vasoconstrictive sprays that must be eliminated before surgery. Also important are the patient's work environment and a history of tobacco or alcohol consumption (either of which may cause nasal congestion) and, more important now than in previous years, cocaine use. Finally, inquire about any nasal areas that the patient does not wish altered and, if appropriate, whether a change in ethnic appearance is desired.

Differences in primary and secondary candidates

Primary and secondary rhinoplasty patients differ in three characteristic ways. First, the secondary patient's scarred, contracted soft tissues will not tolerate aggressive dissection, multiple incisions, or tight dressings. Second, graft donor sites may have already been harvested, necessitating the use of more difficult (distorted septum or concha), painful (costal), or frightening (calvarial) donor sources. Third, the secondary rhinoplasty patient's morale is often more fragile. Having already invested money, time, discomfort, and emotion in one or more unsuccessful procedures, what secondary rhinoplasty patients fear most and need least are additional disappointments. The surgeon should be careful to construct a plan that is based on a clear understanding of what is possible and founded on sound surgical and biologic principles that maximize the airway and respect the patient's aesthetic goals.[67]

The preoperative examination

It is wise to make a habit of examining the internal nose first, so that this most critical functional area is not forgotten in the discussion of aesthetics. Patients are always grateful to breathe well, even when an inadequate airway is not a prominent preoperative complaint; patients who breathe poorly may be unaware of their obstructions. The surgeon must avoid unintentionally decreasing postoperative nasal function; this occurs more often than is often recognized and poor airways frequently dominate the complaints of secondary rhinoplasty patients. The internal nose should be examined without manipulating the airway by asking the patient to breathe deeply and observing areas of collapse or asymmetry in the nasal sidewalls, high septal deviations, distortion of the columella, protrusion of the caudal septum, or alar rim collapse.

Valves

Sidewall collapse with inspiration at one or both of the nasal valves is surprisingly common. It is important to determine why valvular incompetence exists (e.g., prior surgery, intrinsic weakness, or alar cartilage malposition). If sidewall collapse occurs, occlude one nostril and ask the patient to compare flow through the unobstructed airway with and without supporting the collapsing area with a cotton-tipped applicator soaked in 1% Pontocaine hydrochloride for the patient's comfort. Patients with valvular incompetence will notice an obvious and gratifying increase in airway size. The surgeon may observe valvular collapse and substantial airway obstruction, even in the patient with a straight, unoperated septum and without turbinate hypertrophy. Here, septoplasty may be indicated to harvest grafts but by itself will not open the airway; the surgeon must also place appropriate valvular grafts. Reconstruction of the internal and external valves can triple or quadruple airflow in most rhinoplasty patients, even when septoplasty is not simultaneously performed.[8]

Septum

The septum should be palpated for substance, contour, and mucosal cover (indicating the sequelae of allergy, injury, perforation, or chronic cocaine use). It is also important to assess whether a "high" (i.e., toward the anterior edge) septal deviation exists; because hump removal can unmask a high septal curvature, the surgeon should be prepared to camouflage or correct the septal deflection with unilateral or asymmetrically thick spreader grafts.[14,68]

Turbinates

Although the turbinates are time-honored causes of airway obstruction and affect the airways of atopic patients or patients with chronic, severe septal deflection (in which the turbinate contralateral to the septal deviation hypertrophies), clinical and rhinomanometric data indicate that obstructing turbinates are relatively low in the hierarchy of common airway obstruction causes in primary and secondary patients. Because turbinates warm and humidify inspired air, the surgeon should plan conservative resections even in atopic patients. Furthermore, histologic studies have shown that turbinate hypertrophy secondary to septal deviation is characterized by bony, not mucosal overgrowth.[69] Therefore, most patients who have had good septal and valvular reconstruction can be adequately treated by only turbinate crushing and outfracture (or no treatment at all).[70]

External nose

Palpation of the external nose provides important information about cartilaginous size and substance, bony vault length, nasal sidewall stiffness (another assessment of valvular support), and soft tissue thickness. Tip lobular contour is

considered, as is the balance between nasal base size and bridge height (see below). The patient is asked to discuss each nasal area, whether or not it has been mentioned previously: width, length, bridge contour, tip shape, nostril size, columellar and upper lip position, and any asymmetries.

Basic nasal aesthetics

On frontal view, the upper nose should be narrower than the lower nose; symmetric, confluent, divergent lines should connect the two. On oblique view, there should be no regional discontinuities, the supratip should be flat, and tip lobular mass should fall below the levels of the peaks of the alar cartilage domes. On lateral and oblique views, nasal length and base size should balance each other. Ideal parameters have been suggested.[71–75] The practical difficulty in employing many of these guidelines lies largely in the facts that skin sleeve volume and distribution have already been predetermined and that skin contractility is limited, not infinite. Furthermore, ideal aesthetics do not apply to most patients, even most Caucasians.[75] If the surgeon had the latitude of reducing skin volume, the size of the postoperative nose could be altered more radically to a patient's facial measurements, body habitus, or other parameters. In practice, however, the surgeon works within narrower limits. The airway should be patent and stable on forced inspiration. Beyond these basics, the details depend on the patient's skeletal framework and soft tissue cover and his or her aesthetic goals. Rhinoplasty offers, as much as or more than any other aesthetic procedure, the possibility of individualizing an aesthetic goal.

Preoperative photographs

For consultation, formulation of an operative plan, and intraoperative guidance, good photographs are imperative. The patient's photographs should be available before the immediate preoperative visit so that the operative plan on which surgeon and patient have already agreed may be reviewed or modified. Photographs should include full head and close-up frontal views, both oblique views (which often differ, particularly in patients with nasal asymmetry), both lateral views, and an inferior view. Photographs are best taken with a portrait focal length lens (90–105 mm) against a medium–dark background, lit so that symmetries and contours will be depicted accurately. Camera-mounted flash units are inferior to studio systems with umbrella lights or wall-mounted strobes to provide backlighting and to illuminate the face and hair.

Setting goals with the patient

Because practical rhinoplasty strategies may differ from what patients imagine, the patient must understand the logic of the surgeon's plan and prefer it to other reasonable alternatives. Unless the surgeon plans only to reduce the nose, he or she must help the patient understand the benefits of equilibrium or conservative reduction; to this end, words like "balance" and "proportion" often serve better than terms that signify only size. It is best to be specific about the plan down to the last graft and choice of donor sites; this candor places patient and surgeon on the same side of the problem and also ensures that minor postoperative imperfections are more likely to be tolerated by the patient, who understood the necessity of each surgical maneuver beforehand. Recognizing the rationale for grafting is more difficult for primary than for secondary patients; the latter, who have already seen the effects of reduction and disequilibrium on their nasal configurations and airways, are often easier to convince.

Discussion of potential complications and revisions

Patient and surgeon alike must remember that revisions may be necessary, almost predictable, in some difficult configurations if the best possible result is desired. Revisions are frequently minor, but all patients should understand preoperatively what cannot be predicted and therefore not mistake the uncontrollable for the uncontrolled. The patient must know preoperatively that no revision should be undertaken until the end of the first postoperative year. Resolution of swelling and stabilization of the final appearance take at least that long in the primary nose and often longer in patients undergoing secondary rhinoplasty; during that time, irregularities, asymmetries, or poor contours that initially appear to require revision may improve sufficiently without surgery. Nothing should be done until healing is complete. The surgeon should control every possible variable.

Who should perform the revision? To some degree, the answer depends on the same factors involved in the prior rhinoplasty. The surgeon's model and proposed solution should be clear, and the patient's goals reasonable; patient and surgeon must understand each other explicitly. Each operation is geometrically more difficult than the last.

Parameters of rhinoplasty planning

What limits the applicability of most proposed aesthetic ideals is the character, volume, and distribution of the skin sleeve and the limitations that they impose. Three soft tissue parameters can be used to form any rhinoplasty plan,[76,77] and they will therefore apply to both primary and secondary patients.

Skin thickness and distribution

It may be intuitively obvious that skin thickness affects any rhinoplasty plan, but so also does skin distribution. The preoperative large nasal base does not contract into a small nasal base; rather, it contracts to a distorted large nasal base. Skin quality therefore affects both reduction and augmentation. Thicker skin requires more skeletal support and contracts less well; the surgeon must thus be conservative in reduction and will need more substantial grafts to produce a given result (*Fig. 19.10A,B*). Thinner skin allows greater reduction but requires softer grafts to avoid surface distortions (*Fig. 19.10C,D*).

Tip lobular contour

Because the nasal base (the lower nasal third) has a more complex topography than the simpler pyramidal bony and upper cartilaginous vaults, and because the soft tissues are always thicker in the caudal than in the cephalic nose, it follows that the surgeon should select first those maneuvers that provide the best nasal base contours. Ideal tip aesthetics (*Fig. 19.11A*) require a defined point of greatest projection, a flat supratip, and a tip lobular mass that falls below the point of greatest projection. The poorly shaped tip lobule has the opposite characteristics: a poorly defined, low point of greatest tip projection, a convex supratip, and a tip lobular mass that lies cephalad to the point of greatest projection (*Fig. 19.11B*).

Tip lobular contour is important for two reasons. Simple alar cartilage reduction cannot raise the level of the alar dome peaks or redistribute tip lobular mass but instead only produces a smaller replica of the same preoperative tip. To create an aesthetic lobule from a poorly shaped configuration, the surgeon must raise the level of greatest projection and increase

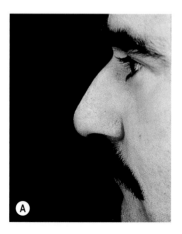
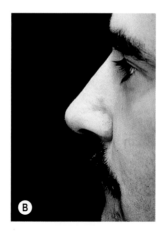
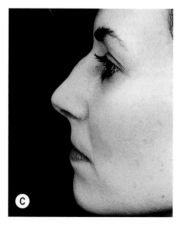
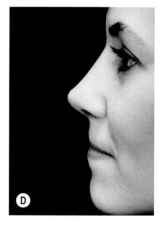

Fig. 19.10 (A,B) Patients with thick nasal skin; skeletal reduction must be more conservative and augmentations more substantial to provide a given result. **(C,D)** Patients with thin nasal skin. Although more soft tissue contraction can be expected, skeletal irregularities and graft visibility are more likely, and techniques must be altered accordingly.

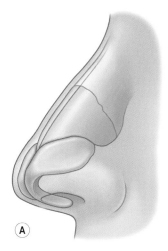 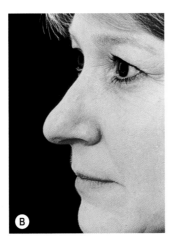 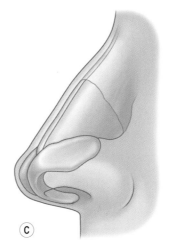 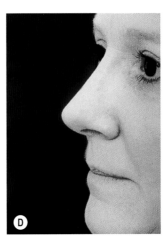

Fig. 19.11 Poorly shaped **(A,B)** tip lobules and well shaped tip lobules **(C,D)**. The poorly shaped tip lobule requires not only a volume change but a configurational change. (B from Constantian MB. Experience with a three-point method for planning rhinoplasty. Ann Plast Surg. 1993; 30:1. D from Constantian MB. Four common anatomic variants that predispose to unfavorable rhinoplasty results: a study based on 150 consecutive secondary rhinoplasties. Plast Reconstr Surg. 2000; 105:316.)

lobular mass caudal to this point, effectively lengthening the middle crural alar cartilage segment. The tip change is one of contour, not only of volume.

The balance between nasal base size and bridge height

Dorsal reduction or augmentation profoundly affects the apparent size of the preoperative nasal base.[77] The higher the dorsum, the smaller the nasal base appears *(Fig. 19.12)*. The reverse is also true: dorsal reduction increases apparent nasal base size. This powerful illusion has its most important practical application in: (1) patients who believe that preoperative nasal base size is excessive, in whom the aesthetic goal may best be reached by a change in balance instead of only size *(Fig. 19.13A,B)*; and (2) patients whose soft tissues are thick, and who therefore may be more successfully treated by the combination of reduction and augmentation *(Fig. 19.13C,D)*, a paradoxical principle that most patients and many surgeons have to see to believe.

Why this author still prefers endonasal rhinoplasty

Endonasal rhinoplasty is an operation designed around changes in the skin surface. The skeleton is only a means to that end. Critical indicators such as skin sleeve movement, balance changes, and the effects of reduction and augmentation all depend on an ability to see the undisturbed nasal surface accurately. This is the anatomy that the patient sees and that determines the success of the surgical result; this is the right-brain part of the operation.

Although not a new operation, open rhinoplasty has enjoyed its resurgence in the past two decades because of the frustration that many surgeons experience in performing the newer rhinoplasty techniques through the endonasal approach. Reinforcing this stimulus is the traditional respect that all surgeons have for anatomy and exposure. The

advocates of open rhinoplasty properly note that binocular vision is possible, that anatomic points obscured by the skin sleeve can be uncovered, that certain techniques can be performed more easily, and that the scar itself is ordinarily imperceptible.

All of these arguments are valid. Open rhinoplasty does, however, impose its own constraints on surgeon and patient. The dissection is slower, and postoperative morbidity may be higher. Poor scars occasionally do occur. Unfortunately, although designed to do so, the open approach has not diminished the incidence or severity of secondary deformities.

These are the common objections, but not necessarily the most important ones. First, by separating columellar skin from the medial crura, the surgeon loses an important component of tip stability and projection, which therefore requires some method (suture fixation or columellar strut) to support the medial crura so that a new nasal tip can be made. The strut can impart rigidity to the columella and increases graft requirements. In primary patients, this consideration may be unimportant, but in secondary patients, whose donor sites are already depleted, every bit of graft material counts. Though incisions are limited, endonasal rhinoplasty is not a blind operation. Most procedures are performed under direct vision with greater access than endoscopic surgery permits. The operative strategy, making skeletal changes through limited incisions and judging progress by feeling the surface, is precisely the same discipline required by suction-assisted lipectomy. Limited pocket dissection minimizes the need for graft fixation and simplifies some procedures. Solid or crushed grafts can be used in ways that would be tedious or impossible by the open approach,[78] although some solutions have been described.[79]

Rhinoplasty is made easier not necessarily by a larger incision but rather by an accurate analysis of the surgical problem and adherence to a strategy that reflects the real biologic processes at work. *Almost all secondary deformities result from inaccurate recognition of anatomic variants, tissue characteristics, or functional/structural interrelationships and almost none occur because the surgeon could not see well.*

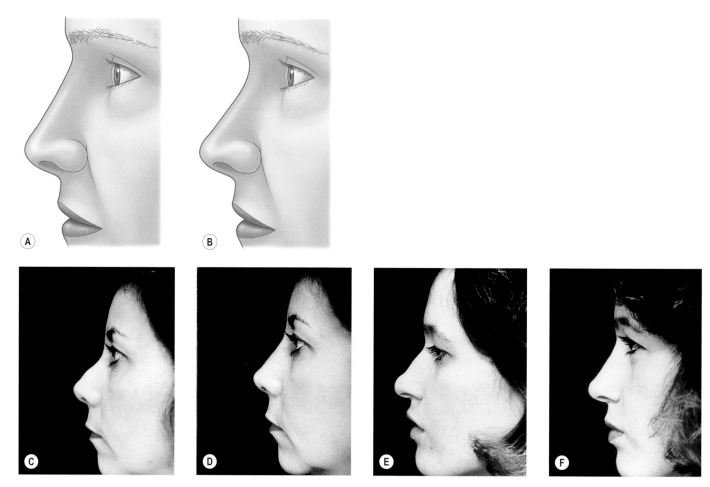

Fig. 19.12 (A,B) The effect of bridge height on apparent nasal base size. Although both nasal bases (lower nasal thirds) are the same size, the nasal base on the right appears larger because the dorsum and nasal root are lower. This illusion provides an important diagnostic and therapeutic tool. **(C–F)** Low radix, in each case, corrected by augmentation. Notice the apparent difference in nasal base size and balance, caused by the alteration in dorsal configuration.

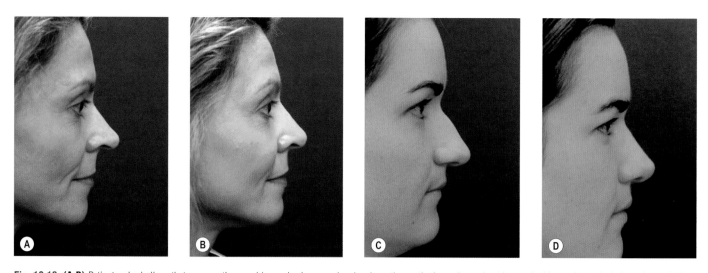

Fig. 19.13 (A,B) Patients who believe that preoperative nasal base size is excessive, in whom the aesthetic goal may best be reached by a change in balance instead of only size, and **(C,D)** patients whose soft tissues are thick, and who therefore may be more successfully treated by the combination of reduction and augmentation, a paradoxical principle that most patients and many surgeons have to see to believe.

The decision to operate

Before agreeing to operate on a patient, the surgeon must be able to answer each of the following questions affirmatively:

1. *Can I see the deformity?* This question eliminates delusional patients or those with minimal defects that may not e surgically correctable.

2. *Can I personally fix it?* This criterion will vary from surgeon to surgeon and must be based on operative experience and ease in correcting specific problems.

3. *Can I manage the patient?* A patient who is unacceptably nervous, impossible to examine, or unwilling to comply with preoperative and postoperative instructions is a poor candidate, even if all other conditions are met.

4. *If there is a complication, will the patient remain controlled and cooperate with treatment?* No patient enjoys a complication, but there are those who, although disappointed, quietly understand and will await the proper time for revision. There are others who become hysterical, angry, disruptive, or accusatory and want an immediate correction. From the author's experience, the personal stress of operating on the latter group and anticipating the outcome if something goes wrong is agonizing. More than that, patients whose emotions are so poorly controlled are in no position to withstand the additional trauma of surgery.

5. *Does the patient accept the margin of error inherent in surgery?* This is the most important criterion. Some patients (and even some surgeons) have unrealistically optimistic opinions about the degree to which any surgeon can control wound healing; the quality and availability of building materials, the patient's immune competence, and the myriad other factors, currently known and unknown, that influence surgical outcomes. The patient's willingness to accept the imperfection that is inherent in surgery is a willingness to accept the imperfection that is inherent in being human.

How to teach yourself rhinoplasty

The following paragraph is from the experience of the author, in the early years of his career.

I recognized early in my career that the rhinoplasty steps that were so neatly drawn in atlases, simply did not apply in the operating room. I soon decided that there had to be a pattern to what I was seeing, but I had no idea what it was or how to recognize it; I needed time to think. I began taking sequential, intraoperative photographs after each critical step, and lateral views at the beginning and end of each of the operations, and silhouettes. Although I no longer take so many intraoperative photographs, at the very least I still photograph the nasal appearance at the beginning and end of every operation, and then at every postoperative visit. Now, after 32 years of practice, these sequences have become the foundation of my rhinoplasty understanding. After surgery, there is ample time to examine each image and decode the feedback that the nose supplies. Each surgeon needs to learn how different augmentations and reductions behave in different noses, and in his/her own hands. Surgeon needs to develop their own judgment; *sequential photographs are the key.*

Surgical technique

Rhinoplasty differs from operations that may be more easily portrayed step-by-step in atlases. Intraoperative feedback is both difficult and unconventional: perspective is limited; skin volume and texture, skeletal structure, and graft material produce constant variations among patients; strategies required for similar deformities differ according to the anatomic details or the patient's desire; and the final postoperative contour depends on soft tissue and skeletal changes and therefore, does not appear immediately. Surgical success will be higher if the surgeon remembers the equilibrium model and therefore interprets the intraoperative nasal appearance as the product of reduction, disequilibrium, augmentation, and skin sleeve movement. This section describes each operative step in the order in which the author ordinarily performs it; depending on the specifics of nasal configuration and surgical plan, some steps may be omitted.

Routine order of surgical steps

The operation is routinely performed under general anesthesia. The patient is placed supine with the arms and legs padded and the knees slightly flexed; the operating table is in 10–15° reverse Trendelenburg position to minimize bleeding. After induction of general anesthesia, the nose is blocked with a freshly prepared solution of 1% lidocaine with epinephrine 1:100 000 (20 mL of 1% lidocaine plus 0.2 mL of epinephrine 1:1000). Infiltration begins at the nasal root, along each lateral nasal wall, into the columella, across the maxillary arch, and into the alar lobules to vasoconstrict the branches of the primary supplying vessels (angular, anterior ethmoidal, superior labial) and the relevant nerves (anterior ethmoidal, infraorbital, infratrochlear). This infiltration usually consumes about 7 mL of the anesthetic solution, the rest of which is saved for the septal surgery. Nasal vibrissae are shaved with a No. 15 blade, and the nose is thoroughly cleansed internally with a povidone–iodine solution. Internal preparation of the nose should be even more fastidious than skin preparation, not the reverse, remembering that the nasal lining is the real operative surface. For hemostasis and anesthesia of the nasopalatine nerve, the internal nasal and posterior nasal branches of the anterior ethmoidal nerve, the internal nasal branch of the nasociliary nerve, and the nasal branch of the anterior superior alveolar nerve, two cotton packs soaked in 4% cocaine solution and squeezed dry with sterile gauze are placed in each airway. Only 4 mL of 4% tinted cocaine solution is made available for each patient (160 mg), safely below the maximum allowable dosage (200 mg). The patient's face is prepared and draped.

Skeletonization

Skeletonization controls access to the underlying structures and also influences skin sleeve movement; by limiting skeletonization, the surgeon can use the undissected soft tissues to immobilize any cartilage grafts. Skeletonize widely over the upper cartilaginous vault to shorten the nose; otherwise limit skeletonization only to those areas that will be changed.

Technical details

The author ordinarily skeletonizes the nose through unilateral or bilateral intracartilaginous incisions *(Fig. 19.14)*, depending on whether alar cartilage modification will be necessary. The incision runs from the lateral end of the caudal reflection of the upper lateral cartilage around the septal angle. With Joseph scissors *(Fig. 19.15)* and then a broad Cottle periosteal elevator, the soft tissues are elevated over the bony and upper cartilaginous vaults only as necessary for access. It is important for the surgeon to obtain smooth elevation of all soft tissues to ensure good cover and avoid dermal injury. If no transfixing incision is necessary, the intercartilaginous incision stops at the junction of the anterior and middle thirds of the membranous septum; if the caudal septum requires shortening, the incision can be carried toward the anterior nasal spine.

Dorsal resection

Producing a straight dorsum from a convex one is not a simple matter. The surgical plan must consider: (1) radix position; (2) dorsal height; and (3) the adequacy of tip support. Dorsal resection can affect nasal length, apparent nasal base size and width, middle vault position, apparent columellar position, and nostril contour. If the radix will be elevated, less dorsal resection is required *(Fig. 19.16)*. Because resection of the bony and cartilaginous vaults alters their dynamic anterior projection, reduced support to the upper nasal skin allows the alar cartilages to rotate cephalad or caudad, depending on the preoperative nasal configuration. Most noses shorten after dorsal resection, but long noses, especially those in which a dorsal convexity has occupied the caudal half, can lengthen after dorsal resection. The surgeon should watch for these intraoperative changes and adjust subsequent steps accordingly. The surgeon must also observe the effect of dorsal resection on middle vault support. If the cartilaginous roof is resected, the middle vault eventually collapses. The surgeon must observe the contour of the middle third to determine the presence of a high septal deviation that may have been masked by a symmetric dorsum or that may have been worsened by dorsal resection. These observations will guide the use of spreader grafts and how they can be used to produce a symmetric result.

Technical details

The author performs the dorsal resection under direct vision using a sharp Fomon rasp. Resection of the dorsal border of the septum is accomplished with a No. 11 blade from which the tip has been broken to avoid lacerating the contralateral dorsal skin. Despite the fact that the rasp and blade permit more conservative resections than saws or osteotomes, the surgeon can still over-resect. The dorsum should feel and appear perfectly smooth through the skin surface after dorsal resection.

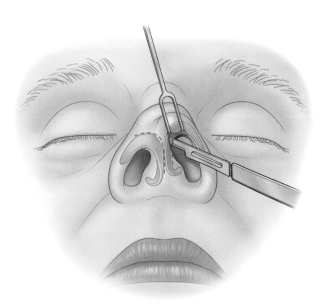

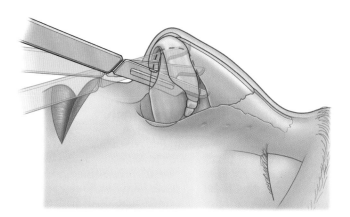

Fig. 19.14 The intercartilaginous incision, which can be lengthened into a transfixing incision if necessary, gives access to the dorsum, upper and lower lateral cartilages, and the septal angle. Dorsal modification; upper and lower lateral cartilage resection; spreader, radix, dorsal, and lateral wall grafts can all be performed through this excellent access point under direct vision.

Fig. 19.15 The intercartilaginous skeletonizing incision begins at the apex and proceeds laterally only as far as necessary. Dorsal access and visualization are easiest for a right-handed surgeon through a left-sided incision, and vice versa. If the surgeon does not need to shorten the upper or lower lateral cartilages, only a single intercartilaginous incision is needed.

Fig. 19.16 (1) Primary rhinoplasty patient with low radix, narrow middle vault, and inadequate tip projection in which radix, spreader, and tip grafts are planned. Preoperative appearance before the incision. **(2)** Nose after skeletonization. Note the difference in columellar position, nasal tip rotation, and apparent flattening of the dorsal hump, all artifacts of skeletonization. **(3)** By elevating the radix skin with a fingertip, the surgeon can estimate the amount of dorsal reduction that is actually necessary, assuming that radix augmentation will be performed. **(4)** Intercartilaginous incision; a similar incision is made on the patient's left side. Both give access to the dorsum, the septal angle, and the alar cartilage lateral crura. **(5)** Transfixing incision for access to the caudal septum. **(6)** Rasp used for roughening the nasal root so that radix grafts will adhere. **(7)** Fomon rasp for lowering the bony vault. **(8)** The bony vault is reduced by careful use of this down-cutting rasp. **(9)** After reduction of the bony vault, the cartilaginous dorsum seems even higher, further demonstrating the importance of the low root on the apparent height of the nasal bridge.

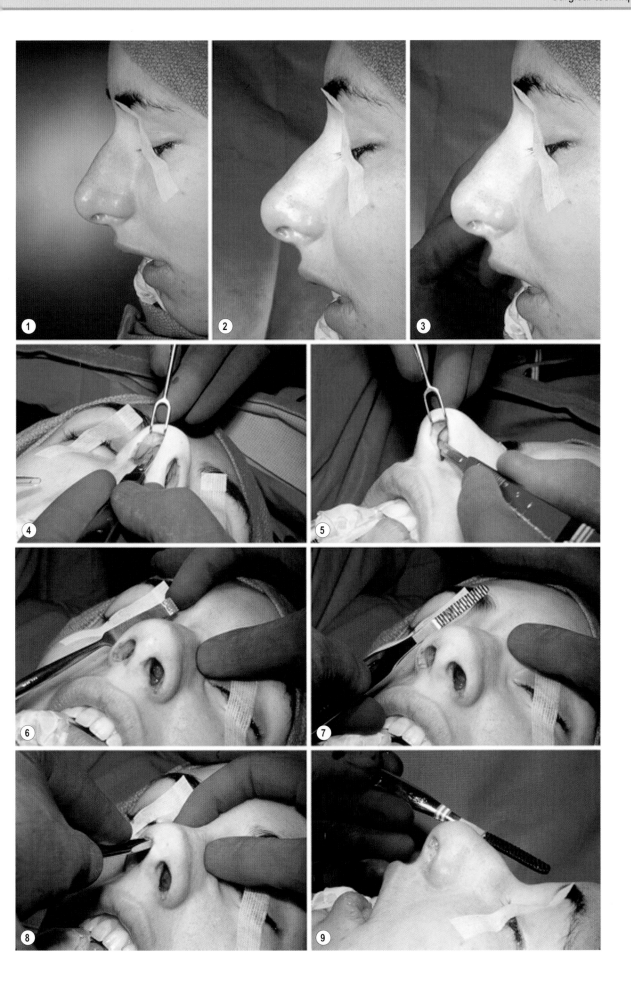

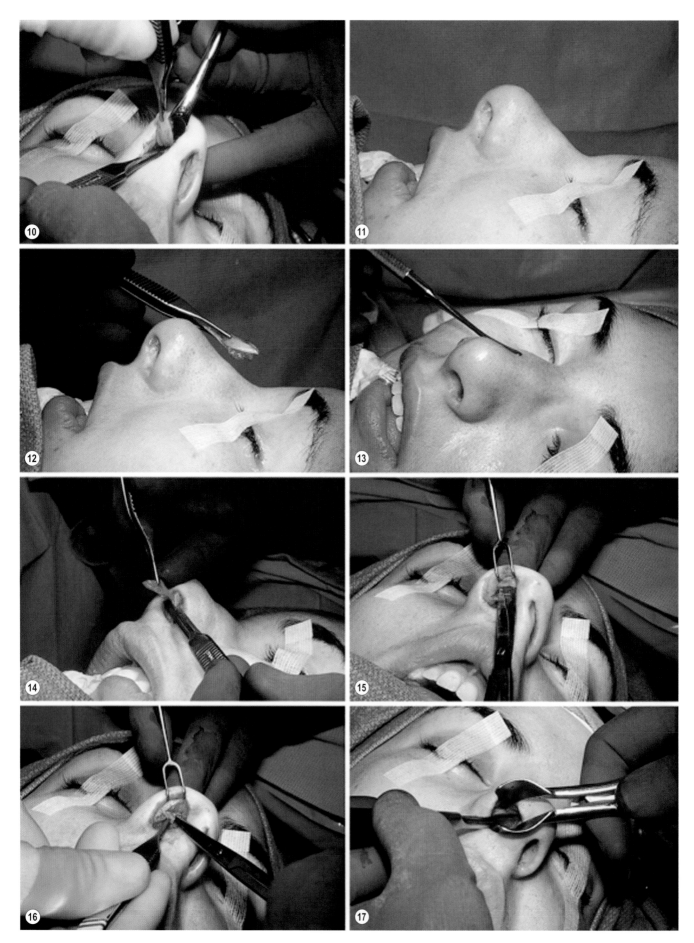

Fig. 19.16, cont'd—*For Legend see p. 428*

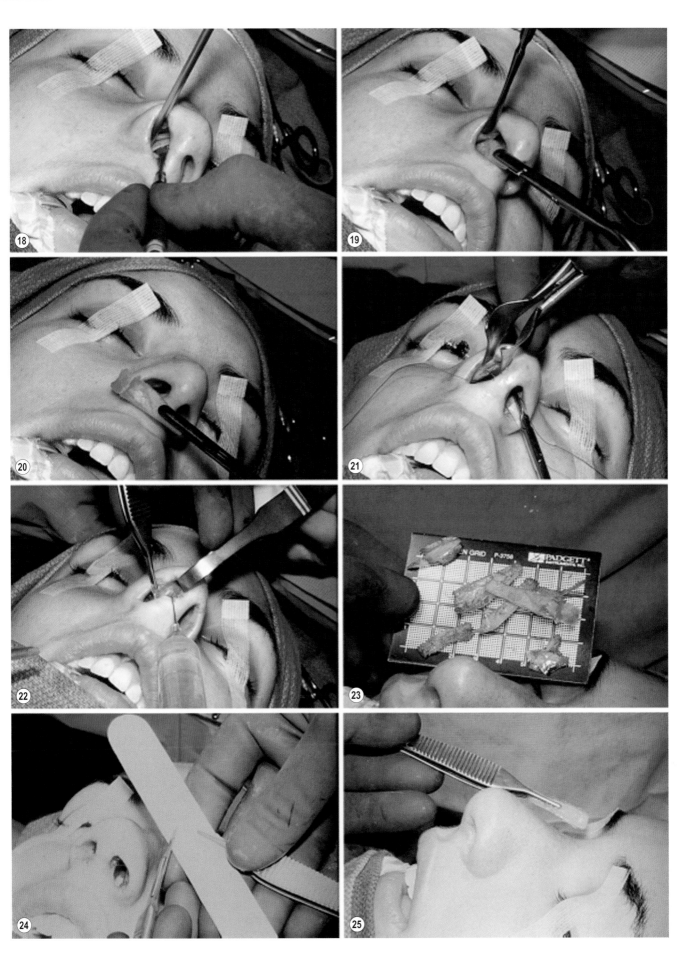

Fig. 19.16, cont'd—*For Legend see p. 428*

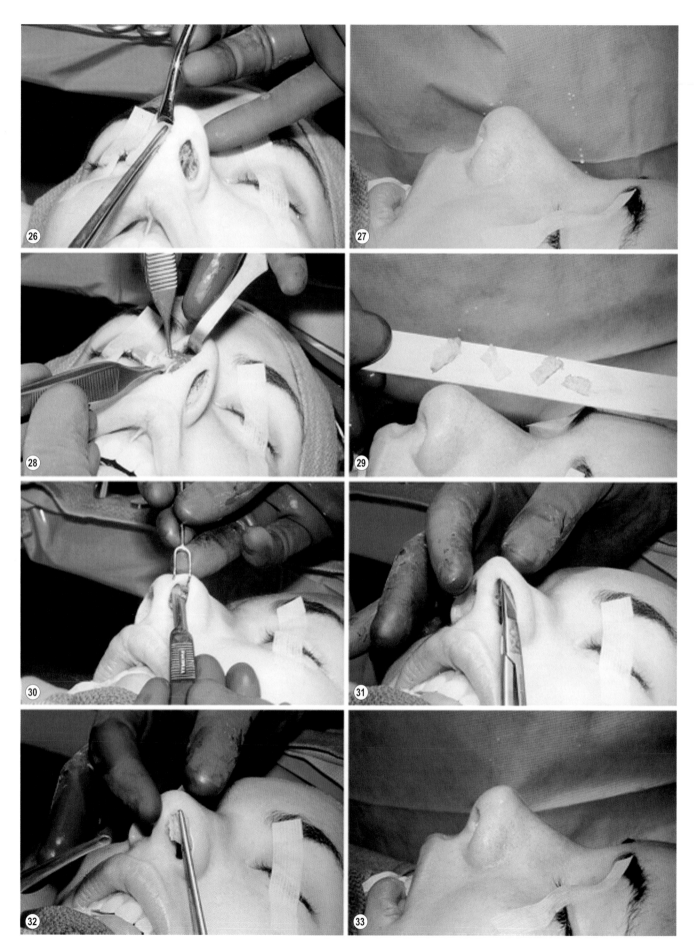

Fig. 19.16, cont'd—*For Legend see p. 428*

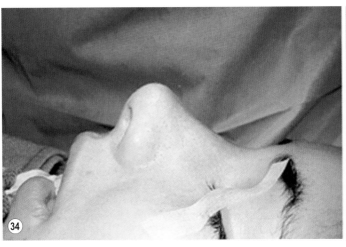

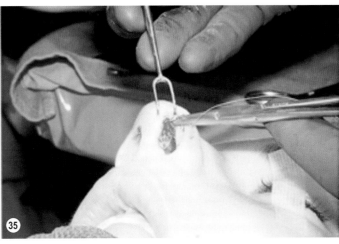

Fig. 19.16, cont'd (10) The cartilaginous roof is resected with a No. 11 blade under direct vision. The knife tip has been broken to avoid perforating the nasal skin. **(11)** The appearance after dorsal resection. Notice the nasal shortening that has occurred simply by dorsal reduction, as well as the change in columellar position and the relative new prominence of the alar cartilages. **(12)** The section of dorsal roof that was resected. Because the radix will be raised, less dorsal resection is necessary. Only a 2 mm resection is needed to open the cartilaginous roof and to destabilize the middle vault. **(13)** After resection of the cartilaginous roof, note the concavity in the upper cartilaginous vault, signifying instability at the internal valves produced by the dorsal resection. **(14)** Caudal septal resection shortens the nose and brings the columella into better relationship with the alar rim. The dimensions and shape of the resection should be altered according to the clinical case. **(15)** The alar cartilage lateral crus is dissected retrograde from the vestibular lining. **(16)** In this patient, the cephalic 2–3 mm is resected, leaving 10 mm. **(17)** Incision through right mucoperichondrium 15 mm above the caudal end of the septum to begin the septoplasty. **(18)** The Freer elevator has lifted mucoperichondrium from both sides of the septum in the area of planned resection; no dissection is performed over the proposed dorsal and caudal struts. **(19)** A cut has been made 15 mm below the anterior edge of the septum, and a second one approximately 10 mm below that. Killian septal forceps are retrieving the first segment of septal cartilage. **(20)** The first strip of septal cartilage has been removed, providing an excellent dorsal graft if necessary. The septum is always resected in the same fashion. Dissection now proceeds toward the vomer to retrieve additional cartilage and bone and clear septal obstructions. **(21)** Several 4-0 chromic mattress sutures repair the septal access incision. **(22)** The septal angle is identified in the transfixing incision, and submucoperichondrial infiltration with local anesthetic facilitates development of spreader graft tunnels. **(23)** Harvested septal cartilage is on the right of the Sheen grid; the resected dorsal roof is in the upper left corner. **(24)** The most suitable segment of septal cartilage is trimmed and beveled to provide the main upper dorsal graft. **(25)** The prepared dorsal graft. A second layer of cartilage has been lightly crushed and placed beneath the first at its cephalic end. Note that the main graft is longer than might be expected to provide continuity into the nasal dorsum; the distal end has been beveled. **(26)** The dorsal graft is placed under direct vision through the right-sided intercartilaginous incision; all other incisions have been closed. **(27)** After placement of the upper dorsal graft, the dorsum has been rendered straight by reduction of the upper and middle thirds and elevation of the root. Note the apparent reduction in nasal base size. **(28)** Placement of the right spreader graft; the left-sided spreader graft has already been positioned. **(29)** Several lightly crushed grafts will recontour the tip lobule. **(30)** An infracartilaginous access incision is made for tip graft placement. **(31)** Dissection is carried into the tip lobule (previously unviolated because of the retrograde lateral crural dissection). The surgeon must dissect only in the areas that require augmentation but widely enough that the tip tissues will drape over the grafts. **(32)** The first tip graft is placed, aiming toward the patient's right alar dome. **(33)** After placement of the first tip graft; compare with 27. The tip is more angular and has been elevated above the supratip; a defined point of greatest tip projection has been developed. **(34)** After placement of a second tip graft, the forces over the lobule are more diffused; the tip looks less angular. **(35)** After placement of all tip grafts, the access incision is closed.

Nasal spine-caudal septum

Caudal septal resection may change the relationship of the columella to nostril rim, nasal length, subnasale contour, and upper lip carriage, an observation that can be confirmed by recalling the appearance of the patient with septal collapse, in whom a sharp subnasale and upper lip retrusion are present even though the nasal spine remains uninjured and unresected.

If the nasolabial angle and upper lip relationships are satisfactory, no transfixing incision and no caudal septal or nasal spine modifications are necessary. If columellar position is satisfactory but the subnasale is full, a short incision can be made in the posterior membranous septum and septal floor, the nasal spine exposed and resected with a small rongeur. If the columella is low but the nasolabial angle is satisfactory, the caudal or membranous septum is resected, paralleling the nostril rims and without shortening the nose. Finally, if the columella is low or the nasolabial angle is acute, more caudal septum and membranous septum is resected anteriorly than posteriorly. Caudal septal and nasal spine resections are two of the most straightforward areas of nasal reduction, in which the intraoperative appearance is often extremely close to postoperative contours. Nevertheless, transfixing incisions should not be made unless some intervention at the caudal septum is required.

Technical details

Be cautious about over-resection; 1 or 2 mm makes the difference between normal columellar position and retraction.

Alar cartilage resection

The aphorism: "as the tip goes, so goes the rhinoplasty", may account in part for the fact that the small, paired alar cartilages have received exhaustive attention in the rhinoplasty literature. Countless techniques have been described to improve alar cartilage contour, most of them constituting various patterns and degrees of resection.[80-88]

As security with tip reconstruction has grown, the author's approach to the alar cartilages has become simpler: preserve as much alar cartilage as possible, consistent with good aesthetics and external valvular support; interrupt the continuity of the alar cartilage arch only if tip projection is excessive or where the arch severely disturbs aesthetics (e.g., the "boxy" or "ball" tip); and use cartilage grafts to restore equilibrium or to improve tip contour.[28,89] Simple observation and anthropometric measurements have repeatedly demonstrated that normal alar cartilage lateral width is 10–12 mm; it is not reasonable to expect that a 2 mm "rim strip" remnant will adequately support the external valves or provide proper tip contour.

The alar cartilages may be altered in one area but not in another. Reduction at the dome decreases tip projection; reduction of the middle crus decreases the length of the tip lobule and the inter-domal distance lateral crural resection decreases the convexity apparent on frontal and oblique views but may weaken the external valves.

Technical details

In the majority of primary rhinoplasties in which only conservative reductions of the cephalic lateral crura edges are necessary, the cartilages are modified retrograde through the intercartilaginous incisions. If the cartilages are distorted, they can be delivered as bipedicle flaps by intercartilaginous and infracartilaginous incisions. If only the arch needs interruption (e.g., to narrow the tip or to resect a "knuckle" at the lateral genu), only that portion of the alar cartilage should be exposed. Finally, if the lateral crus or dome areas are so distorted that a simple reduction or tip grafting will not provide the intended result, the distorting structures can be dissected free from the vestibular and overlying skin and (1) resected and replaced after modification; (2) resected and replaced by septal cartilage grafts; or (3) delivered as a medially based flap, and replaced along the alar rims. Radical freeing of the lateral crura, dome resection, or division of the alar cartilage arch reduces tip projection and so tip grafts are necessary to reconstruct the lobule. Lining should never be resected to avoid vestibular stenoses and iatrogenic airway obstruction.

Upper lateral cartilages: shortening the nose

Resection of the caudal ends of the upper lateral cartilages used to be routine; in fact, this step is unnecessary unless substantial nasal shortening is required.

A variety of interventions shorten the nose. In descending order of their effect, they are dorsal resection, caudal septal resection, resection of the cephalic edges of the alar cartilage lateral crura, and resection of the anterocaudal ends of the upper lateral cartilages. The posterior edges of the upper lateral cartilages should be left to abut the lateral crura; mucosa should never be resected.

Technical details

The caudal edge of the upper lateral cartilage can be drawn downwards by a single hook in its lining, exposing the caudal edge for submucosal resection with Joseph scissors.

Septoplasty, spreader graft tunnels

The deviated nasal septum and its treatment is thoroughly described in Chapter 20. Septoplasty is performed to relieve an airway obstruction from septal deflection and to provide graft material for the reconstruction itself. It is important to inquire about a history of prior trauma because unhealed septal fracture lines may extend to the dorsal septal edge and therefore threaten dorsal strut stability. The surgeon should leave 15–20 mm intact, undissected cartilage along the nasal dorsum and 15 mm caudally in performing any submucous resection to preserve stability and to make spreader graft placement simpler. Recent trauma (within 3 months) is an indication to postpone the rhinoplasty until any fractures have healed and until postoperative edema allows accurate judgment of the aesthetic contours. If significant trauma has occurred, even in the distant past, it is preferable to avoid simultaneous septoplasty and bilateral osteotomies or to postpone osteotomy if the surgeon is not confident of septal support. In practice, the need for bilateral osteotomies in the severely traumatized nose is generally uncommon because a unilateral osteotomy on the outfractured side achieves better symmetry than bilateral osteotomies.

Technical details

If they are needed, spreader graft tunnels are performed before septoplasty. Spreader graft tunnels are facilitated by prior infiltration beneath the mucoperichondrium with local anesthetic. By identifying the septal angle, the surgeon can incise to cartilage beneath each mucoperichondrial flap and develop the tunnels themselves with the sharp end of a Cottle perichondrial elevator. Each tunnel must follow the dorsal septal edge and should extend beneath the caudal edge of the bony arch on each side, leaving a narrow mucoperichondrial attachment along the top edge.

For septoplasty access, the initial mucoperichondrial incision is made 15 mm above (cephalad to) the caudal septal edge; and, using first the sharp and later the blunt end of a Freer elevator in one hand and a Frazier suction in the other, dissection proceeds under the mucoperichondrial flap onto the perpendicular plate of the ethmoid and over any posterior bony obstructions. Once the first flap has been developed, the sharp end of the elevator can cut the septal cartilage at the site of the opening incision; dissection then proceeds on the second side. Elevation of the perichondrium at the junction of septal cartilage and vomer is particularly difficult because the periosteal and perichondrial fibers are interlaced. Because the periosteal fibers are stronger, the mucosal flaps are less likely to tear if the surgeon begins dissection beneath the maxillary and vomerine mucoperiosteum and works cephalad.

The first septal cut is made 15–20 mm below the dorsal septal edge with angled Knight septal scissors, which cut through septal cartilage and ethmoid; make sure that both blades are within the mucoperichondrial flaps before making the cut. A parallel cut is performed 10 mm inferiorly, and using Killian septal forceps, the first graft, now free on three sides, can be twisted so that the ethmoid fractures and is removed in one piece. This maneuver often provides an initial graft 25–30 mm long containing the flattest, thickest, longest piece of septal cartilage, ideal for a dorsal graft. Dissection continues posteriorly and caudally with the sharp end of a Cottle perichondrial elevator. The septal cartilage in the

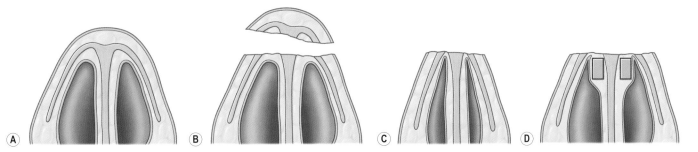

Fig. 19.17 (A) Septal cartilage is not uniform in thickness, but broadens along its anterior edge, where it becomes confluent with the upper lateral cartilages and forms the middle vault roof. **(B)** Any dorsal resection thicker than 2 mm interrupts this cartilaginous arch and removes the widened septal area, regardless of whether the mucosa is intact. **(C)** The surgeon had now created a disequilibrium in which the upper lateral cartilages are no longer held apart by the spreading action of the intact roof. Even if the internal valves were not incompetent preoperatively, they are now. **(D)** Spreader grafts recreate the former intact septal width and reconstitute competent internal valves. Thus spreader grafts are indicated whenever the internal valves are incompetent preoperatively or when the surgeon resects an intact cartilaginous roof, unless the nasal contour independently suggests a substantial dorsal graft (which duplicates the functional effect of spreader grafts).

vomerine groove can often be dislodged by a bit of judicious wiggling with a narrow osteotome. With an osteotome and septal forceps, additional pieces of vomer or perpendicular plate of the ethmoid can be removed if obstructing or if additional graft material is needed, always working under direct vision. In areas of severe deflection, tears in the muco-perichondrial flaps may be unavoidable, but the surgeon should nevertheless proceed cautiously and repair any tears. Close the septal pocket with 4-0 chromic mattress sutures *(Fig. 19.17)*.

Turbinectomy

Partial inferior turbinectomy, defined as a trim of the anterior edge sufficient to obtain 3 mm clearance to the septum or nasal floor, is valuable adjunctive airway treatment if indicated; like all nasal procedures, it has been overdone, and rhinomanometric data suggest that aggressive turbinate treatment is not necessary to achieve subjectively normal airways in most patients if septal and valvular causes have been adequately relieved. Turbinate crushing and out-fracture may suffice in patients whose turbinates contain significant cystic bone and in whom adequate airway size can be achieved without resection. When resection is necessary, biopsy forceps allow smaller, more incremental changes than angled scissors. The raw surfaces left will contract and epithe-lize, further reducing the size of the remaining turbinate; undercorrection is less frequent and much easier to treat than over-resection.

Graft placement and wound closure

Close some of the wounds with 5-0 plain catgut sutures before placing grafts so that their position will be easier to maintain. This sequence keeps grafts from slipping out of one incision as the surgeon closes another.

Osteotomy

Osteotomy achieves two goals: reducing bony vault width and closing the open nasal roof. Because the bony vault may

remain unopened or only partially open after conservative dorsal resections, it is the former of these two objectives that is probably more important. Before performing any osteotomy, the surgeon should be sure that one is necessary. If the lower nasal third is already appropriately wider than the bony vault, narrowing the upper nose further may be counterproductive by making the nasal base appear larger. If there is a high septal deviation, bilateral osteotomies may create a newly asymmetric nose because one nasal bone will move medially farther than the other. In the elderly patient (in whom comminution of the nasal bones may occur), the patient who wears heavy eyeglasses, or the patient with nasal bones extending less than one-third the distance to the septal angle (in whom middle vault width depends partially on bony vault width), the surgeon may wish to omit osteotomy. Finally, osteotomy may lengthen a long nose further by reducing support beneath a large skin sleeve.

Technical details

The gentlest effective technique is preferable. A single lateral osteotomy that begins intranasally, low at the pyriform aperture, and ends higher toward the nasal root (at the attachment of the nasal pyramid to the maxilla) is effective and seems the most anatomically correct. Gentle digital pressure causes a greenstick fracture at the remaining cephalic attachment and will re-form the bony pyramid. I use a guarded osteotome facing the button laterally to constantly assure correct orientation.

Alar wedge resection

Like every other preceding step, reduction of nostril size used to be considered obligatory; it is not. In fact, with more conservative dorsal resections, the degree of surgically developed nostril flare decreases and hence the need for alar wedge resection decreases. In considering the degree of resection, the surgeon should assess the proportion of tip lobular size to nostril length, remembering that tip grafting (if part of the preoperative plan) will increase tip lobular size and may eliminate the need for nostril reduction. Because the alar rim has both external and vestibular skin surfaces, the requirements of each must be assessed and treated individually. If nostril size is excessive, however, it is important to preserve a medial flap at the sill to lessen the possibility of alar notching.[90] Even with the medial flap, excess resection of even 1 mm can notch the nasal floor. Be conservative.

Technical details

An external incision made slightly outside the alar crease is preferable in order not to destroy this important landmark, a unique structure that simple skin repair does not reduplicate. Accurate closure with 6-0 nylon suffices; 5-0 plain catgut is used for the nasal floor. The nonabsorbable sutures should be removed by 5 days.

Prioritizing the septal graft specimen for augmentation

One of the important preoperative unknowns in rhinoplasty is the condition and quality of the graft material needed for the reconstruction. The great appeal of alloplastics lies in their predictability, at least on the day of surgery. This luxury does not accrue to the surgeon using autografts; nevertheless, the longevity and quality of an autogenous result still exceed those of any alloplastic substance yet introduced. The surgeon struggling to complete a reconstruction with poor-quality autografts in barely sufficient or inadequate amounts develops great sympathy for those surgeons who have decided to use alloplastic materials instead. Supplies are limited, so the surgeon must inventory each specimen and prioritize according to the patient's reconstructive needs.

The straightest, smoothest cartilage graft is used for the nasal dorsum to reconstruct this dominant area covered by thin soft tissues. If septum is available, it is used. Failing that, use rib cartilage for the dorsum.

The area of second priority is the nasal tip, for which septal, ear, or rib cartilage work well. Tip graft requirements differ along a spectrum. At the two extremes are the patient with a thick, blunt lobule who desires the greatest postoperative angularity (in whom an ethmoid buttress and several solid cartilage grafts will be needed), and the thin-skinned patient whose well-shaped tip cartilages require only augmentation of the cephalic lobule for refinement. Technical variations help to optimize an insufficient specimen (see below). Rib, ear, or septum each make excellent spreader grafts. Other areas are less demanding: bone that may be unsuitable elsewhere can be used instead for spreader grafts, lateral wall grafts, or alar wall grafts, just as solid or lightly crushed cartilage scraps can fill regional depressions.

Augmenting the most common nasal areas: radix, spreader, and tip grafts

The augmentation phase of any rhinoplasty re-establishes the preoperative nasal equilibrium and alters contours in ways that reduction alone cannot. In selecting each graft, the surgeon should consider areas that may have needed augmentation preoperatively and also those that may now need grafts because of a disequilibrium that the surgeon has created during by reduction (i.e., spreader grafts to support the internal valves after resection of the cartilaginous roof). The nose that is equilibrated at the conclusion of the procedure is less likely to change during healing and therefore gives the surgeon greater control over the result.

Dorsum and radix

The key principle in all augmentation is to match the graft material to the patient's soft tissue characteristics and to his or her aesthetic goals. Unmodified rib cartilage is stiff, ear cartilage is rubbery, and septal cartilage is the most "plastic." Thicker skin needs more augmentation to provide a given result but will hide more underlying flaws: thinner skin requires softer, well contoured grafts that will not show excessively. At the nasal root, where the soft tissue cover is the thinnest and graft visibility or palpability is particularly troublesome, the author layers lightly crushed grafts to fit the defect: usually one longer graft that extends from the radix toward the mid-dorsum, with a second, shorter graft fixed to its cephalic end at the deepest part of the defect. Dorsal and radix grafts are constructed similarly, the former being only a longer version of the latter. The most common errors are to make dorsal and radix grafts too short, too wide, or too rigid; at the cephalic end, neither usually exceeds 5–6 mm. Both dorsal and radix grafts should feel perfect after insertion, without palpable discontinuities or irregularities. If not, remove and revise them. Most grafts are not sutured into position but only fixed with the tape dressing. In a recent review of 100 consecutive radix grafts, and after performing many of them, my revision rate was 3%. It was not that low when started; but with proper technical attention, the augmented dorsum or radix can feel smooth and unoperated; the grafts should be only barely palpable. When a dorsum requires substantial augmentation, the lateral walls may need onlay grafts to properly reconstruct the upper vault pyramid.

Spreader grafts

Although septal cartilage provides the ideal spreader graft (*Fig. 19.17C,D*), strips of costal or conchal cartilage, ethmoid, or vomer may be used instead. Their width should provide confluence between the upper and lower nasal thirds and they must span middle vault length from the bony arch almost to the septal angle. After spreader grafts are placed, caudal slippage can be avoided by a single 4-0 plain catgut transfixing suture placed at the septal angle.

Lateral wall and columellar grafts

Cartilage provides the ideal lateral wall graft, split tangentially or crushed to fit the defect. Where sufficient cartilage is unavailable, ethmoid will correct asymmetries in the deviated nose, or mask the edges of a dorsal graft. Slivers of cartilage that remain can provide "filler grafts" to correct columellar notching from prior open rhinoplasty scars or retraction after trauma or surgery. Augment the columella through a short lateral incision in the membranous septum, limiting cephalic dissection so that the grafts provide adequate augmentation but do not disappear between the medial crura.

Tip grafting

Tip grafting (*Fig. 19.18*) deserves special prominence because of its early appearance as an augmentation method designed to do what reduction rhinoplasty alone could not: alter tip

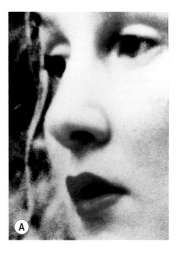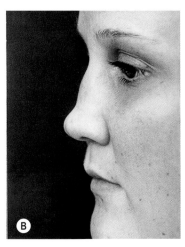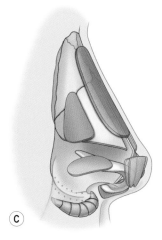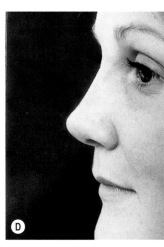

Fig. 19.18 Changes in many nasal regions are "global", not "regional". The saddle nose should affect only supratip height, but it does much more. Patient preoperatively **(A)** and after septal collapse **(B)**. **(C)** Schematic of the surgical plan: Rib cartilage maxillary augmentation, dorsal, caudal support, tip, and lateral wall grafts. All are necessary to correct the protean, "global" effects of loss of septal support. **(D)** Three year postoperative view. (C: Redrawn from Constantian, M.B.: Rhinoplasty: Craft and Magic, St. Louis, Quality Medical Publishing, 2009, p. 1386).

contour and increase tip support. The concept of grafting the primary tip or correcting supratip deformity by augmentation rather than further reduction began the evolutionary thinking from which the modern rhinoplasty paradigm derived.[91] Technical variations have been described,[91–106] but the principle remains the same. The surgeon who uses tip grafts commonly finds that they not only increase tip projection but also alter tip lobular and nostril contour; increase lobular volume (reducing relative nostril size); impart a different ethnic character; and enlarge the nasal base, therefore changing the balance between dorsal height and tip projection. The two most common graft designs are the "shield" graft popularized by Sheen[91,92] and the cephalic transverse onlay graft, with or without a columellar strut, popularized by Peck.[106] The Sheen method effectively lengthens the middle crural segment and therefore increase tip projection; it is therefore an anatomical correction and my favored technique.

The clinical problems that tip graft variations can solve increase with experience, but the following generalities apply:

1. Graft number and substance must suit the soft tissue cover and the patient's aesthetic goals: more substantial grafts are required beneath tissues that are thicker or stiffer (e.g., scarred from prior rhinoplasties), and softer grafts are needed under thinner skin to avoid surface irregularities.

2. Tip angularity varies inversely with the number of grafts used. The normal nasal tip is supported not by the anterior presenting edge of a single rectangular or shield-shaped cartilage but by the broad surfaces of the two alar cartilage domes. A single, solid graft will support only the tip at its single projecting end; in the thin-skinned patient, this design produces an unnatural artifact. The more grafts the surgeon places, the more underlying support diffuses and the less angular the tip becomes. To avoid graft visibility, the surgeon should always use multiple tip grafts *(Fig. 19.19)*.

3. Tip symmetry is paradoxically easier to produce with multiple grafts than with a single graft. Even after

precise midline placement, forces contracting on six graft edges can rotate a single graft and produce an asymmetric appearance. It is easier to place at least two grafts, one angled toward the dome on each side, to distribute forces and to recreate normal anatomy. If the second graft still leaves a deficiency on one side, the surgeon can add more for symmetry without disturbing the first two pieces. Tip grafts are fixed by the dressing.

4. Ethmoid or vomer "buttresses" prevent anterior graft displacement. Augmentation in a lobule whose alar cartilages are intact is different from augmentation in a contracted postoperative lobule from which the alar cartilages have been partially or completely removed. The former case can be treated by selective augmentation of the deficient areas with multiple softened grafts.[28,78] In the latter case, there is no cartilage remnant to act as a "backstop" for any grafts placed anterior to it, and no remaining structure to determine middle crural length and angle. Therefore, an initial buttress graft, usually of ethmoid or vomer and slightly smaller than the primary tip grafts, should be inserted first to define the posterior edge of the pocket and control the anterior position and angle of the main grafts. The same strategy is effective in patients desiring substantial tip projection.

Technical details

Tip grafts are placed through an infracartilaginous incision on the side from which the surgeon operates. It is important to dissect the recipient pocket adequately, but not so liberally that the grafts cannot create the required support and projection. Complete access incision closure is mandatory to minimize infection; the grafts should be manipulated as little as possible and rinsed in saline in an antibiotic solution before insertion. The author now places tip grafts in almost every patient, except for those whose preoperative tip aesthetics are excellent *(Fig. 19.20)*.

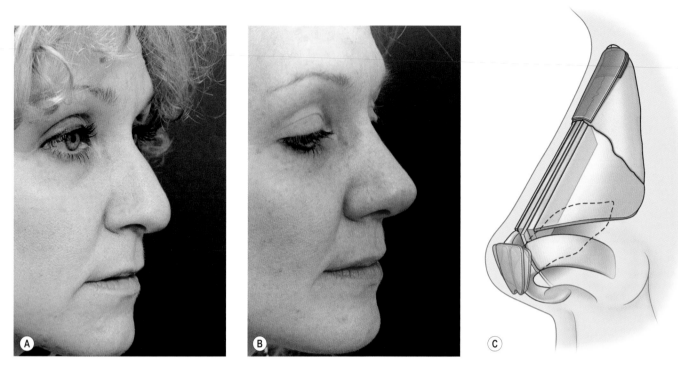

Fig. 19.19 A patient with all four anatomic variants that predispose to unfavorable results: low radix, inadequate tip projection, narrow middle vault, and alar cartilage malposition. Preoperative **(A)** and postoperative **(B)** oblique views. **(C)** Schematic of the surgical correction: dorsal reduction; relocation of the alar cartilage lateral crura; and radix, spreader and tip grafts. This is a common combination of procedures in my primary patients who have dorsal convexities and alar cartilage malposition.

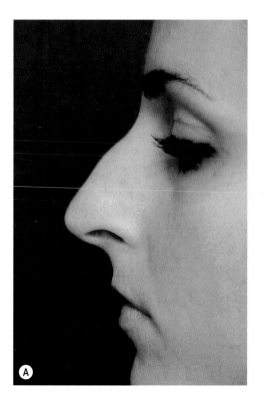

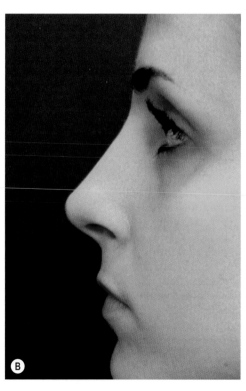

Fig. 19.20 Patient reconstructed by dorsal reduction, relocation of malpositioned alar cartilage lateral crura, and radix, spreader, and multiple tip grafts. Note that tip grafts have increased projection, altered tip lobular shape, and changed the lobular/nostril ratio, appearing to decrease nostril length (no alar wedge resections were performed).

Routine postoperative care

Dressings

Assuming that septal or turbinate surgery has been performed, the nose is packed with 7 cm strips of petrolatum gauze impregnated with bacitracin/mupirocin ointment and layered over No. 18 suction catheters placed in the floor of each nasal airway. Although patency may last only a few days, the tubes do help equalize middle ear pressure and allow some airflow, for which all patients (particularly those anxious about packing) are grateful. Packing and tubes ordinarily remain for 1 week, by which time normal mucus production has returned and the packs can be removed painlessly. The packing should not overstuff the nose, which may dislodge repositioned nasal bones. In the absence of septal resection or turbinectomy, smaller packs can be used and need to remain for only 24–48 h. I prescribe oral antibiotics appropriate for upper airway organisms as prophylaxis against suppurative sinusitis while packs are in place.

The nasal splint is fashioned from layers of ½-inch paper tape placed across the dorsum, tip, and cheeks so that cloth tape of the same width, layered over it, does not touch the skin itself. Several layers of moistened 2-inch plaster are cut to fit and secured with another layer of cloth tape. The splint must be applied precisely but not too tightly; the nasal tip skin is at greatest risk. Particularly in patients whose tip lobules have been expanded by grafts, tip color should be checked frequently in the postoperative period and the tip sling cut and nasal packs or splint removed as necessary. Even in the primary rhinoplasty patient, nasal circulation is not inviolable.

Selection and use of additional graft donor sites and other augmentation materials

Although the nasal septum is the most "plastic" of the autogenous sources for nasal reconstruction, septal cartilage and bone are not always present in adequate amounts even in the primary rhinoplasty patient (i.e., where the septum may be is largely bony). Other autogenous sites are available; each has its particular idiosyncrasies and optimal uses.

Conchal cartilage

Unmodified cartilage from the conchal floor supplies excellent grafts for the nasal dorsum, lateral walls, tip, or internal valves. Although many surgeons harvest conchal cartilage through a postauricular incision, the anterior approach provides the surgeon a better view of the quality and contour of the available cartilage. By either route, it is critical to preserve the posterior conchal wall to avoid deforming the donor ear; even so, substantial donor cartilage can be harvested. The ear should be isolated from the nose during harvesting and gloves and instruments changed prior to returning to the rhinoplasty itself. Such appropriate technical points greatly decrease the

chance of introducing gram-negative organisms from the external auditory canal into the nasal incisions. Conchal cartilage forms an excellent dorsal graft for deep, asymmetric defects beneath a thick soft tissue cover. The method of trimming, rolling, and fixing the graft has been described by Sheen.[107] For shorter, shallower defects or under thinner soft tissue cover, conchal cartilage is not ideal but can be used as a compromise solution. Because of their rubbery consistency and thickness, however, single pieces of solid conchal cartilage will flatten and deform as the overlying soft tissues compress them and so do not make good dorsal grafts.

Calvarial bone

The calvarial outer table supplies grafts well suited for the reconstruction of long, shallow (2–3 mm), symmetric dorsal defects beneath thin soft tissue covers. These grafts must be harvested with exceeding care because intracranial injuries have been described.[108,109] Some surgeons have been discouraged by the long-term results of calvarial bone, but the author has used it frequently with only two (of 50) cases of partial absorption in the supratip. Other surgeons have reported similar success with even larger series.[109] The grafts must be harvested under low speed with use of an electric burr and cold chisel, keeping the bone cool with saline irrigation to avoid overheating its osteocytes. Bony union is the rule. Calvarial grafts need not be immobilized by internal fixation if their position can be maintained by limited pocket dissection and splinting. Where the soft tissues are distorted or the nasal base has collapsed, fixation at the root is necessary, a circumstance that is uncommon in the primary patient unless septal collapse has occurred. However, because of its utility in providing all graft needs, I now use costal cartilage or bone in preference to calvarial grafts.

Costal cartilage

Costal grafts, not commonly necessary in primary rhinoplasty, are nevertheless extremely versatile and available in essentially unlimited quantities. When conchal grafts are too short or calvarial grafts too thin, rib cartilage is excellent for dorsal reconstruction. Slices of costal cartilage (either solid or crushed) can fill the maxillary arch, lateral nasal walls, columella, or tip. The notoriety of rib grafts to warp postoperatively can be avoided by observing their internal stresses as grafts are shaped, and by noting that ribs progressively calcify as patients age (especially beyond 40 years). The more calcification, the more the distorting perichondrial forces are overcome. I always use the smallest rib that will suffice (8th, 9th, or 10th), so that less modification and therefore less disruption of internal stresses occurs; and insert a threaded, longitudinal K-wire as an internal splint in younger, whiter, less calcified, more elastic ribs.[110] Sutured perichondrial/cartilage laminates or crushed slices of rib cartilage provide alternative approaches.[111]

Alloplastics

Except in the single circumstance of maxillary augmentation (described later), this author does not use alloplastic materials for three reasons. First, most reports in the literature share the characteristics of limited, incomplete follow-up of patients and a complication rate defined only as infection or extrusion. Compared with autogenous materials, for which infection, extrusion, and even resorption are rare, such data are not convincing. No alloplastic material has yet demonstrated the success and complication rate that matches autogenous grafts. Second, the rationale for use of alloplastic materials is always their relative ease for patient and surgeon and avoidance of the disadvantages of autogenous grafts. The latter imperfections are perfectly real but largely controllable by the surgeon's experience; the former apply only in the perioperative period. Whereas alloplastic materials offer the convenience of not having to be harvested, they are decidedly inconvenient if they do not achieve their long-term results or need removal for threatened extrusion or infection. Finally, the patient in whom the surgeon most wishes to use alloplastic materials is the one for whom they are least suitable: i.e., the tertiary rhinoplasty patient whose soft tissues are scarred and thin and whose best donor sites have been exhausted. These are the patients who are least likely to benefit from alloplastic materials and whose scarred, hypovascular beds will be least hospitable to them.

Maxillary augmentation

Maxillary augmentation can be an exception to the use of alloplastics in selected patients. Immobile and deep beneath the thick soft tissues of the upper lip, alloplastics are suitable and justifiable unless an autogenous graft is being harvested for other purposes (e.g., rib for the dorsum and maxillary arch). Gore-Tex® (1-mm SAM facial implant brand of expanded polytetrafluoroethylene, WL Gore & Associates, Flagstaff, AZ, 86001) can be rolled and placed through a short incision in the nasal floor. Subperiosteal dissection should be carried high across the maxillary arch tight against the pyriform aperture; the implant must be carefully centralized, and good soft tissue closure must be achieved. The implant can be fashioned so that it augments primarily the central lip or the perialar areas, depending on preoperative lip configuration.

Gore-Tex® is pliable and therefore not noticeable to most patients; the augmentation result appears to be stable. Complications are low. In a current series of more than 350 patients over 17 years, only five implants have required removal (infection). Alloplastic maxillary augmentation should not be performed in patients who have undergone cleft lip repair because of unacceptable extrusion rates: use autogenous materials instead.

The postoperative course

The weeks and months that follow rhinoplasty are critical in several respects. As difficult as nasal surgery is acknowledged to be for the surgeon, it is even more difficult for the patient, who (particularly after primary rhinoplasty) does not know what to expect; has high, perhaps even unrealistic expectations, despite the surgeon's preoperative counseling; and is fearful of complications and anxious for a perfect result. Added to the usual postoperative worries are the unsolicited advice and opinions of interested family members and friends, many of whom have little medical background but who intensify the patient's worries by volunteering their opinions. The postoperative course after rhinoplasty is complex and offers the surgeon an opportunity to make a positive experience out of what otherwise might be a negative one (or vice versa). Surgeons who do not see their patients after the dressings are removed are missing the chance to observe usual and unusual postoperative courses and to develop the skill and experience that might otherwise lead to consistent postoperative success.

The nasal splint and any remaining packing are removed on postoperative day 7. Despite better symmetry, a straighter bridge, or increased tip contour, many patients are disappointed 1 week after surgery and need repeated assurance that the nose is still swollen. The airway, however, should be appreciably better when packing is removed, an instant reward for the patient after a week of bandages. By day 10, the nose has begun to assume a better shape, and it is usually possible to build the patient's increasing confidence from there. Patients should be seen as needed during the first 2 weeks after surgery to clean the nose of secretions that have accumulated around intranasal sutures, to ensure that edema has not displaced the nasal bones, and to educate the patient about changes that will yet occur in the ensuing weeks and months. I see my patients every 3–4 months until the end of the first postoperative year and yearly thereafter, making adjustments for patients who travel from a distance. Patient and surgeon always learn something from each postoperative visit.

Some changes predictably occur during the postoperative period. The degree of change (see above) depends on the degree of disparity between preoperative and postoperative skeletal volume, how well the interdependent skeletal areas have been rebalanced, and how well the re-formed skeleton supports the soft tissues. The bigger the disequilibrium, the greater the postoperative change.

The following sequence occurs in most patients during the first postoperative year:

1. The nose becomes longer and "deskeletonizes" as upper lip edema abates, so that the nasolabial angle decreases and the nostrils become less visible.

2. The nasal base rotates caudally, depending on skin elasticity and the degree of skeletal support; the long preoperative nose has the greatest tendency to elongate postoperatively.

3. The profile assumes its final postoperative shape sooner than the frontal view; the nose narrows on frontal view for at least 12–18 months, particularly in the middle third. During this time, the unsupported middle vault narrows and demarcates from the caudal edges of the bony vault. The nasal skin tries to assume its preoperative shape, a characteristic that has particular implications for tip grafting: the flatter, more contracted preoperative tip will compress tip grafts and alter postoperative contour more than the larger tip with a more pliable soft tissue cover.

4. Skeletal irregularities or asymmetries may appear (and sometimes disappear).

5. Areas of underlying skeletal change or grafts may become visible and suggest the need for revision;

conversely, early postoperative improvement may become obscured by soft tissue contraction and thickening. As the surgeon becomes more experienced, postoperative changes become more interpretable and the surgeon's advice becomes more reliable. As with good physical therapy after hand surgery, at least 50% of the patient's happiness and as much as 90% of the surgeon's intraoperative and postoperative judgment are determined by lengthy and conscientious follow-up.

Variations on the standard

Nasal deviation

The asymmetric nose is common and difficult to correct well. In the acute fracture when bony displacement is the primary defect, closed reduction is effective. However, when the injury has been primarily septal or cartilaginous, closed or even open techniques in the acute situation are often incompletely effective. The surgeon who diagnoses an asymmetric nose as a bony problem alone when septal injury is a substantial component will find that manipulation of the nasal bones or attempts to "twist" the septum into its prior position are incompletely successful and that the prevalence of residual deformity is high.

In the healed deviated nose, the required techniques are identical to those already discussed. Several specific principles should be followed:

1. Asymmetric maneuvers must be done to an asymmetric nose to achieve symmetry. The strategy for correcting nasal deviation should consider the cephalic, middle, and caudal nasal thirds individually. A nose may appear asymmetric despite a symmetric bony vault. In such cases, no treatment of the cephalic third may be indicated, and the surgeon must devote greater attention to the displaced cartilaginous parts. In general, the bony vault is treated by no osteotomy or unilateral osteotomy; the middle third by placement of asymmetrically thick spreader grafts (wider on the side that has collapsed further medially, with or without onlay grafts) and/or onlay grafts for symmetry; and the caudal third by resection of the septal angle and submucosal caudal septal resection and replacement as needed.

2. The strategy for achieving symmetry also depends on whether the nasal dorsum is convex or concave 62. When the deviated nose has a convex bridge, the hump is often its most asymmetric part. By reducing bridge height, the surgeon also removes the area of greatest deflection and therefore makes a straighter nose even before performing any other maneuvers. Conversely, when the nasal dorsum is low and asymmetric relative to a large nasal base, the surgeon can frequently achieve more symmetry by camouflaging the deflection with a straight dorsal graft or by aligning the anterior septal edge with spreader grafts (*Fig. 19.21*).[112–117]

3. Deflection of the septal angle is a frequent cause of misalignment of the nasal base; resection of the septal angle releases the soft tissues at the nasal tip, allowing them to move toward the midline. However, septal angle

or dorsal resection sufficient to correct the asymmetry may simultaneously produce a nasal bridge that is now too low and therefore requires augmentation to re-establish postoperative balance and middle vault support. A deflected caudal septum/septal angle can also be aligned by asymmetrically thick spreader grafts; in this case, placing the thicker graft on the side toward which the septal angle is deflected.

Rhinoplasty in men

Although the diagnostic and technical aspects of rhinoplasty performed on men do not differ from those performed on women, there are other differences. Men have larger frames, heavier bones, thicker skin, and historically have been more likely to involve themselves in contact sports and in work with high physical demands.

Men are also judged to be most attractive when they best represent their phenotype – that is, when they "look male": defined jaws, strong foreheads, and larger noses.[75]

It is also true that men can have turbulent postoperative courses. In my previous survey of 1000 consecutive rhinoplasty patients, men represented 30% of the disruptive or needy patients and 40% of those with body dysmorphic disorder, although men only represented 22% of that population.[118]

This is not to say that men cannot be very good rhinoplasty patients. However, the following generalities almost always apply:

- Men tolerate larger noses than women; that is, shape is more important than size.
- Bridge height is important. Most men prefer a straight (or even convex) dorsal line to one that is concave with retroussé.
- Men want noses that "look male"; not too short, not too narrow, and not too small.
- Secondary male patients most often complain of a bridge that is too low. Be conservative in resections.
- Whereas some women say, "I don't care how well I breathe as long as my nose is pretty," men expect excellent postoperative airways.

Ethnic rhinoplasty

Beauty is subjective. There are patients whose private aesthetics are quite specific, and patients who simply want the surgeon to remove the bump and restore the airway. Thus, ethnic rhinoplasty does not differ from any other type of rhinoplasty.

The point for the surgeon to remember, however, is that for some patients' ethnic background helps determine their aesthetic goals. This determination can work two ways: some patients wish to retain the ethnic characteristics of their noses, and other patients want to lose them. *But the surgeon must ask.* The principles of forming and performing the surgical plan, however, do not differ.

The surgeon trying to correct a low, broad dorsum and a large nasal base covered by thick soft tissues faces the same imbalances and the same challenges regardless of the patient's ethnic background. The interaction with each patient sets the plan. It is only important for the surgeon to determine the

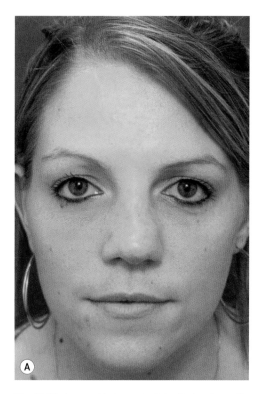 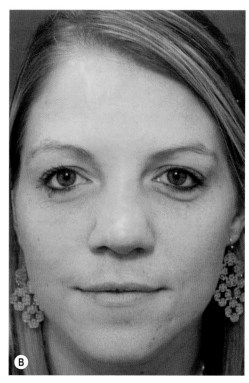

Fig. 19.21 Asymmetrical nose treated with dorsal resection, asymmetrically-thick spreader grafts, dorsal graft, and right lateral wall camouflage grafts. **(A)** Preoperative view. **(B)** 2-year postoperative view.

importance of ethnicity to the particular patient so that all changes are intentional and reflect the patient's aesthetic and ethnic sensibilities.

Cleft lip nasal deformity

Although patients who have undergone lip and nasal repair in infancy (which may have involved only dissection of the lower lateral cartilage on the cleft side) do not strictly speaking constitute a "primary rhinoplasty deformity," they often require definitive corrections during the teen or early adult years. The classic anatomic characteristics have been described elsewhere.[119–124]

The septal, maxillary, nasal base, and alar cartilage abnormalities that typify the unilateral or bilateral cleft lip may be managed by many of the methods designed for aesthetic rhinoplasty. The deformity is always complex and must be analyzed in terms of the symmetry of each nasal third, maxillary arch contour, columellar support, septal obstruction, valvular competence at the internal and (particularly) external valves especially on the cleft side, alar cartilage contour, vestibular webbing or atresia, and tip support. What is frequently characterized as a "short columella" may reflect inadequate tip projection instead and is best managed by increasing the tip projection without columellar lengthening. Also commonly overlooked or unrecognized, is cephalic rotation of the alar cartilage lateral crus on the cleft side. Additional techniques are required for deformities uncommon to the usual primary rhinoplasty: excision of alar rim skin, correction of vestibular webbing, and creation or relocation of the alar crease. The primary repair has frequently often constricted the nostril on the cleft side and may have displaced the alar base medially.

When the alar base is properly positioned, nostril stenosis can be improved by composite grafts from the alar lobule or ear.[125,126] When the nostril stenosis and alar base malposition occur simultaneously, however, an inferiorly based transposition flap lateral to alar base or a crescentic island flap vascularized by subcutaneous and musculocutaneous perforators is effective.[127,128]

Older patients

Older, of course, is relative. Two important considerations for the older patient are (1) how long dissatisfaction with the nose has been present and (2) any structural characteristics that may suggest alterations in the surgical plan.

Older nasal bones are thinner and more brittle, and the bony arch must be able to support eyeglasses. Soft tissues have become atrophic and less elastic, and tend to wrinkle instead of tighten, making some intraoperative judgments more difficult and contraction to a reduced framework less probable. Cartilages may have become more rigid, and many patients believe that their tips have grown larger with time. Whether this reflects actual cartilaginous growth, elongation or thinning of soft tissues or even absorption of the bony vault creating a new imbalance is not yet known. Tips that were adequately projecting in prior years begin to hang from the septal angle, causing an apparent curvature in the lower nose.

It is therefore wise to inquire how long the patient has been unhappy with his or her nasal shape. For some patients, it has been since their teen years. These patients can tolerate more significant changes. Alternatively, the patient whose unhappiness with his or her nasal shape is recent may simply be

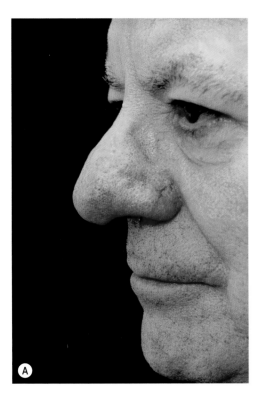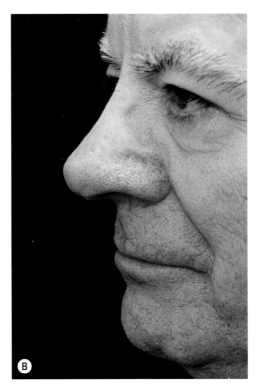

Fig. 19.22 Patient with rhinophyma treated by shaving the external skin, spreader, radix grafts; and a transverse cutaneous excision as a separate procedure. The original premorbid nose is not always well-proportioned.

noticing aging changes. The surgeon's task in these cases is to restore the nose, as far as possible, to its previous, more youthful appearance.[129,130]

Rhinophyma

Rhinophyma *(Fig. 19.22)* is the perfect setting for the reduction rhinoplasty mindset. Rhinophymatous noses really are too large, distorted by sebaceous and vascular overgrowth, chronic inflammation, exudates, and sometimes grotesque soft tissue excesses. The diseased tissues must be reduced, either by tangential or direct excision *(Fig. 19.16)*. While the excised surface heals, skin texture changes, sometimes becoming smoother and sometimes becoming scarred, depending on excision depth. Patients must be forewarned of the latter possibility, but few object because the deformity is so significant and so inaccurately associated ethanol abuse.

Three principles can guide the surgeon treating rhinophyma:

1. Not every nose with rhinophyma was originally small and straight. Before beginning the excision, try to visualize the patient's real underlying contour, and obtain old photographs if possible. The objective is to reduce the nose but produce as little scarring as possible. Compromise may be necessary.

2. Do not assume that every nose was well balanced before it became diseased: some had dorsal humps and low radices, some had inadequate tip projection, and some were already too long. Your patient may need a second rebalancing procedure (e.g., dorsal or tip grafts). Skin excision cannot correct skeletal deformities.

3. Plan excisions according to the nasal planes and aesthetic units to minimize distracting color and contour discontinuities.[131]

The donor site-depleted patient

Although donor site depletion is more common in the secondary patient whose donor sites have previously been harvested, even the primary rhinoplasty patient may be donor site depleted if the septum is bony and yields minimal usable cartilage (a circumstance somewhat more likely in the non-white or post-traumatic nose). In one series,[132,133] 17% of the primary rhinoplasty patients had nasal septa that were at least 75% bony and supplied insufficient donor material for the patient's requirements. A few principles are helpful in such patients:

1. Internal valvular reconstruction can be accomplished by either spreader grafts or dorsal grafts with equivalent functional effects.

2. External valvular reconstruction can be accomplished by battens of cartilage or bone that span the area of collapse, or by composite skin/conchal cartilage grafts.

3. Tip reconstruction may be accomplished by selectively grafting the skeletally deficient lobular parts with use of crushed grafts in limited pockets.

4. Multiple staggered grafts (even with use of tangentially split, crushed ear cartilage) can form a smooth dorsum in patients with an adequate soft tissue cover.

5. Single-unit dorsal grafts are still needed for dorsal defects in thin-skinned patients; not all patients can be treated with minimal donor material.

Problems in the postoperative course

Unlike other plastic surgical operations that are technically or conceptually difficult, rhinoplasty has fewer of the complications that traditionally plague surgeons. Most rhinoplasty surgeons never see lacrimal duct or extraocular muscle injury after rhinoplasty; even septal perforation is relatively infrequent. Because of its very nature, however, rhinoplasty has its own taxonomy of problems, most of which are directly related to an insufficiently complex understanding of the structural interdependencies in the nose, incorrect diagnosis, or technical difficulties. This is actually good news because the most common complications are under the surgeon's control and can be decreased by planning and operative technique.

The following complications are listed in decreasing frequency as they are recognized in the author's own patients and in other surgeons' patients seen in consultation.

Iatrogenic airway obstruction

More common than any of the other complications that will be addressed, and entirely preventable, is a decrease in postoperative airway size, particularly unfortunate if the patient was not obstructed preoperatively. Although attributed by some authors to the use of an intracartilaginous access incision or the narrowing effects of osteotomy,[134,135] more common causes are increased (or new) internal valvular incompetence from resection of the middle vault roof and external valvular incompetence from alar cartilage resection, particularly in cases of cephalic rotation of the lateral crura. Airway obstruction from loss of skeletal support due to surgery may be avoided by a preoperative evaluation that identifies the pertinent anatomy and by maintaining or establishing valvular competence in each patient. Substantial dorsal or spreader grafts correct internal valvular incompetence, with equal efficacy; collapsing external valves can be stiffened by autogenous cartilage.[134] Less commonly, new airway obstruction may be caused by the inadvertent loss of tip support (through septal collapse or excessive dorsal or alar cartilage reduction), excessive alar wedge resection (treated by composite grafts or local flaps), or resection of nasal lining (which should never be performed except at the membranous septum to shorten the nose). Inadequate or excessive nasal shortening misdirects the air stream that should normally flow posteriorly along the nasal floor. Patients with excessively long noses often relieve their airway obstructions by supporting their nasal tips; here, even osteotomy may be counterproductive by decreasing skeletal volume.[135] The over-shortened nose can be improved by dorsal grafts, resection of the posterior caudal septum, composite grafts, "septal extension grafts,"[136] or septal batten grafts. Osteotomy has been indicted as a cause of decreased postoperative airflow, although many authors have now concluded that osteotomy rarely decreases nasal airflow, partly because septal and valvular surgery is so effective in secondary patients. The passion of many patients for "small" noses and the aggressiveness of some osteotomy techniques, however, can produce narrow pyriform apertures, in which case excision of the lateral lips of the pyriform apertures improves the patient's symptoms. Finally, inadequate turbinate resection may leave residual obstruction; more commonly, excessive turbinate resection produces a sense of obstruction (presumably from loss of the normal baffling and resistance functions), nasal dryness, and clear, persistent rhinitis. Insufficient turbinate resection is easy to correct; excessive resection and its sequelae have no current accepted and effective treatment. An improvement in nasal appearance should never oblige the patient to a decrease in airway size; virtually all rhinoplasty patients can maintain or improve function if the surgeon remembers the functional interrelationships that exist and plans the operation accordingly.

Skeletal problems

Irregularities or asymmetries may occur in any modified skeletal structure; their visibility varies with the thickness of the soft tissue cover. Some points should be noted about their interpretation. Irregularities at the caudal edges of the bony vault are often attributed to inadequate reduction but more often represent middle vault collapse, which causes the caudal end of the bony arch to stand out in relief; treatment is spreader or dorsal grafts,[6] not further bony resection.

A palpable or visible low point may appear in the midline of the nasal bridge, either intraoperatively or postoperatively.[137] This "mid-dorsal notch" has been interpreted as an untidy resection of the cartilaginous dorsum. More commonly, however, the mid-dorsal notch is a soft tissue phenomenon that occurs where the thinner, upper nasal skin thickens in its transition to the supratip and therefore represents the cephalic end of the supratip deformity (or the midpoint of the inverted V deformity associated with middle vault collapse) and indicates dorsal over-resection; it should be treated by augmentation.

A new frontal asymmetry may develop when dorsal resection has uncovered a high septal deviation. The high septal deviation can be camouflaged by splinting the anterior septal edge with spreader grafts of unequal thickness, adding any necessary onlay grafts for additional symmetry.

Soft tissue problems

As much as graft quality, soft tissue quality determines the beauty of the final result. Skin that has been damaged by previous surgeries may be unevenly thick, can be assumed to be hypovascular, and may not adapt or cover a rebuilt underlying skeleton (which itself may be constructed of suboptimal materials) evenly. Although the author always uses a closed approach and limited dissection in secondary patients, nasal circulation can never be taken lightly. Surgeons who routinely assume that the wider dissection of the open approach is superior in difficult secondary cases, may wish to rethink their philosophy. Even the best open rhinoplasty surgeons can lose nasal tip or columellar skin, a catastrophe in cosmetic cases and painful for all concerned. The surgeon must always remember the surgical principles that apply everywhere in the body – even the nose.

Graft problems

Skeletal problems caused by grafts rank third only because fewer surgeons augment than reduce. For those surgeons who augment often, graft imperfections are the most common reason for secondary revision. Dorsal grafts must be carefully contoured and placed in pockets that limit their movement. Lateral wall grafts may be indicated to camouflage dorsal graft edges; the bony and upper cartilaginous vaults are pyramidal structures. Similarly, tip grafts may produce unacceptable asymmetries or visible edges, particularly if the surgeon has employed single grafts. Graft visibility depends on the number and substance of the augmentation material as well as the characteristics of the soft tissue cover. The surgeon who uses multiple grafts will find tip symmetry easier to achieve and graft visibility less likely. Suture immobilization of tip grafts can also be performed, although the author prefers not to suture grafts so that they can be manipulated into precise position before the dressing is placed.

Hemorrhage

Most patients, particularly those who have undergone septal or turbinate surgery, have moderate bleeding for the first 48–72 h postoperatively, after which drainage subsides. A total of 3% of patients, however, classically re-bleed between postoperative days 5 and 10. At particular risk are patients who have taken drugs or vitamins that interfere with platelet function. The surgeon's major task is to elicit cooperation from the frightened patient and family; as occurs so often in upper gastrointestinal hemorrhage, the calmed patient frequently stops bleeding. Postoperative hemorrhage cannot be treated by the emergency department staff; the surgeon should see the patient personally, remove previously placed packs, suction the airway, and identify the site of bleeding (which frequently ceases after old blood and clots are removed). When bleeding does not stop, reinsertion of an absorbent pack soaked in phenylephrine hydrochloride is necessary.

The need for posterior packs fortunately occurs less frequently, but the surgeon should be familiar and comfortable with their use before the occasion arises.[138] By examining the posterior pharynx with good lighting, suction, and a tongue blade, the surgeon can extract any clots and estimate the pace of any blood running down the posterior pharyngeal wall. Each drop adds approximately 0.10 mL to the accumulating blood loss. At 1 drop per second (6 mL/min or 360 mL/h), it is easy to see how hematemesis can occur, which naturally frightens the patient further and worsens the bleeding. When an airway suctioned clean of clots and packed with epinephrine-soaked cotton does not promptly stop the bleeding, an effective posterior pack is mandatory. The technique essentially involves passing a small-caliber catheter through the nose and retrieving the end with bayonet forceps through the patient's mouth. The surgeon attaches a tonsil sponge (or the equivalent in commercially prepared packs) to the catheter by its string tethers; by pulling the nasal catheter forward, the tonsil sponge can be drawn posteriorly around the soft palate and snugly against the choanae. The anterior nose is then packed, and the tonsil sponge strings, cut free from the catheter, are tied over ample padding to protect the alar rims. The posterior pack can be removed after 4 days with negligible chance of rebleeding. Any posterior pack is unpleasant to the patient, but not nearly as troublesome as continued bleeding.

Septal perforation

Perforations occasionally occur after difficult septoplasties but can be minimized by cautious dissection over the vomer, by repairing tears in the mucoperichondrial flaps, and by placing 1 mm silicone splints on each side of the septal partition before the nose is packed.

Even with these precautions, the occasional septal perforation may be unavoidable and is usually asymptomatic. Small perforations may cause a curious whistling; larger ones cause crusting, epistaxis, and rhinitis as the turbulent airflow spins through the perforated mucosa. Epistaxis frequently reflects an area of exposed septal cartilage or bone. The repair of septal perforations is difficult; recurrence after local or even distant (labial mucosal) flaps in the largest series approaches 50%. In symptomatic perforations, it is often preferable to identify and eliminate areas of exposed septal skeleton and repair the mucoperichondrial flaps to obtain a perforation with a healed, stable surface. If symptoms can be alleviated in this manner, closure of the perforation itself is not usually necessary.

Rhinitis

Temporary rhinitis may occur for several weeks postoperatively, particularly when an obstructed airway has been improved. Persistent rhinitis, however, is uncommon unless excessive turbinectomy has been performed. The proponents of turbinectomy minimize this sequela,[139,140] but it is a troublesome entity for which there is yet no consistently effective treatment.

Circulatory problems

Circulatory complications occur more commonly after open than after closed rhinoplasty, especially when cautery has been used to control columellar vessels or where excessive retraction has been employed. During primary endonasal rhinoplasty, the surgeon can make inter-cartilaginous and infracartilaginous incisions with or without alar wedge resections without fear of circulatory compromise as long as the incisions are not made longer than is necessary, skeletonization is appropriately limited, the dermis is not thinned, and packs and dressings are not placed tightly. Differentiation of the tip lobule from the dorsum (the desirable "supratip break") reflects not overcorrection of the cartilaginous dorsum but rather adequate dorsal height and tip projection. These factors absent, the surgeon cannot produce a supratip depression by excessively tight taping or steroid injections. But even in the primary rhinoplasty, nasal circulation is not immune to grafts placed under tension, rough tissue handling, or constrictive dressings. The surgeon should plan incisions to provide necessary access and minimize the amount of dissection.

Infection

Bacterial infection is mercifully rare after rhinoplasty and septal surgery[141–149] but has become more common with the emergence and increasing prevalence of methicillin-resistant staphylococcal aureus as a community-acquired pathogen.[150]

The surgeon should remember that the operative surface is not the cutaneous cover but rather the vestibular skin and mucosa and prepare the internal nose thoroughly. Many surgeons use antibiotics while postoperative packing is in place, although their absolute necessity has not been established. Toxic shock syndrome, cavernous sinus and nasofrontal abscess, and even endocarditis are extremely rare but have been reported. Limited but especially troublesome infections occur infrequently in areas of tissue compromise, with excessive manipulation, or where conchal cartilage grafts have been placed carrying gram-negative organisms from the external auditory canals.

Septal collapse

Loss of cartilaginous support has protean effects because the intact septal partition is necessary for normal bridge contour, nasal length, base support, middle vault (and internal valvular) competence, and upper lip carriage. The required reconstruction is therefore predictably complex. The surgeon may minimize the possibility of septal collapse by identifying those patients with unhealed or unstable septal fractures and by leaving a minimum 15 mm width of undissected septum along the dorsum. Those who prefer open septoplasty are similarly wise to preserve undissected mucoperichondrium along the dorsal edge to avoid jeopardizing septal support if unexpected, unhealed fracture lines are encountered.

Red nose

The "post-rhinoplasty red nose" is a cutaneous manifestation of postoperative circulatory readjustment and is displayed varyingly in patients; many never develop this condition, whereas others develop it after the first rhinoplasty. Patients with facial telangiectases develop red noses more frequently; most improve spontaneously during the first postoperative year. When the condition persists, laser treatment is simple and effective.

Nontender discoloration, usually manifested as a "blush" in the nasal tip during the early postoperative period, can signal either low-grade infection or ischemia. Neither can be ignored. Even when the access wound has not been closed under tension, internal pressures caused by grafts, packing, postoperative edema, and taping may render even a carefully placed dressing too tight. The surgeon is wise to remove the tape sling if tip color is not perfectly normal. Even at 24 h, graft position will not be lost; much more can be jeopardized if a tight dressing remains.

Other complications

Lacrimal duct injury (presumably from lateral osteotomy) was described in a 1968 series,[151] in which the incidence of lacrimal obstruction in a 27-patient group was 78%; later studies have confirmed this rare possibility.[152,153] Reports have also appeared of orbital floor and extraocular muscle injury after osteotomy. Such events are unlikely if the surgeon knows and controls osteotome position. Cerebrospinal fluid rhinorrhea, cavernous sinus thrombosis, meningitis, permanent anosmia, recurrent intradermal cysts and blindness after

corticosteroid injection for supratip deformity have been reported but are fortunately uncommon.[154–159]

Serious but rare (0.02% in a pooled series of 12 672 cases) complications have been reported after calvarial bone graft harvesting: hemiparesis; hemiplegia (in a patient with platelet disorder); epidural hematoma; subdural infection; dural, brain, or sagittal sinus lacerations; aphasia; persistent speech defect; and temporal hemianopia. Adverse events are extremely rare in the hands of surgeons experienced with proper bone harvesting technique.[108]

Alloplastics placed during rhinoplasty have their own litany of postoperative problems. The reader is encouraged to become familiar with these misadventures before assuming that alloplastic reconstructions are inherently less troublesome than autogenous materials.[160–169]

The unhappy patient

In a perfect world, the relationship between the surgeon and the aesthetic surgery patient would be even more favorable than in other medical encounters. Although it may be optimal for patient and surgeon to like each other, this is not always necessary or possible for the frightened cancer patient or the intoxicated emergency department patient. In the elective cosmetic case, everything should be different.

Differences do exist in aesthetic surgery, but perhaps not as expected. Where the risks and complications are as real as in nonelective procedures and where the emotional investment may be even greater, patients expect more than passable outcomes without complications. Patients desire excellent results, even "perfect" results, from procedures that are technically difficult, that change appearance and that have profound ramifications for that complex part of the human psyche that we call body image. In aesthetic surgery, as much as or more than in any surgical encounter, it is important for patient and surgeon to understand and (for lack of a better word) "like" each other.

The surgeon–patient relationship is always tested when things do not go as planned. It is these circumstances that measure the surgeon's equanimity and test the degree to which "informed consent" has been obtained. It is here that the patient must understand the difference between the uncontrolled and the uncontrollable. The patient is often seeing a "problem" that he or she cannot necessarily identify but that well-meaning but uninformed friends or family members have interpreted instead. In a sound relationship with the surgeon, education and reassurance will support the patient until the problem resolves or until it can be corrected.

Differences between primary and secondary patients

Two features separate secondary rhinoplasty patients from primary patients: (1) The secondary rhinoplasty patient's tissues have undergone irreversible changes; the diagnosis is more difficult, and the corrective techniques are more demanding; (2) paralleling changes in soft tissues and donor sites, the patients themselves are "depleted." Having undergone one or more unsuccessful procedures, the secondary rhinoplasty patient frequently has a lower tolerance for postoperative problems or disappointments. Thorough preoperative evaluation, counseling, and education of the patient are mandatory. The last thing that a tertiary rhinoplasty patient needs is another unsuccessful result; the surgeon electing to treat such patients must learn the specifics of secondary rhinoplasty problems and perform a biologically sound surgical plan.

Your patient or another surgeon's patient

The identity of the prior surgeon creates distinct differences in management. The surgeon evaluating his or her own unhappy patient has the advantage of knowing the operative circumstances, the characteristics of the donor material, and the patient's personality but has the disadvantage of having to manage both the patient's disappointment and his or her own. Alternatively, the surgeon evaluating someone else's unhappy patient need not overcome disappointment with the current result but has less information about the original deformity, the patient's tissue idiosyncrasies and donor material, the procedures themselves, and the patient's personality and goals. Particularly when a patient is angry with the prior surgeon, it is imperative that the secondary surgeon have confidence that the patient: (1) has realistic surgical goals and understands what is needed to achieve them and (2) appreciates that the original operating surgeon was doing his or her best to produce the patient's original goals.

Until these criteria can be satisfied, the surgeon is wise to delay surgery.

Body dysmorphic disorder in rhinoplasty patients

Body dysmorphic disorder (BDD) is the current name for the disease previously called dysmorphophobia, a term coined by the Italian physician Morselli in 1891 but is really much older.[170] The most common affected body areas are the nose, hair, and genitalia. Strong comorbidity exists between obsessive-compulsive disorder and BDD, and there are associations with major depressive disorder, social anxiety disorder, eating disorder, impulse control disorder and substance abuse;[171–182] and increasing evidence from my own practice series and the mental health literature indicates that a significant number of affected patients have histories of childhood abuse.[183–185] The large body of literature on this topic continues to expand; BDD is important to any discussion of rhinoplasty because across all cultures, the physical feature that most commonly causes emotional distress and for which surgery is most often sought is the nose (45% of cases).

A patient must exhibit three criteria to satisfy the diagnosis of BDD. (1) There must be preoccupation with some imagined defect in appearance; if a slight but real deformity is present, the patient's concern must be markedly excessive; (2) preoccupation must cause clinically significant distress or impairment in social, occupational, or other important areas of functioning; (3) the preoccupation must not be better defined by another mental disorder. Pertinent to rhinoplasty are the following points. Some 72% of BDD patients seek surgery; 48% of such patients have considered suicide, and 27% have a suicide plan.[172–175] Once affected with BDD, men and women are equally likely to undergo aesthetic surgery. Regrettably, surgical and even other medical treatments are generally unsuccessful for BDD patients and may even exacerbate their symptoms. In one study, two-thirds of the patients who had undergone surgery reported no improvement or a worsening of their symptoms.[174]

All of this is not to say that rhinoplasty cannot be performed in patients who share some characteristics of BDD, although those patients with an established diagnosis do not currently appear to be good surgical candidates, even with concomitant psychiatric treatment. In the author's experience, the degree of insight that a patient possesses of his or her "obsession" or overvaluation of a physical deformity has been most helpful in predicting the success of surgical treatment. Unfortunately, the stress of surgery appears to reinforce some patients' belief that their delusional views are undistorted; surgery may make some patients more delusional. Other clinicians have related the same experience.[182]

In a recent review of 1000 consecutive operated rhinoplasty patients in the author's practice, 0.5% of primary patients and 4.5% of secondary patients satisfied the criteria for BDD. The diagnostic difficulty that the surgeon faces is that many non-BDD patients who have had unfavorable results share the more superficial characteristics of patients affected with BDD: understandable apprehension about further surgery; perfectionism; anxiety about every detail of any proposed procedure; fear of complications; depression about their deformities and the financial losses that have been incurred; and the loss of family support. In addition, the deformities for which these patients seek surgery may be subtle but nevertheless real; the fact that a treating physician or even mental health professional may not see the surgical problem does not by itself mean that it does not exist. Thus, the definition of BDD in the mental health literature may be too narrow for the plastic surgeon. The literature provides no simple diagnostic tests, although screening tools have been evaluated.[179,180] The surgeon should nevertheless be wary of the patient with the "minimal defect."

My current thesis, based on data documented elsewhere[183] is this: the degree of difficulty that patients demonstrate to surgeons and staff is partly related to their narcissism in the true sense of the word. In these unfortunate individuals, self-worth is not internal but rather dependent on appearance. The conversion to BDD, in many cases, is related to childhood trauma. There is corroborating evidence to support my theory.[184] These unfortunate patients' childhood experiences have engendered poorly functioning adults who cannot value themselves; who have poor protective capacities (boundaries); who have distorted senses of reality ("my nose is abnormal; therefore I am worthless"); who have difficulty with self-care (particularly during their postoperative courses), as well as with living and behaving moderately. Affected patients often see the surgeon as a rescuer and therefore place unrealistic expectations not only on the surgeon but also on the effect that rhinoplasty will have on their lives preoperatively and postoperatively. These patients may experience an emotional high in the early postoperative period: As one patient told me, "I am never as happy as when I am recovering from cosmetic surgery." However, when the "rescue" does not occur, the fantasy transforms into victim anger and fear of abandonment, not just by the patient but by the plastic surgeon as well. The patient may plan how to entice the surgeon to operate again and re-establish the relationship; leave and find another surgeon; begin a secondary addiction; or think of ways to retaliate, through the medical boards, the internet, destruction of personal property, or even bodily harm. Many of these patients demonstrate and recount significant relational trauma and self-esteem issues that lead them to multiple surgeries, endless revisions, unhappiness with the result, anger against the surgeon, a sense of betrayal, and sometimes a desire to "get even" – hence the importance of recognizing language and behavior that connote victim anger.

This is not to say that every unhappy patient is psychologically disturbed, or even that the patient with a concomitant psychiatric diagnosis cannot undergo successful aesthetic surgery; Edgerton et al.[182] have demonstrated otherwise. However, the surgeon performing rhinoplasty, treating secondary deformities, and trying to understand dissatisfied patients must be conversant with BDD, so that the chances of missing it before surgery are minimized.

The decision to reoperate

The patient counseled properly before surgery knows that resolution of swelling takes time and that the final appearance may not stabilize until the end of the first postoperative year or later. In practice, waiting for the final outcome is a bigger challenge for some patients (and surgeons) than for others.

Accordingly, the surgeon should withhold the decision to reoperate until the postoperative result has stabilized, usually at least 1 year. In some patients or after multiple surgeries, even more time may be necessary. The nature and degree of revision, and who should perform it, depend on the same factors involved in the prior rhinoplasty. Patient and surgeon must understand each other explicitly because secondary surgery itself is often geometrically more difficult than the primary operation. Regardless of the overt indications, patient and surgeon must not abandon the priorities of safety, function, and aesthetics, in that order. Rhinoplasty does not own its reputation by accident.

Secondary rhinoplasty

Space does not permit the discussion of endonasal secondary rhinoplasty. The author's analysis and techniques are available elsewhere.[186] The most common problems requiring secondary rhinoplasty are: iatrogenic or uncorrected airway obstruction, failure to recognize the critical anatomical variants described earlier (low radix or low dorsum, inadequate tip projection, narrow middle vault, or alar cartilage malposition), supratip deformity, problems of length or balance, problems resulting from nasal implants, technical problems related to grafting, or deformities caused by previous open rhinoplasty. Only the last topic will be briefly discussed.

Why primary and secondary rhinoplasty are the same operation

There are surgeons who will perform primary rhinoplasty but not revisions. That is certainly understandable, but for the surgeon who has learned rhinoplasty phenomenology, anatomical variants, principles of balance, grafting techniques, and airway management, the two operations can be viewed as only variations on a surgical theme. If the surgeon is economical in incisions, maintains or establishes equilibrium, removes or repositions deforming parts, maximizes functional support, and uses grafts to create balance, contour and structure, there is really no difference between primary and secondary rhinoplasty except the donor sites.

The secret to good secondary rhinoplasty is good primary rhinoplasty – not only performing but understanding the operation and the genesis of its various postoperative shapes. Because secondary shapes are not limitless but form patterns, the solutions form patterns. With experience, and by studying photos of secondary patients before they had surgery, the surgeon can become facile at recognizing patterns of response and deformity, so that nasal shapes not only indicate the predisposing shapes that produced them but also the procedures that will correct them.

Deformities caused by prior open rhinoplasty

As the open approach has become more common, deformities unique to that surgery are increasing (*Fig. 19.23*). In the author's practice, the incidence of the secondary rhinoplasty patients who had their original surgeries performed through the open approach has risen from 28% to 88% in the past 15 years. The deformities caused by that approach are distinct from those that characterize prior endonasal rhinoplasty and more commonly involve the nasal tip, alar rims, or columella (e.g., a tip that is too narrow or rigid, hard columellar struts, unacceptable columellar scars, alar rim notching, alar collapse, or over-resected nostrils). In contrast, those patients originally treated endonasally most commonly seek secondary rhinoplasty for a dorsum that is too high or a nose that is too long. In a review of 100 consecutive cases,[187] secondary patients treated by the open approach had more presenting complaints (5.6 vs 2.6 for closed rhinoplasty patients) and had undergone more procedures before seeking correction from another surgeon (3.1 vs 1.2 for the closed rhinoplasty patients). The deformities most commonly produced by the open approach are those involving the anatomical parts encountered first during surgical exposure (the columella, alar cartilages, and alar rims) or by those procedures that can be performed more easily or more aggressively through the open approach (e.g., columellar struts and alar cartilage suturing).

Some secondary deformities are easier to correct than others. The nose previously operated through the open approach contains more scar and deep sutures, making the dissection more difficult and the resection of uncorrectable deformities more tedious. Struts may have widened the columella but not produced adequate tip projection; the struts will have to be interrupted or removed and tip projection produced by more anatomic methods. The surgeon should assume that the nasal circulation has been irreversibly damaged, and proceed cautiously. In some cases, the secondary surgeon is operating under skin that may behave as if it had been irradiated. For this reason, the curious strategy of some surgeons to treat the severely damaged tertiary nose by a wide, aggressive, open dissection runs counter to surgical principles followed everywhere else in the body and would

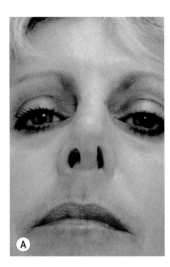
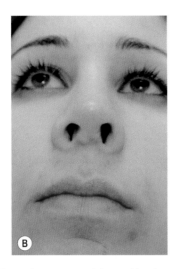
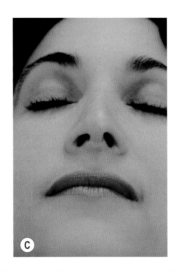
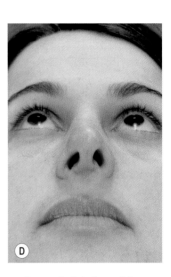

Fig. 19.23 Examples of noses deformed by previous unsuccessful open rhinoplasty. Some deformities are more common after this operation, particularly those of the external valves, nostrils, and columella.

be hard to defend if soft tissue loss occurs. The surgeon who performs both open and closed rhinoplasty in different circumstances would therefore be wise to consider performing the open approach on the primary, unscarred nose, and the closed approach for the scarred, hypovascular, damaged nose, rather than the other way around.

As is so true of all aesthetic procedures, the relationship between patient and surgeon is paramount because perfection is difficult and elusive and because rhinoplasty changes facial appearance. Following the principle that Osler enunciated on treating his famous patient, Walt Whitman: "A doctor does not treat typhoid fever, but he treats the man with typhoid, and it is the man with his peculiarities – his bodily idiosyncrasies – we have to consider".[188]

Like many plastic surgical operations, rhinoplasty is brain surgery.

Access the complete references list online at **http://www.expertconsult.com**

1. Constantian MB. *Rhinoplasty: craft and magic*. St. Louis: Quality Medical; 2009.

   The author's complete text. Covers nasal phenomenology, so that preoperative and postoperative deformities can be seen to form patterns; therefore the solutions are not limitless but also form patterns. The rhinomanometric improvement in airflow is given for each case where the information was available, and analysis and exposition of intraoperative changes are emphasized. Chapters cover not only rhinoplasty analysis and technique but anatomic variants, function, right brain training for rhinoplasty, body dysmorphic disorder, and the author's own complications.

2. Edwards B. *A new drawing on the right side of the brain*. New York: Penguin Putnam; 1999.

   A delightful and instructive adventure into art. Most of us lose the ability to "see" what is really in front of us as the left brain begins to dominate at about age 10, which is why most adults draw at that level of sophistication. Yet plastic surgery, not only rhinoplasty but breast reduction, TRAM flap shaping, forehead flaps, and many other procedures benefit from the ability to call upon right-brain skills at will. This book teaches how, in an entertaining way.

10. Sheen JH, Sheen AP. *Aesthetic rhinoplasty*, 2nd ed. St. Louis: Mosby; 1987:988–1011.

    This two volume text is the 2nd edition of the book that started the revolution in rhinoplasty of the 1980s and beyond. Our entire rhinoplasty lexicon derives from it. Virtually all of the text is still current and any surgeon seriously interested in learning rhinoplasty and its modern roots should own and study a copy.

52. Fomon S, Gilbert JG, Caron AL, et al. Collapsed ala: pathologic physiology and management. *Arch Otolaryngol*. 1950;51:465.

    A classic paper on what we now call external valvular collapse by a pioneer who intuitively understood what the next generation of surgeons forgot: that each airway has two sides.

174. Phillips KA. *The broken mirror: understanding and treating body dysmorphic disorder*. New York: Oxford University Press; 2005.

    A text written by a noted authority on body dysmorphic disorder, intended for the lay public but so well referenced that it can be an introduction and reference work for the interested physician as well.

20

Airway issues and the deviated nose

Bahman Guyuron and Bryan S. Armijo

Access the Historical Perspective section online at
http://www.expertconsult.com

Introduction

The rhinoplasty surgeon's understanding of the anatomy and physiology of the nasal airway and the various causes of obstruction are paramount to making the correct diagnosis and executing the appropriate management. The most common treatment modality in this situation often involves submucous resection of the septum and/or inferior turbinates. Despite being the correct choice in some situations, the decision to perform such procedures should be founded upon a careful analysis of the findings. In addition, the etiology of many nasal airway obstruction problems is not structural. In these scenarios, it is a physiologic obstruction that is amenable to medical management and patience alone. This type of prudent assessment combined with an understanding of the nasal airway anatomy and physiology will lead to successful correction of an often challenging problem.

Anatomy

Nasal anatomy is covered in Chapter 17. Specific anatomy, as it relates to the airway, can be organized into soft tissue and osseocartilaginous categories. Although less commonly involved in nasal airway disorders, the soft tissue envelope with its underlying perinasal musculature plays a vital role in maintaining the patency of the valvular mechanism.

The perinasal musculature can be divided into an intrinsic (having both origin and insertion within the perinasal area) and an extrinsic group containing three paired muscles.[1,2]

The intrinsic group includes the procerus, which elevates the dorsum and lowers the lateral cartilages. Its distal aponeurosis blends with the pars transversa of the nasalis muscle to form the superficial musculoaponeurotic system of the nose. The pars transversa provides lateral wall stability and can also

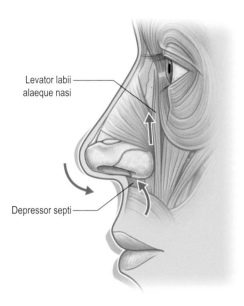

Fig. 20.1 The anatomy of the pertinent perinasal muscles.

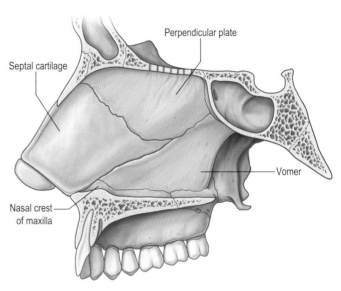

Fig. 20.2 The nasal septum is composed of the septal cartilage, the perpendicular plate of the ethmoid superiorly, the vomer posteriorly, and the maxillary crest inferiorly.

be a dilator. The primary dilatory muscle of the ala is the pars alaris and is responsible for alar flaring. In contrast, the depressor alae or myrtiforme muscle, which originates from the border of the pyriform crest and then rises vertically, like a fan, up to the ala, acts as a depressor and constrictor of the nostrils. Release of this muscle during alar base surgery has a beneficial effect on the external valve.

The three paired muscles of the extrinsic group include the levator labii superioris alaeque nasi, zygomaticus minor, and the orbicularis oris. Of these, the levator labii superioris alaeque nasi is the most important dilator with the zygomaticus minor providing lateral wall stability *(Fig. 20.1)*.

Other soft tissue components involved in airway competence are the nasal alae. Although devoid of cartilage, they are composed of a fibrofatty areolar tissue which is lined by epithelium internally and externally. Collapse of these structures will lead to an airway obstruction.

When considering the structures of the osseocartilaginous vault, the most important central support for the nose is the septum *(Fig. 20.2)*. The perpendicular plate of the ethmoid articulates with the posterior edge of the quadrangular (septal) cartilage and both structures articulate with the vomer inferiorly. The vomer then lays directly on the maxillary crest. The anterior-caudal most portion of the septal cartilage also rests on the maxillary crest, however, in a tongue-and-groove relationship. This point of articulation is unique in that the perichondrium of the cartilage is only partially contiguous with the periosteum of the crest allowing a decussation of fibers which joins the contralateral perichondrium.[2] This crossed configuration can make a seamless submucoperichondrial dissection less than facile. It also lends this portion of the septum susceptible to post-traumatic displacement out of the groove of the crest.

The upper and lower lateral cartilages also play a significant role in nasal support. The point at which the caudal margin of the upper lateral cartilages and the cephalic rim of the lower lateral cartilages overlap is defined as the scroll area. Cartilaginous overlap in this region has been shown to

enhance support at this level.[3] Superiorly, another area of overlap occurs at the junction between the cephalic upper lateral cartilages and the nasal bones. This makes up the keystone area and is characterized by a firm adherence between these structures. Subsequently, trauma to the nasal bones can shift this entire unit. In addition, the upper lateral cartilages are fused to the septum in the mid-vault region and separate as one moves caudally. This is clinically important during placement of spreader grafts, as this region will require sharp dissection to release the upper lateral cartilage from the septum.[2]

Although not of structural significance, the inferior turbinate occupies a large portion of the nasal airway and can account for up to two-thirds of the total airway resistance.[4] It is composed of dense lamellar bone taking origin from the medial wall of the maxilla bilaterally. The turbinates are covered with an erectile mucosal tissue composed of pseudostratified ciliated columnar epithelium. The submucosa contains large quantities of seromucinous glands and vascular channels containing cavernous sinusoids. These channels are under the influence of the autonomic nervous system and thus serve as the end target for decongestant medication. The sympathetic system regulates the resistance vessels (and therefore blood flow) and the parasympathetic system regulates the capacitance vessels (and therefore blood volume) of the nasal mucosa. The submucosa also contains large numbers of mast cells, eosinophils, plasma cells, lymphocytes, and macrophages. Thus, chronic inflammation, secondary to stimulation of these abundant pro-inflammatory cellular constituents can lead to fibrous deposition and chronic hypertrophy of the turbinate.[2]

The internal nasal valve accounts for approximately 50% of the total airway resistance and is the narrowest segment of the nasal airway.[5,6] It is formed by the angle between the junction of the nasal septum and the caudal margin of the upper lateral cartilage and is typically 10–15° *(Fig. 20.3)*.

The external nasal valve is formed by the caudal edge of the lateral crus of the lower lateral cartilage, the soft tissue alae, the membranous septum, and the sill of the nostril and serves as the entrance to the nose. This is an occasional site of obstruction secondary to extrinsic factors, such as foreign bodies, or intrinsic factors, such as weak or collapsed lower lateral cartilages, a loss of vestibular skin, or cicatricial narrowing *(Fig. 20.4)*.[7]

Physiology

As described in Eugene Courtiss *et al.*'s overview on nasal physiology, the nose has seven basic functions: respiration, temperature regulation, humidification, particulate filtration, olfaction, phonation, and as a secondary sex organ. The most vital of these functions is respiration and can be described using some basic laws of physics.[8]

When there is a pressure differential between the external nasal vestibule and the nasopharynx, a gradient is formed and air flows through the nose. Thus, an increase in nasal

resistance (decreases in nasal airflow) can result from such structural limitations as hypertrophied turbinates, septal deviations, valve incompetence, or intranasal masses. The magnitude of nasal airway resistance cannot be underestimated and, in fact, is responsible for approximately half of the total respiratory tree resistance.[5,6]

Bernoulli's principle defines flow through a tubular structure such that the flow at the two ends is constant. In addition, areas of constriction increase flow and areas of dilation decrease flow. In these areas of increased flow, the pressure is decreased and vice versa in areas of decreased flow.[8] This becomes clinically evident in the incompetent internal or external nasal valve. Because these are areas of narrowing/constriction, airflow is increased at the level of the valve, leading to a decrease in pressure. This effectively generates a collapsing force on the valves and is exacerbated upon heavy inspiration or sniffing.[2]

Bernoulli's principle can be mathematically substantiated using Poiseuille's law. This law provides that flow is directly proportional to the difference in pressure multiplied by the radius raised to the fourth power and inversely proportional to the length of the tube.[8]

$$\text{Flow} = \text{Constant (K)} \cdot dP \cdot r^4 / \text{Length}$$

This demonstrates that the longer the tube (nose), the less the flow. Even more dramatic is that a minimal increase in the size of the tube causes an exponential (r^4) increase in flow. This has clinical implications as the cross-sectional area varies throughout the nose. It is narrowest at the internal nasal valve, larger at the level of the mid-turbinates, and largest at the level of the posterior choanae. As a result, minimal changes at the level of the internal nasal valve can have profound changes on nasal airflow and is subsequently cited as the most common cause of nasal airway obstruction.[9–11]

An understanding of laminar and turbulent flow is also essential to a complete understanding of respiration and nasal airflow physiology and dynamics. When laminar flow exists, air moves through a straight tube in a predictable fashion. Air near the walls of the tube is virtually still, whereas flow in the

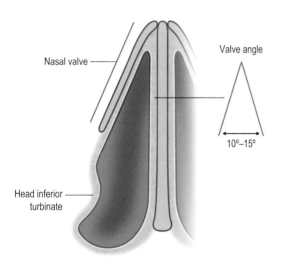

Fig. 20.3 The internal nasal valve is defined by the angle between the junction of the nasal septum and the caudal margin of the upper lateral cartilage and is typically 10–15°.

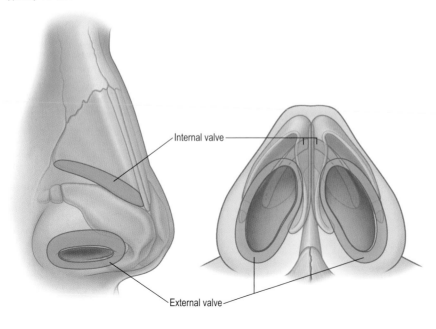

External valve

Fig. 20.4 The external nasal valve is formed by the caudal edge of the lateral crus of the lower lateral cartilage, the soft tissue alae, the membranous septum, and the sill of the nostril.

center moves rapidly. This is in contrast to turbulent flow, where the airflow follows a random path and forms eddy currents and whorls. To overcome turbulence, a greater pressure gradient must be generated. In other words, the less laminar the airflow, the higher the resistance and the lower the airflow. For example, during quiet respiration where pressures are low and under 1.5 cm of water, nasal airflow is considered to be laminar.[12] During inspiration, the main airflow is directed through the middle meatus with a smaller amount coursing through the inferior meatus and an even smaller amount up toward the cribriform plates.[13,14]

Finally, another less well understood factor in nasal airflow is the nasal cycle (cycle of Minz). Approximately 80% of the population experiences cyclical swelling and contraction of the nasal mucosa. While one airway is enlarging, the other is constricting.[15,16] The process requires 30 min to 5 h to complete and total airflow and resistance remains constant throughout this period.[17]

Temperature regulation and humidification

The physiologic nasal regulatory system is so efficient that inspired air is heated almost to body temperature before it even reaches the larynx. Even air at temperatures of −5°C is brought to between 31°C and 37°C. This function typically requires 70–100 calories per day.[10,18]

Regardless of the ambient temperature or humidity, approximately 90% humidification is achieved during inspiration before the air reaches the lungs. This requires 1 liter (L) of water per day.[19] A small amount of this water is recovered during exhalation secondary to cooling of the exhaled air, however a net balance of −250 mL to −500 mL per day still exists.[20]

Particulate filtration

Four mechanisms have been described by which the nasal cavity achieves adequate filtration of inspired air. These include impingement, electrostatic charge, vibrissae, and the mucociliary blanket. Impingement is a phenomenon that occurs when particles suspended in a gas become deposited on the walls of a tube downstream from a bend or constriction. Two such bends exist within the nasal cavity: the internal nasal valve, where the airflow is changed from a column into a sheet, and at the posterior nasopharynx, where the airflow is sharply deflected inferiorly. These two anatomic impingement points are responsible for the deposition/filtration of 85–90% of particulate matter ≥5 μm.[18] The electrostatic charge of the walls of the nasal cavity is positive and produced by the mucociliary blanket. Thus, the negatively charged inspired foreign particles are attracted to the nasal walls and prevented from traveling distally to more sensitive areas of the respiratory tract. Larger particles are trapped within the vibrissae, which are found just within the nasal vestibule. The mucociliary blanket is composed of two layers: the deeper layer is thinner and less viscous and surrounds the cilia, while the superficial layer is thicker and more viscous and houses the cilia tips. As a whole, the mucociliary blanket is a thin, sticky, adhesive sheet with a pH slightly more acidic than serum. It is produced by serous and mucous glands and by the goblet cells of the mucosa at a rate of about 250 mL per day. This blanket ultimately functions, in a rhythmic fashion, to sweep particulate matter to the posterior nasopharynx.[2,18]

Olfaction

Olfaction clearly enhances our sense of taste and aids in memory association. It may also play a protective role by warning of potential environmental dangers when noxious odors are perceived. Causes for an olfactory disturbance are many and include infection, trauma, mechanical obstruction, endocrine disorders and medications to mention a few. In addition, nasal septal surgery can infrequently lead to anosmia; fortunately, this is most often temporary.[8,21]

Phonation

It is well known that the voice is produced via vibrations of the vocal cords with the passage of air. However, the quality of the voice depends on the resonance of air through the mouth, pharynx, and nose. As a resonance chamber, the nose is a necessary component in the formation of certain vowels and consonants alike. Patients may therefore ask if nasal surgery will alter the sound of their voice. To that end, they can be counseled that post-surgical changes in the sound of ones' voice have not been substantiated. Septal perforations, however, change airflow resistance and thus, may change voice quality and/or create a nasal whistle with inspiration.[8]

Secondary sex organ

It has been known for some time that mucosal engorgement occurs during sexual arousal.[16] A relatively recent discovery in nasal physiology is the vomeronasal organ (Jacobson's organ, Ruysch tube). It is composed of bilateral blind ducts in the mucosa of the anterior third of the human septum.[22–25] Their role is not fully understood, but it is felt that they play a part in reproductive behavior by acting as pheromone chemosensory receptors. The external opening of the ducts can be found in the septal mucosa just posterior to the columellar base and 1 mm above the maxillary groove.[25]

Basic science/disease process

With an understanding of the nasal airway anatomy and physiology, one can more easily begin to identify potential sites of obstruction and/or deviation. Although many causes of nasal airway obstruction are "anatomic" in nature, and thus amenable to surgical correction, medical reasons for obstruction cannot be overlooked. Surgical intervention in these instances would be a disservice to the patient. Thus, there may be more than one etiology and therefore, more than one line of treatment. This section will focus on the various etiologies for nasal airway obstruction, with their respective treatment recommendations to follow in a later portion of this chapter.

Rhinitis

Rhinitis can be the result of a number of different causes including infectious, allergic, vasomotor, atrophic, rhinitis medicamentosa, postoperative, hypertrophic, and miscellaneous.

It has even been cited as the number one cause of nasal obstruction.[9]

Infectious rhinitis is the most common type, and presents in two forms: viral and bacterial. Viral rhinitis is more common than bacterial etiologies and is usually the result of the rhinovirus. Bacterial rhinitis is mostly caused by Gram-positive isolates. Regardless of the etiology (viral or bacterial), there is significant mucosal edema during infection and this can last for several weeks leading to a narrowed nasal airway with subsequent obstruction.[26,27]

Allergic rhinitis is said to have prevalence of between 14% and 31% in the United States alone.[28] True allergic rhinitis is mediated by immunoglobulin E in response to an antigen-antibody reaction. This most commonly presents in a seasonal form from environmental factors such as an air-borne pollen or spore. Associated symptoms include sneezing, urticaria, and mucosal swelling.

Vasomotor rhinitis arises when the balance between the sympathetic and parasympathetic nervous systems is disrupted, such that the parasympathetic system is hyperactive. This leads to copious amounts of watery rhinorrhea and mucosal congestion. Although most commonly idiopathic in nature, other potential causes include pregnancy, and endocrine and emotional disorders.[2]

Atrophic rhinitis is a rare condition with its typical onset in puberty and characterized by a slow, progressive atrophy of the nasal mucosa. This results in crusting and often foul smelling drainage.[5] Several organisms have been isolated from patients affected by this condition, however their exact mechanism in the pathogenesis remains unclear.[29,30] A subcategory of atrophic rhinitis, is "empty nose syndrome". This is a poorly understood and highly debated iatrogenic disorder which results from the destruction of normal nasal tissue; specifically the turbinates. The most commonly reported symptoms include a paradoxical nasal obstruction and feeling of intranasal fullness.

Rhinitis medicamentosa (RM) occurs frequently in patients who present with nasal airway obstruction. It is seen with prolonged use of sympathetic agonists such as Afrin or Neo-Synephrine and leads to a rebound phenomenon of mucosal engorgement and profuse rhinorrhea. Patients often try increasing both the dose and the frequency of nasal sprays upon the onset of RM, worsening the condition. The swelling of the nasal passages caused by rebound congestion may eventually result in permanent turbinate hyperplasia.[31]

Postoperative rhinitis or symptoms of nasal obstruction invariably affect virtually all patients after rhinoplasty. This is usually a result of normal postoperative mucosal edema and/or crusting within the nasal cavity. In addition, patients who present with preoperative allergic rhinitis or vasomotor rhinitis may experience a postoperative "flare" and should be counseled as such prior to surgery.

Hypertrophic rhinitis results from chronic mucosal inflammation and can stem from any of the aforementioned types of rhinitis. This chronic inflammation ultimately leads to turbinate hypertrophy, most commonly the inferior turbinate. As would be expected, this is a major cause of nasal airway obstruction.

Miscellaneous causes of rhinitis may include such medications as oral contraceptives, antihypertensives (beta-blockers), and antidepressants. Other causes include Wegener's granulomatosis, polymorphic reticulosis, cystic fibrosis, syphilis, hypothyroidism, and poorly regulated diabetes.[5,32]

The septum

The septum and the nasal bones control the direction of the nose and thus, deviation of the nose can result from malalignment of one or the other or a combination of both. Often, the nasal bones follow the direction of the deviated septum, however these structures may move independently. Midvault deviation consistently accompanies at least anterior and commonly mid and posterior septal deviation. Deviation of the lower nose may involve the caudal septum, anterior nasal spine and lower lateral cartilages. In all types of septal deviation, the middle and/or inferior turbinates may be enlarged. The enlargement is usually juxtaposed to the concave side of the septum. Previous studies have detailed and categorized the types of septal deviation.[33–36]

There are six classes of septal deviation:

1. The most common type is a septal tilt in which the septum itself has no significant underlying curvature, but is tilted to one side. In most cases of septal tilt, the internal deviation of the septum is to the left and the external deviation of the nose is to the right. This is usually accompanied by an enlargement of the inferior turbinate ipsilateral to the external deviation **(Fig. 20.5)**.

2. C-shaped anteroposterior deviation is usually associated with deviation of the vomerine plate. External reflection of the anteroposterior C deviation is often similar to the

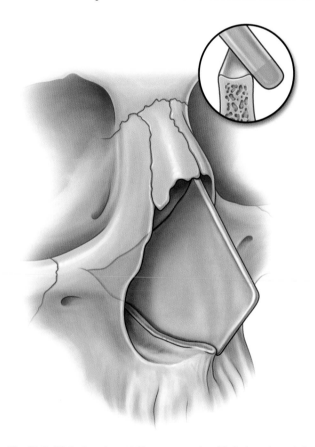

Fig. 20.5 (A) C-shaped septal tilt, anteroposterior. **(B)** C-shaped septal tilt, cephalocaudal.

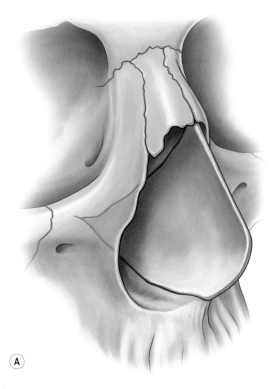

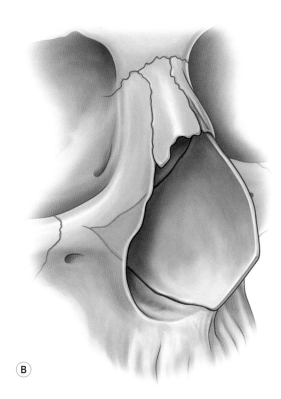

Fig. 20.6 (A) C-shaped septal deviation, anteroposterior. **(B)** C-shaped septal deviation, cephalocaudal.

septal tilt. The middle turbinate is often enlarged as well *(Fig. 20.6A)*.

3. C-shaped cephalocaudal deviation presents externally as a C-shaped appearance of the nose. In reality, the most common form of this deviation is the reverse C with the curve facing the patient's right. The opposing inferior and often the middle turbinates are enlarged *(Fig. 20.6B)*.

4. S-shaped anteroposterior deviation is defined by two curvatures next to each other, in opposing directions. Externally, the anteroposterior deviation will present with a shift of the nose to one side *(Fig. 20.7A)*.

5. S-shaped cephalocaudal deviation is similar to the previous type except that the curvatures combine to form an S-shape in the cephalic to caudal direction. Turbinate enlargement is common with both types of S-shaped deviations *(Fig. 20.7B)*.

6. The last type of septal deviation is a localized deviation or spur. This is a purely functional problem and has no translation to external shape of the nose.[33] Turbinate enlargement is not common with this type of deviation.

The internal nasal valve

The importance of functioning nasal valves in nasal airflow cannot be understated and they have been studied extensively.[9,37,38] The internal nasal valve is a crucial regulator of nasal airflow dynamics and should be preserved and/or reconstructed when performing rhinoplasty. Injury and destabilization of this complex, either from surgery or trauma, may result in collapse and subsequent nasal airway obstruction. For example, in patients undergoing dorsal hump reduction, great care must be taken when separating the upper lateral cartilages and mucosa from the septum as loss of medial support can cause an inverted-V deformity. This effectively narrows the internal nasal valve. In addition, scar tissue may obscure the normal 10–15° angle or cause obstruction by cicatrix or mass effect.[39]

The external nasal valve

Normal function of this valve depends on the structural integrity of the lower lateral cartilages, perinasal musculature, and adequate soft tissue coverage. Functional compromise is seen with encroachment of the nasal spine, and especially the footplates, into the nostril opening. Architecturally weak lateral crura further compound the effects of a widened columella.[33] Other causes for external valve collapse include facial nerve palsy, pinched ala deformity and post-surgical vestibular stenosis secondary to synechiae and over-resection of the lower lateral cartilages.

The turbinates

Mucosal swelling can significantly alter nasal airflow by decreasing the cross-sectional area of the airway. When this becomes chronic, mucous glands enlarge, the basement membrane thickens with interstitial fibrosis and there is eventual hypertrophy of the conchal bone. In fact, previous studies have shown that hypertrophy of the anterior ends of the inferior turbinates is the primary cause of nasal airway

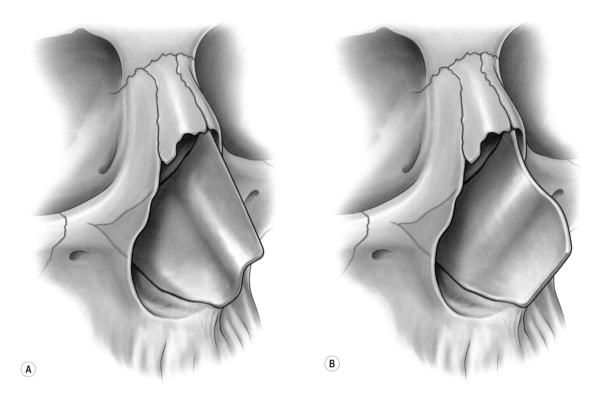

Fig. 20.7 Localized S-shaped septal deviation and septal spur.

obstruction.[39] As alluded to previously, turbinate hypertrophy may also present in the patient with a deviated septum. In these cases, the inferior turbinate on the side opposite the deviation undergoes compensatory enlargement to create equal airway resistance in both airways.

Diagnosis/patient presentation

History

A detailed patient history including history of nasal trauma, previous nasal surgery, airway complaints, allergies, and age is obtained. A negative history of airway obstruction is not a reliable indication of a patent airway, since the patient has no basis for comparison. Symptoms related to environmental agents such as grass pollens or pet dander should be elucidated as this would indicate allergic rhinitis and merit medical management. Complaints of nasal obstruction should also be clarified. Do the symptoms occur during quiet or heavy inspiration or both? A fixed obstruction such as an enlarged turbinate, septal deviation, or mass will manifest in both instances. However, obstruction that occurs only during heavy inspiration may indicate an incompetent valve.

Physical examination

Attention to detail and careful observation are paramount to glean critical information necessary to make the appropriate diagnosis and direct an effective treatment plan. A patient

with dark pigmentation in the lower eyelid and injected conjunctivae may have an atopic component contributing to nasal obstruction.

The external facial/nasal appearance should be critically examined with the patient encouraged to comment on his or her concerns. The nasal aperture is examined during inspiration for possible collapse of the external nasal valve.

Palpation is critical to appreciate the three-dimensional construct and stability of the nose. This portion of the exam should include palpation of the nasal bones, upper lateral and lower lateral cartilages, as well as the membranous and caudal cartilaginous septum. Palpation and percussion over the frontal, ethmoid, and maxillary sinuses is performed to elicit tenderness, which may be indicative of sinusitis. At this point, the patient is asked to occlude one nostril and then the other while taking a breath and state which side is easier to breathe through. If nasal valve incompetence is suspected, the Cottle test is employed. While the patient breathes quietly, the cheek is retracted laterally to open the nasal valve. If breathing is improved, it depicts a positive Cottle test and nasal valve incompetence. Another maneuver allowing independent evaluation of the external and internal nasal valves can be undertaken by simply using a cotton-tip applicator to stent the airway during quiet and heavy inspiration. Facial nerve integrity is also assessed, as paralysis of the perinasal dilators would contribute to a nasal airway obstruction.

Findings noted on the above external nasal exam are corroborated with soft tissue cephalometric analysis of life-size photographs. This is performed in order to assess symmetry of the nose and its relationship to other facial structures. Asymmetry may be present in other facial features, thus affecting the global evaluation of the face. The AP view of the

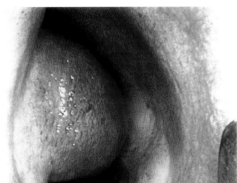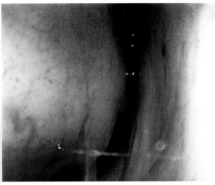

Fig. 20.8 Enlarged inferior turbinates.

face is also used to evaluate the dorsal nasal aesthetic lines as well as the width of the nasal dorsum.

Attention can now be turned to the internal nasal exam which consists of anterior and posterior rhinoscopy. An adequate light source and nasal speculum are required for anterior rhinoscopy. The nasal speculum is held in the dominant hand and spread in a vertical fashion. With this, the examiner will be provided with direct visualization of the anterior third of the nasal cavity, including the external and internal nasal valves, septum, and turbinates. The septum is evaluated for deviation and perforation. Formerly obscure perforations can become apparent after placing the nasal speculum in one nostril and transilluminating from the contralateral nostril. Any crusting, purulence, ulceration or presence of polyps should be noted. The color, size, and character of the turbinates is also documented, as a pale-colored turbinate mucosa may indicate allergy, whereas erythematous mucosa my indicate infection, inflammatory process, or rhinitis medicamentosa *(Fig. 20.8)*.

The above exam maneuvers should be performed before and after vasoconstriction of the nasal mucosa using 0.25% phenylephrine or 1% ephedrine sulfate. These agents can be delivered via an aerosolized misting system or topically with cottonoid pledgets. If available, topical cocaine can also provide potent vasoconstriction as well as local anesthesia.

Posterior rhinoscopy is indicated when the initial survey is negative for a source of nasal airway obstruction and patient history suggests otherwise. Visualization of the posterior nasal airway is best achieved using a 0 or 25° nasal endoscope, however should this apparatus not be available, it can also be done using a warmed dental mirror placed in the posterior oral cavity. This maneuver can reveal pathology such as adenoid hypertrophy, posterior nasal masses and choanal atresia.[2]

Rhinomanometry

Rhinomanometry is a test of nasal function that measures air pressure and the rate of airflow in the nasal airway during respiration. These findings are then used to calculate nasal airway resistance. A more recent advancement has been the introduction of acoustic rhinometry.[40–42] This technique is based on analysis of acoustic reflections from the nasal cavity at a given distance from the nostril. Acoustic rhinometry gives an anatomic/cross-sectional description of the nasal cavity, whereas rhinomanometry gives a functional measure of the pressure/flow relationships during the respiratory cycle. Although technically considered objective tests,

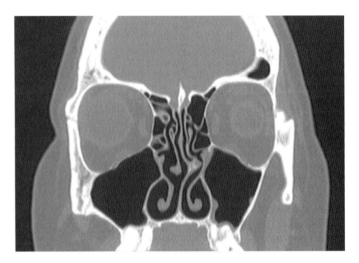

Fig. 20.9 This is a CT scan indicating a large septal spur with deviation as well as a concha bullosa.

rhinomanometry and acoustic rhinometry only provide "snapshot" measurements, which may not be representative of a more chronic condition, since turbinate size and function are dynamic processes that may change considerably over a few hours.[43] As such, these tests are commonly not part of the standard preoperative evaluation and should not replace a comprehensive history and physical examination.

Radiology

The radiographic standard of care for diagnosing paranasal sinus disease and the structural integrity of the nasal vault has become computed tomography and/or magnetic resonance imaging. These scans can very accurately detect air-fluid levels indicative of sinus disease or anatomic abnormalities such as septal deviations, spurs and bullosae, and concha bullosa; all of which can cause nasal airway obstruction *(Fig. 20.9)*.[44]

Patient selection

Paramount in the process of patient selection is a commanding knowledge of the nasal airway anatomy and physiology. This, coupled with a skillfully directed history and physical exam will significantly augment the surgeon's repertoire for addressing the subtleties of the deviated nose and its untoward effects on both form and function while allowing for more predictable results. To that end, the surgeon must first be able to identify between those patients who will best be served by medical therapy alone and those who will require a surgical intervention for the most favorable results. Once this crucial step has been satisfied, the following steps and descriptions in this chapter can be utilized for optimal patient care.

Treatment/surgical technique

Treatment of rhinitis based on sub-type

Infectious rhinitis

Viral rhinitis is most commonly self-limiting and treated symptomatically. Oral and topical decongestants should be used sparingly (limit to no more than 3 days at a time) to avoid rhinitis medicamentosa.[45] Rarely, a patient may become secondarily infected with a bacterial isolate in which case antibiotics would be warranted.

Bacterial rhinitis/sinusitis should be treated with a 2–3 week course of directed antibiotic therapy. Decongestant use should again be limited to a short duration only and as symptoms demand.[45,27] The reasoning for the extended antibiotic course is based on studies citing the bacterial (and viral) damage to cilia requires a regeneration period of approximately 2–3 weeks.[46,47] Empowered with this knowledge, it is clear why a short course of antibiotics will likely fail secondary to persistent mucostasis, which is followed by reinfection.

Allergic rhinitis

Allergic rhinitis, as previously mentioned, is quite common and as such, has entire specialties devoted to its diagnosis and treatment. Although the rhinoplasty surgeon should be able to recognize and diagnose allergic rhinitis in an effort to avoid an unnecessary operative intervention, these patients would best be served by a specialist, such as an allergist.

Vasomotor rhinitis

This troublesome autonomic imbalance is most commonly treated with oral decongestant modalities. A less common but more aggressive option in recalcitrant cases is division of the vidian nerve. The vidian nerve carries parasympathetic and sympathetic fibers from the greater superficial petrosal nerve and deep petrosal nerve, respectively. Access is transnasal and the nerve is transected at the level of the sphenopalatine foramen. It should be noted that there is a steep procedural learning curve and the results may be transient.[48–51]

Atrophic rhinitis

The treatment of this malady is symptomatic in nature, with frequent nasal saline lavage. Should foul drainage ensue, such things as alkaline nasal douches and/or 25% glucose in glycerine can be applied to the nasal mucosa, as these agents inhibit the growth of the foul smelling proteolytic organisms.

Rhinitis medicamentosa

The treatment for rhinitis medicamentosa is simply stopping the offending agent. Patients should be counseled that complete resolution may not occur for several weeks after cessation. In the meantime, corticosteroids on a tapering dose (a Medrol dose pack) can be instituted for symptom control.

Hypertrophic rhinitis

The treatment of hypertrophic rhinitis leading to turbinate hypertrophy will be discussed in the section on 'turbinate disorder treatment'.

Correction of deviated nasal bones

The deviated nasal bone can be unilateral depression of one nasal bone or a bilateral deviation. The unilateral deviation can be corrected with an onlay graft if the problem is not functional. This is accomplished using a layer of septal cartilage or a layer of diced cartilage graft. Under general anesthesia and with adequate local anesthetic infiltration to achieve the desired nasal vasoconstriction, an inter-cartilaginous incision is made and the target nasal bone is exposed. The periosteum is elevated using a Joseph's periosteal elevator. A septal, or conchal cartilage graft, in the form of a single or double layer or diced cartilage, depending on the degree of the nasal bone shift, is applied and the incision is repaired loosely to allow for drainage. More commonly however, a visible shift of the nasal bone will induce some medial transposition of the ULC and thus compromise the ipsilateral internal nasal valve function. Under this scenario a unilateral out-fracture of the nasal bone will produce a better functional and aesthetic outcome. Through a small vestibular incision at the piriform aperture, the periosteum is elevated using a Joseph's periosteal elevator. A low to low osteotomy is made and the nasal bone is out-fractured. To avoid return of the nasal bone to the previous position, a folded Adaptic saturated in bacitracin ointment is placed between the nasal bone and the septum and kept in position for at least 1 week. During this time, the patient is maintained on systemic antibiotics.

Treatment of the deviated septum

Surgical correction of the deviated septum can be accomplished through an open technique if concomitant rhinoplasty is planned or through an L-shape (Killian) type incision if the correction of the deviated septum is the sole surgical goal. When the open technique is used, the mucoperichondrium is elevated off of the left side of the septum starting from the caudal septal angle. A small incision may be needed anteriorly in order to visualize the correct subperichondral plane. Once in the correct plane with the glistening, grayish cartilage in view, the blunt end of a periosteal elevator is used to raise the mucoperichondrial flap. Dissection is continued posteriorly and cephalically. When the dissection reaches the junction of the quadrangle cartilage and the vomer bone, it could prove easier to start the dissection from the posterocaudal septum and extend it anteriorly. The fibrous attachments are firm anterocaudally, rendering the dissection arduous. The technique of septal correction is contingent upon the type of septal deviation.

Septal tilt

The septal tilt is corrected by initially removing the posterocaudal portion of the septum, leaving an L-strut septum anteriorly and caudally. The sharp end of the septal elevator is used to incise the septal cartilage and the dull end is used to elevate the mucoperichondrium. At least 15 mm of cartilage is maintained anteriorly and caudally. The mucoperichondrium and periosteum caudal and posterior to the L strut are elevated off the septum on the left side. The remainder of the posterocaudal septum is disengaged from the perpendicular plate, the vomerine groove and anterior nasal spine. The deviated portion of the cartilaginous septum, the vomer and perpendicular bone are removed as radically as needed. The septum must then be repositioned after removal of a small segment of the overlapping cartilage and fixated in the midline. This is performed with a figure-of-eight suture using 5-0 PDS. Prior to repositioning of the septum, it is imperative to ensure that the anterior nasal spine be in the midline, otherwise correction of the septal deformity will not be adequate. The nasal spine may be repositioned with an osteotomy, if needed *(Fig. 20.10)*.

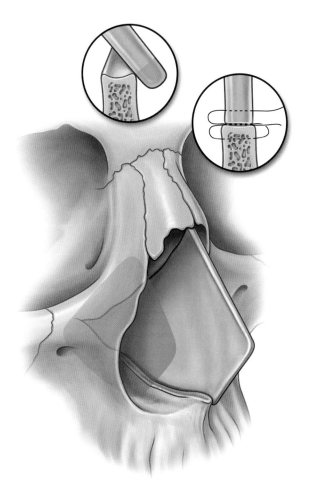

Fig. 20.10 Correction of septal tilt. The posteriocaudal portion of the septum is removed, leaving an L-strut septum anteriorly and caudally. The septum is repositioned after removal of a small segment of the overlapping cartilage and fixated in the midline with a figure-of-eight suture.

C-shaped anteroposterior deviation

Correction of the anteroposterior deformity first requires resection of the posterocaudal portion of the septum, as described for septal tilt. An osteotomy of the anterior nasal spine and residual vomerine plate is often necessary in order to place this structure in the midline. Also, partial disjunction of the perpendicular plate of the ethmoid and quadrangle cartilage is done only if deemed beneficial to correct the deviation in the cephalic third of the nose. Finally, the L-shaped frame is scored in a cephalocaudal direction on the concave surface if the other measures do not result in straightening the septum. This seldom becomes necessary. However, the effects of scoring are not predictable. Therefore, in order to control the response to scoring, bilateral extramucosal stents are placed and fixed in position with a through-and-through suture. Stents are left for 3 weeks. The anterior deviation is corrected by separation of the ULCs from the septum, osteotomy, reposition of the frame and possible placement of spreader grafts *(Fig. 20.11A)*.

C-shaped cephalocaudal deviation

Correction of the cephalocaudal deformity also requires resection of the posterocaudal septum. Complete separation of the junction between the cartilaginous septum and the maxillary crest is performed, as well as a partial release of the cephalic portion of the quadrangular cartilage from the perpendicular cartilage if deemed necessary. An anterior nasal spine osteotomy may be needed to correct deviation at this level. The dorsal L strut cartilage is scored in an anteroposterior orientation on the concave side of the deformity, only if release of tension caudally does not correct the deformity. Spreader grafts are also utilized anteriorly to guide and control the response from the scoring. If deviation only involves the caudal septum, bilateral spreader grafts and a septal rotation suture may suffice. Internal extramucosal stents are then placed if the caudal portion of the septum has to be scored *(Fig. 20.11B)*.

S-shaped anteroposterior deviation

This type of septal deviation is corrected by removal of the posterior portion of the cartilage and bone, bilateral cephalocaudal scoring of the cartilage on the concave surfaces if necessary, and osteotomy, with repositioning of the nasal spine and vomer bone. Cartilage memory is directed with the extramucosal stents and spreader grafts anteriorly if it is scored *(Fig. 20.12A)*.

S-shaped cephalocaudal deviation

This type of septal deviation is corrected with removal of the posterocaudal portion of the septal frame, bilateral anteroposterior scoring of the concave portion of the cartilage, release of the septum from the maxillary crest, and partial release from the perpendicular plate. The anterior portion of the septum is then supported with bilateral spreader grafts, and the cartilage memory is guided with bilateral extramucosal stents posteriorly, when the cartilage is scored *(Fig. 20.12B)*.

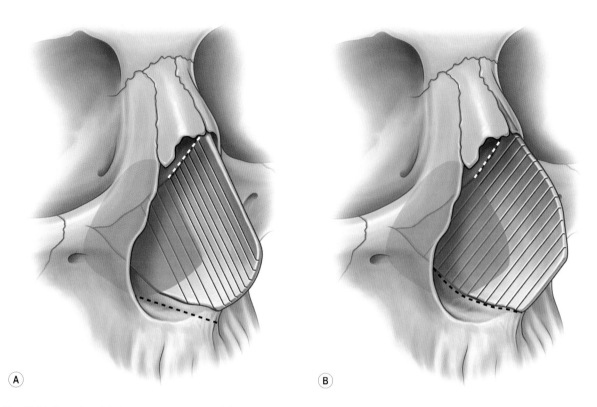

(A)   (B)

Fig. 20.11 Correction of C-shaped septal deviations. **(A)** Anteroposterior. Shown in this illustration are the resection of the posteriocaudal portion of the septum, partial disjunction of the perpendicular plate of the ethmoid and quadrangle cartilage and the scoring of the L-shaped frame in a *cephalocaudal* direction on the concave surface, only if necessary. **(B)** Cephalocaudal. Shown in this illustration are the resection of the posteriocaudal portion of the septum, partial disjunction of the perpendicular plate of the ethmoid and quadrangle cartilage and scoring of the L-shaped frame in an *anteroposterior* direction on the concave surface. An anterior nasal spine osteotomy may also be used to correct deviation at this level.

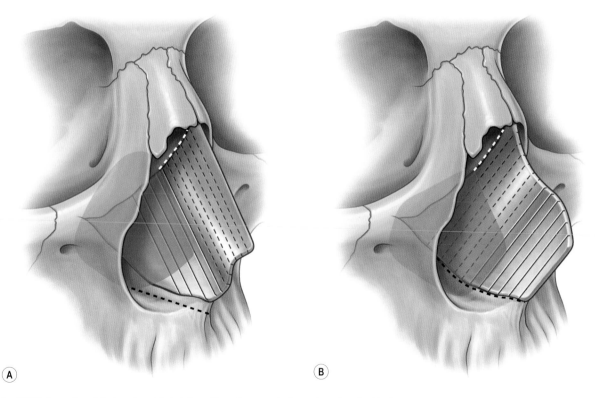

(A)   (B)

Fig. 20.12 Correction of S-shaped septal deviations. Corrections are similar to those described in the correction of C-shaped septal deviations. Scoring of cartilaginous deviations is performed on the concave surfaces. **(A)** Anteroposterior. **(B)** Cephalocaudal.

Localized deviation

Correction simply involves removal of the deviated portion of the cartilage and bone, while taking care to maintain a sufficient amount of L-strut for structural integrity. This is followed by application of extramucosal Doyle stents for 4 days.

Treatment of the incompetent internal nasal valve

Several techniques have been described to reconstruct the incompetent internal nasal valve. These have included placing conchal cartilage over the nasal dorsum and securing this to the upper lateral cartilages or a suture technique, which traverses over the nasal dorsum to secure either upper lateral cartilage. Both techniques serve to flare or widen the upper lateral cartilages and thus, open the angle.[52,53]

Likely the most significant contribution in this area is the spreader graft which has been popularized by Sheen. A precise submucoperichondrial plane is created between the upper lateral cartilages and septum for placement of bilateral rectangular pieces of cartilage. These pieces should extend from the osseocartilaginous junction to a point just caudal to the anterior septal angle and tapered at each end for contouring. The spreader grafts main purpose served is widening of the nasal valve angle with an increase in both cross-sectional area and overall airflow. Other benefits include added structural support, improvement of the dorsal aesthetic lines, and nasal bone stabilization after osteotomy *(Fig. 20.13)*.[38,54,55]

Spreader flaps could also be used and are created by folding the free anterior margins of the upper lateral cartilages.[56,57]

The upper lateral splay graft, as described by Guyuron spans the dorsal septum but is deep to the upper lateral cartilages. The intrinsic spring in the splay graft elevates each upper lateral cartilage with the septum as the fulcrum, thus correcting any middle vault collapse and opening the internal valve.[58]

Treatment of the incompetent external nasal valve

Treatment varies with the exact pathology, however the basic premise is based on reinforcing the lateral crura, alar rim, and soft tissue envelope thereby stenting the valve. This increases the overall cross-sectional area and maximizes airflow. A number of techniques have been written about and include lateral crural strut grafts,[59] lateral crural spanning grafts,[60] cephalic trim grafts,[61] suture techniques, and alar batten grafts *(Fig. 20.14)*. Any supportive cartilage graft placed in the region of the alar lobule or rim will tend to support the external nasal valve and prevent collapse, provided the soft tissue envelope is supple. If there is a shortage of alar skin and/or significant vestibular stenosis, more advanced options such as a composite auricular graft, V-Y advancement[62] or alar base flap may be required.[63–65]

Treatment of turbinate disorders

Although the primary goal of management of the turbinate; maximize nasal airflow, sounds simple, it has been an area of vigorous debate and controversy for over 100 years. There are myriad medical (discussed previously) and surgical treatments available for approaching the hypertrophic turbinate. Unfortunately, upon review of the literature, there is a paucity of comparative data analyzing the different techniques. The range of surgical treatments can be divided into the following categories: mechanical procedures, destructive procedures, and turbinate resection procedures.[66]

Mechanical procedures

The mainstay in this category is turbinate outfracture. This technique has the advantage of being quick and easy to perform with relatively no morbidity. The downside is when this procedure is performed in isolation, recurrent turbinate hypertrophy is common with eventual relocation of the turbinate back to its original position. In addition, simple outfracture does not address the turbinate with hypertrophic mucosa, which is either associated with, or even the primary pathology responsible for the enlarged turbinate.[67] Thus, this technique is often combined with other procedures.

Destructive procedures

Destructive procedures aim to reduce the bulk of the turbinates by direct destruction and/or introducing scar. The first method, electrocautery, can be done in a superficial or submucous plane with monopolar or bipolar diathermy. It too, has the advantages of being technically facile and quick. However, surface electrocautery can be associated with edema and crusting for up to 3–6 weeks, as well as, adhesions in 20–30 percent of cases.[68,69] In addition, in submucous and bipolar electrocautery, the conchal bone must be avoided to prevent long-term edema, erythema, and sequestrum.[67]

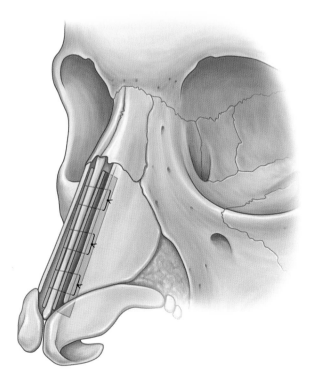

Fig. 20.13 The proper location of a spreader graft is illustrated.

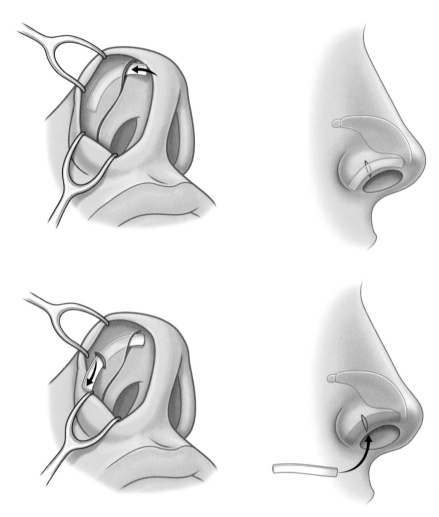

Fig. 20.14 The proper placement of an alar batten graft is shown.

Cryosurgery works by inducing mucosal injury by causing intracellular crystal formation. Thus, its main affect is seen in the water-laden goblet cells and therefore only addresses hypertrophic mucosa.[70] Prolonged crusting, late hemorrhage and the need for multiple treatments are reported complications.

Laser turbinate reduction is not novel and has been in use since the early 1970s, in Europe.[71] Many lasers have been used including CO_2, Nd:YAG, argon, and the potassium-titanyl-phosphate laser. As with the previous techniques, lasers are fast and easy with a relatively low complication profile (i.e., hemorrhage). Like electrocautery and cryotherapy, lasers only address the mucosa and not the underlying bone.[66]

Turbinate resection procedures

Complete turbinectomy has largely fallen out of favor secondary to multiple reports citing severe complications as well as an increase in our knowledge and understanding of the important physiologic role the turbinate plays. If too much turbinate is removed, the excessively patent nasal airway can lead to pharyngeal dryness, increased sensitivity to cold air, ozena, and a paradoxical sensation of nasal obstruction.[72] Thus, when approaching turbinectomy, most agree a conservative approach is best.

Submucous turbinate resection has been advocated by many. However, this does not eliminate the hypertrophic soft

tissues. Partial turbinectomy is likely the most versatile option, as it addresses both the hypertrophic mucosa and underlying bone while leaving a normal sized turbinate behind. It also portends less morbidity and greater success than complete turbinectomy. Despite removing conchal bone and potentially some mucosa, this procedure is designed to spare turbinate mucosa and, thus, its important physiologic function of warming, humidifying and cleansing inspired air.[13] Partial turbinectomy should be done evenly across the full length of the turbinate, rather than only anteriorly or posteriorly as advocated by a few. Otherwise, the intact portion of the turbinate undergoes compensatory hypertrophy and requires additional surgery. For the submucous resection, as described by Mabry, a medial mucoperiosteal flap is created using Bovie electrocautery and the turbinate is outfractured with an elevator. Takahashi forceps are then carefully used to grasp, rotate, and resect the exposed conchal bone. The remaining mucosal flap, barring over-resection, naturally drapes over the resected conchal bone. Judicious cauterization is then used for hemostasis of the mucosal edges.[73]

Postoperative care

Following the completion of the procedure, a dorsal splint is applied if a rhinoplasty is part of the plan. The dorsal splint reapproximates the free tissue envelope to the corrected

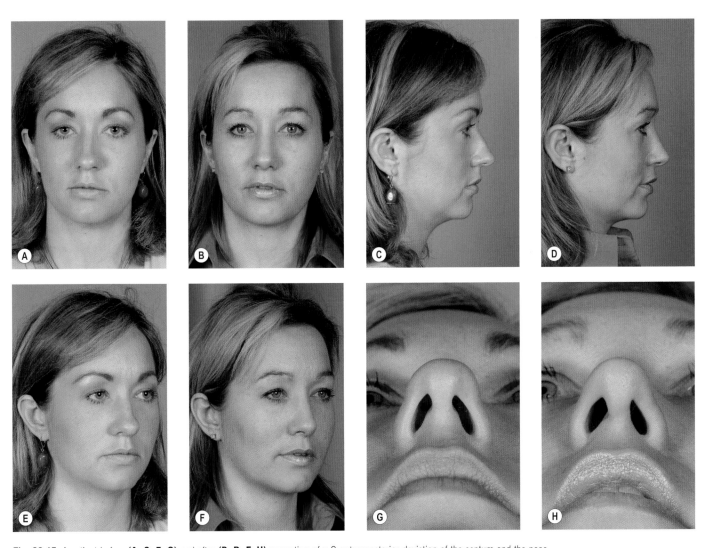

Fig. 20.15 A patient before **(A, C, E, G)** and after **(B, D, F, H)** correction of a C-anteroposterior deviation of the septum and the nose.

framework. A combination of metal splints and Aquaplast over Steri-Strips is preferred by the authors. The Aquaplast provides stability, whereas the metal portion allows precise molding of the Aquaplast splint. Doyle splints are also placed within the nostrils in an extramucosal fashion. The use of the Doyle splints allows further stabilization of the septum. The external splint is left on for 8 days, while the internal Doyle stent is removed in 3–4 days.

The simple extramucosal internal stents that are placed after any septal correction surgery are kept in for 2–3 weeks. The patient is kept on a first generation cephalosporin for the duration that the Doyle internal splints are used. A Medrol® dose-pack is also prescribed if a nasal bone osteotomy is part of the surgical plans, to minimize swelling and bruising. However, corticosteroids are avoided in patients with active acne. Heavy physical activity is curtailed for 3 weeks.

Outcomes/prognosis/complications

Without adequate preoperative and intraoperative assessment of the deviated nose, an incomplete correction of the nasal deformity and function is inevitable. Inadequate

straightening of any one or combination of structures may contribute to the recurrent or continued nasal deformity. One must address the septum, bony framework, upper lateral cartilages, lower lateral cartilages, internal valve, external valve, and turbinates. Minor discrepancies may be corrected with taping or continued splinting, but unfortunately, most will ultimately need surgical revision. Other possible complications include synechia, septal hematoma, septal perforation, infection, bleeding, and atrophic rhinitis *(Figs 20.15, 20.16)*.

Secondary procedures

The prevailing goal of any rhinoplasty surgeon is to achieve the best result with the first operation. However, even the most skilled surgeon with the best intentions will care for patients requiring secondary procedures to achieve improved results. Each patient's pathology is unique and should be managed on a case-by-case basis. Specific techniques are discussed within this chapter and throughout the text. Adherence to these principles will minimize the need for secondary procedures.

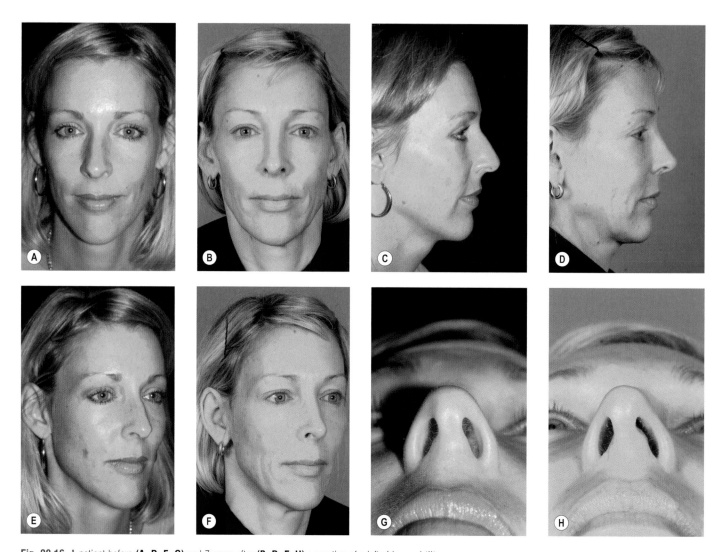

Fig. 20.16 A patient before **(A, D, E, G)** and 7 years after **(B, D, F, H)** correction of a left side nasal tilt.

Access the complete references list online at **http://www.expertconsult.com**

2. Howard BK, Rohrich RJ. Understanding the nasal airway: principles and practice. *Plast Reconstr Surg.* 2002;109:1128.

  The authors present a thorough review of the nasal airway beginning with pertinent nasal anatomy and moving onto physiology, pathology and treatment. It is well cited and discusses in detail the key concepts and principles in the practical management of the nasal airway.

8. Courtiss EH, Gargan TJ, Courtiss GB. Nasal physiology. *Ann Plast Surg.* 1984;13:214.

9. Constantian MB, Clardy RB. The relative importance of septal and nasal valvular surgery in correcting airway obstruction in primary and secondary rhinoplasty. *Plast Reconstr Surg.* 1996;98:38.

33. Guyuron B, Behmand RA. Caudal nasal deviation. *Plast Reconstr Surg.* 2003;111:2449.

  The authors begin by describing the anatomic structures that define the caudal nose. They go on to discuss the specific structures and their associated abnormalities as they relate to

abnormalities of the caudal nose and nasal airway. The discussion includes a description of the surgical technique necessary to address each deformity. In particular, six types of septal deviation are described in terms of diagnosis and treatment.

34. Gunter JP, Rohrich RJ. Management of the deviated nose: The importance of septal reconstruction. *Clin Plast Surg.* 1988;15:43.

35. Byrd HS, Salomon J, Flood J. Correction of the crooked nose. *Plast Reconstr Surg.* 1998;102:2148.

37. Constantian MB. The incompetent external nasal valve: Pathophysiology and treatment in primary and secondary rhinoplasty. *Plast Reconstr Surg.* 1994;93:919.

39. Chand MS, Toriumi DM, Landecker A. Surgical management of the nasal airway. In: Gunter JP, Rohrich RJ, Adams WP Jr. *Dallas rhinoplasty.* 2nd ed. St. Louis: Quality Medical; 2007;909.

  The authors begin with a discussion on the preoperative assessment of a patient who requires surgical management of the nasal airway. This includes the history, physical examination, and appropriate diagnostic studies. This is followed by a detailed discussion regarding the treatment strategies of the various components making up the nasal airway.

58. Guyuron B. Nasal osteotomy and airway changes. *Plast Reconstr Surg.* 1998;102:856.

The author provides a prospective investigation involving 48 consecutive patients who underwent various nasal bone osteotomies during rhinoplasty procedures. The author concluded that the nasal osteotomy does constrict the nasal airway in most incidences. The length of the nasal bones, the

degree of nasal bone repositioning, the position of the inferior turbinates, and the type of osteotomy are definite factors contributing to airway narrowing after nasal bone osteotomy.

66. Jackson LE. Management of the inferior turbinate hypertrophy. *Plast Reconstr Surg.* 1999;104:1197–1198.

The author provides a critical appraisal in the medical and surgical management of the inferior turbinate. Acknowledgement is made regarding the continued debate in the treatment of inferior turbinate pathology. Advantages, disadvantages, complications and controversies of each form of treatment are reviewed and discussed. A staged protocol of increasingly invasive interventions is proposed.

21

Secondary rhinoplasty

Ronald P. Gruber, Simeon H. Wall Jr., David L. Kaufman, and David M. Kahn

SYNOPSIS

- Secondary rhinoplasty may be done to correct a complication, to correct an untoward result, or simply to pursue further improvement.
- Secondary rhinoplasty is more difficult than primary. All measures to help the surgeon should be used, including such measures as preoperative imaging and the intraoperative use of models.
- Open and closed rhinoplasty techniques can both be used effectively in secondary rhinoplasty. All cases are individualized.
- In many secondary cases, problems are due to deficiencies in the cartilaginous or bony framework of the nose. Cartilage grafting is the mainstay for the correction of these problems.
- A useful algorithm for suture-based nasal tip plasty is: (1) hemi-transdomal suture; (2) lateral crural mattress suture; (3) interdomal suture; and (4) columella-septal suture.
- Airway compromise is a frequent problem which must be addressed in secondary rhinoplasty.

Introduction

Definitions

Secondary rhinoplasty is by definition a reoperation of a nose previously operated upon by a prior surgeon. We distinguish this from a "revision", which is a reoperation by the same surgeon on his/her patient. Usually, the secondary operation is more extensive than the revision. Secondary rhinoplasty and revision rhinoplasty are done for reasons that include complications of surgery or unsatisfactory results or the need for further improvement. For legal reasons, it is important to distinguish between: (1) a complication; (2) an untoward result; and (3) the need for further improvement. A complication may or may not be attributable to an action taken by the

surgeon. For example, a true saddle nose deformity is most likely the responsibility of the surgeon. However, a supratip deformity is usually an untoward result, even though more often than not we think it can be prevented. Seeking "further improvement" is done on a satisfactory result when both the surgeon and patient feel that more can be done to obtain an even better result.

Why secondaries are difficult

If rhinoplasty is the most difficult operation in aesthetic rhinoplasty then surely secondary rhinoplasty is even more difficult.[1] The overall revision rate of 20% suggests that this is the case. Whereas, the patient who needs a revision rhinoplasty is willing to let the first surgeon perform it, he/she is much less likely to allow a third procedure by that surgeon if, for whatever reason, there is dissatisfaction once again. It behooves the surgeon therefore in a revision rhinoplasty to do everything possible to avoid an unhappy patient with its concomitant problems (law suit and public complaining on the internet).[2]

Patient presentation

Dealing with the secondary rhinoplasty patient requires more skill and patience than a primary case. The patients are often unhappy, skeptical and need more reassurance than they did prior to their first surgery. The operation is often more complicated but not necessarily so. It is important to acknowledge the patient's complaints. But one must always remember not to be judgmental of the first surgeon. Untoward and unsatisfactory results are a part of rhinoplasty. The nose is an unforgiving part of the anatomy. Unlike a breast augmentation, a 1 mm discrepancy can easily be noticeable and objectionable. The very best rhinoplasty surgeons in the world have had to contend with this fact.

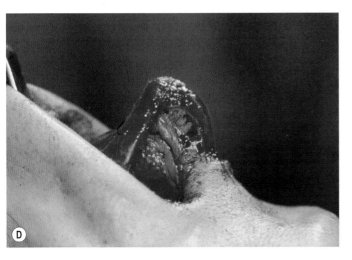

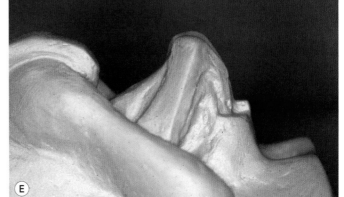

Fig. 21.2 (D,E) After suture techniques, excisional techniques and grafts are complete.

Patient selection

Nasal evaluation

JP Gunter[3] has probably done more than any other surgeon to emphasize the importance of analysis. Kim and Toriumi[4] have a complete review on this subject and Pessa and Rohrich cover this subject in Chapter 17. We would like to emphasize what we consider the most important aspect of analysis in our practices: the use of digital imaging.

It behooves the surgeon to use imagers *(Fig. 21.1)* for preoperative planning for each patient. Imagers are widely available and economical. It is helpful to demonstrate to the patient what you think should to be done and eliciting their feedback as to what they think should be done. The patient needs to know what can and cannot be realistically achieved. In the process of imaging, the surgeon him/herself learns what problems may exist. Sometimes, the process of morphing can be enlightening. Often what may appear to be the problem when judging the patient sitting in the examining chair is not the problem as seen by the camera on the monitor. Conversely, some anatomic problems only become obvious when on the monitor. Patients with unrealistic expectations can be weeded out by this process. Above all, morphing with an imager is a form of mock surgery. FIG **21.1** APPEARS ONLINE ONLY

Operative techniques

Artistry in rhinoplasty

It is not enough to have the knowledge of nasal anatomy.[5] Rhinoplasty is sculpting with a biological medium (cartilage and some bone). As such, we need to employ an artist's principle: copying. It is much easier to copy a beautiful structure than it is to create it from memory. Commercial artists rely on this concept. Unless you are a naturally gifted artist, you will find this to be the case. Few of us can draw a decent picture of a cat from memory, but even an artistically challenged individual can copy a reasonable facsimile of a cat from a photograph. Consequently, we recommend the use of an intraoperative model of the ideal or prototype nasal framework

(Fig. 21.2). It saves the effort of memorizing facts (e.g., how much the tip should be elevated above the dorsum; what the width of the lateral crus should be; what the angle of divergence is, etc.). Magnifiers and loupes make it difficult to see the nose from a distance and get the proper perspective. Therefore, it is also helpful to have a video camera in the operating room (which gives a profile view of the patient (from a distance) at all times). It is not surprising that some surgeons are on occasion perplexed to see that the patient's nose has nostril exposure the next day or at the time of splint removal. They may have neglected to judge that angle accurately when the patient was in the supine position. Stepping back to evaluate the patient, or using a video camera, gives a better perspective and helps avoid this problem. FIG **21.2A–C** APPEARS ONLINE ONLY

The open versus closed approach in secondary rhinoplasty

The decision to open the nose or not in a secondary can be more difficult than in the case for a primary rhinoplasty.[6] If there is little to do, e.g., rasping the dorsum or attaching a rim graft, there is no question that a closed approach is ideal. And if it appears that visualization will be beneficial to completing the task, e.g., straightening the nose, or straightening out a twisted tip, there will be little questioning that an open approach will permit greater accuracy and therefore a better final result. However, there are many less clear cut cases. For example, if the patient has had multiple prior surgeries with a thick round fibrous tissue filled ill-defined tip the decision is much more difficult. That is because opening the nose (whether there is an existing columellar scar or not) has the potential for even more edema and subsequent fibrosis to the tip. In the nose with thick skin, fibrous tissue deep to that skin can be a surgeon's nightmare *(Fig. 21.3)*. Further surgery, no matter how precise in terms of achieving a finely sculpted framework, can aggravate the thickness problem and give a worse result. The best approach in these kinds of cases is to select a surgical plan that minimizes surgical trauma and undermining. It is best to consider an open approach in this case, only if it is felt necessary that some surgical maneuvers will be impossible to achieve without it, e.g., lengthening the nose.

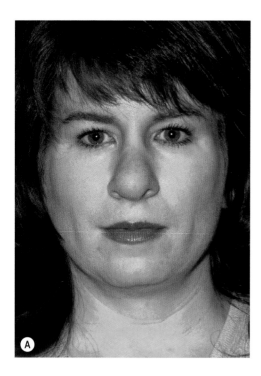
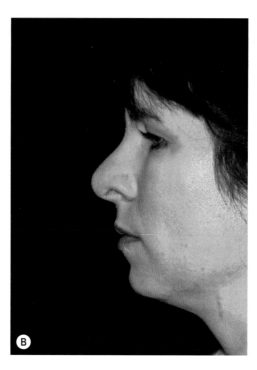

Fig. 21.3 (A,B) A patient who has extraordinarily thick skin should be a strong warning that the open approach and/or wide undermining procedures can aggravate the thick skin condition.

Anesthesia

Most of our patients receive conscious intravenous sedation because it is less costly to the patient. The overall benefits of conscious sedation are reviewed elsewhere.[7] Unfortunately, many residency programs do not train surgeons to use it, forcing them to learn it following their formal training. Patients are instructed to take Flurazepam (Dalmane) 60 mg 1 h prior to arriving at the surgery center. On arrival, the relaxed patient then receives IM Hydroxyzine (Vistaril), 100 mg and IM Nalbuphine (Nubain) 10 mg. Demerol 50 mg can be used as an alternative to Nalbuphine. In the operating room, the patient is sedated with incremental 1 mg doses of Midazolam (Versed). When the patient has difficulty counting backwards from 100, Ketamine 30 mg is given slowly over 30 s. For larger female patients and males, 50 mg is employed. Additional incremental doses of Versed (1 mg) are used if the patient should not enter that desired "dissociative state" that Ketamine is known to produce, which lasts for approximately 5 min.

Local anesthetic is injected into the nose during that time. It consists of a solution containing a 50/50 mixture of Xylocaine 1% and Bupivacaine (Marcaine) 0.25% with an epinephrine concentration of 1/200 000. A total solution of 30–50 mL is used in a hyperinfiltration technique. When general anesthesia is used, the epinephrine concentration is increased to 1/100 000. Injection of the dorsal septum provides most of the anesthesia to the septum although supplementary anesthesia is given to other areas. The inferior turbinates are injected to provide anesthesia for a subsequent lateral osteotomy and to be able to tolerate the pledgets that are inserted to absorb blood that would otherwise run down the patient's nasopharynx and cause intermittent coughing. Using the above approach has avoided the need for topical anesthetics such as cocaine.

If one is going to undertake conscious anesthesia, it is imperative that he/she be familiar with airway management. It is a good idea to mask-ventilate the patient for a few breaths during Ketamine to appreciate what the patient's potential airway difficulty might be during the case. It is also important to have an oral airway immediately available should it be necessary to insert it if the oximeter indicates that the patient is hypoventilating or his/her jaw has fallen back causing a partial airway obstruction. In addition, it is important to have available reversal agents including Narcan (Naloxone) for the narcotics and Flumazenil (Romazicon) for the benzodiazepines.

Suture techniques versus grafts

Suture techniques

The universal horizontal mattress suture[8,9] is a suture that can be applied to any unwanted convex or concave cartilaginous structure of the nose in a secondary rhinoplasty. A short learning curve is necessary because if the gap between purchases is too little, no effect results but if the gap between purchases is too large, the cartilage will buckle *(Fig. 21.4)*. Our studies have shown that one suture can increase the strength (biplanar modulus in engineering terms) of the cartilage by approximately 35%, whereas scoring the cartilage to achieve the same degree of correction can weaken the cartilage by as much as 50% *(Fig. 21.5)*. The lateral crural mattress suture is the most obvious example. However, the universal horizontal mattress suture is also useful for wanted curvatures of the septal L-shaped struts. Ear cartilage is much more usable when it is straightened and stiffened with this particular suture. When the concha cymba is removed from behind the ear, it is split down the middle, pinned to a silicone block, concave side down. A 5-0 PDS horizontal mattress suture is applied at each

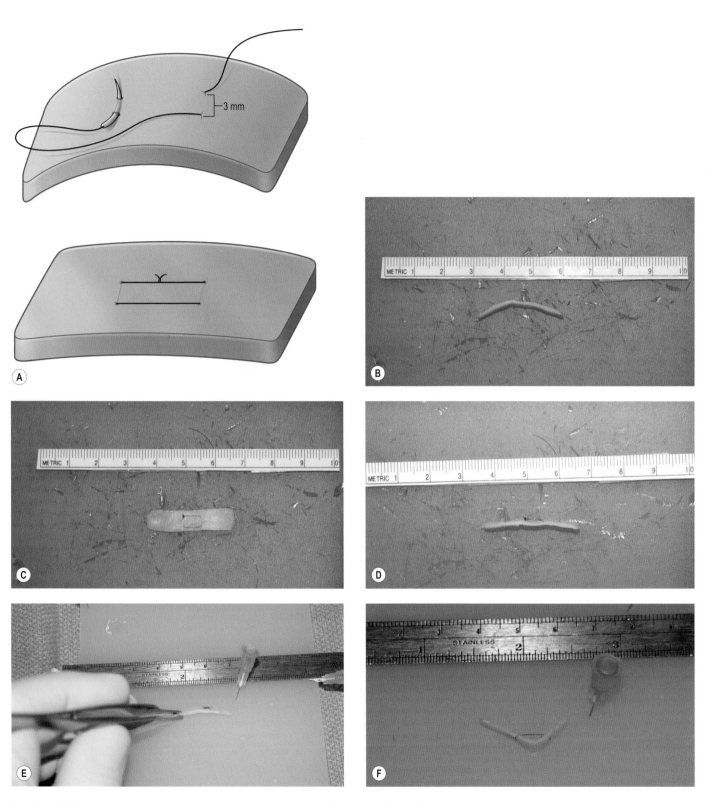

Fig. 21.4 (A) The universal horizontal mattress suture corrects convexities of strip cartilages. **(B–D)** When the spacing between bites is approximately 6 mm, most of the convexity is removed. More than one such suture may be needed. **(E,F)** If the spacing between bites is too small, no effect is seen; if the spacing between the bites is too large, buckling occurs.

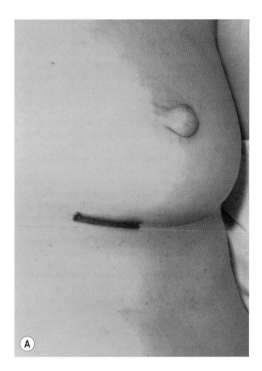

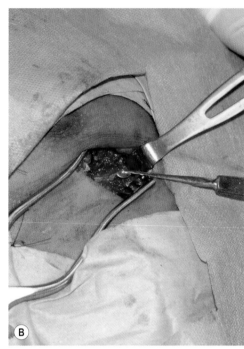

Fig. 21.7 (A,B) Rib is relatively easily obtained by making an inframammary incision and exposing the nearest available cartilaginous rib (usually the 5th rib). Often, only the anterior surface of the rib need be removed with the aid of a slightly curved osteotome or septal knife.

end of the cymba to straighten it and stiffen it *(Fig. 21.6)*. Such a suture reinforced graft makes a good columellar strut and can even replace the entire lateral crus if it is missing.

✂ FIGS **21.5, 21.6** APPEARS ONLINE ONLY

Grafts

Most secondary rhinoplasties demand grafts to either replace missing cartilage that has been excessively removed or to provide support for weak structures. Septal cartilage is preferred. However, it is usually unavailable in sufficient quantities. Therefore either ear or rib is required. For small amounts of cartilage, we prefer ear cartilage. Since it can be straightened and stiffened as described above, it is useful for almost ever situation where septal cartilage would ordinarily be used. However, when large amounts of cartilage are required, we prefer rib.[10,11] In particular we prefer the 5th rib that is accessible from an inframammary incision *(Fig. 21.7)*. The entire rib need not be removed. The anterior half is relatively easily removed with a slightly curved 1 cm osteotome and/or a septal knife.

If structural support is not needed, cartilage grafts need not be solid in order to reconstruct noses. Diced cartilage has a vital role, especially if it is wrapped in a substance like fascia to give it shape. This technique was developed primarily for dorsal augmentation by Daniel.[12] Erol[13] demonstrated that diced cartilage in a Surgicel wrapping could be useful. However, the authors prefer fascia to avoid the possibility of absorption due to the slight toxic effect of Surgicel. The cartilage is cut into small bits approximately 1 mm in size and placed in a blanket of fascia (on a silicone block). The fascia is simply folded over and secured with 5-0 plain catgut suture. It is helpful to have applied a silicone sizer in the patient's dorsum, to get an idea as to how long and thick to make the diced cartilage graft (DCF) graft *(Fig. 21.8)*.

One option we do consider for reconstruction in secondary cases is the use of irradiated allograft rib cartilage. This can

be useful when the patient is resistant to harvesting autogenous material. The main problem with allograft, of course, is the potential for absorption. Although some reports of long-term survival exist,[14] one must be prepared for absorption approximately 10 years postoperatively. An option we never consider for secondary rhinoplasty is the use of implants of any material. We recognize that many surgeons have found them helpful because they are easy to employ and economical for the patient. However, occasional failures (risk of skin necrosis and implant exposure) although unlikely, can be exceedingly difficult to correct when they happen.

Common problems

Broad, bulbous, round tip

General approach

One of the most common frustrations in secondary rhinoplasty is the broad, or bulbous or round tip.[15] Patients complain about this most often and most vigorously. Fortunately, there are some good solutions. It is important to decide whether to use the open or closed approach for the reasons mentioned above. Most of the time, the cephalic part of the lateral crus has been resected at the first surgery. In fact, too much has often been removed. The first goal is getting to the abnormal tip anatomy. In the open approach, careful elevation of the flap is necessary. In the closed approach, it may be necessary to deliver the tip cartilages with an intercartilaginous and marginal incision. The second goal is to establish a lateral crus that is approximately 5–6 mm wide and render it straight. Usually, suture techniques will convert the existing tip framework into something that is more normal and stronger.

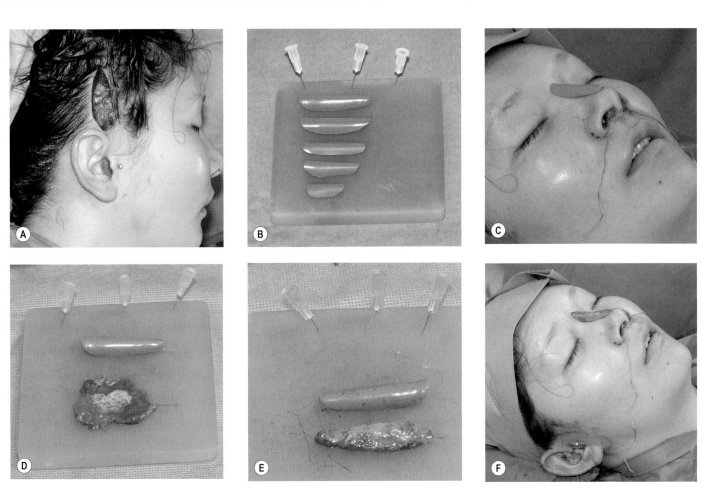

Fig. 21.8 (A) Deep temporalis fascia is harvested using a vertical incision beginning at the root of the ear. **(B)** Silicone dorsal nasal sizers are helpful to sculpt a dorsal graft when doing secondary rhinoplasty. **(C)** The silicone sizer is applied to the dorsum to see if it is the appropriate size. It is then applied internally to see if it is the proper size. **(D)** Cartilage of any type is diced into 1 mm sizes and placed in the deep temporalis fascia. It is easiest to work on the cartilage on a silicone block with pins to stabilize the fascia. **(E)** The fascia is rolled over like make a cigarette and sutured down one side with 5-0 plain catgut. The sizer acts as a model to determine the width and length of the graft. **(F)** The diced cartilage graft is lying on the dorsal surface of the nose.

Tip-plasty by suture techniques *(Fig. 21.9)*

Suture techniques are one of the main means by which the framework is modified.[15–20] The many types of suture techniques that apply to the primary rhinoplasty apply equally to the secondary rhinoplasty, although fewer are necessary because some of them have usually been applied at the first surgery. Guyuron and Behman *et al.*[15,16] have reviewed most of the common techniques. Daniel[17] has a useful algorithm and we have one that deals with most problems. Our own suture algorithm for tip-plasty involves four basic sutures: (1) hemi-transdomal; (2) lateral crural mattress suture; (3) interdomal suture; and (4) columella-septal suture. The hemi-transdomal suture[21] is a variation of the transdomal suture that narrows the dome. It is placed at the cephalic end of the dome so that it everts the caudal rim and prevents rim collapse or concave rims. The hemi-transdomal suture minimizes the need to use rim grafts which are often used to maintain a straight nostril rim or prevent concave rims. Daniel[17] and Toriumi[22] were aware of the importance of having a suture at the cephalic end of the dome. The lateral crural mattress suture removes any residual convexity of the lateral

crus. One, two or even three such sutures will flatten out the lateral crus and make it strong. This is especially useful in secondary cases because the lateral crurae are often weak from the first surgery with residual convexity. The interdomal suture brings the domes together and provides a small amount of tip rigidity and symmetry. The columella septal suture secures the tip to the caudal septum. One can adjust the height to some degree with this suture, although it is not a substitute for the columellar strut. All of these suture techniques require either 5-0 nylon or PDS. If one is certain there is good soft tissue coverage, a permanent suture such as nylon is a reasonable choice. *Figure 21.9* is an example of a patient who had multiple prior surgeries and grafts. She required sculpting of the tip cartilages with suture techniques. In addition to the four suture algorithms described above, she required a humpectomy and osteotomies. 🔗 FIG **21.9** APPEARS ONLINE ONLY

Closed approach

Some secondary noses simply do not warrant the extensive dissection associated with closed method of tip delivery or the open approach. Some patients are unhappy with their existing scar and are nervous about another open approach. These cases are benefitted by cephalic resection of the lateral crus alone. This is done by way of an intracartilaginous incision. All the cartilage (of the lateral crus) cephalic to the incision is removed. The decision is guided by what the minimal surgery is necessary to achieve the goal. *Figure 21.10* is a good example of a broad tip problem *(Fig. 21.10)*. The patient exhibited a broad tip, supratip deformity, and radix deficiency. Because of the very thick skin and her nervousness about the scar, it was decided to use a closed approach. The tip cartilages were delivered. The patient received cephalic trim of the lateral crus along with interdomal and lateral crural mattress sutures (5-0 PDS). A radix graft was used and the caudal septum was shortened. A lateral osteotomy was also performed. 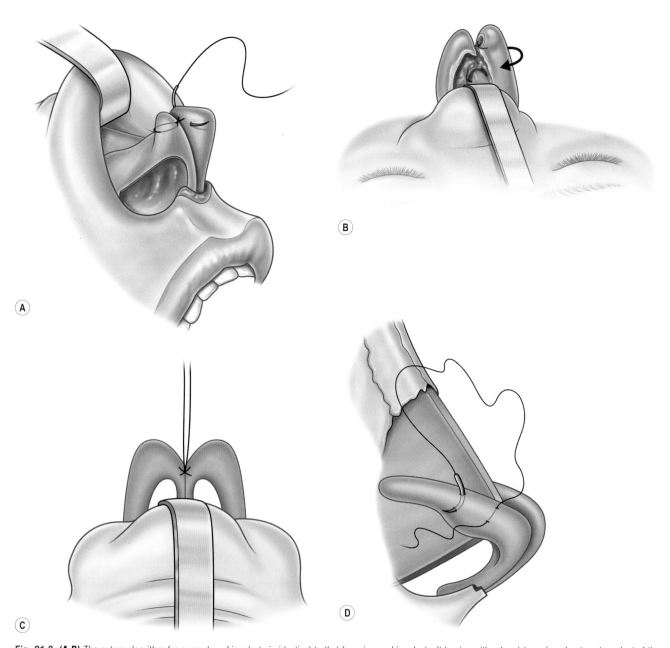 FIG **21.10** APPEARS ONLINE ONLY

Deficient tip *(Fig. 21.11)*

The tip can be deficient (underprojected) either because the infratip lobule is small or the columella is short or both. When the tip is deficient a tip graft is in order; when the columella is short a columellar strut is in order; if both are deficient both grafts are used. Deficient tips benefit enormously from a tip graft because the tip graft provides structure and definition. We prefer the "anatomic tip graft,"[23] similar to the classic Sheen shield graft[24] and Daniel's golf tee graft[25] whether via

Fig. 21.9 (A,B) The suture algorithm for secondary rhinoplasty is identical to that for primary rhinoplasty. It begins with a hemi-transdomal suture (a variant of the transdomal suture). It is a single suture that narrows the cephalic side of the dome and everts the rim of the lateral crus to minimize rim deformities. **(C)** An interdomal suture brings the tips together for symmetry and increased strength. **(D)** A lateral crural mattress suture reduces convexity of the lateral crus and thereby removes unwanted bulbosity or increased width of the tip. Often 2 to 3 such sutures are needed to do the job.

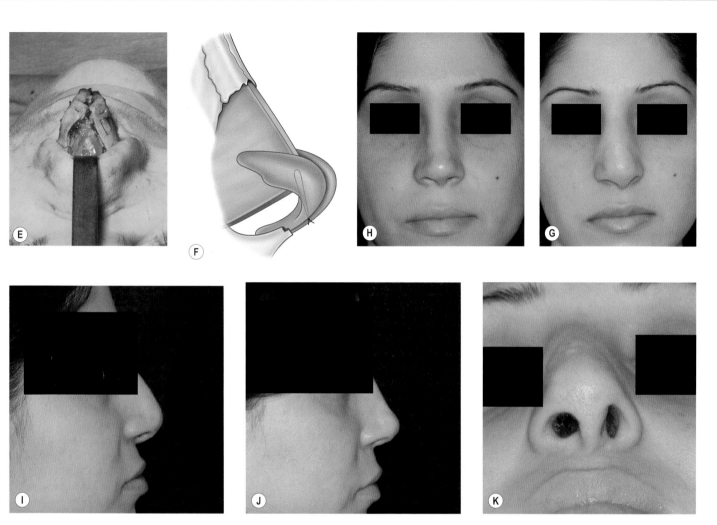

Fig. 21.9, cont'd **(E)** Intraoperative view of a lateral crural mattress suture. Note how it converts a convex lateral crus to a straight one and gives it additional strength. Two or three such sutures are often necessary. Typically 5-0 PDS is a good suture for this purpose. **(F)** A columella-septal suture secures the tip complex to the caudal septum. It can either provide a small amount of projection or deprojection, depending on the direction that the suture is oriented. Care must be taken not to tie the knot too tightly in order to avoid a retracted columella. **(G,I,K)** is an example of a patient who had multiple prior surgeries and grafts. She required sculpting of the tip cartilages with suture techniques. In addition to the four suture algorithms described above, she required a humpectomy and osteotomies. **(H,J,L)** At 17 months postoperatively, she exhibits considerable improvement.

the open or closed approach. The graft has a shape that simulates the normal surface anatomy of the middle crus and domes. Septal cartilage is ideal, although it needs to be scored slightly to avoid a tombstone effect. Concha cavum makes an excellent tip graft because it has just the right amount of curvature and requires no scoring and is almost always available. More often than not, additional tip projection is needed and is provided by a "support graft" (cap graft) which is a two or three layered graft that is placed deep to the tip graft for three purposes: (1) to provide more projection; (2) to immobilize the tip graft; and (3) to fill the dead space deep to the tip graft. Suturing tip grafts in place is not necessary. The patient in *Figure 21.11I–N* is a good example of a deficient tip problem. The patient exhibited a narrow over resected tip, inverted V deformity and alar retraction. At surgery, through an open approach, the tip cartilages had to be separated and an interdomal graft put between them. An anatomic tip graft was laid on the surface (ear acting as donor) and small rim grafts were also required. She also received a dermis graft to augment the lips. 🔗 FIG **21.11** APPEARS ONLINE ONLY

Collapsed middle third of nose

One of the more frequent problems requiring secondary or revision rhinoplasty is middle vault collapse. All too often when a humpectomy is performed in a primary rhinoplasty, some surgeons neglect to reconstruct the middle third (internal valve) of the nose with either spreader flaps[26,27] or spreader grafts.[28] Failing to do so results in an inverted V deformity that is not only unaesthetic but is a functional problem in terms of airway obstruction. Fortunately, the solution is relatively simple. Spreader flaps open up the internal valve and recreate the normal width of the middle third of the nose. These maneuvers are covered in Chapters 18, 19, and 20. In addition to a tip deficiency the patient *(Figure 21.11I–N)* required spreader grafts.

Alar rim deformities (Figs 21.12, 21.13A,B)

Secondary noses often exhibit pinched or collapsed rims. Some part of the lateral crus is either weak or absent causing

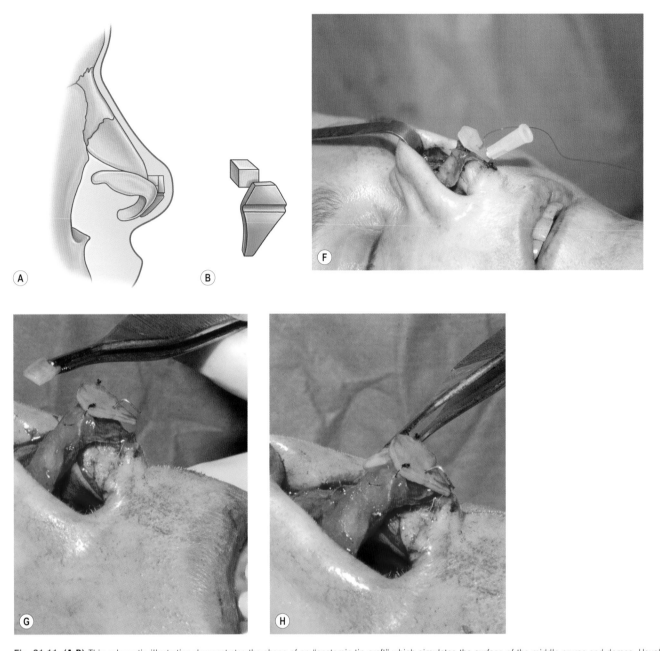

Fig. 21.11 (A,B) This schematic illustration demonstrates the shape of an "anatomic tip graft" which simulates the surface of the middle crurae and domes. Usually, a support graft (appearing as a block of cartilage) is placed deep to the tip graft in order to enhance the effect of tip augmentation. **(F)** The cartilaginous tip graft itself is pinned to the existing tip complex to see what the best location for it is. **(G,H)** After securing the posterior end of the tip graft to the existing tip complex a support graft (in this case only a one layer graft) is applied to the deep side of the tip graft. So doing helps secure the tip graft at the proper angle and fill the dead space.

the collapse. Patients not only complain of the appearance but also of inspiratory airway obstruction. Restoring the integrity of the lateral crus is the goal. In many cases a lateral cural strut as described by Gunter[29] is the solution *(Fig. 21.12)*. A small piece of thin cartilage usually 3–4 × 15–20 mm in size placed just deep to the cephalic edge of the existing lateral crus will provide structural integrity and restore aesthetic appearance. If the problem is small a simpler procedure is the use of the alar rim contour graft as described by Troell *et al.*,[30] Rohrich *et al.*[31] and Guyuron[32] *(Fig. 21.13C–F)*. Typically, the graft is the size of a matchstick and is placed either from the

medial side (in the approach) or through a separate incision posteriorly in the closed approach. FIG **21.13** APPEARS ONLINE ONLY

If the posterior (lateral) aspect of the lateral crus is collapsed the patient may complain of feeling it and seeing it in his/her nostril. It may even be a cause of airway obstruction *(Fig. 21.13G–J)*. Fortunately, the treatment is relatively simple. Part of much of the lateral crus can be delivered through the nostril by making a U-shaped incision. A medially based composite flap is elevated; one or more horizontal mattress sutures are placed on the convex cartilage deformity. These sutures will straighten and stiffen the lateral crus and in most cases, avoid the need for a graft in this region, which is often thick and annoyingly palpable to the patient.

Another class of sutures that are helpful to prevent alar collapse is the suspension sutures that secure the lateral crus to a more cephalically located structure and prevent it from collapsing into the vestibule, e.g. the suspension suture of Davidson and Murakami[33] and that of Lieberman and Most[34] which secure the lateral crus to the nasal bone with a screw.

Thin skin tip

Thin skin noses *(Fig. 21.14)* have the advantage that the surgeon can show off his/her sculpting skills, acquire definition and great detail. It has the disadvantage, however, that any imperfections can be seen through the thin skin. Any small changes of cartilage warping or absorption or shifting can show through thin skin and mar the result. One of the best paddings is fascia. A one-layer sheet of deep temporalis fascia can be enormously helpful in correcting the thin skinned secondary rhinoplasty patient.[35] *Figure 21.14G,H* demonstrates a patient whose thin skin adversely affected her result. However, a one-layered fascial graft placed over the entire tip framework softened the result. One important caveat is that temporalis fascia can thicken to three times its original thickness (and shrink in total overall area) during the first postoperative week.[36] Therefore it needs to be sutured in place to prevent that from happening. An alternative tissue padding is a dermafat graft taken from behind the ear.

FIG **21.14** APPEARS ONLINE ONLY

Short nose

The short nose *(Fig. 21.15)* used to be one of the most difficult cases to correct.[37–43] Here, too, modern techniques have made this problem much less formidable. The algorithm we employ today is the one introduced over a decade ago and has not changed in any significant way. Through an open approach (which is almost a must) the upper lateral cartilages are released from the dorsal septum. Any available septal cartilage is harvested for a septal extension graft. If none is available, concha cavum will work but is somewhat thick. A double hook is placed on the tip cartilages and pulled caudally. After

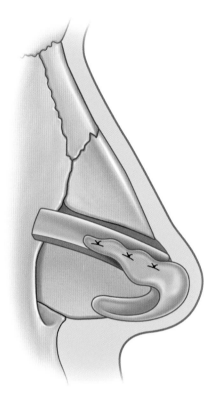

Fig. 21.12 Schematic of lateral crural strut that corrects either concave rim deformities, collapsed alae and pinched alae. Note that the graft is placed just deep to cephalic side of existing lateral crus. Often it is helpful to have it extend laterally (posteriorly) for even more support.

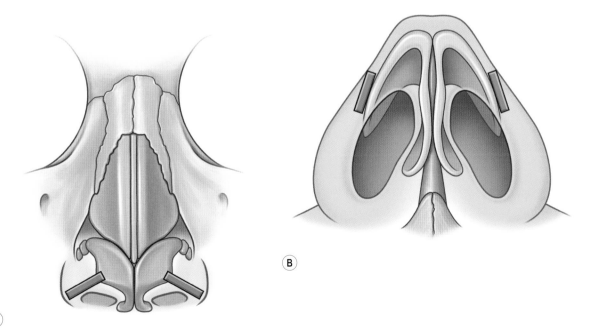

Fig. 21.13 (A,B) Alar rim deformities are best corrected with rim grafts. The Guntergram indicates the nonanatomic position of this graft along the alar rim.

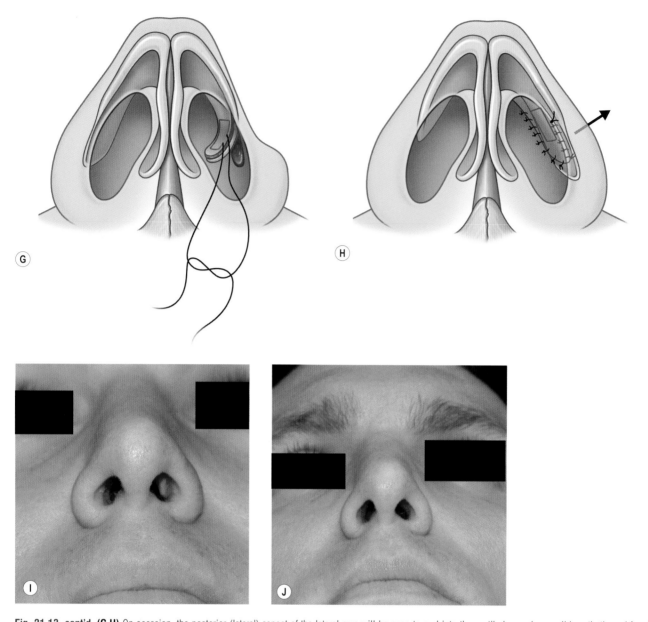

Fig. 21.13, cont'd (G,H) On occasion, the posterior (lateral) aspect of the lateral crus will be seen to curl into the vestibule causing a mild aesthetic and functional (airway) problem. However, correction can be achieved by creating a medially based U-shaped composite flap. One or more universal horizontal mattress sutures are then applied to the undersurface of the flap to remove that curvature. An alternative is the lateral crural strut graft. **(I,J)** Pre- and postoperative basal views of a patient who had such a deformity of the lateral (posterior) aspect of the lateral crus corrected by mattress sutures applied to the undersurface of a composite lateral crus flap.

infiltrating the vestibular skin of the lateral crus a releasing incision is made between the upper lateral cartilage and lateral crus. Small scissors are used to expand the gap between these two cartilages which lengthens the side wall of the nose. The septal extension graft is applied either on the horizontal or vertical component of the L-shaped strut to maintain the tip cartilages in a caudally displaced location. If the gap between the upper lateral cartilage and lateral crus is significant, an intercartilaginous graft[44] is placed between the two and is sutured in place. Septal cartilage is ideal as it is thin and will not produce unnecessary thickening. The patient in *Figure 21.15K,L* is a good example of a secondary short nose problem. She had a silicone implant at the first surgery and still had a severely short nose. At surgery, the implant was

removed. A rib graft was required to make a dorsal graft, a columellar strut and septal extension graft. Ear cartilage was used for the tip graft. FIG 21.15 APPEARS ONLINE ONLY

Broad nasal base

Some secondary noses still have a broad nasal base *(Fig. 21.16)*, despite having received a nasal base excision. In some cases, further nasal base excision may help. But in many others, further skin removal will either make the nostrils stenotic or the ala so small that they appear unnatural. One solution is to perform an alar base release and secure the alae medially with an interalar suture,[45] a procedure developed by many surgeons over the years.[46] This procedure is particular

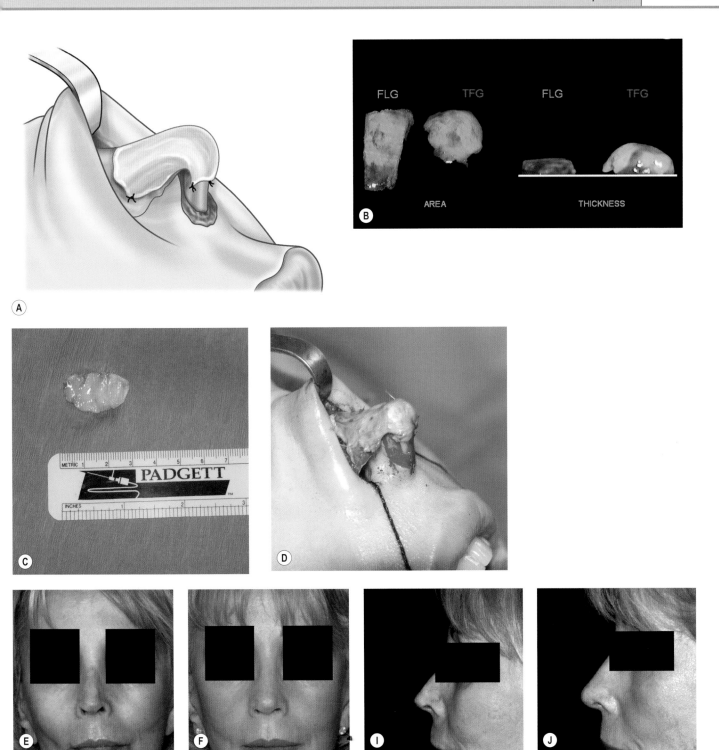

Fig. 21.14 **(A)** The schematic demonstrates how a one-layer graft, e.g., fascia, or dermis, is applied to the entire surface of the tip cartilages whose overlying skin is exceptionally thin. **(B)** A temporalis fascia graft (TFG) will demonstrate a thickness increase of up to three-fold during the first postoperative week if not sutured down. A tensor fascia lata graft (FLG) on the other hand, does not experience that kind of contraction and thickening. (Courtesy of Indorewala S. Dimensional stability of the free fascia grafts: an animal experiment. Laryngoscope 2002; 112:727.) **(C,D)** An intraoperative view of deep temporalis fascia and its application to the surface of the nose. **(E,F)** Pre- and postoperative frontal views of a secondary rhinoplasty patient with thin skin that shows many irregularities. **(I,J)** Pre- and postoperative side views of a secondary rhinoplasty patient with thin skin that shows many irregularities.

useful in those patients who have a vertically oriented alar axis (parenthesis alae). Further narrowing at the alar alone has the potential in those patients to make the alae assume a bowling pin appearance. By mobilizing the entire ala (including the cephalic aspect) that problem can be minimized.

Before executing the procedure, one should perform the pinch test. The examiner should bring the alae together with two fingers to see if the nasolabial angle becomes more obtuse than desired. If so, a limit should be placed on how much alar release is performed or one should plan to resect some of the

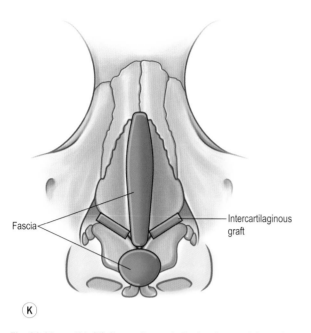

Fig. 21.14, cont'd (K) Gunter diagram indicating the use of fascia for the tip and dorsum to improve the thin skin condition.

anterior septal spine region to prevent an abnormally obtuse nasolabial angle postoperatively. 🔗 FIG **21.16** APPEARS ONLINE ONLY

Through a buccal sulcus incision a Joseph periosteal elevator is used to free the soft tissue off the maxilla. The surgeon is also releasing the recently described pyriform ligament by Rohrich et al.[47] sweeping the instrument along the horizontal pyriform rim. If necessary the release can extend into the floor of the nasal vault. A 2-0 nylon interalar suture is then passed from the dermis of one ala to that of the other. Alternatively, two smaller sutures can be used. Care must be taken to avoid placing the large suture knots too close to the skin surface. The patient in *Figure 21.17* had a prior nasal base excision but not enough improvement. Further excision would have only distorted her alae and possibly nostrils. Alar release was performed to get further improvement. 🔗 FIG **21.17** APPEARS ONLINE ONLY

Nasal dorsum irregularities

One of the most common problems requiring secondary or revision rhinoplasty is dorsal irregularities *(Fig. 21.18)*. Often this is because of a failure to accurately sculpt the dorsum. The dorsum may not have been rasped properly or small particles of cartilage may have been left behind inadvertently. Often it is due to cartilage graft warping which is not uncommon when ear cartilage grafts are used. Despite what appears to be a very smooth graft at the primary surgery the graft may shift and form small excrescences that are either visible or palpable in the upper dorsum where the skin is very thin. It

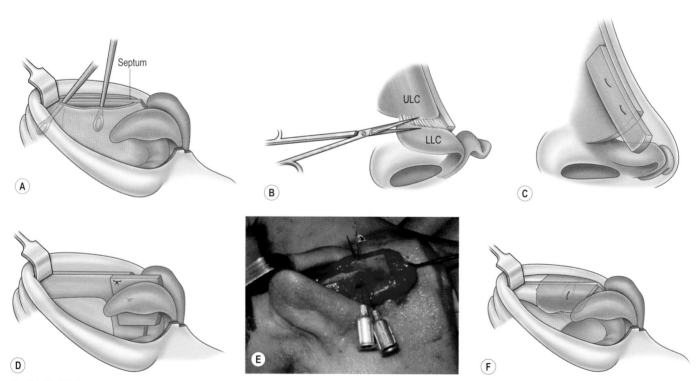

Fig. 21.15 (A) Schematic of elevation of the mucoperichondrium as a first step to correcting the short nose. **(B)** A gap is created between the upper lateral cartilage (ULC) and lateral crus (LLC), keeping the lining in tact. This maneuver lengthens the side wall of the nose and may require an intercartilaginous graft to fill the gap. **(C)** A horizontally oriented batten (septal extension graft) is applied to the dorsal septum to lengthen the nose. **(D)** Schematic of vertically oriented batten applied to caudal septum will work also. **(E)** An intraoperative view of vertically oriented septal extension graft applied to the vertical component of the L-shaped strut. **(F)** When necessary, an intercartilaginous graft is applied to the gap created between the upper lateral cartilage and lateral crus to maintain the length of the side wall of the nose.

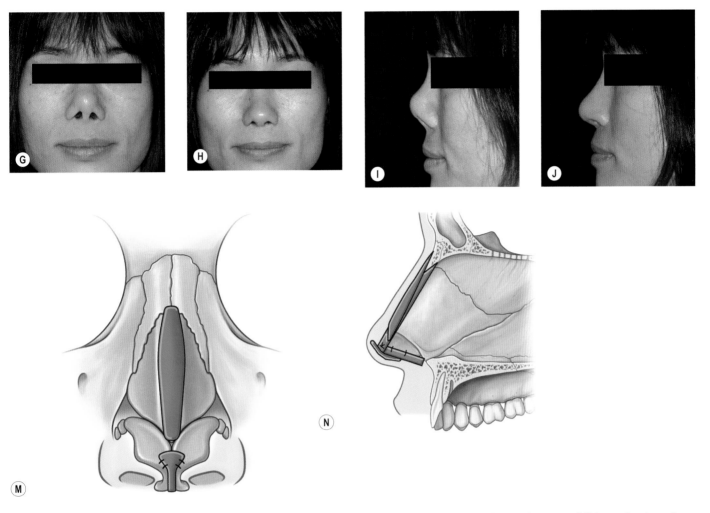

Fig. 21.15, cont'd (G,H) Pre- and postoperative frontal views of a patient with a short nose who has a silicone implant from a prior surgery. **(I,J)** Pre- and postoperative side views of the patient with a short nose. **(M,N)** Guntergram demonstrating that the patient with a short nose needed a dorsal graft columellar strut and septal extension graft of rib origin. The tip graft was of ear origin. The silicone implant was removed.

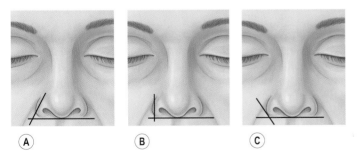

Fig. 21.16 (A–C) The nose has an alar axis. When it points straight down and the two axes are parallel, the patient is said to have parentheses alae. It is a potential problem, in that if an alar base excision is performed, the axes may turn inward giving the patient a bowling pin deformity.

is for this reason that fascia and diced cartilage in fascia grafts are used today more than ever before as a means of treating dorsal deficiency in primary rhinoplasty. The treatment of choice for small irregularities is a simple rasping of the dorsum. So doing, however, can cause a slight dorsal deficiency and the surgeon should be prepared to put in a soft tissue filler such as fascia or even a dermafat graft. A small dermafat graft can often be harvested from behind the ear by de-epithelializing that area first and removing a segment that is often 3 × 1 cm in size. It is mostly fat, of course, but will make a satisfactory padding of the dorsum when minimal augmentation is needed. 🔗 FIG **21.18** APPEARS ONLINE ONLY

Septoplasty

The fundamentals of septoplasty are discussed in Chapter 20. An important caveat to be mentioned however, is that in a secondary case, the lining of the septum is often frail and difficult to elevate from the cartilage. Perforations are easy to acquire unless one is extra careful. For this reason, the open approach is imperative when doing septal work on secondary cases. Also, we have found that the easiest way to approach the septum is to: (1) hyperinfiltrate the soft tissues immediately prior to dissection techniques, and (2) split the dorsum and tip cartilages *(Fig. 21.19)* down the middle until the anterior septal angle is reached. The anterior septal angle is a structure that can be seen and palpated even in the most difficult secondary cases. From there, elevation of the mucoperichondrium can be done under direct vision. Sharp dissection is often necessary. A suction elevator that is fairly sharp is

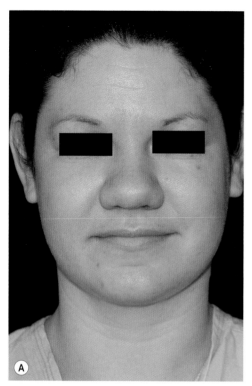

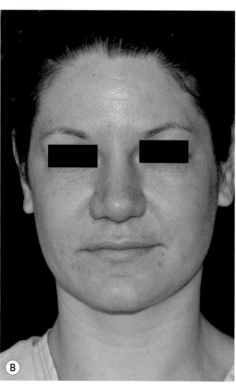

Fig. 21.17 (A,B) Pre- and postoperative frontal views of a patient who received alar base excision and thinning of the alar wall but incomplete correction of the broad nasal base.

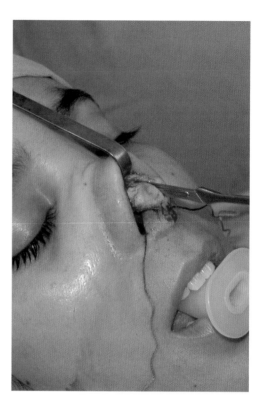

Fig. 21.19 Secondary cases are usually filled with scar that conceals the anatomy. The best approach is to split the dorsum and tip down the middle, ignoring the anatomy. So doing will reveal the anterior septal angle, a relatively constant anatomic finding. The tip cartilages and septum will be easier to dissect from this point on.

Postoperative care

Early care

At approximately 6 days postoperatively, the patient is seen for splint and suture removal. Postoperative edema can be quite alarming to some patients *(Fig. 21.20)* and therefore the patient will need reassurance. The patient will also benefit from taping (flesh colored tape) of the nose for a few more days *(Fig. 21.21)* so that they adjust better to the changes that have occurred. FIGS **21.20, 21.21** APPEARS ONLINE ONLY

Early bad result

Results[48,49] are never perfect but the patients' nose should have a very satisfactory appearance in the early postoperative period. On occasion, the nose may appear unusually unaesthetic the day after surgery or several days later when the splint is removed *(Fig. 21.22)*. The most common problem seen at this time after the operation is that the nose has an extremely obtuse nasolabial angle. Hoping for a resolution and waiting several months to a year in anticipation of eventual correction can be a poor option. The patient will not be happy to wait that long, with a gross deformity. The patient is very likely to become hostile during that watch and wait period. Giving the patient false hope that the problem will correct itself will not help either.

indispensible. This is the type of surgical dissection that will tax the surgeon more than any other because there is an ever present risk of septal perforation. Small perforations should be repaired immediately with plain catgut as one proceeds to expose the septal cartilage.

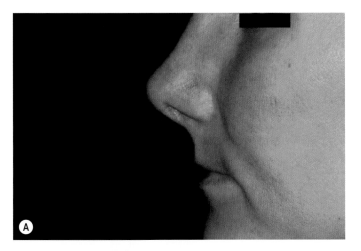

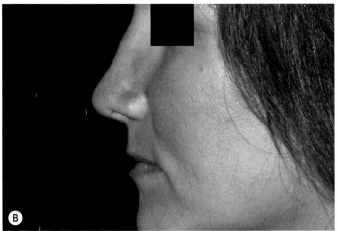

Fig. 21.22 (A,B) This patient was seen 1 week after surgery and noted to have a severely obtuse nasolabial angle. Because this problem was not likely to abate, it was advised that she return to surgery and have it adjusted before the tissues had a chance to heal.

The treatment of this condition is to return to the operating room and correct the problem before the tissues heal. Early return should be done only if it is obvious that there is an easily correctable and significant anatomic error (e.g., an obviously displaced graft). It is easier to tell the patient that an immediate adjustment is necessary than to see the patient repeatedly and deal with the frustration of an obviously poor result. For us, re-exploration as late as 12 days after surgery has been successful at making a surgical adjustment of this type. There is no significant increase in edema or induration by so doing.

Fillers

Some patients experience problems early after their surgery due either to absorption of autogenous material placed in the nose or a failure to fully correct the deformity. These patients may have small depressions. Rather than waiting until the 8–12 month period has passed when they will receive permanent filler, e.g., dermis or fascia or crushed cartilage grafts, it is often useful to give the patient temporary filler such as a collagen or hyaluronic acid product. This will relieve the

patient's anxiety during the healing phase and "buy time" until a more permanent solution can be provided.

Corticosteroids

Secondary patients in particular have swelling. Triamcinolone is a useful means of reducing that edema and induration and helps to get the patient through that difficult period when the nose (particularly the tip) can be alarmingly large. Starting at 4–6 weeks postoperatively, the patient is seen for the possible use of Triamcinolone. An initial low dose is used (1 mg). Great care must be taken not to inject it intradermally (as would be evidenced by a wheel) in order to avoid dermal atrophy.[50] This injection technique is repeated q.3 weeks as many as six times if necessary.

Complications and untoward results

Skin necrosis after the open approach

There is a rare but major potential complication[51,52] after open rhinoplasty – flap necrosis *(Fig. 21.23)*. Fortunately, this complication is not likely to occur in secondary rhinoplasty when the first operation was open because the skin has been conditioned by the first procedure. There are several potential causes of this problem: smoking, poor circulation of the skin due to prior trauma or surgical scars; defatting of the flap, such that the dermal circulation is damaged; and extensive alar excisions. To avoid flap necrosis, patients are asked to stop smoking 10 days before surgery. In the patient that has significant surgical scars on the nose, atrophy of the skin or severely discolored skin, the open approach is deferred. The skin flap is never defatted other than to pull away any soft tissue that is hanging from the dorsal skin with a pair of forceps. FIG **21.23** APPEARS ONLINE ONLY

There is a potential for interference with the nasal circulation if the ala is completely detached from the face. Rohrich *et al.*[53] demonstrated the circulation of the nasal skin and how branches of the lateral nasal artery near the upper ala are significant contributors to the blood flow of the nasal tip. To avoid interference with the circulation in the open approach alar base excisions should be conservative, i.e., they should not extend along the entire alar groove.

The treatment of necrosis requires conservative management. Excision of the wound with grafting should not, in general, be employed. The nose has a remarkable ability to heal without much scarring in most cases. Whatever scarring does occur is almost always less conspicuous than a skin graft. The surgeon will want to wait at least a year before deciding if any surgical measure should be done *(Fig. 21.24)*. FIG **21.24** APPEARS ONLINE ONLY

Columellar scar

Fortunately, columellar scars *(Fig. 21.25)* are seldom a problem requiring secondary correction. However, there will be occasions when surgical correction will be necessary. The problem is often a thickening of the soft tissue (due to scar deposition) just anterior to the actual scar. The design of the scar is seldom the cause of the problem, however. Another problem is a notching along one side of the columella due usually to inadequate apposition of tissues at the time of the original closure. Rather than excising the entire scar, it is usually best to deal with the specific problem as if there were no columellar scar. For example, in the case of notching, it is best to simply excise the bulge along the side of the columella as if it were a small

growth. In the case of a bulging fibrotic columellar flap, it is often best to leave the scar as it is (assuming it is flat) and simply open the side of the columella and debulk the soft tissue (*Fig. 21.25*).

Post-rhinoplasty fibrotic syndrome

Occasionally, we will see a patient for a secondary rhinoplasty who requires either an open or closed approach and has a satisfactory intraoperative course in terms of being able to achieve a nicely sculptured framework. However, for one reason or another, the patient goes on to have increased edema, fibrous induration and ultimately a thickened nose that is wider, thicker and worse than the original preoperative condition. The patient in *Figure 21.26* is such a case. She had multiple prior surgeries resulting in a short nose with nostril show. A secondary rhinoplasty was performed, including a septal extension graft, tip graft and rim graft. Despite early improvement, the patient went on to have a wider nose than before. The increased width of the nose, which was the most distressing to the patient, was undoubtedly due to fibrous deposition. This problem is best dealt with avoiding or minimizing surgery. If surgery has to be done because the deformity is very obvious, it is best to use a minimalist approach. In particular, it is wise to avoid undermining, which tends to lead to edema and subsequent fibrosis.

The difficult patient

As is the case for all types of aesthetic surgery, there is a group of patients who are difficult to please. Postoperative management requires patience and tolerance. The patient's concerns should be acknowledged and not ignored. The

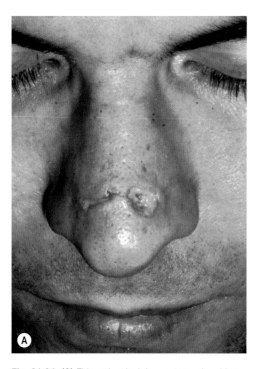

Fig. 21.24 (A) This patient had three sutures placed between the dermis and dorsal septum for the purposes of minimizing a supratip fullness. Unfortunately, it caused three areas of necrosis that coalesced.

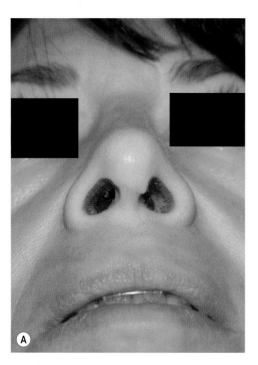
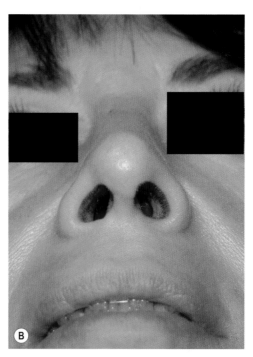

Fig. 21.25 (A) Columellar scars, if not retracted, occasionally appear as irregularities along the side of the columella. **(B)** Rather than excising the whole scar and starting afresh, it is often best to enter the side of the columella to debulk any fullness or excise whatever is protruding on the side, as was necessary in this case.

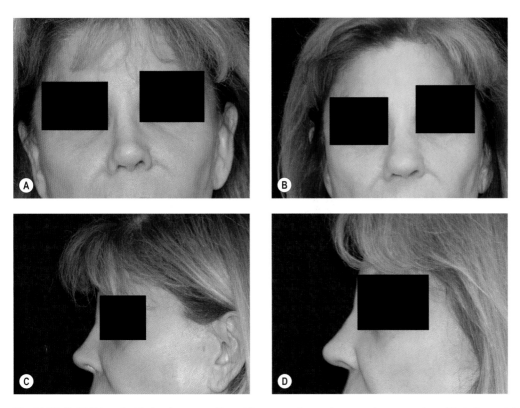

Fig. 21.26 (A–D) This patient had a short nose with nostril exposure. A secondary procedure was performed including septal extension graft, tip graft and rim graft. Unfortunately, the fibrous deposition postoperative left here with a thicker nose than preoperatively – a condition that is reasonably called the post-rhinoplasty fibrotic syndrome.

patient should be reassured that everything will be done that can be done to give the best result possible. As soon as it is obvious that the patient's condition is not going to improve and that a revision is likely in the future, it should be discussed with the patient. The patient will fare better if they know that they can look forward to an improved result. Getting a second opinion for the patients can also be very

helpful. A second opinion from a colleague assures the patient that everything possible is being done and often provides the surgeons with some alternative ideas that he or she had not considered. Waiting for the patient to get his/her own second opinion is problematic because that surgeon may not be familiar with you or your work and may be unnecessarily critical.

Bonus images for this chapter can be found online at **http://www.expertconsult.com**

Fig. 21.1 Imaging is a key to successful analysis and patient communication. It is also a way to perform mock surgery.

Fig. 21.2 (A) This autoclavable model of the prototype ideal framework for the nose makes it easy for the surgeon to perform his/her biological sculpting. Copying from a model is much easier than memorizing the angles and relationships between various parts of the tip complex. The **(B)** nasal tip should **(C)** ideally look something like the prototype model. **(D,E)** After suture techniques, excisional techniques and grafts are complete.

Fig. 21.5 A single universal horizontal mattress suture can increase the strength of cartilage by 35%. Scoring the cartilage to achieve the same degree of straightness can reduce the cartilage strength by 50%.

Fig. 21.6 (A–E) The ear is a great source of donor cartilage. This concha cavum/cymba graft is applied to a silicone block where it

will be divided into two units: cymba and cavum. As individual units, they are easily straightened with horizontal mattress sutures and made into usable units of cartilage to reconstruct various parts of the secondary nose.

Fig. 21.9 (L) At 17 months postoperatively, she exhibits considerable improvement.

Fig. 21.10 This patient is a good example of a broad tip problem. **(A,C,E)** She exhibited a broad tip, supratip deformity, and radix deficiency. Because of the very thick skin it was decided to use a closed approach. The tip cartilages were delivered. The patient received cephalic trim of the lateral crus along with interdomal and lateral crural mattress sutures (5-0 PDS). A radix graft from the septum was used and the caudal septum was shortened. A lateral osteotomy was also performed. **(B,D,F)** At 14 months postoperatively, considerable improvement

was obtained.

Fig. 21.11 (C) Tip graft sizers are made of silicone. They come in three sizes. **(D,E)** The sizer is held in place to the existing tip complex with a needle. When the appropriate size is chosen it is placed on the donor cartilage and used as a cookie cutter like device to carve a tip graft. **(I,K,M)** This patient is a good example of a deficient tip problem. She exhibited a narrow over-resected tip, inverted V deformity and alar retraction. At surgery, through an open approach, the tip cartilages had to be separated and an interdomal graft put between them. An anatomic tip graft was laid on the surface (ear acting as donor) and spreader grafts were inserted. Small rim grafts were also required as indicated in the Guntergram. She also received a dermis graft to augment the lips. **(J,L,N)** The postoperative result at 22 months shows considerable improvement.

Fig. 21.13 (C,D) Pre- and postoperative frontal view of a patient who exhibited a collapse alar rim, corrected by an alar contour rim graft; **(E,F)** basal view also shows the improvement.

Fig. 21.14 (G,H) Pre- and postoperative basal views of a secondary rhinoplasty patient with thin skin that shows many irregularities.

Fig. 21.15 (K,L) Pre- and postoperative basal views of the patient with a short nose.

Fig. 21.16 (D–F) The pinch test is done to be sure that bringing the alar together does not cause an abnormal nasolabial angle when an alar release and interalar suture procedure is performed. **(G)** An incision is made at the junction of ala and nostril sill. An elevator is used to release the ala from the maxilla and pyriform groove. **(H)** Intraoperative view of buccal sulcus entry to release the ala from its maxillary attachments. **(I)** Cadaver demonstration to emphasize that when performing an alar release, it is often necessary to elevate the periosteum off the nasal vault in addition to releasing the Pessa/Rohrich ligament.

Fig. 21.17 (C,D) Pre- and postoperative basal views of a patient who received alar base excision and thinning of the alar wall but incomplete correction of the broad nasal base. **(E,F)** Pre- and postoperative frontal view of the same patient who received further reduction of nasal base width, using the alar release method including interalar sutures. **(G,H)** Pre- and postoperative basal view of the same patient who received further reduction of nasal base width, using the alar release method including interalar sutures.

Fig. 21.18 The patient exhibited dorsal deficiency **(A)**, treated with ear cartilage augmentation **(B)**. Late postoperatively, one can see dorsal irregularities on the profile view **(C)** and frontal view **(D)**.

Fig. 21.20 An unhappy patient is first noticed when the splint is removed and the patient stares in the middle. If the patient says nothing as he/she looks at her new nose, it is an ominous sign. The patient may be reluctant to criticize her/his surgeon and yet is unwilling to give a compliment.

Fig. 21.21 (A–C) One half-inch flesh colored tape is frequently applied to the nasal tip shortly after the splint is removed on day 6. The tape helps reduce the edema but more importantly, gives the patient more time to adapt to the new nose as the swelling recedes.

Fig. 21.23 One of the worst disasters in primary or secondary rhinoplasty is tip necrosis. Often, this is from defatting the flap when performing the open approach. It is less likely in a secondary rhinoplasty, however, because the flap has been conditioned as a result of the first operation.

Fig. 21.24 (B) This patient had three sutures placed between the dermis and dorsal septum for the purposes of minimizing a supratip fullness. Unfortunately, it caused three areas of necrosis that coalesced. **(C,D)** Skin necrosis should be treated conservatively and usually heals better than one would think. The preoperative patient **(C)** exhibits a broad tip and alar retraction. The skin necrosis he developed eventually faded to a thin transverse scar **(D)** that, although slightly perceptible, was in a favorable location and it did not end up with a totally distraught patient.

 Access the complete references list online at **http://www.expertconsult.com**

1. Byrd HS, Constantian MB, Guyuron B, et al. Revision rhinoplasty. *Aesthet Surg J.* 2007;27:175.

2. Gruber RP. Use of the internet by patients. How it affects your practice and what to do about it. In: Korman J, ed. *Practice management.* In press, 2011.

3. Gunter JP, Rohrich RJ, Adams WP. *Dallas rhinoplasty: Nasal surgery by the masters.* St. Louis: Quality Medical; 2008.

4. Kim DW, Toriumi DM. Nasal analysis for secondary rhinoplasty. *Facial Plast Surg Clin North Am.* 2003;11:399.

5. Oneal RM, Bell RJ Jr, Schlesinger J. Surgical anatomy of the nose. *Clin Plast Surg.* 1996;232:195.

6. Daniel RK. Secondary rhinoplasty following open rhinoplasty. *Plast Reconstr Surg.* 1995;96:1539.

9. Gruber RP, Nahai F, Bogdan MA, et al. Changing the convexity and concavity of nasal cartilages and cartilage grafts with horizontal mattress sutures: part II. Clinical results. *Plast Reconstr Surg.* 2005;115(2): 595–606.

15. Guyuron B, Behmand RA. Nasal tip sutures part II: the interplays. *Plast Reconstr Surg.* 2003;112(4): 1130–1145.

   The authors submit that nasal tip sutures produce subtle but significant morphological alterations. Nine such suture techniques are discussed.

17. Daniel RK. Rhinoplasty: a simplified, three-stitch, open tip suture technique. Part II: secondary rhinoplasty. *Plast Reconstr Surg.* 1999;103(5):1503–1512.

   The author emphasizes the importance of nasal tip sutures in secondary rhinoplasty. Strut sutures, domal equalization sutures, and columella septal sutures are described, and case studies are presented.

18. Gruber RP, Weintraub J, Pomerantz J. Suture techniques for the nasal tip. *Aesthet Surg J.* 2008;28(1): 92–100.

23. Gruber RP, Grover S. The anatomic tip graft for nasal augmentation. *Plast Reconstr Surg.* 1999;103(6): 1744–1753.

   A nasal tip graft mirroring aesthetic surface morphology (hence "anatomic") is described.

29. Gunter JP, Friedman RM. Lateral crural strut graft: technique and clinical applications in rhinoplasty. *Plast Reconstr Surg.* 1997;99(4):943–952.

   Strips of cartilage are affixed deep to the lateral crura to create the lateral crural strut graft. These grafts are useful in reshaping and repositioning the lateral crura. The authors describe the details of this technique.

31. Rohrich RJ, Raniere J Jr, Ha RY. The alar contour graft: correction and prevention of alar rim deformities in rhinoplasty. *Plast Reconstr Surg.* 2002;109(7):2495–2505.

   The authors describe a rhinoplasty graft inserted into an alar-vestibular pocket, useful as a buttress in managing alar rim deformities. In addition to defining an aesthetic alar contour, a patent external valve is established.

38. Gruber RP. The short nose. *Clin Plast Surg.* 1996;23(2): 297–313.

22

Otoplasty

Charles H. Thorne

SYNOPSIS

- Analysis. Analyze the problem in thirds.
- Endpoint. Know what normal looks like, so you know your surgical endpoint.
- Do not be destructive. Do not do anything to the ear that cannot be reversed.
- Skin is precious but weak. Preserve skin in the sulcus and do not rely on skin tension to maintain ear position.
- Lobule. Consider lobule setback in every case.
- Asymmetry. In asymmetric cases, operate on both ears most of the time.
- Facelifts are otoplasties. Do not deform the tragus, lobule or sulcus.

 Access the Historical Perspective section online at
http://www.expertconsult.com

Introduction

The term "otoplasty" refers to surgical changes in the shape or position of the ear. The most common indication is the patient with prominent, but normally shaped, ears. In this situation, otoplasty is an enormously rewarding procedure for the surgeon and the patient/family, because good results and satisfied patients can be expected in most cases. In addition, the technical maneuvers required are among the simplest in all of plastic surgery.

The complexity of the otoplasty procedure increases as the deformity of the ear increases. If correction of prominent ears is at one end of the otoplasty spectrum, then reconstruction of congenital microtia with rib cartilage grafts is at the other. Surgical reshaping of the ears, or otoplasty, is best conceptualized with the whole spectrum of ear deformities in mind; that way, the surgeon will avoid the pitfall of learning a single recipe and attempting to apply it in every situation.

The single most important exercise for the surgeon, before performing any procedure in the otoplasty spectrum, is to have the characteristics of a normal ear firmly in his/her mind. With proper choice of technique, the surgeon can usually avoid the uncorrectable problems of over-correction and unnatural contours.[1]

Basic science/disease process

The cause of ear deformities is not known. Some articles in the literature suggest that ear deformities are the result of absent or misplaced muscles around the ear. Some newborn children have extremely soft, pliable ears. When these children have prominent ears and they lie on their sides, the ears tend to fold forward against the cheek, rather than back against the head, tending to make them more prominent as the years go on.

Diagnosis/patient presentation

Overall size and shape

The overall size and shape of the ear is evaluated to determine if the ear is prominent with an otherwise normal size and configuration, or if there are abnormalities in addition to the prominence. Excessively large ears, Stahl's ears, cryptotia, underdeveloped shell-like helical rims, postoperative deformities, cauliflower ears, elongated lobules or earring-related or facelift-related deformities are noted.

Upper third

The upper third of the ear is evaluated to determine if it is prominent, if the antihelix/superior crus of the triangular fossa is well formed and if the helical rim is well defined.

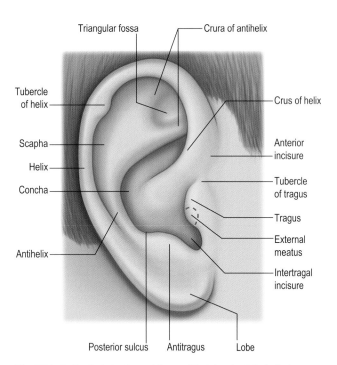

Fig. 22.1 Anatomical structures of the ear. The tubercle of the helix is synonymous with Darwinian's tubercle (Reprinted with permission from Janis JE, Rohrich RJ, Gutowski KA. Otoplasty. Plast Reconstr Surg. 2005;115(4):60e–72e.)

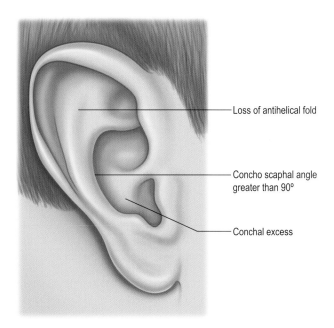

Fig. 22.2 Main components of the prominent ear. (Reprinted with permission from Janis JE, Rohrich RJ, Gutowski KA. Otoplasty. Plast Reconstr Surg. 2005;115(4):60e–72e.)

Middle third

The middle third of the ear is evaluated to determine if the concha is overly deep or protruding. In addition, the relationship between the antihelix and the helix is examined to determine if, e.g., the underdevelopment of the antihelix/superior crus in the upper third extends into the middle third or if it is confined to the upper third.

Lower third

The lobule is evaluated to determine if it is prominent. It is important to note that even if the lobule is not particularly prominent on initial examination, it may be excessively prominent once the upper two-thirds of the ear have been corrected intraoperatively.

Asymmetry

Asymmetry is noted, mostly because patients and families will always comment on it. In asymmetric cases it is usually preferable to operate on both ears rather than attempt to set back only the prominent ear to match its less prominent counterpart *(Fig. 22.1)*.

Patient selection

Since otoplasty is perhaps the only cosmetic procedure that can be performed in childhood, additional considerations come into play. The fact that parents and grandparents may be involved in surgical decision making for a patient who cannot yet express himself or herself alters the doctor–patient relationship.

The degree of prominence/deformity and the age at presentation will determine when a surgical recommendation is made. For young children with very prominent ears and whose parents desire early correction, otoplasty is recommended as early as age 4 years. While there may be situations when earlier intervention is warranted, it is reasonable to view the age of 4 years as a minimum for most otoplasty procedures and its variations. In situations where the entire ears require reconstruction, as in microtia, this author prefers to follow the recommendations of Firmin[6] and wait until approximately the age of 10 years.

In other cases, the parents may want the child to participate in the decision process and that will necessitate later intervention. General anesthesia or deep sedation by an anesthesiologist is usually required up until the early teenage years, especially in boys. Occasionally, there are girls who are mature enough to request and tolerate the procedure under local anesthesia without an anesthesiologist, but this is rare. It is also common to have patients present at approximately 18 years of age, when they are legally independent, or later when they have earned the money for the procedure. Finally, it is not unusual for adults at almost any age to request correction, either because they have wanted it all their lives or because their desire to, e.g., have a facelift, has led to the realization that their ears are also prominent.

Families frequently ask about the effect of early surgical treatment on growth of the ears. For whatever reason, this has never been an issue in this author's experience. For one thing, there is a large variation in acceptable ear size. It has also never been shown that an otoplasty retards auricular growth. Finally, many prominent ears are on the large side and some growth retardation would be welcomed by the patient and/or the family *(Fig. 22.2)*.

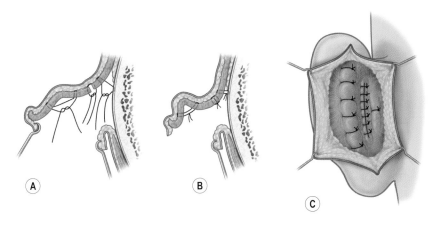

Fig. 22.3 Technique for the standard otoplasty. The combination of Mustarde sutures, conchal resection/closure and conchal-mastoid sutures is shown. **(A)** Suture placement. **(B)** Suture tightened and ties appropriately. **(C)** Position of sutures as shown from the surgeon's vantage point.

Treatment/surgical technique

While the delicate, complex contours of the ear may be difficult to create *de novo* (i.e., microtia), anatomic considerations are minimal in standard otoplasty. There is abundant blood supply, making almost any combination of incisions acceptable without the risk of necrosis. There are no motor nerves in the neighborhood. The terminal branches of the great auricular nerve will always be injured but normal sensory function usually returns.

The one anatomic structure that can be compromised in otoplasty is the external auditory canal (conchal setback narrows the meatus). Otherwise, the anatomic considerations of otoplasty are those of preservation: preservation of the sulcus, preservation of the natural softness of the auricular contours, and preservation of the normal landmarks such as the posterior wall of the concha (that is, the middle third of the antihelix.)

Standard otoplasty for prominent ears of normal size

Incision

The incision is made in the retroauricular sulcus. In the upper third of the ear, the incision can be extended up on to the back of the ear to provide adequate exposure to place Mustarde sutures between the triangular fossa and scapha. While an incision placed higher, on the back of the ear, will make the dissection easier, this author prefers the depth of the sulcus where the ultimate scar will be better hidden.

Dissection

No skin is excised, except a small triangle from the medial surface of the lobule (not the retrolobular skin), taking care to preserve enough tissue for a normal earlobe and retrolobular sulcus. This skin excision on the lobule is frequently necessary for repositioning of the lobule at the end of the procedure. The cartilage is exposed on the posterior (medial) surface of the ear and soft tissue is excised from deep to the concha. In the region of the earlobe, deep dissection is performed under the concha in preparation for lobule repositioning. Branches of the great auricular nerve will be seen and divided.

Correction *(Fig. 22.3)*

Mustarde concha-scapha and triangular fossa-scapha sutures are placed using 4-0 clear nylon sutures on an FS-2 needle.[7] The number of sutures depends on the how far into the middle third of the ear the antihelical deficiency extends. In some cases the sutures will only be required in the upper third of the ear. In other cases, they will extend through the middle third as well. These sutures are placed in order to create a soft curvature to the antihelix and no attempt is made to correct the prominence of the ear at this point. The Mustarde sutures are not parallel to each other but, instead, are arranged like spokes on a wheel, all pointing toward the top of the tragus (center of the wheel). Care is taken to create a superior crus that curves anteriorly such that it terminates almost parallel to the inferior curs. If the superior crus is created such that it is a direct, cephalad extension of the antihelix (straight line), the result will appear unnatural and amateurish.

A small crescent of cartilage (≤3 mm at its widest point) is excised from the posterior wall of the concha, at its junction with the conchal floor. The defect in the concha is closed primarily using numerous 4-0 nylon sutures. It is important that the conchal resection be placed precisely. If it is too large or if it is too far up the posterior conchal wall, then it will irrevocably deform the antihelix. If it is too far anterior, in the floor of the concha, it will not decrease the height of the posterior conchal wall and the closure may be visible. Lack of attention to the placement of the conchal resection is a common cause of complications. A conchal setback suture (Furnas suture) is then placed between the reduced concha and the mastoid fascia using a single 3-0 nylon or 3-0 PDS suture.[8] The author prefers not to tie this suture until after lobule repositioning has been performed. This combination of a small conchal resection and a small conchal setback avoids the distortion of a large conchal resection and the unreliability of a large conchal setback. This author avoids conchal setback alone in all but the mildest cases. The other problem with reliance on a conchal setback (Furnas suture) alone is that the external auditory meatus can be narrowed to the point of significant stenosis *(Fig. 22.4)*.

The earlobe is repositioned by closing the triangular defect on the medial surface of the lobule created by the skin excision *(Fig. 22.5)*. The 5-0 PDS sutures do not just approximate the skin; rather, they approximate the skin AND take a bite of the concha deep in the sulcus (similar to Gosain and Recinos[9]).

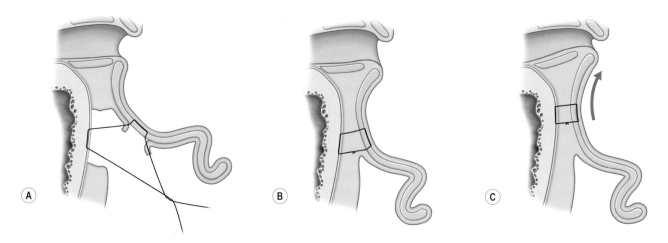

(A)   (B)   (C)

Fig. 22.4 Placement of Furnas concho-mastoid sutures. Note that suture placement too close to the external auditory canal can constrict the canal. (Reprinted with permission from Janis JE, Rohrich RJ, Gutowski KA. Otoplasty. Plast Reconstr Surg. 2005;115(4):60e–72e.)

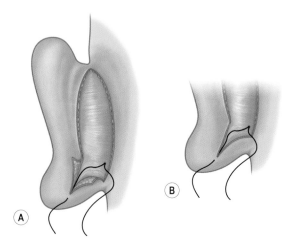

(A)   (B)

Fig. 22.5 Lobule repositioning. The technique for lobule repositioning is shown. A triangle of skin is excised on the earlobe, never compromising the appearance of the lobe or the ability for the patient to wear earrings. Sutures are placed close to the skin defect while catching a bite of the concha deep in the closure.

When these sutures (usually two) are tied the earlobe position will be corrected. Ideally, the endpoint of earlobe repositioning should be slight over-correction because the skin will stretch over time. The author has not had success when repositioning of the helical tail is used as the sole method of earlobe repositioning, as described by Webster.[10]

Endpoint

Otoplasty surgery is all about the endpoint. How do you know how tight to make the Mustarde sutures? That is, how do you know how sharp to make the antihelix? How do you know how tight to tie the Furnas conchal-mastoid suture? Or the earlobe correction sutures? The answers to these questions lie in the knowledge of a normal ear. If the surgeon remembers the following regarding how the ear should look from various vantage points it will aid tremendously in the intra-operative decision-making:[11]

1. From the front, the helical rim should be visible, poking out from behind the antihelix.

2. From the side, the contours of the ear should be round and soft, never sharp.

3. From behind (and this is the most helpful to the surgeon who is sitting behind the patient intraoperatively), the contour of the helical rim should be a straight line, not a "C", or a "hockey stick", or any other shape. If the helical contour is a straight line, it almost ensures that a harmonious correction will be achieved. Regardless if the ultimate correction is slightly under- or slightly over-corrected, a harmonious correction will read as "normal" to the outside world and almost all patients will be happy. This is perhaps the single most important lesson from this chapter.

The last judgment is how close to the head the ear should be placed. This is determined by tying the Furnas suture, which is the last maneuver that the author performs (other than wound closure). The final position of the ear should be over-corrected minimally to allow for some relapse, but not enough to create an unsatisfactory result if no relapse should occur.

Closure

The skin is approximated using 5-0 plain gut sutures without excision skin (**Figs 22.6, 22.7**).[12]

Otoplasty for large ears or ears with inadequate helical rim definition

Incision

An incision is made on the lateral (visible) surface of the ear, just inside the helical rim (or where the helical rim would be if it is underdeveloped).[13] In addition, an incision in the retro-auricular sulcus may also be required depending on what additional maneuvers are required.

Dissection

The lateral incision is extended through the cartilage. The posterior surface of the cartilage is dissected, just as if a standard posterior incision had been made.

Correction

In the case of excessively large ears, the scaphal cartilage (and perhaps some scaphal skin) are trimmed to the desired size and shape. Care is taken to excise more cartilage than skin. At this point the helical rim will be too long for the new scapha and will require shortening at the end of the procedure. Mustarde sutures are placed if necessary through this anterior access. Conchal resection/setback and earlobe repositioning are performed through a separate incision in the sulcus if necessary *(Fig. 22.8)*.

Closure

A wedge is then removed from the helical rim so that it will fit the scapha, which is now of lesser circumference. The amount of helix removed is important and should be determined precisely. The desired resection will leave the helix the correct length for the new scapha and allow closure without excess tension. However, in the case of ears with inadequate formation of the helical rim, it is precisely the slight tension on the helical closure which will cause the helical rim to turnover and form a more natural contour. The helix is reapproximated carefully using horizontal mattress sutures of 5-0 nylon sutures attempting to evert the skin edges to avoid notching. The lateral incision is closed with a combination of a few interrupted 5-0 plain sutures and a running 6-0 plain suture. The author believes the running closure is desirable because this skin edge is highly vascular and has a tendency to ooze or even bleed actively when the adrenaline in the local anesthesia solution wears off.

Otoplasty for constricted ears

Constricted ears are tremendously variable and no single technique is applicable to all. Tanzer[14] divided constricted ear deformities into three types: type I – involving only the helix; type II – involving the helix and scapha; and type III – extreme cupping of the ear. In the author's opinion, they are also the most difficult deformities to correct. The simplest appearing example of the constricted ear is the "lop ear", in which the upper pole of the ear is turned over. There is always deficiency of tissue in this region. In other words, even if you could pick up the lopped part of the ear it would still be slightly smaller than the normal ear on the other side. In some cases, it is adequate to excise directly the leading edge of the overhanging skin and cartilage to create a less hooded appearance. In more significant deformities (Tanzer type II) it is necessary to expand the overhanging cartilage with radial cuts and reinforce the area with a conchal graft.

Other constricted ears appear prominent, but unlike standard prominent ears, they are prominent because the helical circumference is inadequate. It is as if the helix has been tightened excessively like a drawstring, forcing the ear forward. In other words, the ear cannot lie flat because the excessively short helical rim draws the auricle into a cup. Any attempt to

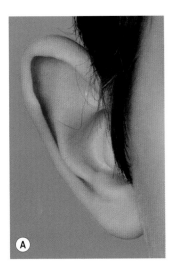
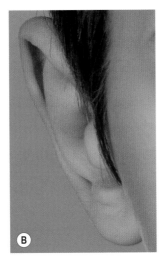

Fig. 22.6 Otoplasty. The patient is shown before **(A)** and after **(B)** standard otoplasty. The upper, middle, and lower thirds of the ear have been set back in a harmonious fashion. The contours are soft and natural.

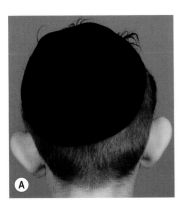
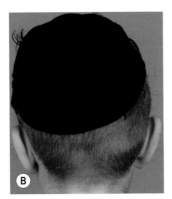
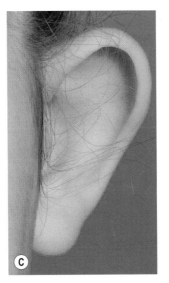
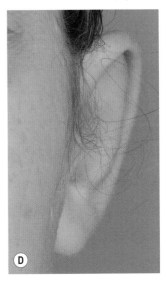

Fig. 22.7 Otoplasty. **(A,B)** Posterior view before and after otoplasty. The helical rim contour is straight and the scars are hidden within the sulcus. **(C,D)** Frontal view of the same patient showing a harmonious correction and soft natural contours.

set back a constricted ear must be accompanied by elongation of the helix. The most common technique for elongating the helix is by a variation of the incision described above for large ears. The incision is made inside the helical rim and extended anteriorly around the crus of the helix into the preauricular region to the junction of the ear and the temporal scalp. The crus of the helix is then mobilized and when standard otoplasty maneuvers are performed, the crus of the helix is recruited into the helical rim. The donor site in the concha is closed primarily as if the crus of the helix had been taken for a composite graft to the nose. Any excess or unusable crus of the helix is discarded.

In the case of more severely constricted ears (Tanzer type III), it is preferable to discard the cartilage and construct a framework as if the patient had classic microtia.

Otoplasty for cryptotia

The term cryptotia is used to describe the rare condition where the upper potion of the ear is buried beneath the temporal scalp. The ear can literally be pulled out of the scalp to examine it. The correction is performed by pulling the ear out of its bed in the scalp, incising around it in order to release it fully, and resurfacing the defect behind the upper pole of ear with a skin graft or a local flap. In some cases the auricular cartilage is normal in contour and only requires the soft tissue rearrangement described above for correction. In other cases, the cartilage is misshapen, as in a lop ear, and requires cartilage grafting to augment the deficient native cartilage framework in addition to the soft tissue considerations. The deformity must be much more common in Asian patients since almost all the publications on this deformity come from Asian countries and the author of this chapter has seen very few cases in a 20-year practice.[15]

Otoplasty for Stahl's ears

The Stahl's ear deformity consists of an abnormal crus extending superolaterally, as shown in *Figure 22.9*. The deformity is variable. In the mildest cases, the extra crus is barely noticeable and can be ignored and the otoplasty performed as if it were a standard case of prominent ears. More severe deformities include excess scapha in the region of the abnormal crus and termination of the abnormal crus in a point ("Mr Spock" ears). In the most severe cases, there is also complete absence of the normal superior crus.

Correction of the deformity mandates resection of the abnormal crus.[16] The author makes an incision inside the helical rim as described above but *not* through the cartilage.

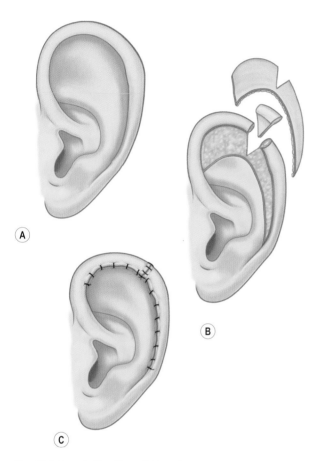

Fig. 22.8 Ear reduction. The technique of ear reduction is shown. (Redrawn from Argamaso RV. Ear reduction. Plast Reconstr Surg. 1990; 85(2):316.)

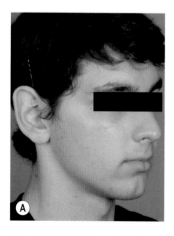
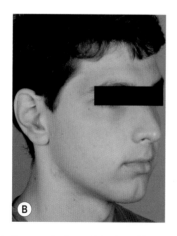
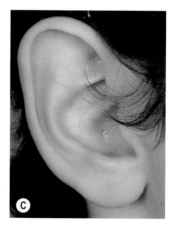
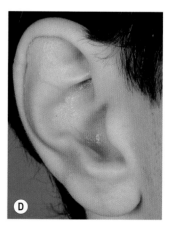

Fig. 22.9 (A,B) Oblique views before and after ear reduction and otoplasty. The scaphal reduction is apparent. **(C,D)** Close up oblique views showing the scar in the helical rim where the wedge was removed.

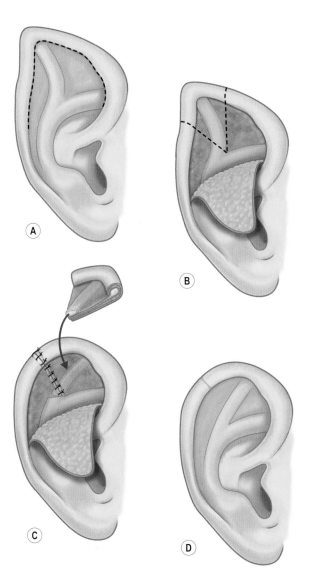

Fig. 22.10 Correction of Stahl's ear. The lateral skin is reflected, the abnormal crus is excised, the cartilage defect is closed primarily and the cartilage from the excised crus is used as an onlay graft to recreate the normal superior crus. **(A)** The skin incision is shown inside the helical rim. **(B)** The abnormal crus is excised. **(C)** The cartilage defect is reapproximated and the excised cartilage is placed as an onlay graft to reconstruct the superior crus. **(D)** The final result. (Redrawn from Kaplan HM, Hudson DA. A novel surgical method of repair for Stahl's ear; a case report and review of current treatment modalities. Plast Reconstr Surg. 1999; 103:566–569.)

The skin is carefully dissected off the lateral surface of the cartilage *(Fig. 22.10)*. Note this is an entirely different plane from that described for macrotia or underdeveloped helical rims and must be performed carefully, so as preserve the viability of the skin. The lateral skin of the ear is more firmly attached to the cartilage and there is much less subcutaneous tissue than on the back (medial surface) of the ear. The abnormal crus is resected and placed as an onlay graft to reconstruct the absent superior crus. The cartilaginous defect left by the resected crus is closed primarily. The skin is then reapproximated. The Stahl's ear deformity can be severe and patients are usually quite happy, even if the result falls short of completely normal.

Correction of aging, elongated ear lobes

Earlobe reduction can be remarkably rejuvenative in a patient with droopy, inelastic, elongated earlobes. The procedure is also occasionally warranted in younger patients who have congenitally enlarged earlobes. Earlobe reduction can be performed concomitantly with a facelift or as an isolated procedure. A number of techniques have been described. The anatomy of the individual patient dictates the design. The most common procedure in the author's hands, however, is amputation of the caudal border of the lobule. The author goes to some trouble to place the scar on the back side of the earlobe where it is not visible.

Incision

The ideal contour is drawn on the lobule. The excision is designed asymmetrically so that the incision is made caudal to this line on the lateral surface and cephalic to it on the medial surface. In addition the ends of the excision are located slightly medial to the margin of the lobule. The idea is to excise more tissue from the medial side of the ear lobe and to create a longer skin flap on the lateral surface. This lateral flap is thinned so it is more mobile than is medial counterpart.

Closure

The combination of the asymmetric design, the thinner lateral flap and the fact that the ends of the defect are not located precisely on the margin of the lobule but rather slightly medial to it, result in the ultimate scar being hidden on the medial surface of the lobule. Numerous sutures, meticulous tapering and some patience are required for the best outcome.

Correction of earring-related complications

Earring-related complications are extremely common. These complications are most common in the lobule but the more serious complications occur where the cartilage of the ear has been pierced. While a number of procedures have been described for correction of elongated piercings, the author has found that simple excision and closure is most effective. This technique applies to both elongated earring holes and those that have torn completely through the lobule margin. In the latter case, a Z-plasty can be added in an effort to avoid a notch. In reality, an everted closure using horizontal mattress sutures seems to yield equivalent results at the lobule margin. The medial and lateral skin are closed with nylon sutures, and no deep, absorbable sutures are used. The earlobes can be re-pierced in 6 weeks, depending on how stiff and fibrotic they are after the repair. Avoiding absorbable sutures in the subcutaneous tissue of the lobe seems to minimize the inflammation and shorten the recovery and the waiting period before re-piercing.

Correction of facelift deformities around the ear

After 20 years of hard labor in this area, the author has concluded that a facelift is just one type of otoplasty. Facelift deformities of the ear are frequently unfixable, leading to lesson number one in facelifting: AVOID THEM. Such problems fall into the following categories:

1. Deformities of the lobule (pixie ear)
2. Deformities of the tragus
3. Deformities of the retroauricular sulcus
4. Unsightly hypertrophic or poorly placed periauricular scars.

Earlobe deformities

Earlobe deformities after facelift are the result of excessive anterior and inferior traction on the lobule due to inexpert trimming of the facelift flap. Such deformities are completely avoidable but difficult to correct. The facial skin should be trimmed so that the ear can barely pulled out from under it. In other words, it is far better to have the facelift flap tucked up under the earlobe (even elongating the earlobe), than to have it too low where the closure will visible or even deforming. As anyone with experience will verify, secondary lifting may generate a disappointing amount of skin advancement and a pixie ear may be improvable but not totally correctable. Be careful about promising a patient that you can repair it entirely.

Tragal deformities

Tragal deformities consist of either anterior traction on the tragus, amputation of some of the tragal cartilage or excess facial skin at the bottom of the tragus that serves as an across-the-room surgical signature. There is little that can be done for the first two conditions, since too much tissue has been removed. In fact, further lifting attempts may only make them worse: when the facial skin is rotated cephalad, there may be even less skin available for tragal coverage than there was originally. The latter deformity, lack of definition of the caudal tragus, however, can be corrected. As Connell has emphasized, the tragus should have a well-defined top and bottom. Imperfect trimming of the facelift flap often results in an oblique fold at the caudal edge of the tragus and a gradual transition from the tragus to the lobule rather than the normal right angle. Removal of a triangle of skin can correct the problem and make it much less obvious that the patient has had a facelift.

Retroauricular deformities

Surgeons seem to feel that it is necessary to place the facelift incision up on the back of the ear. If that is excessive or is done a few times, there may be little skin remaining behind the ear. If the incision is placed in the sulcus or minimally on the auricular cartilage, it will not migrate if the flaps are trimmed judiciously. Once the deformity is created, there is no solution except release of the ear and placement of a full thickness skin graft.

Scars

Unsightly scars can frequently be improved by excision and additional facelifting maneuvers as long as no tension is placed on the closure. Although axiomatic in facelifting it bears repeating: the facelift flap should be redraped and trimmed so the edges are touching. While a few sutures are placed, no sutures should really be necessary in the preauricular region or the post-auricular sulcus. Hypertrophic scars are more problematic. It they are due to tension, they may be improved, if they are due to the patients' intrinsic scar forming idiosyncrasies, they will not be. The problem is that a surgeon evaluating such scars may not know in advance which category the scars fit in. Therefore, revision of scars should be approached with trepidation. Kenalog injection is helpful and eliminates the need for revision in many cases. If recurrent hypertrophic scars or real keloids develop, the author recommends scar revision with postoperative radiation beginning immediately on the day of the scar revision.

Postoperative care

A piece of Xeroform and a soft bulky dressing are placed on the skin. The purpose of the dressing is to protect the repair, keep the skin of the ear moist, and to absorb drainage. No attempt is made to put pressure on the ear. A doughnut of gauze is placed around each ear specifically to avoid pressure. The author has seen significant abrasions of the ear from dressings that were excessively tight, in one case an ulceration with exposed auricular cartilage.

The dressing is left in place 3–5 days depending on when the most convenient day for an office visit occurs. No further dressings are used. Since absorbable skin sutures are employed, no sutures require removal in the standard otoplasty case. In the case of ear reduction, there are a few nylon sutures in the helical rim that require removal.

The patient or family is instructed to wear a loose headband at night only. The goal is to have no pressure on the ear during the day and only enough at night to prevent inadvertent pulling forward of the repaired auricle. The nocturnal headband is continued for 4–6 weeks, although most patients confess to discarding it much sooner than that. Remember, the head band should only be tight enough that it does not fall off.

Outcomes, prognosis, and complications

Most patients who undergo otoplasty are satisfied with the results, making the procedure gratifying for the surgeon as well. The technique for standard otoplasty described above largely eliminates the worst of the otoplasty complications: over-correction, sharp edges, unnatural contours, inharmonious setback, telephone deformity, and infection.

However, any technique has its complications and the technique recommended is no exception. Suture complications are relatively common. The nylon mustarde sutures may eventually protrude through the posterior skin. This may occur within the first few weeks or not for years. In some cases, the sutures are associated with inflammation or a granuloma. Suture removal immediately cures any apparent infection and does not seem to lead to recurrence of the prominent ear.

The second complication that is more common with this technique is under-correction or recurrence. While this in not ideal, it is far better in this author's opinion than over-correction or distortion. Although the literature suggests that the Mustarde technique is associated with an unacceptable rate of undercorrection/recurrence, the author has had two cases of undercorrection/recurrence requiring reoperation in his career.

Secondary procedures

Unfortunately, patients requesting secondary procedures are not uncommon. The most common complaints of these patients are:

1. Over-correction
2. Visible cartilage irregularities or unnatural contours
3. Unpleasing shape of the ear (e.g., telephone ear, protruding lobules)
4. Under-correction, usually of the upper pole of the ear.

Over-correction can usually be improved by removing sutures, undermining skin and occasionally placing a skin graft. Some otoplasty techniques however do not lend themselves as well as others to reversal. Visible cartilage irregularities are extremely difficult to correct. Firmin[6] has the best and most impressive series of patients in this category in whom she has removed the damaged cartilage and placed expertly carved pieces of rib cartilage. Unpleasing shapes of the ear such as telephone ear can usually be improved significantly. Even if the over-corrected areas cannot be completely repaired the disharmony can be corrected. In the case of telephone ear, e.g., where the middle third of the ear is over-corrected relative to the upper and lower poles, there may be nothing that can be done about the overcorrected portion. The ear will look substantially improved, however, if the upper third and lower thirds are setback so that the overall impression is one of harmony and, when viewed from behind, the helical rim forms a straight line contour.

References

1. Thorne CH. Otoplasty. *Plast Reconstr Surg*. 2008;122(1): 291–292.
   The author of this chapter demonstrates his preferred otoplasty technique in a video and emphasizes the role of endpoint visualization when performing the procedure.

2. Luckett WH. A new operation for prominent ears based on the anatomy of the deformity. *Surg Gynecol Obstet*. 1910;10:635.

3. Converse JM, Wood-Smith D. Technical details in the surgical correction of the lop ear deformity. *Plast Reconstr Surg*. 1963;31:118–128.

4. Stenstroem SJ. A "natural" technique for correction of congenitally prominent ears. *Plast Reconstr Surg*. 1963;32:509–518.
   The technique of otoabrasion is described. The technique was fully embraced by a large number of surgeons.

5. Matsuo K, Hirose T, Tomono T, et al. Nonsurgical correction of congenital auricular deformities in the early neonate. A preliminary report. *Plast Reconstr Surg*. 1984;73:38–51.
   This is the first report showing the enormous potential for neonatal molding of congenital ear deformities.

6. Firmin F. Ear reconstruction in cases of typical microtia. Personal experience based on 352 microtic ear corrections. *Scand J Plast Reconstr Surg Hand Surg*. 1998;32(1):35–47.

7. Mustarde JC. The correction of prominent ears using simple mattress sutures. *Br J Plast Surg*. 1963;16: 170–178.

8. Furnas DW. Correction of prominent ears by concha mastoid sutures. *Plast Reconstr Surg*. 1968;42:189–193.

9. Gosain AK, Recinos RF. A novel approach to correction of the prominent lobule during otoplasty. *Plast Reconstr Surg*. 2003;112(2):575–583.

10. Webster GV. The tail of the helix as a key to otoplasty. *Plast Reconstr Surg*. 1969;44(5):455–461.
    This paper describes a technique for repositioning the lobule that is a classic but with which the author of this chapter has not had success.

11. McDowell AJ. Goals in otoplasty for protruding ears. *Plast Reconstr Surg*. 1968;41:17–27.

12. Spira M. Otoplasty: what I do now – a 30-year perspective. *Plast Reconstr Surg*. 1999;104(3):834–840.

13. Argamaso RV. Ear reduction with or without setback otoplasty. *Plast Reconstr Surg*. 1989;83(6):967–975.

14. Tanzer RC. The constricted (cup and lop) ear. *Plast Reconstr Surg*. 1975;55:406–415.

15. Kajikawa A, Ueda K, Asai E, et al. A new surgical correction of cryptotia: A new flap design and switched double banner flap. *Plast Reconstr Surg*. 2009;123(3): 897–901.

16. Kaplan HM, Hudson DA. A novel surgical method of repair for Stahl's ear: a case report and review of current treatment modalities. *Plast Reconstr Surg*. 1999;103(2):566–569.

23

Hair restoration

Jack Fisher

SYNOPSIS

- Techniques have evolved in the last 50 years, resulting in more natural (and aesthetically pleasing) hair transplants. The discussion of transplantation refers to micrografts or minigrafts or, more specifically in current nomenclature, follicular grafts.
- The true objective of hair restoration must go beyond artificial results to a point where the patient who has had hair restoration does not look like he has had any procedure done at all. The final result should be a natural-appearing hairline and natural-appearing density.
- Rather than continuing the trend of using techniques such as flaps, microsurgery, tissue expansion, and scalp excisions, most surgeons today doing hair restoration have gone to refined, anatomic, naturally occurring miniature grafts in the majority of patients.
- Hair restoration is one of the most common aesthetic procedures performed in the male population.

Introduction

In order to identify the ideal technique for hair restoration, numerous methods have come and gone during the past 50 years. Most patients undergoing hair restoration today, however, undergo hair transplantation because of the significant refinements of this specific technique. In a patient in whom it is obvious that a procedure such as hair transplant has been performed, the result is less than satisfactory. Techniques such as flaps, excision of bald areas, and expansion no longer dominate this field in the era of small, natural-appearing grafts. The discussion of transplantation refers to micrografts or minigrafts or, more specifically in current nomenclature, follicular grafts. Follicular units refer to the naturally occurring clusters of, typically, one to three hairs that emerge from the scalp.[1]

In the past, results were frequently mediocre to poor, and the use of technically challenging flaps and intricately designed scalp excisions, rather than enhancing results, caused an unnatural appearance that was often difficult to correct. Although these patients had significant amounts of hair transferred, the hair often looked artificial.

The true objective of hair restoration must go beyond these artificial results to a point where the patient who has had hair restoration does not look like he has had any procedure done at all. The final result should be a natural-appearing hairline and natural-appearing density.

Rather than continuing the trend of using techniques such as flaps, microsurgery, tissue expansion, and scalp excisions, most surgeons today doing hair restoration have gone to refined, anatomic, naturally occurring miniature grafts in the majority of patients. The reason for this change is not only physician-directed: patients today are demanding and expecting better results.

Another critical issue is the large number of patients who in the past had hair plug procedures and want corrective surgery, which requires a sophisticated approach for correction of these difficult problems. Some of the least satisfactory results of all types of male aesthetic surgery are in hair restoration. This can be attributed to poor technique and poor selection of patients.

A successful hair restoration requires a sense of aesthetics just as demanding as in any other aesthetic procedure. This chapter discusses those factors necessary for a successful outcome, focusing primarily on the status of current hair transplantation. At the beginning of the 21st century, hair transplantation with use of small grafts is where the field appears to be headed, with less flap surgery and less scalp excision.

Hair restoration is one of the most common aesthetic procedures performed in the male population.[2] However, of all the fields of aesthetic surgery, it has suffered one of the worst reputations for producing unnatural results and unhappy patients.

Basic science: anatomy of hair

The embryologic origin of hair is both ectodermal and mesodermal. The ectoderm forms the hair and pilosebaceous follicle; the mesoderm forms the dermal papilla.

Hair consists of a shaft and a root. The shaft is the visible portion above the scalp surface; its diameter varies from 60 to 100 μm. The three layers of the shaft – the cuticle, cortex, and medulla – consist of keratinized cells. The root or bulb is the follicle and sits at an oblique angle in the scalp (*Figs 23.1, 23.2*).

Hair grows at different angles, depending on the site of the scalp, and the proper angulation of the hair is key in hair restoration surgery to effect a natural result. In androgenic alopecia, the follicle reduces in size and the number of dormant follicles increases. These atrophic follicles take a more superficial location, and the visible hair shaft thins. Hair follicles are still present in these bald areas, but they are atrophic and essentially nonfunctional.

The hair shaft itself is composed of keratin, a fibrous protein produced by the hair follicle. The keratin is an end product of the hair matrix, which exists at the base of the hair follicle canal within the subcutaneous tissue. Within the matrix are rapidly dividing cells, and above this area of rapid cell division lies the zone of keratinization, which makes the hair shaft. The layering of these newly keratinized cells at the base of the shaft causes the process of hair growth as the shaft moves up through the surface.

Anatomy of a normal hairline

A discussion of the anatomy of hair could not be complete without also discussing the anatomy of the normal hairline.

A critical anatomic landmark in the mature male hairline is the frontal–temporal recession. This landmark is formed by the emergence of two convex lines making up the frontal and the temporal hairlines. Design of the frontal–temporal recession is critical to a natural result (*Fig. 23.3*). A hair restoration in which this rule has not been observed leads to an extremely unaesthetic appearance, especially in the mature adult. Young males usually do not have this recession, and this is one characteristic that distinguishes the child from the adult pattern. As baldness progresses, the frontal–temporal recession increases, forming an acute angle. Both women and children tend to have a continuous line between the frontal and temporal areas without this recession. Another important characteristic of a natural hairline is the transition from fine hair to more dense hair with a degree of irregularity along the margin. Natural hairlines are not straight and regular. Many of the unsatisfactory results in hair restoration demonstrate a fundamental lack of knowledge of these critical points. Other important factors are that the hair follicle sits about 3–3.5 mm below the surface of the scalp and that scalp thickness varies between 5.5 and 6.5 mm. These factors are important in

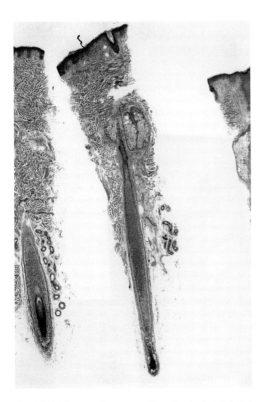

Fig. 23.1 Microscopic cross-section of a single hair follicle unit.

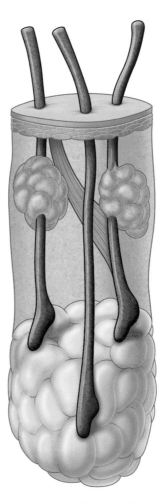

Fig. 23.2 Anatomy of hair unit with terminal follicles, sebaceous glands, and insertion of erector pili muscle.

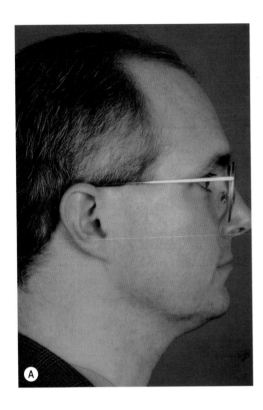

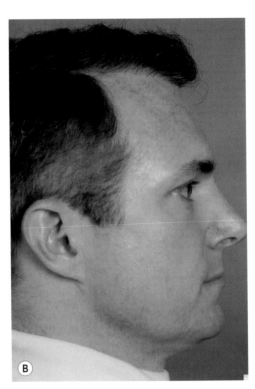

Fig. 23.3 **(A)** Preoperative and **(B)** postoperative appearance of a patient who had undergone hair transplantation in the frontal area in which the acute frontal–temporal angles were maintained, resulting in a normal-appearing recession. Maintenance of this recession is critical for a natural appearance.

considering the placement of the grafts in the scalp, the thickest layer of skin on the human body.

Characteristics of hair

There are two primary types of normal adult hair. Vellus hair is soft, short, lightly pigmented or hypopigmented hair that can be almost invisible. It can be found over the entire body. On the scalp, it is primarily seen in the frontal area on the forehead, and it also makes up a large area of the bald scalp. Terminal hair is the coarser, long hair and is pigmented. Within the terminal hair group are subgroups, such as those on the scalp, pubic area, and eyebrows. As an individual who is destined to lose hair ages, the terminal hairs can be replaced by vellus hairs. It is usually a progressive evolution in which the terminal hairs are lost and the thinner, shorter hairs slowly replace them until it converts to a vellus-type pattern. This process continues until, eventually, baldness is evident in the area. It is an interesting phenomenon that biopsies, even of bald areas, show that hair follicles are present, but they are atrophic in nature and are no longer producing significant amounts of hair in these individuals.

There is great variation in all aspects of hair, which is determined in each individual on the basis of race, sex, and area of the scalp. There is also variation in thickness between races: whites have thinner hair than both blacks and Asians do. The shape of the hair also varies greatly. The differences correspond to cross-sectional characteristics. For example, wavy hair is oval on cross-section, whereas stiff or straight hair tends to be round. An important variable is the density of hair per square centimeter. The density of adult hair can vary between 200 and 400 hairs per square centimeter. In the

presence of androgenic alopecia, the number of hairs drastically drops off. Large plug grafts, in which 20–60 hairs could be contained in each graft, often led to an unnatural appearance in many patients, resulting in cornrows. The transplantation of these grafts led to a clustering and unnatural look. Normally, one to three hairs emerge from a single orifice, and this fact is critical in obtaining a natural result in hair transplantation. Once this number is exceeded, that is, more than one to three hairs, there is the risk of a visible, unnatural result, especially along the frontal hairline.

The other critical variable is the angle at which the hairs exit the scalp normally. A violation of this principle also leads to an unnatural appearance. In the frontal area, the hair is angled forward; on the temporal and parietal areas, it tends to be angled slightly forward and downward. In the vertex, a spiral pattern is present; below the occipital area, the hairs are angled downward toward the neck. The two factors, thickness and density of hair per square centimeter, are important variables in the visual appearance of the hair. Whereas dark hair is effective in covering areas, fair hair is less effective. The converse is true, however, in designing a natural appearance. Blond or salt-and-pepper hair gives a more acceptable result when it is transplanted versus dark hair, especially in light-skinned individuals. This is especially obvious with dark plug grafts, in which thick hair clusters give a particularly unnatural result in contrast with light-colored skin.

Hair growth cycles

A discussion of the hair follicle cycles of growth and degeneration is relevant in considering hair restoration surgery. These cycles will have an impact on the time it takes for newly

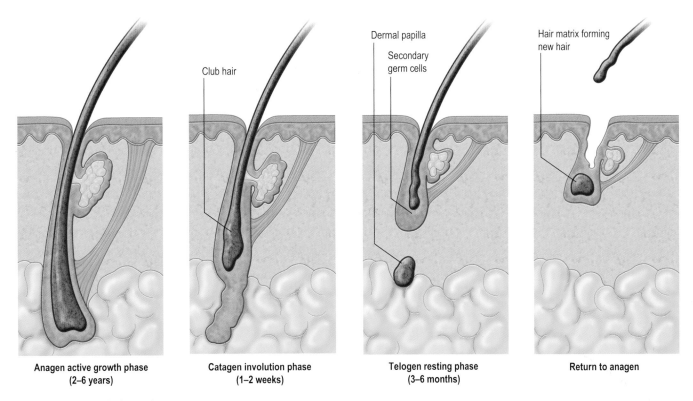

| Anagen active growth phase (2–6 years) | Catagen involution phase (1–2 weeks) | Telogen resting phase (3–6 months) | Return to anagen |

Fig. 23.4 The cycles of hair growth.

transplanted hair to begin to grow and also on the period necessary to see the final result.

There are essentially three cycles – anagen, catagen, and telogen. During the growth phase, referred to as anagen, the follicular cells are actively reproducing, and matrix keratinocytes are producing cells that differentiate into the different hair components. It is estimated that approximately 90% of the hair on the scalp is in the anagen phase, which lasts approximately 2–5 years. During the regression phase, called catagen, there is a degeneration of the keratinocytes, and special mesenchymal cells, referred to as dermal hair papillae, cluster and separate. This phase typically lasts 2–3 weeks (*Fig. 23.4*). The final resting phase, called telogen, lasts approximately 3 months. During the 3–4-month phase of telogen, the follicle is inactive and hair growth ceases. Approximately 10% of hairs are in telogen phase at any one time. In the telogen phase, the dermal papilla releases from its epidermal attachment, and eventually there is a reforming of a growing bulb. The old hair is shed, and as the cycle goes back to anagen, a new hair will come up and grow in this area. This information is relevant in discussing hair transplantation with patients. After the follicle has been transplanted, one usually sees a resting or telogen phase, and the patient should not expect any significant hair growth for 3–4 months. Although some of the hairs transplanted occasionally seem to continue to grow immediately after the surgical procedure, this can be misleading. This early growth frequently leads to a shedding of the hair shaft before the telogen phase. Therefore, the patient needs to wait several months before any significant hair growth is seen.

Diagnosis/patient presentation

Types and patterns of baldness

The most common type of hair loss in both men and women is referred to as androgenic alopecia. The mechanism of androgenic alopecia is inherent in each individual hair follicle as it responds to external stimuli, essentially androgens. The progressive loss of hair is predetermined by genetic characteristics associated with these responsive scalp follicles. In regions of the scalp susceptible to androgenic alopecia, androgens reduce the growth rate, the hair shaft diameter, and the length of the anagen phase. The mode of action of androgens on the target cells occurs at the bulbar region of the follicle. Testosterone is converted to dihydrotestosterone (DHT) by 5 ox-reductase. DHT acts on the target cells, and as discussed in the section on the role and effectiveness of medications, below, it is on this mechanism that finasteride acts in attempting to reduce hair loss by blocking the formation of DHT. It appears that androgenic alopecia is under the control of a single dominant sex-linked autosomal gene. However, this may be influenced by other modifying factors, and there is probably a polygenic component to the expression of male-pattern hair loss. In most men with hair loss, the hair follicles in the frontal and crown regions of the scalp appear most likely to be affected by androgenic alopecia. Although there is considerable variation among ethnic groups as far as the average number of hairs, and also variation among the different hair colors, it is typical that the average individual with a relatively full head of hair has approximately 100 000–150 000 or more hairs growing from the scalp.

Hair loss in women is frequently of a diffuse nature, and thus, most women may not be ideal candidates for hair restoration. The pattern of hair loss, because of its diffuseness, often results in a lack of appropriate donor hair. However, there is a subgroup of women who demonstrate hair loss similar to the male pattern.[3] The hair loss in these women frequently begins at the vertex and progresses anteriorly as they approach their 30s and 40s. The family history in these women is also compatible with a male-pattern type of hair loss, with many of the male and female family members reporting balding in both the vertex and superior portions of the scalp. It is this subgroup of women who may be the most appropriate candidates for hair transplantation because the posterior scalp area has adequate donor hair. The history these women give is fairly typical and is one of slow but progressive hair loss, and it is most evident on the superior scalp with good density on both sides and posteriorly. The other interesting characteristic in many of these women is that they maintain a low frontal hairline with a margin of hair anteriorly. This is unlike the male counterpart with progressive elevation of the frontal hairline and increasing temporal recession as the patient ages. Women with this primary type of alopecia characteristically will maintain that frontal hairline for life, and therefore transplantation needs to begin in this relatively low frontal area and progress posteriorly.

In many women, however, the cause of hair loss is secondary to numerous factors, such as surgery, metabolic disorders, chemotherapy stress, and autoimmune disease. This type of hair loss is often of an acute nature, and most of these patients are not candidates for transplantation. On occasion, in the patient who has had hair loss after chemotherapy, if enough time has transpired to allow recovery and there still has been no regrowth, transplantation may be appropriate. However, the take of the grafts has not been ideal in these patients. In many women, the cause of hair loss is secondary to cosmetic surgery, and the mechanism is traumatic hair loss.

Traumatic alopecia is primarily secondary to ischemia of the hair bulbs, although it can be secondary to direct tissue loss, as in postburn alopecia.[4] Numerous factors can lead to this ischemia. Prolonged pressure on the scalp in a single area, such as in a patient who lies in a comatose position for hours at a time, can cause enough ischemia to the scalp that there can be hair loss without loss of the actual scalp soft tissues. In addition, patients undergoing prolonged surgical procedures under general anesthesia can sustain pressure in an isolated area of the scalp, leading to hair loss.

One of the most common causes of traumatic hair loss is aesthetic surgery of the face and scalp area. Temporal hair loss is probably the most common of this group. It may be due to damage of the hair bulb from a subcutaneous dissection in the temporal area or excess skin traction with resulting ischemia. This also is seen in patients undergoing a coronal forehead lift, with hair loss in the area of a coronal scar. In most of these patients, the alopecia is temporary, and hair will regrow after several months. In some patients, however, the hair loss is permanent, and hair transplantation may be appropriate.[5,6] In addition, the scar itself in the scalp or facial area may widen, and because of the absence of hair follicles within the widened scar, a visible area of hair loss is seen.

Significant ischemia, which reduces blood flow to the follicles, can explain the temporary loss of hair in hair transplantation. The same phenomenon is seen in patients undergoing facelift and other aesthetic surgery, especially with closure under tension or with compromised flaps. With severe ischemia, death of the bulb can lead to permanent alopecia. Interestingly, an increase in growth due to enhanced blood flow may explain the effects of minoxidil, in which there is vasodilatation of the scalp and tissue surrounding the hair follicle. Whatever the exact mechanism, decreased blood flow affects hair loss, both temporarily and permanently.

Classification

Numerous classifications of hair loss have been described on a morphologic basis, which compares the hair-bearing with the nonhair-bearing areas. The first attempts to classify patterns of baldness were described in 1950 by Beck[7] in male white patients and in 1951 by Hamilton,[8] who analyzed patterns of hair loss in both white and Chinese patients. Later, others, including Norwood, suggested modifications of Hamilton's classification *(Fig. 23.5).*[9] Most of these classifications divide the patterns of baldness into six or seven main groups with subgroups. These classifications may be difficult to apply because so many variations can be seen from patient to patient. Another classification system developed by Bouhanna and Dardour[10] distinguishes three stages, with variances in stage 1 and stage 2, thus defining five basic patterns. Ludwig[11] devised a classification system for types of androgenic alopecia in women. All classification techniques have some limitations but can be useful tools in planning hair restoration.

Evaluation of the patient

Compared with other areas of aesthetic surgery, hair restoration is unique in that hair loss is not only progressive but also unpredictable. In aesthetic surgery there are generally areas of the face where one can predict with some accuracy the effects of the aging phenomenon. In male-pattern baldness, although there is some ability to predict hair pattern changes on the basis of family history, there is also a great deal unknown as far as the evolution of any particular patient's hair loss. Therefore, evaluation of the patient must take into consideration the progressive nature of hair loss postoperatively during the ensuing decades. It is critical in the early phases of a patient's evaluation to design a hair pattern that will be appropriate not only as the patient ages but also on the basis of progressive hair loss. It is not unusual for a young patient in his late teens or early 20s who has significant hair loss to wish to redesign the hairline to a juvenile appearance. It is important that the physician explains to the patient the long-term ramifications and problems that will occur if a juvenile hairline is attempted and what the results will be as the patient ages. Young patients can be dissatisfied on hearing that their transplanted hairline should be placed high with a temporal recession. Patients who demand an inappropriate hairline should be rejected for surgery because they are unrealistic and will be dissatisfied later when they realize that they

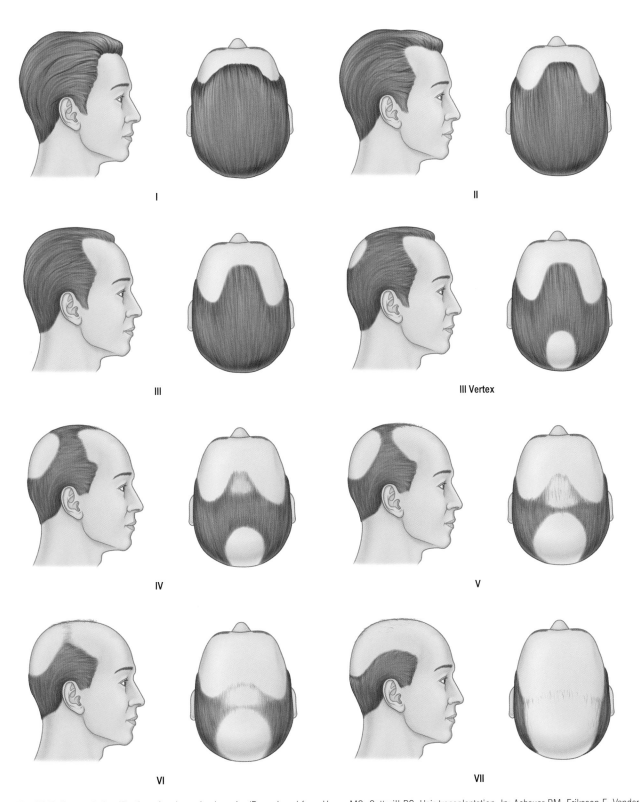

I

II

III

III Vertex

IV

V

VI

VII

Fig. 23.5 Norwood classification of androgenic alopecia. (Reproduced from Unger MG, Cotterill PC. Hair transplantation. In: Achauer BM, Eriksson E, Vander Kolk C, *et al.* (eds) Plastic Surgery, vol. 5. St. Louis, Mosby, 2000, p. 2487. Redrawn from Norwood OT. Male pattern baldness: classification and incidence. South Med J 1975;68: 1359–1365.)

are going to undergo extensive further surgery. Many of these patients wind up wearing a hairpiece for the rest of their lives to cover an area that is unsatisfactory or that often looks bizarre because of the progressive nature of the hair loss. As in any area of aesthetic surgery, having a patient with realistic expectations is critical, especially since many hair restoration patients will be seen in a practice for years because of progressive hair loss. The patient with hair loss in his 20s is going to have to deal with the ramifications of surgical procedures for the next 5–7 decades. Unfortunately, the young patient can find someone who will do hair restoration for him. Typically, such patients come back a decade later, now in their late 20s or early 30s, often regretful, wishing to have the work either undone or modified. Besides the young patient, one must also be cautious with the extensive hair loss patient with only a lateral and posterior fringe who wants complete coverage of alopecia. These patients can be given an adequate framing of the face; however, the posterior occipital area in some cannot be grafted or at least should be grafted sparingly.

In the initial consultation with a patient, certain variables or parameters can be evaluated that assist the physician in decision-making and help the patient establish a set of realistic expectations. A family history is useful, especially of the maternal side of the family, although hair pattern inheritance can represent a mosaic of family characteristics. When a patient presents a history of brothers, uncles, and a maternal grandfather with significant baldness, one can predict with some certainty that this patient is also likely to have extensive hair loss. Thus, designing the hair restoration pattern for this patient should take into consideration this family history. Another factor is the great variation in available donor hair. One can see patients with an abundance of donor hair ranging from 240 to 400 hairs per square centimeter who can undergo multiple future procedures. There are also patients with far less donor hair, and a conservative approach must be entertained. This is particularly important in discussing with the young patient replacement of hair in the occipital area. One of the most difficult areas to deal with at a later point in life after hair transplantation is the occipital region. The individual who had overly aggressive transplantation in the occipital area at a young age and then proceeds to have significant hair loss around the transplants, resulting in a halo of alopecia, presents with a bizarre appearance. These patients require either further grafting, chasing the halo of hair loss, or possible excision of the previously grafted areas. However, the individual who has significant donor hair density and reports stabilization of hair loss may be an appropriate candidate for occipital grafting.

In young patients the best approach is to graft the frontal and superior regions first and wait until their hair pattern is more mature before working on the occipital area. This is particularly important for patients with limited or fine donor hair, when there is a finite number of grafting procedures in the future. The amount of donor hair in the posterior scalp is a critical component in the assessment of these patients.

It is useful to draw a specific pattern on the scalp to demonstrate as the patient is looking in a mirror where you think the most appropriate hairline pattern should be *(Fig. 23.6)*. If a high, appropriately designed hairline with temple recession is unacceptable to the patient, this may be the patient who should not be considered for any type of hair restoration. Although you may make the patient happy initially, if both the plastic surgeon and the patient live long enough, both will have to deal with any problems that were caused by poor design or poor planning.

The classification of hair loss is a useful tool in planning the hair pattern. The individual who has a Norwood II or III pattern and has stabilized is more likely to obtain an excellent result, without worrying about continually chasing further hair loss. Because of the progressive nature of male-pattern hair loss, it is critical to set goals for the patient so the patient understands what may be required several decades later.

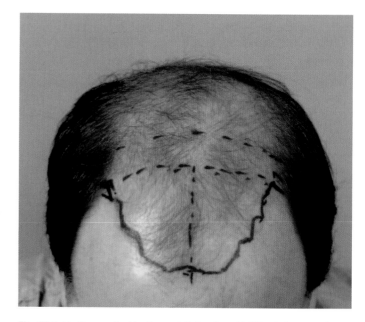

Fig. 23.6 Marking a patient to demonstrate location of hairline during consultation. Note the irregularity of the hairline to avoid an unnatural straight-line appearance.

Unlike facelifts or other aesthetic procedures, which can be repeated years later, hair restoration may not be able to be repeated because of limited donor hair.

A thorough examination of the patient requires an assessment not only of the pattern of hair loss but also of characteristics such as color, texture, density, curling, and straightness. Curly hair tends to appear denser because it covers up the underlying scalp. However, straight, dark hair, unlike curly hair, may not appear to have as much density because of the scalp's visibility between the straight dark hairs, especially if the skin is light. In addition, straight, dark, thick hair on light-colored skin can look unnatural if several hairs exit at a single site because of the contrast between the skin and hair. The same number of fine or light-colored hairs exiting together on light skin, however, may look natural because of this lack of contrast. This phenomenon, in which multiple hairs exit at a single site and appear packed together at the base, spreading out distally, is called compression. This tufted look may occur when a graft with several hairs is placed in a small or tight recipient site, compressing the base of the graft. This problem is more evident in black-haired individuals on light skin, and micrografting is critical in these patients to avoid this problem. White, blond, or salt-and-pepper hair has far less of a problem with visible compression because of the lack of contrast. In African Americans with dark hair against a dark skin background, compression is less likely because of little or minimal contrast. All these variables must be taken into consideration to give as natural-appearing a result as possible. Hair color, hair texture, and skin color play important roles in the aesthetics of the result.

The goal is to design a hairline in harmony with the mature face and to re-establish a balance between the scalp and the other facial features. A natural hairline should be aesthetically invisible and age-appropriate. In other words, the patient should not look like a hair transplant has been done *(Fig. 23.7)*. This is accomplished by a relatively high mature hairline with temporal recession at the proper height. In addition,

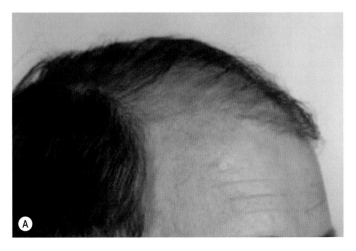

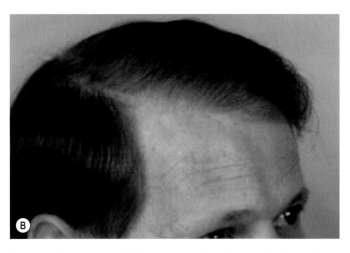

Fig. 23.7 (A) Preoperative view of a 46-year-old man who underwent two sessions of follicular hair transplantation. **(B)** Postoperatively, the patient has a hairline that is appropriate for his age with a temporal recession at the frontal–temporal angle. The other important aspect is the design of irregularity of the hairline along the frontal margin as well as placement of the finest available grafts anteriorly. Thin or light-colored hair also facilitates design of a natural appearance. A successful hair transplantation should not be recognizable.

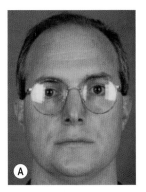
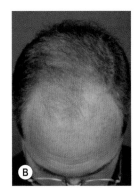
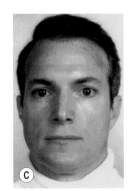
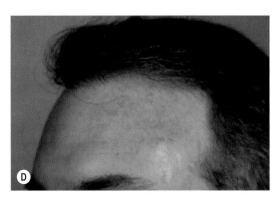

Fig. 23.8 A 40-year-old patient with salt-and-pepper hair who underwent a total of 2800 follicular grafts in two sessions. **(A,B)** Preoperative appearance. **(C)** Appearance after the second session of follicular grafting. **(D)** The patient's salt-and-pepper hair helps facilitate the naturalness of the frontal hairline. Other points include the appropriate distance between the glabella and the anterior hairline, which should be at least 8–10 cm, and maintenance of the hairline parallel to the ground with a normal temporal recession.

graft direction is important for the correct angulation of the individual hairs consistent with their location on the hairline. The hair in the frontal area of the scalp has an anterior angulation normally. Too oblique an angle is unnatural; posterior angulation is also typically inappropriate.

During the aging process, there is simultaneous recession of the frontal hairline upward or superiorly and movement of the temporal hairline posteriorly. Maintenance of this frontal–temporal angle is critical to a natural appearance in hair restoration. Procedures, whether grafting or flaps, that blunt or fill in the frontal–temporal angle not only will cause an unnatural appearance but will lead to significant problems later as the hairline recedes, leaving a bizarre appearance.

In most patients, the anterior level of the hairline in the midline should be at least 8–10 cm above the glabella. In addition, the anterior hairline appears more natural if it runs parallel to the ground when viewed from a lateral vantage point *(Fig. 23.8)*. Some patients with significant hair loss maintain a frontal forelock, and if it sits too low on the forehead, it may be more appropriate to begin the grafting process slightly posterior to the centrally located tuft of existing hair. Trying to chase an isolated frontal forelock that is sitting low on the forehead can result in too low a hairline with an unnatural

appearance. In addition it is always possible secondarily to place grafts lower if necessary; however, the converse is not true. In other words, grafts originally placed too low because of chasing a low frontal forelock are difficult, if not impossible, to modify.

An appropriate term to discuss with patients, especially young patients, is what is referred to as "framing the face." Patients in their 20s and 30s frequently dislike going bald, not because of the hair loss itself, but because they think they look several decades older than their stated age. We tend to associate balding with the aging process. In many of these patients, it is natural to transplant only half or a third of the area of male-pattern baldness and give the patient an adequate result without necessarily treating the posterior or vertex area. Again, if the patient has limited donor hair, is relatively young, and by family history is going to continue to have progressive hair loss, a conservative approach is much safer. There are several criteria that one can use when rejecting a patient, including inadequate donor hair and too low a density, especially in patients with class VI or VII Norwood patterns. In addition, there are patients who may have little available usable donor hair because of too much scarring from previous grafting that was healed by secondary intention.

Finally, the patient who has unrealistic expectations, especially if young and demanding a procedure that the physician considers inappropriate, should be rejected for surgery. There are also patients with medical problems that can interfere with grafting, such as hypertension, which can cause bleeding, but this usually can be corrected with the appropriate antihypertensives.

Role and effectiveness of medications

Both minoxidil in a local application and finasteride administered orally have been used in the medical management of hair loss.[12] It is believed that minoxidil works primarily by increasing blood flow, which promotes hair regrowth or hair stabilization in those follicles that are being affected genetically by androgenic alopecia. Finasteride, which is an oral medication, is a selective inhibitor of 5 alpha reductase type II. It was originally developed for the treatment of benign prostatic hyperplasia; however, it has been available in the US since 1997 for use in treatment of male-pattern baldness. The mechanism of finasteride relates to the effect of androgens on the hair follicle of patients with a genetic predisposition to male-pattern baldness. There is an uptake of circulating testosterone by scalp hair follicle cells, in which it is converted by the enzyme 5 alpha reductase to DHT. DHT binds to an androgen receptor. It is considered that hair follicles in areas susceptible to male-pattern hair loss are sensitive to the effects of testosterone. Finasteride inhibits 5 alpha reductase, thereby having an impact on DHT and the androgen receptors of the hair follicles. Studies document that 1 mg/day finasteride not only reduces hair loss but, in a limited percentage of patients, can cause some growth of hair. This is usually more effective in the younger population, and once true baldness has occurred, it is unlikely that finasteride will have any significant effect.

The use of finasteride has clearly been shown to stabilize hair loss, and there can be some reversal, although it primarily has its best effects on the vertex area of the scalp. Although both finasteride and minoxidil can be effective, finasteride may be more useful in younger patients and therapy must be long-term. Most of the studies have shown that it requires at least 6 months to 1 year for some significant improvement to be seen from the use of finasteride.

Technique

Video
1–9

The instrumentation for hair transplantation is relatively simple. Although many instruments and devices have been developed during the last few decades, the current technique as developed by Carlos Uebel[13,14] in Brazil and others has significantly simplified the technical aspects of the procedure. The donor site is harvested as a transverse strip by use of a standard no. 10 knife blade from the posterior scalp. Proper angulation of the knife blade is critical in harvesting the donor site to avoid damaging the donor hair follicles. Multiblade knives that cut multiple strips at the same time are available but can cause significant transection of follicles if the angulation is incorrect.

The width of the strip can vary from 1.5 to 2 cm; the length is purely dependent on the number of grafts needed and can vary from 12 to more than 20 cm. Because of the mobility of the posterior neck and lower scalp skin, it is relatively easy to close this area primarily. Excision of the original donor scar, when donor tissue is reharvested in subsequent procedures, avoids the problem of multiple incisions and leaves the patient with a single transverse donor scar. On occasion, if the patient has had previous surgery or if there is scarring, it may be necessary to elevate the flap inferiorly to allow closure without tension. Hemostasis is obtained with the cautery, and the incision is approximated with several stay sutures for alignment. Several strategic buried 3-0 Vicryl sutures are placed, and then the closure is followed with a running 3-0 nylon suture. The donor site can rapidly be closed with the stapler, which many consider a superior technique. The key factor in harvesting the donor site is proper angulation of the knife to prevent inadvertent transection of the hair follicles and damage to the donor grafts *(Fig. 23.9)*. The donor strip is cut into multiple breadloaf sections, which are then cut by the assistants into the grafts.

The remaining instrumentation for insertion of the hair grafts with the technique published by Uebel requires nothing more than a no. 11 blade and a fine pair of pick-ups. In this technique, an assistant is lifting the follicular grafts off a towel or tongue depressor and positioning them for the surgeon, who is making an incision with a no. 11 blade. The key to this technique is in the timing and dexterity of the maneuver. The assistant holds the small graft adjacent to the no. 11 blade; an incision is made, the blade is withdrawn, and then the assistant puts the graft at the beginning of the orifice that has been made and the surgeon finishes pushing it in *(Fig. 23.10)*. With two individuals who are experienced with this technique, it is not unusual to put in 500 or more grafts per hour once the technique is mastered.

There is a great deal in both the dermatologic and hair transplant literature about the use of numerous sophisticated and complex instruments for hair transplantation; however, Uebel's technique has made most of this equipment unnecessary. In the past, different types of punches and electrical coring devices were used to take out punch grafts, but because the larger grafts are traditionally no longer used by most individuals, a lot of this instrumentation is no longer required.

The grafts are placed on a moist towel, which is sitting in a metal tray with ice-chilled saline *(Fig. 23.11)*. They are kept cold during the entire process before implantation. In the technique of Uebel, the assistant holds on the towel the grafts that have been presorted to size and hands them to the surgeon and they implant them together. The recipient area has already been anesthetized with both supraorbital and supratrochlear blocks and the tumescent solution. Typically, the grafts are placed as close together as possible, working either from anterior to posterior or posteriorly proceeding up to the proposed anterior hairline. This order of placement of grafts depends on the surgeon's preference. The only drawback to advancing posteriorly is that, when there is significant bleeding, it runs down into the fields; however, with the use of tumescent technique, bleeding us usually minimal.

The key to this technique is training the surgeon and assistant in proper handling of the grafts. This method requires development of the assistant's dexterity to place the graft at the edge of a small incision made by the no. 11 blade. With

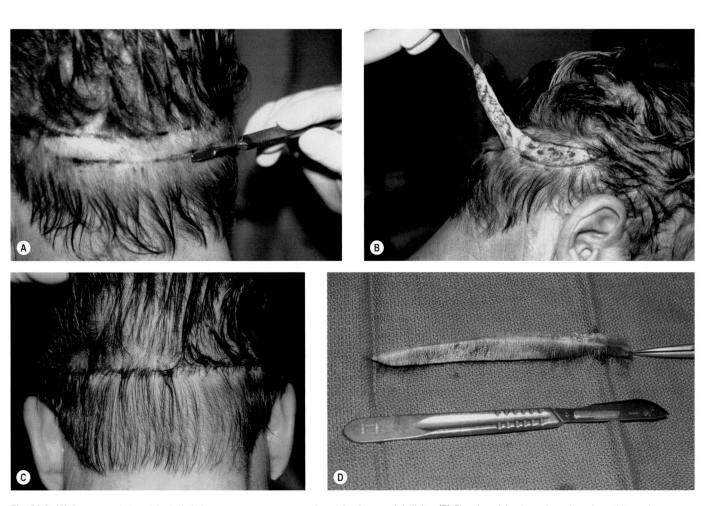

Fig. 23.9 (A) Proper angulation of the knife is important to prevent transection of the donor graft follicles. **(B)** Elevation of the donor tissue is performed in a subcutaneous plane, taking care to avoid transection of the base of the hair follicles. **(C)** Closure with a running suture. The donor site is easily closed because of laxity of tissues in the posterior scalp and neck area. **(D)** The harvested donor strip before it is cut into transverse breadloaf sections. These are then cut into individual follicular grafts.

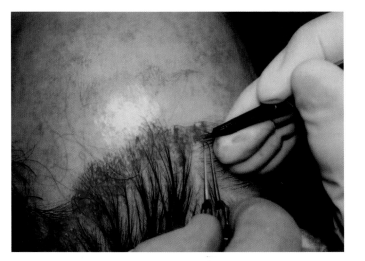

Fig. 23.10 The Uebel technique of graft insertion. The no. 11 blade is used to make a small incision and then partially withdrawn as the assistant places the graft at the beginning of the orifice. The surgeon then inserts the graft into the hole that has been made.

this technique, the implantation of 1500–2500 grafts can go quickly *(Fig. 23.12)*. This transfer of large numbers of small grafts at one time is an important concept. Limmer[15] and others advocated covering the entire area of alopecia with small grafts, and the technique described makes the concept feasible. After the insertion of the grafts, a dressing is applied, usually for 24–48 hours. Mineral oil covered by a Curlex dressing gives good protection for 24 hours without any adherence of the dressing to the grafted area. The patient is seen the next day, the dressing is removed, and the patient is instructed on careful washing of the hair. At approximately 10 days the patient is seen in the office, and the sutures in the donor area are removed.

Anesthesia

Anesthesia used in hair transplantation is relatively simple. Most procedures can be performed with just local anesthesia, with use of nerve blocks in both the donor and recipient areas. Both of these areas are also distended with a dilute saline–lidocaine–epinephrine solution for hemostasis. Scalp blood vessels do not contract well because of their attachment to the surrounding connective tissue. Therefore, the scalp blood

The anatomy of the nerves of the scalp is relevant in hair restoration in considering local anesthesia and reducing damage to the nerve during the surgical procedure. The procedure is begun with occipital nerve blocks in the donor area by use of lidocaine with epinephrine, followed by a tumescent solution that allows both adequate anesthesia and good hemostasis. The supraorbital nerve, a branch of the frontal nerve, provides sensory innervation to the forehead. During the implantation of the grafts, both supraorbital and supratrochlear blocks are performed as well as tumescence of the recipient area. This gives excellent anesthesia and hemostasis during this surgical procedure and frequently does not need to be repeated during the operation.

Outcome, prognosis, and complications

Number of procedures

An important issue to discuss with patients is the number of sessions necessary to obtain the desired result. A patient who thinks that one procedure is going to be the total solution will be disappointed. An assessment of how many procedures during what time period is important to establish a good physician–patient relationship.

With current techniques of 1500–3000 grafts, many patients with limited hair loss require only two procedures. The patient with more extensive hair loss, however, may require as many as three or four procedures. Some patients will be pleased after only one procedure with limited hair loss; but usually with one procedure, the frontal hairline lacks adequate density. It is appropriate to prepare most patients for at least two sessions to give a refined result.

Complications are relatively few for most patients. In healthy individuals with unscarred recipient sites, it is reasonable to expect 90–95% of the grafts to grow successfully. Hematoma and infection are extremely rare in hair transplantation and can be readily managed. Cysts can form after graft implantation when the recipient scalp epithelium grows over the transplant epithelium, forming an epidermal inclusion cyst. Positioning the transplant epithelium level or slightly above the surrounding recipient epithelium reduces this problem. When cysts occur, unroofing and warm soaks usually resolve the problem.

The patient who requires a great deal of evaluation and thought, besides the young or potentially unrealistic patient, is the one who has an unsatisfactory result and is seeking a secondary revision. These patients are hair cripples and frequently wear hairpieces for the rest of their lives to cover either disfigurement or a bizarre appearance. Many of these secondary revision patients had grafting at too young an age with a low hairline and then went bald behind the grafted area. Also, a high hairline or temple recession was not designed, so the patient has a juvenile hairline in a mature face. This disparity causes a disharmony between natural facial aging and the hair pattern. Many of these patients can be dramatically improved with regrafting or with a combination of excisions and reuse of the previously grafted hair. Some of these patients can have their grafts removed along the frontal hairline if they are bald behind this frontal fringe as long as they understand that there will be some visible

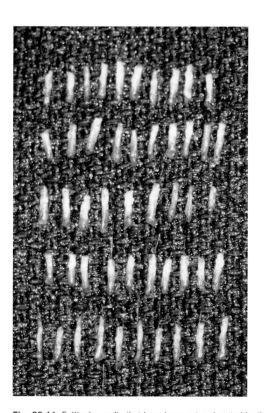

Fig. 23.11 Follicular grafts that have been cut and sorted by the number of hairs in each. The towel is soaked in ice-chilled saline kept in a metal tray. The grafts are sorted in rows of 10. During the implantation process, the assistant holds the towel and hands the grafts to the surgeon, following the Uebel technique.

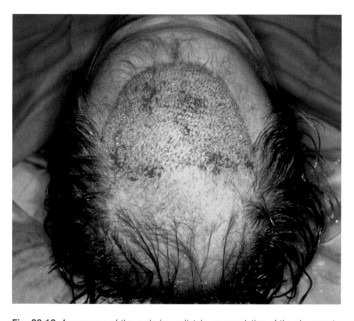

Fig. 23.12 Appearance of the scalp immediately on completion of the placement of approximately 1200 follicular grafts. Small incisions were made with the tip of a no. 11 blade, and the grafts were immediately inserted.

vessels are less likely to undergo rapid spontaneous hemostasis compared with other areas of the body.

In selected patients, it may be necessary to add sedation with midazolam and fentanyl. Because it is not unusual to put in 2000 or more grafts per patient, which can take 3–4 hours, selected patients can benefit from light sedation.

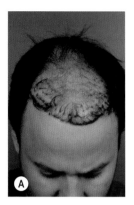
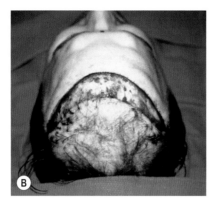
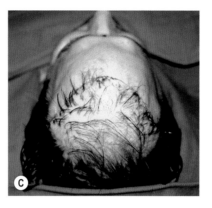
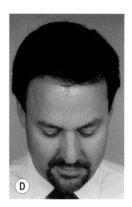

Fig. 23.13 (A) This patient demonstrates all three problems of an unsatisfactory result. First, the patient had grafting at an early age before a mature hairline was established and the grafts were placed too low, with progressive hair loss posteriorly. Second, the hairline was poorly designed and showed little knowledge of the natural evolution of androgenic alopecia. Third, the patient had large hair plugs, which resulted in an unnatural cornrow appearance once the surrounding hair was lost. No attempt was made to design a proper frontal–temporal recession, causing an unnatural rounding-off of the angle. **(B)** Excision of the frontal hairline with removal of the large plug grafts and elevation of the forehead accomplished by suture fixation to the periosteum. **(C)** Closure of the defect. **(D)** Final result after a total of 2700 follicular grafts in two sessions.

scarring. This can often be preferable to a few rows of unsightly plugs in an unusual location. The other possibility is to do an excision with an aggressive forehead lift to put the scarring in a more superior and natural location. During the clinical evaluation process, especially with the secondary revision patient, it is useful to draw the areas on the patient that you think should be either treated or grafted. This is particularly important in the patient who comes in wearing a hairpiece covering up unsightly grafted areas. The patient can then return for a second consultation to make sure not only that there is a realistic expectation but also that the physician is comfortable the patient's goals can be met.

The other important issue in the patient who has had multiple previous procedures, especially with a plug coring technique, is the scarring of the donor site, which healed by secondary intention. These can be some of the most difficult reconstructions because of limited available donor hair surrounded by dense scarring. A great deal of time and evaluation is required to find the best available donor hair, and this often requires an intricate design, taking donor strips from multiple sites. An appropriate assessment of risk and complications with these patients is required. The morbidity from hair transplantation in general is relatively low because bleeding and infection are fairly rare. However, a major problem is difficulty healing the donor area in patients who have had multiple plug graft procedures with secondary healing of the donor site. These patients are often badly scarred, and there can be difficulty healing the donor site, even when it is harvested with the strip technique and closed carefully in a linear fashion.

Secondary procedures

Most patients with an unsatisfactory result fall into three major groups. First is the patient who had grafting at an early age before a mature hairline was established in whom the grafts were placed too low, with progressive hair loss behind the grafts. Second, the hairlines were poorly designed and showed little knowledge of the natural evolution of androgenic hair loss. Third, the unsatisfactory result was due to use of large hair plugs, causing the typical cornrow appearance.

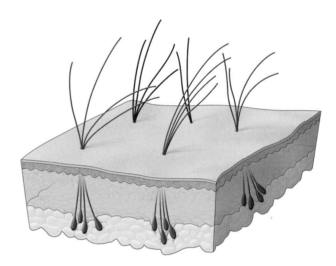

Fig. 23.14 Graft compression. Grafts containing multiple hairs are placed in tight incisions, leading to bouquet formation.

Figure 23.13 demonstrates a patient in whom all three of these problems occurred. This patient had large plug grafts inserted at an early age. The grafts were placed too low on the forehead. No attempt had been made to design a frontal–temporal recession, thus abnormally rounding off the frontal–temporal angle. Finally, large plug grafts had been inserted, and the natural progression of hair loss posteriorly resulted in the patient wearing a hairpiece to cover his significant deformity.

Correction of this problem requires a thorough analysis of the deformity with a specific surgical plan. The patient's hairline is too low, and any further grafting around the existing patient plugs to disguise them would not correct this situation. The first step was elevation of the hairline by excision of the anterior row of plugs combined with a superior advancement of the forehead. The forehead was fixed to the frontal bone by Mitek suture fixation to maintain the forehead height. The removed grafts were recycled, and after the scar healed, the patient underwent two sessions of grafting for a total of 2700 follicular grafts.

Other patients may have problems related only to the cornrow appearance, which can be corrected by plug reduction and recycling in association with follicular grafting along the frontal hairline.[16,17] Besides the cornrow problem associated with large grafts is the problem of compression. When large grafts with multiple hairs are placed in small recipient holes, constriction at the base of the graft leads to bouquet formation *(Fig. 23.14)*.

Even with proper attention to detail, problems will occur because of the progressive nature of male-pattern hair loss.

One such problem is the development of a temporal alley. This occurs when a patient who had transplantation in the frontal and superior scalp undergoes hair loss laterally, leaving a gap or alley between the frontal hair and temporal area. This can usually be corrected by further grafting in the gap as long as sufficient donor hair remains.

Correction of the unsatisfactory hair restoration requires a systematic analysis for proper surgical correction. With the techniques currently available, these patients can be significantly improved.

Access the complete references list online at **http://www.expertconsult.com**

1. Bernstein RM, Rassman WR. Follicular transplantation, patient evaluation and surgical planning. *Dermatol Surg* 1997;23:771.

   This paper identifies the basic units in which hair naturally grows; there are 1–3 follicles in a unit.

3. Halsner U, Lucas M. New aspects in hair transplantation for females. *Dermatol Surg* 1995;21:605.

   The unique characteristics of female hair loss are presented, including the specific pattern of hair transplantation unique to creating a natural female hairline.

4. Barrera A. The use of micrografts and minigrafts for the treatment of burn alopecia. *Plast Reconstr Surg* 1999;103:58.

   The ability of hair grafts to grow successfully in burn scar is presented. The specifics for successful management of hair loss after burns are discussed in detail.

5. Seyhan A, Yoleri L, Baruteu A. Immediate hair transplantation into a newly closed wound to conceal the final scar on the hair bearing skin. *Plast Reconstr Surg* 2000;105:1866.

   The ability to place hair follicles into acute incisions is presented in order to minimize visible scars. The authors demonstrate that hair follicles will successfully grow when placed directly into a fresh incision.

16. Vogel JE. Correction of the cornrow hair transplantation and other common problems in surgical hair restoration. *Plast Reconstr Surg* 2000;105:1528.

    Various options and techniques are discussed for the treatment of previous unsatisfactory hair transplantation. The author details the different techniques available to the surgeon for the secondary restorations.

24

Liposuction: A comprehensive review of techniques and safety

Jeffrey M. Kenkel and Phillip J. Stephan

SYNOPSIS

- Incorporation of a diet and exercise program in conjunction with liposuction will allow patients to achieve their optimal shape and contour. Patients who do not adhere to diet and exercise are least happy with their results.

- A thorough history and physical exam should be performed and a preoperative clearance obtained, especially for large volume or long combined cases.

- Marking the patient in front of a mirror allows both the surgeon and patient to see and understand the areas of concern and intended treatment. Cellulite and other contour irregularities can be pointed out preoperatively to the patient.

- Over-the-counter herbal and diet medications may have unfavorable interaction with surgery and/or anesthesia and should be discontinued 3 weeks prior to surgery.

- Knowledge of the differing thickness and consistency of fat throughout the body is crucial to determining proper depth and technique for each region of the body.

- Superficial liposuction should be reserved for significant superficial irregularities and be performed by those experienced in liposuction techniques.

- Wetting solutions should always be used and a strict record of volume infused and aspirated should be kept by the operating room personnel.

- Surgical access sites should be concealed, often asymmetric, and utilized to allow the best access and treatment results. Excessive use of a single access incision may result in a deformity.

- Patients with surgical scars on their abdomen must be thoroughly examined to rule out the presence of a hernia.

- Treatment with UAL begins superficially and ends in the deeper plane. In contrast, evacuation proceeds from the deeper layers to the more superficial layers.

- Postoperative contour deformities should be clinically evaluated, and if mild, can respond to lymphatic massage or other non-invasive methods. A systematic approach should be used to correct contour deformities when they occur.

Introduction

Suction-assisted lipectomy, lipoplasty, or more commonly referred to as liposuction, originally introduced by Illouz in the early 1980s, continues to be one of the most popular means of body contouring and overall treatment modalities offered in aesthetic surgery today.[1] Annually, according to the American Society of Plastic Surgery and American Society for Aesthetic Plastic Surgery, it consistently ranks among the top procedures performed in plastic surgery for the last 10 years.[2] With greater understanding of the biochemical and physiologic properties of liposuction, as well as bio-medical technological advancements, suction-assisted lipoplasty has undergone tremendous evolution leading to overall improvements in technique, patient safety, and outcomes. Over the past two decades, it has grown from a procedure that facilitates small or spot reductions to one that has become an almost irreplaceable tool in the aesthetic surgery armamentarium in neck, breast, and circumferential body contouring. Liposuction has become a useful adjunct to other areas of plastic surgery, including breast reconstruction, and postoperative contouring in upper and lower extremity reconstruction. A number of important innovations and modifications to the standard suction-assisted liposuction (SAL) have progressively refined the procedure; these include: the use of wetting solutions; advances in cannula design; ultrasound-assisted liposuction (UAL); power-assisted liposuction (PAL); vaser-assisted liposuction, and laser-assisted liposuction (LAL). There has been a strong movement concentrated on defining appropriate safety guidelines for liposuction and other body contouring procedures focusing on deep venous thrombosis prophylaxis and fluid resuscitation ensuring safety and efficacy of the different treatment modalities for our patients.

Even with these refinements, liposuction, as with all invasive procedures is not without risk. Aesthetic body contouring with liposuction requires a complete knowledge of the anatomic, biochemical, and physiological components of the different modalities and their limitations and indications in order to perform the procedure in a safe, controlled manner. Using a coordinated approach along with a thorough understanding, liposuction can be performed safely with relatively predictable results and outcomes.

Basic science and anatomic considerations

Anatomy texts divide subcutaneous fat throughout the body into superficial and deep layers or compartments separated by Scarpa's fascia, or the superficial fascial equivalent.[3] However, for the purposes of liposuction and body contouring, subcutaneous fat is arbitrarily divided into three layers: superficial, intermediate, and deep *(Fig. 24.1)*.[4,5] The importance of this distinction is that the superficial layer is one that rarely is violated. If this layer is treated, there may be vascular compromise and/or a significantly increased risk for contour irregularities. The relative consistency and thickness of each of these separate layers varies for different anatomic areas. For example, the fat of the back has a more fibrous, compact superficial and intermediate layer, with an underlying loose, areolar layer. This contrasts with the fat of the inner thigh, which is not as fibrous and is less compact.[3] This is critical information for the aesthetic surgeon in order to perform safe

and appropriate suctioning of the targeted area minimizing potential contour irregularities and skin necrosis. The variation in fat consistency and depth will be discussed further as it relates to safe suctioning techniques and the choice of modality which may be preferred for the most effective treatment.

Anatomic "zones of adherence,"[6] which are present in both men and women, are important to identify and mark during the preoperative consultation. These are areas of relative dense fibrous attachments to underlying deep fascia, which help define the natural shape and curve of the body. There are gender-specific variations with respect to each of these zones *(Fig. 24.2)*. It is important to recognize these zones, as they are identified as high-risk areas for contour irregularities after surgical intervention if not properly respected. However, these are not areas to avoid in all cases, and on occasion, help guide the surgeon in establishing "contour goals" for surgical intervention. Regardless of the tool used for liposuction, it is helpful to consider the treatment area in terms of the three surgical layers. These arbitrary layers help delineate areas of safety when performing liposuction. The most common areas treated are the intermediate and deep layer. Treatment of these layers allows uniform reduction without risk of injury to the subdermal plexus and unwanted skin injury.

Classification

It is helpful to classify patients based on the three types of lipodystrophy and skin redundancy *(Fig. 24.3)*.

Type I: *Localized lipodystrophy.* Often younger patients with good skin tone and minimal skin irregularities.

Type II: *Generalized lipodystrophy.* These patients tend to have slightly diminished skin tone with some skin irregularities and circumferential lipodystrophy throughout their trunk and extremities.

Type III: *Skin redundancy and lipodystrophy.* Patients displaying significant skin redundancy that would be more amenable to excisional surgical techniques to improve shape and contour. If necessary, liposuction may be a useful adjunct in order to achieve an optimal result.

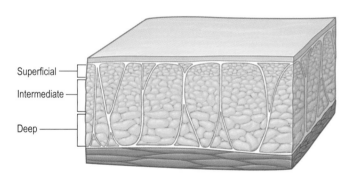

Fig. 24.1 Surgical layers of subcutaneous fat: superficial, intermediate, and deep.

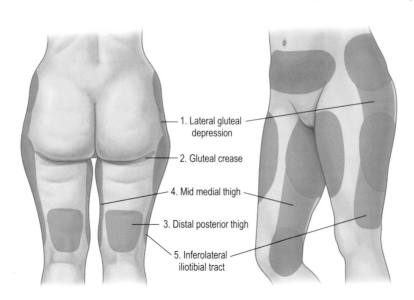

1. Lateral gluteal depression
2. Gluteal crease
4. Mid medial thigh
3. Distal posterior thigh
5. Inferolateral iliotibial tract

Fig. 24.2 The zones of adherence are areas where the fibrous support structures of the subcutaneous fat and skin are adherent to the underlying deep fascia. These attachments create adherence and depressions contributing shape of the body's surface.

Cellulite is a skin condition that is often seen when evaluating patients for liposuction. Cellulite is a dimpling of the skin, particularly in the areas of thighs and buttocks. It has a poorly understood pathophysiology but is thought to be related to fibrous, dermal attachments to the underlying fascia and surrounding hypertrophied fat.[3,7] It has a hormonally mediated component. There is no predictable, long-term treatment of cellulite. Liposuction in areas of overlying cellulite may soften or accentuate the superficial deformity. This should be clearly delineated to the patient as the goals of surgery are reviewed.[8]

Diagnosis, operative indications and patient selection

Liposuction patients often present with a variety of expectations, concerns, and/or complaints. In order to achieve optimal contour with liposuction, appropriate patient selection is imperative. As a general rule, liposuction is performed in healthy patients who maintain realistic goals and expectations. Studies have shown that patients who undergo proper long-term lifestyle changes will in fact achieve the highest

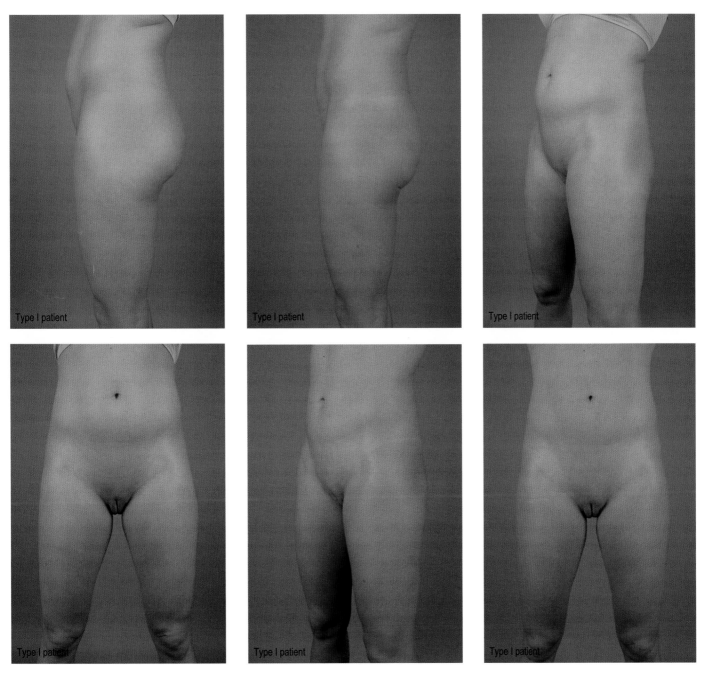

Fig. 24.3 Patient examples of three types of patients (I–III).

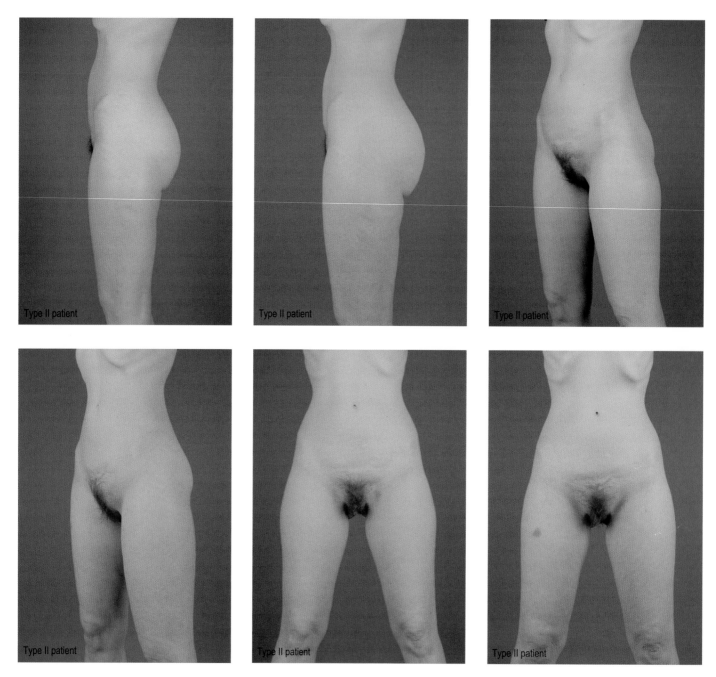

Fig. 24.3, cont'd

level of postoperative satisfaction from their liposuction-assisted body contouring procedure. Rohrich *et al.*[9] concluded that those patients who were committed to a positive lifestyle change involving a healthy diet and regular exercise, or who were already practicing a "healthy lifestyle" that continued postoperatively, experienced the best self assessment and satisfaction scores with liposuction postoperatively *(Fig. 24.4)*. A successful body contouring patient must satisfy four key elements to achieve and maintain optimal results:

1. Lifestyle change
2. Regular exercise
3. Well-balanced diet
4. Body contouring.

Appropriate candidates for liposuction are not morbidly obese, are of a stable weight, and have incorporated the above lifestyle changes into their preoperative regimen. It is preferable for patients to commit to the necessary changes in diet, exercise, and lifestyle modification before undergoing surgery. It is the responsibility of the surgeon to address all concerns, expectations, and goals prior to the procedure in order to establish realistic expectations of the procedure to the patient. Preoperative consultation with a dietician may prove

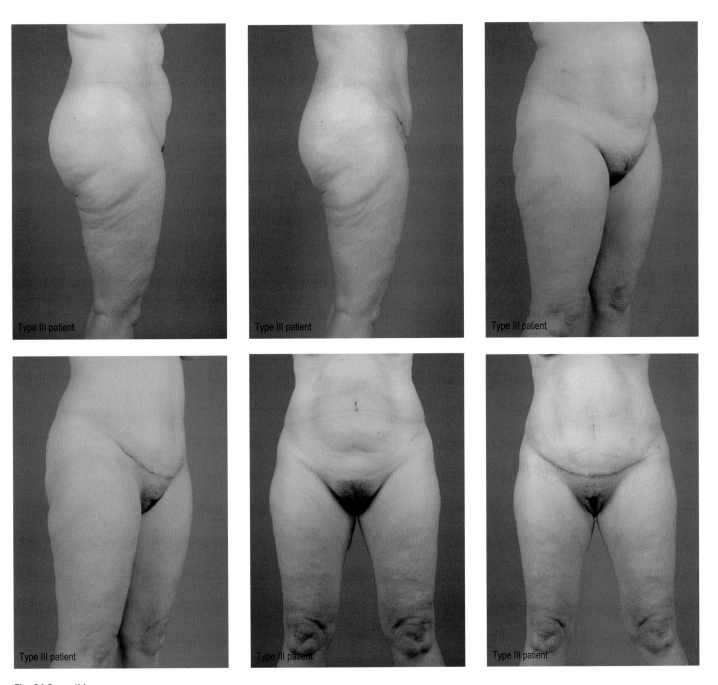

Fig. 24.3, cont'd

beneficial for long-term patient satisfaction. Liposuction is contraindicated in patients who are pregnant, or in poor general medical health. Patients with morbid obesity, cardiopulmonary disease, body image perception issues, unrealistic expectations, wound healing difficulties, or have extensive or poorly located scars should be excluded from consideration for liposuction.

Preoperative assessment

Initial evaluation

During this initial interaction, it is imperative that the plastic surgeon be able to assess the patients' goals of surgery and be able to determine if the patient has realistic expectations regarding outcome and postoperative body image. It may be useful to have the patient prioritize the body regions that they are most concerned with, while focusing on specific complaints within these areas. A detailed medical history should be obtained, including any medications, allergies, and tobacco use. Especially important are notations in the medical history of diabetes, massive weight loss, previous surgery, previous liposuction, and a full detailed list of medications and supplements. Any concerns about a patient's medical suitability to undergo anesthesia and/or an operative procedure should result in referral for preoperative clearance with either an internist or cardiologist. The patients need to be asked specifically about herbal and over-the-counter medications, because

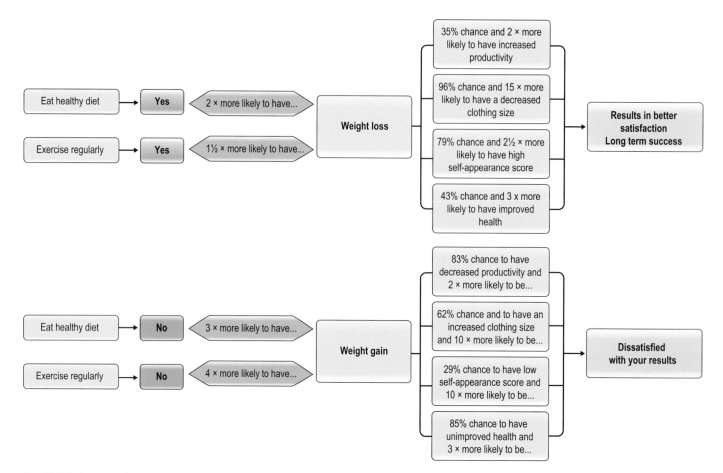

Fig. 24.4 Patients committed to a healthy lifestyle are more likely to be satisfied with the result of liposuction. (From Rohrich RJ, Broughton G, Horton JB, et al. The key to long term success in liposuction: a guide for plastic surgeons and patients. Plast Reconstr Surg 2004; 114:1945–1952.)

these are frequently omitted. Nonessential medications should be discontinued at least 3 weeks before surgery. In selected patients, a preoperative evaluation by a primary care doctor, internist, or cardiologist may be warranted. This typically includes anyone with a significant medical history, or patients older than 50 years of age.

It is often prudent to notify the consulting physician of expected operative times and the amount of expected aspirate and infiltrate. Often, our medical consultants view liposuction as a very benign operation with minimal operative time and morbidity, when in fact a large-volume liposuction case can have significant fluid shifts and time under general anesthesia.[10] Massive weight loss patients should undergo the same preoperative evaluation and clearance for liposuction as they would for any excisional type body contouring procedure (including nutrition, hemoglobin, iron, B12, etc.).[11] It is safest to refrain from operations until these lab results are normalized. Herbal remedies and supplements are not regulated by the Food and Drug Administration (FDA) and thus may place the patient at potential risk of untoward complications, including bleeding or hypercoagulability and should be avoided in the perioperative period.[12] Avoiding aspirin, NSAIDs, and hormonal therapy can help prevent such complications as well. It is the authors' policy for patients to discontinue use of all NSAIDs, aspirin products, fish oil, and supplements, 3 weeks prior to surgery. Of course, if there is a medical indication and necessity for these drugs, consultation

with the primary physician or appropriate specialist should be completed before discontinuation of the medical therapy. A frank discussion of the risk of oral contraceptives and estrogens is held with the patient regardless of the magnitude of the procedure. We strongly recommend that these medications be discontinued 1 month prior to the operative procedure.[13]

Physical exam

A detailed physical exam is performed at the first visit and consultation. Specific attention to prior scars, presence or absence of hernias, evidence of venous insufficiency, and presence of pre-existing asymmetry or contour irregularity should be discussed and noted in the chart. At the initial and subsequent visits, height and weight with calculation of body mass index (BMI) is paramount for safety, as well as for observation of long-term trends during follow-up. For liposuction candidates, six key elements are documented[4–6]:

1. Evaluation of areas of lipodystrophy and contour deformities
2. Skin tone and quality
3. Asymmetries
4. Dimpling and cellulite
5. Myofascial support
6. Zones of adherence.[6]

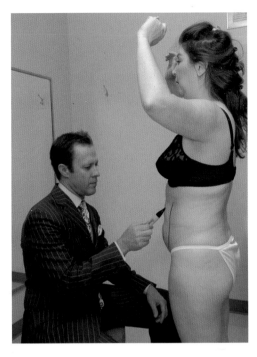

Fig. 24.5 Patient examination in front of a mirror.

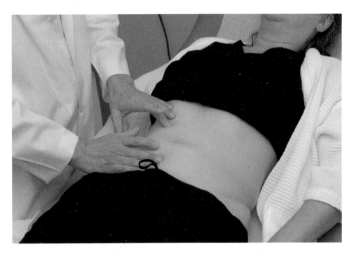

Fig. 24.6 Patient examination in the supine position confirming integrity of the abdominal wall.

The physical exam is best performed in front of a full-length mirror *(Fig. 24.5)*. This allows an open dialogue between patient and physician, wherein the patient's concerns can be addressed and previously unrecognized problem areas can be assessed and addressed. Any areas of cellulite should be pointed out to the patient, and a specific discussion of expected outcome in these areas should be noted. At the initial evaluation, high-quality medical images should be obtained, with anterior, posterior, lateral, and oblique views. This will allow for documentation of results, as well as objective evaluation of outcomes by both patient and physician. Professional medical photography can be a very useful tool for accurate and consistent pre and postoperative documentation.[14]

While the patient is in a supine position with the head elevated, abdominal integrity is examined *(Fig. 24.6)*. This is helpful for detecting hernias or myofascial diastases. Findings may be difficult to interpret in larger individuals, males, or patients with multiple scars. An ultrasound examination or CT scan may further clarify this region and prevent potential intra-abdominal injury in these patients. During the initial consultation, when the patient is in front of the mirror, it is important to point out potential problem areas that may cause less than optimal results, so the patient may visualize and appreciate these areas.

A follow-up visit is typically scheduled 2–3 weeks after the initial consultation. During this visit, computer images *(Fig. 24.7)* are reviewed, which allows the patient to establish realistic expectations. These objective images portray the advantages, disadvantages, and limitations of body contouring surgery. The patient should understand that imaging is for educational purposes only and is *not* a guarantee of the final result. The second visit allows further dialogue between the patient and physician so that all questions may be answered and issues addressed. For example, a second opportunity to address any last minute concerns by the patient in regards to

recovery time, pain control, bruising, and postoperative changes will help strengthen the patient's confidence in the procedure and decrease the likelihood of any uncertainties or surprises within the perioperative period.

Patient education and informed consent

Patient education is stressed throughout the course of the initial evaluation, physical examination, and follow-up visit so that the patient has sufficient information about the procedure, postoperative course, and long-term results to make a truly informed decision. The patient and physician should discuss the procedure itself, alternative treatments, financial obligations (including further surgeries if required), and complications and risks. The risks for liposuction include, but are not limited to, bleeding, infection, pain, thermal injury, seroma, dyspigmentation, paresthesias, contour irregularities, and dysesthesias. Large volume liposuction carries increased risks of fluid shifts, volume overload, and anesthesia complications.[10] These problems are discussed under "Complications", below. Informed consent is vitally important in the evaluation and management of liposuction patients both to protect the surgeon and the patient from unexpected outcomes or patient dissatisfaction. This important process should be performed by the operative surgeon (not a nurse or staff) and clearly documented in the medical record.

Operative considerations

Video 1

Preoperative marking

Guiding marks are performed prior to surgery with the patient in the erect position. In patients undergoing total body liposuction or contouring in combination with excisional surgery, marking can be done in the office the day before surgery. This allows for a more private environment and ample time to review the plan with the patient. Marking is done in front of a mirror, thus allowing the patient to contribute to the process and further confirms exactly what will be addressed during the procedure. Areas to be suctioned are marked with a circle; zones of adherence and areas to avoid

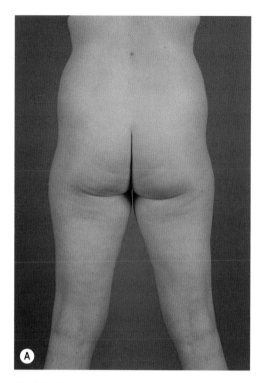
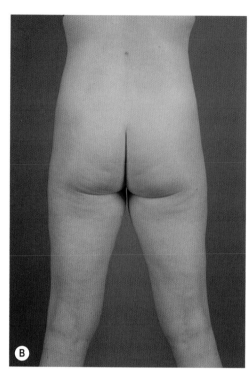

Fig. 24.7 Computer imaging aids in preoperative discussion with the patient.

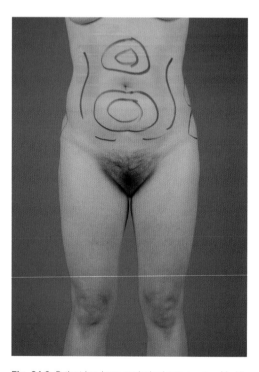

Fig. 24.8 Patient has been marked prior to surgery. Markings demonstrate the contours of the areas to be suctioned as well as the planned incision sites.

are marked with hash marks. Asymmetries, cellulite, and dimpling are marked for their respective treatment and to allow patients to see problem areas. When complete, the marks are once again reviewed with the patient to ensure that all areas of concern are addressed.[4,5] Access incisions are also marked at this setting. Often two incisions are needed per area to be suctioned, the incisions should be placed adjacent to

suctioned areas and not too distant. With liposuction, it is beneficial to choose access points that can treat multiple areas. Care should be taken to prevent access incision placement in or adjacent to zones of adherence. The suctioning may cross the zone and disrupt it. Incisions should also allow each area to be treated from different directions for optimal contouring. Incisions should be no longer than 3–4 mm in length and placed in well-concealed areas. Of note, the incisions utilized for ultrasound-assisted liposuction are slightly longer (5–6 mm) than for standard liposuction to account for the placement of skin protectors when utilized. The surgeon should not hesitate in placing additional incisions if access is insufficient with the existing markings.

Figure 24.8 shows the preoperative markings and preferred placement of access incisions based on areas to be suctioned. Cosmetically, it is preferable to stagger incisions in an asymmetric fashion to camouflage their appearance.[4,5]

Anesthesia technique/location of operation

It is up to the surgeon to determine the optimal surgical setting for each patient undergoing liposuction. Factors which influence this decision are: the amount of expected lipoaspirate, length and extent of procedure, patient positioning, operating surgeon preference, anesthesiologist preference, and overall health of the patient. Depending on the geographical location, there are differing regulations for the location of liposuction procedures, usually based on the type of anesthesia and the size of the liposuction procedure. For example, one recommendation is to avoid epidural and spinal anesthesia in office-based settings because of potential hypotension and volume overload issues.[15]

As a general rule, small-volume liposuction cases can be performed with local anesthesia, with or without mild sedation. Complex, large-volume liposuction and combined cases should be performed under general anesthesia. Our institutional preference has been to perform the majority of cases under general anesthesia. Deep-sedation cases and general anesthesia procedures are performed under supervision of board-certified anesthesiologists in licensed surgery centers or hospitals. All prone cases are performed with general endotracheal anesthesia for airway control. Operative location should be determined after careful patient evaluation, assessment of the complexity of operation, and appropriate evaluation of medical co-morbidities. The anticipated postoperative course and the need for possible overnight observation both factor into choice among inpatient, observation, or outpatient hospital settings.

Awake liposuction has been performed in the office-based setting with a tumescent technique. The authors prefer to do such procedures only for single area treatments or in small revisions. Detailed patient assessment and strict limitations on volumes infiltrated and amount of lipoaspirate expected should be reviewed prior to performing in an unmonitored office-based setting.[16] Although there is some convenience and cost-saving to office-based surgery, with the recent advancements and attention to patient safety, this should be discouraged except for small localized areas and limited volumes.

Special importance should be given to medical co-morbidities such as obstructive sleep apnea. Current American Society of Anesthesiology recommendations are: for patients with signs or symptoms suggestive of moderate to severe obstructive sleep apnea, surgery should be performed in a hospital setting with extended recovery and observation to prevent postoperative respiratory complications.[17] It is recommended that liposuction procedures, whether inpatient or outpatient, if under anesthesia care, should be performed in an accredited facility with the capability to manage any postoperative insult.[18] During the liposuction procedure, it is useful to have the circulating nurse maintain an accurate liposuction data sheet to facilitate consistent and accurate communication among the surgeon, the anesthesiologist, and the operating room team (*Fig. 24.9*).

Maintenance core body temperature and immediate preoperative care

The patient is placed in a forced air, warming blanket 30–60 min prior to the procedure. Additionally, pedal or calf compression devices are also applied in the holding area. This should be instituted as part of preoperative orders to assist in DVT prophylaxis and prevent the patient becoming cold during the procedure. During the procedure, all areas not being treated should be covered by the forced warm air blanket. The wetting solutions should be warmed and not administered cold.

Patient positioning

Prone/supine

Once marked, the patient position is determined. The cadence of the operation usually begins with the patient in the prone position followed by supine. This necessitates prepping and draping the patient twice. If the team works together, turnaround time should be limited to <10 min. An alternative method is to prep the patient circumferentially while standing and to then position the patient on a sterile table with position changes not necessitating a reprep. We dislike this technique as it may be embarrassing for the patient and increases the likelihood of hypothermia. Once in the operating room, the compression devices are applied to the patient before being placed under general anesthesia. In the majority of our liposuction cases, we prefer to position the patient prone first. A soft hip roll is placed beneath the iliac crests to elevate the treatment areas off the bed, and either pillows or longitudinal rolls are used to support the upper chest (*Fig. 24.10*). The breasts should be placed medially and nipples protected.

The patient's arms are extended on padded arm boards at <90° from the long axis of the table. The face must be appropriately padded, including placing the cervical spine in a neutral position and protecting the globes. Patients in the prone position are subjected to pressure changes over the

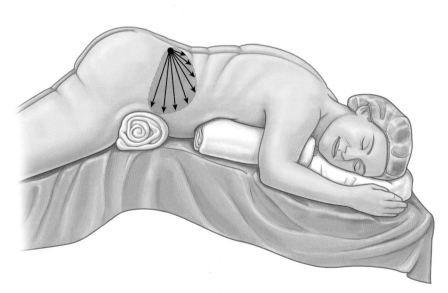

Fig. 24.10 The patient in the prone position. A large proportion of a liposuction procedure can be performed in this position. Appropriate padding and arm position is important to avoid intraoperative complications.

forehead, malar areas, iliac crest, and bony prominences of the arms and legs. Special attention also needs to be given to the female and male genitals. In the prone position, up to 70% of the contouring can be performed and may include liposuction of the arms, back, hips/flanks, lateral, posterior, and medial thighs.

With the patient in the supine position, the remainder of the trunk and extremities can be addressed. This may include treatment of the arms, abdomen, anterior medial thighs, and knees. This position does not have significant effects on the cardiopulmonary systems. Brachial plexus injuries can occur if the arm is abducted >90°. The hips and knees should be flexed at approximately 30° with a pillow. Pressure points in the supine position include the occiput, scapula, posterior iliac crest, sacrum, and heels.

Lateral decubitus positioning

Although rarely used in our hands, the lateral decubitus position can access the flanks, lateral back, buttocks, thighs, and lower legs. A disadvantage of this method is that a side-by-side comparison to the contralateral area is not available to assess symmetry.

Wetting solutions and perioperative fluid management

When first described, liposuction was performed without the use of any infiltrated wetting solution which resulted in blood loss of up to 45% of aspirate in some areas.[19,20] In an effort to reduce blood loss, the practice of infiltrating wetting solutions (saline or LR mixture with dilute amounts of epinephrine and lidocaine) was developed. Liposuction has continued to evolve to include the addition of infiltrating subcutaneous wetting solutions prior to suctioning in order to provide hydro-dissection, improve hemostasis, and potentially provide some perioperative analgesia.

There are four different terms used to describe the types of wetting solution: *dry, wet, superwet, and tumescent.*[19] These terms are based on the volume of infiltrate as a ratio of the volume suctioned *(Tables 24.1, 24.2)*. The dry technique uses no wetting solution and has few if any indications in liposuction. The wet technique involves pre-infiltrating 200–300 mL of solution per region to be treated, regardless of the anticipated amount to be aspirated. The superwet technique employs an infiltration of 1 mL of solution per estimated 1 mL

of expected aspirate, and finally the tumescent infiltration, popularized by Klein *et al.*, involves extensive infiltration of wetting solution that creates significant tissue turgor and results in total infiltration of ~3 mL of wetting solution per 1 mL aspirated.[19–23] Regardless of the technique used, the infiltrate should be allowed to set for 7 min and no longer than 30 min prior to suctioning because of the estimated onset of action of the anesthetic and vasoconstrictor in the solution. As detailed in *Table 24.2*, there is negligible blood loss (<1% of the lipoaspirate) when the superwet technique or tumescent techniques are utilized.

Many authors have popularized different variations of these solutions, but all formulations include some variant of fluid (NS/LR), epinephrine, and lidocaine.[19–22] Marcaine should be avoided because of its potential cardiac effects and duration of action; it has yet to be proven clinically as a suitable anesthetic in wetting solutions.[24] The most common solution mixtures are shown in *Table 24.3*.

Table 24.2 Techniques of liposuction and infiltrates[19]

Technique	Infiltrate	Volume aspirate
Dry	No infiltrate	To treatment endpoint
Wet	200–300 mL/area	To treatment endpoint
Superwet	1 mL infiltrate:1 mL aspirate	1 mL aspirate/infiltrate (treatment endpoints)
Tumescent	Infiltrate to skin turgor	2–3 mL aspirate/mL

(Data from Fodor PB. Wetting solutions in aspirative lipoplasty: a plea for safety in liposuction. *Aesthet Plast Surg.* 1995;19(4):379–380.)

Table 24.3 The most common formulations of wetting solutions

Wetting solution contents	Quantity
Klein's formula	
Normal saline solution	1000 mL
1% lidocaine	50 mL
1:1000 epinephrine	1 mL
8.4% sodium bicarbonate	12.5 mL
Hunstad's formula	
Ringer's lactate solution	1000 mL at 38–40°C
1% lidocaine	50 mL
1:1000 epinephrine	1 mL
Fodor's formula	
Ringer's lactate solution	1000 mL
Aspirates <2000 mL 1:500 epinephrine	1 mL
Aspirates 2000–4000 mL 1:1000 epinephrine	1 mL
Aspirates >4000 mL 1:1500 epinephrine	1 mL
UT Southwestern formula	
Ringer's lactate solution	1000 mL at 21°C
Aspirates <5000 mL 1% lidocaine	30 mL
Aspirates >5000 mL 1% lidocaine	15 mL
1:1000 epinephrine	1 mL

Table 24.1 Estimated blood loss with different liposuction techniques[19]

Technique	Estimated blood loss as % of volume aspirated
Dry	20–45
Wet	4–30
Superwet	1
Tumescent	1

(Data from Fodor PB. Wetting solutions in aspirative lipoplasty: a plea for safety in liposuction. *Aesthet Plast Surg.* 1995;19(4):379–380.)

Lidocaine

Most wetting solutions utilize lidocaine as the local anesthetic component to be included in the wetting solution. It has been reported to provide analgesia for up to 18 h postoperatively when injected in dilute concentrations into the subcutaneous space.[25] Initially with the large volumes of solution injected, there was concern about lidocaine toxicity. Toxicity from lidocaine affects the heart and central nervous system most commonly. The initial signs and symptoms of lidocaine toxicity include circumoral numbness, tinnitus, and lightheadedness. Increasing levels can yield tremors, seizures, and eventually cardiopulmonary arrest. Intraoperative findings would include arrhythmias, and cardiac irregularities.[26] The traditional recommended maximum dose of lidocaine with epinephrine is 7 mg/kg;[27] however, in the liposuction setting, numerous studies have documented the safety of lidocaine in concentrations >35 mg/kg and as high as 55 mg/kg in large volume cases.[22,28] These higher doses have proven to yield peak plasma levels below the toxic range. It is theorized that this margin of safety is due to the dilute nature of lidocaine solutions used in liposuction, slow infiltration, the avascular plane injected and a high lipid solubility of lidocaine. There are many other variables that one must consider when incorporating lidocaine into a wetting solution. First and foremost, the lidocaine absorption rate is extremely variable and dependent on multiple factors including the activity of the cytochrome P450 system, drug interactions, fluids, and concentrations of the drug administered. Medications that tend to increase lidocaine levels include oral contraceptives, beta blockers, and tricyclic antidepressants.

Recently, there has been significant attention addressed to the importance of *monoethylglycinexylidide* (MEGX). MEGX is an active metabolite of lidocaine that is less protein-bound and thus pharmacologically more active. It has been reported to be up to 83% active, meaning that it will contribute to the overall activity of lidocaine and ultimately its potential toxic effects. Studies have been performed which show that the peak levels of the metabolite MEGX occur within 8–32 h after initial infiltration.[29] The peak systemic levels was greater than initially thought but still below the level of toxicity. Based on a recent study, this may increase levels up to 1 mg/mL.

A recent study published showed that tissue levels of lidocaine beyond 8 h postoperatively are sub-therapeutic. A well designed study by Hatef et al.[30] prospectively randomized liposuction patients to receive preoperative subcutaneous infiltration of 10, 20, or 30 mg/kg of lidocaine wetting solution prior to the procedure observing intraoperative anesthesia requirement, postoperative pain, and the need for postoperative analgesia. Surprisingly, no significant difference was evident between any of the three groups. Some people argue this as a reason to eliminate lidocaine altogether in wetting solutions, stating the possibility of minimal effect is not worth the small risks it poses in patients under regional or general anesthesia. Further studies are warranted.

Additionally, further investigation on the use of bupivacaine in low doses may provide another alternative for postoperative analgesia. A recent publication by Failey et al.[31] demonstrated no significant difference in the incidence of adverse events or postoperative length of stay for patients who underwent liposuction with bupivacaine, compared with other wetting solutions.

Epinephrine

The epinephrine contained in wetting solutions, with its vasoconstrictive properties is the key to minimal blood loss during liposuction. This effect also decreases the rate of vascular absorption of lidocaine, potentiating the local anesthetic effect. Epinephrine toxicity can result in tachycardia, hypertension, and arrhythmias. Many investigators have studied the doses of epinephrine in wetting solutions. It has been reported to have an upper safety limit of 15 mg per surgical procedure. Regardless, it is known that epinephrine, even in small concentrations, may still have a profound effect on the cardiovascular system. Most commonly, epinephrine in 1 mg with 1/1000 dilution is injected into a 1 L bag of infiltrate either NS/LR.

In a study evaluating the hemodynamic effects of epinephrine during liposuction surgery, the authors found a linear correlation between epinephrine concentration and cardiac index.[10,29,32] While the doses of epinephrine are low and its half life is <2 min, peak concentrations do not occur until around 5 h after infiltration. In larger volume cases, it is recommended that infiltration be staged decreasing the "peak" effect of epinephrine and its subsequent effect on the cardiovascular system. Regardless, a thorough patient evaluation with special attention to the presence of cardiovascular disease should be performed to avoid the untoward effects associated with epinephrine infiltration in some patients.[33]

Although rarely used, halothane may sensitize the heart to catecholamines, resulting in ventricular arrhythmias. Despite the protective effect of lidocaine against arrhythmias, halothane should not be used during liposuction procedures.

To maximize its effect, the infiltrate should be allowed to set for a minimum of 7 min and no longer than 30 min prior to suctioning because of the estimated onset of action of the anesthetic and vasoconstrictive properties of the solution.

Current recommendations for perioperative fluid management

The intraoperative data sheet *(Fig. 24.9)* is useful, especially in large volume cases to guide the intraoperative and postoperative fluid requirements. Perioperative management guidelines previously published were developed after a thorough review of 100 consecutive procedures using the superwet technique. Perioperative fluid management during liposuction procedures requires attention to maintenance intravenous fluids, third-space losses, wetting solution infiltration, and lipoaspirate.[34–36] Liposuction is considered a moderate surgical stress; therefore 3–5 mg/kg per hour of crystalloid solution is adequate volume for maintenance replacement and third-space losses. Additional fluid may be given during procedures in which the lipoaspirate amount is more than 5 L. The ratio of 0.25 mL of crystalloid solution for each aspirated milliliter over 5 L is considered.

Fluid resuscitation

Body contouring procedures can result in significant fluid shifts and intravascular volume changes for the patient. The operating surgeon should maintain a dialogue with the anesthesia provider, so that patients receive adequate replacement volume and proper fluid resuscitation during the intraoperative period. As mentioned above, awareness of four key elements will guide the intraoperative fluid management of liposuction patients: intravenous (IV) fluid maintenance (body weight dependent), third space losses, volume of wetting solution infiltrated, and total lipoaspirate volume. Large-volume liposuction patients can present an especially difficult challenge for fluid resuscitation.[37,38] Strong consideration should be given for placement of a Foley catheter in patients undergoing large-volume aspiration to assist in resuscitation.

As previously mentioned by Rohrich *et al.* in 1998 (updated in 2006), the following formula aids in fluid management for these patients.[36]

1. Replace losses from preoperative oral intake loss as needed
2. Maintain fluid throughout the procedure and manage it based on vital signs and urine output
3. Employ the superwet infiltration technique
4. Administer crystalloid replacements, 0.25 mL for each mL of lipoaspirate over 5 L.

As always, the fluid management of any patient should be based on sound surgical judgment and with all intraoperative considerations, patient factors and co-morbidities accounted for. The safety of procedures, especially large volume liposuction, demands vigorous attention to detail to keep patient volume status appropriate and prevent instances of severe fluid shifts during intraoperative and postoperative resuscitation.

Treatment options

After appropriate preoperative planning and informed consent, there are now multiple options for which type of liposuction to perform. Selecting the appropriate modalities requires a knowledge of and familiarity with the recent advances in liposuction. Factors that influence the selection of a particular type of treatment include surgeon preference, target area, expected aspirate, and history of previous liposuction. Currently, the most commonly utilized options include: *traditional liposuction*, as popularized by Illouz,[1] commonly referred to as suction-assisted liposuction (SAL); *power-assisted liposuction* (PAL); *ultrasound-assisted liposuction* (UAL); *vaser-assisted liposuction*; and *laser-assisted liposuction* (LAL). The traditional SAL still remains the most common and popular modality for lipoplasty among plastic surgeons.

Suction-assisted lipoplasty uses a two-stage technique whereby the site is infiltrated with a predetermined wetting solution and then evacuated after allowing time for the solution to set and take effect. Patients are marked as previously described and incisions 3–4 mm in size are made for access. Advantages of this technique include the ease of use, malleable cannulas, a wide variety of cannulas, and decades of experience and results. The disadvantages of SAL include being more difficult to use in fibrous areas and secondary liposuction. There is more physical work involved to break up and remove fat with traditional SAL.

Power-assisted liposuction uses an externally powered cannula, which is variable in size and flex, and oscillates in a 2–3-mm reciprocating motion at rates of 4000–6000 cycles/min. Advocates of PAL contend that it is best used for large volumes, fibrous areas, and revision liposuction.[39,40] Because the PAL cannula breaks up fibrous fat much more readily, the procedure is significantly faster and less labor intensive for the surgeon than traditional SAL. Suction is still a major component of PAL, and most units are compatible with standard aspiration equipment. Both the power source, and the suction are attached to the proximal end of the handpiece. If the surgeon prefers, syringe suction is a useful adjunct and can be used with an adapter. As with SAL, a wide variety of probe tip configurations and diameters are available. PAL systems have multiple power settings; they can be programmed for a variety of areas, tissue types and according to the preferences of performing surgeon. Some of the disadvantages of earlier PAL systems was the significant noise generation and the mechanical vibration experienced by the operating surgeon. However, these modalities are now run on electrical power sources decreasing the degree of vibration and noise. PAL is touted for its ability to reduce surgeon work in liposuction and perform liposuction in all body areas and types with ease and speed above traditional liposuction.

Ultrasound-assisted liposuction utilizes ultrasonic energy to break down fat and facilitate suction-assisted removal. Its mechanism of action is also primarily mechanical in nature, but cavitation and some thermal effects are purported to occur. With this technique, fat is emulsified, which allows removal through traditional liposuction cannulas. UAL comprises three stages: (1) infiltration, (2) emulsification, and (3) evacuation and contouring.[41] Skin protection may be utilized to help protect the skin from thermal injury. Limiting the application of energy and bathing the access site with saline will help prevent untoward injury to skin and dermis. A towel should cover the region behind the access site to prevent direct contact of the probe with the skin during excursion. As with the other technologies, a variety of probe tip configurations and lengths are available, including hollow and solid technology. For UAL, the treatment is begun at a depth of approximately 1–2 cm, depending on the body area. The plane is treated uniformly, beginning at one side of the area and moving in a radial fashion to the contralateral side *(Fig. 24.11)*. This is continued in this manner until the endpoint is reached. When this occurs, the probe is moved to a deeper plane. Most treatment sites will have a minimum of two planes and sometimes three. When the last plane is completed, evacuation begins in the deeper plane *(Fig. 24.12)* to remove the emulsified fat. Next, the operating surgeon begins

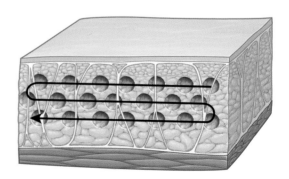

Fig. 24.11 UAL superficial to deep.

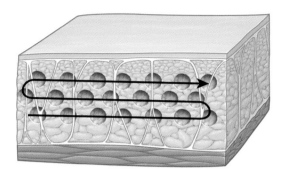

Fig. 24.12 UAL deep to superficial.

final contouring, if necessary. Standard cannulas for final contouring are used. Smaller cannulas are less efficient at evacuating fat but decrease the likelihood of contour irregularities. It is important that UAL endpoints be respected to avoid overzealous resection of fat. Advantages of UAL include less surgeon fatigue, as well as improved results in fibrous areas and in secondary procedures. By utilizing ultrasound-assisted liposuction advocates report more uniform treatment of fat layers and improved contour with less revision. Disadvantages include increased equipment cost, slightly larger incisions, longer operative times, and the possibility of thermal injury.[4] Thermal injury is not typically seen with the application times currently being used today. UAL requires a superwet environment and cannot be performed without a wetting solution. Finally, UAL requires continuous movement to prevent excessive exposure of the tissues to heat *(Fig. 24.13)*.

Vaser-assisted liposuction employs a newer generation ultrasound-assisted liposuction device that incorporates less energy with more efficient, solid probes. The grooves on the end of probes allow better lateral fragmentation of tissue with lower energy. The probes come in an array of sizes and grooving, depending on tissues in which they will be used. The system uses less energy, decreasing its thermal component to the tissues.[42,43] After treatment with either continuous or intermittent energy the fat broken down is then evacuated with a traditional liposuction cannulas. An article by Garcia and Nathan advocates the use of VASER in large volume liposuction to reduce blood loss especially in fibrous fatty areas where blood loss is likely to increase *(Fig. 24.14)*.[44]

Laser-assisted liposuction has been at the forefront of marketing hype at the time of this publication. The treatment involves insertion of a laser fiber via a small skin incision. Depending on the manufacturer, the fiber may either be housed within a cannula or as a separate fiber. There are several commercially available lasers on the market under different trade names. The most common available wavelengths in the United States are 924/975 nm, 1064 nm, 1319/1320, and 1450 nm. Many of these devices utilize more than one wavelength during treatment. Most companies and physicians utilizing these devices employ a four-stage technique: infiltration, application of energy to the subcutaneous tissues, evacuation, and finally subdermal skin stimulation. The laser fiber purportedly acts to disrupt fat cell membranes and emulsify fat.[45] Evacuation then commences via traditional liposuction cannulas. For smaller regions (such as the neck), some vendors suggest skipping the evacuation phase, allowing the body to absorb the liquefied contents. These devices have been marketed for purported skin-tightening effects.

The belief is that the heating of the subdermal tissue may provide a skin tightening effect. No large, prospective trials have been undertaken to examine the benefits of LAL over existing technologies, so unfortunately, these reports remain anecdotal and lack scientific validation. Dibernardo and colleagues evaluated skin tightening and skin shrinkage after treatment with a 1064/1320 nm laser in the abdomen of five patients, and found a 26% improvement in skin elasticity and an average reduction in area of 17%.[46,47]

A previously published randomized, double-blinded, controlled study by Prado et al.[48] showed no difference in the outcomes of LAL versus traditional SAL. In that study, each patient served as his or her own control. Factors evaluated included cosmetic result, postoperative pain, length of operation, lipocrit, and free fatty acids. Besides the lack of difference in the cosmetic outcome of LAL versus SAL, the authors also reported a longer operative time with LAL, less early postoperative pain with LAL, and elevated free fatty acids/triglycerides in the laser-treated lipoaspirate. Regardless of its efficacy in tightening skin, we must recognize that there is a fine line between dermal contraction and full thickness injury when applying heat to the subdermis. There are manufacturer claims about tissue contraction and skin tightening but there have been no clinical papers supporting this claim.

Surgical endpoints

Longstanding endpoints have been established for traditional liposuction such as skin pinch, final contour, and volume of aspirate. However, with the advent of new technology the operating surgeon must be aware of the differences in surgical endpoints for this new technology in order to prevent significant injury or complications and allow for the best aesthetic results. These endpoints have been divided into primary and secondary endpoints. Skin pinch and final contour are the most critical end points in traditional liposuction and account for the best determination of final result.[5,49] A reduction in convexity to a smooth contour is the ultimate goal with the endpoint being surgical judgment. Other indicators such as treatment time, blood in aspirate and amount of aspirate are important factors to consider. Measured volume aspirated is a good indicator for bilateral procedures in order to judge symmetry and contour comparing each side to the opposite. However, recognizing preoperative asymmetries is important because lipodystrophy is not usually perfectly symmetrical. In UAL, the most important endpoint is reached when one encounters a loss of tissue resistance, which is appreciated through the treatment hand as well as the nondominant guiding hand. Additionally, the aspirate, when used, may become more blood tinged, indicating adequate emulsification of the treatment site. Furthermore, experience helps dictate energy application times in particular regions of the body. Secondary endpoints for UAL include site-specific treatment time and volume to allow for comparison of size and symmetry of treatment on either side. Contour should not be judged during emulsification or the evacuation phase. Once evacuation is complete, contour may be assessed. Alternatively, treatment with SAL or PAL uses final contour and symmetrical pinch test results as their primary endpoints. Treatment time and volume, similarly, can be used to help ensure that treatment is symmetrical *(Table 24.4)*.

Table 24.4 Surgical endpoints for UAL and SAL/PAL[4]

Endpoint	UAL	SAL/PAL
Primary	Loss of tissue resistance	Final contour
	Blood aspirate	Symmetrical pinch test results
Secondary	Treatment time	Treatment time
	Treatment volume	Treatment volume

(Data from Rohrich RJ, Beran SJ, Kenkel JM. *Ultrasound-assisted liposuction*. St Louis: Quality Medical; 1998.)

Table 24.5 Typical cannula size and location utilized

Site	Evacuation (mm)	Contouring (mm)
Neck	2.4	2.4 and 1.8
Arms	3.7	3.0 and 2.4
Back	3.7	3.0
Hips	4.6 (deep plane only)	3.7 and 3.0
Abdomen	3.7 (deep plane only)	3.7 and 3.0
Thighs	3.7 (deep plane only)	3.0
Knees	3.0	2.4
Calves/ankles	3.0	2.4

The operating surgeon should not hesitate to add multiple sites for evacuation and final contouring to create a smoother, more uniformly treated area and minimize the risk for contour deformities. As a general rule, superficial liposuction should not be performed routinely and is reserved for patients who have significant superficial irregularities. Only surgeons with extensive experience in liposuction should perform this procedure due to the high propensity for skin injury and contour irregularities of the superficial soft tissues.

Finally, when contour irregularities are recognized intraoperatively, they can be treated with autologous fat grafting immediately at the site of the deformity. Trying to feather edges of the defect most often leads to an even greater problem, further complicating its treatment. This will be discussed more under complications.

Cannulas and probes

Suction of fat is achieved through cannulas (hollow tube with opening(s) at tips). Cannulas have changed significantly over the years. They are available for multiple different purposes, modalities and specific regions. The cannulas come in a wide variety of size (diameter of the tube), tip configuration (number and location of holes at the tip), and length of cannula. Each factor alters the amount, speed and viability of fat removed.[50]

Tip configuration

The tip of the cannula has a bearing on the speed, efficacy and safety of liposuction. Most tips are blunt with multiple apertures (openings) set back from the end to allow suctioning. The sharper the tip of the cannula the more likely the operating surgeon is to penetrate unwanted structures, i.e., fascia, peritoneum, etc. Cannulas can be found with a variety of openings and configurations.

Cannula diameter

The most common cannula sizes utilized in liposuction are between 2.5 and 5.0 mm. However, cannula sizes are available down to 1.8 mm and up to 1 cm in size. There are very limited uses for the large or very small specialized cannulas. As cannula size increases, the amount and speed of tissue removal increases, however the risks of causing contour deformities and tissue damage also increases. In general large cannulas are used for deeper fat deposits and the smaller cannulas are utilized for superficial deposits and final contouring. See below for common cannula sizes for various areas.

Cannula length

Length of the cannula can vary from 10 cm to 30 cm. As the length increases, the ability to finely control evacuation is more limited. With longer cannula length more areas can be suctioned with fewer access incisions. However, the surgeon should never compromise on number of access incisions to allow adequate suctioning and contouring (*Table 24.5*).

Cannulas utilized in traditional SAL

Most traditional liposuction cannulas used for SAL have rounded and somewhat tapered tips to allow easier movement through the tissues. The majority of cannulas have multiple distal openings that are set back from the tip to avoid contour irregularities. These openings vary in size and are generally proportionate to the diameter of the cannula. Multiple openings allow improved efficiency in fat removal. Single- and double-aperture cannulas are safe because the opening can be directed away from the skin; however, they do aspirate fat at a slower rate. The most common cannula type is the Mercedes type, which has three apertures set back from the tip to allow efficient circumferential fat removal. There are multiple variations with either larger or smaller opening which can be tailored to the surgeon's preference or the desired effect.

Cannulas utilized in PAL

An array of cannulas is also available for the PAL systems (Microaire Surgical Instruments, Charlottesville, VA). These cannulas are small and malleable, which is very useful when working along curved surfaces. They are comparable in length and diameter to SAL cannulas, permitting the use of small access incisions.

UAL

Ultrasonic technology uses either a hollow cannula or a solid probe. VASER probes (Sound Surgical Technologies, Louisville, CO) are solid and have rings circumscribing them. The rings allow for lateral fragmentation; therefore the greater the number of rings, the more lateral fragmentation that is possible.

Two or three ring probes are generally used in areas that have soft, nonfibrous fat, and the single ring probe is reserved for more fibrous secondary areas. The golf tee-shaped tip cannula provides a sharp edge allowing for a more aggressive treatment of the tissues and great tissue fragmentation.

Treatment areas

Arms

The liposuction of arms is covered in Chapter 29.

Back

The anatomy of the subcutaneous fat and skin is unique from other regions of the trunk and extremities; it has a very thick dermis and a dense, fibrous characteristic to the underlying fat, more superficial in location. Beneath this, there lies a loose, areolar plane of fat on top of the deep fascia. The preferred position to treat these patients is in the prone position with the bed in a head down flexed position. The fibrous nature of the fat and the dense tissue make the utilization of UAL and PAL extremely useful for this area. The quantity of fat removed can be moderate, but improved results are often observed with release of folds and attachments to deeper tissue. Access incisions will depend on the distribution of fat and/or skin rolls and should often be placed medially and laterally; if at all possible the incisions should be placed in the bra/bathing suit line for the best cosmetic result.[49,50] Women will often complain of fat along the roll of bra-line and large pockets of lipodystrophy can be seen *(Fig. 24.15)*. This area responds especially well to UAL allowing the fold to be broken up and excess fat removed. When suctioning the back, forceful excursion of the cannula should be avoided, as fibrous areas may redirect the cannula to an unsafe location. Suctioning from areas off of the thoracic cage (hip region) towards the posterior back should not be performed to obviate intra-abdominal and intra-thoracic penetration of the cannula *(Fig. 24.16)*.[4,5]

Abdomen

Liposuction of the abdomen, its limitations and benefits are often misunderstood by patients. Contouring the body in any area requires the physician to evaluate that area circumferentially. This is particularly true in the lower trunk where the final contour not only depends on the abdomen but also the area of the hips or flanks. Furthermore, many patients seeking contouring of the abdomen may not be candidates for liposuction alone and require excisional techniques to allow them the best possible change in contour.

The abdomen is bordered superiorly by the xiphoid process and costal margin, the pubis and inguinal ligament inferiorly,

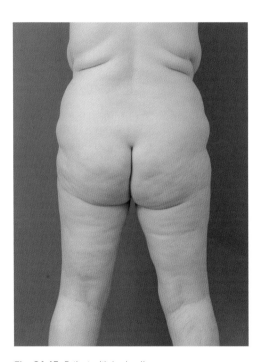

Fig. 24.15 Patient with back rolls.

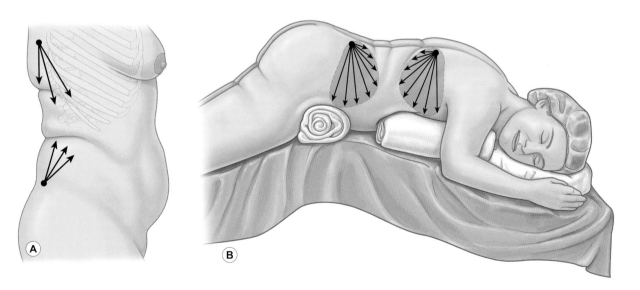

Fig. 24.16 Patient in position for suction of back rolls.

and the anterior superior iliac spines laterally. Careful pre-operative evaluation and physical exam is essential. This includes detail pertaining to the distribution of fat, scars, skin laxity, and the presence or absence of hernias. The physical examination may be challenging on patients who are over-weight, with a large pannus, or with extensive scarring necessitating preoperative imaging to rule out any abdominal wall defects or hernias. Patients with diastasis, abdominal wall laxity, or significant intra-abdominal fat should be counseled on the possible benefit and/or need for skin excision, or plication in order to achieve an optimal contour and aesthetic result.

The subcutaneous abdominal fat is amenable to all of the various modalities of liposuction and continues to be one of the most popular and desired areas for liposuction. Suctioning the deep two-thirds of the fat is safe and effective. The sub-scarpal fat below the umbilicus is loose while the area above the umbilicus tends to be more compact and fibrous.[51] The operating surgeon should reserve superficial liposuction for the linea alba or for the correction of secondary deformities, and only then with extensive experience and care. There have been published reports of superficial sculpting of the abdomen, but this should only be attempted by experienced hands.[52]

Access to the abdominal region may be gained through an umbilical incision, bilateral lower abdominal incisions, and/or suprapubic incisions. It is also useful to extend the table at the waist up to 15 or 20° to allow excursion of the cannula away from the suprapubic region and specifically the pubic ramus. In patients with a long torso and a moderate degree of lipodystrophy overlying their costal margin, an inframammary fold incision can be made to access this fatty area. As with other body regions, the surgeon should never approach an area of convexity from an area of concavity to avoid intraabdominal or thoracic penetration *(Fig. 24.16)*. In the abdomen, it is imperative that short, controlled strokes be

used to avoid the potential for inadvertent fascial perforation, particularly when working in and around scars. Finally, the distribution of fat in the abdomen can vary; people with large volumes of intra-abdominal fat will not respond well to abdominal liposuction and should be counseled accordingly to prevent unwanted outcomes and disappointment.

The skin of the abdomen can be prone to contour irregularities. Constant feedback from the tissues by means of manual palpation, pinch, and symmetry assessment helps decrease the likelihood of contour irregularities.[51]

Hips/flanks

As mentioned earlier in this chapter, the authors prefer to treat the hips and in the prone position, as this position allows for simultaneous treatment of both sides and for comparison. This is a common area of suctioning in males and females and is accessible through the bilateral or single midline paraspinous region and/or an incision in the lateral gluteal fold. This is determined by the location of the fat. On very rare occasions, in patients with only lateral fullness, treatment can be adequately perform in the supine position with the patient rotated. Suctioning in this area can provide excellent results, and all modalities have proven effective. The fat is loose and in some cases fibrous, with thick overlying skin. Significant striae may be seen in patients with weight fluctuations or in postpartum women. Liposuction in these patients may reduce the lipodystrophy but may result in superficial contour irregularities or skin redundancy. When performing liposuction of the hips and flanks, knowledge of the differing aesthetic consideration of the hips and flanks in males and females is crucial to preventing inappropriate masculinization or feminization. In general, males tend to have fullness in the superior and lateral region, while females usually exhibit prominence more inferiorly and posteriorly *(Fig. 24.17)*.[53] In

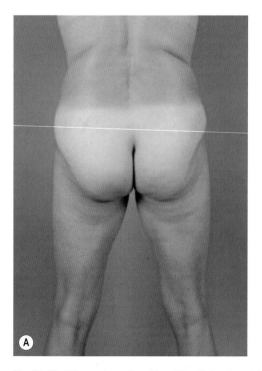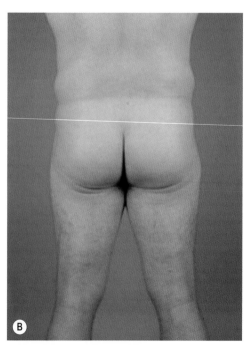

Fig. 24.17 Difference in configuration of the **(A)** female and **(B)** male hip region.

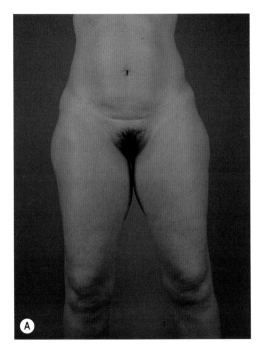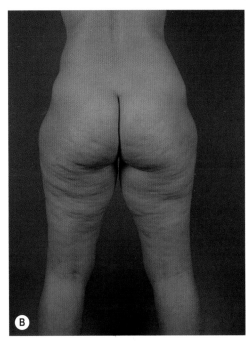

Fig. 24.18 The violin deformity may require fat grafting to the zone of depression in addition to liposuction of the surrounding areas of excess fullness.

male patients the term *flank* describes an area immediately superior and posterior to the iliac crest. It begins in the paraspinous area and enlarges as it expands laterally. Anteriorly, the flank blends with the tissue of the lower abdomen. The inferior margin is defined by the zone of adherence along the iliac crest. In contrast, the female hip is located more inferiorly and typically centered over the posterior iliac crest. The hip extends down to the level of the lateral greater trochanteric adherent zone. The fat in this region is typically loose but fibrous as it becomes more superficial due to the thickness of the overlying dermis. It is essential to mark the lateral gluteal depression prior to liposuction, as violation of this important area can lead to either a persistent or exacerbated, irregular contour and deformity. Often, this adherent zone is a landmark to which both the hips and lateral thighs are reduced. In some patients, this area may represent an area of significant depression and may benefit from autologous fat transfer *(Fig. 24.18)*.

Access to the hip and flank can be achieved via two inferiorly placed lateral paraspinous incisions that are easily concealed by undergarments or bathing suits. With more laterally displaced lipodystrophy, incisions may be moved more laterally. In contrast, patients with more posteriorly oriented fat may be adequately treated through a lower midline access incision. This may be moved more superiorly if the fat overlies the area of the inferior-posterior costal margin. Alternatively, the area overlying the distal, posterior costal margin can be approached from a "bra-line" access site in patients undergoing back contouring. The midline incision typically does not heal as well as paraspinous incisions and thus should be discussed with the patient. The lateral gluteal fold access incision may also contour the more inferior portion of the hip/flank, which allows for a nice blending between the lateral thigh and hip/flank area. This incision, in combination with a single midline access site, allows for effective

contouring and avoidance of incisions overlying the buttock area, which may have a tendency to dimple. However, caution should be used when contouring via the lateral gluteal fold incision, as overzealous resection through the trochanteric adherent zone has a high likelihood of resulting in a contour deformity.[4,51]

Buttocks

The buttock area must also be approached with caution. There are widely varying ideals on the appearance of an aesthetically pleasing buttock. These change with time and vary across age groups, ethnicity, and geography. It is important to discuss preoperatively, the expectations and outcomes desired from a patient requesting buttock contouring/liposuction. A uniform reduction of the buttock can be achieved through cautious treatment of the intermediate layer resulting in a decrease in buttock projection in an anterior/posterior dimension. Access incisions are placed asymmetrically, to avoid an operated look. Avoiding deep, aggressive suctioning and ensuring the length, position, and integrity of the inferior gluteal crease is of critical importance. Overzealous treatment in the deep or superficial plane may result in buttock ptosis.[53] This area is most easily accessed via paraspinous or gluteal access incisions. These should be well concealed by clothing and/or bathing suits. Additionally, excessive contouring of the lateral proximal posterior thigh may result in an extension of the gluteal fold in the female patient and masculinization of the gluteal area *(Fig. 24.19)*. Often patients requesting buttock contouring actually desire increased shape and projection and will require augmentation and or fat transfer. This should be discussed thoroughly in the preoperative evaluation to ensure both the patient and operating surgeon's expectations are identical. Augmentation of the buttock with a variety of techniques is covered in Chapter 28.

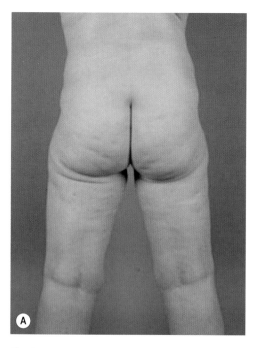 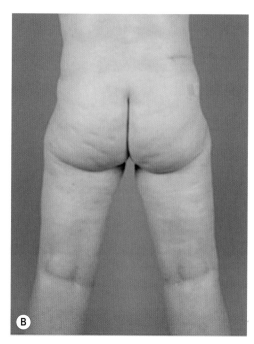

Fig. 24.19 Masculinization of the female buttock.

Thighs

Males and females have varied distributions of fat in the thigh region. Women tend to accumulate the fat either in a diffuse, circumferential manner or in significant amounts medial and lateral. Cellulite may also be seen in women, as are superficial irregularities and preoperative contour problems. In general, men tend to accumulate more compact fat in the proximal thighs. The fatty layer tends to be more fibrous. The dense fibroconnective tissue tends to prevent extensive superficial contour irregularities and cellulite. It should be noted that these are generalizations and any patient can present with either diffuse or focal accumulations of lipodystrophy and the operating physician should thoroughly evaluate with exam and photographs. Common terms for deformities related to the thigh and hips include: *saddlebag* (a trochanteric bulge lateral to gluteal crease); *banana roll* (preoperative or postoperative roll inferior to the gluteal fold), and *violin deformity* (female contour of narrow waist, full hips, full lateral thighs, and depression in the zone of adherence between the hips and thighs).

Cellulite is very common in the thigh region and may be the presenting complaint of some patients; this needs to be addressed early with patients. Informed consent should include the fact that cellulite will not improve with suctioning, may worsen and that no improvement in superficial contour irregularities is possible with liposuction. To date, there are no published studies suggesting a treatment modality for cellulite.

In many instances, patients undergoing contouring of the thigh are best suited for a circumferential approach in the prone/supine position.[3,4,51] Although patients may present with an isolated medial or lateral deformity, we have found this less common in our patient population. The degree of contouring of specific regions of the thigh is dependent on the analysis and needs of each patient. The adherent areas of the thigh to recognize include: the gluteal crease; the lateral gluteal depression; the posterior, inferior, and distal lateral thigh; and the area of the mid-inner thigh *(Fig. 24.2)*.[6]

Lateral and posterior thighs

Suctioning the lateral thigh is done in the prone position or occasionally the lateral decubitus position.

The prone position allows the operating physician to work both sides and assess for symmetry. Incisions are often placed in the lateral gluteal crease. Occasionally, a patient may benefit from a midlateral incision. The lateral thigh is amenable to all forms of liposuction; both the intermediate and deep planes can be suctioned. The lateral thigh is likely the site of the most contour irregularities in our experience; the visibility of the lateral thigh as well as the possibility for skin laxity contribute to this. Extreme caution is advised in the superficial plane for fear of worsening preexisting contour irregularities. Commonly cannulas in the 3.0–4.6 range are used for lateral thigh suctioning. Often final contouring or transitioning from lateral to anteriorly is performed in the supine position to remove any "shelf" that may exist following the prone position.

Suctioning the posterior thigh should be approached with caution. In many patients, the skin is adherent to the underlying tissues with a paucity of fatty tissue. Overzealous suctioning in this area results in loss of the adherent zone and rolling and redundancy of the skin. Special care should be taken when addressing the proximal posterior thigh. Problems in this area can be very difficult to correct, requiring either autologous fat transfer or skin excision. In females overtreatment of this area may elongate the gluteal fold, masculinizing the female silhouette. Suctioning of the lateral thigh and posterior thigh is easily facilitated via the previously described lateral gluteal fold access incision and or a more medial gluteal fold access incision.[53]

Medial

The medial thigh is the most unpredictable and difficult area to treat in our view. Patients often present with complaints of legs rubbing together when walking, or difficulty with clothing in the medial upper thigh. Fat in the medial thigh is loose and soft and the overlying skin is thin and often lax.[51] The plane of suctioning is intermediate fat, and smaller cannulas such as 3.0 and 2.4 are generally utilized. This area can be treated in both the prone and supine position together or supine with legs "frogged". Realistic expectations must be established with the patient and certainly the possibility of skin redundancy or laxity should be reviewed.

Anterior thigh

The anterior thigh is characterized by compact fat of limited thickness. Patients often have more fullness proximally compared with the distal anterior thigh. Contouring of this area helps eliminate step off or transition points from the medial and lateral thighs and helps decrease the projection of the thigh in the posterior to anterior view. The anterior medial thigh can often be addressed through the same access site as the medial thigh. Laterally, we often make an accessory access incision on the proximal anterior thigh. Fine cannulas should be used in this area as it is compact and fairly thin. Irregularities can occur frequently in inexperienced hands.

Knees/ankles

Lipodystrophy around the knees is usually confined to the areas of medial and anterior leg. Treatment is relatively straightforward with small stab incisions to obtain easy access. The posterior knee should be avoided. Suctioning proceeds with small cannulas in the supine positioning/frog-leg position. There is often a tendency to over-resect the medial knee and not address the anterior portion; visualization is the best way to determine the end point. Volume is usually small. The goal of contouring in this region should be to help improve and taper the distal thigh.

The treatment of the calves and ankles remains challenging and requires more prolonged recovery. Patients may complain of a lack of definition and poor tapering from the bulkier calf to the ankle. Patients must be aware of the increased morbidity associated with treatment of this region. Specifically, contour irregularities are much more common and difficult to correct. In our experience, treatment of this region doubles the recovery time of liposuction (from 3 to 6 months). Small, fine cannulas are essential, utilizing multiple access sites to decrease the risk for access site deformities.[51]

Neck

Patients with minimal to mild skin laxity and lipodystrophy of the neck may be candidates for liposuction of this region. All liposuction devices may be used in this region, but care must be taken to avoid contour irregularities, skin injury, and nerve injuries.

The patient is positioned with their neck hyper-extended with a shoulder roll or pill beneath the upper back. For centralized lipodystrophy a single submental access incision may be used. For most, lateral access with a lobular incision allows for transitioning laterally.

An appropriate amount of wetting solution should be placed and ample time utilized to allow for the epinephrine effect. Direct subdermal suctioning should be avoided. In our hands, key pinch is the critical endpoint allowing for symmetry. Continuous assessment of contour is important. Overzealous treatment of this area may result in hallowing and skeletonizing the neck or potential neurapraxia of the marginal mandibular nerve.[54,55] Fortunately, this usually resolves within a few weeks.

Postoperative care

At the conclusion of surgery, liposuction patients are placed in a compression garment which is customized based on surgeon preference and procedure performed. Some type of compression foam) may also be used under the garment for the first week to assist in contouring; this also helps diminish bruising and edema in our hands. In our practice, patients who have undergone any large-volume procedure (>5000 mL aspirate), liposuction of multiple areas, or liposuction in addition to abdominoplasty or other excisional body contouring procedure are kept overnight for 23-h observation.[53] Patients are asked to ambulate the day of the surgery, and sequential compression devices are placed on the patient in the preoperative holding area and continued until discharge. Patients are allowed to shower as early as 1 or 2 days postoperatively and are instructed to keep the compression garment on 24 h a day for 2 weeks. The patient may remove the compression garments for bathing. Initial postoperative visits are scheduled for 5–7 days postoperatively; return to activity/work can occur as early as 3–4 days or at 2 weeks, depending on the procedure. Walking is encouraged immediately, and light activity is allowed 2 weeks after surgery, unless the patient has undergone an associated abdominoplasty or other invasive procedure. Patients should expect to initially gain some weight after liposuction due to volume shifts and postoperative swelling. Edema tends to peak from 3 to 5 days after surgery. Bruising should be minimal and dissipate by 7–10 days after surgery. Patients should begin to see contour changes in their waist by 2 weeks and at 6 weeks, be able to appreciate significant changes in their shape. As patients' activity level improve and necessary lifestyle changes proceed, further changes may be noticed. The final aesthetic result can be seen 3–6 months after surgery, depending on the patient. These postoperative volume changes and swelling are often a source of angst for patients and are best discussed in the preoperative consultation to alleviate any post-surgical complaints/worries and allow for appropriate patient expectations. Postoperative lymphatic massage is encouraged to help with swelling and induration and is often started prior to surgery and resumed shortly after the procedure.

Complications

Although viewed by many people as a simple and benign procedure, liposuction, especially large volume liposuction, can be associated with significant morbidity and should be performed by appropriately trained physicians. Much attention has been directed toward outcomes and prevention in the

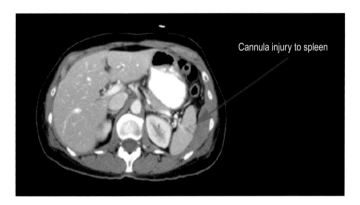

Fig. 24.20 CT scan showing a canula injury to the spleen.

past few years, with the ultimate goal of improved results while maintaining patient safety. Complications can vary from mild postoperative nausea and vomiting to deep venous thrombosis (DVT)/pulmonary embolism (PE) and even death. Postoperative complications occur in three different windows. These are: the perioperative period (0–48 h); early postoperative period (days 1–7), and late postoperative period (1 week to 3 months). In a questionnaire to board-certified members of the American Society for Aesthetic Plastic Surgery, a significant increase in complications was observed when liposuction was combined with other contouring procedures, most notably when paired with abdominoplasty.[56] Perioperative complications can include anesthesia and cardiac complications, cannula trauma to skin and/or internal organs, and volume loss/overload from bleeding or excess fluid administration. Cannula injury to blood vessels, bowel and other solid intra-abdominal organs have been reported in the literature.[53] Although rare, these complications are related to incomplete preoperative examination (hernia) and overaggressive suctioning or penetration by the infiltration cannula (*Fig. 24.20*).

Liposuction surgery, especially when it involves multiple areas, places the patient at risk for hypothermia. Hypothermia is generally defined as a core body temperature of <36.4°C. In anesthetized patients, the pathophysiology of hypothermia is related to an inter-threshold shift in thermoregulation. Its risk is amplified in larger volume cases, where a greater surface area of the patient is exposed at one time and patients are under anesthesia longer. Studies have shown the core body temperature can drop up to 2.8°C in the first hours of surgery as a result of the anesthesia effect on autonomic regulation of core temperature.[57] Preventative measures include warming of the wetting solutions and prep, increase of the ambient room temperature, and use of preoperative and intraoperative warming devices (Bair Hugger®, Arizant, Eden Prairie, MN). Prewarming the patient with forced air for 1 h has also been shown to significantly reduce the incidence of hypothermia and should be considered, particularly for longer body contouring cases and those involving multiple areas.

In the perioperative period, fluid shifts occur, which if improperly managed can lead to hypovolemia or volume overload. As a general rule, we require our patients to obtain preoperative medical clearance when they are over 50 years of age or have any concomitant risk factors, such as cardiopulmonary disease. As stated previously, careful management

of intraoperative and postoperative fluids, as well as use of an intraoperative data sheet[58], helps prevent volume-related complications from liposuction. The tumescent liposuction technique has been implicated in volume overload and pulmonary edema; however, this can often be attributed to incorrect patient selection and/or poor fluid management.[59,60] Fluid overload and untoward sequelae from large-volume liposuction (>5 L) prompted a warning by the American Society of Plastic Surgeons that physicians performing liposuction should be trained in comprehensive fluid resuscitation and the physiology of large-volume liposuction.[61]

Other early postoperative complications can include venous thromboembolism, infection, and skin necrosis. The incidence of DVT in liposuction has been reported at <1%, but a marked increase in this percentage is demonstrated when liposuction is combined with other surgery (abdominoplasty/belt lipectomy).[62] Physicians should familiarize themselves with the American College of Chest Physicians (ACCP) current recommendations and a scoring system to assess risk such as the UT Southwestern Modification of the Davison–Caprini Risk Assessment model currently available.[13,62,63] Administration of enoxaparin has resulted in a decreased incidence of DVT, but has been associated with an increased risk of perioperative bleeding and hematoma.[62] Classical clinical signs such as lower extremity swelling, Homan's signs, shortness of breath, chest pain, and/or tachycardia should alert the provider to the possibility of DVT/PE and warrant immediate evaluation and treatment (*Table 24.6*).

Wound infections, including necrotizing fasciitis are serious complications known to occur in lipsuction.[64] Fortunately, they are rare. Complaints of persistent postoperative fevers and/or cellulitis should be closely monitored and aggressively treated. As a preventative measure, first-generation cephalosporins are administered perioperatively within 30 min of the incision unless the patient has a known history of methicillin-resistant *Staphylococcus aureus* (MRSA), in which case vancomycin is administered preoperatively. There is no indication for routine postoperative antibiotics after the perioperative dose in standard liposuction.

Late complications of liposuction include delayed seroma formation, edema and ecchymosis, paresthesias, hyperpigmentation, and contour irregularities. Seromas following aggressive liposuction are rare and thought to be secondary to overzealous treatment of an area, which denudes the fascia. It appears to be technique-dependent rather than technology specific. A loose closure of cannula sites, postoperative compression garments, and expressing residual fluid over liposuction areas at the end of procedure all can potentially reduce the incidence of seroma formation.[53] Postoperative edema and ecchymosis occur to a varying extent, in all patients. Prolonged edema can occur up to 3 months post-surgery and is best treated with supportive care and lymphatic massage. Significant ecchymoses may result in hemosiderin deposition and ultimately hyperpigmentation. This can be challenging to eliminate. Postoperative paresthesia/dysesthesia can occur in all forms of liposuction. The sensory changes are usually reversible and can take up to 10 weeks to recover, but recovery is generally felt to be quicker with SAL than with UAL.[65] There is no current data addressing the sensory changes associated with new technology or laser-assisted liposuction.

With regards to aesthetic outcomes, the most common late postoperative complication from liposuction is contour

Table 24.6 UT Southwestern modification of Davison–Caprini model[62]

Step I: Exposing risk factors

1 Factor	2 Factors	3 Factors	5 Factors
Minor surgery	Major surgery (general anesthesia or time >1 h)	Previous MI/CHF	Hip/pelvis/leg fracture
	Immobilization	Severe sepsis	Stroke
	Central venous access	Free flap	Multiple trauma
	BMI >30	Circumferential abdominoplasty	

Step II: Predisposing factors

Clinical setting (factors)	Inherited (factors)	Acquired (factors)
Age 40–60 (1)	Any genetic hypercoagulable state (3)	Lupus anticoagulant (3)
Age >60 (2)		Antiphospholipid antibody (3)
History DVT/PE (3)		Myeloproliferative disorder (3)
Pregnancy (1)		HIT (3)
Malignancy (2)		Homocystinemia (3)
OCP/HRT therapy (2)		Hyperviscosity (3)
Total of Step I and Step II:_____		

Step III: Orders

1 Factor	Low risk	Ambulate TID
2 Factors	Moderate risk	Intermittent pneumatic compression device and elastic compression stocking on patient at all times while not ambulating
3 Factors	High risk	Intermittent pneumatic compression device and elastic compression stocking on patient at all times while not ambulating
>4 Factors	Highest risk	Intermittent pneumatic compression device and elastic compression stocking on patient at all times while not ambulating + Lovenox 40 mg SQ daily postoperative

(Data from Hatef DA, Kenkel JM, Nguyen MQ, et al. Thromboembolic risks assessment and the efficacy of Enoxaparin prophylaxis in excisional body contouring surgery. *Plast Reconstr Surg.* 2008;122(1):269–279.)

deformity or irregularities. Up to 20% of patients can present or will complain of some sort of contour irregularity.[66,67] Mild irregularities are often present after suctioning and are treated conservatively with lymphatic massage as swelling and edema resolve. Once a contour deformity is identified, it is best to define the etiology. Blind suctioning of the surrounding areas is not often the correct treatment and can significantly worsen the problem. Once a proper assessment of the etiology is made, then treatment can either be directed at re-injecting the fat in the over-resected region or suctioning the adjacent areas in order to reduce the prominence of the concavity and blending the adjacent areas. The most comprehensive data on treating contour deformity is from Chang, where he presents a multimodality approach to assessing and treating contour deformity to achieve long-term results.[66,67] UAL has a decreased incidence of contour deformities versus traditional SAL in our hands. It is the preferred method for secondary liposuction cases in which fat grafting is not indicated. Careful preoperative analysis, planning, and proper informed consent all help to minimize the risk of postoperative contour irregularity.

Emerging technology

The noninvasive dissolution of fat is an extremely attractive concept for patients. Many new technologies are being developed to facilitate this, with varied reports of success. The earliest version was "mesotherapy" or "lipolysis", an evolving technology, the goal of which is a reduction in fat by dissolution.[68] The concept dates back to 1952 and involves injection of phosphatidylcholine, deoxycholate, and/or other agents which are purported to dissolve fat. Widespread marketing and patient desire to avoid anesthesia have allowed mesotherapy and its variants to gain popularity because of their "noninvasive" nature. However, large scale studies are not available for evaluation. Park *et al.*[69] showed no discernible difference in the treatment in lower extremities with mesotherapy by measurement or CT scan evaluation.

"Lipodissolve" is considered by some, but not all, practitioners to be a variant of mesotherapy. It is the injection of a standardized solution into the subcutaneous fat, rather than the mesoderm. The use of these products in the United Sates is controversial and not supported by the US Food and Drug Administration (FDA). Warnings from the FDA caution providers against its unproven use and false marketing claim.[70] Several studies on safety and efficacy are available for review. Common side-effects reported include hyperpigmentation and persistent pain, and 12% of patients had cosmetic outcomes that were less favorable than expected.[71] Due to lack of scientific data and adequate studies and outcome results, the use of mesotherapy or its variants is not currently recommended, unless performed in conjunction with a clinical trial.

'Low level laser therapy' has recently emerged as a treatment for lipodystrophy. This is considered an "off label" use of this technology. It involves a low level laser therapy done in conjunction with a modest diet and exercise regimen. The application is percutaneous and reportedly painless. There is a single randomized controlled double blind study reporting reduction in lipodystrophy circumference.[72] No further studies or long-term data is available on the efficacy of low level leaser therapy at this time.

Noninvasive fat removal with ultrasound technology has received significant attention. The focused external ultrasound therapy is one of the most popular fat reducing technologies currently being evaluated and has considerable popularity in Israel, Spain, and Japan. There are currently two competing technologies attempting fat destruction by thermally or nonthermally ultrasound-mediated (via cavitation) mechanisms. There is no "evacuation" phase and the technology relies primarily on fat removal by the body's own phagocytic mechanisms. The 'UltraShape' device is a nonthermally mediated (cavitation) mechanism and is currently being marketed outside of the United States. Preliminary data by Brown *et al.*[73] have shown it to be effective in treatment in a preclinical porcine model, in which the UltraShape device was target specific for the adipocyte, preserving the surrounding neurovasculature. Clinical studies have validated its safety.[74] At the time of this publication, the company is performing a multicenter, prospective, randomized, blinded study evaluating its safety and efficacy.

'LipoSonix' technology uses high-intensity focused ultrasound (HIFU) to disrupt fat in a thermally mediated mechanism. The device is currently undergoing clinical trials outside of the United States and also is being marketed in Europe. LipoSonix disrupts fat via a thermocoagulation mediated mechanism (versus UltraShape, which acts via cavitation, causing disruption of fat cell membrane). LipoSonix is currently being marketed outside of the United States. Neither the UltraShape nor LipoSonix is FDA approved or available in the US.

Liposuction combined with radiofrequency ablation of fat cells is currently being investigated under the trade name 'BodyTite' (New York). The purported benefits are thermal destruction of fat cells, removal via aspiration cannula, and sub-necrotic heating of the dermis for skin tightening. This device is not currently approved by the FDA.[75]

'Cryolipolysis' is a new and vastly different technology currently being evaluated for fat destruction under the trade name 'Zeltiq' (Pleasanton, CA). The concept is a controlled cooling of the subcutaneous fat, with destruction of selective fat cells without epidermal or dermal injury. It is undergoing use within the United States.[76–79]

We firmly believe that nonsurgical body contouring will be validated and ultimately approved in many different forms in the upcoming years. We do not believe it will replace liposuction but will be another option that appropriate patients may choose. It is important to keep in mind until adequate scientific validation of these novel devices is performed outside of manufacturer influence any discussion of potential benefit is strictly advertisement and market driven. As new technology is continually being introduced, we must temper our enthusiasm and base treatment on solid, scientific evidence. Device manufacturers often provide scant, if any, objective data to support claims such as skin tightening, reduced pain, and improved aesthetic results.

Conclusion

Over the past three decades, the procedure of liposuction has evolved and become consistently one of the most popular cosmetic procedures performed around the world. As evidenced by the large numbers of devices in clinical development and active clinical use, there remains a duty by the clinician to monitor not only the safety of the device but also the true efficacy. Although touted as a relatively simple procedure, the process of liposuction/liposculpture is as much an art as science. As such, the physician must understand the pathophysiology of both the patient and disease process in order to effectively treat the patient and achieve safe and aesthetically pleasing results. The authors are confident that liposuction will remain one of the most popular procedures performed in the years to come, and we must thus remain committed to the common goals of patient safety and improved aesthetic outcomes.

Bonus images for this chapter can be found online at
http://www.expertconsult.com

Fig. 24.9 The intraoperative data sheet records essential information from the operative procedure.
Fig. 24.13 Liposonix ultrasonic liposuction machine.
Fig. 24.14 The Vaser system.

 Access the complete references list online at **http://www.expertconsult.com**

1. Illouz YG. History and current concepts of lipoplasty. *Clin Plast Surg.* 1996;23:721.

3. Lockwood TE. Superficial fascial system (SFS) of the trunk and extremities: a new concept. *Plast Reconstr Surg.* 1991;87(6):1009–1018.

This landmark paper describes anatomical studies detailing the anatomy of the SFS. The findings of this report form the basis for widely accepted surgical strategies in body contouring.

6. Rohrich RJ, Smith PD, Marcantonio DR, et al. The zones of adherence: role in minimizing and preventing

contour deformities in liposuction. *Plast Reconstr Surg.* 2001;107(6):1562–1569.

9. Rohrich RJ, Broughton 2nd G, Horton JB, et al. The key to long term success in liposuction: A guide for plastic surgeons and patients. *Plast Reconstr Surg.* 2004;114: 1945–1952.

10. Kenkel JM, Lipschitz AH, Luby M, et al. Hemodynamic physiology and thermoregulation in liposuction. *Plast Reconstr Surg.* 2004;114(2):503–513.

Hemodynamic parameters during large-volume liposuction procedures were assessed. Metrics generally remained within safe ranges, but low body temperature was uniformly observed.

15. Iverson RE, Lynch DJ, and the ASPS Committee on Patient Safety. Practice advisory on liposuction. *Plast Reconstr Surg.* 2004;113(5):1478–1490.

This document represents the findings of the ASPS's Committee on Patient Safety with regards to liposuction.

20. Rohrich RJ, Beran SJ, Fodor PB. The role of subcutaneous infiltration in suction-assisted lipoplasty: a review. *Plast Reconstr Surg.* 1997;99:514.

22. Klein JA. Tumescent technique for regional anesthesia permits lidocaine doses of 35 mg/kg for liposuction. *Dermatol Surg Oncol.* 1990;16(3):248–263.

This paper addressees the pharmacokinetics that permit the use of high concentrations of lidocaine in tumescent liposuction. Tumescent liposuction is advocated as sustained analgesia and minimal blood loss are achieved with this technique.

34. Rohrich RJ, Raniere J Jr, Beran SJ, et al. Patient evaluation and indications for ultrasound-assisted lipoplasty. *Clin Plast Surg.* 1999;26(2): 269–278; viii.

36. Rohrich RJ, Leedy JE, Swamy R, et al. Fluid resuscitation in liposuction: a retrospective review of 89 consecutive cases. *Plast Reconstr Surg.* 2006;117(2): 431–435.

56. Hughes 3rd CE. Reduction of lipoplasty risks and mortality: an ASAPS survey. *Aesthet Surg J.* 2001;21:120.

This survey was designed to examine changes ASAPS member surgeons have made in response to the 1998 recommendations from the 1998 Lipoplasty Task Force. A major complication rate of 0.2602% and a mortality rate of 0.0021% were reported.

57. Young VL, Watson ME. Prevention of perioperative hypothermia in plastic surgery. *Aesthet Surg J.* 2006;26:551–571.

25

Abdominoplasty procedures

Dirk F. Richter and Alexander Stoff

SYNOPSIS

- The abdominal area is the one of the most common areas treated in plastic surgery procedures. Mostly after pregnancies or weight changes, patients desire improvement of the abdominal wall, including the repair of additional ventral hernias.

- Assessment of the abdominal region includes a detailed medical and physical history, including pregnancies, prior surgeries especially in the lower truncal area, and weight changes. Preoperative identification of any existing ventral hernia including diastasis recti is imperative.

- Essential issues of abdominal findings are the existence and localization of vertical and horizontal tissue excess, the relation of fatty and skin excess, the examination of the umbilical stalk with exclusion of umbilical hernia. Further perioperative issues are preoperative bowel evacuation for reduction of intraabdominal pressure, careful intraoperative handling, maintenance of an adequate body temperature, sufficient medical thromboembolism prophylaxis, precise intraoperative preparation with respect to anatomical key points, postoperative compression treatment and early management of postoperative complications such as seromas.

- The "fleur-de-lis" abdominoplasty allows an improvement of the entire abdominal area with simultaneous tightening of the waist circumference. It is essential to initially assess and temporarily close the vertical line prior to resection of the lower abdominal redundant tissue. Care should be taken to avoid extending the vertical incision line cranially between the breasts.

- In patients with massive weight loss (MWL), aesthetic outcome will improve by high-lateral-tension and fleur-de-lis abdominoplasty, and in most cases, circumferential truncal procedures are necessary for superior results.

- The preparation epifascial to the Scarpa fascia allows a preservation of subfascial lymphatic vessels for prevention of seroma formation and enables an additional tightening of Scarpa fascia for improvement of the inner thigh region.

- It is mandatory to analyze any suspected skin tumor in the area of excised tissue.

Access the Historical Perspective section and Figure 25.1 online at
http://www.expertconsult.com

Introduction

Abdominoplasty is one of the most commonly performed aesthetic procedures, which encompasses not only aesthetic features but also structural reconstruction of the abdominal wall. Aesthetic enhancements include improvement in abdominal wall contour, reconstruction of a natural appearing umbilicus and optimal placement of the resulting abdominal scar. The reconstructive component includes recreation of the original fascial and muscular anatomy as well as the restoration of any other anatomical deformations, which may be present.

The primary goals in abdominoplasty procedures are to achieve an optimal resection of abdominal skin and subcutaneous tissue in a three-dimensional manner, with a resulting wound tension that is distant from the area of tissue resection; the purpose of keeping wound tension distant from the resection is to prevent an impairment of perfusion. In addition, the abdominal musculoaponeurotic layer should be restored to prevent abdominal hernias, diastasis and consequent muscular imbalance of the trunk, while at the same time, improving the abdominal wall contour.

Due to the number of variations and modifications of abdominoplasties, it is key to select the appropriate technique in every individual case, determining the best procedure by minimizing morbidity and postoperative disability for desirable and predictable results.[1]

Anatomy

Knowledge of the anatomy of the abdominal wall is essential for aesthetic and reconstructive abdominal procedures. The abdominal wall is embryonically derived in a segmental manner, reflected in blood supply and innervation. The formation of the abdominal wall is initiated by the transition of the embryo from a trilaminar disk to a three-dimensional structure on the 22nd day of gestation. The further intrauterine development of the abdominal wall has multiple crucial stages, which can lead to congenital defects of the abdominal wall. After separation of the umbilical cord the abdominal wall becomes a definitive structure.

Abdominal skin and fat tend to be distributed in the lower abdomen with aging and pregnancy. Especially as a result of multiple pregnancies, striae become common, resulting in a rupture and separation of dermal collagen with consequent skin thinning.[18] At this time, the therapy of striae is exclusively by surgical excision *(Fig. 25.2)*.

The umbilicus

As one of the most visible and aesthetically recognized landmarks of the abdominal wall, the umbilicus is situated in the midline, approximately 9–12 cm above the top of the mons pubis. The periumbilical area is characterized by a round or ellipsoid shape with a slight depression of 4–6 cm in diameter. The fascia surrounding the umbilicus can be unstable with an increased incidence for hernias, resulting in a risk of bowel injury during umbilical dissection. The blood supply to the periumbilical area is supplied by branches from the subdermal plexus, from both deep inferior epigastric arteries as well as a blood supply from the median umbilical ligament.

Skin, muscle, and fascia

The skin of the abdomen has areas of increased adherence to the underlying fascia ("zones of adherence"), such as the anterior superior iliac crest and the linea alba. The abdominal subcutaneous tissue is divided by two layers of fascia, the superficial Camper's fascia and the deep Scarpa's fascia, a strong fibrous layer of connective tissue, which is continuous with the fascia lata of the thigh.[19]

The superficial fat layer has a more compact character, with smaller lobules and a rich vascularization, while the deeper fat layer contains larger lobules with a more scattered pattern.

Since patients presenting for abdominal wall surgery often have musculoaponeurotic laxity, the knowledge of these anatomical structures is crucial. The abdominal musculature includes four paired muscles, which are the rectus abdominis, connected in the median linea alba, the external oblique and internal oblique and the transversus abdominis muscle, which incorporate into the anterior and posterior rectus sheath at the linea semilunaris. The rectus abdominis muscles are enclosed by an anterior and posterior sheath, originating at the infracostal margin and attaching at the symphysis pubis. Above the arcuate line (or semicircular line of Douglas, situated approximately midway between umbilicus and pubic symphysis), the anterior rectus sheath is formed by the external oblique and internal oblique aponeurosis, while the posterior rectus sheath is formed by the internal oblique and transversus aponeurosis. Below the arcuate line, the posterior rectus sheath is absent, except for the transversus fascia and the peritoneum, which are found posteriorly. At the inferior aspect of the rectus muscles, the pyramidalis muscles are present in 80–90% of patients *(Fig. 25.3)*.

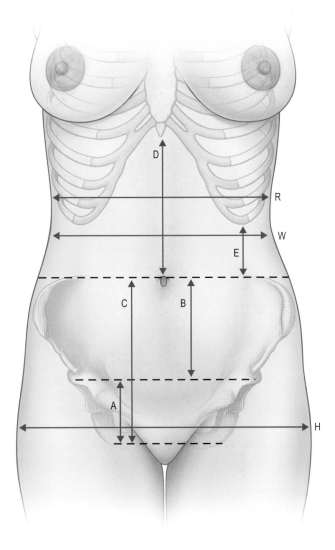

Fig. 25.2 Anatomical landmarks. Normal abdominal anatomic proportions. The approximate measurements for an average female abdomen are listed. These vary according to individual height and bone structure. The umbilicus is located in line with the most superior point of the iliac crest in 99% of patients. **(A)** Distance between top of mons and anterior valvar commissure. Average height is 5–7 cm. **(B)** Distance between umbilicus and top of mons. Average height is 11–13 cm. **(C) = (A + B)** Distance between umbilicus and top of anterior and vulvar commissure **(C = D)**. **(E)** Distance between the costal marginal and the iliac crest. The proportion of this distance to the width of the base of the rib cage **(R)** determines whether the patient is long waisted or short waisted. The normal proportion (E : R) is roughly 1 : 3 (long waisted approaches 1 : 2, short waisted approaches 1 : 3).The rib cage tapers inferiorly. A narrower lower rib cage relative to the width under the armpits helps to emphasize the waist by creating a subtle V. **(H)** Hip width. A wider pelvis than rib cage emphasizes the waist; the waist is more defined when R<H. **(W)** Natural waist – the narrowest point of the torso. (Note that the umbilicus usually sits below the natural waist by about 1–4 cm). Relative to the hips, this waist-to-hip (W : H) ratio in healthy women is roughly 0.72 : 1; in healthy men, it is roughly 0.83 : 1. Note that the natural contour of the healthy abdomen reveals a subtle epigastric sagittal depression transitioning to a mild infraumbilical convexity. A subtle vertical sulcus at 'eh' lateral rectus border, which is more distinct in a muscular person, may also be seen.

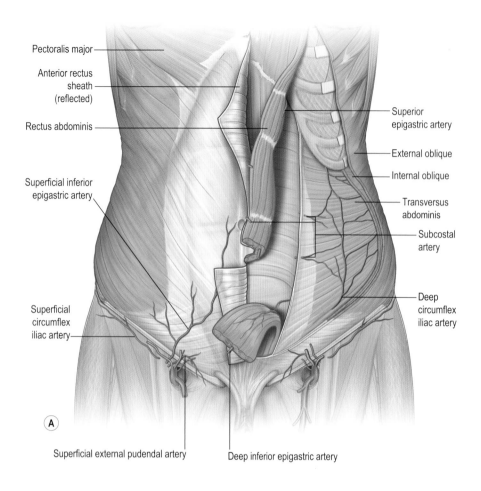

Pectoralis major

Anterior rectus sheath (reflected)

Rectus abdominis

Superficial inferior epigastric artery

Superficial circumflex iliac artery

Superior epigastric artery

External oblique

Internal oblique

Transversus abdominis

Subcostal artery

Deep circumflex iliac artery

(A)

Superficial external pudendal artery

Deep inferior epigastric artery

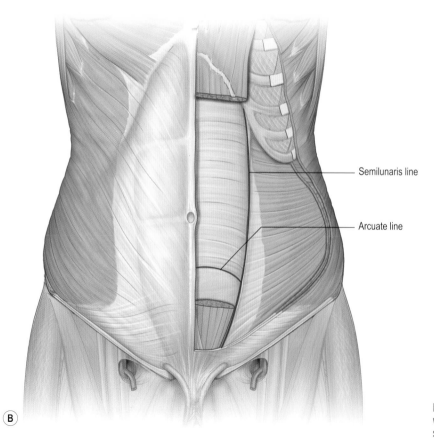

Semilunaris line

Arcuate line

(B)

Fig. 25.3 (A) Anatomy of the musculature of the abdominal wall with arterial supply. **(B)** Arcuate line and linea semilunaris.

The correction of frequently accompanying rectus diastasis with consequent muscular imbalance is an important step in abdominal wall surgery in order to avoid back complaints.

Lymphatic system

The lymph vessels collect the subdermal accumulated lymph fluid and drain into the deeper fat layer, passing into larger vessels. The abdominal lymphatic system is divided into supraumbilical drainage into the ipsilateral axillary lymph nodes and infraumbilical drainage into the superficial inguinal lymph nodes. The lymph vessels in the infraumbilical area pass through the sub-scarpal plane, explaining the importance of Scarpa's fascia preservation in abdominal wall surgery.[18]

Blood supply

The blood supply to the abdominal wall comes from numerous major arteries of the thorax and pelvic region, which communicate through many anastomotic interconnections. Taylor and Palmer introduced the concept of angiosomes, or vascular territories of the body.[20] They describe two types of cutaneous blood supply: (1) direct vessels that directly supply the skin and (2) indirect vessels that "emerge from the deep fascia as terminal spent branches of arteries whose main purpose is to supply the muscles and other deep tissues." In a subsequent study in 1988, Moon and Taylor were able to demonstrate connections between the deep superior and deep inferior epigastric systems and their relationship to the cutaneous circulation.[21–23]

A detailed knowledge of the arterial supply of the abdominal wall is important for abdominal wall surgery, especially in cases of prior abdominal or chest wall surgeries. Huger described different zones of the abdominal blood supply, which should guide the surgeon in planning and performing a safe operation *(Fig. 25.4)*.[22] Huger defined zone I of the abdominal wall as the area that is fed anteriorly by the vertically oriented deep epigastric arcade. Zone III was defined as the lateral aspect of the abdominal wall (flanks) that are fed by the six lateral intercostal and four lumbar arteries. The lower abdominal circulation is provided by the superficial epigastric, superficial external pudendal, and superficial circumflex iliac systems (zone II). A rich plexus between these systems allows collateral flow.

In standard abdominoplasty procedures, after mobilization of the abdominal flap in the lower abdominal area and midline region up to the xiphoid, the cutaneous blood supply to zone

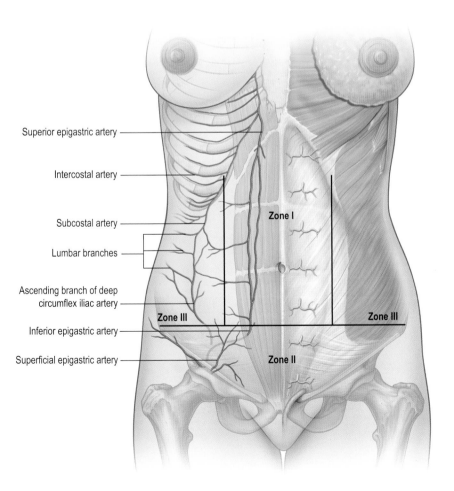

Fig. 25.4 Zones of blood supply.[22]

I and a main part of zone II is disrupted, resulting in an abdominal flap perfusion mainly supplied by zone III. Since the mobilized abdominal flap is dependent on the lateral perforating branches from the lateral intercostals and lumbar arteries, it is imperative to preserve these vessels. Therefore, it is crucial to study any preoperative existing scar, such as subcostal cholecystectomy incisions. In certain circumstances, even a vertical midline incision can jeopardize flap perfusion.

Nerves

Cutaneous sensation of the abdominal wall is derived from the anterior and lateral cutaneous branches of the intercostal nerves 8–12, which pass between the internal oblique and transversus abdominis muscles, entering the rectus abdominis

muscle and reaching the overlying fascia and skin. The lateral cutaneous branches penetrate the intercostal muscles in the midaxillary line, ending in the subcutaneous layer. Both branches are responsible for the overlapping of the sensory dermatomes T5–L1. The motor branches of the oblique and transversus abdominis muscle derive from lower thoracic and lumbar dorsal nerves, while the rectus abdominis muscle is innervated from branches of the intercostals nerves 5–12, which pass behind the rectus muscles and enter the muscles at the junction of the lateral one-third and medial two-thirds.[23]

As peripheral nerves with either motor nor sensory innervations to the abdominal wall, the iliohypogastric and iliohypogastric have to be mentioned, since their course can be disrupted in lateral transverse lower abdominal incisions, resulting in consistent loss of sensory in the area of the groin and medioventral thigh *(Fig. 25.5)*.

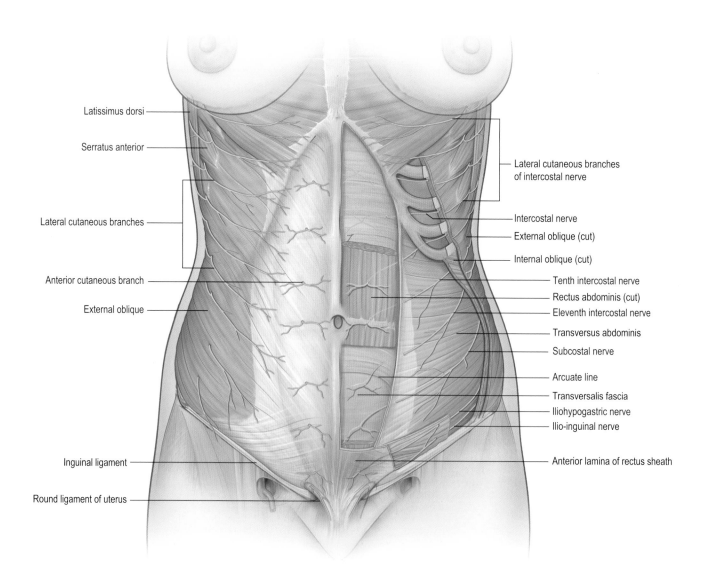

Latissimus dorsi

Serratus anterior

Lateral cutaneous branches of intercostal nerve

Lateral cutaneous branches

Intercostal nerve

External oblique (cut)

Internal oblique (cut)

Anterior cutaneous branch

Tenth intercostal nerve

External oblique

Rectus abdominis (cut)

Eleventh intercostal nerve

Transversus abdominis

Subcostal nerve

Arcuate line

Transversalis fascia

Iliohypogastric nerve

Ilio-inguinal nerve

Inguinal ligament

Anterior lamina of rectus sheath

Round ligament of uterus

Fig. 25.5 Abdominal nerves.

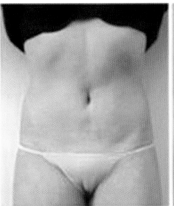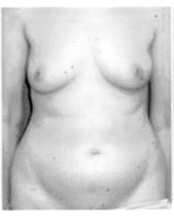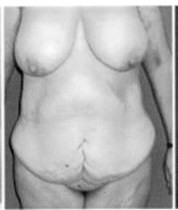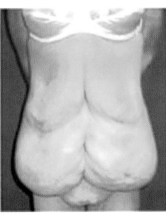

Fig. 25.6 Pittsburgh rating scale for abdominal deformities.

Pathology

Pregnancy is the commonest cause of abdominal wall deformities because the skin and musculoaponeurotic structures are stretched beyond their biomechanical capability to retract. Consequently, there is thinning and loss of elasticity of the skin with possible striae and diastasis of the rectus muscles. Postpartum weight loss contributes to the process of abdominal wall deformities, because of limited skin retraction. Massive weight loss after dieting or bariatric surgery results in similar pathophysiologic changing of the abdominal wall, including excess skin and subcutaneous tissue and a laxity of the abdominal wall musculature. Increasing demand of these specific patients for abdominal wall restoration has extended the abdominal surgery to lower circumferential procedures. These problems are reviewed in Chapter 27 and 30.

Fat accumulation occurs in a distribution pattern that varies according to the gender. With weight gain, women tend to add local adiposity in the lower trunk and hip region, while men see an increase in abdominal girth. In women, fat accumulation commonly in the posterior thigh region can result in cellulite, induced by fibrous septa within the subcutaneous tissue.[24]

Diastasis recti results from a hyperextension of the rectus sheath with a widening of the aponeurosis at the linea alba, presenting as a supra- and/or infraumbilical protrusion. This abdominal wall weakness can occur in conjunction with ventral hernias, including postoperative incisional, congenital epigastric, and umbilical hernias. Preoperative diagnosis of hernias is crucial to avoid intraoperative bowel injury.

Infections in the abdominal wall have to be treated meticulously, since they can escalate to a bacterial gangrene and necrotizing fasciitis with life-threatening conditions. Benign and malignant tumors in the abdominal area are quite uncommon. Possible wide resections can lead to larger substantial defects with the requirement of microsurgical tissue transfer.

Congenital abdominal wall defects distant to the umbilicus are relatively uncommon and based on structural defects of the abdominal wall. Omphalocele, a defect in the group of persistent fetal ducts, resolve spontaneously in 80% of children within the first 12 months.[25] Gastroschisis, one of the more common congenital abdominal wall defects, results in herniation of fetal abdominal viscera into the amniotic cavity, which has to be surgically corrected in most cases by primary closure or staged silo repair. A discussion of abdominal wall reconstruction appears in Volume IV, Chapter 12.

Classification of problems

In 1988, Bozola and colleagues published a classification including five different groups of aesthetic deformities of the abdomen with assigned operative procedures.[26,27] Group I comprised younger nulliparous women with normal elastic skin and good muscle tone but excess adipose tissue in the subcutaneous layer in the abdominal area. Group II patients usually had at least one pregnancy, mild lower abdominal skin laxity, diastasis recti, and excess adipose tissue most often present inferior to the umbilicus. Group III includes patients with significant infraumbilical skin, excess adiposity, and abdominal muscle laxity with diastasis of the rectus and oblique muscles. In addition, patients often have striae after multiple pregnancies. Patients in group IV and V have severe skin and fat excess superior and inferior to the umbilicus, accompanied by mild to severe diastasis of the rectus and oblique muscles. Group V patients present with an umbilicus which is below the ideal height.

To attempt the correlation of appearance and physical examination findings to appropriate surgical interventions in patients after massive weight loss, Song *et al.* designed the "Pittsburgh Rating Scale", a classification system that addresses the full range of post-weight loss deformities found in this unique population *(Fig. 25.6)*.[28]

Patient selection and indication

The preoperative evaluation of intra-abdominal content and the resulting pressure is important to avoid a postoperative pressure increase or abdominal compartment syndrome. In cases of elevated intra-abdominal pressure, in the supine position, the abdominal wall elevates above the costal margin and the level of the iliac crest *(Fig. 25.7)*. Abdominoplasty procedures with or without rectus plication, have to be performed cautiously in such cases.

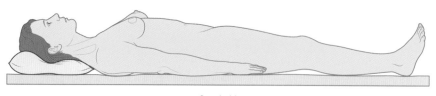

Scaphoid

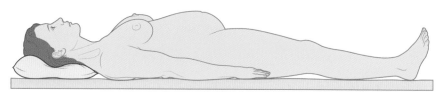

Nonscaphoid

Fig. 25.7 Assessment of intra-abdominal pressure in the supine position. The nonscaphoid abdomen will be prone to pressure increase after abdominoplasty.

History and physical examination

During the first consultation, a review of the patient's medical history and a physical examination is done. The evaluation of medical history should include the weight history with the current BMI, weight fluctuations and constancy, possible bariatric procedures, nutritional disorders, medication, the number of pregnancies and children, history of caesarean section, abdominal surgeries and abdominal hernias, the frequency of exercise, gastrointestinal, cardiac and pulmonary history, and a smoking history. Previous liposuction in the abdominal area has to be documented. Women wishing to become pregnant should be advised to postpone abdominal contouring, however. Future pregnancy does not demonstrate a contraindication.

The physical examination covers the entire abdominal wall, including the skin and fat layer, the musculoaponeurotic layer and the intra-abdominal volume. Examination of the skin and fat tissue is done by pinching and measurement of the subcutaneous layer thickness. Skin quality and the presence of striae are assessed, noting that supraumbilical striae commonly are not resected in abdominoplasties. Studies on skin quality in post-bariatric patients have demonstrated damage to collagen structures.[29,30]

The lower and occasionally upper abdominal pannus have to be evaluated and measured, with the fold areas examined for eczema and consequent hyperpigmentation. The skin excess in the areas below the lower abdominal fold, in the area of the lateral and upper abdomen, the waist, hips and thighs as well as the lower chest have to be included into the preoperative assessment, during upright standing, supine as well as sitting positions.

Any scar in the abdominal area can impair the blood supply, especially subcostal and midline scars. Horizontal upper abdominal scars will limit the choice of procedure, perhaps leaving reverse abdominoplasty as the only viable option. Vertical midline scars can be included into the fleur-de-lis technique.

The knowledge of abdominal zones of adherences in the supraumbilical midline and the inguinal area is crucial for the surgical planning. Upper abdominal rolls arise from a zone of adherence at the waist level.

Lastly, the abdominal wall has to be critically examined for bulging due to a rectus diastasis or due to incisional, epigastric or umbilical hernias. In cases of diagnostic uncertainty, a computed tomography (CT) or magnetic resonance imaging (MRI) can be helpful.

The following documentation is recommended:

- Quality of skin
- Thickness of adipose tissue
- Number and location of folds
- Location of abdominal wall defects
- Patient's favored clothing
- Pre-existing scars
- Status of abdominal musculature

The following measurements are recommended:

- Distance from umbilicus to top of mons
- Distance from umbilicus to sternal notch
- Distance from anterior vulva commissure to top of mons
- Waist and hip measurement, waist-to-hip ratio
- Thickness of abdominal adipose tissue by pinching.
- Due to an increased risk of thromboembolism and seroma formation, indication for abdominal surgery should be made critical in cases of a BMI higher than 30 or an estimated weight of resection above 1500 g. Further, a higher preoperative BMI restricts the postoperative aesthetic results.

Photographic documentation

It is important to ensure complete photographic documentation pre- and postoperatively, consisting of at least five and if possible eight views, including: anterior, oblique anterior, side, oblique posterior and posterior views. Additional photographic documentation should include the patient in a forward bending position from side and front views as well as the patient in sitting position. Commonly accepted postoperative time points for photography are at 3, 9, and 12 months.

The area to be photographed should extend from the submammary fold down to the symphysis pubis; adjoining areas can be included in additional photographs. Also helpful are views with abdominal muscles contracted and relaxed. One photo-set is made in the upright position with the patient's arms down and another with raised arms. Furthermore, patients can be photographed in the sitting position to demonstrate redundant upper abdominal laxity and tissue excess. Supplementary images can be obtained with patients grasping and holding up excess abdominal tissue in the central and waist region, as well as pinching of excess tissue in the central abdominal area with front and side views in a bent forward position.

Informed consent

Patient education and consultation on the operative procedure, possible alternative techniques, as well as the risks and benefits are a crucial part of preoperative management. Besides regularly available standard consent forms, which have to be reviewed with the patient, an audio-visual demonstration is useful for improved understanding and recollection later. As with any cosmetic procedure, patients have to be informed ruthlessly about any imaginable complication; this can include seeing photographs of major wound complications such as flap necrosis with subsequent skin grafting. Additionally, standard and individual consent forms have to be explained and documented. Ideally, the informed consent should be signed by the patient and the consulting surgeon at the earliest opportunity, followed by a second consent shortly before surgery. Patients have to be informed about their postoperative care, including their expected level of activity. Patients must clearly understand the limitations of the surgical result in cases of existing variables of bone structure, intra-abdominal fat, and existing scars. Lastly, patients must be aware that like any aesthetic or reconstructive procedure, their abdominoplasty may require an operative revision at a later date.

Patients' preoperative instructions

Patients are required to stabilize weight for at least 12 months preoperatively; any desired weight loss should be implemented prior to the surgery. Patients are strongly advised to stop smoking 6 weeks prior to the surgery, and at a minimum, at latest 2 weeks prior and for at least 2 weeks postoperative. Patients should take antiseptic showers in the evening and morning prior to the surgery, the abdominal folds and the umbilicus should be cleaned thoroughly with cotton sticks and antiseptic solutions.

If perioperative blood transfusion is a possibility, patients are informed preoperatively, as this will require blood typing and an informed consent.

Anticoagulant drugs must be avoided 10 days prior to surgery. The patient should also avoid perioperative use of various homeopathic drugs and nutritional supplements, which can induce bleeding.

Due to an expected increase of intra-abdominal pressure, surgery is generally performed with bowel purgation the night before surgery. In severe cases, patients can be restricted to a fluid diet for 24 h prior to surgery.

Patients should be well informed about the intraoperative procedures, including any adjunct activities such as positioning, antithrombotic arrangements, Foley catheter, drain and garment placement, and patient-controlled analgesia.

Patients must be instructed about the postoperative course, regarding thromboembolism prevention, respiratory exercises, early mobilization, avoidance of high abdominal pressure, the schedule for drain and suture removal and the minimum time required off work and away from exercise.

Preoperative markings

The expected markings should be demonstrated and discussed with the patient during the initial consultation, to allow enough time for patients to be concerned with the future scar course. Preoperative markings should be carried out as close as possible to the time of surgery. We recommend the photographic documentation of operative markings for reference later in cases of the patient's discontent. Reviewing the preoperative markings after the surgery will also aid the surgeon in a personal program of quality improvement.

The scar course in male patients should generally run flatter and lower than in female patients with respect to a reduced waist tightening.

Aesthetic procedures

Markings and scar-position – measurements

We commence the marking with a partially dressed patient in the upright position in order to mark the borders of the underwear. The future scars should then be evaluated and discussed with the patient. In this context, it is important to inform the patient that tractive forces and tissue excess may cause asymmetric results and aberrant scar positions. We mark the future scar line with a different coloured felt pen. This procedure has proved its value, since the patient gets involved in the preoperative planning, and thus feels jointly responsible for the future scar course (*Fig. 25.8*).

The expected resection is then evaluated by careful pinching of the tissue (*Fig. 25.9*). According to the physical equilibrium of forces, we mark the lower incision line about one to two finger-breadths below the expected scar line. The patient is asked to evaluate the redundant tissue for precise positioning.

The lower incision line will run parallel to the scar line and is normally 1–2 cm below the abdominal fold. It is essential to respect a minimum distance of 6–7 cm superior to the anterior vulva commissure. In cases of mons pubis hypertrophy or ptosis the lower incision line must be adapted (see *Fig. 25.29*).

Subsequently, we estimate the upper incision line, which will be checked intraoperatively prior to the abdominal flap resection to ensure wound closure.

Finally, we evaluate the abdominal wall for local fat depots; these are marked for adjunctive liposuction. The markings end with measurement for symmetry and a marking of the midline.

Pre-, intra-, and postoperative management and general considerations

All important steps in pre-, intra-, and postoperative management should be documented in a standard check lists.

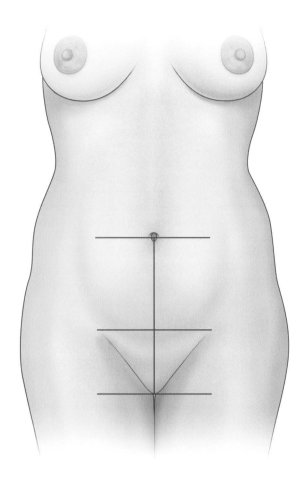

Fig. 25.8 Markings are to be performed with respect to the anterior vulva commissure and the umbilicus.

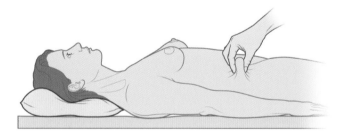

Fig. 25.9 Pinching of the abdominal tissue in upright and supine position.

Special preoperative care is recommended in patients with dry skin with stretch marks, using lipid balancing cream, massage of the abdominal tissue and avoiding UV-exposition at least 14 days prior to the operation. Two days prior to surgery patients are advised to use antiseptic lotions for body wash, with special focus on regions of surplus skin.

Preoperatively, patients should always be prewarmed by using convective warming devices immediately prior to surgery and active warming should be used in surgeries longer than 1 h. Numerous studies have shown a significant reduction of postoperative complaints and complications due to systemic warming.[31]

Perioperative thromboprophylaxis with sequential compression devices or stockings should be implemented in all patients having abdominal wall surgery. In many cases, the intraoperative and postoperative use of heparin may also be indicated. Antibiotic prophylaxis is not necessarily recommended, although in patients with prolonged umbilical stalk or impaired body hygiene with distinct abdominal fold, a single dose of antibiotic prophylaxis may be indicated.

Patient positioning in the operating room should involve, adequate padding of feet, knees, buttocks, back (especially for hyperlordosis cases), shoulders and head. A change of intraoperative positioning to the "beach chair" position should be previewed at the start of the procedure because it will be used for reduction of wound tension at the time of wound closure.

Before the patient awakes from anesthesia, a compression girdle should be fitted in order to avoid the rupture of fascial sutures on awakening. Coughing and increased abdominal pressure should be avoided during extubation, a process which should be handled gently and with great care. Postoperative patients are immediately transferred into a preheated bed. Core temperature should be measured in the recovery room and active warming should be started when patients are hypothermic or if they feel cold. Adequate hydration is an essential condition for good wound healing and for support of the circulatory system.

Wound closure

- For optimal wound closure, the patient has to be intraoperatively flexed at the level of the hips. As mentioned previously, this maneuver should be checked prior to preparation and draping.
- Larger wound cavities superior and inferior to the umbilicus may be reduced using progressive tension sutures, utilizing slow absorbable suture material. This is done to help prevent seroma formation.
- Wound closure is performed by reapproximation of each layer. It is recommended to insert drains before deep fascial closure. We usually prefer to insert one drain on each side.
- Continuity of the Scarpa's fascia is achieved with slow absorbable sutures in a single knot or running technique. A new generation barbed suture may be used (in a running manner) for a shortened closure time and less tissue damage. The subdermal layer is closed using slow absorbable sutures in single knot or running technique or alternatively, using barbed sutures in a running technique. We facilitate a minimum of tension at the dermal layer by everting both wound edges; this helps to ensure optimal coaptation of the wound in order to avoid using intracuticular sutures. Nevertheless, for reasons of wound security, an intracuticular absorbable barbed suture can be used *(Fig. 25.10)*. Alternatively, a two component wound closure device consisting of an adhesive mesh tape and new generation cyanoacrylate (PRINEO™, Ethicon Inc., Somerville NJ) has shown to be equally safe but faster than intradermal sutures in a multicenter study.[32] We currently favor this closure

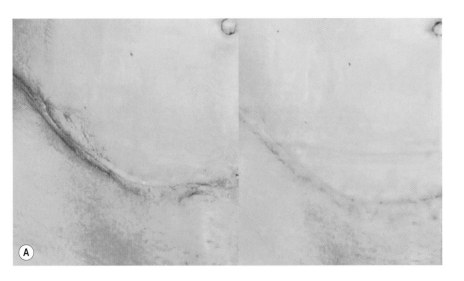

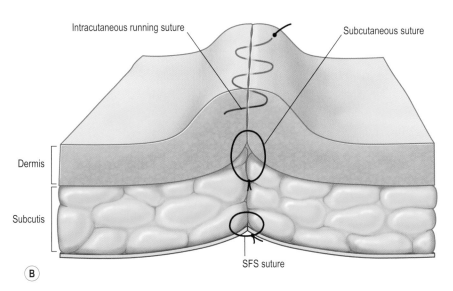

Intracutaneous running suture

Subcutaneous suture

Dermis

Subcutis

SFS suture

Fig. 25.10 Schematic and postoperative (3 weeks and 3 months) view of an everted skin closure for optimal scarring. Patients have to be forewarned about the initially unpleasing appearance.

system, since it reduces operating time, it acts as a germ barrier and is easily removable.

Documentation

In addition to standard information, operative records should document the presence and extent of abdominal wall weakness and hernias, including their repair and reconstruction. The management of the umbilicus should be carefully documented, as should the use of absorbable and nonabsorbable sutures and any other reconstructive material. Furthermore, it is essential to document the weight of the resected abdominal tissue and ideally to photo-document the specimen. Any skin or tissue abnormalities should be recorded, and the cutaneous perfusion of the wound edges should be documented. If liposuction has been done, the type of technique should be recorded (vibration-, ultrasonic-, laser-assisted or manual), along with the amount of and type of fluid infiltrate, and the type and diameter of the canula used. The areas of liposuction should be documented along with the amount of fluid and fat after the aspirate has settled.

Surgical techniques and results

Surgical techniques and results are shown in *Table 25.1*.

Mini-abdominoplasty

Introduction

The mini- or short-scar abdominoplasty is characterized by a transverse incision that is shorter than the incision used in full abdominoplasty procedures. Originally, the results of the short scar technique were limited, but with the development of liposuction and endoscopy, the mini-abdominoplasty has experienced a renaissance.

Indication and patient selection

The mini- or short-scar abdominoplasty is indicated in patients with a mild to moderate skin laxity and tissue excess of the lower (infraumbilical) abdomen, together with a sufficient distance between the symphysis and the umbilicus. It is common for young women with a pre-existing Pfannenstiel incision to benefit from this technique. Liposuction of the

Table 25.1 Indication for different techniques

	Mini	Modern	Short-T	Standard	HLT	Anchor	Circular	Reverse
Lower abdomen	+	++	++	+++	+++	+++	+++	0
Periumbilical	(+)	+	+	++	++	+++	++	+
Upper abdomen	0	(+)	+	++	++	+++	++	+++
Diastasis/hernia	(+)	+	++	++	++	+++	++	+
Flanks/hips/thighs	0	0	0	(+)	+	++	+++	0

upper abdomen and flanks has a supportive effect by improving abdominal contour. In addition, by utilizing endoscopy, or a long lighted retractor, a co-existing diastasis recti or an epigastric hernia can be treated. The exact position of the incision is quite flexible, depending in large part upon the patient's personal preference With respect to vascular anatomy, the mini-abdominoplasty is a safe procedure because only *Huger zone II* is compromised.

Markings

As mentioned above, the patient most suited for a mini-abdominoplasty will have a moderate problem confined to the lower abdomen.

Markings are made with the patient in the upright position. The borders of the patient's underwear are initially marked. The patient is asked to pull up the abdominal tissue symmetrically to evaluate the lower incision line in relation to the future scar position. A critical measure is the width of skin preserved between the umbilicus and the upper skin incision after skin excision: a distance of at least 9 cm between the upper resection line and the umbilicus should be strictly respected to avoid an unaesthetic appearance. If, after skin resection, the distance is expected to be <9 cm, an inverse T-scar with umbilical transposition should be preferred.

How long should the scar be planned? In this context, the fat distribution in the region of the iliac crest should be evaluated and a comprise reached between lateral elongation of the scar and the potential of a dog ear deformity. Always the cosmetic outcome should be optimized, despite the final scar length *(Fig. 25.11)*.

Anesthesia

This procedure may be performed under local anesthetic with or without sedation in slim patients. If surgery includes a reconstruction of the anterior rectus sheath, local anesthesia may be inadequate, since adequate anesthesia of this layer is difficult to obtain. In this situation, we recommend general anesthesia or spinal anesthesia.

Preoperative care

Preoperative considerations have been discussed above. Since the extent of preparation and resection as well as the resulting wound size are limited, perioperative risks are less frequent. General principles should be followed, including preparation for intraoperative beach-chair positioning, bowel purgation, and thrombosis prophylaxis.

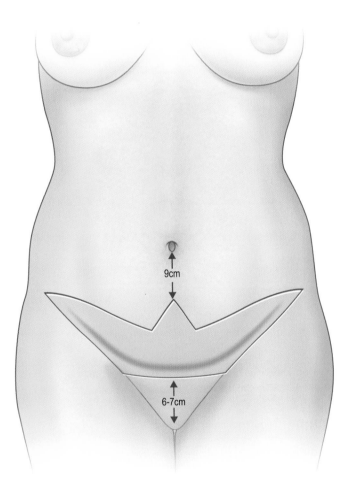

Fig. 25.11 Preoperative markings for a short scar abdominoplasty. The red line demonstrates the resulting scar line. It is essential to respect the umbilico-pubic distance. The distance from the upper resection line to the umbilicus should be at least 9 cm.

Operative technique

Preoperative infiltration of lactated Ringer's solution with epinephrine can be performed before preparation and draping to allow ample time for the epinephrine to achieve proper vasoconstriction. Any supportive liposuction of the abdominal wall should be performed prior to the abdomino-plasty in order to sufficiently thin out the different layers, including the epifascial layer. Techniques such as ultrasonic- or vibration-assisted liposuction may generate shrinking of the skin for additional skin tightening effect. Thus, in young patients with an elastic skin tone and a long distance between symphysis and umbilicus, an umbilical transposition may be omitted.

The procedure is initiated by making the inferior trans-verse incision. The dermis can be divided utilizing a cold blade or electrocautery, preferably with a Colorado® micro-dissection needle for optimal dermal hemostasis. It is manda-tory to move the Colorado® needle in a precise and rapid manner to avoid burn injuries and consequent wound healing disorders, which are usually very rare. Dissection continues downwards to Scarpa's fascia. The surgical assistant has to ensure a careful upward pull of the abdominal flap in order to facilitate a clear layer definition of Scarpa's fascia, which in general is strongly developed and simple to identify. Appropriate preservation of Scarpa's fascia requires a learn-ing curve. Dissection proceeds cranially on the epifascial surface of Scarpa's fascia to a point which is two or three finger-breadths inferior to the umbilicus. At that point, Scarpa's fascia is incised and dissection is carried down to the anterior rectus sheath. Preservation of major lym-phatic vessels in the inferior abdomen and a consequent reduction of postoperative seromas is fostered through this approach.[21,41]

Even if rectus fascial reconstruction is unnecessary, the abdominal flap is raised cranially up to the level of the umbili-cal stalk. If a supraumbilical rectus diastasis is diagnosed preoperatively, we recommend detaching the umbilical stalk from the abdominal wall fascia and continuing the dissection to the xiphoid and costal margins. The umbilical base should be marked for re-fixation.

The plication of the anterior rectus sheath from the xiphoid to the symphysis is accomplished using nonabsorbable suture material in a single knot technique. In this regard, a second layer of fascial suturing may be applied (Pitanguy technique). The same suture material can be used for the refixation of the umbilicus. Markings should be done on tensed skin and adhere to a distance of minimum 9 cm between umbilicus and upper incision line.

The first incision is performed in the midline with placing a bullet forceps subdermally. This enables the surgeon to evaluate the lateral vectors of tension and amount of resec-tion. The marked superior line of skin and tissue excess is checked and if appropriate, is adjusted to the level of the inferior incision-line. A Pitanguy type flap demarcator can be utilized. The resection of skin and tissue excess is performed oblique to the wound edge in a 45° angle to enable a precise adaptation of different layer thicknesses for optimal wound closure.

Further, patients are bent into beach-chair position and temporary wound closure is performed with bullet forceps starting laterally to medial. In order to avoid dog-ears, the longer superior wound edge is shifted slightly medially to adapt to the shorter inferior. Forceps are removed consecu-tively from lateral to medial and an immediate closure of Scarpa fascia and subcutaneous tissue is performed using absorbable suture material. Final approximation of wound edges can be ensured during subcutaneous closure. Wound closure ends with an intracuticular suture or application of PRINEO™.

Drains can then be inserted, although in mini-abdomino-plasty procedures without fascial reconstruction and without liposuction, they may be dispensable. After dressings are placed and a compression garment is fitted, the patient is transferred into the beach-chair position.

Postoperative care

The operation can be performed as outpatient or inpatient surgery. Early ambulation is mandatory. Drains are left in place until discharge is <30 mL in 24 h. The patient should rest in a relaxed position with a flexion of approximately 30° at the hip joint. This position should be retained for 2–3 weeks postoperatively, in order to assure a tension free healing of the scar. Showering is generally permitted after drain removal. Postoperative clinical examination should investigate the pos-sibility of seromas. Patients should be asked about bowel function; abdominal auscultation and percussion is advisable, especially when a reconstruction of the fascial system or a herniotomy has been performed.

Decreased bowel sounds, a postoperative fever, or other signs of illness should lead to investigation for the possibility of intra-abdominal incidents. An ultrasound scan may be helpful.

Suture material or PRINEO™ should be removed after 3 weeks postoperatively. After suture removal, we recommend the use of silicon patches for at least 3 months, which may improve scar quality and maturation.

Sporting activities should be omitted for 6 weeks postop-eratively, and in cases of fascial reconstruction, for 8 weeks. Patients should be advised to avoid saunas and tanning beds. A compression garment should be worn for the same period of time.

Outcomes and results

As mentioned earlier, patients with mild to moderate skin and tissue excess of the lower abdomen are good candidates for a short scar mini-abdominoplasty. Patients with a pre-existing cesarean scar can have this scar excised or revised in conjunc-tion with a mini-abdominoplasty.

Patients with a pot belly due to diastasis recti and mild skin excess are also appropriate candidates for this technique, with considerable improvements after concurrent plication of the anterior rectus sheath (Fig. 25.12).

The primary limitation of this procedure is the presence of upper abdominal skin folds and rolls; these patients will require one of the more extensive procedures described sub-sequently in this chapter.

"Modern" abdominoplasty with umbilical transection

Introduction

Abdominoplasty with a pre-fascial release and transposition of the umbilicus without circumferential release from the abdominal flap presents another effective procedure that can accomplish astounding results, especially in combination with liposuction and fascial plication. This enables mainte-nance of umbilical appearance without a periumbilical scar.

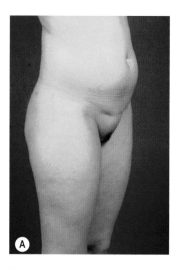 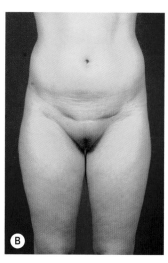 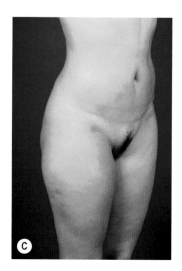 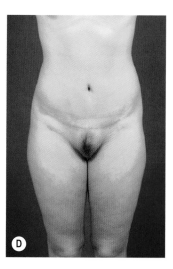

Fig. 25.12 A 31-year-old patient after two pregnancies with two cesarian sections. **(A,B)** Pre- and **(C,D)** postoperative oblique and front views of a short scar abdominoplasty without umbilical transection. Note the low placement of the previous scar and the high-riding umbilicus as well as the infraumbilical diastasis recti.

Indication and patient selection

This abdominoplasty represents an extension of mini-abdominoplasty procedures for patients who suffer from surplus skin in the area of the lower abdomen, as well as a modest amount of looseness in the periumbilical area. A sufficient distance of at least 14–18 cm between the symphysis and the umbilicus as well as a good elastic skin tone with limited stretch marks is essential for superior results, since the amount of resectable skin is comparable with mini-abdominoplasty procedures. By transposing the umbilicus caudally, a tightening of the periumbilical skin is created without a scar of the umbilicus itself. Additionally, this approach enables excellent visualization for rectus diastasis or hernia repair.

Therefore, this technique represents a good alternative between mini-abdominoplasty and standard abdominoplasty procedures. In addition to patients with periumbilical looseness, this abdominoplasty is well suited for patients who will not accept umbilical scars or who would be at risk of developing hypertrophic or keloid scars. Lastly, this technique is helpful in the candidate for a mini-abdominoplasty in whom a tension free closure cannot be ensured, or in where there is concern about vascularity due to smoking.

Markings

In contrast to mini-abdominoplasty procedures, this technique is suited for patients with longer distances of 14–18 cm between the umbilicus and symphysis; this will be seen in patients who have an unnatural high umbilical position. The principles of the scar-line assessment and positioning are similar to mini-abdominoplasty and demonstrated earlier. In general, the scar-line is slightly longer, since more tissue can be resected compared with the mini-abdominoplasty.

Certain aesthetic principles should be understood and followed. The aesthetic relation of 60% upper to 40% lower abdomen as well as a distance of at least 9 cm between the umbilicus and the symphysis have to be respected.

Preoperative care

This is covered under 'Patient selection and indication', above.

Operative technique

The operative technique is in general aspects, identical with the mini-abdominoplasty described above. Common features include the infiltration of lactated Ringer's solution with epinephrine, adjunctive liposuction, and flap dissection with preservation of Scarpa's fascia in the lower abdomen. However, the base of the umbilical stalk is detached from the anterior rectus sheath. As the flap is migrated caudally, the umbilical stalk is then reattached at an inferior position. The umbilicus should not be moved inferiorly any closer than 9 cm from the pubic symphysis *(Fig. 25.13)*.

Postoperative care

This has been discussed earlier.

Outcomes and results

Abdominoplasty with umbilical transection represents a good alternative between mini-abdominoplasty and standard abdominoplasty. This technique is suitable for patients with mainly periumbilical skin wrinkles without the degree of tissue surplus necessitating a full abdominoplasty procedure *(Fig. 25.14)*.

Standard abdominoplasty

Introduction

The standard abdominoplasty is one of the most common plastic surgery procedures performed worldwide. Prime advantages are the simultaneous treatment of the upper abdomen, periumbilical area and lower abdomen with concealable scars.

Traditional abdominoplasty involved widely mobilizing the abdominal wall up to the costal arch or even higher in order to ensure a tension-free wound closure. Wound healing disorders and wound edge necrosis were often misinterpreted as a result of too much wound tension. Multiple studies have since demonstrated that circulatory disturbance of the abdominal skin flap is the result of extensive undermining and destruction of the lateral perforators of the *Huger zone II*.

Modern abdominoplasty techniques respect these circulatory principles. The main principle is to operate with the most minimal invasive technique which will yield the best achievable aesthetical result. Undermining is mainly performed in the midline area anterior to the linea alba and both rectus muscles, including the median zones of adhesion first described by Lockwood and specified by Aly.[33,34] The lateral abdominal regions may be released indirectly using additional liposuction or the Lockwood-dissector for discontinuous undermining, preserving the lateral perforators and the lateral attachment to the rectus abdominis muscles. This is important for the overall aesthetic outcome

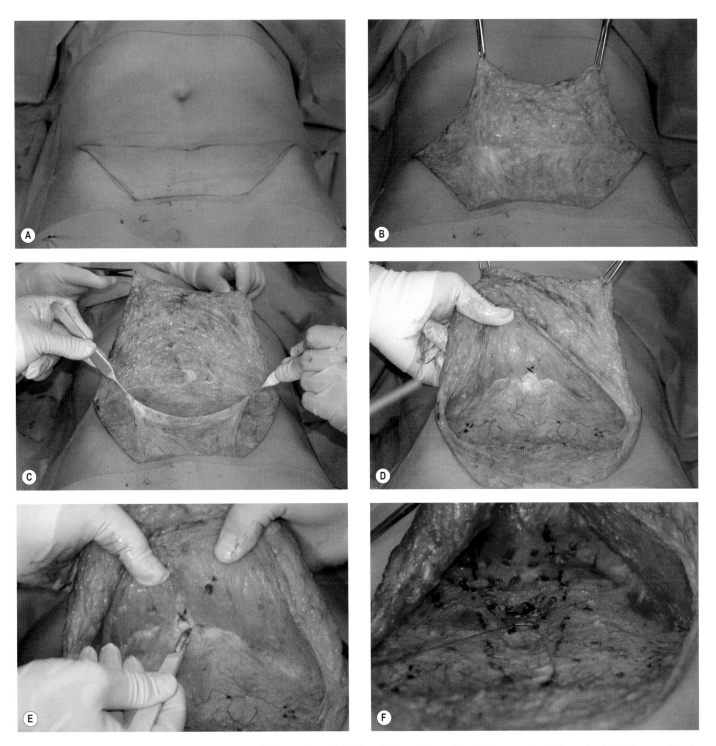

Fig. 25.13 Intraoperative view of abdominoplasty with umbilical transection. **(A)** Markings in the supine position; **(B,C)** preservation of Scarpa fascia; **(D,E)** preparation of the umbilical stalk **(F)** closure of the umbilical base with nonresorbable suture material;

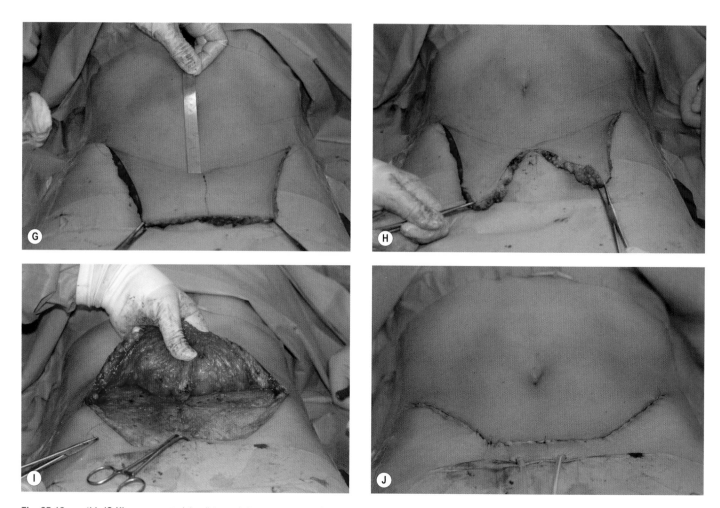

Fig. 25.13, cont'd (G,H) assessment of the distance between upper resection line and the umbilicus with resection of the redundant tissue; **(I)** refixation of the umbilical stalk to the anterior rectus sheath and **(J)** the intraoperative result.

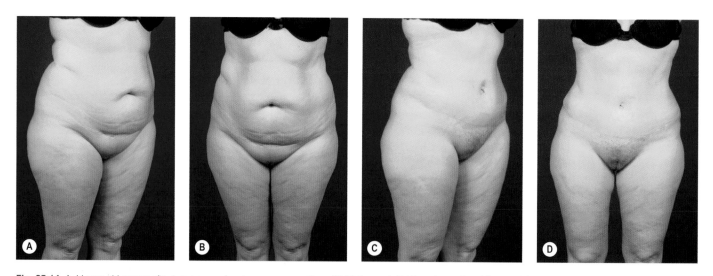

Fig. 25.14 A 44-year-old woman after two pregnancies, two cesarean sections. **(A,B)** Pre- and **(C,D)** postoperative oblique and front views of an abdominoplasty procedure with umbilical transection and fascial plication.

in cases of a pre-existing diastasis. In this context, the contour of the rectus muscle may be restored by midline plication of the rectus fascia. Ideally, the superficial fascial system should remain connected to the rectus muscle aponeurosis. If divided, the upper abdomen will appear tent-shaped, with an elevated risk of seroma.

The disadvantage of midline rectus fascial plication may be a midline gathering of soft tissues. This tissue excess can be easily and safely reduced through the open excision or with additional liposuction without the risk of circulatory disturbance. Occasionally, extended lateral undermining may be necessary.

Indication and patient selection

This operation is indicated in patients presenting skin and soft tissue excess of the upper and lower abdomen with acceptance of a circular periumbilical scar.

Suitable patients typically demonstrate a localized and diet-resistant adiposity of the abdominal wall in combination with co-existing slack and atonic skin. Such patients have often been through multiple pregnancies. A pot-belly deformity of the upper abdomen may be misinterpreted as tissue redundancy rather than a fascial diastasis. In such cases, liposuction can be dangerous if there is an epigastric hernia. Due to the relatively long incision in the lower abdominal fold, excellent access is available for diastasis or hernia repair. Also, with this incision, a considerable amount of excess tissue may be removed. Smokers have an elevated risk for wound healing disorders.[35,36] Diabetics are predisposed to suffer from postoperative wound infection. Apart from that, diabetics represent a group of patients who may benefit from this procedure by preventing chronic and potentially life-threatening infections within the abdominal fold.

Markings

As described earlier, the border of the patient's underwear is first marked. Then we mark the expected and desired scar position.

In the upright position, we precisely mark the midline. The patient is asked to elevate the redundant abdominal tissue for identification of the abdominal fold. A vertical distance of 7 cm is measured from the labial commissure to the lower incision, followed by marking of the lower incision line parallel to the abdominal fold, considering any ptosis of the mons pubis. Then in the supine position, the expected amount of resection is assessed and marked. Particular attention is paid to the midline area to assess for the potential necessity of an inferior inverse "T" incision, including an umbilical circumcision. This upper incision is drawn as a preoperative estimate. Normally, the upper incision is not made until the end of the procedure after intraoperative assessment of the correct tissue resection.

Evaluation of possible pre-existing hernias and diastasis should be repetitively performed in the supine position, marking the extent of the diastasis recti. We measure and document the length of the scar-line bilaterally starting from the midline to ensure symmetry.

Choosing an appropriate incision-line, we need to be aware that a longer inferior incision will lead to a gently curved, upward course of the scar (Baroudi) and a longer superior incision will cause a straighter or downward course of the scar (Pitanguy).

Respecting this simple principle, the scar course may individually be matched to the age and fashion style of the patient. An exceptional scar course should be discussed critically with the patient, since fashion changes occur at short intervals. For example, a high-cut-bikini approach may later cause problems for the fashion-conscious patient wearing hipsters or a bare midriff T-shirt.

Preoperative care

Preoperative considerations have been discussed above. In patients who are candidates for a standard abdominoplasty, the wound size and operating time are greater and patients may have a surplus of weight as well as other co-morbid factors. For all these reasons, as compared with minimal procedures, the full abdominoplasty patient will have a higher risk for complications.

Prophylaxis for pulmonary embolism and deep vein thrombosis is an essential consideration, especially in patients taking birth control medications or hormone replacement therapy, since they have an increased risk. The patient should be counselled about this preoperatively; risks will be decreased if hormonal replacement is discontinued 3–4 weeks prior to surgery.[37]

In cases of an extended diastasis or hernia, the reconstruction of the fascia results in an increased intra-abdominal pressure, which may be a source of respiratory difficulties. Preoperative breathing exercises (utilizing an incentive spirometer) beginning 1–2 weeks prior to and continuing for 2 weeks after the operation are advisable to the patient. A cold, dry cough or any kind of respiratory infections should lead to postponement of surgery, since fits of coughing may provoke a rupture of the fascial sutures with consequent secondary bleeding.

It can be helpful to recommend placing the patient into a tight compression girdle for 2 weeks day and night preoperatively, to accommodate to the increased intra-abdominal pressure postoperatively.

Smoking cessation for 6 weeks preoperatively is suggested to patients. In case of failure, cessation or at least a drastic reduction of smoking for at least 2 weeks prior to the operation is recommended. Diabetes may be a relative contraindication to this procedure, especially in poorly-controlled patients. Furthermore, it is important to exclude any skin irritation or inflammation in the area of the abdominal folds and umbilicus. An inspection of these areas immediately prior to the operation is strongly advised. Diabetics should receive a single-shot antibiotic immediately prior to surgery.

Operative technique

Preoperative infiltration of lactated Ringer's solution with epinephrine can be performed before preparation and draping to allow ample time for the epinephrine to achieve proper vasoconstriction. Any adjunctive liposuction of the abdominal wall should be performed prior to the abdominoplasty, in order to sufficiently thin out the different layers, including the epifascial layer. We commence the operation with a final check of the measurements and markings. Points of references may be tattooed using methylene blue, especially the midline inferior and superior to the estimated resection area.

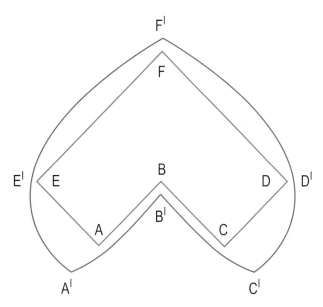

Fig. 25.15 Excision pattern of the umbilical stalk from the previous abdominal wall (red line A–F) and the incision pattern at the new umbilical insertion (blue line A'–F').

- The lower incision line may be additionally infiltrated with local anesthetics to reduce postoperative pain and the consecutive risk of blood pressure increase. The lower incision line is cut, utilizing the Colorado needle with careful superficial coagulation. During downward dissection, the frequently large superficial epigastric vessels should be ligated.
- The surgical assistant has to ensure a careful upward pull of the abdominal flap using bullet forceps in order to facilitate a clear layer definition to preserve Scarpa's fascia. By staying above Scarpa's fascia, the subjacent lymphatic vessels are preserved. In previously operated patients, identification of the appropriate dissection layer may be difficult. Dissection superficial to Scarpa's fascia continues cranially up to a level two to three finger-breadths inferior to the umbilicus. At that point, Scarpa's fascia is incised, and dissection continues along the anterior rectus sheath.
- The umbilical stalk is then circularly transected from the abdominal flap and may be temporarily sutured closed for asepsis. Surrounding perforators may be ligated with maximal awareness, since they tend to retract after dissection beneath the anterior rectus sheath. Dissection continues superior to the umbilicus along the rectus fascia up to the xiphoid. The linea alba can easily be identified, as it is distinctively connected to Scarpa's fascia. The lateral perforators should be preserved *(Fig. 25.15)*.
- Plication of the anterior rectus sheath from the xiphoid to the symphysis is accomplished using nonabsorbable suture material in the technique described by Pitanguy (see above). In the case of a diastasis of the lower abdomen located beneath Scarpa's fascia, the tissue may be bluntly mobilized to allow for midline fascial plication. In some patients, there may be a pronounced fat layer beneath Scarpa's fascia, something which can be thinned using liposuction. Since lateral dissection is

avoided up to the costal arch for preservation of the lateral perforators, medial rectus plication may cause soft tissue bulging in the midline. This may be treated by one of three ways: discontinuous separation of lateral adhesions using the Lockwood-underminer; performing an open excision of fatty tissue, or doing liposuction after wound closure.

- The abdominal flap is then pulled down and several progressive tension sutures are placed, followed by an incision of the flap in the midline. Utilizing a bullet forceps or Pitanguy tissue demarcator, the upper resection line can be estimated for a tension-free wound closure. Further evaluation of resection volume may be facilitated by additional vertical incisions and temporary wound closure using bullet forceps. The upper incision line is then marked and the resection of skin and tissue excess is performed oblique to the wound edge in a 45° angle to enable a precise adaptation of different layer thicknesses for optimal wound closure. After meticulous coagulation, the wound is closed temporarily. The new umbilical position is estimated and marked. Several umbilical incision patterns have been described (we prefer the V inverted incision). The umbilical section of the abdominal flap is then circumferentially defatted to achieve a surrounding depression around the umbilical stalk. The supraumbilical midline may also be accentuated by midline liposuction or open excision.
- Paramedian plication of the anterior rectus sheath may facilitate a correction of an asymmetrically located umbilical stalk or for accentuation of an hourglass figure with further waist tightening.
- As an option, the upper side of the umbilical incision may be fixed to the cranial base of the umbilical stalk and the anterior rectus sheath, using a nonabsorbable suture in order to create a periumbilical depression and for reduction of tension within the umbilicus *(Fig. 25.16)*.
- Wound closure, drains and compression garment application have been described earlier (see Wound closure, above).

Postoperative care

General postoperative care has been discussed with mini-abdominoplasty. For the standard abdominoplasty, we prefer to perform the operation on an inpatient basis with a 2–3-night hospital stay.

Patients with pre-existing umbilical scars from previous surgery such as herniotomy or laparoscopy should be observed for possible disturbances of blood supply. A slight postoperative discoloration of the umbilicus is usually not precarious. A complete necrosis of the umbilical stalk is very uncommon and may be treated conservatively, with satisfying results.

Outcomes and results

Patient satisfaction after standard abdominoplasty is consistently high, since it enables a treatment of the entire abdomen. The legacy of a long scar with limited treatment effects to the hips and the back region, is an unfortunate aspect of this procedure.

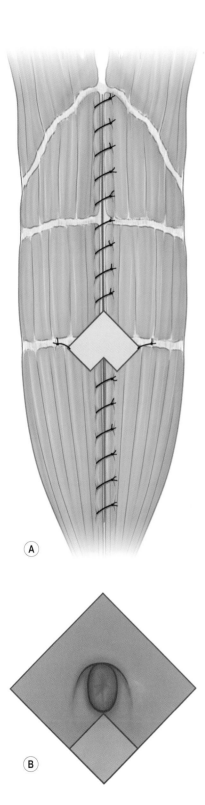

(A)

(B)

Fig. 25.16 Fixation of the umbilical stalk to the anterior rectus sheath after midline plication. The blue line indicates the umbilical stalk incision pattern, the red area has to be provided from the abdominal flap in terms of an inverted V-flap.

Patients often ask how the operative benefits may be affected by future pregnancies. If they are able to control weight, continue exercise and treat their abdominal skin with topical agents, the benefits of the abdominoplasty procedure may persist after pregnancies *(Figs 25.17, 25.18)*.

High-lateral-tension (HLT) abdominoplasty

Introduction

This extended modification of abdominoplasty procedures not only treats the abdomen, but also the hips and the lateral thigh. A modified incision pattern is used.

In the 1990s, Lockwood recognized that many patients, particularly those after massive weight loss who received a standard abdominoplasty showed good results in the central abdominal region. However, the flanks showed no improvement or were made worse due to a gathering of excess tissue in the flank region. This led to the concept of shifting tension from the central abdomen to increased tension laterally. Lockwood enumerated several surgical principles that were in many ways diametrically opposite to the ones of a standard abdominoplasty, namely, an extensive discontinuous undermining and a more conservative resection centrally with wider excision of the lateral skin.

Indication and patient selection

The HLT abdominoplasty is suitable for patients that expect more than an abdominal tightening and is often applicable for patients after massive weight loss. Women usually suffer from an additional skin laxity in the lateral thigh region, whereas men often complain about the typical love handles. The experienced surgeon may be confronted with abdominoplasty procedures that result with lateral dog-ears, despite the extent of lateral tissue excision and scar elongation. Additional liposuction may be supportive, although often insufficient due to a surplus of skin.

Even though this procedure may address only a minority of patients, this technique represents a good solution for patients for whom an abdominoplasty is deficient and a lower body-lift is beyond their needs.

Markings

Markings are made with the patient in an upright position. As described earlier, the borders of the underwear are initially marked. Like a standard abdominoplasty, the patient is asked to elevate the redundant abdominal tissue for identification of the abdominal fold. A vertical distance of 7 cm is measured from the vulva commissure, followed by marking of the lower incision line parallel to the abdominal fold. The inferior incision line is drawn laterally towards the anterior axillary line and continues upwards to the mid-axillary line following an angle of 45°. In a next step, a second line is drawn starting at the highest point of the umbilicus running parallel to the lower incision line. When this marking reaches the anterior axillary line, it turns downwards in an angle of 45° meeting the lower line in the mid-axillary line forming an angle of 90° at the end of the resulting scar *(Fig. 25.19)*.

Preoperative care

This is discussed in detail above. In addition, for this procedure, it is helpful to position patients on additional soft

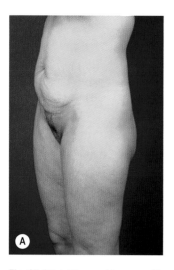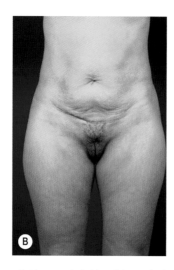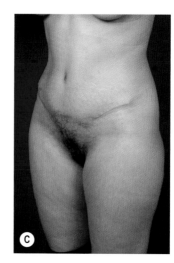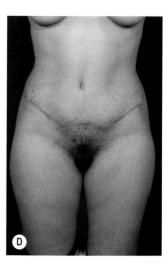

Fig. 25.17 A 42-year-old woman with a remarkable amount of striae distensae in the periumbilical region after a single pregnancy. **(A,B)** Pre- and **(C,D)** postoperative oblique and front images of a standard abdominoplasty procedure with incomplete elimination of striae.

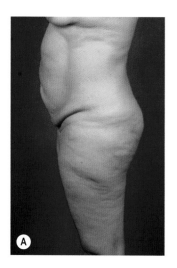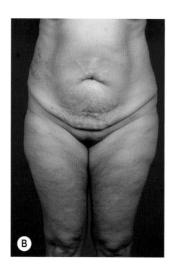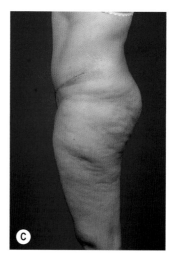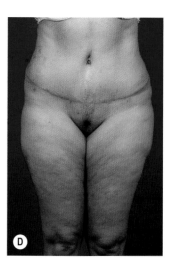

Fig. 25.18 A 43-year-old patient with a poor skin tone after previous liposuction. **(A,B)** Pre- and **(C,D)** postoperative oblique and front images of a standard abdominoplasty procedure with fascial tightening and externus belt procedure.

cushion pillows in the gluteal area for elevation of the flanks and the lateral thighs. This will facilitate access for the more lateral extension involved in this procedure. Alternatively, a change to the lateral position can be done.

Operative technique

The operative technique is similar to a standard abdominoplasty, although flap mobilization in the midline area is performed as far lateral as necessary for rectus plication. Further flap advancement can be achieved through vertical discontinuous undermining utilizing the Lockwood dissector. However, the skin resection pattern with a significant lateral resection further laterally is performed with high-tension wound closure. In the lateral area of the right angle incision, it is recommended to reduce subdermal fat and lengthening of the abdominoplasty incision in order to avoid dog-ears.

Postoperative care

Postoperative care has been discussed previously.

Outcomes and results

The HLT abdominoplasty presents a treatment concept with additional focus on hips and thighs. A laterally elongated scar has to be accepted for a convincing result, which is mostly well accepted by the patient. Since the lateral abdominal perforators are generally not injured, a safe and constant perfusion can be ensured and therewith an extensive liposuction of the entire abdominal wall may be securely performed *(Fig. 25.20)*. In some cases, limited benefit may be noted at the lateral aspect of the thighs.

Fleur-de-lis abdominoplasty

Introduction

The fleur-de-lis or anchor abdominoplasty was first popularized in 1985 and is derived from techniques previously described by Regnault[9] (classic W technique) or Kelly (1910) and Babcock (1916).[1-4] The principles and the power of this procedure is the ability to eliminate horizontal and vertical redundant tissue of the lower and upper abdomen, with a maximum improvement of body shape and reduction of waist circumference. It is also possible to combine this technique with a high lateral tension abdominoplasty, thus accomplishing impressive changes. General principles such as preservation of the lateral perforators, discontinuous undermining with elimination of dead spaces, are mandatory. The primary disadvantage of this procedure is the increased scar length.

Indication and patient selection

This technique is suitable for patients suffering from a tissue surplus of the lower and particularly of the upper abdomen, often after massive weight loss. One unique indication is the patient who presents with a pre-existing abdominal midline scar.

Another special case is the patient who presents, having already undergone an abdominoplasty, but who is still concerned about tissue excess, often in the upper abdomen. This can be demonstrated with the patient in a sitting position, or bending over slightly in the upright position.

Bariatric surgery is discussed in Chapter 30. When considering a vertical midline scar, it is important to ask about the presence of a gastric band as transverse tissue resection may reposition a gastric band access port.

Markings

The key in planning this procedure is to independently assess the horizontal and vertical surplus of skin and fat tissue. The estimate of tissue surplus is accomplished through accurate pinching of the skin, while the patient is in upright and relaxed supine position.

We usually commence in the upright position with the marking for a standard abdominoplasty or more frequent HLT abdominoplasty incision pattern. Then the horizontal tissue surplus of the upper abdomen is estimated and the marking may be performed in a single or double-ellipse technique as previously described by Aly[34] to avoid an over-resection *(Fig. 25.21)*. Markings usually result in an omega-like figure *(Fig. 25.9B)*.

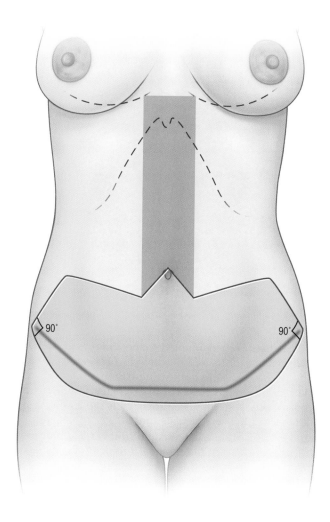

Fig. 25.19 HLT abdominoplasty pattern.

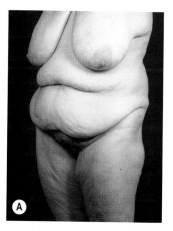
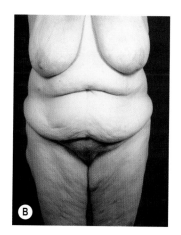
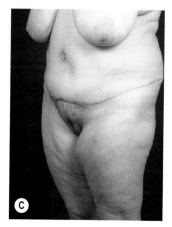
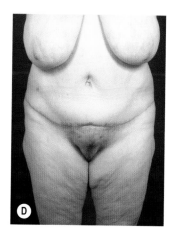

Fig. 25.20 A 54-year-old patient with a massive skin and soft tissue redundancy at the abdominal and flank region. **(A,B)** Pre- and **(C,D)** 3 months' postoperative oblique and front images of an HLT abdominoplasty procedure with fascial tightening without any additional liposuction.

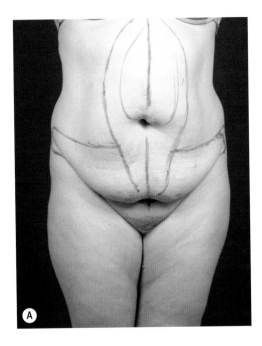
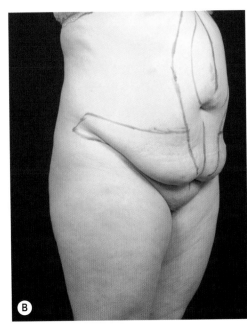

Fig. 25.21 (A,B) Fleur-de-lis markings.

It is important to clarify to the patient the height of the vertical scar, since it may extend up between the breast after final closure. In order to prevent this, we recommend a precise marking below the xiphoid and treatment of any possible dog-ear primarily by local superficial liposuction rather than a more superior excision.

Symmetry is controlled during the entire examination and marking. Finally the upper and lower incision-line as well as the vertical incision-lines may be measured and compared. Markings should be checked in the upright, supine and sitting position.

Preoperative care

Preoperative care is as discussed previously. If a simultaneous high lateral tension abdominoplasty is planned, the additional padding discussed for that procedure is used.

Operative technique

The general operative technique is as for standard abdominoplasty.

- Abdominal flap mobilization is done as for standard abdominoplasty. Principles include staying above Scarpa's fascia inferiorly, dissecting superiorly on the anterior rectus fascia and laterally to the lateral rectus margin (linea semilunaris), preserving lateral perforators.
- For lateral flap mobilization, we prefer the Lockwood-underminer for careful discontinuous lateral undermining. Before final tissue resection may be accomplished, the entire estimated vertical and transverse resection area has to be temporarily closed utilizing bullet forceps.
- Precise closure of each wound layer is the key for adequate wound healing and discreet scarring. In this technique, the umbilicus must be integrated into the vertical scar. At the appropriate umbilical height, a transverse incision is made on both abdominal flaps with the circular fat excision in the periumbilical region. The

umbilical stalk is then adapted to the abdominal flaps, allowing skin excisions for optimal incorporation. A secondary aesthetically unpleasing trumpet-like widening of the umbilicus may result from extensive skin removal. To control this, a step-by-step excision is done, observing the effects of transverse tensile forces.
- Wound closure at the cranial end of the vertical scar may be difficult because of the frequent problem of a dog-ear in this region. To avoid this complication, an open excision of the subdermal fat tissue or even additional "Burow-triangles" on the level of the inframammary fold may be indicated. A primary correction by superficial liposuction may be attempted.
- After finalizing wound closure, an adjusting liposuction may be performed.
- We regularly insert three to four drains.
- Before the patient wakes from anesthesia, the compression garment has to be applied. Patients are transferred0 into the beach-chair position.

Postoperative care

Postoperative care has been discussed previously.

The hospitalization period is usually slightly prolonged, since patients frequently demonstrate a prolonged drainage from the upper abdominal area. Special attention should be given to breathing exercises.

Single-shot antibiotic prophylaxis should be mandatory in this procedure. Optionally, a broad-spectrum 5-day regimen may be used.

Outcomes and results

If basic principles such as maximal preservation of perforators and minimal undermining with minimal dead space are followed, wound healing should be unproblematic and rapid. The aesthetic effects to the hip and waist are dramatic and not comparable with any other technique. The midline incision most often heals without excess scarring. Additionally, a

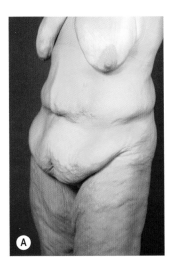
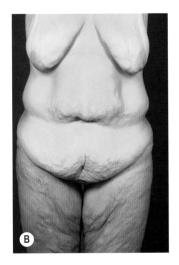
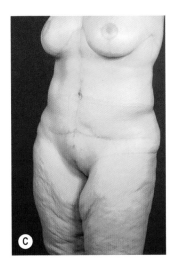
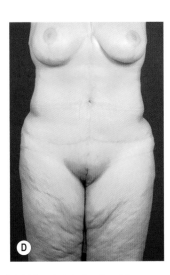

Fig. 25.22 A 45-year-old patient with weight reduction of 80 kg, with circumferential skin excess in the abdominal, flank, lateral/medial thigh and gluteal region. After rejecting a lower bodylift, the patient underwent a fleur-de-lis abdominoplasty. **(A,B)** Pre- and **(C,D)** 3 months' postoperative oblique and front images of a fleur-de-lis abdominoplasty procedure with fascial tightening and breast reshaping.

significant improvement is achievable to the back and flank folds due to an extreme recruitment of lateral skin.

Patients with massive tissue surplus in the upper abdomen are good candidates for this procedure, providing they can accept the visible scar *(Fig. 25.22)*.

Abdominoplasty in MWL patients

The number of patients after massive weight loss (MWL) has increased dramatically within recent years, mainly due to a changed health consciousness, as well as modern and popularized techniques in bariatric surgery. Both men and women often suffer from massive deformations of the abdominal wall, which cause significant hygienic and functional discomfort.

Because of remarkable perioperative problems in this patient group, the MWL patient and bariatric surgery are reviewed in Chapter 30.

Abdominoplasty with Scarpa's lift

Introduction

During abdominoplasty, the accurate dissection and preservation of Scarpa's fascia enables an adjunctive intraoperative maneuver utilizing fascial tightening, without impairment of the lymphatic drainage. Because Scarpa's fascia continues caudally into Colles' fascia, traction placed on Scarpa's fascia can result in a transition of traction into the medio-ventral thigh region. This in turn can facilitate a limited indirect subcutaneous lifting effect on the medial thigh.[38]

Indication

Patients after mild to moderate weight loss may suffer from minor skin laxity at the inner thigh region, which does not require an additional direct tightening procedure. As an intraoperative adjunctive procedure to the vertical skin tightening during an abdominoplasty, the subdermal tightening of Scarpa's fascia might additionally help the inner thigh region. It has to be emphasized that only a limited group of patients can be addressed by this maneuver. Patients with massive

surplus of skin generally have to undergo traditional horizontal and vertical procedures.

Operative technique

After preparation and preservation of Scarpa's fascia to the level of the arcuate line it can be vertically tightened to the anterior rectus sheath utilizing nonabsorbable sutures in single knot or running technique. Effects to the inner thigh region may be checked and demonstrated intraoperatively.

Outcomes

The main advantage in terms of providing a simultaneous indirect lift of the medial thigh region by fascio-fascial transition from the Scarpa to the medial thigh inguino-cruralis fascia has gained our attention. Since patients after a mild to moderate weight loss are often impatient with their medial thigh skin laxity and decline an additional medial thigh procedure with additive medial thigh and groin scars and their consequent potential complications, this additional intraoperative maneuver enables an extension of surgical offers to our patients in this rapidly growing field of plastic surgery *(Figs 25.23, 25.24)*.

Circumferential abdominoplasty

Introduction

The original idea of circumferential abdominoplasty was to deal with lateral dog-ears extending around to the back from an abdominoplasty. Since the early 1990s however, the circumferential abdominoplasty has been adapted to an increasing demand for circular lower trunk dermatolipectomies involving an extended preparation and resection of the entire lower trunk.[39–41] This topic is reviewed in Chapter 27.

Reverse abdominoplasty

Introduction

The majority of patients presenting with excessive truncal tissue suffer from redundant skin and soft tissue of the lower

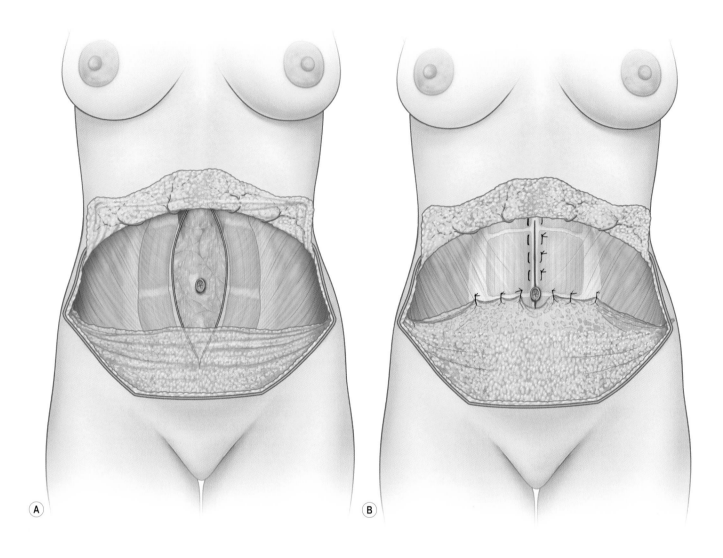

Fig. 25.23 (A) Intraoperative preservation of Scarpa fascia and **(B)** fascial tightening to the anterior rectus sheath.

abdomen. These patients can normally be treated with one of the procedures described in this chapter. In certain individuals, however, tightening of skin in the upper abdomen alone may be indicated.

Indication

The indication for this procedure is not as common as other abdominoplasty procedures and is rarely performed solely. It may be performed either during a reduction mammaplasty or in combination with a standard abdominoplasty. The most common indication in our practice is the MWL patient who has undergone a conventional abdominoplasty and may suffer from persistent skin and soft tissue excess of the upper abdomen.

Patient awareness and acceptance of the resulting scar line is mandatory for the performance of this procedure. Since the majority of patients are female, a positioning of the scar in the inframammary fold is achievable, although patients must be aware of a visible scar between the breasts. The indication for

male patients is limited, because the scar in this region cannot be concealed.

In selective cases, the excess tissue of the reverse abdominoplasty may be utilized for autologous augmentation of the breast as part of a mastopexy procedure. The abdominal flap of the upper abdomen is de-epithelialized and rotated cranially for tissue augmentation. A secure fixation to the periosteum of the ribs is performed with permanent sutures.

Markings

The marking is performed with the patient in the upright position. The patient is asked to slightly bend forward for demonstration of tissue excess. This enables an optimal assessment of the vertical and horizontal tissue excess. The inframammary fold is then marked extending laterally to the anterior axillary line. The patient in the supine position facilitates the examination of the inframammary fold mobility, which can be considerable in patients after massive weight loss. The surplus of tissue and the consequent lower incision

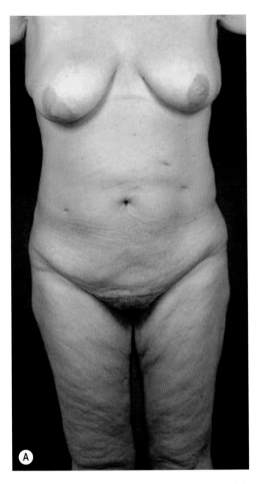
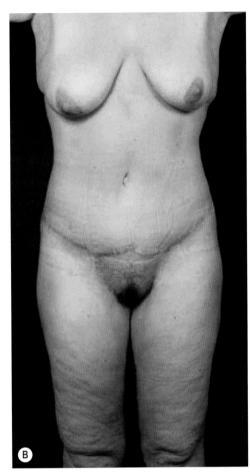

Fig. 25.24 A 41-year-old female patient after 22 kg weight loss and two pregnancies. **(A)** Preoperatively and **(B)** 3 months postoperatively after a standard abdominoplasty, including a bilateral scarpa lift. The inner thigh region could be improved, preventing the patient from an additional inner thigh scar. (Printed with kind permission from Springer, Richter DF, Stoff A. The Scarpa lift – a novel technique for minimal invasive medial thigh lifts. Obes Surg. 2011;21:1975–1980.)

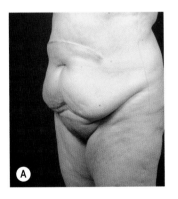
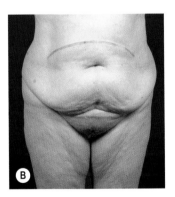
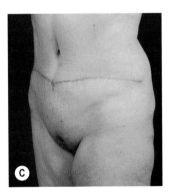
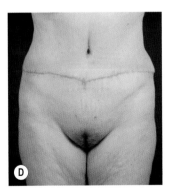

Fig. 25.25 A 52-year-old patient after an atypical open laparotomy procedure with a transverse scar. **(A,B)** Pre- and **(C,D)** postoperative front view following an abdominoplasty procedure with a pre-existing scar.

line is assessed by accurate pinching. It is recommended to include a V-shaped scar course at the midline to avoid an apparent décolleté scar. Vertical markings for orientation may be helpful to ensure a symmetric wound closure. The width of resection is generally <15 cm *(Fig. 25.25)*.

Vertical abdominoplasty

The vertical abdominoplasty refers to a purely vertical incision with lateral mobilization of abdominal soft tissue. This procedure is primarily indicated in patients with a pre-existing

scar in the abdominal midline who seek an improvement of the abdominal contour without additional transverse scars. Especially in patients with a request for vertical fascial tightening due to pre-existing diastasis recti or scar hernia, this procedure may improve the abdominal contouring.

Umbilicoplasty

For umbilical preservation and recreation, multiple techniques have been published to date. The reconstructed

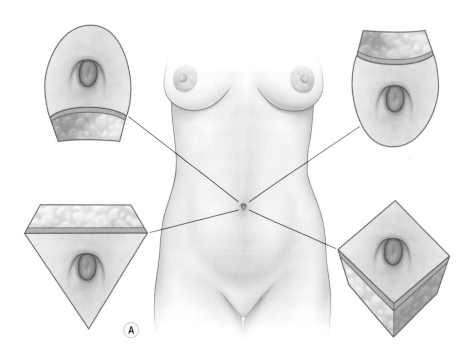

Fig. 25.26 Mutiple umbilicoplasty techniques.

umbilicus should be fairly small, vertically oriented, superiorly hooded, and with a slight circular depression of 4–6 cm diameter. Additionally, it is advantageous to accentuate the natural abdominal midline.

When raising an abdominal flap, the umbilicus is released with a circumumbilical incision made in a round or rhombic shape; the stalk is then prepared and separated from the abdominal flap. Re-insetting the umbilicus is done first by attaching the umbilical stalk to the anterior rectus sheath with four point fixation sutures at 3, 6, 9, and 12 o'clock, using long-term resorbable sutures. The abdominal flap is then drawn over the umbilicus and temporarily closed.

After determination of the new umbilicus location by utilizing the Pitanguy type flap demarcator (or Lockwood marker) or measurement of the umbilicopubic distance below and above the abdominal flap, the umbilical incision can be made in different patterns, depending on the surgeon's preference. The horizontal crescent-shaped incision with the convexity up or the similar inverted V inverted are the most frequent used incision patterns with in our experience the best achievable results *(Fig. 25.26)*.

In MWL patients, it is usually necessary to shorten the umbilical stalk to avoid a stalk herniation, despite sufficient subcutaneous tacking sutures. It is also crucial to grasp stable tissue of the umbilical stalk at an appropriate height for fixation at the anterior rectus sheath to avoid any herniation and improve the hollow appearance.

When the new umbilical location is determined, a circular area of 4–6 cm diameter is defatted and the abdominal flap thickness subsequently reduced in the supraumbilical midline cranially to the level of the xiphoid. This can be performed either through liposuction or direct excision of a 1–2 cm measuring subcutaneous wedge for creation of a midline groove.

A main aspect of umbilical accentuation in our experience is emphasizing the supraumbilical abdominal flap depression. This is accomplished through fixation of the abdominal flap dermis to the anterior rectus fascia slightly above the umbilical stalk origin.

Attention has to be taken regarding a sufficient size of abdominal flap incision for reinsertion of the umbilical stalk. If the incision is performed too small, a contracting scar with small appearance of the umbilicus results. In contrast, an overly large incision can result in a huge, unfavorable umbilicus. In this regard it is recommended to perform the incision while the abdominal flap is closed temporarily to take into account the conditional umbilical enlargement from increased tension.

Externus belt

In cases of severe abdominal muscular wall laxity, a simple anterior rectus sheath plication can be insufficient for waist accentuation. In these instances, a supraumbilical externus belt can be applied for enhancement of the waist contour.

After midline plication of the anterior rectus sheath, two fascial reins of external oblique aponeurosis about 2–3 fingerbreadths wide are incised, overlapped across the midline and sutured. To aid with dissection of the fascia, hydrodissection with saline solution can be helpful. Under maximal tension the fascial reins are fixated to the below external oblique fascia using nonresorbable sutures.

If this procedure results in secondary relaxation of the median plication of the anterior rectus sheath, the central plication can be retightened with a second layer of sutures *(Figs 25.27, 25.28)*.

Techniques with previous scars

In the era of minimal invasive surgery with multiple short scars, we frequently observe patients with atypical scars,

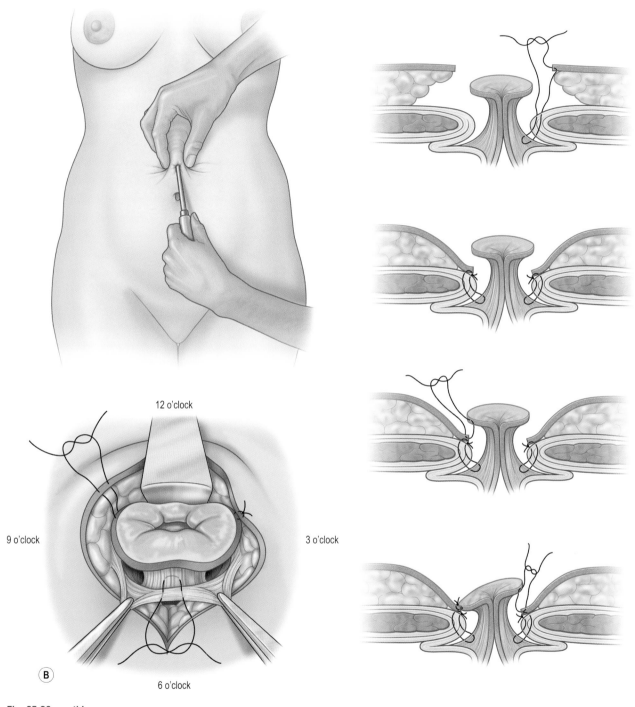

12 o'clock

9 o'clock

3 o'clock

B

6 o'clock

Fig. 25.26, cont'd

which restrict the choice of abdominoplasty technique. Of note, horizontal scars near the costal margin can complicate operative planning, since they cannot be included into the preferred lower abdominal approach.

As a rough guide to avoid complications from impaired perfusion, if a scar will not be removed in the resected specimen, surgeons should at most indirectly undermine or if possible, completely avoid, any undermining in the scar area.

Ideally, the pre-existing scar should be integrated into the proposed incision course, regardless of a possible impaired aesthetic appearance. Impaired perfusion of the abdominal flap may result in necrosis of the dermal and fat layer with consequent wound dehiscence.

In cases of cranial transverse scars after abdominal laparotomy, the lower incision should be planed higher to be included in the final abdominoplasty scar *(Fig. 25.25)*.

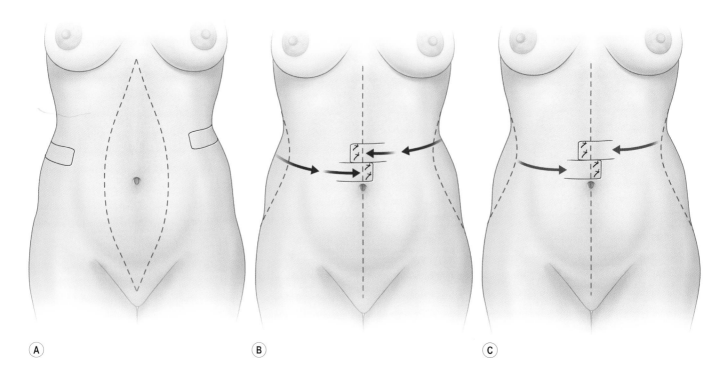

Fig. 25.27 Intraoperative schematic view of an externus belt procedure with preservation and fascial tightening.

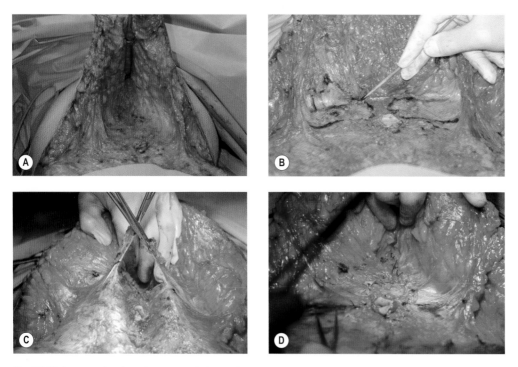

Fig. 25.28 Intraoperative view of an externus belt procedure with preservation and fascial tightening. After release of midline adhesions the fascial flap is designed. Following diastasis recti plication, the flaps are crossed and fixated with reconstructiion of fascial layers.

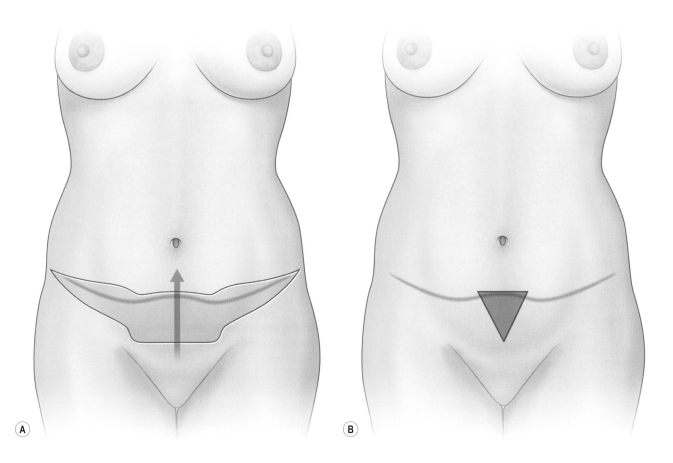

Fig. 25.29 Horizontal and vertical monsplasty.

Management of the mons pubis

Secondary findings in patients with abdominal wall laxity and tissue excess are often hypertrophy or mild to severe ptosis of the mons pubis. Especially in MWL patients, the mons pubis is deflated not only in a vertical but also horizontal vector. Patients may complain about a pseudo-hypertrophy of the mons pubis which is created by an imbalance between abdominal flattening and mons pubis laxity. This can be accentuated by the disruption of lymphatic drainage to the mons.

Additive liposuction of the mons pubis is sufficient in most abdominoplasty cases without local skin excess. In patients particularly after MWL with hypertrophy and surplus skin in the mons pubis region, we routinely perform a horizontal monsplasty, which is integrated into the lower abdominal incision. It is recommended to respect a distance of 6–7 cm from the incision line to the anterior vulva commissure.

In cases of severe hypertrophy and ptosis of the mons pubis, as may be seen in MWL patients, a combined horizontal and vertical monsplasty is indicated. In this context, an additional V-shaped excision at the midline can be conducted. Surgical dissection should be carried out cautiously due to the ilioinguinal nerve which innervates the mons pubis and inguinal crease together with a very anteroproximal part of

the root of the penis or labia majora.[42] In cases of extreme surplus skin, a bilateral monsplasty can be included into a medial thigh plasty, which is frequently performed in MWL patients, preferably as second stage procedures following abdominoplasty or lower circumferential trunk procedures *(Fig. 25.29)*.

Complications

Patients can expect postoperative pain or soreness, numbness of the abdominal flap, bruising, general fatigue and discomfort due to increased abdominal tension for many weeks.

Complications can be localized or systemic. Local complications include hematoma, seroma, wound infection, fat necrosis, wound dehiscence, paresthesias and persisting numbness. Of these, seromas are the most common problem and are usually handled with serial punctures and drainage. Persistent seromas may require an indwelling drain, or in the case of a late encapsulated seroma, a secondary surgical procedure. If a seroma pocket becomes infected, cellulitis will first be apparent and the patient may become febrile and systemically ill. If suspected, an infected seroma must be surgically drained. In general, if seromas are detected in time, a simple aspiration may preserve from a deteriorating course.

Minor wound dehiscence is common and is normally a self-limiting problem. Significant dehiscence may be due to excess tension or marginal wound necrosis. If necrosis occurs, it is usually in the distal portion of the abdominoplasty flap near the midline where tension is greatest. Appropriate treatment is conservative wound care, although once a significant area of necrosis has demarcated, it should be surgically debrided. If secondary wound healing is ineffective, a skin graft may be necessary for wound closure. It is seldom possible, and almost never indicated to attempt additional flap advancement to close a postoperative wound healing defect.

Many local problems of a cosmetic nature can result from abdominoplasty. These include lateral dog-ears, widened or hypertrophic scars, malpositioned scars, and numerous cosmetic problems directly related to the umbilicus. Most of these problems can be avoided with proper preoperative planning and attention to surgical detail. If liposuction has been done simultaneously, issues pertaining to that procedure include contour irregularities and dermal tethering.

Systemic complications include deep vein thrombosis, pulmonary embolism, respiratory compromise due to increased intraabdominal pressure, and systemic infections including toxic shock syndrome. All of these complications are potentially lethal and must be dealt with expeditiously. Surgeons should be aware that abdominoplasty, especially when combined with other procedures such as liposuction, has a higher systemic complication rate than any other type of routine cosmetic surgical procedure.

Contraindications

Patients with significant health risks, with unrealistic surgical goals and body dysmorphic disorder are primary contraindications for an elective abdominoplasty procedure. Relative contraindications to abdominoplasty include: right, left, or bilateral upper quadrant scars; further severe co-morbid conditions (e.g., heart disease, diabetes, morbid obesity, cigarette smoking); eventual future plans for pregnancy; a history of thromboembolic disease, and morbid obesity (BMI >40). Patients with disposition to keloids or hypertrophic scars have to be informed, and must accept the postoperative scarring associated with these conditions.

 Bonus images for this chapter can be found online at **http://www.expertconsult.com**

Fig. 25.1 Development of abdominoplasty procedure, demonstrating the different types of abdominoplasty and the historical highlights.

 Access the complete references list online at **http://www.expertconsult.com**

1. Hunstad JP, Repta R. *Atlas of abdominoplasty*. Philadelphia: Saunders Elsevier; 2009.

   This major work on all current abdominoplasty procedures is written by a leading authority on this subject, covering all topics from patient selection, incision placement, ancillary procedures up to all possible complications by highlighting key considerations for a safe and successful performance.

8. Pitanguy I. Abdominolipectomy. An approach to it through an analysis of 300 consecutive cases. *Plast Reconstr Surg*. 1967;40:384.

13. Dellon AL. Fleur-de-lis abdominoplasty. *Aesthet Plast Surg*. 1985;9:27.

   Dellon first published, in 1985, his approach to a vertical and horizontal restoration of the abdominal wall through a combined resection, the "fleur-de-lis" technique.

15. Lockwood T. High lateral-tension abdominoplasty with superficial fascial system suspension. *Plast Reconstr Surg*. 1995;96:603–608.

   This article describes the principles and details of this new approach to abdominoplasty. It offers an alternative technique, especially in patients after massive weight loss with limited treatment of the flanks.

16. Saldanha OR, Pinto EB, Matos WN Jr, et al. Lipoabdominoplasty without undermining. *Aesthet Surg J*. 2001;21(6):518–526.

21. Costa-Ferreira A, Rebelo M, Vásconez LO, et al. Scarpa fascia preservation during abdominoplasty: a prospective study. *Plast Reconstr Surg*. 2010;125(4): 1232–1239.

22. Huger Jr WE. The anatomic rationale for abdominal lipectomy. *Am Surg*. 1979;45(9):612–617.

27. Bozola AR. Abdominoplasty: same classification and a new treatment concept 20 years later. *Aesthet Plast Surg*. 2010;34(2):181–192.

28. Song AY, Jean RD, Hurwitz DJ, et al. A classification of contour deformities after bariatric weight loss: the Pittsburgh Rating Scale. *Plast Reconstr Surg*. 2005;116(5): 1535–1546.

   Rubin, as a currently "leading postbariatric surgeon" has published an interesting work on the different deformities in patients after bariatric weight loss, which may serve as a guideline for plastic surgeons during preoperative planning and for evaluation of their postoperative outcomes.

34. Aly AS. *Body contouring after massive weight loss*. St Louis: Quality Medical; 2006.

   This work is published by a currently "leading postbariatric surgeon." Aly has composed a unique work on all reliable techniques for body contouring of patients after massive weight loss.

26

Lipoabdominoplasty

Osvaldo Ribeiro Saldanha, Sérgio Fernando Dantas de Azevedo, Osvaldo Ribeiro Saldanha Filho, Cristianna Bonneto Saldanha, and Luis Humberto Uribe Morelli

SYNOPSIS

The results of lipoadominoplasty include:

- Better body contour, because liposuction decreases abdominal measurement.
- Less morbidity due to preservation of the perforating vessels and the absence of dead space.
- Low percentage of complications.
- It is easy to perform because all surgeons perform liposuction and abdominoplasty.
- Rejuvenated abdomen with a more natural profile.
- Preservation of suprapubic sensitivity.
- Quick postoperative recovery and shorter scar.
- It can be associated with vibroliposuction or ultrasound liposuction.
- Safe in smokers and postbariatric patients.

 Access the Historical Perspective section and Figure 26.1 online at **http://www.expertconsult.com**

Introduction

Functional and aesthetic deformities of the abdominal wall due to skin flaccidity, lipodistrophy, and diastasis of the fascia and muscles cause many negative psychological, physiological, and aesthetic effects.

Abdominoplasty and liposuction attempt to correct those problems. For many years abdominoplasty was considered to be a relatively easy procedure to perform, but its results were not always satisfactory from a cosmetic point of view. In the evolution of aesthetic abdominal surgery many surgical treatments have been proposed, as surgeons searched for innovations.[1–17] The goals have been an improvement of shape with minimal morbidity and a low complication rate. For the past few years, there has been considerable progress in

methods to undermine the abdominoplasty flap and treat abdominal wall fat.

Lipoabdominoplasty was developed as a safe aesthetic and functional option combining complete abdominal liposuction and full abdominoplasty in the same surgical procedure, promoting the benefits of both techniques. It was the result of clinical–surgical observation, anatomic cadaver studies, and scientific research of the abdominal perforating vessels. There are two components: (1) superficial liposuction, which undermines the flap, making it free to slide to the pubis; and (2) preservation of the abdominal perforating vessels.

This technique is more than simply using liposuction while performing abdominoplasty. It is a wider concept which respects abdominal anatomy and substitutes cannula undermining instead of traditional undermining. As a consequence, blood supply from abdominal perforating vessels is preserved. In addition, this procedure creates a narrow central tunnel which makes possible safe and direct plication of the rectus abdominis muscles.

Basic science/disease process

Anatomic principles of the lipoabdominoplasty

Lipoabdominoplasty is based on an understanding of the vascular anatomy of the abdominal wall, particularly the perforating vessels, which come from the deep epigastric arteries. Many studies have evaluated the vascular anatomy of this region based on cadaver dissections, clinical observations, and noninvasive radiological examinations.[27–29]

Taylor et al. (1991) studied skin vascularity, describing the angiosomes which separate the abdominal area into superior, inferior, and lateral regions.[29] In the superior region, the superior epigastric vessels are responsible for blood supply. In the lateral region, the superficial and deep circumflex vessels and branches of the intercostal vessels provide blood supply.

Abdominoplasty

Lipoabdominoplasty
'Saldanha's technique'

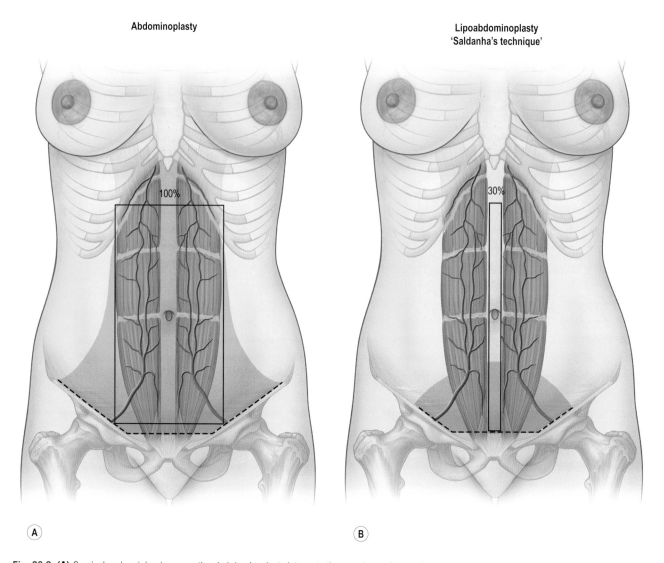

(A)

(B)

Fig. 26.2 (A) Surgical undermining in conventional abdominoplasty interrupts the vascular perforators from the rectus muscles. **(B)** Lipoabdominoplasty preserves vascular perforators from the rectus muscles but allows for a relatively avascular midline tunnel to perform rectus plication. The broken lines indicate the incisions; note that they are shorter in lipoabdominoplasty.

In the inferior region, the main vascularity comes from the inferior deep epigastric vessels *(Fig. 26.2)*.

According to Huger,[30] in classical abdominoplasty, normal vascular flow is interrupted by section of the perforating vessels coming from the rectus abdominis muscle. Consequently, the vascularity of the remaining flap is supplied by the intercostals, subcostal and lumbar perforating branches, situated superiorly and laterally. Therefore when combined with liposuction, extensive traditional undermining may damage the vascularity of the flap, increasing the risk of tissue necrosis. This anatomy is described in Chapter 25.

An important paper published by Graf,[31] using Doppler flowmetry, looked at perfusion in the periumbilical perforating vessels on the 15th day after lipoabdominoplasty, showing that liposuction did not damage vessels whose diameters were 1 mm or more. Furthermore, there was a 9% increase in the caliber of the arteries and a 56% increase in the flow of these perforators. The explanation for this increase in flow is uncertain, but may be due to the physiopathology of surgical trauma generating vasodilatation.

Munhoz *et al.*[32] identified and quantified the perforating vessels, which allowed for a comparative evaluation of the blood supply of the flap in the pre- and postoperative periods of patients who had undergone lipoabdominoplasty. In this study more than 81.21% of perforating vessels were preserved.

Another relevant paper was published by De Frene *et al.*,[33] in which the authors performed breast reconstruction using flaps based on vessels which perforate the rectus abdominis muscles, in patients who had previous abdominal liposuction. The successful outcomes demonstrated that liposuction had not harmed the larger perforating vessels.

Fundamental principles of the technique

The two fundamentals of this technique are preservation of abdominal wall perforating vessels and the use of superficial liposuction. In this anatomic location, superficial liposuction, originally introduced by De Souza Pinto, involves aspiration of fat superficial to Scarpa's fascia.[7,26] The key finding which makes lipoabdominoplasty possible is that superficial cannula liposuction significantly mobilizes the abdominal wall flap. The flap can then be advanced inferiorly to the pubis, without the need for classical undermining in the area of the vascular perforating vessels. A narrow central tunnel between the vascular perforators can then be safely opened in order to accomplish rectus plication.

This technique makes it possible to preserve at least 80% of blood supply to the abdominal wall, to preserve sensory nerves and lymphatic vessels, and to have fewer complications than with traditional abdominoplasty

Diagnosis/patient presentation

Preoperative ultrasound

Although a careful clinical abdominal examination may detect small abdominal masses suspected to be hernias, not all hernias are totally palpable. The systematic use of ultrasound in the preoperative phase of lipoabdominoplasty improves safety by identifying the presence of a hidden ventral hernia before carrying out liposuction of the abdominal wall.

Although the incidence of incisional hernia is low (about 4.3%), taking into consideration that the mortality index is 50%, when intestinal perforation occurs due to liposuction the use of preoperative ultrasound is justifiable.

Patient selection

All patients with the traditional indications for abdominoplasty are candidates for lipoabdominoplasty. Typical findings are lipodystrophy of the abdomen, flaccidity of the abdominal wall skin, and the possibility of rectus muscle diastasis.

Smokers require special care, but the conservative principles inherent in this technique make lipoabdominoplasty possible in these patients.

Treatment/surgical technique

Marking

The abdomen is marked in the traditional manner, as described by Pitanguy,[5] with a 12–14-cm horizontal component, and 7–8-cm oblique components on each side, inclined approximately 40–45° in the direction of the iliac crests. The distance from vaginal furcula to the horizontal marking is 6–7 cm *(Fig. 26.3)*.

For better orientation at the beginning of tunnel undermining, the rectus diastasis is marked *(Fig. 26.4)*. If indicated, dorsal areas to be aspirated are marked.

Infiltration

The wet or superwet technique is used, infiltrating the abdominal wall fat with a solution of saline and epinephrine (1 : 500 000), using an average infusate of 1.0–1.5 litres.

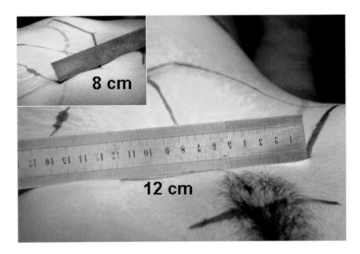

Fig. 26.3 Horizontal marking (12–14 cm), oblique marking (7–8 cm), and initial distance from the pubis (6–7 cm).

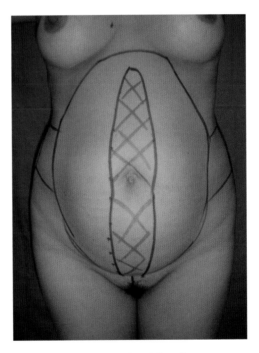

Fig. 26.4 Previous demarcation of diastasis.

Epigastric and subcostal liposuction

In order to perform liposuction safely, the patient is placed in a hyperextended position on the surgical table. Liposuction is started in the supraumbilical region with a 3- and 4-mm cannula, removing the fat of the deep and superficial layers, going out to the flank *(Fig. 26.5)*. As in classic liposuction, enough fat thickness is maintained to avoid vascular impairment and contour deformities.

Lower abdomen

Before removing excess skin, in order to facilitate the visualization and the preservation of the Scarpa's fascia, all fat in the superficial layer is aspirated along with partial removal in the deep layer, using a 6-mm caliber cannula *(Fig. 26.6)*. The flap

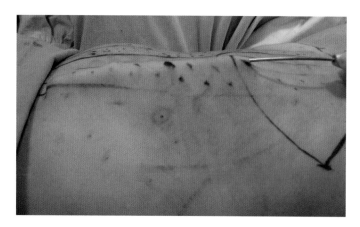

Fig. 26.5 Superior abdominal liposuction.

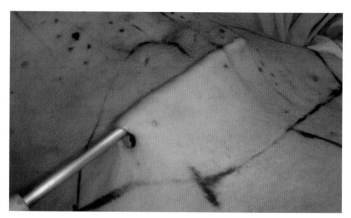

Fig. 26.6 Lower abdominal liposuction.

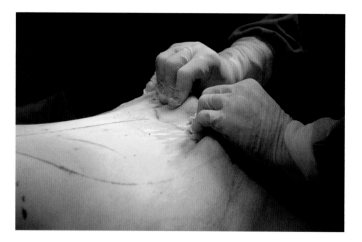

Fig. 26.7 The flap descent evaluation.

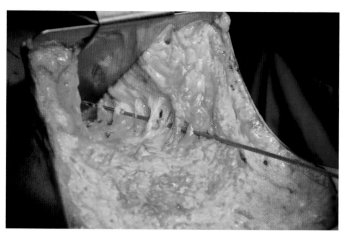

Fig. 26.8 Perforating vessels and Scarpa's fascia preservation.

mobility is assessed before the umbilicus is isolated and resection of the infraumbilical skin is done as in a traditional abdominoplasty *(Fig. 26.7)*. When necessary, complementary open liposuction is performed, removing more fat below the Scarpa's fascia in order to create a homogeneous surface to accommodate the superior flap, which becomes thinner in its descent.

Selective undermining

A tunnel is then undermined in the midline of the upper abdomen between the internal borders of the rectus abdominal muscles, avoiding the midportion of these muscles which is an area of the perforating vessels *(Figs 26.8, 26.9)*.

Tunnel undermining may reach the xiphoid process, depending on the degree of plication necessary. For a better view of the anatomic structures, and to facilitate the plication, a special retractor has been created that exposes the surgical area and avoids trauma on the edge of the flap *(Fig. 26.10)*. The larger the diastasis, the larger the undermining of the tunnel, because the vessels will be further apart, emanating from the substance of the rectus abdominis muscles.

Preservation of Scarpa's fascia

In the lower abdomen all the superficial fat layer should be aspirated to facilitate the visualization and preservation of

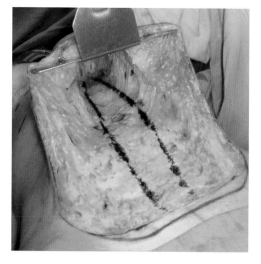

Fig. 26.9 Selective undermining of the tunnel.

Scarpa's fascia, leaving it intact after the removal of the lower abdominal skin.

The preservation of Scarpa's fascia is important for many reasons. There is less bleeding due to preservation of the inferior perforating vessels; there is homogeneous support for the upper flap, which becomes thinner on its descent; it

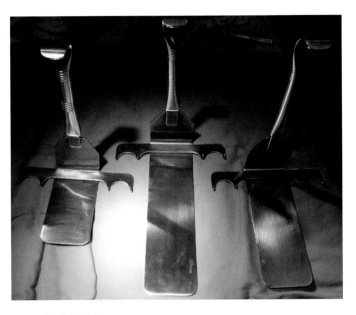

Fig. 26.10 Saldanha's retractor.

provides shorter scars laterally because the preservation of Scarpa's fascia and the rectus muscle plication produce a centripetal retraction, reducing the final surgical scar in 30% of cases to shorter than the initial incision. It also offers a better adherence between the flap and the deep layers *(Fig. 26.11)*.

Resection of the infraumbilical tissue and rectus abdominal muscle plication

In the infraumbilical midline, a vertical strip of soft tissue containing Scarpa's fascia and adipose tissue is removed. This will expose the medial edges of the rectus abdominis muscles which are then plicated from the xiphoid appendix to the pubic symphysis *(Figs 26.12, 26.13)*.

Omphaloplasty

A star-shaped omphaloplasty technique is used, with an incision shaped like a cross on the abdominal wall and a rectangular shape outlined on the umbilical pedicle. The cardinal points of the umbilical pedicle are sutured, approximating

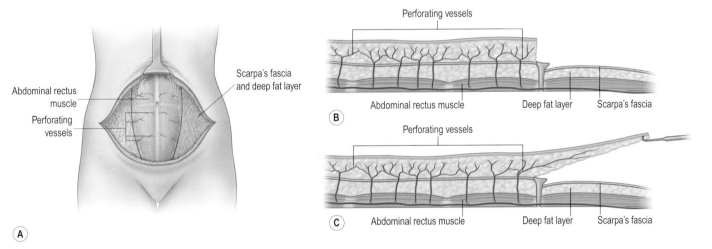

Fig. 26.11 (A–C) Preservation of Scarpa's fascia and partial deep fat layer in the lower abdomen to accommodate the abdominal flap.

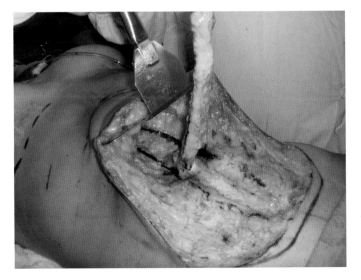

Fig. 26.12 Resection of the infraumbilical fuse.

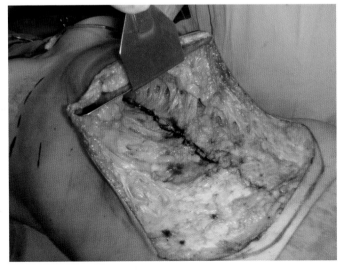

Fig. 26.13 Plication.

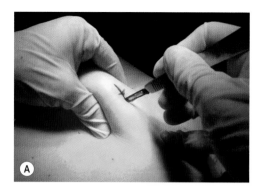
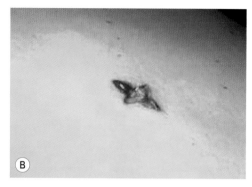

Fig. 26.14 (A) Marking and **(B)** incision: the "star technique" omphaloplasty.

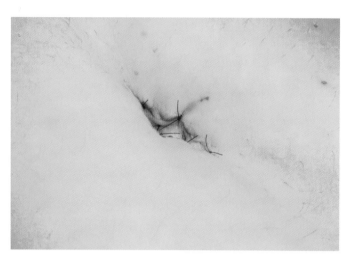

Fig. 26.15 Final appearance of umbilicus.

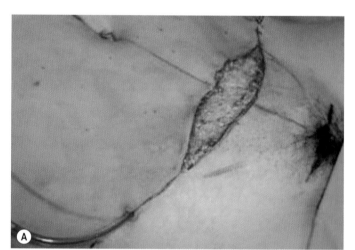

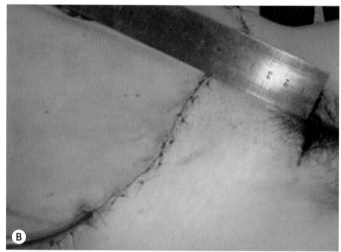

Fig. 26.16 (A,B) Suture of the layers and lowering the scar.

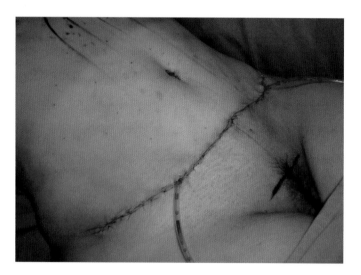
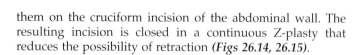

Fig. 26.17 Scar 6–8 cm from the vulvar commissure and aspiration drain.

them on the cruciform incision of the abdominal wall. The resulting incision is closed in a continuous Z-plasty that reduces the possibility of retraction *(Figs 26.14, 26.15)*.

Suture of the layers and drain

Suturing is done in two layers, with 3-0 Monocryl in the deep layer and 4-0 in the subdermis, trying to take the tension off the midline skin closure by placing more tension laterally, as recommended by Lockwood.[12,13] The skin is closed with interrupted 5-0 nylon stitches. At the end of the procedure, if there is decreased abdominal tension, it is possible to remove 2–3 cm more of pubic skin, putting the scar lower *(Fig. 26.16)*. A continuous aspiration drain (4.2 mm) is used for 1–2 days *(Fig. 26.17)*. The surgery takes about 2 hours and the patient stays in hospital for 1 day.

Intermittent pneumatic pressure of the legs, adjusted between 30 and 40 mmHg, is used throughout the procedure and in the immediate postoperative period, until the patient is able to mobilize actively.

Dressings and postoperative care

The dressing consists of paper surgical tape on the suture line. These tapes are changed on the third postoperative day, and again on the eighth day, at which time the stitches are removed. The umbilical stitches are removed on the 12th day after surgery.

The patient is instructed to use a compressive garment for 20 days after surgery.

In addition, patients can benefit from lymphatic drainage, which is started on the fourth day of the postoperative period.

Patients who undergo lipoabdominoplasty present an intermediary recovery between an abdominoplasty and a liposuction because the lipoabdominoplasty is less invasive, causes little vascular and nerve trauma, and leaves a smaller dead space. These factors altogether result in less morbidity and a faster return to social and professional activities than is the case with traditional abdominoplasty.

Outcomes

In the first 10 years of the author's series, there was an increase of 100% in the abdominal procedures: before 2000, averaging 35 patients per year and in 2009, averaging 75 patients per year. In the same time period, there was a 50% reduction in the need for surgical revisions. Late in the series there were two cases of traditional abdominoplasty, chosen because the patients primarily had skin excess after bariatric surgery.

There was a decrease in the final scar extension when compared to the initial marking in 30% of patients. The initial line always measured 28 cm in length – 12 cm horizontal and 8 cm oblique on each side. In 602 patients, 180 had a final scar between 25 and 27 cm, with an average reduction of 2 cm from the initial marking. This is due to the traction that the Scarpa's fascia makes on the skin.

The graceful shape of the umbilicus scar was independently evaluated and rated as good or excellent *(Figs 26.18–26.23)*. ⊚ FIGS **26.19–26.23** APPEAR ONLINE ONLY

The overall results were rated as good to excellent in almost all cases, with better body contour, and a decrease in the abdominal measurements.

On the 7th or 14th day after surgery, the operated area is edematous, including the abdomen and other aspirated areas; however, after 1–2 months, the edema recedes.

Lipoabdominoplasty achieves the results possible with both traditional abdominoplasty and liposuction. The combined procedure achieves a better body contour with reduced morbidity. For most surgeons, there is a fast learning curve because they will be familiar with traditional abdominoplasty and liposuction techniques when done independently.

Complications

In the author's series, the complication rate for traditional abdominoplasty was compared to that with lipoabdomino-plasty. From 1979 to 2000 there were 496 traditional abdomi-noplasty surgeries, and from the year 2000 to 2010 there were 602 cases of lipoabdominoplasty, as shown in *Table 26.1*. The lipoabdominoplasty cases consisted of 12 males and 590 females, with an average age of 36.

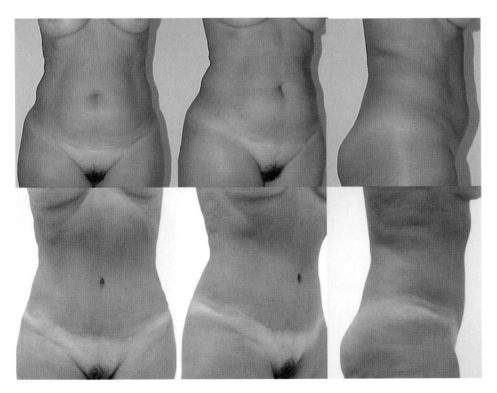

Fig. 26.18 Case 1: pre- and postoperative views.

Table 26.1 Personal statistics of abdominal surgery

	1979–1999	2000	2001	2002	2003	2004	2005	2006	2007	2008	2009	Total
Abdominoplasty	469	25	–	–	–	–	–	–	1	–	1	496
Lipoabdominoplasty	–	15	45	55	64	62	65	68	71	75	82	602

Table 26.2 Surgical revision in lipoabdominoplasty

	2000	2001	2002	2003	2004	2005	2006	2007	2008	2009
Total = 602	15	45	55	64	62	65	68	71	75	82
Scars	3	5	4	3	4	3	3	4	2	1
Skin flaccidity	–	–	1	2	1	1	1	2	–	1
Insufficient liposuction	–	–	1	2	2	1	1	1	1	–
Excessive liposuction	–	–	–	–	–	–	–	–	–	–
Infection	–	–	–	–	–	–	–	–	–	–
Other causes	–	–	–	–	1	–	–	–	–	–
Total = 51	3	5	6	7	8	5	5	7	3	2
Percentage (%)	20	11	11	11	13	8	7	10	4	2

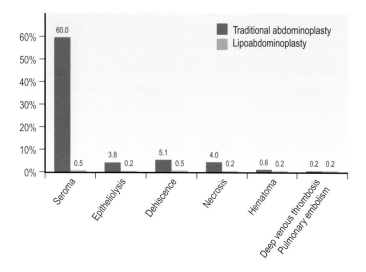

Fig. 26.24 Complications graph comparing traditional abdominoplasty with lipoabdominoplasty.

Figure 26.24 shows the 10-year statistics in the performance of lipoabdominoplasty with selective undermining, compared to the percentage of complications with traditional abdominoplasty.

Table 26.2 shows the percentage of surgical revisions in lipoabdominoplasty. This decreased from 20% with

traditional abdominoplasty to 10% with lipoabdominoplasty. The cases of surgical revision due to complementary liposuction and postoperative skin flaccidity (3%) corresponded to patients who had undergone previous bariatric surgery and presented a great amount of flaccidity. There was a need for surgical revision of scars in 5.3%, which represents 63% of all surgical revisions for lipoabdominoplasty.

A reduced incidence of seroma (from 60% to 0.5%, $P < 0.0001$), epitheliolysis (3.8% to 0.2%, $P = 0.0003$), wound dehiscence (5.1% to 0.5%, $P < 0.0001$) and necrosis (4% to 0.2% $P = 0.0002$) has statistical significance. It is hypothesized that the reduction in flap necrosis may be due to improved vascularity on the arterial side, or possibly due to better venous return.

Although the reduced incidence of hematoma (0.6–0.2%) and the incidence of deep venous thrombosis/pulmonary embolism remained the same (0.2%), the small numbers involved are not statistically significant.

 Bonus images for this chapter can be found online at
http://www.expertconsult.com

Fig. 26.1 Undermining evolution in abdominoplasty from 1899 to 2009.
Fig. 26.19 Case 2: pre- and postoperative views.
Fig. 26.20 Case 3: pre- and postoperative views.
Fig. 26.21 Case 4: pre- and postoperative views.
Fig. 26.22 Case 5: pre- and postoperative views.
Fig. 26.23 Case 6: pre- and postoperative views.

Access the complete references list online at http://www.expertconsult.com

4. Callia WEP. *Dermolipectomia abdominal (operação de Callia)*. São Paulo: Carlos Erba; 1963.

5. Pitanguy I. Abdominoplasty: Classification and surgical techniques. *Rev Bras Cir.* 1995;85: 23–44.

11. Illouz YG. A new safe and aesthetic approach to suction abdominoplasty. *Aesthetic Plast Surg.* 1992;16:237–245.

12. Lockwood T. High-lateral-tension abdominoplasty with superficial fascial system suspension. *Plast Reconstr Surg.* 1995; 96:603–608.

16. Saldanha OR, de Souza Pinto EB, Matos W, et al. Lipoabdominoplasty without undermining. *Aesthet Surg J*. 2001;21:518–526.

   In 2001, using the term "lipoabdominoplasty" for the first time and with the publication of this technique, Saldanha standardized a selective undermining along the internal borders of the rectus abdominal muscles, corresponding to 30% of the traditional undermining, thus preserving the abdominal perforating vessels, performing liposuction and abdominolipoplasty in the same surgical time, safely.

20. Saldanha OR, de Souza Pinto EB, Matos W, et al. Lipoabdominoplasty with selective and safe undermining. *Aesthetic Plast Surg*. 2003;22:322–327.

   The aesthetic treatment of the abdominal region using the principles of liposuction associated with traditional abdominoplasty. Lipoabdominoplasty is different from other techniques because it has the advantages of conserving perforator vessels of the abdominal wall.

22. Saldanha OR. *Lipoabdominoplasty*. Rio de Janeiro, Brazil: Di-Livros; 2006.

   In this book the author describes the anatomical concepts, history, and evolution of the technique of lipoabdominoplasty. Saldanha describes each detail of this surgery.

24. Saldanha OR, Azevedo SF, Delboni PS, et al. Lipoabdominoplasty: the Saldanha technique. *Clin Plast Surg*. 2010;37:469–81.

   The incidence of complications was compared in traditional abdominoplasty to that in lipoabdominoplasty. From 1979 to 2000 the author performed 496 traditional abdominoplasty surgeries, and from the year 2000 to the present date lipoabdominoplasty was performed on 602 patients.

26. De Souza Pinto EB. *Superficial Liposuction*. Rio de Janeiro: Revinter; 1999;1–4.

   Superficial liposuction, introduced by Souza Pinto, was one of the fundamental principles of lipoabdominoplasty because it made its performance possible and easier. This procedure gives more mobility to the abdominal flap so that it can slide down easily and reach the suprapubic region.

29. Taylor GI, Watterson PA, Zelt RG. The vascular anatomy of the anterior abdominal wall: The basis for flap design. *Perspect Plast Surg*. 1991;5:1.

27

Lower bodylifts

Al Aly, Khalid Al-Zahrani, and Albert Cram

SYNOPSIS

- The subcutaneous abdominal fat is divided into a superficial and deep layer by the superficial fascial system, which in the abdomen is called Scarpa's fascia.
- The skin/fat envelope is tethered to the underlying musculoskeletal anatomy in zones of adherence. These include the spine, the sternum, the linea alba of the abdomen, the inguinal area, the suprapubic area and the area between the hip and lateral thigh fat.
- Massive weight loss (MWL) patients make up the majority of patients who undergo lower bodylift/belt lipectomy surgery. Second are females with a BMI in the range of 26–28. Third are normal weight females who wish a more dramatic improvement than an abdominoplasty alone.
- Three factors affect patient presentation: the BMI, the fat deposition pattern, and the quality of the skin/fat envelope.
- Bodylift/belt lipectomy procedures can be thought of as a circumferential wedge excision of the lower trunk. One end of the spectrum of procedures is the lower bodylift type II (Lockwood technique) and the other end is the belt lipectomy/central bodylift (Aly and Cram technique).
- Patients presenting for this surgery require a complete medical assessment and a thorough physical examination.
- In planning a bodylift/belt lipectomy, scar position can be approximated by simulating the tissue dynamics at the time of closure. Anteriorly, the inferior marks control scar position and posteriorly, the superior marks control the scar position.
- The operative sequence usually involves anterior surgery first, followed by posterior surgery and closure.
- Postoperative care requires hospital level nursing with attention to patient positioning, early ambulation, fluid infusion and pain control.
- Major complications are possible, but the commonest problem is seroma.

Access the Historical Perspective section online at
http://www.expertconsult.com

Introduction

Body contour deformities of the lower trunk can range from "anterior only" to "circumferential" deformities. If the problems are restricted to isolated moderate lipodystrophy deposits then liposuction may be the only treatment modality needed. Anteriorly, if skin laxity and/or abdominal wall weakness are encountered, then abdominoplasty techniques are needed to create the best contour. If, in addition to the anterior deformities, lateral and posterior lipodystrophy is present, then liposuction may be added to abdominoplasty so that the best possible contour is attained. If the deformities involve skin and subcutaneous laxity circumferentially, then bodylift/belt lipectomy procedures are usually required to adequately address the issues. Thus, in looking at the treatment of a large range of patients presenting with lower truncal deformities, there is a transition from liposuction only, to "anterior only" excisional procedures, to "circumferential" excisional procedures. The decision as to which procedure or procedures to utilize in a particular patient will vary based on the patient's desires as well as the surgeon's philosophy and experience. This chapter addresses circumferential lower truncal excisional procedures, which will be referred to by a number of names including bodylift, belt lipectomy, and circumferential dermatolipectomy.

Basic science and disease process

Anatomy

It is important to have a clear understanding of the blood supply of the abdomen, when contemplating circumferential dermatolipectomy of the lower trunk. The anatomy of abdominal wall blood supply is thoroughly reviewed in Chapter 25.

The subcutaneous abdominal fat is divided into superficial and deep layers by the superficial fascial system, which in this

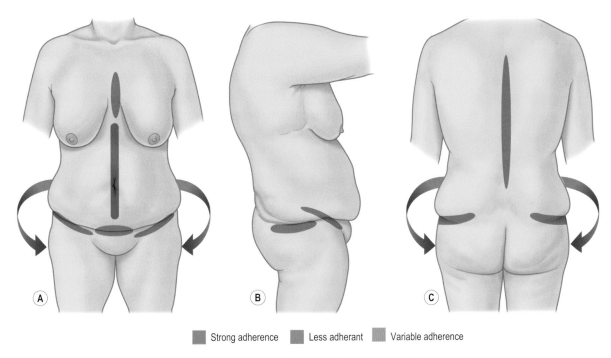

Strong adherence   Less adherant   Variable adherence

Fig. 27.1 The zones of adherence of the trunk. Note the inferomedial descent of tissues that occurs with aging and/or weight loss.

region of the body is called Scarpa's fascia. In thin patients the two layers are fairly close to each other in thickness. In patients who have a high BMI the superficial layer is often much thicker than the deep layer.

There are areas within the trunk where the skin/fat envelope is tethered to the underlying musculoskeletal anatomy, restricting either descent or elevation, which can occur with aging, weight fluctuation, or surgical manipulation. These areas are called "zones of adherence" and act like "hooks" for the skin/fat envelope to hang on to as it falls down, especially after the skin has been stretched by excess weight and then deflated by weight loss. It is important to understand where these zones of adherence are located and how they affect tissue draping *(Fig. 27.1)*. The zones of adherence overlying the spine and the sternum are both strong areas of adherence and are always present, while the zone of adherence overlying the midline linea alba of the abdomen is often week to nonexistent. There are strong zones of adherence overlying the inguinal region bilaterally that play an important role in controlling final scar position during bodylift/belt lipectomy. A more variable zone of adherence is located in the horizontal suprapubic area which when present leads to a suprapubic crease. Its strength and attachment is quite variable from individual to individual. This zone of adherence, along with the inguinal zones of adherence, is responsible for a panniculus hanging over the mons pubis.

Another important zone of adherence is located between the hip and lateral thigh fat deposits. This is an important attachment because it acts like a stop gap of the lateral thighs preventing movement of tissues, either in the superior or inferior direction, especially during manipulations at surgery. In some procedures, such a "lower bodylift type II", as described by Lockwood,[1,2] this zone of adherence is intentionally destroyed to allow for significant elevation of the lateral thighs.

Overall, the soft tissue skin/fat envelope of the lower trunk tends to fall inferomedially, seemingly around the sacrum.

The disease process

There are three groups that can potentially benefit from bodylift/belt lipectomy.[3] Although all of these groups will share some of the same indications and principles in design of the operations, they differ and should be considered here.

Massive weight loss patients

Issues specific to this patient group are reviewed in . Massive weight loss (MWL) patients make up the majority of patients who undergo bodylift/belt lipectomy.[3] The lower trunk of MWL patients can be thought of as a balloon. As patients gain weight and then lose it, the balloon is initially stretched by the weight gain then deflated as weight loss ensues. Like a balloon that has been inflated for a long time, the intrinsic elasticity of the skin is irreversibly altered during this process, leading to redundant lax skin, which is almost always circumferential in nature. The usual pattern is of an inverted cone *(Fig. 27.2)*.

The 20–30 pounds overweight group

Women who are 20–30 pounds overweight (BMI range of 26–28) who have never lost any significant weight despite reasonable exercise and nutritional habits are the second group that can potentially benefit from bodylift/belt lipectomy.

Body mass index (BMI) = Weight in kg/height in meters squared

These patients present with lipodystrophy of the lower trunk that is circumferential in nature which leads to generalized lack of definition of the lower trunk *(Fig. 27.3)*.

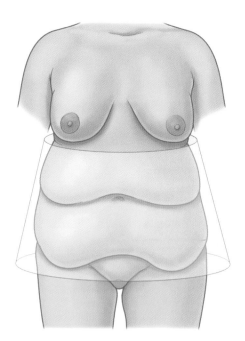

Fig. 27.2 The figure demonstrates the typical shape of the lower trunk after massive weight loss; a three dimensional "inverted cone".

Normal weight patients group

A third group that may benefit from bodylift/belt lipectomy are normal weight patients who ordinarily would be considered candidates for an abdominoplasty, but desire more dramatic improvements in lower truncal contour. These patients often desire a remarkable improvement in their anterior thighs, lateral thighs, buttocks and lower back. In many similar patients, liposuction can improve all of these areas when combined with an abdominoplasty, however, if patients desire significant lifting and contour delineation, then a circumferential excisional procedure is required *(Fig. 27.4)*.

A subgroup of normal weight patients that can benefit from a bodylift/belt lipectomy is made up of older patients whose skin will not contract with liposuction due to skin laxity and will require the pull created by the circumferential excision *(Fig. 27.5)*.

Diagnosis and patient presentation

Most of the subsequent discussions will be centered around the MWL patients and the other groups will be mentioned when appropriate. Although MWL patients are grouped together they are quite variable in their presentation *(Fig. 27.6)*. Three factors seem to affect the presentation; the BMI at presentation, the fat deposition pattern and the quality of the skin/fat envelope.

BMI level at presentation

Massive weight loss patients will present to the plastic surgeons at different BMI levels. For some, this level is still very high, BMIs of ≥35; for others it may be intermediate, BMIs of 30–35; and for others, the BMI may drop to the mid or low 20s *(Fig. 27.6)*. If the patient loses weight through bariatric

surgery, then the type of bariatric operation utilized is likely to affect their final BMI. Lap-band patients tend to lose the least weight, while gastric bypass patients tend to lose more weight, and gastric sleeve patients loose an intermediate amount. Duodenal switch patients are uncommon, but tend to experience the largest drops in BMI.

Fat deposition pattern

The type of deformity that a MWL patient presents with also depends on their particular fat deposition pattern. Humans are born with a genetically controlled pattern of fat deposition, as well as a fat loss pattern. For example, females tend to store fat in the extraperitoneal space, the lower abdomen, hips and thighs; a pattern often referred to as "pear-shaped" *(Fig. 27.7)*. Males on the other hand tend to store fat more centrally in what is often referred to as "apple-shaped", where fat is deposited intraperitoneally and in the flanks (or "love handles"), and less fat is deposited in the thighs *(Fig. 27.7)*. The "pear' and "apple" patterns are only a couple of the many potential fat deposition patterns present in the population.

The skin/fat envelope

The skin/fat envelope is what a plastic surgeon operates on and its intrinsic properties are especially important. Some patients present with very pliable and thin skin/fat envelopes, while others will present with very thick nonpliable tissues. A concept that the authors have found very helpful in examining these patients is the "translation of pull" *(Fig. 27.8)*. For example, when examining the patient prior to surgery the lateral abdominal tissues are pinched simulating the effects of the lateral abdominal resection of a bodylift/belt lipectomy on the distal thigh, which can be predictive of the final result with a certain degree of accuracy. Conversely, if the pinch demonstrates very little translation of pull to these areas, as in the case of patients who present with high BMIs and thick, nonpliable, skin/fat envelopes, this also can be used to predict the final result. As a general rule, the greater the BMI drop, the more translation of pull will be present. Thus, a patient who drops from a BMI of 60–30 will demonstrate a greater translation of pull than a patient who drops from 35 to 30.

Commonalities of presentation

Almost all massive weight loss patients present with a *"hanging panniculus"*. The size and shape of the panniculus will vary from one patient to the other based on their intrinsic fat deposition pattern *(Fig. 27.9)*. Almost every massive weight loss patient will present with a *"ptotic mons pubis"*. The most obvious deformity is vertical excess with varying degrees of horizontal excess.

The waist, which is the narrowest aspect of the lower trunk between the ribs and the pelvic rim, can be blunted in many massive weight loss patients by the hanging skin/soft tissue envelope as it drapes from the ribs to below the pelvic rim. Often, there are remaining fat deposits in the hip and lower back that also contribute to this blunting. With a few exceptions, the thighs are greatly affected by the weight gain/loss process. The anterior and lateral thighs are usually ptotic. In patients that belong to the "20–30 pound overweight group"

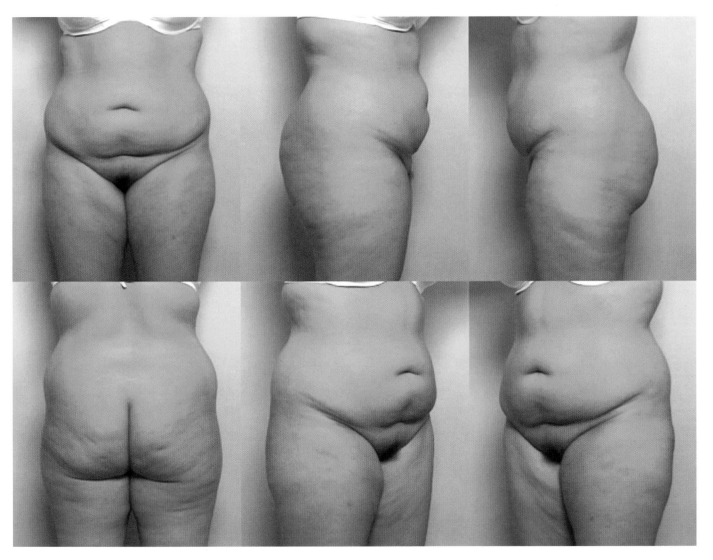

Fig. 27.3 This patient is typical of the "20–30 pound overweight" group. Note the generalized circumferential lipodystrophy of the lower trunk.

and "the normal weight group", the thighs are not as dramatically affected but are still areas of concern.

As with the thighs, the buttocks in the massive weight loss patient are usually ptotic due to the effects of the weight gain/loss process. Those that present with a high BMI, above 35, will most often present with overly projected buttocks. Patients that stabilize at a low BMI of ≤26, will often present with fairly flat underprojected buttocks. Many massive weight loss patients also present with a lack of demarcation between the lower back and buttocks *(Fig. 27.10)*.

Many patients present with back rolls that are bothersome. Some back rolls are located in the lower back and those are generally amenable to improvement through bodylift/belt lipectomy. Superior back rolls, usually contiguous with breast rolls, or just below them, are not affected by bodylift/belt lipectomy procedures and must be addressed through upper bodylift procedures *(Fig. 27.11)*. A small subset of patients will present with "intermediate back rolls" which are located in what the authors call "no man's land" between the upper and lower back rolls. These are very difficult to treat because they may not be eliminated by a bodylift/belt lipectomy or an upper bodylift. Fortunately, these are rare presentations.

Patient selection

Although a "bodylift/belt lipectomy" can be thought of as a circumferential wedge excision of the lower trunk there are variations of the procedure.[4] We have categorized what we feel to be the ends of the spectrum of bodylifts and will go over the differences so that the reader may understand what each can accomplish. On one end is the "lower bodylift type II", as originally described by Lockwood.[1,2] On the other end, there is the "belt lipectomy" as described by the authors, originally in Iowa.[3] It is not the intent of the authors to suggest that one type of bodylift should be utilized over the other. Rather it is hoped that the surgeon would be familiar with these techniques and be able to individualize the particular procedure to the needs of their particular patient.

Lower bodylift type II (Lockwood technique)

In this type of bodylift, the overall circumferential wedge of resection is located lower onto the lower trunk. The procedure can be thought of as a truncal-thigh lift, not just a truncal lift.[5]

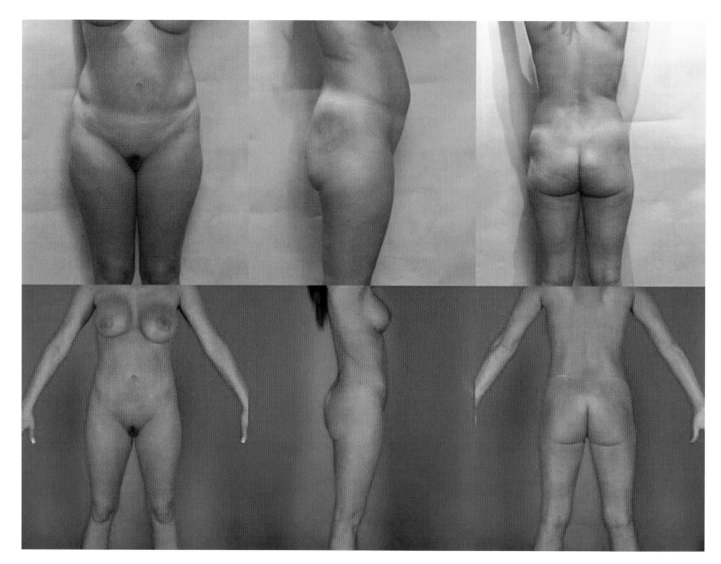

Fig. 27.4 This patient presented in her mid-30s with a desire to improve her abdominal contour but also desired the best possible contour of her entire lower trunk which included better waist definition, lifting of her anterior and lateral thighs, as well as a buttocks lift.

The bilateral zones of adherence located between the hip and trochanteric fat deposits are intentionally destroyed to allow the surgeon to lift the lateral and anterior thighs very aggressively. This is made easier by extensive circumferential liposuction of the soft tissue envelope of the thighs. These steps discontinuously undermine the thighs from the underlying musculoskeletal system allowing for a vigorous elevation of the entire thigh complex, with the exception of the posterior thigh. The posterior thigh can not be lifted directly because of the infra-buttocks zone of adherence which prevents such elevation.

The results of a lower bodylift type II are impressive in its elevation of the thighs. Since the circumferential wedge of excision is low, it creates a fairly low scar that can be covered by most underwear or swimwear patterns *(Fig. 27.12)*. There are disadvantages and limitations of lower bodylift type II. Since the final scar is intentionally created below the widest aspect of the pelvic rim, the waist is not narrowed as much as it would if the final scar is created above. The authors call this the "sundress effect" because it brings the upper truncal tissues across the widest aspect leading to blunting of the waist, rather than narrowing. Anteriorly, the scar is

considerably lower than the anterior superior iliac spine (ASIS), which poses no significant problem if the abdominal flap that is brought down to the level of the scar is thin. However, if the abdominal flap is thick, as in higher BMI patients, it will add to the prominence of the ASIS region, which should be flat, not convex. A disadvantage of a posterior low scar in a lower bodylift type II, which runs across in the midst of the upper third of the buttocks unit, violates the unit principle. This is not problematic in patients who value hiding the scar within low underwear lines and do not require demarcation between the lower back and buttocks, i.e., a male patient. On the other hand, most female patients desire as much buttocks definition as possible and demarcation between the lower back and buttocks (see Box 27.1 for the main advantages and disadvantages of the lower bodylift type II).

Belt lipectomy/central bodylift

Belt lipectomy/central bodylift procedures overall have a more superiorly based wedge of excision when compared with a lower bodylift type II.[6] There is some weakening of the

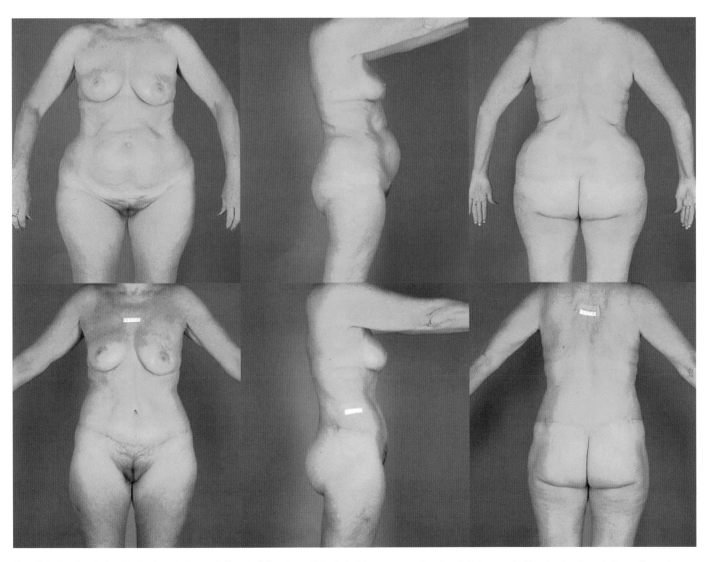

Fig. 27.5 A patient in her 60s is shown before and after a belt lipectomy. Patients in this age group often do not attain enough skin retraction through liposuction and may require an excisional procedure to attain the best possible contour.

Box 27.1 **Lower bodylift type II**

Advantages

- Lifts the trunk.
- Very aggressive thigh lift.
- Reduces the amount of surgery that maybe subsequently needed on the thighs.
- Low scar position to be covered by low lying swim/underwear.

Disadvantages

- Blunts the waist in most patients.
- Scar violates the buttocks unit posteriorly.
- Lack of demarcation between lower back and buttocks.
- Bulge over the ASIS in patients with thick panniculi.

zone of adherence between the hip and lateral thighs but no attempt is made to completely destroy them, as in a lower bodylift type II. These differences lead to a more superiorly positioned scar, circumferentially around the lower trunk. Posteriorly, the scar is ideally positioned at the natural junction between the lower back and buttocks, which promotes more attractive buttocks, demarcates the lower back from the buttocks, and in most patients creates a narrower waist. Anteriorly, the scar positioning above the ASIS further promotes narrowing of the waist by "cinching" above the widest aspect of the pelvic rim. This is especially helpful in patients who present with thick abdominal flaps, which will fit in a depression above the ASIS, rather than over it. Because the zones of adherence are only weakened during this technique, the thighs are not as aggressively lifted as in a lower bodylift type II.

There are disadvantages of belt lipectomy/central bodylift, with the superiorly positioned scar being the primary one. Fashions at the time of the writing, cover a lower position on the torso than most belt lipectomy/central bodylift scars, especially the posterior aspect. Although this may change with fashion trends, it is a legitimate problem, especially in male patients who generally do not care for waist narrowing or buttocks definition. Another disadvantage of this technique is that the extent of thigh elevation is not as great as that attained with a lower bodylift type II technique. Thus, the

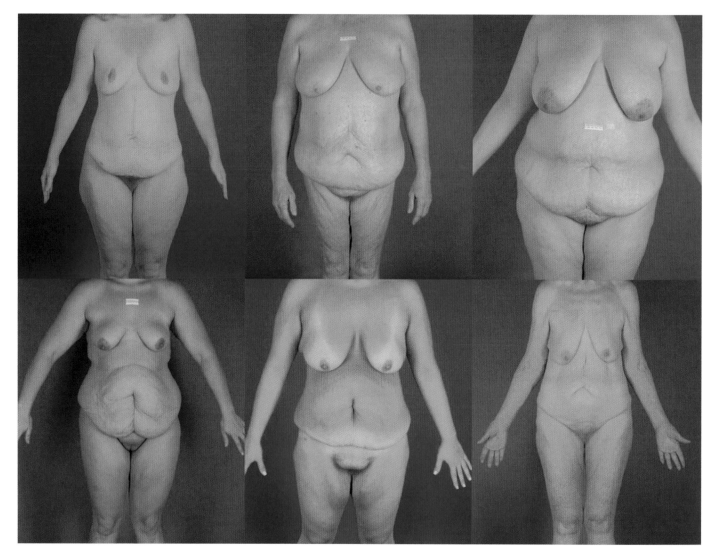

Fig. 27.6 Six massive weight loss patients are shown at presentation after weight stabilization. Note the significant amount of variability in BMI, fat deposition pattern and quality of the skin/fat envelope.

extent of thigh reduction that may need to be performed after the belt lipectomy/central bodylift is usually more extensive than after a lower bodylift type II.

It is important to note that a plastic surgeon who treats MWL patients on a regular basis should be familiar with both the lower bodylift type II and belt lipectomy/central bodylift, so that they may mix and match these techniques to create the best possible outcome for a particular patient (see Box 27.2 for the main advantages and disadvantages of belt lipectomy/central bodylift).

Selection criteria

Significant cardiopulmonary disease is a contraindication for bodylift/belt lipectomy procedures. Smoking is considered a contraindication by most surgeons. Some surgeons operate on smokers and accept a higher complication rate. Diabetes certainly can have detrimental effects on healing and increases the risk of infection. The surgeon has to determine if the overall medical condition of the patient can tolerate these

---

Box 27.2 **Belt lipectomy/central bodylift**

Advantages

- Lifts the trunk.
- Leads to waist narrowing.
- Improves buttocks contour.
- Demarcates the lower back from buttocks.

Disadvantages

- High position of scar outside of normal swim/underwear.
- Thigh reduction is not as aggressive as other technique.
- May result in more extensive thigh reduction surgery than other technique.

---

added risks. The authors of this chapter have for many years avoided operating on diabetics but recently started including some well selected patients. Patients with collagen vascular disease should also be approached with extreme caution. The authors have operated on a few and have had difficulty with healing and infection.

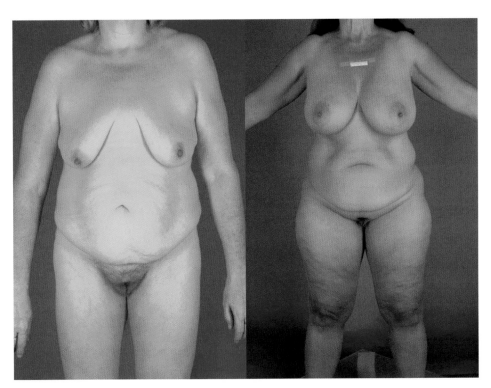

Fig. 27.7 Two patients demonstrating the two most common fat deposition patterns. On the left, the "apple" shape is shown, most often encountered in males, although demonstrated in a female here. On the right, the typical "pear"-shaped female pattern of fat deposition is shown.

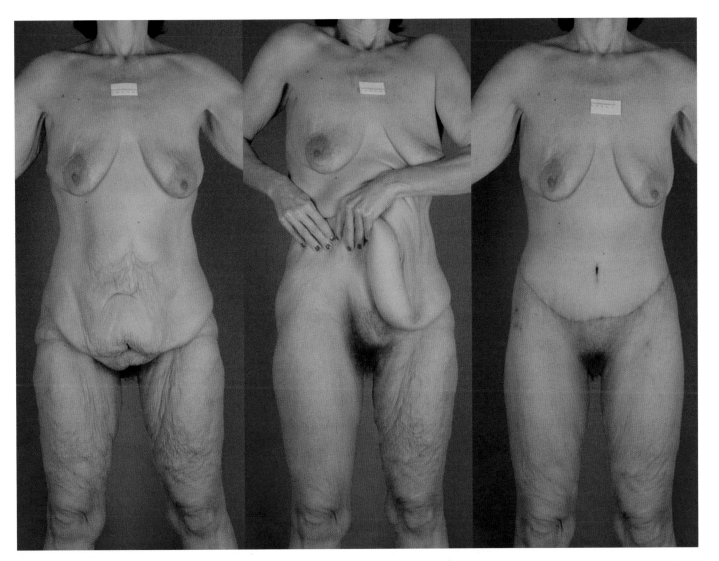

Fig. 27.8 The "translation of pull" is demonstrated in this figure. The patient in the middle picture is demonstrating the potential distant effects of the proposed resection, simulated by the pinching hands. Note the postoperative anterior thigh contour is fairly similar to the preoperative pinch.

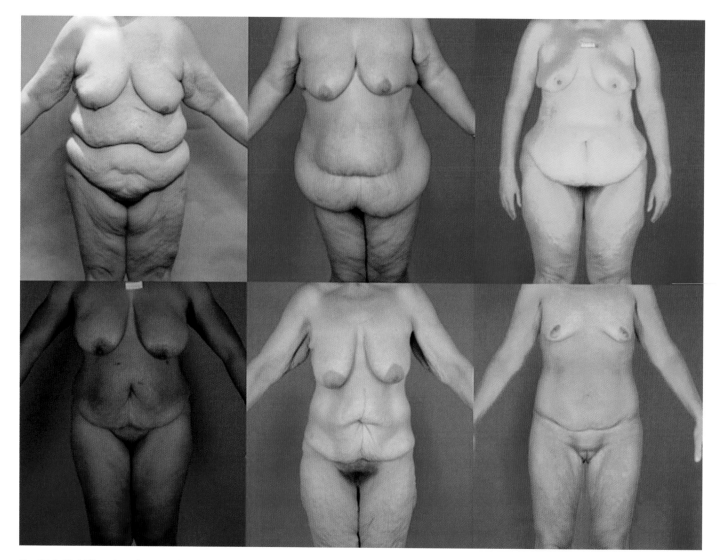

Fig. 27.9 Six MWL patients demonstrating the variety in shape and size of their presenting panniculi.

The BMI at presentation should be a very important factor in determining whether a plastic surgeon should operate. As will be discussed later in this chapter, complications increase with increasing BMIs.[7] Many plastic surgeons do not operate on patients that present with a BMI >32. This is a reasonable level, especially for those surgeons who are new to MWL body contouring surgery and/or circumferential procedures. The authors of this chapter routinely operate on patients in higher BMI ranges but they accept a much higher complication rate, especially if the BMI is >35, where the complication rate is around 100%.

Ideally, it is best to delay body contouring procedures until patients have stabilized their weight loss. It is important that weight stabilization is reached without "heroic efforts", like starvation diets and extreme exercise regimens. The weight loss process in many patients will often have "false plateaus" where the patient will stabilize, but then start to drop again. It is important that the surgeon determine whether the patient has reached their true plateau, which is not always easy. If the patient has had bariatric surgery it is beneficial to engage the bariatric surgeon to help answer that question. The longer the time of stabilization the more likely the patient will be able to maintain that weight loss, thus increasing the chances of long-term success. Most surgeons feel that a minimum of 3 months of stabilization is required. The length of time it takes to reach maximum weight loss, and 3 months of stabilization differs from one bariatric procedure to the other. For lap-bands, the average time is around 2 years. For gastric bypass and gastric sleeve procedures, the average is around 18 months. And for duodenal switch procedures the average is 12–14 months. These numbers are not absolute and may vary considerably from individual to individual.

If a patient presents with too much intra-abdominal content to allow flattening of abdominal contour by muscle wall plication, then the result of a circumferential procedure is very similar to that attainable by panniculectomy.[8] It would thus be prudent to avoid the increased risk of the circumferential excision and limit the procedure to a panniculectomy.

The recovery period after a circumferential dermatolipectomy can be quite challenging both physically and psychologically. Choosing a patient with unstable psychological problems to go through the prolonged and arduous recovery can result in disastrous consequences. (Criteria for patient selection are given in Box. 27.3.)

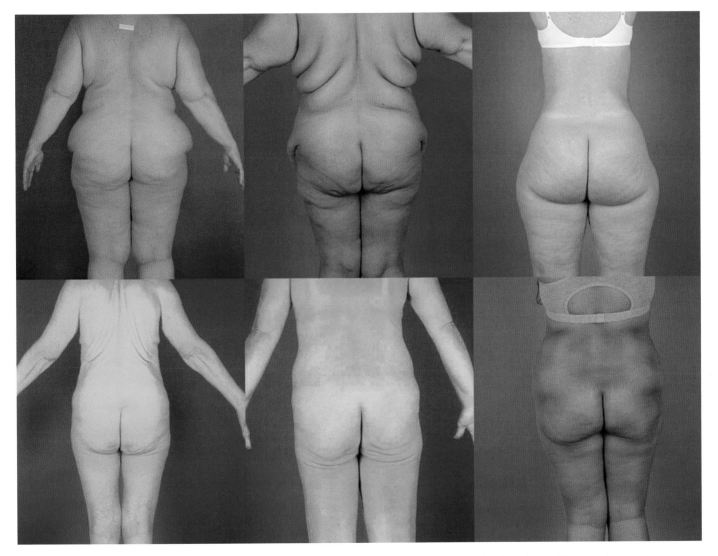

Fig. 27.10 The variety in shape and size of the buttocks is demonstrated in these six MWL patients. The accompanying lipodystrophy of the hip region, as well as the descent of the buttocks, often contribute to a lack of buttocks definition and demarcation from the lower back.

Box 27.3 **Patient selection**

- Medical stability.
- Psychiatric stability.
- Nonsmoker (most surgeons but not all).
- Low intra-abdominal content.
- Weight stability.

Preoperative evaluation

Massive weight loss patients will present with multiple areas of deformity and they include arms, breasts, upper back rolls, thighs and face. The lower trunk and hanging panniculus is usually the chief complaint.

A detailed weight history is essential in patients that present for lower truncal contouring. It is important to ascertain the etiology of their lower trunk abnormalities, which include aging, child birth, skin laxity due to sun exposure and MWL. If the main cause is weight loss, then the following questions should be answered:

- What was their greatest weight?
- How did they lose weight?
- What was their lowest weight?
- How long have they been at their present weight?
- Do they think they are going to lose more weight?
- Are they prone to "heroic methods" of weight loss?

A careful history of all significant medical problems should be ascertained. Specifically, patients should be questioned about diabetes, cardiovascular disease, high blood pressure, collagen vascular disease, bleeding disorders, smoking history, history of deep venous thrombosis/pulmonary embolus, previous abdominal scars, bariatric surgery, bariatric surgeon/primary care physician follow-up and psychiatric problems. A history of nutritional habits should be collected. Post-bariatric surgery patients that are not on vitamins indicate a lack of appropriate follow-up and probable nutritional deficits. This should alert the plastic surgeon to pursue their laboratory examinations very carefully. Other important information that should be ascertained in the MWL patient is their history of anemia, hypocalcaemia, iron deficiency, vitamin B deficiency, low albumin/protein, low magnesium,

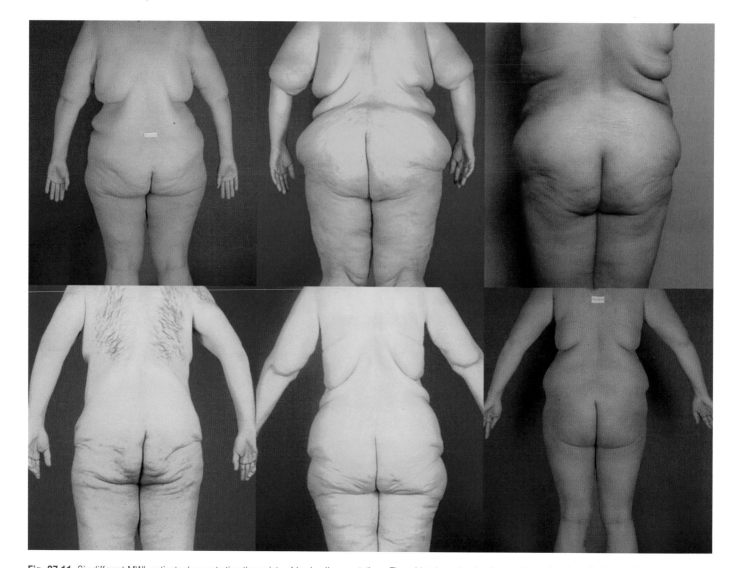

Fig. 27.11 Six different MWL patients demonstrating the variety of back roll presentations. The mid to lower back rolls are often reduced or eliminated after bodylift/belt lipectomy, but the upper back rolls are not.

elevated liver function tests and thiamine deficiency. It is also important to determine abnormalities of their bowel habits such as frequent diarrhea, which can predispose the patient to nutritional abnormalities as well as potential intraoperative contamination of the wounds should it occur during surgery.

Many MWL patients have extensive psychiatric histories. The authors have found it necessary to obtain psychiatric clearance for each belt lipectomy/bodylift patient. This is done to emphasis the extensive nature of the surgery to the patient as well as alerting the mental healthcare provider that their services may be required in the postoperative period.

The following points should be carefully noted on physical examination:

- The degree of skin laxity
- The amount of subcutaneous fat
- The translation of pull, as described above
- The presence of scars: subcostal cholecystectomy scars may jeopardize the flap vascularity and vertical midline scars may limit abdominal flap inferior mobility
- Waist definition
- The presence of abdominal or back rolls

- The degree of rectus diastasis and/or the presence of hernias
- The amount of intra-abdominal content must be noted. The traditional "diver's test" is not effective in most MWL patients because of the thickness and laxity of the abdominal wall fat. The authors utilize the more effective method of laying the patient in the supine position and evaluating their abdominal contours. If the contour is scaphoid and the abdominal wall falls below the rib cage, then it would be expected that rectus fascia plication will be effective in flattening the contour.[9] If the abdominal tissues are above the level of the ribs, then it can be presumed that intra-abdominal contents are large enough to prevent effective plication (see **Fig. 25.7**)
- The degree of buttocks projection and ptosis
- The degree of anterior and lateral thigh lipodystrophy and ptosis.

In the MWL patient, the altered absorption or restriction of food can create significant abnormalities of laboratory values, leading to potential problems at surgery.[10] Thus an extensive set of labs should be obtained as early as possible in the care

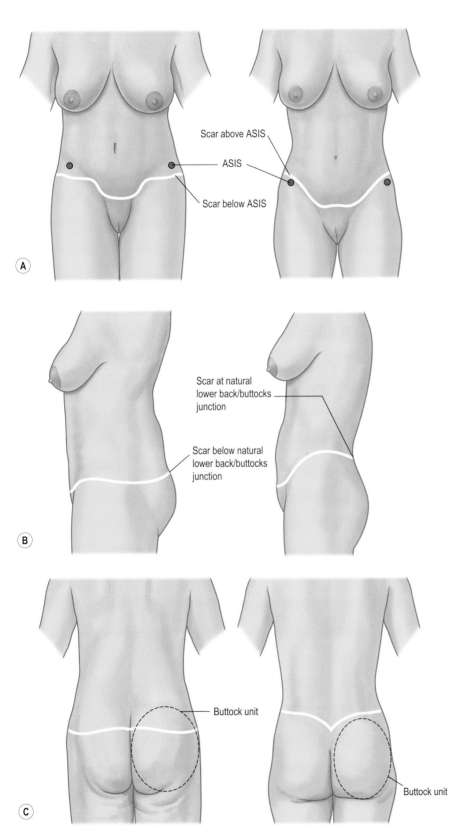

Fig. 27.12 Overall, the scar in a lower bodylift type II is more inferiorly placed than in a belt lipectomy. Anteriorly, the final scar is below the ASIS in a lower bodylift type II (**A,** left), and above it in a belt lipectomy (**A,** right). Laterally and posteriorly, the scar is below the natural junction of the lower back with the buttocks (**B,C** left), whereas it is located at, or just above, the natural junction in a belt lipectomy (**B,C** right).

of the patient because it may take some time to correct abnormalities. Those labs include: CBC, blood urea nitrogen, creatinine, electrolytes, glucose, urinalysis, liver function tests, iron, calcium, albumin, pre-albumin, total protein, vitamin B, magnesium and thiamine. Chest X-ray and EKG are obtained if indicated.

Treatment/surgical techniques

Rational for circumferential excisional procedures

A basic tenet of plastic surgery is that "Tension is bad". It is true that tension is bad for scarring and blood supply but it is essential for improving body contour in excisional procedures. In abdominoplasty, the elliptical excision creates the greatest amount of tension in the central zone of the abdomen. The areas above and below this region, superiorly the epigastric region and inferiorly the mons pubis, demonstrate the greatest amount of improvement. As the elliptical excision is followed laterally, the amount of tension decreases, reaching zero at its lateral edges *(Fig. 27.13)*. Thus the improvements above and below the excision, the anterior thighs and lateral abdomen, also decrease in magnitude as the elliptical excision is traversed from medial to lateral. In an ordinary low BMI patient with "anterior only" deformities, there is little need for improvement above and below the excision, outside of the

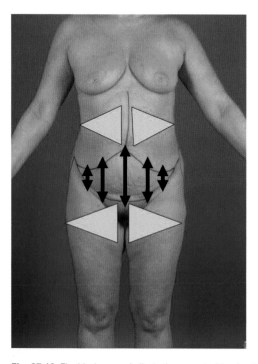

Fig. 27.13 The black arrows indicate the amount of tension that will be created at closure after the proposed resection of the abdominoplasty ellipse. The greatest amount of tension is central and trails off to zero at the lateral edge of the elliptical closure. The extent of body contour improvement, above and below the resection is directly related to the amount of tension. Thus the extent of improvement, light blue, above and below the final scar will also be greatest centrally and fizzle to zero, laterally. This patient does not need improvement laterally, above and below the proposed excision, thus is an ideal candidate for an abdominoplasty.

anterior abdomen. However, in most massive weight patients, many 20–30 pound overweight patients, and some normal weight patients, there is a need for significant improvements above and below the level of excision circumferentially around the entire lower trunk *(Fig. 27.14)*. Thus, with the tension maintained circumferentially, the improvement is also maintained circumferentially above and below the excision.

If the concept of maintaining tension around the trunk is ignored in patients who need improvements circumferentially, either by doing an abdominoplasty or a T type (fleur-de-lis) resection, the results are less than ideal with the lateral and posterior aspects of the lower trunk remaining unchanged after surgery *(Fig. 27.15)*.

Belt lipectomy

What will be described here is a belt lipectomy or central bodylift technique because it is what the authors perform most often, based on the fact that most of their patients are female.

Goals

Overall, a bodylift/belt lipectomy procedure treats the lower trunk as a unit and should address most of the patients concerns in this region. Keeping the patient's presenting deformity and desires in mind, Box 27.4 shows the general goals which should be sought after.

Markings

The markings in bodylift/belt lipectomy surgery are the "road map" to success. Although there are decisions to be made intraoperatively, the majority of planning and decision-making should be done during the marking process. It is wise to look at the patient's photographs prior to starting the marking process to delineate areas of special concern, potential pitfalls, and level of the desired final scar. It is important to photograph the markings and use them in two ways. First, evaluate them prior to surgery and make needed adjustments. Second, compare the patient's final contour, usually at 12 months after surgery, to the markings. It is the only way to improve one's technique.

The abdomen is the patient's greatest concern and the surgeon should strive to attain the best possible abdominal contour, not compromising that for lateral or posterior contour. It should be remembered that there is a general inferomedial rotation of tissues around the sacrum as a fulcrum, and to reverse this deformity, fairly aggressive lateral resections are required to attain harmonious truncal contour.

The marking instructions in this chapter are only guidelines. It is impossible to impart the knowledge required to

---

Box 27.4 Goals

1. Elimination of the panniculus/flattening the abdomen.
2. Elimination of mons pubis ptosis and redundancy.
3. Creation of waist definition (usually a desire in females).
4. Lifting the anterior and lateral thighs.
5. Elimination of lower back rolls, and in some patients mid back rolls.
6. Lifting the buttocks.
7. Creation of better buttocks contour.

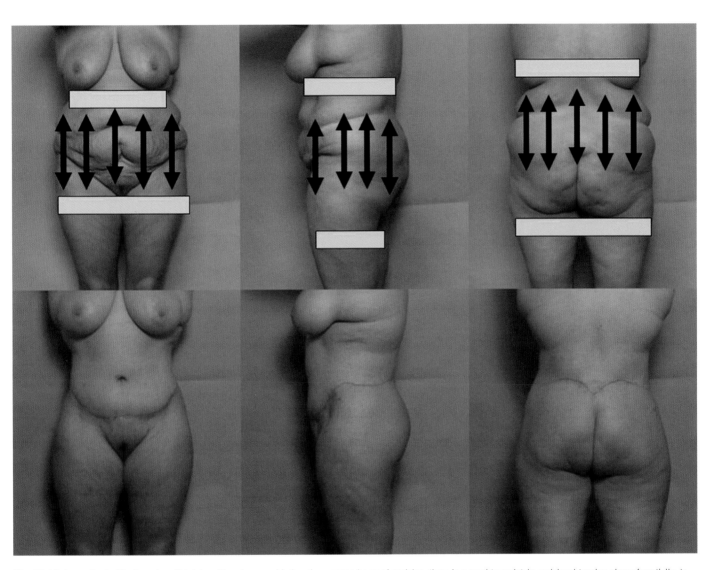

Fig. 27.14 In a patient with circumferential deformities above and below the proposed area of excision, there is a need to maintain excisional tension circumferentially, to attain the appropriate improvements in all the involved areas.

mark each and every patient, with all the variety that these patients present. Although a lot of technical details will be dealt with here, it is more important to learn the principles behind those details so that they can be applied under varying conditions.

Controlling scar position is something that every surgeon should aspire to attain. As a general principle, *"scar position can be approximated by simulating the tissue dynamics at closure"*. Because different techniques, i.e., lower bodylift, central bodylift, as well as different surgeons approach things differently, it is important for the surgeon to figure out how to simulate these dynamics using their own particular technique details. However, some basic principles apply to all techniques and we will attempt to cover these in the following discussion.

Marking the vertical midline

It is sometimes difficult to find the anterior midline. The villous hair pattern in the epigastric region can be helpful to delineate the midline. Inferiorly, the vaginal fourchette in the female, and the midline of the penis in males, are helpful in delineating the midline.

Horizontal mons pubis marking

Essentially all MWL patients have vertical excess of the mons pubis and varying degrees of horizontal excess. Thus, it is important to eliminate as much of the vertical excess as possible during bodylift/belt lipectomy. Since the mons pubis is "V" shaped, a low resection well within the hair-bearing skin, will leave behind a much narrower final mons pubis.

This eliminates the need for removing horizontal excess, in the form of lateral excisions, in most patients. If there is a need to address horizontal excess it is the preference of the authors that it is addressed in a later procedure to avoid the possibility of mons pubis permanent lymphedema. Many other authors prefer to take care of it in the same surgery.

The horizontal marking of the mons is done while the patient is lying supine, with the tissues retracted superiorly utilizing the nondominant hand to create a pleasing appearance of the mons. The midline bony prominence is palpated and 1–3 cm above it the horizontal mark is made from one lateral edge of the mons to the other. This maneuver simulates the dynamics at the time of closure with the hand simulating the superior pull of the resected abdominal flap on the

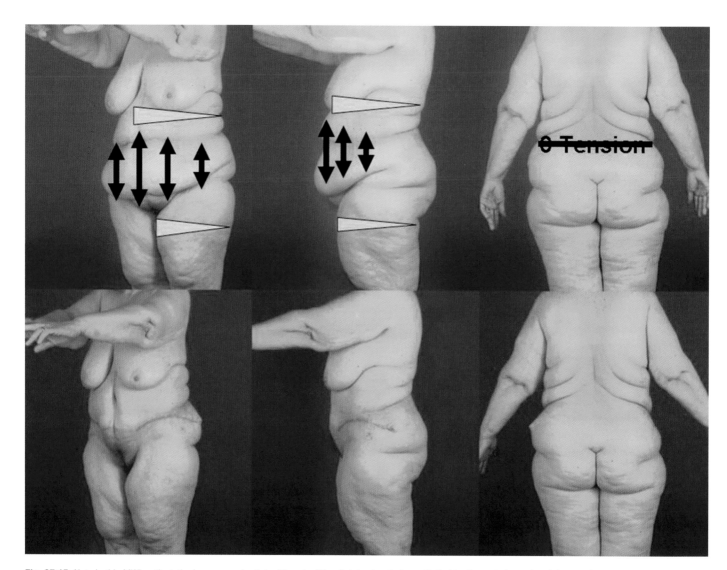

Fig. 27.15 Note in this MWL patient, the improvements attained by a traditional abdominoplasty are limited to the central anterior abdomen, shown below. Because there is no tension created by the abdominoplasty laterally and posteriorly, shown by the loss of light blue color, above, there is no improvement in these areas.

resistance of the mons to rise created by supra-pubic fascial attachments. If measured, the distance from the vaginal fourchette to the top of the proposed superior aspect of the mons, under tension, is usually 6–8 cm *(Fig. 27.16)*. The mark is measured on either side of the midline to maintain symmetry.

Mark from lateral mons to ASIS

The horizontal mark from the mons pubis to the ASIS is done with the patient in a slightly flexed position. To simulate tissue dynamics at the time of closure, the nondominant hand pushes the abdominal tissues superomedially in a fairly aggressive manner to simulate the pull of the resected abdominal flap on the closure in this area *(Fig. 27.17)*. The traction created by the hand is resisted by the zone of adherence in the inguinal area. The mark is then made where the surgeon desires the final scar to be. If the surgeon desires a high "French Bikini" angled scar, then the ASIS is palpated and the mark is aimed just superior to it. This is the preference of the authors because it creates a scar at the natural junction between the abdominal and thigh units and it promotes a

narrower waist. If the surgeon prefers a lower scar, the same maneuver is performed but the line is drawn in a lower position depending on where the surgeon wants it to be.

Superior horizontal abdominal marks

With the patient in a semiflexed position the superior proposed line of excision is marked, usually a few centimeters above the umbilicus in MWL patients, and less so for patients who are 20–30 pounds overweight or normal weight patients. These marks, unlike the inferior marks described above, are guidelines that are adjusted intraoperatively based on tissue mobility and desired contour. Generally, the resection is fairly aggressive in MWL patients because this will achieve the best possible contour and because there is no need to temper the vertical resection to prevent a lateral dog-ear. The circumferential excision frees up the surgeon to be as aggressive as he/she needs to be to attain the best possible contour. This is one of the major advantages of circumferential excisions over anterior only procedures. The authors prefer to match the distances of the upper marks to those of the lower marks to help alignment at closure. Centrally, matching the mons pubis

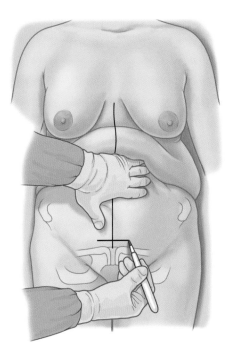

Fig. 27.16 The horizontal mark of the mons pubis. Note the mons pubis is elevated to a pleasing appearance and the mark is made 1–3 cm above the pubic bone.

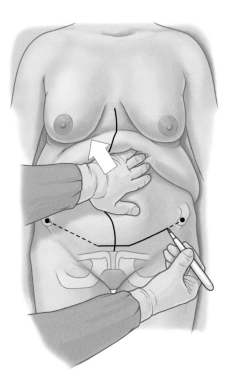

Fig. 27.17 The mark from the lateral edge of the mons pubis to the ASIS. The mark is made with the nondominant hand pushing the tissues superomedially to simulate the pull of the resected abdominal flap on the inferior line of resection.

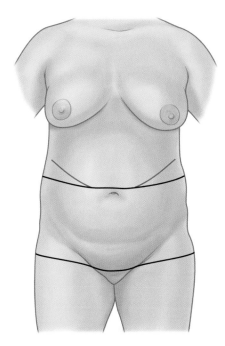

Fig. 27.18 The superior lateral mark should be marked without much angulation, especially if the patient is marked in the supine position. A severely angulated mark, shown in red, could lead to central abdominal flap necrosis due to a significant reduction in the remaining blood supply.

horizontal mark, the superior marks are flat or slight V shaped, especially if one wants to avoid a "W" shape to the final scar *(Fig. 27.18)*.

To match the lower line from the mons pubis to the ASIS, there is a tendency, especially in the supine position to angulate the superior lateral mark when the surgeon prefers the

"French Bikini" angle. This should be avoided because it leads to less remaining intercostal, subcostal and lumber vessels reaching the midline, resulting in potential tissue necrosis centrally. When the patient stands up, the superior lateral marks, which were made fairly flat in the supine position, will become angulated because the panniculus gravitationally descending more in the midline. Thus, if the marks were to be angulated in the supine position they will be even more dangerously angulated, leading to potential complications.

It is important to note that anteriorly, the inferior marks control scar position due to the fact that the inferior zones of adherence are far less mobile and act to keep the scar closer to them, rather than the fairly mobile abdominal flap.

The posterior vertical midline is marked

The posterior markings are performed with the patient standing.

The posterior midline extent of resection is marked

Examination of the back on either side of the midline reveals that in most MWL patients the lower back tissue is fairly smooth and then it transitions to wrinkled skin, at varying distances down the buttocks unit. Generally, the transition can be thought of as the top of the buttocks, which has descended secondary to the deflation of weight loss. The inferior point of the midline extent of resection is marked close to this level, especially if the midline buttocks crease is fairly low and needs to be elevated. Once the inferior point is decided upon,

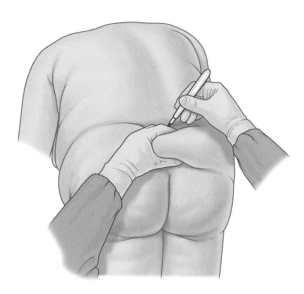

Fig. 27.19 Marking the extent of central midline of the back excision is done with the patient in the flexed position to simulate the position that the patient will be in after their abdominoplasty component is completed. This will reduce the risk of dehiscence because it accounts for the competing anterior and posterior tensions at the end of the entire procedure.

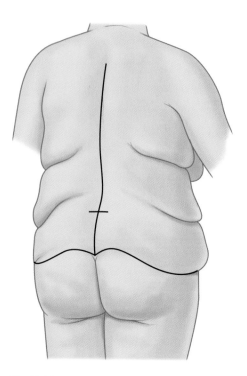

Fig. 27.20 The inferior posterior mark is made in a smooth shallow "S"-shaped fashion. Because the greatest descent occurs out laterally, at the posterior axillary line, this shape of excision allows for the greatest resection at this level.

the tissue superior to it is pinched while the patient is flexed at the waist, to simulate the position they will be in after their abdominoplasty component is completed. The superior midline mark is then made *(Fig. 27.19)*. This maneuver is essential to reduce the risk of dehiscence.

At this point, the surgeon has to evaluate the level of the lateral aspects of the anterior superior and anterior inferior marks and compare them to the position of the midline back marks. Obviously, the anterior superior lateral mark will eventually have to connect to the superior midline mark while the lateral aspect of the anterior inferior marks will have to connect to the inferior midline mark. If there are great discrepancies, adjustments can be made at this point.

The inferior back marks

The inferior back marks, from the midline of the back to the lateral extent of the anterior marks, are made in a smooth shallow "S" fashion *(Fig. 27.20)*. This mark is made first by the authors, rather than the superior mark because it is helpful in creating the shape of the resection, which is important in controlling contour. The lowest aspect of the S should be located at the posterior axillary line because that is the area of greatest vertical descent of the lower trunk due to aging and/or weight loss.

The superior back marks

To create the superior back mark, from the midline of the back to the lateral extent of the anterior markings, the inferior mark is pinched, bringing the buttocks and lateral thigh tissues up as high as needed to create the desired lateral buttocks/thigh contour *(Fig. 27.21)*. The top of the pinch is marked at a number of points, which are then connected to each other, from the midline to the lateral aspects of the anterior mark. The authors prefer the final midline scar to have a "V" shape to create the scar at a natural junction between the lower back, sacrum and buttocks. Others prefer a straight line closure, while very few surgeons prefer an inverted "V" pattern.

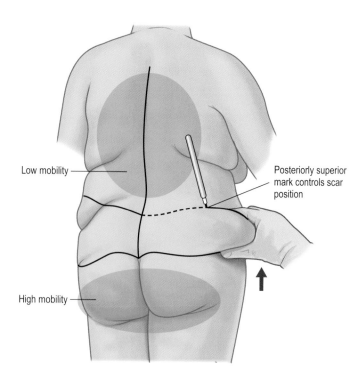

Low mobility

Posteriorly superior mark controls scar position

High mobility

Fig. 27.21 The posterior superior mark is made by lifting the inferior mark at a number of points, noting the appropriate buttock contour created by the lift, and then connecting these points. It is important to note that the superior mark is what controls final scar position because it is located in a less mobile area than the highly mobile buttocks.

The superior marks of the back control scar position in a belt lipectomy because the superior back tissues are much less mobile than the buttocks tissues below.

Thus, if the markings are performed for a belt lipectomy/central bodylift, with an intended scar at or just above the widest aspect of the pelvic rim, the final scar is usually within 2–3 cm of the superior mark. If a lower bodylift is being performed, this rule may not apply because the area of resection is further away from the zones of adherence in the lower back and the final scar position may be more than 3 cm inferior to the original superior mark. Prior to surgery, the authors evaluate and adjust the position of the posterior superior mark and determine if it is in the correct place, based on the knowledge of how far the final scar tends to be from it.

Vertical alignment marks

Vertical alignment marks are made circumferentially. The authors like marks to be made on the lateral aspects of the mons pubis, and at the level of the ASIS. The remaining marks positions are determined based on the size of the patient and should be left up to the desire of the operating surgeon. It is important to note that in most patients, there is a significant diameter mismatch between the superior and inferior circumferential marks. The inferior marks are almost always longer in diameter, up to 15 cm per side in larger patients, than the superior mark, necessitating adjustments, or "cheating" during the closure. This can often lead to little puckers that almost always resolve in the long term.

Surgical technique

Positioning sequence

There are many potential positioning sequences that can be utilized to perform a bodylift/belt lipectomy. As long as the desired contour is attained, it matters little what sequence is utilized. Whatever position sequencing is chosen, it is very important that there are enough operating personnel available to complete the turns efficiently and in a coordinated fashion.

Prone/supine positioning is the most commonly utilized sequence. This sequence has the advantage of one turn, an ability to judge symmetry of the back excision, and it allows for augmenting the buttocks in a natural position. Its disadvantages include more risk of positioning injuries, especially if operative times are prolonged in this position, which include potential respiratory difficulties, shoulder injuries, ulnar nerve injuries, and increased potential for eye injury.

Supine/prone positioning is also a single turn sequence with the added advantage of making sure that the highest priority of contour is the anterior resection. Its increased disadvantage over the above mentioned sequence is that turning the patient to the prone position after the anterior resection is completed is more difficult because of the risk of dehiscing the anterior closure during the turn.

Supine/lateral decubitus/lateral decubitus positioning is the preferred sequence of the authors because of the need to create the best possible anterior contour and then adjust the remainder of the resection to it. Other advantages include the ability to abduct the legs in the lateral decubitus position and to allow for greater lateral resection of excess tissue. Disadvantages include an inability to visualize the entire

back/buttocks during the resection potentially leading to a greater chance for asymmetry. Augmenting the buttocks in the lateral position is more challenging and harder to judge. Another potential disadvantage is that there are two turns required, with an added turn at the end prior to transferring the patient to the hospital bed. Although the authors are able to accomplish these turns very efficiently and without over exposure and heat loss, they have a very well trained team with extensive experience. Less ideal situations may not produce such ideal conditions.

Anesthesia and DVT/PE prophylaxis

The majority of surgeons performing bodylift/belt lipectomy utilize a general anesthetic. The authors of this chapter utilize a general anesthetic with a thoracic epidural placed prior to surgery which has been found to be very effective in decreasing postoperative discomfort.[11] At the time of writing of this chapter, the authors are compiling data which point towards a significant reduction in DVT/PE when an epidural is utilized. Although the orthopedic and anesthesia literature is supportive of the notion that epidural use reduces the risk of DVT/PE, it is too early to definitively claim that in the field of plastic surgery. If an epidural is not utilized, the reader has to make a decision as to whether they should add chemoprophylaxis to the routine of lower extremity alternating compression stockings and early ambulation. It is not clear at this point what is the best chemoprophylaxis regimen if it is to be utilized.

Surgical technique

The technique that is described here is a belt lipectomy procedure as performed by the authors.

In the operating room, the patient is put in the supine position on a bean bag, arms are abducted at 90°. The markings are reinforced and methylene blue tattooed to prevent fading with the prepping of the patient. After insertion of an indwelling urinary catheter and application of sequential compression boots the patient is prepped and draped.

Traction sutures are placed at the 6 and 12 o'clock positions, at the appropriate depth within the umbilicus, to facilitate a circumumbilical incision. The umbilicus is incised, and the umbilical stalk is freed from surrounding tissues using scissors. Some patients may have an undetected periumbilical hernia so care must be taken while dissecting the stalk.

The inferior lower abdominal mark is then incised and the dissection is taken down to, or just deep to, Scarpa's fascia. Some patients have very well defined Scarpa's fascia, while others have a less distinct layer. Scarpa's fascia is preserved from the incision line and upward toward the umbilicus (*Fig. 27.22*). The authors believe that leaving some fatty tissue on top of the rectus fascia reduces the risk of seroma.

The type of supraumbilical dissection performed is dependent on the thickness of the presenting abdominal flap. If the flap is thin, then a more traditional elevation towards the costal margins and xiphoid is performed. The authors try to leave a very thin layer of fat on the rectus fascia to help reduce seroma. The extent of abdominal flap elevation should be just enough to attain the proper advancement of the flap, create the best possible contour, and preserve as many vascular perforators as possible. If the abdominal flap is thick, then a

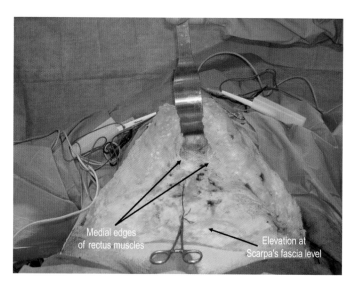

Fig. 27.22 All infraumbilical elevations are performed at, or just deep to, Scarpa's fascia level. This figure demonstrates flap elevation in a "thick panniculus" patient, where the authors routinely liposuction the supraumbilical flap. To avoid vascular supply issues, this type of patient has a very limited supraumbilical elevation, just to the medial edges of the rectus muscle, to allow for a full complement of rectus perforators to remain intact.

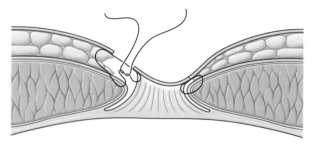

Fig. 27.23 Three point fixation sutures that are utilized to create inversion of the umbilicus and a final periumbilical scar that is located internally to avoid external scar prominence. Note the authors do not defat the umbilical defect because it is felt that this may lead to an increased risk of flap necrosis.

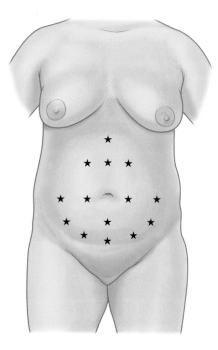

Fig. 27.24 The figure demonstrates the pattern of quilting sutures utilized by the authors.

very limited dissection tunnel, up to the xiphoid, is performed to expose the medial edges of the rectus muscle, and concomitant liposuction of the flap is performed to thin the flap *(Fig. 27.22)*.

Abdominal wall vertical plication is then performed from xiphoid to pubis. Some authors prefer a single layer, while others, including the authors, prefer a two layer plication. The choice of suture is based on surgeon preference. The authors utilize long lasting, nonpermanent, barbed, running sutures. Horizontal plications are performed if deemed necessary.

In order to achieve maximum flap advancement, the patient is flexed at the waist and the flap is advanced inferiorly. The flap is then tailored with the upper mark used as a guide. When resecting the excess flap, it is often necessary to bevel the resection if the flap is thick.

If the mons pubis is deemed too thick, it can either be reduced by liposuction or by direct excision of sub-Scarpal fat. Direct excision usually requires tacking down of the mons Scarpa's fascia to the underlying rectus fascia at the appropriate level.

With the abdominal flap tailored and temporarily tacked in place, a 1.5–2 cm vertical incision is made in the midline overlying the umbilical stalk. A path for the umbilical stalk to be brought through is created by blunt dissection, with no fat removal. The authors feel that fat resection in the neoumbilical region may lead to vascular compromise of the flap. The desired inversion of the umbilicus is attained through "3 point fixation sutures", placed at 3, 6, and 9 o'clock. These are inverted 3–0 nonpermanent mono-filament sutures that are placed through the abdominal wall fascia, the subcuticular layer of the abdominal flap and the subcuticular layer of the umbilicus *(Fig. 27.23)*. When these sutures are tied, they will create as much, or as little, inversion as the surgeon desires as well as pulling the scar inside the umbilical depression. The remainder of the umbilicus is sutured to the surrounding abdominal flap with interrupted inverted subcuticular

sutures. No external sutures are utilized to avoid suture marks. It is important to note, that there are many umbilicoplasty techniques that have been reported and most are effective. What has been presented here is just the authors' preference. What is important is that whatever method is utilized creates an umbilicus that is relatively small, somewhat vertical (because it tends to widen with time) and that the scar does not have track marks associated with it. The scar should also be located on the inner aspect of the umbilical depression so that it is well hidden.

Quilting sutures, placed between the abdominal flap and the underlying abdominal wall, are utilized by some surgeons, including the authors, to obliterate potential dead space in the hopes of reducing the risk of seroma formation.[12] Other names utilized for these sutures are progressive tension sutures as well as Baroudi stitches. *Figure 27.24* shows the pattern of quilting sutures utilized by the authors when combined with a limited supraumbilical dissection.

Abdominal closure is usually accomplished over one or more closed suction drains. The authors prefer to bring out

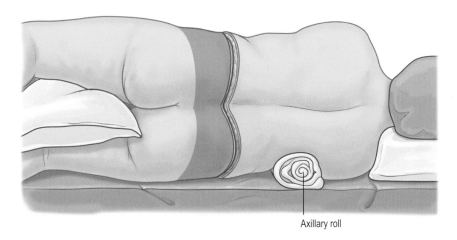

Axillary roll

Fig. 27.25 The authors prefer the lateral decubitus position to excise the tissues from the lateral dog-ear created by the anterior resection to the midline of the back. This position allows for maximal hip abduction and easy access for lateral thigh liposuction. It is essential that the patient is appropriately padded, including an axillary roll.

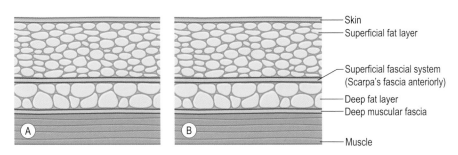

Skin
Superficial fat layer

Superficial fascial system
(Scarpa's fascia anteriorly)

Deep fat layer
Deep muscular fascia

Muscle

Fig. 27.26 The level of elevation of the inferiorly based flap during the back resection is dependent on the presenting anatomy and the desired goals of the patient. In patients with high BMIs and/or over-projected buttocks at presentation, the dissection is deepened to the just above the muscle fascia to allow for narrowing of the waist and reduction of buttocks projection **(A)**. In patients with low BMIs and/or under-projected buttocks at presentation, the dissection is deepened to the superficial fascial system level to maintain fullness and increase final projection **(B)**.

these drains laterally, at about the lateral level of the ASIS, because pubic area drains tend to become quite uncomfortable if left in place for longer than a week, which is not an infrequent occurrence in MWL patients. Closure involves re-approximation of Scarpa's fascia and one to two superficial layers for skin closure. The lateral dog-ears created by the anterior resection are temporarily closed with staples to allow for the upcoming turns.

Turning of the patient to the lateral decubitus position should be accomplished by the coordinated effort of the anesthetist and at least four other operating room personnel. It is very important to keep the waist flexed at all times and the best way to insure that is to assign one person to this task. All pressure points need to be padded, including an axillary roll. The hips are abducted to allow for the maximum excision of the lateral tissues, which can be accomplished with pillows placed between the knees *(Fig. 27.25)*.

With the patient re-prepped and draped, the back excision from the lateral dog-ear to the midline of the back is undertaken. Most patients will undergo liposuction of the lateral thighs, which is performed at this juncture.

The authors prefer to make the superior mark incision first. The level to which the dissection is deepened is dependent on the desired amount of fat to be left in the buttocks. In patients with over-projected buttocks, the desired goal is to reduce the projection and create a depression at the waist by cinching above the hip. This is best accomplished by dissecting down to just above the muscle fascia and then elevating an inferiorly based flap down to the level of the proposed excision line *(Fig. 27.26)*. When tailoring the flap, the resection is beveled to further create narrowing of the waist.

In patients that have normal or deficient buttocks projection, the goal of surgery is to maintain as much projection as possible. Thus, the superior mark incision is deepened to the superficial fascia level and the flap is dissected inferiorly to the level of the proposed excision at this level *(Fig. 27.26)*. During the tailoring process, the inferior flap is not beveled.

The inferior dissection of the lateral thigh region of this segment of the procedure is usually limited to the proposed inferior excision line, when performed by the authors. Other investigators will directly undermine over the entire lateral thigh region in an effort to completely release the zone of adherence and allow for greater elevation of the lateral thigh tissues. This is combined with deep permanent sutures that grab the superficial fascial system of the lateral thighs and advance it onto the muscle fascia superiorly.

After tailoring the inferiorly based flap, closure is performed in a similar manner to the anterior closure. A drain is inserted prior to closure. Closing one side will lead to a midline dog-ear which is temporarily closed with staples to allow for the next turn. The patient is then turned and the same steps are repeated for the other side.

The patient is then turned to the supine position while making sure they are maintained in the flexed position and transferred to a flexed hospital bed under the supervision of the operating surgeon.

Autoaugmentation of the buttocks for patients who present with underprojected buttocks is advocated by some investigators. In these procedures, the proposed tissue to be excised from the back is de-epithelialized and rotated into the buttocks region to create bulk. There are a variety of flap designs and techniques that have been proposed. The authors do not utilize these flaps for a variety of reasons. First, these flaps can augment the buttocks in the wrong position, lead to malposition of the back scar, and most often are not needed at all. The authors are a referral center for complications associated with body contouring after MWL and some very difficult problems have been encountered with these flaps. These include fat necrosis, major skin necrosis, chronic pain, chronic seromas, major dehiscence, and sepsis. The added time in the operating room to autoaugment the buttocks also increases the time of a procedure that is already long, worsening the potential for complications. It is the authors' opinion that these flaps should not be attempted by the novice body contouring surgeon because even very experienced surgeons who perform these techniques are selective in whom they choose to perform them on.

Postoperative care

A sign is placed on the patient's bed which reads "Patient is not to be moved in any way till completely awake and alert". The reason for the sign is that while the patient is drowsy from anesthesia, simple body position movements by the nursing staff can lead to dehiscence. Once the patient is awake and alert, they can sense tension and will be able to prevent dehiscence on their own. The patient is educated prior to surgery about the ability to sense tension and how they are to help the nursing staff with this aspect of their postoperative care. This is especially relevant when the patient is ambulated. It is a standing order for the authors that all patients are walked the same day of surgery, with assistance, even if it is just a few steps. The epidural catheter anesthetic infusion is managed by the anesthesiologist and is left running until the morning of the second postoperative day. The infusion is then discontinued, but the catheter is left in place. If the patient is unable to tolerate discomfort without the epidural infusion, then it is restarted but in the majority of cases, the epidural catheter is removed. The urinary catheter is removed 4–6 h after the epidural infusion is discontinued. The authors recommend a 2-day minimum stay in the hospital because almost all major problems tend to occur within this time period. Criteria for discharge include the ability to ambulate with only one person's help, tolerance of pain with oral medication, the ability to take food and drink by mouth, and the ability to urinate without a urinary catheter. Most patients are able to go home between the second and third day.

For the first week, the patient is ambulated bent at the waist and then allowed to slowly straighten up over a couple of days. Activity is slowly increased as tolerated over the first 3–4 weeks, with most patients being able to return to non-physical work in 4 weeks. A compression garment is worn by the patient starting a few days after surgery when the surgeon feels comfortable that it will not compromise blood supply of the abdominal flap. Subsequently, the patient is asked to wear the garment for as long as they can tolerate it. The garment helps reduce swelling and speed up the attainment of final contour and it may reduce seroma formation. Drain removal is based on ≤40 cc/day, with most drains removed at 2 weeks, even if this criteria is not met. A postoperative care summary is given in Box 27.5.

Box 27.5 Postoperative care summary

- "Patient is not to be moved in any way till completely awake and alert" should be posted on the patient's bed.
- Ambulate the same day of surgery with assistance.
- Do not allow patient to straighten up for 1 week postoperatively.
- A 1–2 day monitoring period is highly recommended.
- Garments should be worn for extended periods of time.
- Maturation of results take at least 1 year.

Most patients will not attain their final contour for at least 1 year, with a few patients continuing to improve for up to 2 years.

Outcomes/prognosis/complications

As with the patient presentation, the prognosis after belt lipectomy depends on the patient's BMI, fat deposition pattern, and the quality of their fat/skin envelope. Of these factors, the patient's BMI is the most important. As a general rule, the lower the BMI at presentation, the better the result and the lower the complication rate. Conversely, the higher the BMI, the less attractive the result, and the higher the complication rate. In MWL patients, the authors have categorized patients by BMI level: group I BMI ≥36; group II BMI 30–35; and group III BMI ≤29. Although the cut-offs between groups are arbitrary, the intent of the categorization is to help the surgeon and patient predict, in a general manner, the expected results. Thus group I patients (*Figs 27.27, 27.28*) will demonstrate less improvement and more complications after bodylift/belt lipectomy than those in group II. Group II (*Figs 27.29, 27.30*) will demonstrate less improvement and more complications than those in group III (*Figs 27.31, 27.32*). This rule holds as long as one compares these patients in groups. Within each of these arbitrarily chosen BMI ranges, patients do not necessarily follow the rule that a lower BMI automatically guarantees better results or lower complication rates because other factors such as fat deposition pattern and the amount of skin laxity also play a role.

It is important to explain to patients, *prior to surgery*, that their contour is improved significantly after bodylift/belt lipectomy *but their skin quality is unchanged*. Thus, once the swelling associated with surgery is resolved, skin elasticity on palpation is unchanged from its preoperative characteristics, especially in the epigastric region. Both the inexperienced surgeon and the patient may desire more tissue excision, but this will lead to failure.

A subject that has not been addressed in the literature is the sensory loss associated with circumferential dermatolipectomy procedures. Traditional abdominoplasty sensory loss is usually located inferior to the neo-umbilicus in a triangular pattern, with the base straddling the midline at abdominal scar and the apex at the neo-umbilicus. Over a 1–2 year period, sensation tends to return to this area with the apex descending and the base becoming narrower. Although the authors have not performed prospective studies to delineate the sensory loss associated with circumferential procedures, informal retrospective observations have demonstrated a lack of

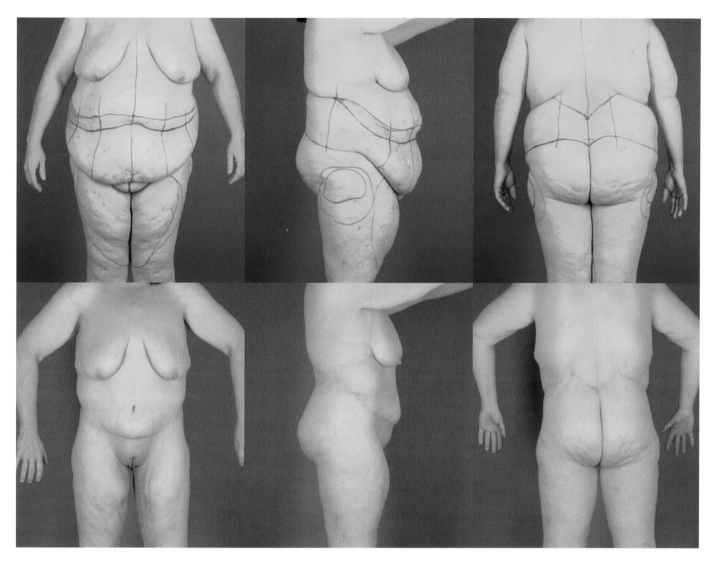

Fig. 27.27 This figure demonstrates preoperative (above) and postoperative (below) photographs of a patient that presented with a BMI >35, a group I patient, who underwent a belt lipectomy/bodylift. Because the abdominal flap at presentation was thick and required thinning, the supraumbilical tissues, shown above the proposed superior marks, were liposuctioned and a limited central flap dissection was performed to maintain the rectus perforators blood supply. Note there were two proposed lines of excision marked in the hopes of reaching the more superior one, but if not then a more inferior one would have been utilized. The scar was intentionally kept high in order that a "cinching" at the waist could be accomplished. Posteriorly the inferiorly-based buttocks flap was elevated at the level of the underlying muscle fascia, in order to "cinch" around the waist and create a depression above the buttocks proper, which increases the apparent projection of the buttocks. Note that group I, which when compared with groups II and III, demonstrates less overall improvement in lower truncal contour.

consistency in a "typical pattern" such as that seen with the abdominoplasty. What has been observed is that the area of sensory loss is usually circumferential and that it improves from 6 months to 1 year. Often the pattern is quite asymmetric. Anteriorly, the pattern often follows the traditional abdominoplasty pattern, while over the lateral thighs the patterns are quite variable, and can be extensive in some. Posteriorly the patterns are again quite variable, sometimes including half the buttocks surface area, while in others the pattern is almost no sensory loss in the back. In most patients, the pattern straddles the circumferential scar but interestingly in some patients, the loss is completely below the scar, which means that the scar itself is sensate. The authors suspect that these varying patterns are due to both the varying anatomy of the patient and the different surgical approaches, i.e., liposuction or no liposuction of an area.

It is also important to warn the patients prior to surgery that should they gain significant weight, most or all of their body contour improvement can be reversed.

Complications

Circumferential bodylift/belt lipectomy procedures performed on normal weight patients tend to have similar complication profiles to their abdominoplasty counter parts. On the other hand, MWL patients that undergo bodylift/belt lipectomy have significant risk of complications, more so than in any other area of aesthetic surgery. This is especially true if the surgeon chooses to operate on patients presenting in the higher BMI ranges. *As a general rule, the higher the BMI the higher the complication rate.*

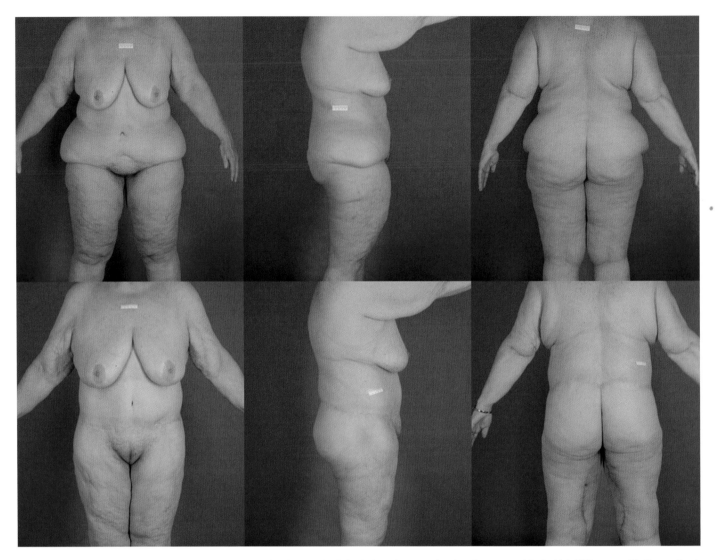

Fig. 27.28 The figure demonstrates pre (above) and postoperative photographs (below) of another group I patient that presented in the high BMI range, >35. She previously underwent an unsuccessful "anterior only" abdominoplasty to treat her circumferential lower truncal excess. A belt lipectomy/bodylift was performed on this patient, which required a complete redo of the abdominal region.

Seromas

The most common complication of bodylift/belt lipectomy, outside of small nonhealing areas along the incision line, is seroma. As a matter of fact, if the surgeon elects to operate on patients presenting with BMIs >35, they should expect a seroma in almost all cases. The surface area of the operative field, concomitant liposuction, the shearing forces on the lower trunk during normal movement, and the intrinsic nature of MWL patients may all contribute to the high rate of seroma. Unfortunately, there is little scientific knowledge of what makes up a seroma, its etiology, how to prevent it, or how to treat it. Most of what is known is based on anecdotal evidence. Currently, the authors leave a layer of fat on the rectus fascia in the infraumbilical dissection of the abdominal flap and utilize quilting sutures in the hope of reducing seroma frequency. When a seroma is encountered, the authors serially aspirate it and if that is not successful, they will inject the pocket with a sclerosing agent, doxycycline, in the hopes of closing down the pocket. It has become apparent that the presence of a seroma capsule is not an indication for operating on a seroma, as is traditionally believed. The authors have found that on re-operating on these patients, for reasons unrelated to seroma, a seroma type capsule is almost always present, but it is empty. It has also become apparent that if a fluid filled pocket is small and nonexpanding, it does not need treatment, because it will eventually resolve on its own. Thus, the authors will watch a small fluid collection, rather than aspirate it.

If a seroma should become infected, it usually requires incision and drainage, antibiotic coverage, and making sure the pocket closes from deep to superficial by the use of a "wick" type dressing.

Wound separation

The long incisions in circumferential dermatolipectomy combined with the high level tension created by the procedure very often lead to small wound separations. Most often they will heal without much difficulty or negative sequelae but

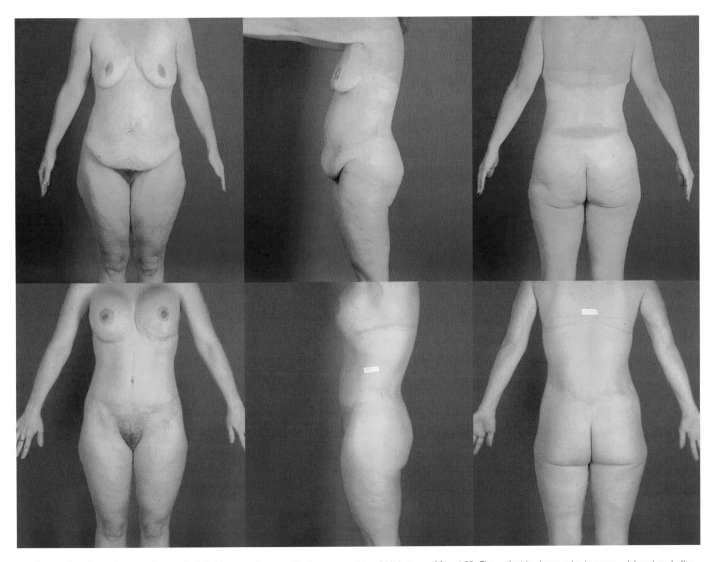

Fig. 27.29 This figure demonstrates a patient that belongs to group II, who present with a BMI between 30 and 35. The patient is shown prior to surgery (above) and after belt lipectomy/bodylift (below). Patients in this group will generally demonstrate more improvement than group I, but less than group III.

they can be bothersome to the patient. Thus, it is best to warn patients about these areas prior to surgery. Treatment is usually conservative, allowing secondary intention healing to occur.

Dehiscence

A dehiscence is defined as a wound separation at the superficial fascial system level or deeper. Circumferential procedures are more prone to dehiscence because of the competing tensions, especially the anterior and posterior closures. Fortunately, dehiscences are fairly rare if a number of issues are addressed. Dehiscence may occur within the immediate postoperative period or a few weeks after surgery when the patient has presumably healed. Three strategies will help reduce the risk of dehiscing in the early postoperative period. First, the extent of the back midline resection is preoperatively marked with the patient in the flexed waist position attained

after the anterior resection is completed. Second, the sign placed on the patient's bed that warns all healthcare personnel to avoid manipulating the patient until they are awake and alert is essential because "*an awake patient can sense tension and protect themselves*". Third, preoperatively patients and nursing staff are coached on how a patient is be "rolled out of bed" with the aid of the patient "sensing tension" and avoiding body positions that strain the closures. A late dehiscence usually occurs when the patient quickly bends at the waist, presumably after they feel they have healed. It is important to advise patients that all their movements, for the first 3 months after surgery, should be slow and deliberate, which will lead to a sense of tension before the tension reaches the level required to dehisce. Should a dehiscence occur, treatment is based on the particular situation. Early dehiscence can be treated by a return to the operating room for attempted closure, closure in the emergency room, or the application of a wound-vac. The area involved may require a scar revision in the long run.

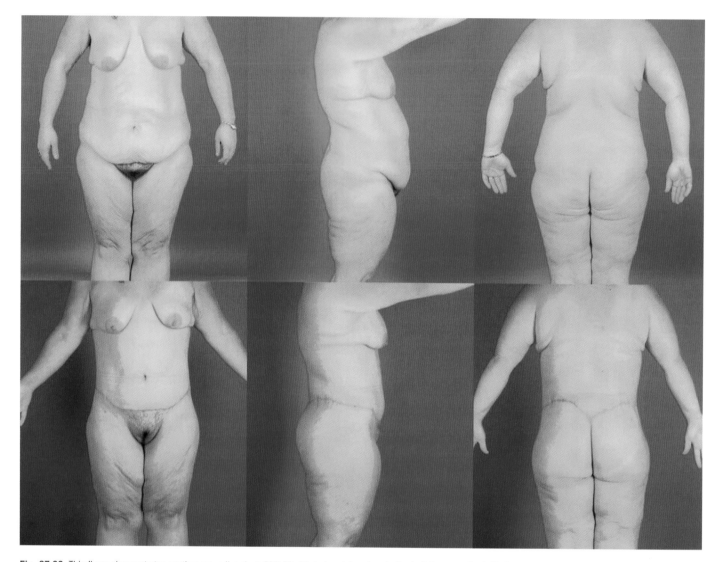

Fig. 27.30 This figure demonstrates another group II patient, BMI 30–35, before (above) and after belt lipectomy/bodylift (below). Note the patient subsequently also underwent an upper bodylift.

Infection

The most common cause for infections after a bodylift/belt lipectomy is undetected seromas. It is wise to see these patients for at least a year after surgery to make sure that there are no undetected seromas. As mentioned earlier, the authors do not treat small nonexpanding fluid collections but they do keep a close watch on them in case they become infected. The treatment of an infected seroma is described above. Occasionally a patient will develop a skin cellulitis, which is unrelated to a seroma. Those are treated as in any other cellulitis encountered after a surgical procedure, usually with appropriate antibiotic coverage.

Tissue necrosis

Tissue necrosis can occur after bodylift/belt lipectomy, especially in the anterior midline of the inferior aspect of the abdominal flap, due to a variety of factors which include smoking, excessive tension on the closure, acute angulation of the supero-lateral excision line of the abdominal flap, and old abdominal scars interfering with the normal blood supply. The authors avoid operating on smokers, but other surgeons choose to do so. Usually those surgeons will adjust their technique by limiting the midline supraumbilical elevation and utilizing discontinuous undermining to mobilize the flap. Excessive tension on closure can also lead to vascular compromise. It is difficult to determine the right amount of tension that will attain the best contour but avoid vascular compromise. Quilting sutures can help reduce tension on the closure but it is best to avoid too much tension in the first place.

There is a tendency to over angulate tailoring of the lateral abdominal flap in an attempt to match the inferior incision line, especially if it is angulated sharply, as in a "French Bikini" line *(Fig. 27.18)*. Since the main blood supply of the abdominal flap is the intercostals, subcostal, and lumbar vessels, sharp angulation of the superior incision will violate these feeding vessels and thus may lead to necrosis of the midline inferior flap. Since the inferior line marks are what controls final scar position, not the superior line marks, there

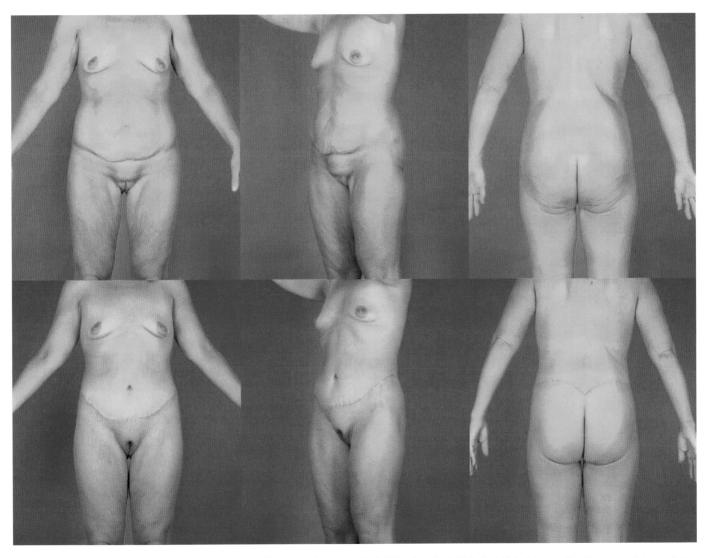

Fig. 27.31 This figure demonstrates a group III patient, BMI <30, before (above) and after belt lipectomy/bodylift (below). Note that group III patients, overall demonstrate a greater degree of body contour improvement than either group I or II patients.

is no need to angulate sharply, which avoids this potential complication.

As in traditional abdominoplasty, subcostal scars can and will interfere with the remaining blood supply of the flap after a traditional elevation. As mentioned above, the remaining blood supply of the flap includes intercostals, subcostal, and lumbar vessels, which can be interrupted by a subcostal scar, or any upper abdominal horizontal scar leading to potential necrosis of the tissues left behind inferior to the scar.

If a subcostal scar is encountered, there are a number of strategies that can be employed to decrease the risk of necrosis. In some MWL patients, their subcostal scar is so low that it can be used as the upper limit of the resection, thus eliminating any tissue that may be compromised. Another potential manner by which a subcostal scar can be handled is to perform a T type resection with the subcostal scar used as one of the vertical limbs brought together in the midline. The authors have no experience with this option. The most common way for the authors to handle subcostal scars is to

alter the sequence of surgical steps by making the superior mark incision first and conservatively elevate the supraumbilical flap, while evaluating the blood supply of the tissue at risk, which is immediately infero-medial to the scar *(Fig. 27.33)*. If those tissues are deemed ischemic, they are resected and the inferior flap is advanced superiorly, as in a reverse abdominoplasty. Obviously, this will lead to a fairly high final scar position, which the patient should be warned about prior to surgery. On the other hand, if the sub-scar tissues are found to have an adequate blood supply, then the supraumbilical flap is advanced inferiorly to the proposed inferior mark and the inferior flap is tailored accordingly.

Deep vein thrombosis and pulmonary embolism (DVT/PE)

Patients undergoing bodylift/belt lipectomy have more than one factor that increases the risk of DVT/PE. Some patients may undergo the belt lipectomy while in the obese state,

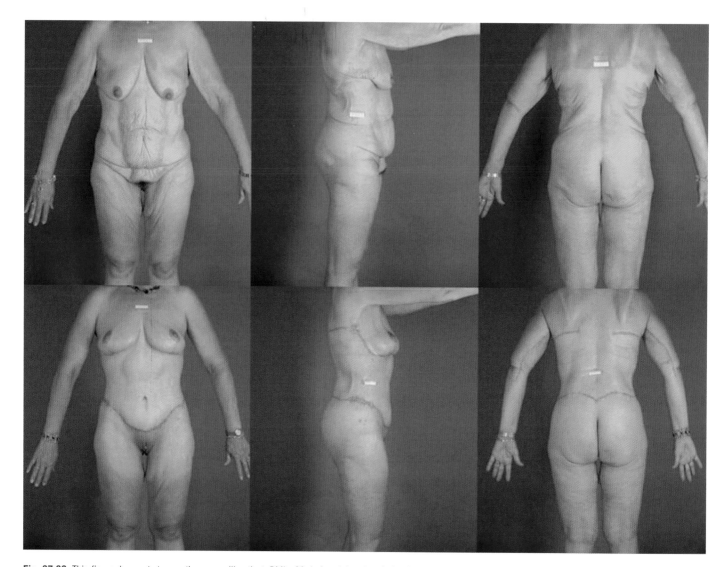

Fig. 27.32 This figure demonstrates another group III patient, BMI <30, before (above) and after belt lipectomy/bodylift (below). Note the greater overall improvement over group I or II patients.

which increases their risk. Plication of the abdominal wall increases intra-abdominal pressure and may potentially lead to decreased venous return, which potentiates DVT/PE. Another important factor is the prolonged operative time for these procedures. To prevent DVT/PE standard prophylaxis includes early mobilization and the use of sequential compression stockings. At the time of writing, there is a significant amount of discussion about other means of reducing DVT/PE. The majority of these discussions are centered around adding chemoprophylaxis to the standard regimen. There are many suggested rating scales that surgeons may utilize to stratify patients' risk potential. Under most of those scales, a circumferential dermatolipectomy would place patients in the high risk group, thus requiring chemoprophylaxis. The difficulty is in deciding which chemoprophylaxis regimen to utilize and to deal with the occasional bleed that may accompany such treatment. The authors have never utilized chemoprophylaxis but over the last 10 years have utilized postoperative epidural analgesia to both control pain and

reduce the risk of DVT/PE, with excellent success. More randomized trials need to be conducted on chemoprophylaxis, as well as epidural analgesia, before definitive recommendations can be made.

Psychological difficulties

Massive weight loss patients often have psychological issues that either result from their obesity or helped cause the obesity.[13] Massive weight loss helps relieve patients of many of their medical problems but often does not eliminate the psychological issues. This combined with the fact that the postoperative recovery from a bodylift/belt lipectomy can be quite stressful psychologically, MWL patients may deteriorate after their bodylift/belt lipectomy. If this psychiatric deterioration leads to problems that interfere with their postoperative treatment, major complications can occur. The authors obtain psychiatric clearance on all bodylift/belt lipectomy

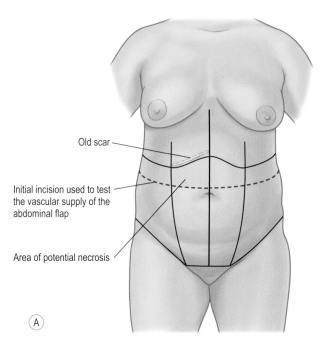

Old scar

Initial incision used to test
the vascular supply of the
abdominal flap

Area of potential necrosis

(A)

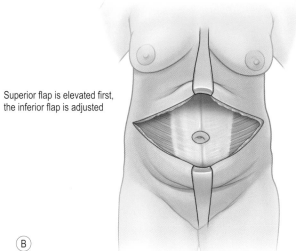

Superior flap is elevated first,
the inferior flap is adjusted

(B)

Fig. 27.33 This figure demonstrates the most common approach that the authors utilize when a "chevron" cholecystectomy scar is encountered. The superior proposed line of excision is incised first. The supraumbilical elevation is limited to the medial edges of the rectus muscles. The shaded area, inferior to the chevron scar, is then evaluated at this point and if it is found to be vascularly compromised, the superior flap is tailored at the level of the old scar. The inferior flap is then elevated and tailored to that resection line. On the other hand, if the shaded area demonstrates good vascularity, which fortunately occurs in most situations, then the superior flap is advanced inferiorly in the usual manner and the inferior flap is tailored accordingly, resulting in a scar located in the usual position.

Box 27.6 An upper bodylift does the following

- Eliminates vertical and horizontal excess of the upper trunk.
- Elevates the inframammary crease, especially its lateral component.
- Eliminates upper back excess/rolls.
- Creates breast contour based on a correctly positioned inframammary crease.
- If needed, eliminates upper arm excess.

patients and have found this to be very helpful in reducing the rate of psychological problems postoperatively.

Secondary procedures

Upper bodylift

Bodylift/belt lipectomy surgery treats the lower trunk, from the rib cage to the pelvic rim and should improve the mid-upper back, anterior thighs, lateral thighs, and medial thighs. It does not improve upper back rolls/lateral breast rolls, breast contour, or arm contour.[14] The upper trunk which starts at the inferior border of the neck and ends at the inferior border of the breast, thus is untreated by a bodylift/belt lipectomy. To treat this anatomic unit, the authors advocate the use of an "upper bodylift" procedure. The key factor in deciding if the patient needs an upper bodylift is the position of the lateral inframammary crease. In many MWL patients, the entire inframammary crease has descended with the weight gain/loss process, but especially the lateral aspect because the two midline zones of adherence, located over the sternum anteriorly and the spine posteriorly, tether tissues centrally but allow descent laterally *(Fig. 27.34)*. These patients thus present with lateral descent of the inframammary crease, which is perceived as upper back rolls/lateral breast rolls, anterior and posterior inverted "V" deformities, and both vertical and horizontal excess of the entire chest.

In patients that do not present with lateral descent of the inframammary crease the breasts and the arms are treated as separate entities. If the lateral inframammary crease is found to be inferiorly positioned then some form of upper bodylift is required to treat the entire upper truncal unit. Some upper bodylift results are shown in *(Figs 27.35, 27.36)*.

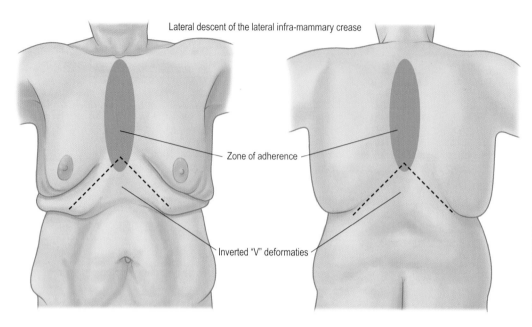

Lateral descent of the lateral infra-mammary crease

Zone of adherence

Inverted "V" deformaties

Fig. 27.34 This figure demonstrates the typical deformities encountered in the upper trunk after massive weight loss. Note that lateral descent of the inframammary crease is just another name for upper back/lateral breast excess.

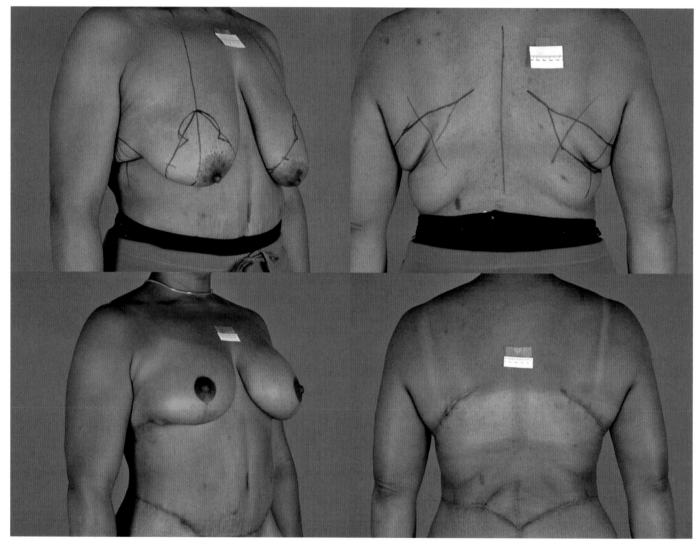

Fig. 27.35 This figure demonstrates a patient prior to surgery (above) and after an upper bodylift (below). Note the upper back rolls and the lateral descent of the lateral inframammary crease prior to surgery. The inframammary crease is lifted to its proper position, the upper back excess is eliminated, and the lifted breasts are shown after surgery.

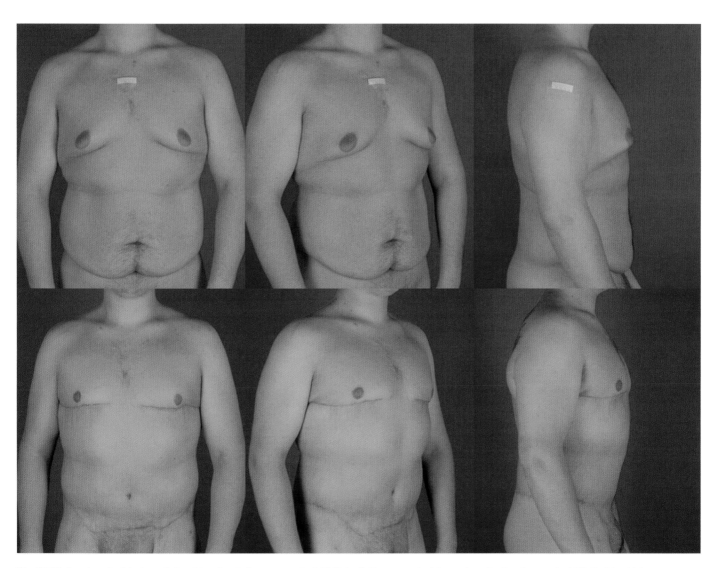

Fig. 27.36 A male patient is shown before (above) and after an upper bodylift (below). The same principles apply as the female upper bodylift; the lateral inframammary crease is lifted to its proper position, upper back/lateral chest excess is eliminated, and the breast reconstruction is built upon a properly positioned inframammary crease.

Access the complete references list online at **http://www.expertconsult.com**

1. Lockwood T. Lower bodylift with superficial fascial system suspension. *Plast Reconstr Surg* 1993;92: 1112–1122.

2. Lockwood T. Lower bodylift. *Oper Tech Plast Reconstr Surg* 1996;3:132–144.

3. Aly A, Cram AE, Chao BS, et al. Belt lipectomy for circumferential truncal excess: The University of Iowa experience. *Plast Reconstr Surg* 2003;111(1): 398–413.

   This is the first article ever published that describes the use of circumferential lower truncal lipectomy/belt lipectomy in the treatment of massive weight loss patients. It also describes four groups, including the massive weight loss group, where circumferential procedures can be utilized.

4. Aly AS. Option in lower truncal surgery. In: Aly AS, ed. *Body contouring after massive weight loss*. St Louis: Quality Medical; 2006:59.

   This chapter describes the differences between the different types of circumferential procedures both in technique and philosophy.

5. Lockwood TE. Lower bodylift and medial thigh lift. In: Aly AS, ed. *Body contouring after massive weight loss*. St Louis: Quality Medical; 2006:147.

   This chapter describes Lockwood's original technique, which differs significantly from belt lipectomy. It describes the use of the superficial fascial system in excisional truncal contouring as well as describing his technique for medial thigh lifting.

6. Aly AS, Cram AE. The Iowa belt lipectomy technique. *Plast Reconstr Surg* 2008;122(3):959–960.

7. Aly AS, Capella JE, Staging, reoperation and treatment of complications after body contouring in the massive weight loss patient. In: Grotting JC, ed. *Reoperative aesthetic and reconstructive plastic surgery*. St Louis: Quality Medical; 2007:1701.

8. Aly AS. Belt lipectomy. In: Aly AS, ed. *Body contouring after massive weight loss*. St Louis: Quality Medical; 2006:83.

This chapter goes in detail over the authors' approach to contouring the lower truncal area. It covers patient presentation, physical examination, markings, operative technique, results, and complications.

9. Aly AS. Belt lipectomy. In: Aly AS, ed. *Body contouring after massive weight loss*. St Louis: Quality Medical; 2006:86.

11. Michaud AP, Rosenquist RW, Cram AE, et al. An evaluation of epidural analgesia following circumferential belt lipectomy. *Plast Reconstr Surg* 2007;120(2):538–544.

The article describes the authors' regimen for epidural anesthesia, which the authors believe to be essential, not only alleviating postoperative pain, but also in reducing the risk of VTE/PE.

28

Buttock augmentation

Terrence W. Bruner, José Abel de la Peña Salcedo, Constantino G. Mendieta and Thomas L. Roberts III

SYNOPSIS

Micro fat grafting

- Ideal candidates for augmentation by micro fat grafting (MFG) have sufficient liposuction donor sites to provide adequate fat for grafting.
- Fat grafting <1000 cc per buttock markedly decreases the risk of complications.
- Buttock augmentation by micro fat grafting is extremely technique-dependent and requires meticulous attention to sterility and even distribution of grafted fat over hundreds of passes, from bone to skin.
- The synergistic effect of augmentation combined with concomitant liposuction is the optimal method to achieve ideal proportions.
- No sitting is allowed for the first 2 weeks after surgery.
- Preoperative markings are crucial in guiding the surgical procedure and should be performed with the patient in the standing position.

Implants

- Ideal candidates for buttock implants are thin patients with an athletic build and little or no ptosis.
- Determine the patient's expectations and evaluate the size of the proposed implant with templates.
- Make two paramedian incisions, one for each implant, leaving two centimeters between them inferiorly; 5 cm superiorly, as they curve laterally.
- Subcutaneous undermining in the sacral area must be minimal and the skin and underlying tissue at the midline must remain untouched.
- Create both pockets before placing the implants.
- If infection of the pocket occurs, treatment usually requires temporary removal of the implant for 3–6 months.
- Always use closed-suction drains.
- Implants will not correct gluteal ptosis.

Access the Historical Perspective section online at
http://www.expertconsult.com

Introduction

- Buttock augmentation is major surgery, with the potential for significant complications.
- The overall goal of buttock augmentation is to achieve a more youthful appearance and contour and to create the ideal waist-to-hip ratio of 0.7.
- There are three acceptable methods of buttock augmentation: (1) silicone implants placed in the intramuscular plane; (2) silicone implants placed in the subfascial plane; and (3) autologous micro fat grafting (MFG).
- A fourth method of buttock augmentation, subcutaneous placement of buttock implants, is solely mentioned so it can be condemned due to the unacceptably high complication rate.
- Each method of buttock augmentation carries its own set of indications, risks, surgical equipment needs, and complications.
- Preoperative planning and the surgical technique used should be patient-specific with regard to individual anatomy and patient desires.
- Preoperative markings are crucial in guiding the surgical procedure and should be performed with the patient in a standing position.

Basic science

Gluteal aesthetic ideals

The attractiveness of the buttocks is not judged in isolation, but in proportion to the waist. According to Singh,[2] there is one female body shape that men universally find most attractive (full buttocks, narrow waist). These ideal female proportions are summarized as a waist-to-hip ratio of 0.7 (measuring the waist at its narrowest and the buttock at the level of maximum circumference). In addition to this overall

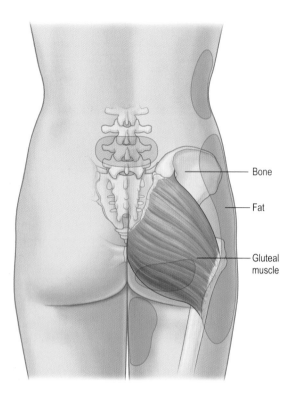

Fig. 28.1 Anatomy of the gluteus maximus muscle.

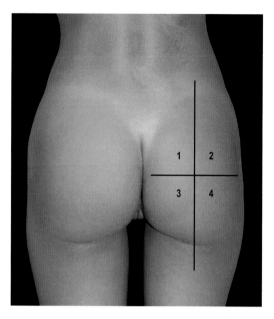

Fig. 28.2 Ideal gluteal aesthetics based on quadrant analysis.

proportional relationship, there are various characteristics associated with attractive youthful buttocks. These include: (1) A smooth inward sweep of the lumbosacral area and waist; (2) a very feminine cleavage as the buttocks separate superiorly and inferiorly; (3) maximum prominence on the vertical axis at the level of the mid to upper buttock, and on the transverse axis, at the junction of the medial and central thirds of the buttocks; (4) minimal infragluteal crease; and (5) no ptosis.[13]

Topographical anatomy

A thorough grounding in anatomy and aesthetics is essential when dealing with the gluteal aesthetic unit.[17] We can all recognize attractive buttocks, but translating these aesthetics into words becomes a challenge. Dr Ralph Millard[18] emphasized in his book, *Principalization of Plastic Surgery*, that in order to be successful in our surgical design, approach and ultimate results, we must first understand the beautiful – in this case, the ideal buttock.

The gluteus maximus muscle originates primarily along the lateral margin of the sacrum and, to a lesser extent, from the coccyx and sacrotuberous ligament. The origin continues in an upward curvilinear fashion to the posterior iliac spine (identified as bilateral dimples in the parasacral zone); traditional teaching tells us that the muscle attaches all along the superior iliac crest, but in reality it only follows the crest for one-third of its initial distance. The superior limit of the gluteus maximus muscle is the posterior iliac spine. The gluteus maximus inserts into the iliotibial tract, and to a lesser degree, the greater trochanter *(Fig. 28.1)*.

Knowledge of the superior aspect of the gluteus maximus origin is essential in describing the ideal buttock. However, buttocks aesthetics are not solely dependent on the gluteus

muscles; the overall buttock shape is also influenced by bony pelvic anatomy, fat distribution, and to a lesser degree the tightness of skin. The skin will influence the appearance if there is laxity or ptosis, as is the case in massive weight loss patients. In fact, the attractiveness of the female buttock is primarily dependant on the thickness and distribution of the fatty layer, which is usually 50–60% of the volume of the buttock. Confirmation of this can be easily obtained by looking at the shape of the buttocks in a woman's fitness magazine. The women who exercise and diet competitively to make their muscles maximally full and visible accomplish this also by losing body fat. This loss of fat makes the buttocks look gaunt and unfeminine.

Aesthetic analysis

To evaluate the buttock, it is helpful to divide it into quadrants by drawing an imaginary line down the center of the buttock. The ideal buttock has equal volumes on either side of this line and has the shape of a football.

To further assess volume distribution, a horizontal mid-buttock line is added to divide the buttocks into four quadrants *(Fig. 28.2)*. The ideal buttock also has equal volumes above and below this horizontal line. If we evaluate each quadrant individually, then the lower quadrants, three and four are equal, but tend to be slightly wider than one and two. In determining the best procedure for a particular patient, all four quadrants are evaluated as either sufficient or deficient.

Once volume has been assessed, there are three other zones that surround the buttock, which become important in our evaluation: the upper inner gluteal/sacral junction, the lower inner gluteal fold/leg junction, and mid-lateral gluteal/hip junction.

Upper inner gluteal/sacral junction: ideal presacral space shape

The inner gluteal/sacral space should be well defined so that a V-shape is apparent; this lower presacral space is appropriately called the "V" zone *(Fig. 28.3)*. As the "V" zone becomes more visible, the buttock has greater aesthetic appeal. In the ideal buttock, the gluteal muscle edge should be well defined and have a semicircular upward turn. If this space is not well defined, the buttock becomes blunt and appears flat, especially on the lateral view.

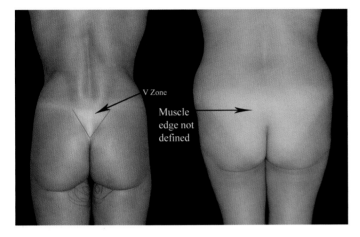

Fig. 28.3 The "V" zone. Visible muscle fullness versus loss of definition from excess fat and back of muscle volume.

Lower inner gluteal fold/leg junction

To describe this relationship, the intergluteal crease will be referred to as the midline. The upper aspect of the crease is easily identified; however, the inferior aspect is defined at the point where the buttock begins to separate from this midline. In the ideal buttock this occurs at about the bottom two-thirds to three-quarters of the muscle. The separation widens until it meets the inner leg junction. At this point the lower gluteal fold has a 45° take-off from the center intergluteal crease line and the inner gluteal fold/leg junction should create a diamond shape space *(see Fig. 28.4)*. This is a key point in gluteal aesthetics.

As the lower inner gluteal fold and inner leg become fuller, it changes the 45° sloping line to a more horizontal position, which causes the diamond shape space to turn into a straight line, losing its aesthetic appeal *(Fig. 28.4)*. As the fullness increases, it develops an inverse relationship creating an upward slope (negative angle) *(Fig. 28.4)*. Improvement of this zone will depend on the severity of the fullness.

Lateral mid-buttock/hip contour

In the aesthetic buttock, the lateral mid-buttock is an area without any depression. This zone is categorized as having; no depression, mild depression, moderate or severe depression *(Fig. 28.5)*.

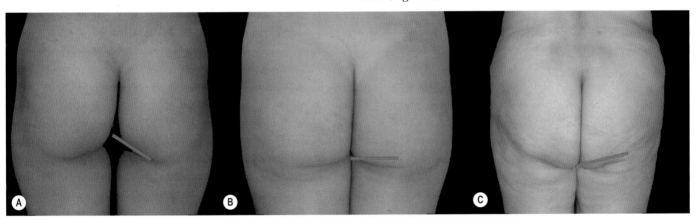

Fig. 28.4 Red lines indicate how the fullness increases at the lower inner gluteal fold and the diamond zone turns from a 45° into a straight line. **(A)** Downward slope; **(B)** horizontal line; **(C)** upward slope.

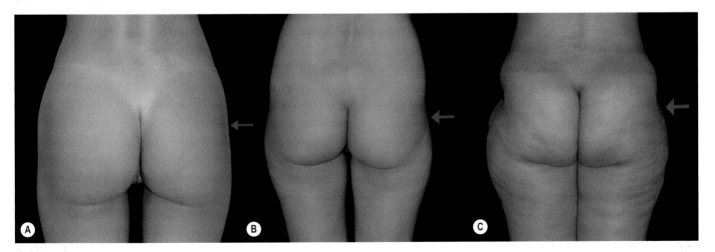

Fig. 28.5 Variation in lateral mid-buttock depression. **(A)** None to mild; **(B)** moderate; **(C)** severe.

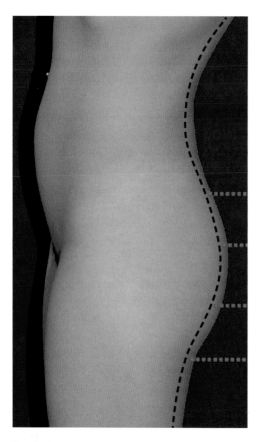

Fig. 28.6 Aesthetics of the gluteal region – lateral view.

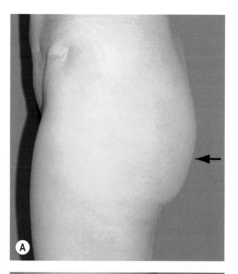

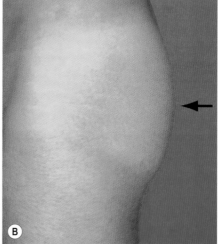

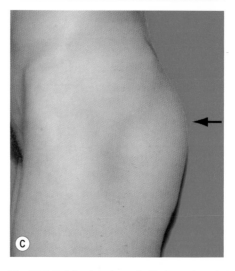

Lateral view aesthetics

On lateral view, the presacral area should have a sweeping curve that has a lazy S shape (from the back to the bottom of the gluteus) *(Fig. 28.6)*. Most of the gluteal volume is central and has equal distribution in the upper and lower gluteal zones, giving a C-shape curve. It has been suggested that the peak of the central mound should be at the level of the pubic bone *(Fig. 28.7)*.

Determining where most of the volume lies (upper, central or lower buttock) will be important in deciding what procedure is best used to augment the buttock *(Fig. 28.8)*.

Fig. 28.7 Variation in volume distribution on lateral view.

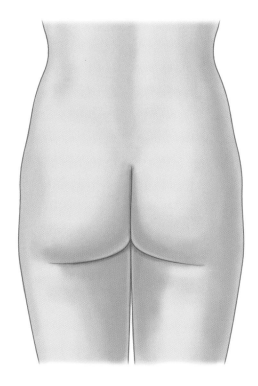

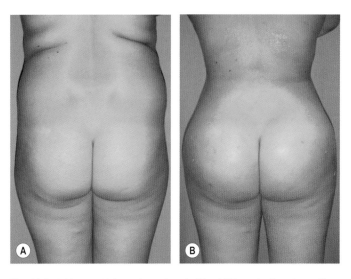

Fig. 28.9 A 22-year-old Caucasian patient desiring full buttocks throughout. After buttock augmentation with 900 cc of fat grafted per side.

Fig. 28.8 Ideal gluteal aesthetics. One can see that the upper aesthetic unit of the gluteus follows its origin; it begins at the midsacral line, continues as a semicircular line that connects to the posterior iliac spine (identified as *bilateral* dimples in the parasacral zone) and peaks at 2–3 cm above this point. In a well-developed buttock with very little lower presacral fat, a visible "V" zone is apparent, which further accentuates the upper inner muscle anatomy; the muscle has a football shape with nearly equal volumes in all four quadrants (quadrants three and four tend to be slightly wider than quadrants one and two). The gluteal unit is marked superiorly by its attachment to the iliac ridge (easily palpated) and inferiorly by the inferior gluteal crease. Without a doubt, the most important contributor to gluteal aesthetics is the volume of distribution in all four quadrants. When this volume is adequate, all other aesthetic points can be overlooked and still render an attractive buttock. The inferior gluteal aesthetics is defined by a diamond shape at the intergluteal/leg junction, the medial buttock cheeks have a 45° take-off from the intergluteal line and flows into the inferior gluteal crease which terminates at or just beyond the mid-buttock line. On lateral view there is an S-shaped curve from the lower back as it comes into contact with the buttock and most of the gluteal volume is located in the central zone.

Table 28.1 Ethnic ideals of beautiful buttocks

	Buttocks size	Lateral buttocks fullness	Lateral thigh fullness
Asian	Small to moderate, but shapely	No	No
Caucasian	Full, but not extremely large	Rounded (voluptuous) or hollow (athletic)	No
Hispanic	Very full	Very full	Slight fullness
African-American	As full as possible	Very full	Very full

Diagnosis/patient presentation

Patients present with a desire to improve their body contour/proportions, due to aging or general soft tissue deficiency. Specific patient desires can be affected by ethnic background and social relationships. There are six zones where augmentation is requested: upper medial buttocks, mid medial buttocks, lower medial buttocks, lateral hollow/ trochanteric depression, lateral thigh, and various localized depressions.

Ethnic ideals need to be taken into consideration regarding patient desires *(Table 28.1)*.[13] Some Caucasian patients may desire full, but not overly large buttocks which are rounded laterally *(Fig. 28.9)* or a trim, athletic appearance with hollow lateral buttocks. Some Asian patients may desire buttocks that are relatively small, whereas some Hispanic patients may

prefer buttocks that are full and rounded medially and laterally, with lateral buttocks that are relatively full *(Fig. 28.10)*. Some African-American and Caribbeans of African descent *(Fig. 28.11)* may desire larger buttock size, with fullness in the lateral buttocks and lateral thighs ("hips").

Gluteal augmentation is not just about making the buttock bigger, but rather accentuating, contouring, and reshaping. The focus becomes *volume redistribution*; shifting volume from an unattractive zone to a more desirable position. With this perspective, even the full-figured woman becomes a candidate since, on closer examination, the large buttock has maldistributed adiposity, with deficient volume in pertinent aesthetic zones *(Fig. 28.12)*. The question is no longer who is a candidate, but rather, what reshaping method is best for each particular patient? Liposuction is for sculpting, while fat transfers and/or implants are used for volume expansion.

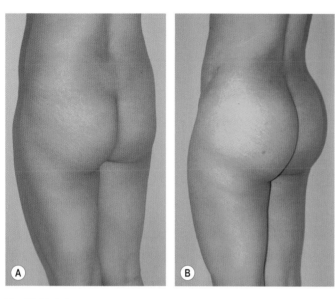

Fig. 28.10 A 25-year-old Hispanic patient desiring more fullness to the lateral buttocks. After 780 cc of fat grafted per side.

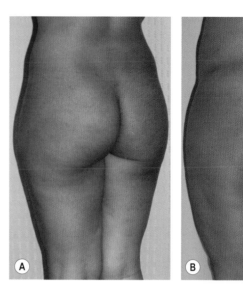

Fig. 28.11 A 36-year-old African-American female status post-buttocks augmentation with 890 cc of fat grafted per side.

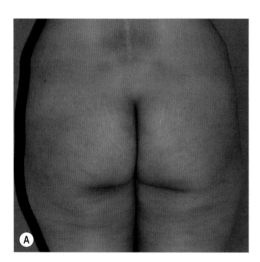

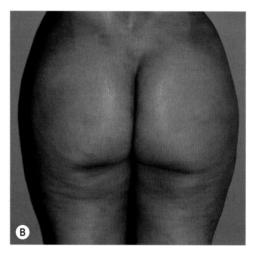

Fig. 28.12 Improvement of the gluteal region with overall volume redistribution.

Patient selection

The ideal patients for implant-based augmentation are young, with an athletic build with little or no ptosis. Morbidly obese patients are not candidates for this surgery unless they lose weight, after which the laxity of tissues converts them into good candidates if they undergo excisional procedures to correct the back and gluteal regions.

Early series on implant-based augmentation documented unacceptably high rates of would dehiscence and implant exposure. As patients requested greater augmentations, larger implants were used, resulting in higher complication rates. Patients were retrospectively stratified into various groups of body frames, based on size/BMI *(Figs 28.13–28.16).*[9] The larger the body frame, the greater the risk of wound dehiscence and implant exposure ✂ FIGS **28.13 28.14 28.16 28.16** APPEAR ONLINE ONLY

How do we distinguish the frames?

As surgeons, we would like some sort of scientific method to help guide and standardize these four body frames. While the approach used was very subjective, in an attempt to cement a standard tool, several evaluation methods were examined: percentage body fat, body mass index, dress size, and presacral fat measurements. The small frame is usually a BMI of ≤20 (US dress size 0–2); the medium frame is a BMI of 21–27 (US dress size 3–9); the large framed patient is a BMI of 28–31 (US dress size 10–14) and finally, the extra large frame usually has a BMI of ≥32 (US dress size >15).

Conclusion

If the BMI is ≤20, the patient will usually not have enough fat for augmentation and implants are the volume enhancer of

Table 28.2 Advantages and disadvantages of various techniques of buttocks augmentation[a]

	Autologous fat grafting: current technique (excluding >1000 cc/buttock) (n = 74)	Intramuscular or submuscular implants	Subfascial implants (semisolid, textured)
Possible to consistently obtain ideal proportions (WHR = 0.7) in one operation?	Yes	No	No
Can this technique meet all ethnic shape requests?	Yes	No	No
Area of buttock that can be augmented	Any and all areas	Upper and mid-buttock only	Lower and mid-buttock only
Augment lateral buttock?	Yes	No	Minimally
Augment lateral thigh?	Yes	No	No
Can liposacral area at same time?	Yes	No	No
Shifting of implant possible?	No	Yes	Yes
Can this technique consistently deliver as large a size as the patient desires?	Yes[b]	No	Often, but not always
Edge of implant visible?	No	Occasionally "double bubble"	Occasionally
Implant palpable (firm)?	0%	10%	100%
Foreign body concerns for patient?	No	Yes	Yes
Future silicone litigation possible?	No	Yes	Yes
Wound dehiscence	0% (but 4% have <2 cc sterile drainage/day for 1–6 weeks)	About 30%	About 30%
Seroma around implant	0%	2–4%	19%
Length of operation	5–6 h	2–4 h	4 h
Infection	2.7%	1.4%	7%
Total major complications	2.7%	15–25%	35%

[a]See also Bruner and colleagues.[18]
[b]Unless patient requests extremely large augmentation >1000 cc.

choice. Patients with a BMI of ≥28, usually have abundant lipodystrophy and are best augmented with fat.

What has been most helpful in patient selection has been "presacral fat measurements"; anyone with 6–7 cm presacral thickness will usually have the body type that has sufficient fat for transfers. There is an excess layer of fat over the sacrum which makes these patients a set up for wound dehiscence if implants are used. There is no foolproof system that will individualize each patient, given all the variables discussed. As a general rule, we should start considering fat transfer as the preferred choice for augmentation in patients that have a BMI of ≥24, a US dress size above 8, or a 5–6 cm presacral fat thickness. However, physicians' judgment and experience remain the standard.

Aesthetic goals

Research by Singh, as well as other authors, has documented the importance of an ideal waist-to-hip ratio of 0.7.[2] There is a tremendous synergistic effect of liposuction of the lower back, waist and flanks in conjunction with buttock augmentation to achieve this ideal waist-to-hip ratio. This is clearly evidenced by the fact that fuller, more shapely buttocks

appear more attractive when the waist is slender rather than fuller.

In attractive female buttocks, there is beautiful cleavage as the buttocks separate superiorly. Furthermore, there is an inward sweep of the lower back, lumbar and sacral area, which accentuates this cleavage. It is also important to make the buttocks shorter vertically, than one would think. A short full buttock is attractive. A vertically long buttock simply appears big. (For a detailed summary of advantages and disadvantages of the various techniques for buttock augmentation see *Table 28.2*.)

Principles of buttock implants

Implant placement and selection

There are three main issues that need to be decided when selecting implants: implant location, shape, and size. The implant content can be a solid silicone elastomer or silicone cohesive gel. The gel implants are used in the international circles whereas, in the US, at the time of this writing, surgeons are limited to the elastomer implants.

Anatomic planes of dissection for implant placement: advantages and disadvantages

Subcutaneous plane (of historical interest)

Subcutaneous placement of a gluteal implant has serious disadvantages. Since the system that maintains the skin attachment to the gluteal region is composed of aponeurotic expansions running from the gluteal aponeurosis to the dermis, the creation of a subcutaneous pocket will damage these expansions leaving skin that is without fixation, thereby resulting in implant migration *(Fig. 28.17)*. Furthermore, in this plane, the implants are highly visible; the skin envelope can become ptotic, and severe capsular contracture can occur,

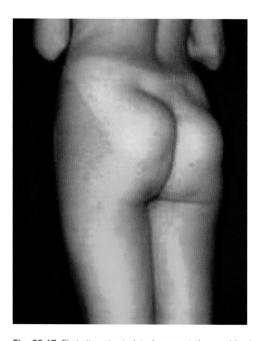

Fig. 28.17 First attempts at gluteal augmentation used implants designed for breast augmentation. Implants are positioned in a subcutaneous plane, have capsular contracture and have the wrong dimensions needed for a natural and visually pleasing result.

giving the shape of a large mushroom *(Fig. 28.18)*. There is *no* indication for use of the subcutaneous plane.

Submuscular plane (rarely used today)

In 1984, Robles and colleagues described the submuscular approach.[10] This approach preserves the aponeurotic system that holds gluteal skin in position and has the advantage of reducing the formation of capsular contracture. However, it introduced a new anatomic problem with the potential risk of injury to the sciatic nerve. This is the largest peripheral nerve in the body, emerging from the pelvis via the greater sciatic foramen, entering the surgical plane below the bottom edge of the piriformis muscle *(Fig. 28.19)*. It then wraps tightly superiorly and laterally around the ischial tuberosity. As the dissection of the submuscular plane is carried inferiorly, the sciatic nerve can be injured. Even if the nerve is not injured during dissection, if the lower edge of the implant extends below the mid-buttock, it will be resting on the nerve and may cause symptoms. The submuscular position also has the disadvantage of being a small space and therefore limits the use of larger implants. Consequently, implants should rarely be placed in this submuscular plane.

Intramuscular plane (location of choice)

This plane disrupts the muscular fibers of the gluteus maximus. The goal is to have 2–3 cm of muscle over the pocket and to leave 3 cm thickness of gluteus maximus deep to the pocket to protect the sciatic nerve. Because the implant is placed within the muscle, there are no anatomical landmarks. Once at the right depth, the surgeon must remember that this plane is curved like the surface of a globe, so the dissection must be curved downward as it is carried superiorly, laterally and inferiorly. A common problem is to break out of this plane during superior dissection, perforating into the subcutaneous tissue. Then when the patient sits, the implant shifts upwards, causing pain at the iliac crest. Another technical difficulty is the lack of a natural tissue plane within the gluteus maximus, which means that the dissection produces disruption of the muscle fibers, promoting a higher incidence of seroma and hematoma.

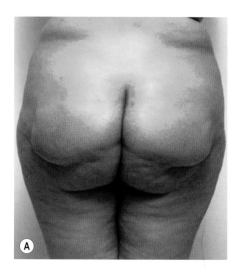
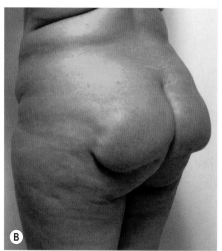
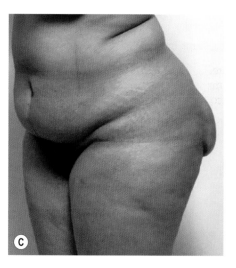

Fig. 28.18 Subcutaneously placed implants with mushroom-like encapsulation.

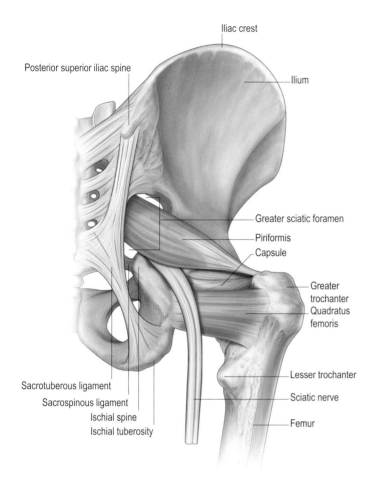

Iliac crest

Posterior superior iliac spine

Ilium

Greater sciatic foramen

Piriformis

Capsule

Greater trochanter

Quadratus femoris

Lesser trochanter

Sciatic nerve

Femur

Sacrotuberous ligament

Sacrospinous ligament

Ischial spine

Ischial tuberosity

Fig. 28.19 Anatomy of the sciatic nerve.

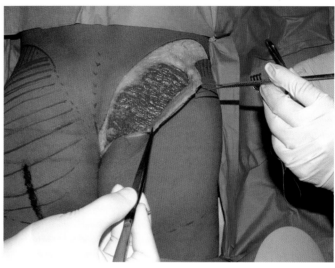

Fig. 28.20 Cadaver dissection showing the rasing of a fasciocutaneous flap. Subfascial undermining starts at the site of the fascial incision.

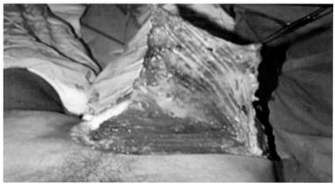

Fig. 28.21 Cadaver dissection showing the gluteal aponeurosis as a viable dissection plane for gluteal augmentation.

Although the initial thinking with the intramuscular placement was to keep the implant more superficial to avoid compression of the sciatic nerve, it has been shown that by keeping all poles of the implant inside the muscle, sciatic symptoms are quite rare. Since the gluteus maximus extends almost to the infragluteal crease, this has facilitated the development of elliptical implants which convey maximal fullness at the mid-buttock level. A double bubble deformity can also occur, especially if the implant is not low enough to add volume to the lower pole.

Subfascial plane

This is an excellent technique developed by De La Pena, but requires textured gel implants, which at the time of this writing are not available in the United States.

This technique is based on extensive anatomical analysis of the gluteal layers. The gluteal fascia is very strong *(Figs 28.20, 28.21)*. It covers the entire gluteus maximus muscle, from origin to insertion.

Implant shape selection

Choice of implant *shape for the intramuscular plane requires evaluating* two aspects:

1. The muscle height to width relationship in the PA view
2. The volume of distribution in the lateral view.

Muscle height to width ratio

To find this relationship, identify the superior and inferior points of the gluteus muscle as well as the most medial and lateral points. At a glance you will notice a height to width relationship which will fall into one of three ratios: 1:1 (short muscle), 2:1 (tall muscle), or 1.5:1 (intermediate). The ideal buttock is intermediate but leans more towards a 2:1 relationship *(Fig. 28.22)*.

Implant selection

In intramuscular implant augmentation, the size is determined intraoperatively with the aid of sizers so as not to create muscle tension at closure. Implant shape selection is based on the muscle height to width ratio; the tall buttock (2:1 height to width ratio) is best augmented with the anatomic implant. The short buttock (1:1 ratio) is best augmented with the round implant, while the intermediate buttock (1.5:1 ratio) may require the lateral view to make the final determination *(Fig. 28.23)*.

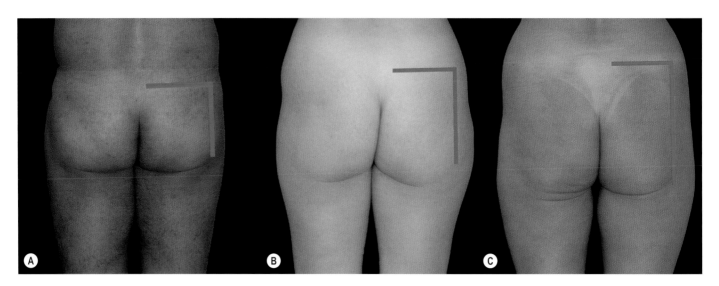

Fig. 28.22 Variations in height to width ratios in buttock anatomy. **(A)** Short, 1 to 1; **(B)** Intermediate, 1-2 to 1; **(C)** Tall, 2 to 1.

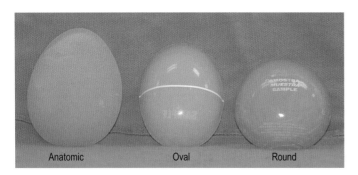

Fig. 28.23 Standard buttock implant shapes.

The lateral view

The lateral view will evaluate where most of the bulk of the gluteal volume is located; lower, central (midbuttock) or upper buttock.

If the buttocks are fuller inferiorly, a round implant will look best since the round implant adds most of its projection in the upper and central zones, equalizing the volumes throughout the buttock. If the buttocks have no significant projection superiorly or inferiorly, we prefer the oval implant for the intermediate or tall muscle. If the maximum fullness is *in the upper buttock*, an anatomic implant (maximum prominence inferiorly) will have the best result since the anatomic design adds most of its volume inferiorly. If a round implant is used in these cases, it will accentuate the already full upper buttock which in turn will accentuate the lower gluteal deficiency making the buttock look very disproportionate.

Implant size selection

Selecting implant size involves the fine balance of trying to obtain the size the patient desires, yet preventing the complications of implant exposure and wound dehiscence. Often these are in conflict, as the tissues will not allow as large an augmentation as the patient desires. In these cases, fat transfers can be combined to further increase volume.

Since each patient's anatomy is different and implant exposure rates rise as tension increases, implant size cannot be determined prior to surgery. Sizers are used intraoperatively to identify the largest implant the buttock will accommodate, without creating excessive muscle tension at closure. If the patient desires a larger augmentation, the implants can be exchanged with larger implants at 3–6 months, or fat transfers can be performed. Fat transfers have also been performed at the same time as the implant augmentation, taking great care to avoid grafting fat particles in the implant pocket, which greatly increases the risk of infection. Cannula trauma to the implant pocket (liposuction or grafting) can increase the risk of seroma, and creates the potential for fracture of the implant.

Micro fat grafting surgical technique

Pre-surgical markings

There are two essential points regarding appropriate marking for buttock augmentation by micro fat grafting. The first is to thoroughly sculpt the flanks, lumbar area and lumbosacral area to create an inward sweep, which will synergistically emphasize the new fullness of the buttocks after fat grafting. This includes performing liposuction to create a deep sacral "V", which will enhance the superior gluteal cleavage. This is further accentuated by grafting the upper medial buttocks, immediately adjacent to the sacrum. Second, it is important to have adequate donor sites. Clinically, we have discerned no difference of fat survival from the various areas that are used donor fat. The vast majority of buttock augmentation procedures range from grafting 600–1000 cc per buttock or 1200–2000 cc of graftable fat. Up to one-third of the fat that is harvested may become damaged during the harvesting process, meaning 1800–3000 cc must be available for the body.

The areas of maximum prominence should be at the junction of the middle and central thirds transversely and the mid and upper poles of the buttocks. The patient is asked to bring a favorite bathing suit and markings are made outlining the borders of the swimwear and, during the surgical procedure, every effort is made to place liposuction incisions within the boundaries of these markings.

Surgical technique

After marking, the patient undergoes a standing circumferential povidone–iodine prep. Antibiotic prophylaxis is ampicillin/sulbactam (Unasyn) 3 g Q.6 h; Gentamicin 5 mg/kg, and Cefazolin (Ancef) 1 g Q.4 h. After general anesthesia is initiated, a povidone–iodine soaked sponge is then place over the anus.

Maximum effort is made to maintain sterility and prevent infection. With the patient in the supine position, tumescent solution is infused to all of the fat donor sites and is warmed up to 110–115° Fahrenheit just prior to infusion. This is an excellent method of maintaining the patient at appropriate body temperature during the surgical procedure.

Harvesting and preparing fat is a multiple step process. A 4 mm harvesting cannula is used with the power assisted liposuction device (Micro-Aire™). Since incorporating the use of the PAL hand held device, the authors feel there has been a reduction in the time required to harvest the appropriate amount of fat without compromising fat survival. It is essential that the vacuum used to provide negative suction be maintained at <22 inches of mercury, otherwise "gassing-out" of oxygen and nitrogen, can disrupt cell membranes and markedly decrease fat survival.

Once harvested, the fat is then quickly processed. This begins with instilling 10 cc of an antibiotic solution (3 g ampicillin/sulbactam and 80 mg Gentamicin plus 1 g Cefazolin in 1000 cc of saline) into each canister (200–300 cc asp. rate). The fat is placed into 60 cc syringes and centrifuged at 2000 rpm for 3 min. Any tumescent fluid is then poured off and any oil is decanted from the fat. The fat is transferred to 60 cc injection syringes or 5 cc hand-held syringes. Any grafting to the anterolateral areas is performed at this time with the patient in the supine position to complete the liposuction of the flanks, lower thoracic and lumbosacral areas.

The 15 cm grafting cannula is 3 mm diameter with a single side hole and "bullet" tip. The majority of fat is grafted with the use of 60 cc syringes. Fat is grafted to all anatomic layers from the periosteum up to the subcutaneous. It is essential to maintain an awareness of the course of the sciatic nerve and avoid compression or trauma to it.

Final contouring is performed by judicious liposuction to achieve the desired contour. Liposuction of the infra-gluteal bulge ("banana roll") is absolutely avoided because it functions as a support for the buttock, and liposuction of this area can result in sagging of the inferior pole. Virtually all areas that are dimpled or flat and resist distension are tethered down by a fascial band to the muscle. Even if you can hydraulically pump these areas up, they will reappear postoperatively unless the tethering bands are selectively released. This is performed with a J-shaped dissector and should only be done after fat has been forcefully grafted into the area. The J-dissector may need to be passed extensively, but only in a radial fashion; a sweeping motion can accomplish complete sub scission and must be avoided, as this can result in a bulge. Two 10-French round, multiperforated TLS drains are routinely placed across the sacrum and flanks bilaterally and exiting the stab incisions made through the bra strap area.

This has markedly decreased the incidence of postoperative seroma formation and need for serial aspiration. A compressive garment is applied. A 3-inch thick gauze triangle made from Kerlix rolls is applied to the lower lumbar/sacral area to help facilitate skin adherence to the sacrum and maintain the superior gluteal cleavage and inward sweep of the lumbo sacral area. Any fluid accumulation to this pre-sacral area will result in loss of the superior gluteal cleavage.

Intramuscular implant surgical technique

Markings

The areas to have liposuction or fat transfers are marked in the preoperative area with the patient in the standing position. The intraoperative markings are minimal, identifying only the tip of the coccyx and infragluteal crease (this helps identify the drain exit points).

Preparation

Preoperative medicines include Decadron 10 mg IV and Cleocin 600 mg IV. The pneumatic stocking compressions are placed and functioning prior to induction. The surgical procedure is only 2–3 h, therefore a Foley catheter is not necessary.

Anesthesia/positioning

The procedure can be performed under general anesthesia, spinal, or IV sedation.

The gluteal area is prepped from the knees to the upper back and as far lateral as possible. Draping should leave the entire gluteal zone and lower back exposed; a Betadine soaked gauze is placed over the anus and secured with 2-0 silk so as to avoid contamination. A sterile towel is placed over the gauze to cover the anus and the inner gluteal zone.

Incision design/selection

A vertical inter-gluteal midline incision extending 8 cm up from the tip of the coccyx has been widely used, but given a dehiscence rate of 10–25%, has been supplanted by *bilateral parasacral incisions*. These incisions avoid the sacral midline with its poor blood supply, thereby decreasing dehiscence rates to <10%.

These incisions are designed as follows: with the patient in the prone position, the tip of the coccyx is palpated and marked; staying exactly in the sacral midline the central inter-gluteal crease is drawn from the tip of the coccyx 8 cm cephalad. The future incisions are marked 1 cm on either side of this midline, so that both incisions are 2 cm apart in the inferior and middle portions. If these lower distances are not respected, central skin necrosis may occur. As the incision reaches the upper buttock, it follows the upper gluteal curvature (this occurs at about the 6 cm mark from the coccyx), becoming 4–5 cm apart *(Fig. 28.24)*.

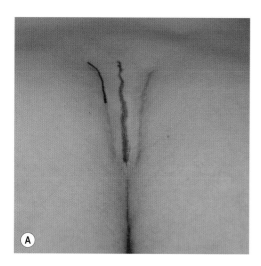
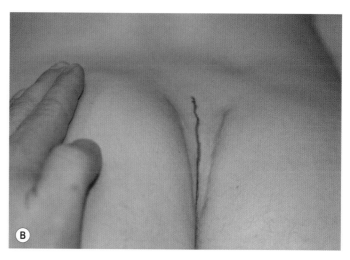

Fig. 28.24 Bilateral para-sacral incisional markings for implant placement.

Skin flap dissection

The incision sites are infiltrated with 10 cc of 1% lidocaine with Epinephrine 1:100 000. Tumescent fluid is injected into the intramuscular and subcutaneous tissues, as well as the areas to be suctioned. The incision is made down to the gluteal fascia. Using hooked retractors, the tissues are placed under upward traction. The dissection is performed, making sure to preserve the fascia on the muscle. The dissection can be done with a gauze pad wrapped around the thumb, digitally elevating the subcutaneous tissues with an upward sweeping motion. The goal of the initial subcutaneous dissection will be to expose just enough of the muscle and fascia to allow implant placement. This usually means a subcutaneous tunnel 8 cm wide and about 6 cm long.

Muscle dissection

Using the mid-sacral level as the reference point, the fascia is opened following the direction of the muscle fibers for a length of 5 cm.

The intramuscular dissection is started by using a long curved hemostat (tonsil or Kuettner), perforating the muscle for a depth of 1 cm and spreading widely so that a ring forceps can be inserted with the other hand. This is then pushed 1 cm into the muscle, spread, and the tonsil clamp is inserted, alternatively spreading the muscle to a total depth of 2.5–3 cm. This dissection creates only a small muscular opening which must be enlarged. With the use of the cautery, the muscle incision is opened medially and laterally to its full fascial incision length. Once the correct depth of dissection is achieved the Deaver retractors are introduced on both sides of the muscle and spread. This is an intramuscular procedure; no plane exists, and you must create a pocket curved like the surface of a globe. The closed ring forceps is used to bluntly push and create the muscle pocket; the muscle pocket should be kept at 3 cm thickness throughout. It is best to start the pocket dissection in the superior lateral direction (a key point to this portion of the dissection is to tilt the tip of the ring forceps down to about 45° and keep curving deeper as dissection proceeds laterally. The pocket is further defined with the Aiache gluteal muscle dissector (serrated instrument).

Dry long narrow lap pads are packed in the wound for 1–2 min. This wait is rewarded by a remarkably dry field.

Expander

To help define the pocket further, a 300–400 cc breast implant expander is placed and over-inflated until no further expansion can be obtained (at least 500–600 cc). The expander will stretch the muscle and help indicate areas that need further dissection. The inferior dissection extends 3–5 cm below the coccyx, placing the implant in a more anatomic location with improved aesthetic contour. To ensure safety, the inferior dissection is performed with the aid of the expander in place; blunt finger dissection is used to push muscle fibers away from the implant in an inferior direction. The expander is left over inflated in the first side, while dissection is carried out on the second side to allow maximum time for intraoperative expansion.

Sizers/implant size

Once the surgeon is satisfied with the dissection, a sizer is inserted to determine the appropriate implant that can be used. When the implant is in place, the edges of the muscle incision should be in close proximity with very little tension at closure. *It is mandatory to have a variety of sizers and implants available in the operating room to help assess what is the largest implant that can be placed with minimal tension.*

Drains

Once the implant size has been determined, a Jackson Pratt drain is introduced in the pocket and brought out through a separate stab incision in the infragluteal crease. The use of a drain has decreased the incidence of seroma formation.

Implant placement/closure

The implant pocket is irrigated, the surgical field is reprepped and redraped, and the implant is introduced with the use of a sterile sleeve to avoid implant contact with the skin. The muscle is closed with 2-0 Monofilament absorbable suture. The subcutaneous wound is closed in layers with a final running 3-0 Vicryl. The opposite side is then completed in a similar fashion. The wounds are further reinforced with Dermabond to seal the incision and prevent contamination.

There are three key points to this operation:

1. Incision selection.
2. Keeping the gluteal fascia on the muscle during dissection, allowing for better purchase of the tissues during closure, limiting muscle dehiscence.
3. Proper implant size selection to minimize wound tension at closure.

Subfascial implant surgical technique

Markings

With the patient in a standing position the markings are made using custom designed templates (Silimed®). The template must be centered over the gluteal region leaving at least 2 cm between the template and the infragluteal fold and 2 cm from the border of the sacrum (*Figs 28.25, 28.26*).

Positioning and incisional markings are the same as the intramuscular technique.

Technique

The initial incision and dissection is as for the intramuscular technique. When reaching the muscular aponeurosis at the lateral border of the sacrum, an 8–10 cm incision into the aponeurosis is made parallel to the sacrum border entering the subfascial dissecting plane. Tumescent solution, 100–150 cc, is instilled with a tumescent cannula. This enables the identification of the avascular plane deep to the fascia

and facilitates sharp dissection of the septa in the subfascial plane, permitting the elevation of an intact fasciocutaneous flap.

The septae parallel the direction of the muscle fibers and, therefore, radiate out in a fan-like pattern (*Figs 28.27, 28.28*).

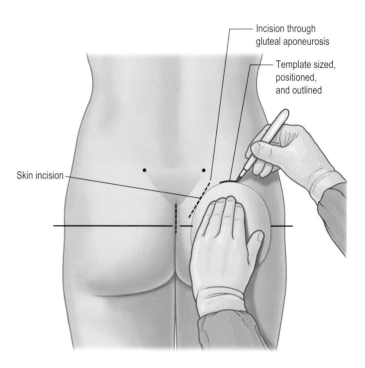

Fig. 28.26 The planning for surgery should entail the incision, which at the present time has been replaced from a single midline incision to two incisions in the intergluteal crease, therefore isolating completely one pocket from the other. Then, the fascial incision and creation of the subfascial pocket using the gluteus maximus muscle as a platform for the implant. The horizontal line across each buttock will be matched to a comparable line on the permanent implant to help guarantee correct implant alignment.

Fig. 28.25 Illustration showing the correct placement of the implant. Markings must follow the anatomic shape of the gluteal region and ensure that the implants will be lateral to the sacrum and positioned at least 2 cm above the infragluteal fold.

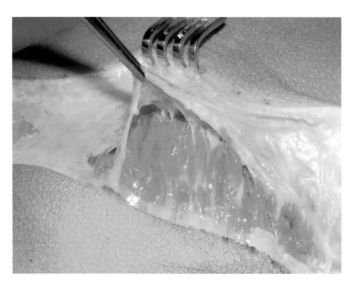

Fig. 28.27 Fascial incision and elevation of the gluteal aponeurosis to create the implant pocket.

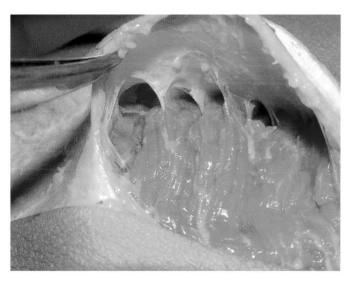

Fig. 28.28 Aponeurotic expansions traverse the superior layer of the gluteal maximus muscle. Dissection between the aponeurotic expansions is essential for creation of the implant pocket. This view gives a sense of the uniformity of the space that is shaped like the gluteus maximus muscle below.

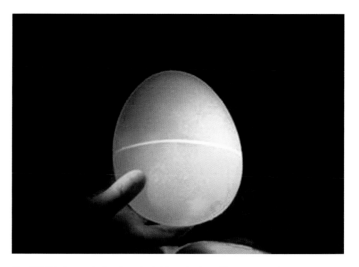

Fig. 28.29 Anatomically shaped, highly cohesive silicone filled gel gluteal implant. The transverse line ensures perfect positioning and alignment inside the pocket.

Hints and tips

1. To facilitate visibility while undermining, it is advisable to dissect from medial to lateral and from cephalic to caudal. Maintain a wide field of exposure without going beyond the skin markings.
2. Create both pockets before introducing any implants, so the volume of the buttock plus an implant on one side does not interfere with dissection of the contra lateral pocket.
3. Once the pockets are dissected, a sizer is used to evaluate the volume and shape of the pocket and confirm the correct implant size for the patient.

Drains are placed exiting the infra gluteal fold. The solid elastomer or cohesive gel implant is then inserted, making sure that the implant is perfectly aligned on its axis *(Fig. 28.29)* and fitting loosely inside the pocket *(Figs 28.30, 28.31)*.

Once the implants have been inserted, begin the closure by reattaching the gluteal aponeurosis at the same level where it was cut making sure that no tension is placed in the suture line. Then separately close the deep and superficial subcutaneous layers over the sacrum. Finally, each incision is closed using a running 4-0 Monofilament and sealed with Dermabond.

Postoperative care

Micro fat grafting

Buttock augmentation by micro fat grafting is performed on an outpatient basis. The patient must meet standard criteria for appropriate discharge, as outlined by accrediting organizations. It is essential that each patient have a competent caregiver for the first 3–4 days postoperatively. A Foley catheter is left for the first 24 h and postoperative antibiotics of Augmentin and Ciprofloxacin are used for 5 days.

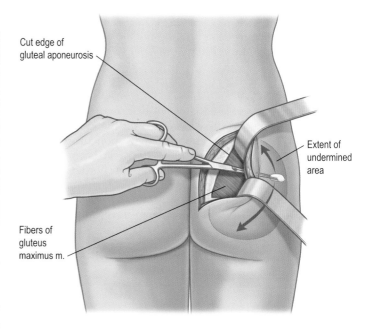

Cut edge of gluteal aponeurosis

Extent of undermined area

Fibers of gluteus maximus m.

Fig. 28.30 Undermining of the subfascial plane of dissection must extend 2 cm beyond the periphery of the implant.

Activity and follow-up

Patient activity is significantly limited for the first 1–2 weeks after surgery. No sitting is permitted except for a bowel movement. The patient must sleep in the prone position and is encouraged to ambulate as much as possible starting the evening of surgery. A full body compression garment is left in place until postoperative day 4 or 5. Close and frequent follow-up is required for the 2-week period after surgery for surveillance of possible infection. A buttock examination is performed by the patient on a daily basis to check for any areas of redness or tenderness. The suction drains are removed once their output is <30 cc/day. After 2 weeks, minimal sitting is allowed for up to 15–20 min at a time. The compression

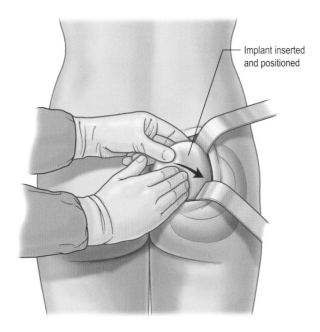

Fig. 28.31 Once the pocket is created, insert a sizer, evaluate the pocket and assess implant size and positioning. The implant should fit loosely in the pocket.

garment is worn for a total of 11 weeks. Patients can resume regular exercise at 6 weeks. The patient may resume unrestricted activity at 12 weeks postoperatively.

Implant-based augmentation

Activity

Since most wound dehiscences occur between days 12 and 16, patients are instructed to minimize activities that cause wound pressure or friction. They are asked to sleep prone for 3 weeks. They are allowed to sit only when going to the bathroom. After 2 weeks, the patient may return to normal activities, except for exercise and prolonged sitting. For the first 4 weeks, driving is not permitted.

Patients usually return to work after 3 weeks. Patients can resume physical exercise after 6–8 weeks. If wound dehiscence occurs, an additional 6 weeks of restricted activity may be required. The patient may resume unrestricted activity at 12 weeks postoperatively. The implants will initially feel very firm (like sitting on rocks) and it will take 3 months for them to soften.

Garments

If liposuction was performed, patients wear compressive garments for 6 weeks. If no liposuction was performed, an abdominal binder is used for 2–3 weeks, to place pressure in the upper part of the buttock. This theoretically helps decrease tension on the incision.

Drains

While drains are in place, the patient is kept on prophylactic antibiotics. Antibiotic ointment should be applied to the drain sites daily. The drains are removed when the output is <30 cc/day. They are usually not kept for more than 7–10 days.

Postoperative pain management

Most of the discomfort occurs between days 3 and 10. The discomfort is greatest in the early mornings. In order to help with the postoperative discomfort, Medrol dose packs and Neurontin 100 mg p.o. bid are helpful. Muscle relaxants are also prescribed as well as anxiolytic medications.

Outcomes, prognosis, and complications

Buttock augmentation by either micro fat grafting or implants can restore a more youthful appearance to the female buttocks and better approximate the aesthetic ideal waist-to-hip ratio of 0.7. Outcomes are patient specific and dependent upon how well the surgical procedure achieves the patient's desires. This requires taking into consideration the ethnic identity of the patient and incorporating this into the surgical procedure. Overall, patients are extremely satisfied with the surgical results and often comment about their improved self-image. In general, autologous micro fat grafting provides greater flexibility in obtaining the desired degree of augmentation, as well as achieving the various ethnic ideals, as previously described.

Complications associated with buttock augmentation are highly dependent on the technique that is used. An in depth analysis of the diagnosis, management and prevention of complications associated with buttock augmentation has been previously described.[19]

Complications of micro fat grafting

The complications associated with buttock augmentation by micro fat grafting are diverse and very in acuity and severity. There are specific factors that predispose patients to developing postoperative complications. These include high-volume fat grafting (>1000 cc per buttock) and undergoing extensive liposuction (>5 L of lipo-aspirate). Interestingly, BMI does not appear to correlate with the overall incidence of both major and minor complications. Potential complications associated with substantial augmentation by micro fat grafting (500–1000 cc per buttock) include:

Infection

There are certain pre-disposing factors associated with micro fat grafting that make infection a significant concern. These include potential contamination of the fat during the harvesting, preparation and grafting process. The presence of the anus within the operative field and in close proximity to the operative incisions, and the generally poor vascularity of the recipient site (the buttock being primarily comprised of fat) for placement of nonvascularized fat grafts into a warm, moist environment. The most common cultured bacteria associated with infections are Gram negative bacteria and skin flora. Management of an infection includes culture-specific antibiotics. Localized abscess formation can occur, and usually requires drainage and local wound care.

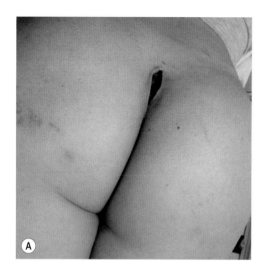

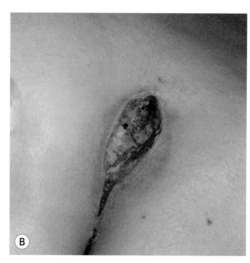

Fig. 28.32 Intramuscular implant augmentation with dehiscence of the intergluteal incision 10 days postoperatively.

Seromas

Because extensive liposuction of the flanks, lower lumbar, and sacral area is performed to achieve gluteal cleavage and an inward sweep of the lower back, this area is prone to accumulation of fluid postoperatively. Seroma formation in the postoperative period generally requires serial aspiration and optimization of compression. Percutaneous placement of a pigtail drain may be needed for larger, recurrent seromas.

Neuropraxia

There is a small, but significant risk of patients developing neuropraxic injury or sciatic nerve compression. Management includes both medical and surgical options. The administration of Neurontin and steroids, as well as NSAIDs, will markedly improve the symptoms that the patients are experiencing. Should more severe sciatic compression be of concern, surgical management consists of liposuction of any fat grafted around the sciatic nerve.

Hematologic and metabolic disturbances

Symptomatic hypovolemia may present during the first couple of days postoperatively and is best managed with PO fluid intake, and in more severe cases, administration of IV fluid. To prevent any metabolic and electrolyte disturbances, patients are encouraged to drink a gallon of sport electrolyte drink on a daily basis.

Complications of implants

Wound dehiscence

By changing the surgical incision from mid-sacral to separate bilateral parasacral incisions, the resultant improved blood supply has decreased wound dehiscence from 30% to approximately 5%. Should wound dehiscence occur, management includes meticulous local wound care and serial dressing changes. The result is wound closure via secondary intention. Any scar revision can be performed 3–6 months after the wound is healed *(Fig. 28.32)*.

Implant exposure

If no tension is placed during muscle closure the incidence of exposure is approximately 2%. If an excessively large implant is placed or the patient has extremely tight muscle fibers with very little stretch, the incidence can be as high as 30%.[20] If implant exposure occurs, surgery is necessary to irrigate the wound and exchange the implant. Patients are told that these are implant salvage techniques and implant removal may be required.

Infection

This is rare with an incidence of approximately 1%. If an infection develops, treatment usually requires temporary removal of the implant. Infections most commonly occur around the 10th–14th day postoperatively, but can occur as late as 3 months. However, implants have been salvaged with implant exchange using a closed antibiotic irrigation system. The pocket is irrigated for several days. Ultimately, implant removal may be required.

Seroma

Both ultrasound and MRI can be helpful with diagnosis of peri-implant seroma. If a seroma occurs, it must be evacuated. The use of drains has decreased the incidence of seroma in the immediate postoperative period. Late seroma has an incidence of 3% and is usually seen around 3–6 months postoperatively. It has mainly been seen with the use of textured implants. Resolution requires implant exchange (substituting for smooth implants), partial capsulectomy, and drainage.

Capsular contracture

Capsular contracture has a 1% incidence; it is improved with implant exchange and partial capsulectomy.

Neuropraxia

Hesitation by surgeons with this technique revolves around concerns for sciatic nerve injury. Understanding the anatomy

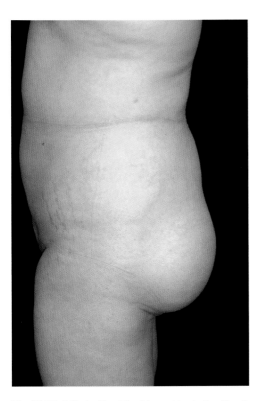

Fig. 28.33 Patient with subfascial round implants with subsequent inferior malpositions.

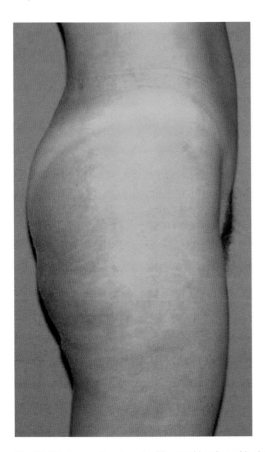

Fig. 28.34 Preoperative view of a 38-year-old patient with gluteal hypoplasia. The patient was subjected to a gluteal augmentation 2 years before using a small intramuscular implant. Note the high sitting implant and double contour of the buttock profile.

is crucial, however, one must realize that these structures are deeper than our intended 3 cm muscle thickness dissection. Patients will complain of sciatic type discomfort and decreased sensation in the first 4–6 weeks following surgery due to swelling. In these patients symptoms are improved with physical therapy, oral NSAIDS and Neurontin. Most of these symptoms will improve and eventually resolve over the next 2–4 months. Until full recovery occurs, the patient must be cognizant of the decreased sensation, as any trauma or ischemia may go unnoticed by the patient.

Implant rotation

This is not an issue with the round implants; however there is a small, <1%, incidence of implant rotation with the anatomic implants.

Implant malposition

Over time, the pocket and capsule may widen, thereby displacing the implant *(Fig. 28.33)*. This is about 1–2% incidence. If this occurs, capsulorrhaphy sutures will help close the pocket *(Figs 28.33, 28.34)*.

Hyperpigmentation/skin discoloration

Skin discoloration can occur, especially in the medial quadrants. The etiology is unknown but may be associated with a subclinical hematoma. This may be followed by wound dehiscence, drainage, and exposure, and require reoperation and implant removal. If the discoloration persists and the wound remains intact without issues, topical skin lighteners may help.

Skin ulceration

This is rare but seen more in subcutaneous and subfascial placements. This will require the removal of implants and waiting 3–6 months for correction.

Chronic pain

Chronic pain is rare. Possible causes include: myositis, fasciitis, capsular contracture or nerve impingement. On some occasions, the implant may be too large and results in pain on sitting as the implant shifts superiorly against the muscle attachments to the posterior iliac crest. In these cases, decreasing implant size or exchanging from an anatomic to a round implant may help.

Secondary procedures

Secondary revisions may be necessary in order to achieve the desired result for our patients. Some secondary procedures are technique dependent, while others apply to buttock augmentation patients as a whole, regardless of the primary procedure that was performed. These procedures include the following.

Scar revision

Following initial buttock augmentation surgery, the final appearance of the scars required for the surgical procedure may be suboptimal. This would include the midline or paramedian sacral incisions for buttock implants or the incisions for liposuction or lipo-injection for micro fat grafting. Regarding micro fat grafting, the injection sites may have widened or become hyperpigmented, or, usually more concerning to the patient, is some contour abnormality associated with these sites. Mild contour indentations may be attributed to the repeated trauma to the subcutaneous fat at the sites of injection from repeated motion during the initial fat grafting procedure. These contour deformities are best addressed by micro fat injection to these areas, thereby achieving a more aesthetic appearance. Once the contour or dimpling is corrected, then any scar revision can be performed as an adjunct procedure.

Additional augmentation

Whether a patients' initial buttock augmentation was performed by either micro fat grafting or implant-based augmentation, there are some inherent limitations regarding the amount of augmentation that can be performed. There are limitations regarding the size of the implants that can be placed in either the subfacial or intramuscular plane.

Likewise, for fat grafting, there may be limitations regarding the amount of fat available from donor sites, or the quantity of fat grafted in a single setting. Should a patient desire additional augmentation, this is usually performed by micro fat grafting regardless of the technique used for the initial surgical procedure.

Liposuction

Patients may desire additional improvement in contour of the lower lumbar and sacral areas to further accentuate the gluteal cleavage. It is not recommended that patients undergo aggressive lipo-sculpting of the lower lumbar and sacral areas at the time of implant-based augmentation due to concern for wound healing and adequacy of blood supply. Aggressive lipo-sculpting to this area may be performed once the patient has fully recovered from the initial procedure.

Bonus images for this chapter can be found online at
http://www.expertconsult.com

Fig. 28.13 Small frame BMI <20.
Fig. 28.14 Medium frame BMI 21–27.
Fig. 28.15 Large frame BMI 28–31.
Fig. 28.16 Extra large frame BMI >32.

Access the complete references list online at **http://www.expertconsult.com**

1. Chajchir A, Benzaquen I, Wexler E, et al. Fat injection. *Aesthetic Plast Surg.* 1990;14:127–136.
3. Singh D. Universal allure of the hourglass figure: an evolutionary theory of female physical attractiveness. *Clin Plast Surg.* 2006;33:359–370.
4. Roberts TL, Toledo LS, Badin AZ. Augmentation of the buttocks by micro fat grafting. *Aesthet Surg J.* 2001;21(4): 311–319.
7. Mendieta CG. Intramuscular gluteal augmentation technique. *Clin Plast Surg.* 2006;33(3):423–434.

   The best available description of this technique, including planning, intraoperative decision-making, perioperative management, complications and their management, based on the largest American experience.

8. De La Peña JA, Rubio OV, Cano JP, et al. Subfascial gluteal augmentation. *Clin Plast Surg.* 2006;33(3): 405–422.

   The most comprehensive paper on this technique by its developer. These excellent results depend on the use of the author's silicone gel implant, which is not available in the United States; the available elastomer complications preclude this technique.

9. Mendieta CG. Classification system for gluteal evaluation. *Clin Plast Surg.* 2006;33(3):333–346.
13. Roberts 3rd TL, Weinfeld AB, Bruner TW, et al. "Universal" and ethnic ideals of beautiful buttocks are best obtained by autologous micro fat grafting and liposuction. *Clin Plast Surg.* 2006;33(3):371–394.

   The largest series of augmentation by fat grafting with the technique well-illustrated. The authors report for the first time, the importance of ethnic variations in the perception of ideal shape, and how to obtain these ideals. Also documented for the first time, is the importance of the ideal 0.7 waist-to-hip ratio, and a fascinating appendix summarizing Singh's theory of why it is truly universally acknowledged as the ideal female shape.

17. Centeno RF, Young VL. Clinical anatomy in aesthetic gluteal body contouring surgery. *Clin Plast Surg.* 2006;33(3):347–358.

   An outstanding and well-illustrated description of the anatomic relationships that must be understood to safely perform the various techniques of buttocks augmentation.

18. Millard R. *Principalization of plastic surgery.* Boston: Little, Brown; 1986.
19. Bruner TW, Roberts 3rd TL, Nguyen K. Complications of buttocks augmentation: diagnosis, management, and prevention. *Clin Plast Surg.* 2006;33(3):449–466.

   A comprehensive and honest review of complications of all current techniques gleaned from the world literature (minimal information) and in-depth analysis of the author's own large experience (300+ cases) of fat grafting and implant augmentation. A "must read" before a surgeon begins to learn buttocks augmentation.

20. Mendieta CG. Gluteoplasty. *Aesthet Surg J.* 2003;23(6): 441–455.

29

Upper limb contouring

Joseph F. Capella, Matthew J. Trovato, and Scott Woehrle

SYNOPSIS

- Upper limb contour is often of great concern to individuals following weight loss.
- Correction of contour deformities of the axilla and forearm and in some instances the lateral thoracic region as well as the arm are critical to maximizing the aesthetics of the upper extremity.
- Liposuction often plays an important role in brachioplasty.
- Scar placement is an important element of upper extremity contouring.
- Upper limb contouring is associated with few serious complications.

 Access the Historical Perspective section online at
http://www.expertconsult.com

Introduction

The rapid growth in bariatric surgery over the last decade has led to an increase in demand for surgical procedures to address the contour deformities of the arm following weight loss. According to the American Society of Plastic Surgeons, from 2000 to 2008, there has been a 4059% increase in the number of brachioplasty procedures performed in the US.[1] While weight loss affects the entire body, for some individuals the arms are often of greatest concern because of their visibility in everyday activities. The combination of a patient desire for improved aesthetics of the upper limb and the ready visibility of the arms in routine activities creates a special challenge for plastic surgeons considering upper limb contouring.

Basic science/disease process

The arm deformity associated with weight loss is often dramatic and is influenced by multiple factors, including patient body mass index (BMI), highest BMI ever obtained, change in BMI, age, and sex *(Figs 29.1–29.5)*. In the morbidly obese individual, fat deposits are usually most prominent along the axilla, anterior, posterior and medial arm *(Fig. 29.1)*. With weight loss, these regions of the upper extremity manifest the greatest excess in soft tissue. Patients presenting at a lower BMI and particularly those who had reached a very high BMI prior to weight loss are likely to have more soft excess than an individual who has had smaller change in weight *(Figs 29.2 and 29.3)*. Patients in their fifth decade and beyond, particularly women, perhaps because of attenuated connective tissue, often present with large amounts of excess tissue despite relatively small changes in BMI *(Fig. 29.4)*. Men tend to have the majority of their deformity limited to the proximal arm and axilla *(Fig. 29.5)*. Women may have this appearance as well, but are more likely to have a deformity extending to the elbow and forearm *(Fig. 29.4)*.

Diagnosis/patient presentation

For some individuals following weight loss, the arms are their primary concern. More often, however, the arms are one of many concerns. Specific to the upper limb, patients usually present with multiple complaints, including a "bat-winged" appearance, arm stretch marks, large size of the arm relative to the forearm, excess skin and fat at axilla and lateral thoracic region and, for some individuals, loose skin along the proximal forearm.

The average age in our postbariatric population is 39.[29] Most of these individuals are very active and eager to minimize time off work and time away from family obligations. It is therefore quite common for a patient who expresses

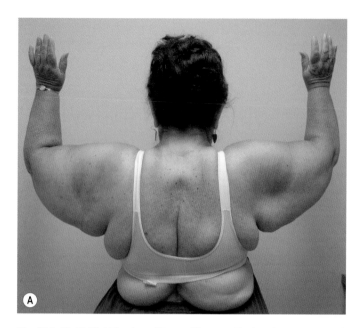

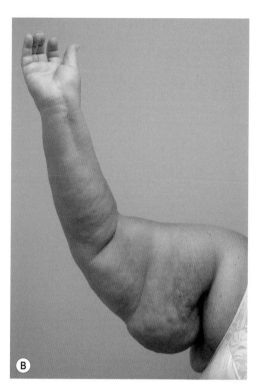

Fig. 29.1 **(A, B)** Morbidly obese 69-year-old woman. Fat deposits are most prominent along axilla and posterior arm and, to a lesser degree, anterior arm.

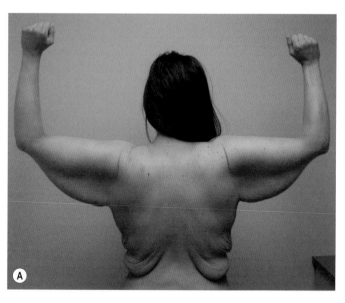

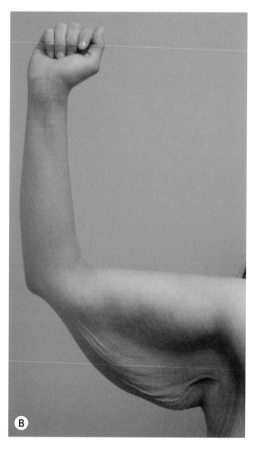

Fig. 29.2 **(A, B)** A 28-year-old woman, 6 years following 185 lb (84 kg) weight loss. Her current weight and body mass index are 188 lb (85 kg) and 27 respectively. Note extreme degree of soft-tissue excess.

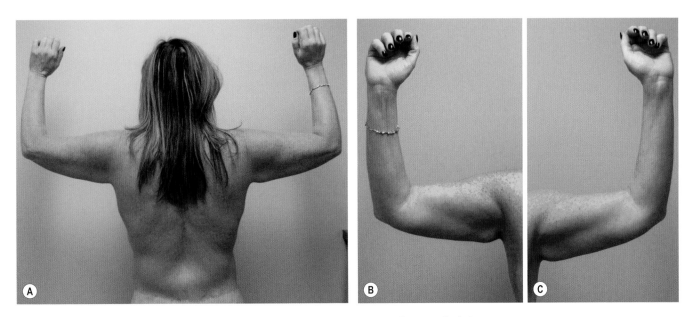

Fig. 29.3 (A–C) A 37-year-old woman following 60 lb (27 kg) weight loss. Note relatively small amount of soft-tissue excess.

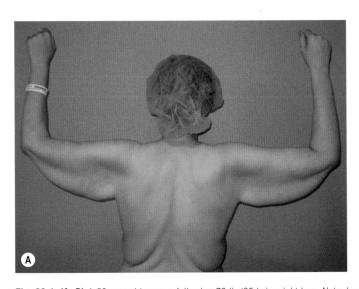

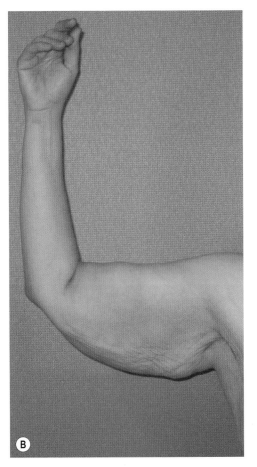

Fig. 29.4 (A, B) A 52-year-old woman following 78 lb (35 kg) weight loss. Note degree of soft-tissue excess despite relatively small amount of weight loss.

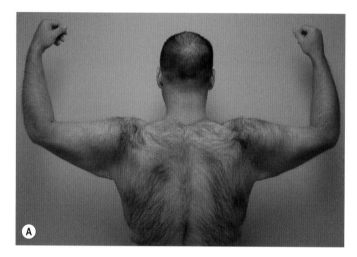
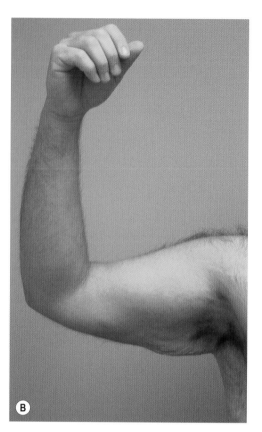

Fig. 29.5 (A, B) A 35-year-old man following weight loss of 128 lb (58 kg). Note that the contour deformity is primarily limited to the axilla and proximal half of the arm.

concerns about multiple areas of the body to request that all areas be addressed as soon as possible. One of the most important components of patient assessment is determining in what order and with what other procedures a brachioplasty should be performed. The patient's goals should be carefully considered in formulating a plan. With regard to the arm specifically, it is important to gain a clear understanding from patients of their tolerance for scars and of the degree of contour improvement they are expecting. A postbariatric patient anticipating an optimum result from a limited procedure in the proximal arm is likely to be disappointed.

Patient selection

Candidates for brachioplasty should undergo a thorough history and physical examination. Like all postbariatric patients, special attention should be directed toward weight history. Critical information includes the patient's height, current weight, and maximum weight. The time interval between their maximum and current weight and length of time at the current weight should be documented. If weight loss was achieved through bariatric surgery, the technique and when it was performed should be noted. Other important weight-related information includes whether the individual is being followed by a bariatric surgeon, the time of the last visit, whether supplemental medication has been prescribed, and if it is being taken regularly. Problems potentially related to bariatric surgery should be explored, i.e., frequent vomiting, abdominal pain, weakness, light-headedness, and

frequent bowel movements. For patients who have lost weight through lifestyle changes, some discussion should be take place as to how this was accomplished, i.e., exercise, diet and exercise, medication, and whether they are being supervised by a professional.

Examination of the postbariatric brachioplasty candidate should be thorough, with particular attention directed toward the upper body. Along with the degree of soft-tissue excess present along the forearm, arm, and axilla, an assessment should be made of the breasts, lateral thoracic region, and back. The fat content of all these areas should be noted. A standardized exam form is helpful *(Fig. 29.6)*. Notation is made as to whether intertriginous dermatitis is present, potentially along the axilla. Lymphedema and/or stigmata of lymphedema should be documented, as should the presence of arterial or vascular insufficiency. Existing scars, transverse arm bands, and striae along the upper extremity should be noted.

The best candidates for brachioplasty are healthy individuals who have achieved a stable weight, have a BMI less than 28, and who have lost substantial weight, generally over 50 lb (23 kg). Individuals with a BMI greater than 28 can obtain dramatic results; however the final aesthetic result is less likely to be ideal. The value of performing a brachioplasty depends greatly on the extent of the deformity to be corrected, which in turn usually depends primarily on the degree of weight loss. Variables representing relative contraindications to brachioplasty are high patient BMI and small BMI change from highest weight, significant patient reservations regarding arm scars, a history of hypertrophic or hyperpigmented scars, and unrealistic patient expectations, particularly with

Arms	Left: Striae	Yes	No		Skin excess	None	Mild	Moderate	Severe
	Lipodystrophy	None	Mild	Moderate	Severe				
	Scars	Yes	No						
	Transverse bands	Yes	No		Lymphedema	Yes	No		
	Right: Striae	Yes	No		Skin excess	None	Mild	Moderate	Severe
	Lipodystrophy	None	Mild	Moderate	Severe				
	Scars	Yes	No						
	Transverse bands	Yes	No		Lymphedema	Yes	No		

Axilla/flank	Lipodystrophy	Left	None	Mild	Moderate	Severe
		Right	None	Mild	Moderate	Severe
	Intertriginous dermatitis	Left	None	Mild	Moderate	Severe
		Right	None	Mild	Moderate	Severe
	Skin excess	Left	None	Mild	Moderate	Severe
		Right	None	Mild	Moderate	Severe

Breast	Current breast size		Desired breast size						
	Excess grams of breast tissue		Left		Right				
	Diameter of NAC		Left		Right				
	Distance from sternal notch to nipple (normal 23–25 cm)		Left		Right				
	Distance from IMF to nipple (10–12 cm)		Left		Right				
	Distance from midline to nipple (10–12 cm)		Left		Right				
	Scars	Left	None	Biopsy	Inverted T	Vertical	Periareolar	IM	Axillary
		Right	None	Biopsy	Inverted T	Vertical	Periareolar	IM	Axillary
	Breast ptosis	Left	None	Grade I	Grade II	Grade III	Pseudoptosis		
		Right	None	Grade I	Grade II	Grade III	Pseudoptosis		
	Lymphadenopathy	Left	None	Grade I	Grade II	Grade III	Pseudoptosis		
		Right	None	Axillary	Supraclavicular				
	Palpable mass	Left	Yes	No					
		Right	Yes	No					
	Palpable mass	Left	Yes	No					
		Right	Yes	No					
	Nipple discharge	Left	Yes	No					
		Right	Yes	No					

Fig. 29.6 Physical examination form.

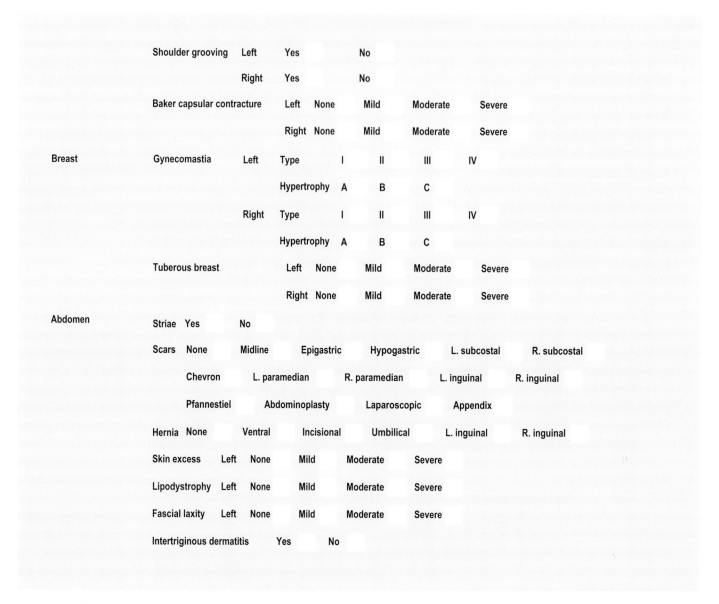

Fig. 29.6, cont'd

regard to short scar versions of brachioplasty. Absolute contraindications in our practice at this time are a history of lymphedema and/or arterial or venous insufficiency of the upper extremity. A related contraindication is a patient who is at high risk of developing one of these conditions. Examples include patients who have undergone axillary lymph node dissection or axillary radiation.

Plan formulation

The information gathered from the patient history and physical exam is instrumental in formulating a preliminary plan. For patients expressing concerns only about their arms, the plan is clear. For these patients, it is important to clarify the importance of addressing the axilla in rejuvenating the arm. Following massive weight loss, most patients express concerns about more than just their arms; usually the breasts,

lateral thoracic region, back, abdomen, thighs, and buttocks are of issue as well. The options available to the plastic surgeon are multiple. Our preference is to perform a body lift first, as a single procedure, and then to follow with a combination mastopexy/lateral thoracoplasty/brachioplasty not before 3 months.[30] A medial thigh lift, if necessary, would take place at least 3 months later. Our rationale for this sequence and combination of procedures derives from the observation that the body lift procedure greatly affects the rolls frequently present along the upper and lower back. In the vast majority of patients, any remaining rolls along the back and flanks following a body lift can then be addressed by the combination mastopexy/lateral thoracoplasty/brachioplasty.

While the upper body procedures may be performed prior to the body lift, it is often difficult to estimate accurately the appropriate amount of tissue to be excised at the lateral thoracic region. The vast majority of postbariatric patients are candidates for a body lift; however, a discussion of the criteria for this procedure is not within the scope of this chapter.

Before being considered for any procedure, certain criteria must be met and issues addressed. The patient should be at a stable weight for at least several months. This will vary depending on bariatric procedure. Operating during a period of active weight loss may result in an early recurrence of soft-tissue laxity and, from a safety perspective, the patient is unlikely to be nutritionally and metabolically optimized. Patients with symptoms suggestive of problems related to bariatric surgery should be evaluated by their surgeon. Individuals with a history of major mental illness or acute mental illness are asked to be evaluated by an appropriate health professional. Patients are advised to maintain the supplemental regimen prescribed by their bariatric surgeon. Individuals with a history of tobacco consumption are urged to stop as soon as possible. The risks of tobacco, including impared wound healing and thromboembolic phenomena, are clearly established in the literature and are relayed to the patient.[29,31] My preference is for patients who are on medications for weight loss, to stop them. All patients are referred for medical clearance. While weight loss dramatically improves the health of morbidly obese individuals, not all conditions are eliminated.[32] A careful medical evaluation of health is imperative.

After discussing a possible plan with the patient, I review several topics. Many individuals are eager to lose more weight prior to surgery, feeling that their surgery would be safer and that more skin could be removed if they are at a lower weight. My feeling is that most people whose weight is stable at the time of consultation are at the weight they are most likely to maintain over the long term. While many postbariatric patients can lose weight for relatively brief periods of time, long-term additional weight loss following bariatric surgery or through lifestyle change is difficult to achieve. Individuals losing weight in a short period of time can lead to several undesirable outcomes. First, they may become nutritionally and metabolically unbalanced just at the time surgery is to be performed. Secondly, weight gain in the future will in most instances diminish the aesthetic results of a procedure. I advise patients to eat a balanced diet and maintain a stable weight. On the other hand, I do explain that a certain amount of excess soft tissue will be removed during surgery. Their new weight following surgery should be their current weight minus the weight of the tissue removed. A 3-month postoperative weight similar to their weight at consultation suggests a significant weight gain. I also explain that the long-term results of this surgery are best maintained by weight stability, minimizing exposure to sun (ultraviolet light), and no tobacco consumption.

Laboratory

A patient history can often be suggestive of problems; however, a thorough laboratory work-up is critical for identifying existing deficiencies or abnormalities. It is not unusual for menstruating women to have few, if any, symptoms despite having severe anemia following bariatric surgery. Along with a complete blood count and other studies, our routine includes a complete metabolic panel. Abnormal laboratory values are acted on as they are made available.

Individuals found to be malnourished with a total protein less than 6 g/dL and/or albumin less than 3 mg/dL may be referred to their bariatric surgeon for re-evaluation and possible nutritional supplementation. Those findings may be corroborated by edema on physical exam. Protein-depleted patients may demonstrate difficulty healing wounds. Severely anemic patients with hemoglobin less than 10 g/dL are referred to their primary physician and/or hematologist. Patients with hemoglobin above 10 g/dL are advised to continue on iron, folate, and B$_{12}$ supplementation and to have their blood cell count repeated in a week. Our preference is for patients to have hemoglobin above 12 g/dL before surgery. Patients are advised of the possible need for a blood transfusion. My practice has not been to have patients bank their own blood. In most institutions, blood can only be given within 1 month of surgery. One month may not be adequate time for anemic patients to replenish their blood levels.

Preoperative visit

At the preoperative visit, usually 2 weeks before surgery, the planned surgical procedure is reviewed in detail, as are the potential complications. Requested consultations and recommendations are discussed with the patient. Another critical function of the preoperative visit is to review images taken at the first consultation. Patients rarely have a completely accurate sense of their deformities. Key elements of this discussion are to highlight existing asymmetries, the presence of bands, which in many cases cannot be completely corrected, review the extent of their deformities, and to explain the degree to which the planned procedure or procedures will address their deformities. I prefer not to do image morphing, but rather show examples of individuals with similar body types who have had the same procedures. Perhaps more than any other postbariatric body-contouring procedure, candidates for brachioplasty must have a very clear understanding of the scar involved with the procedure.

The process of scar maturation must be discussed, as should the potential risks for hypertrophic and hyperpigmented scars. A failure to discuss the full spectrum of scar quality can lead to a disappointed patient despite an excellent result in contour. Restrictions and recovery guidelines are reviewed. Patients often have the sense that recovery from surgery should involve significant bed rest. I emphasize the importance of frequent ambulation. Medications that should be avoided prior to surgery are reviewed; these include medications that increase the risk of bleeding (aspirin and nonsteroidal anti-inflammatory agents) and those that increase the risk for deep-vein thrombosis (oral contraceptives or hormone replacement therapy). Patients are advised not to take either for 2 weeks before or after surgery. I conclude with a plan for deep-vein thrombosis prophylaxis.

Thromboembolic disease prophylaxis

Thromboembolic disease has been very rare in our brachioplasty series. All patients undergoing brachioplasty have activated lower extremity sequential compression devices in place prior to surgery, during surgery, and until ambulation is regular. Following surgery patients are encouraged to ambulate shortly after the conclusion of the procedure. Patients with a BMI of greater than 32 are given 5000 units of

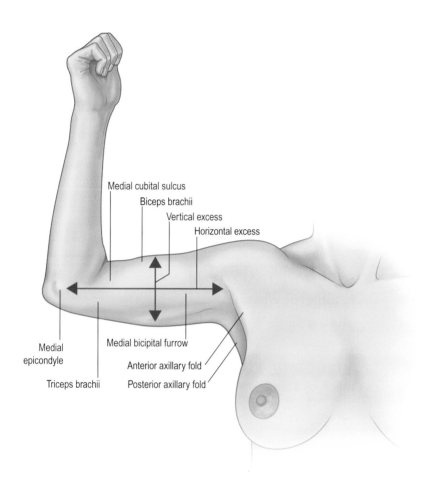

Medial cubital sulcus

Biceps brachii

Vertical excess

Horizontal excess

Medial
epicondyle

Medial bicipital furrow

Triceps brachii

Anterior axillary fold

Posterior axillary fold

Fig. 29.7 Arm surface anatomy. Medial arm perspective, highlighting location of bicipital sulcus, medial cubital sulcus, medial epicondyle, and components of axilla.

heparin subcutaneously prior to surgery. Individuals with risk factors other than obesity are treated on a case-by-case basis. Thromboembolic disease prophylaxis for patients undergoing brachioplasty and additional procedures, particularly abdominoplasty, is outside the scope of this chapter.

Video 1

Treatment/surgical technique

Anatomy

When considering the posteromedial approach to brachioplasty, identification of several superficial anatomic landmarks is critical for consistent scar placement *(Fig. 29.7)*. Important surface anatomy includes the anterior and posterior axillary folds, biceps and triceps muscles, medial epicondyle, medial bicipital furrow, and medial cubital sulcus. A posteromedial approach to brachioplasty in virtually all instances involves the axillary dome. An incision in this region should remain superficial, involving only skin and a small amount of subcutaneous fat. Liposuction is not usually performed in this region. The superficial-lying intercostobrachial nerve can sometimes be encountered and inadvertently sacrificed. The result is numbness along the proximal, medial aspect of the arm. This condition is well tolerated by patients and rarely noted. Liposuction prior to dissection of the medial and posterior arm should provide an easily identifiable plain immediately deep to the superficial fascial system and

superficial to the deep fascia of the arm. Along the entire arm and elbow, vital structures remain deep to the deep fascia and are unlikely to be injured. Along the proximal two-thirds of the medial and posterior arm, superficial to the deep fascia, are the medial and posterior brachial cutaneous nerves and small superficial unnamed veins *(Fig. 29.8)*. The cepahalic vein and anterior brachial cutaneous nerve should remain out of the field of sharp dissection. Prior liposuction and careful dissection should spare the medial and posterior brachial cutaneous nerves. Injury to these nerves would result in corresponding numbness to these areas of the arm. Along the distal one-third of the arm and in the region of the elbow, the basilic vein and medial antebrachial cutaneous nerve are superficial to the deep fascia and vulnerable to injury *(Fig. 29.9)*. Once again, liposuction prior to sharp dissection in this area is helpful in visualizing these more important structures. Zones of adherence along the arm are limited primarily to the lateral arm and elbow region *(Fig. 29.10)*. The posteromedial approach does not involve sharp dissection along the lateral arm and fat deposits in this area are not common. Liposuction along the medial and posterior arm addresses fat deposits commonly encountered along the posterior elbow and facilitates sharp dissection along the medial elbow.

Marking

The goal of our technique is for the scar to lie along the posteromedial arm, approximately at the level of the triceps

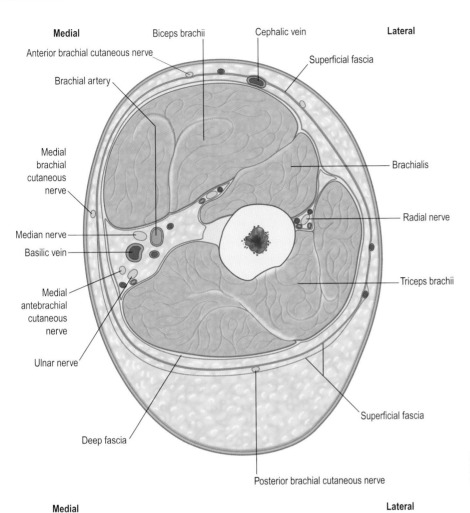

Medial

Anterior brachial cutaneous nerve

Brachial artery

Medial brachial cutaneous nerve

Median nerve

Basilic vein

Medial antebrachial cutaneous nerve

Ulnar nerve

Deep fascia

Biceps brachii

Cephalic vein

Lateral

Superficial fascia

Brachialis

Radial nerve

Triceps brachii

Superficial fascia

Posterior brachial cutaneous nerve

Fig. 29.8 Sagittal view of arm anatomy. Sagittal view of midportion of arm, highlighting nerves, arteries, veins, and fascial planes at this level.

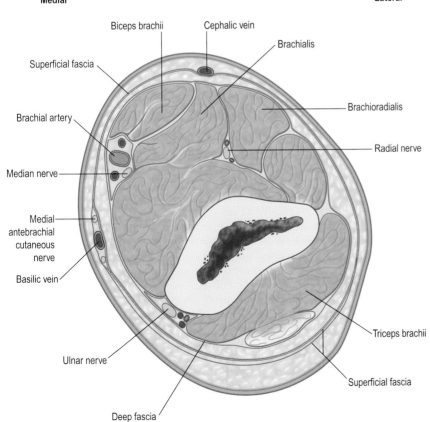

Medial

Lateral

Biceps brachii

Cephalic vein

Brachialis

Superficial fascia

Brachioradialis

Brachial artery

Radial nerve

Median nerve

Medial antebrachial cutaneous nerve

Basilic vein

Triceps brachii

Ulnar nerve

Superficial fascia

Deep fascia

Fig. 29.9 Sagittal view of arm anatomy. Sagittal view of distal portion of arm, highlighting nerves, arteries, veins, and fascial planes at this level.

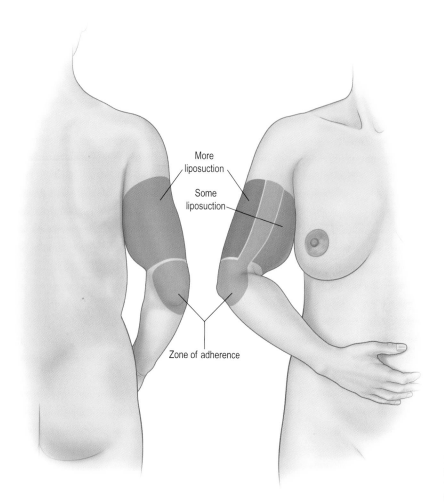

More
liposuction

Some
liposuction

Zone of adherence

Fig. 29.10 Zones of adherence. Medial and lateral view of arm surface, highlighting with shading areas of greatest tissue adherence: medial, lateral, and posterior elbow region and lateral and anterior arm.

muscle. At the axilla, the scar should lie within the axillary dome. Marking begins with the patient standing and the arm extended perpendicularly from the body *(Fig. 29.11)*. A line is drawn along the lateral inferior border of the pectoralis major muscle from point A, the superior portion of the axillary dome to point B, the inferior portion of the dome. A point C is found, usually at the level of triceps muscle that can be advanced easily to a point D at the most superior portion of the axillary dome. The points at A, B, and C are connected to complete the ellipse at the axilla. The preceding steps determine the soft-tissue excess to be excised from the axillary dome. A dotted line is then drawn from the medial epicondyle, point E, to the lateral aspect of the axillary dome over the triceps muscle, point F. In heavier individuals, the posterior portion of the arm may need to be grasped to determine the location of the triceps muscle. Finally, an area G above the dotted line E–F is identified corresponding to the region of maximum soft-tissue excess on the posterior aspect of the arm. Moderate downward traction is placed on the area using multiple digits, typically the index, long, ring, and small finger to identify a level H, which descends to the height of point E or the medial epicondyle. A line is then drawn from point E through H and on to the lateral aspect of the ellipse, point I. The line from E through level H–I should mirror the corresponding soft-tissue excess of the posterior arm in that region. Typically the line rises gradually over the distal arm and more so as it reaches

the proximal one-third of the arm and descends slightly towards the axilla.

Operative technique

Sterile drapes are placed on the operative table and arm boards. With the patient in the supine position, a sequential compression device is placed on one leg and a blood pressure cuff on the other. An intravenous catheter is placed in the dorsal aspect of the hand or wrist. Intravenous antibiotics are given, typically a first-generation cephalosporin. A pulse oximeter device is placed on the ear. Following general anesthesia, often with a laryngeal mask, the forearm, arm, axilla, flank, and chest are prepped with Betadine. A sterile towel is wrapped around each hand and proximal forearm and secured to itself and the patient with staples. A drape is stapled to the patient along the upper chest and over the midclavicular portion of the shoulders. Drapes are placed over the patient's body from the lower chest and inferiorly *(Fig. 29.12)*. The previously made markings along the axilla, points A to B and back to A through C are scored with a knife blade. Similarly, the line from E through H and on to the lateral limb of the axillary ellipse is scored. Beginning with the right arm and using a no. 15 blade, four stab wounds are made: (1) along the proximal medial forearm; (2) just proximal to the medial

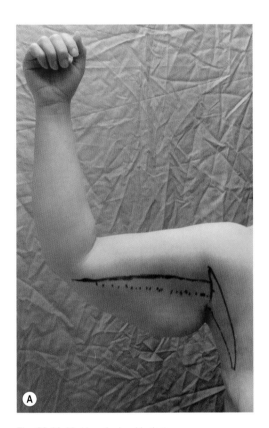

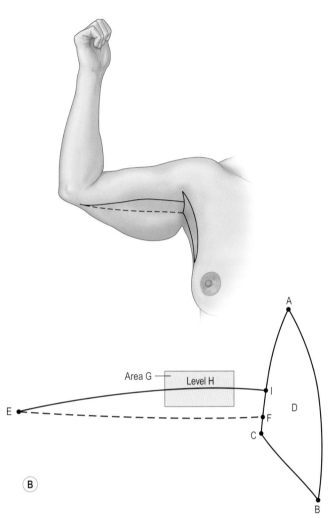

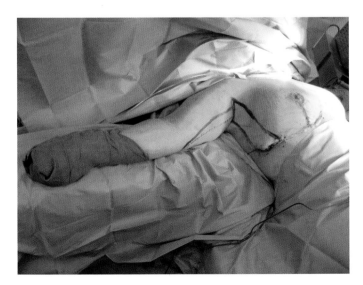

Fig. 29.11 Markings for brachioplasty.

epicondyle; (3) in the proximal and mid posterior arm; and (4) in the distal lateral arm. Via these stabs wounds tumescent fluid (1 liter of saline, 1 cc of 1/1000 epinephrine, 50 cc of 1% lidocaine) is injected into the subcutaneous tissues of the medial and posterior arm. If fatty deposits are to be addressed along the anterior and lateral arm, fluid should be injected into these areas as well. Our preference is to inject at a 1:1 ratio of fluid injected to the volume of aspirate removed. Excessive fluid injection may compromise control over excision.

While the tumescent fluid is setting, the ellipse at the axilla is excised. Only a small amount of subcutaneous fat is removed with the skin to avoid any deeper structures. Liposuction is then performed with a 3–4-mm cannula beginning through the stab wound along the proximal medial forearm. Via this approach, the medial arm is suctioned with particular attention directed towards the distal medial arm where the skin is more firmly adherent to the underlying fascia. The arm is typically resting on the arm board during this maneuver. Suction is then performed along the posterior and posterolateral arm via the stab wound along the distal lateral arm. The surgeon is standing and the forearm is elevated off the arm board by an assistant.

Fig. 29.12 Draping for bilateral brachioplasty. In this case, brachioplasty is being performed along with lateral thoracoplasty and mastopexy

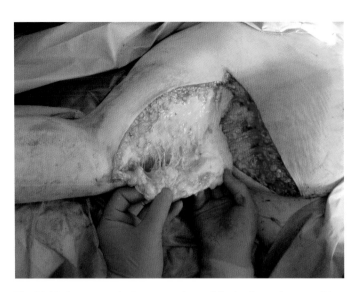

Fig. 29.13 Appearance of subcutaneous tissues following liposuction to medial and posterior arm. Plane of dissection readily visible.

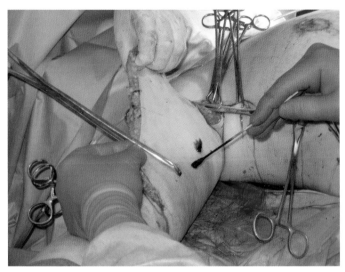

Fig. 29.14 Use of Pitanguy large-skin demarcator to determine amount of soft-tissue excess.

Finally, liposuction is performed to the entire posterior arm via the posterior stab wounds. The surgeon is standing and the arm medially rotated over the patient's chest. With the arm resting on the arm board, the skin from point E through H–I at the axilla wound is incised. The subcutaneous tissues are divided to reach the "honeycomb"-appearing plane produced by the liposuction. Dissection is easily performed in this plane to the posterolateral aspect of the arm *(Fig. 29.13)*. The supporting ligaments to the skin in the region of the elbow are thicker and slighter more difficult to divide.

With the dissection complete, a towel clamp or Adair is used to approximate the lateral skin edge of the axillary ellipse, point I, to a point directly across the wound along the skin edge A–B. Point C or a point either slightly above or below C along the lateral aspect of the ellipse is found which, when attached to the medial skin edge A–B, immediately below where point I has been attached to the skin edge A–B, creates the desired contour of the proximal arm and axilla. Additional towel clamps are then used to approximate the lateral and medial skin edges of the axillary ellipse.

Once the desired points along the axillary ellipse have been approximated, attention is directed towards the arm. Towel clamps are placed along the upper divided skin edge, E through H–I. Beginning in the region of greatest tissue excess of the arm, typically slightly proximal to the midarm, a Pitanguy long skin demarcator is secured to a towel clip. The surgeon and assistant then apply upward traction on the entire lower skin flap edge. Advancement of the demarcator posteriorly towards the lower flap will cause it to glide posteriorly for 1 cm or more before stopping. The lower flap is drawn into the jaws of the demarcator under moderate tension. Once mild resistance is reached, the lower flap is released by approximately 1 cm. This point is then marked *(Fig. 29.14)*.

The same technique is repeated along the arm three or four times to develop an outline of the flap to be excised. The dots are connected and the flap excised. Careful hemostasis is gained. No drain is placed. Towel claps are used to approximate the flap edges along the axilla and arm. At the axilla, 2-0 Vicryl interrupted sutures are used to approximate the

superficial fascial system and deep dermis, approximately 0.5 cm from the flap edge. Incorporated in this approximation is a superficial bite of the deeper tissues to help eliminate dead space. A 3-0 Monocryl intracuticular suture is then placed. A similar closer of 2-0 and Vicryl and 3-0 Monocryl is used along the arm, however, the deeper tissues are not incorporated in the closer. ABD pads are placed on the wounds of the axilla and arm, followed by a loosely applied elastic wrap to the arm. To support the dressings at the axilla, an upper pole breast binder is placed or, if breast surgery is being performed concomitantly, a bra is placed.

In our practice, the lateral thoracic region is often addressed in combination with a brachioplasty and mastopexy. The sequence of procedures in these cases is for the mastopexy to be performed first. From the lateral extent of the inframammary wound closure, the taylor-tack technique is then utilized to assess the excess skin and soft tissue along the lateral thoracic region and to the dome of the axilla. Once this assessment has been made, the excess skin and a small amount of subcutaneous fat from the lateral thoracic region and axilla are removed. The arm portion of the brachioplasty procedure can then begin as described above from the step where liposuction is performed. The remainder of the procedure is the same, except for the final wound closure which will extend inferiorly from the axilla to the lateral thoracic region and terminate at the lateral extent of the mastopexy inframammary wound closure. In cases where large areas of skin and soft tissue have been removed from the lateral thoracic region, the dermal sutures can placed to incorporate a superficial bite of the tissues at the base of the wound or a drain can be left in place for several days *(Fig. 29.15)*. These efforts may diminish the likelihood of a seroma or persistent fluid drainage from the axilla.

In addition to the arm, the proximal forearm may be a concern for some patients, particularly women in their fifth decade and beyond. Management of the proximal forearm begins with the routine brachioplasty as described above, up to the point just before the final intracuticular layer of 3-0 Monocryl is placed. With the 2-0 Vicryl suture in place, the taylor-tack technique is used to assess the excess skin and soft

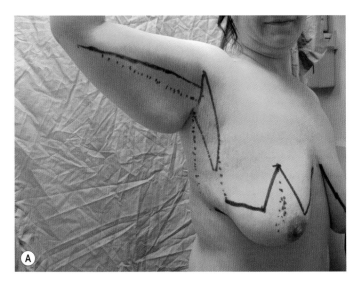

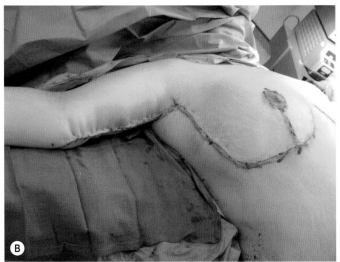

Fig. 29.15 (A) Markings for planned combination mastopexy, lateral thoracoplasty, and brachioplasty. **(B)** Final closure of combination mastopexy, lateral thoracoplasty, and brachioplasty.

tissue along the proximal forearm beyond the medial epicondyle. The skin and a small amount of subcutaneous fat from the pattern created along the proximal medial forearm are removed. The final closure begins with 2-0 Vicryl in the forearm and is then followed by the 3-0 Monocryl along the forearm, arm, and axilla.

Postoperative care

Ambulation is encouraged as soon as possible after surgery. Brachioplasty is nearly always performed in an ambulatory setting, particularly if it is the only operation being performed. Discharge home is usually within several hours of the conclusion of the procedure. Dressings are removed 2 days postoperatively. Showering is permitted at this time. Patients are advised to keep their axillae dry at all times when not showering and to avoid perspiring excessively or lifting their arms (not forearms) above shoulder level for 2 weeks following

Table 29.1 Complication rates associated with brachioplasty	
Brachioplasty complication rates *n* = 350 cases (700 arms)	
Skin dehiscence	25%
Seroma	10%
Infection	2.6%
Hematoma	0.6%
Skin necrosis	0.6%
Deep-vein thrombosis	0.3%

surgery. This still allows the forearms and hands to be used for grooming. No garments are required to be worn. Lower-body vigorous activities may be resumed 2 weeks following surgery. Upper body vigorous activities, including arms, may be resumed at 6 weeks. Patients are encouraged to take narcotics as needed but to minimize them as soon as possible. Routine follow-up is at 1 week, 6 weeks, 3 and 6 months, and yearly thereafter. Images are usually taken at the 3-month follow-up.

Outcomes, prognosis, and complications

The vast majority of patients following brachioplasty are very pleased with their results when proper screening and preoperative education have been performed. Patients most likely to approach an aesthetic ideal and to have a high level of satisfaction are those with a presenting BMI of less than 28 and those who have had a preoperative BMI change of greater than 20. Patients presenting at a higher BMI, greater than 28, and who have also experienced very substantial weight loss prior to surgery are also very likely to be satisfied but are less likely to achieve an aesthetic ideal *(Fig. 29.16)*. Candidates for surgery presenting a higher BMI, greater than 32, and who have had relatively little weight loss prior to surgery and patients with a BMI change of less than 5 are usually the least satisfied and have small aesthetic improvement *(Fig. 29.17)*. Critical to achieving the best results with arm-contouring surgery is addressing the upper body as a whole. Patients are unlikely to be satisfied with their arms if their forearms, axilla, or lateral thoracic region have not been addressed and are contributing to their upper body concerns.

Major complications from brachioplasty are few *(Table 29.1)*. In our review of 350 brachioplasty cases (700 arms), skin dehiscence was the most frequent complication, at 25%. Few of the dehiscences occurred acutely (within the first 24–48 hours of the procedure), but rather became evident approximately 2 weeks following the procedure. Of the dehiscences, 95% occurred at the intersection of the closure of the dome and the arm. Like any triangular-shaped skin flap, the tip of the flap has compromised blood supply. The typical course is for the tip of the flap to take on a dusky appearance in the first few days following the procedure, and by about 2 weeks wound separation occurs. The majority of skin dehiscences are less than 2 cm in size. Avoiding this complication is

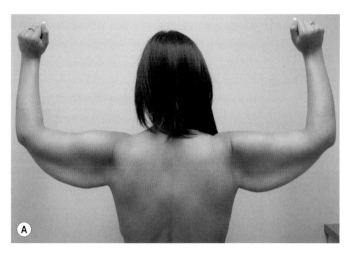
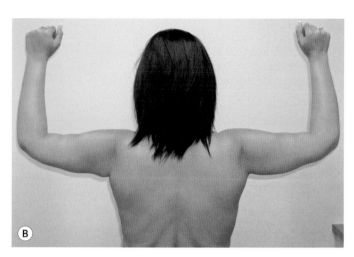
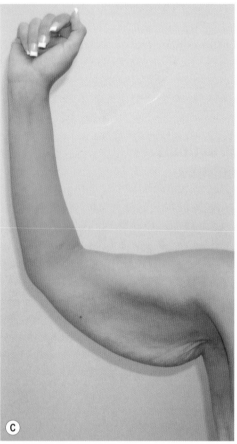
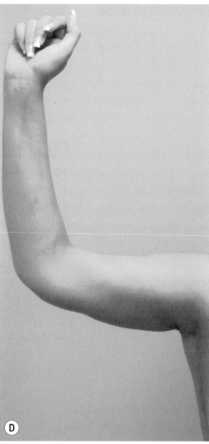

Fig. 29.16 (A, C) A 27-year-old woman 3 years following weight loss of 164 lb (75 kg) Current weight and body mass index (BMI): 202 lb (92 kg) and 37 respectively. Highest weight and BMI: 366 lb (166 kg) and 67. **(B, D)** Six months following brachioplasty with concomitant liposuction and posteromedial scar placement.

challenging because some form of Z-plasty must be present for the closure to extend from the axilla to the arm and prevent scar contracture. While advising the patient to limit extension of the arm may be helpful, it is unlikely to prevent this problem entirely.

The dehiscences are treated with dressing changes. In some instances, hypergranulation tissue may arise in the area of skin dehiscence. Nitrate application is an effective treatment for this. In our series, seromas are the second most frequent problem, occurring in 10% of cases. The vast majority, approximately 90%, occur along the distal medial one-third of the

arm, immediately beneath the scar. Most become evident at about 3 weeks postoperatively and range in diameter from 1 to 4 cm.

Initially we manage seromas with needle aspiration. This technique unfortunately has a very high recurrence rate. The technique of marsupialization, incising the skin over the seroma, draining the seroma, and suturing the seroma cavity to the skin, is 100% effective but results in a scar that may be wider than the adjoining scar and prolong the healing of the wound. Our preference at this time is to drain the seroma via the scar and place a secured Penrose-type drain into the

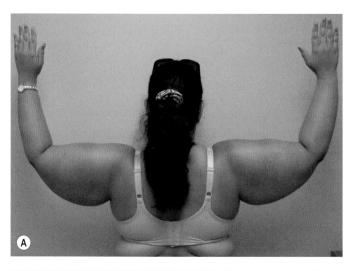

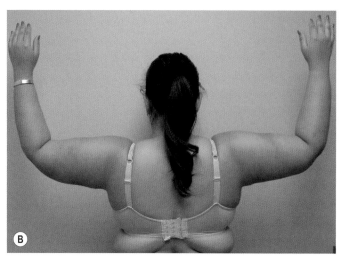

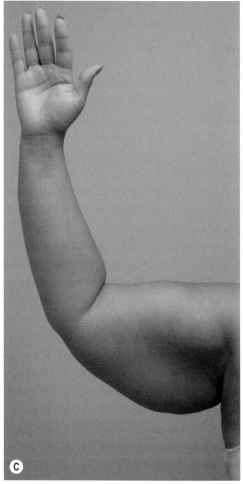

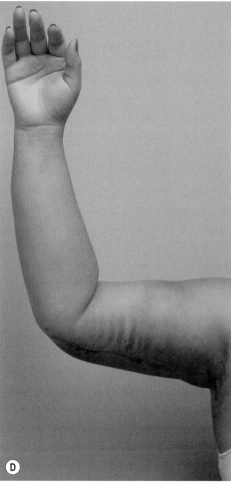

Fig. 29.17 (A, C) A 37-year-old woman 7 years following weight loss of 45 lb (20 kg). Current weight and body mass index (BMI): 220 lb (100 kg) and 37 respectively. Highest weight and BMI: 265 lb (120 kg) and 44. **(B, D)** Six months following brachioplasty with concomitant liposuction and posteromedial scar placement.

seroma cavity. Patients are maintained on antibiotics while the Penrose is in place. This simple technique has proven to be very effective. Infections have been very infrequent, as have bleeding and hematomas. Complaints of dysesthesia beyond 3 months have been few, and rare beyond 6 months. Skin necrosis has also been very infrequent, despite liposuction being performed in virtually all cases. We have only one

documented instance of deep-vein thrombosis in a patient undergoing brachioplasty. The patient presented with a palpable cord extending from the forearm to the arm, suggestive of superficial thrombophlebitis. An upper extremity venous Doppler study revealed involvement of the deep system of the arm. There have been no instances of pulmonary embolism.

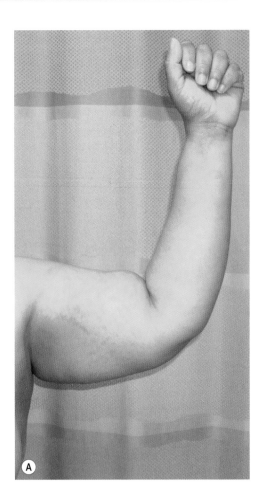

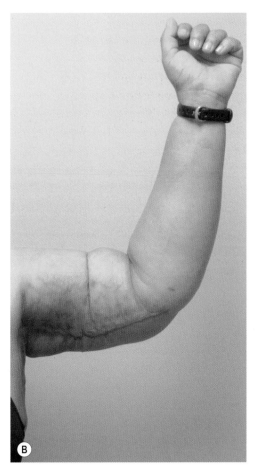

Fig. 29.18 (A) A 40-year-old woman following weight loss of 30 lb (17 kg). Current weight and body mass index (BMI): 150 lb (68 kg) and 28 respectively. Highest weight and BMI: 180 lb (82 kg) and 34. **(B)** Three months following brachioplasty with concomitant liposuction and posteromedial scar placement. Note hypertrophic scar and increased perceptibility of transverse band.

Secondary procedures

Patients seeking improvement following brachioplasty surgery typically have concerns about scar quality or location, or overall upper limb contour. Complaints about scar quality include wide, pigmented, or hypertrophic scars. Some patients, concerned about scar perceptibility, may seek a more posterior or more anterior position for their scars. Concerns about contour include excess skin and/or fat and irregular contour or the presence of transverse bands *(Fig. 29.18)*. We have found that the vast majority of brachioplasty arm scars mature to become similar in color to the patient's adjoining skin.

As has been noted regarding scars in general, arm scars of patients of a lower Fitzpatrick rating are likely to have a quicker and more complete dissipation of pigment than individuals higher on the scale. Aside from strongly advising the avoidance of ultraviolet light to scars during the period of maturation, we have not required patients to apply or consume any of the multitude of available products purporting to improve scar quality. We have not had a positive experience with steroid injections for treatment of hypertrophic scars. In most instances, steroid injection has substituted the hypertrophic scar with an equally conspicuous area of abnormal-appearing, attenuated skin. Our approach to wide, hypertrophic, or hyperpigmented scars is to encourage patients to allow time for the natural process of scar maturation to take place. We have found that virtually all arm scars become increasingly less perceptible over time, either through depigmentation or with the resolution of hypertrophy. In instances where the patient is unwilling to wait an extended period of time, we advise patients to wait at least 8–10 months before seeking any kind of intervention. Requiring that patients delay intervention allows for some relaxation of skin and soft tissue to take place.

Our treatment of poor scars is to excise them and reapproximate the soft-tissue edges. In the vast majority of cases we have found some improvement in scar quality with this protocol. Our rationale for this approach is that tension appears to be one of the most important variables affecting scar quality. The wound tension at scar revision is likely to be less than at the time of the approximation of the flaps at the primary procedure. If at the time of the planned scar revision minimal soft-tissue excess exists and remaining arm fat is present, liposuction will be performed prior to scar revision in an effort to diminish arm volume and minimize wound tension at closure.

Patients and plastic surgeons have different opinions about the ideal and least perceptible location for brachioplasty scars.

Regardless of preference, scar location can be adjusted as long as some soft-tissue redundancy is present. Once again, as with scar revisions, significant soft-tissue excess can be produced with liposuction. Secondary procedures for complaints regarding generalized soft excess are treated with an approach similar to that described above for primary procedures, as are generalized irregularities secondary to a primary liposuction, nonexcisional procedure. Secondary procedures for focal irregularities following liposuction can be more challenging.

A common area for oversuctioning of fat is in the distal one-third of the arm, just proximal to the elbow. Treatment of this condition can involve liposuction alone or direct excision of the surrounding areas of the arm. The presence of transverse bands remains an occasional but recurrent complaint for patients following brachioplasty. The bands are usually evident prior to brachioplasty, are more noticeable among higher-BMI individuals and are typically found on the anterior aspect of the arm, proximal to the elbow. In some instances, the band appearance may be made more noticeable by brachioplasty, particularly if the scars are hypertrophic (*Fig. 29.18*). Repeated flexion of the elbow over time appears to produce a permanent band of scar tissue in the soft tissues of the arm. While liposuction of the anterior aspect of the arm on either side of the band significantly diminishes the perceptibility of the band, it does not address the band itself. Z-plasty of the band has been suggested, but should be approached cautiously because of the more anterior scar location.

Access the complete references list online at **http://www.expertconsult.com**

1. American Society of Plastic Surgeons. 2000/2002/2003 /2004/2005/2006/2007/2008 National Plastic Surgery Statistics. Available at: http://www.plasticsurgery.org/ public_education/loader.cfm?url=/commonspot/ security/getfile.cfm&PageID=16158. Accessed December 1, 2009.

10. Hallock GG, Altobelli JA. Simultaneous brachioplasty, thoracoplasty and mammoplasty. *Aesthetic Plast Surg.* 1985;9:233.

13. Lockwood T. Brachioplasty with superficial fascial system suspension. *Plast Reconstr Surg.* 1995;96:912.

    Anatomic studies are reported by the author that reveal that the posteromedial soft tissue of the arm in youth is firmly suspended to the clavipectoral periosteum by means of the clavipectoral and axillary fasciae. Loosening of these structures leads to ptosis of the posteromedial arm. On the basis of this anatomic concept, the brachioplasty technique proposed provides anchoring of the arm flap to the axillary fascia and repair of the superficial fascial system to reduce the risk of scar widening or migration and unnatural arm contours. The series included five cases. While the series is small, the article highlights the importance of the superficial fascia system and in body-contouring surgery.

17. Abramson DL. Minibrachioplasty: Minimizing scars while maximizing results. *Plast Reconstr Surg.* 2004;114:1631.

    A short-scar brachioplasty or minibrachioplasty technique is described by the author that limits the scar to the axilla and proximal arm. Eight patients were treated with the technique. Brachioplasty techniques with scars limited to the proximal arm are likely to have a limited scope of utility in the massive weight loss patient.

20. Capella JF. Brachioplasty. Baker, Gordon Symposium. February 1, 2005.

21. Pascal JP, Le Louarn C. Brachioplasty. *Aesthetic Plast Surg.* 2005;29:423.

    A technique for brachioplasty is described where the scar is placed along the posteromedial arm and concomitant liposuction is used to help preserve both deep and superficial lymphatics, reduce damage to vessels and nerves, reduce volume, and allow for better tissue mobilization. The series includes 21 patients. The concepts presented in this article are similar to the techniques discussed in this chapter and those I presented in February 2005 in Miami, Florida at the Baker, Gordon Conference. Liposuction is a particularly important component of brachioplasty.

27. Gusenoff JA, Coon D, Rubin JP. Brachioplasty and concomitant procedures after massive weight loss: a statistical analysis from a prospective registry. *Plast Reconstr Surg.* 2008;122:595.

    The authors analyze data from a prospective registry of massive weight loss patients who underwent brachioplasty alone or with concomitant operations to identify statistically significant complications. Outcome measures included operative time, time since gastrc bypass, need for revision, arm liposuction, and complications such as seroma, dehiscence, hematoma, infection, and nerve injury. Patients with a greater change in body mass index had a higher chance of wound infection. Longer operative time was associated with increased rates of surgical complications at the operative site. There was a trend toward increased complications when arm liposuction was combined with brachioplasty. The series included 101 cases. This article is particularly important in that it reviews a relatively number of cases and makes conclusions based on data.

29. Nemerofsky RB, Oliak DA, Capella, JF. Body lift: An account of 200 consecutive cases in the massive weight loss patient. *Plast Reconstr Surg.* 2006;117:414.

30. Aly AS, Capella JF. Staging, reoperation and treatment of complications after body contouring in the massive-weight-loss patient. In: Grotting J, ed. *Reoperative aesthetic and reconstructive surgery*, 2nd ed. St. Louis: Quality Medical Publishing; 2007:1701-1740.

31. Geerts WH, Heit JA, Clagett GP, et al. Prevention of venous thromboembolism. *Chest.* 2001;119: 132S-175S.

30

Post-bariatric reconstruction

Jonathan W. Toy and J. Peter Rubin

SYNOPSIS

- Obesity is a widespread issue. With the rise in bariatric surgical procedures, there has been a concomitant increase in the demand for plastic surgical reconstruction after massive weight loss (MWL).
- Assessment of the MWL patient begins with a complete history and physical exam. Weight history, past surgical history, and nutritional status are key.
- Psychiatric co-morbidities are common in the MWL population presenting for body contouring. Preoperative identification is imperative.
- Essential elements of patient management include intraoperative positioning, maintaining body temperature, venous thromboembolism prophylaxis, and medical optimization.
- The abdominal area is the most common area of treatment in MWL patients. Ventral hernias are common – a high index of suspicion must be maintained.
- In the MWL patient, circumferential truncal body contouring procedures are necessary in many cases to achieve good aesthetic outcomes.
- Multiple body contouring procedures may be performed safely in combination, depending on patient preference, assistants in the operating room, length of anesthesia time, and the patient's overall medical condition.

  Access the Historical Perspective section online at
http://www.expertconsult.com

Obesity

Definition and epidemiology

Overweight and obesity refer to ranges of weight that are greater than that generally considered healthy for a given height. The primary measurement for obesity used to categorize patients is the body mass index (BMI).[6] According to the World Health Organization (WHO), overweight is defined as a BMI between 25 and 29.99 kg/m². Obesity begins at 30 kg/m² with obese class I equivalent to 30–34.99 kg/m².[7] Modifications to the classification have been added, including the categories of super obese (50–60 kg/m²), and super, super obese (>60 kg/m²) *(Table 30.1)*.[8]

In the United States, obesity is increasing at an alarming rate.[9] In 2008, the prevalence of obesity among American adult men and women was 32.2% and 35.5%, respectively. However, the prevalence of overweight and obesity combined was an alarming two-thirds of the adult population.[3] Approximately 5% of the American population is considered morbidly obese.[10] A rise in obesity among children and adolescents has also been noted in the past three decades.[9] Worldwide, the overweight and obesity population is estimated to be approximately 1.7 billion people.[11]

Obesity is an independent risk factor not only for all-cause mortality, but also for major diseases including coronary heart disease, type II diabetes, hypertension, certain malignancies, and musculoskeletal disorders.[2] One cannot ignore the psychosocial ramifications of obesity.[12] Disturbingly, obesity is predicted to overtake smoking as the leading cause of death in the United States.[13] Not only does obesity result in lower societal productivity and higher healthcare costs, rises in patient morbidity and mortality have spurred governmental interventions.[14–16]

The etiology of obesity is more complex than originally thought. Although some simplify the problem to "more calories in than out", other factors, including genetics, environment, and psychological factors are influential.[12] Certain medical conditions may also play a role: Cushing's disease, hypothyroidism, systemic steroids all cause increases in weight.

Notoriously difficult to treat, obesity is often resistant to many forms of therapy. Gastric bypass procedures have been shown to provide cost-effective, durable long-term weight control in the moderately to morbidly obese.[17,18] Improvements in safety as well as a decrease in morbidity associated with

Table 30.1 BMI and obesity classification[7,8]

BMI (kg/m²)	Classification
<18.5	Underweight
18.5–24.9	Normal weight
25.0–29.9	Overweight
30.0–34.9	Class I – Obesity
35.0–39.9	Class II – Obesity
40.0–49.9	Class III – Morbid obesity
50.0–59.9	Class III – Super obesity
≥60.0	Class III – Super, super obesity

bariatric surgery have led to a concomitant rise in bariatric surgical procedures, resulting in growing numbers of patients seeking removal of the excess skin and fat remaining following weight loss.[19,20]

MWL from surgery or diet and exercise alone, may be described as weight loss in excess of 50 pounds. Plastic surgeons have had to modify traditional surgical approaches and techniques in order to appropriately treat the unique deformities found in this emerging patient population.

Methods of weight reduction

Diet and exercise

Diet and exercise play an integral role in any weight loss regimen. Simplified, in order to lose weight, caloric intake must be less than total body expenditure of energy in order to consume endogenous triglycerides.[21] Caloric restriction may take the form of generalized reduction in calories, but may be aided by adjustments in the types of macronutrients eaten (e.g., fats, carbohydrates).[22,23] A recommended diet of between 1000 and 1200 kcal/day for women, and 1200–1600 kcal/day for men is commonly followed for a target weight loss of 1–2 pounds per week. In most cases, an initial weight loss of 10% of body weight over a 6-month period is suggested.[24] Unfortunately, long-term studies have found diet therapy alone is ineffective in the treatment of obesity.[24,25]

Often coupled with a reduction in caloric intake is physical activity or an exercise regimen. Physical activity is valuable, primarily aiding in long-term weight loss maintenance.[26,27] Isolated physical activity with no changes in a high calorie diet is insufficient to cause significant amounts of weight loss.[28]

Pharmacotherapy

The anorectic agents fenfluramine and phentermine have both in the past, been approved by the Food and Drug Administration (FDA) as individual agents. However, these drugs are not commonly used to treat obesity due to associations with the development of primary pulmonary hypertension and valvular heart disease.[29–32]

Currently, weight loss drugs are approved by the FDA for patients that have a BMI ≥ 30 kg/m², or a BMI between 27 and 29.9 kg/m² in conjunction with an obesity-related medical complication.[21] The majority of weight loss medications are anorexiants. Most are only approved for short-term use, and patients typically regain weight once discontinued.[33]

Two drugs are approved for long-term treatment of obesity. Orlistat (Xenical), a noncentrally acting anti-obesity agent, inhibits triglyceride digestion in the gastrointestinal tract. In combination with a hypocaloric diet, Orlistat promotes weight loss over a 1-year period.[34] Adverse effects of orlistat are primarily gastrointestinal with complaints of oily stool (including fat-soluble vitamin malabsorption) and fecal incontinence.[35] Sibutramine (Meridia) inhibits the reuptake of neurotransmitters in the brain, thereby increasing satiation. Weight loss in clinical trials with sibutramine has been shown to be greater than with placebo alone.[36,37] Currently, there are no pharmacologic anti-obesity agents that are truly effective against morbid obesity.[24,25]

Bariatric surgery

Bariatric surgery in the morbidly obese has been shown to ameliorate, and even cure some chronic diseases that have long been considered refractory to medical management. Perhaps the most profound effect of bariatric surgery is the reduction in type II diabetes. In 1995, a landmark study by Pories et al. was the first to report significant improvements in glucose control following bariatric surgery.[17] Further studies have demonstrated 83% and 86% resolution rates of type II diabetes following bariatric surgery.[38,39] Diabetes resolution was found to occur only days following surgery, well before weight loss was achieved.[17]

Diabetes is not the only disease improved by bariatric surgery. Sjostrom et al., demonstrated that hyperlipidemia was lowered by 10-fold following either gastric bypass, gastroplasty, or gastric banding as compared with controls.[40,41] Hypertension and sleep apnea have also been shown to improve following bariatric surgery.[10] Increases in life expectancy have been noted in patients following weight loss.[40,42,43] Bariatric surgery results in durable and stable weight loss within 1 year following surgery, that is three to four times superior to that achieved with nonsurgical treatment.[10,44]

Indications for bariatric surgery as a treatment of obesity include: BMI >40 kg/m², or BMI between 35 and 40 kg/m² with a high-risk comorbid condition, failed medical management, multidisciplinary evaluation, a motivated and well-informed patient with realistic expectations, and a commitment to long-term follow-up.[45–47]

Multiple surgical techniques have been described to treat obesity. The plastic surgeon should understand the various procedures and the effects they may have. Three main categories exist: restrictive, malabsorptive, and a combination restrictive malabsorptive.

Restrictive procedures produce satiety with the surgical creation of a small gastric pouch with a restricted outlet, thereby restricting food intake.[48] The advantage to restrictive procedures is the reduction in the malabsorption of nutrients seen long-term in malabsorptive procedures. Vertical banded gastroplasty involves the creation of a circular window made in the stomach a few inches below the esophagus. A small vertical pouch is made. Complications include esophageal reflux, stomal narrowing or widening, and less successful

Table 30.2 Advantages and disadvantages of various methods of weight loss

Method of weight loss	Advantages	Disadvantages
Diet and exercise	Noninvasive	Diet modification alone not usually effective in long term
Pharmacotherapy	Noninvasive	Oily stool Malabsorption of fat soluble vitamins Fecal incontinence
Bariatric surgical procedure	May ameliorate or improve many chronic diseases	Invasive
VBG	Decreased rates of nutrient malabsorption	Esophageal reflux Stomal narrowing/widening Less successful stable weight loss vs other bariatric surgical procedures
LAGB	Adjustable through port Decreased rates of nutrient malabsorption Absorptive surface of gastrointestinal tract unaltered	Lesser degree of weight loss vs other bariatric surgical procedures Erosion of device into stomach Removal requires surgery
BPD	Both restrictive and malabsorptive mechanisms	Protein-calorie malnutrition Anemia Bone demineralization Stomal ulcer formation Frequent/foul smelling stools Dumping syndrome
RNYGB	Both restrictive and malabsorptive mechanisms Many variations possible	Nutritional deficiencies Dumping syndrome

VBG, vertical banded gastroplasty; LAGB, laparoscopic adjustable gastric banding; BPD, biliopancreatic diversion; RNYGB, Roux-en-Y gastric bypass.

results with stable weight loss compared with gastric bypass, which has caused this procedure to fall out of favor.[49–52]

The more popular purely restrictive bariatric surgery is laparoscopic adjustable gastric banding (LAGB), where a band is placed around the upper stomach 1–2 cm below the gastroesophageal junction, creating a 20–30 cc upper gastric pouch.[50] The degree of constriction is adjusted with the alteration in the amount of saline in the band through the subcutaneous port. Because the absorptive surface of the gastrointestinal tract is unaltered, there is a decreased risk of nutritional deficiencies. Excess weight lost ranges from 52% to 68%.[53–56] The disadvantages of LAGB are less weight loss compared with combination restrictive malabsorptive procedures and a permanent intraabdominal foreign body. One of the most serious complications of LAGB is erosion of the device into the stomach, requiring surgical intervention, including removal of the band.[57] As evidence accumulates regarding the safety and efficacy of LAGB, it is anticipated that the use of these devices will dramatically increase.[51,58]

Purely malabsorptive procedures divert nutrients and interrupt the digestive process. More common techniques involve both restrictive and malabsorptive mechanisms, rather than malabsorption alone. Biliopancreatic diversion (BPD) has evolved to include a limited gastrectomy to reduce stomach size, as well as the creation of a malabsorptive limb, with a 50 cm common channel for absorption. Major complications from BPD include protein-calorie malnutrition, anemia, and bone demineralization.[49,50,52] Although the greatest degree of malabsorption occurs with this procedure, there is also a risk of stomal ulcer formation, frequent and foul smelling stools, and dumping syndrome.[57,59]

Currently in America, the most popular bariatric surgical procedure is the gastric bypass, or roux-en-Y gastric bypass (RYGB). Both the size of the stomach and the gastric outlet are restricted. This is a restrictive and malabsorptive combination procedure in which the degree of malabsorption is determined by the length of the jejunum attached to the gastric outlet.[60] Many variations of RYGB are possible.

Late complications of bariatric surgery are most relevant to the plastic surgeon.[57] These include inadequate weight loss, psychiatric conditions, dumping syndrome, and most importantly, nutritional deficiencies.[49,59,61] Adequate calorie intake and nutrition is the cornerstone of postoperative healing. Folate, calcium, vitamin B_{12}, and iron deficiencies may be seen following bariatric surgery. Daily supplemental vitamins reduce the risk of neurological and hematologic complications.[62] The incidence of peripheral neuropathy following bariatric surgery was 16% in one study.[63] A summary of the advantages and disadvantages of various methods of weight loss are shown in *Table 30.2*.

Diagnosis/presentation/evaluation

History

Patient evaluation includes a complete medical history. A distinction must be made in the mode of weight loss. Key information to obtain regarding the patient's weight includes:

- Date and nature of bariatric surgical procedure
- Maximum, lowest, and current weight and BMI

- Goal weight
- Recent (past 3 months) changes in weight status.[64]

  Other important history required includes:

- Past or current tobacco use
- Prior surgeries
- Prior pregnancies, plans for future pregnancies
- Breast history, including prior surgeries, history of cancer, family history, mammographic history, breast biopsies
- Prior deep venous thrombosis/pulmonary embolism, or coagulopathy
- Psychiatric history
- General medical issues.

Many patients will have had numerous medical co-morbidities prior to weight loss, that have improved significantly or since resolved. These benefits commonly occur within 2–5 months following bariatric surgery.[65] Sequelae of gastric bypass must also be assessed, including history of past or current dumping syndrome, or prolonged emesis.

Screening for nutritional status is important.[66] Protein intake by history is considered adequate if 70–100 g of protein per day is reported, although serum protein measurement is indicated before post-bariatric body contouring. Following bariatric surgery, protein is one of the major nutrients affected and may be reflected as hypoalbuminemia, anemia, and edema. Although seen in Roux-en-Y gastric bypass, the most common procedures associated with protein deficiencies are malabsorptive in nature such as the biliopancreatic diversion.[46,66] Protein intake is essential for wound healing especially if multiple contouring procedures are performed. Pre-albumin and albumin levels elucidate issues with protein intake and absorption. Protein supplementation may be required preoperatively.

Deficiencies in nutrients and vitamins, such as thiamine, folate, B_{12} and iron are common.[67,68] A history of current or past supplementation may screen for this. Nutritional deficiencies are most common in malabsorptive procedures including Roux-en-Y gastric bypass and biliopancreatic diversion.[66]

Anemia is not uncommon in the MWL population and may be related to generalized or specific nutrient deficiencies. Although iron deficiency is most common, micronutrients such as B_{12}, folate, copper, fat-soluble vitamins A and E, or zinc may be deficient and contribute to anemia.[69,70] A complete hematological work-up, including measurement of iron stores should be performed, especially in high-risk patients. In some cases, iron deficiencies may be refractory to oral therapies and require more aggressive treatment with parenteral iron, blood transfusions, or surgical interventions.[67] Iron deficiency may be seen in association with any gastric bypass procedure.

Physical examination

A generalized physical assessment of the degree of skin excess, distribution of fat, number and location of rolls, and the quality and elasticity of the remaining skin indicates which areas of the body would benefit from contouring surgery. Characteristically patients will present with predictable patterns of tissue descent around the body.

Zones of adherence, which are tight, nonyielding areas of fascial attachment to the underlying muscular system act as tethering points from which skin laxity will hang. These areas of restriction are located in the midline of the anterior and posterior trunk, and around the pelvic rim. Areas of skin and soft tissue that are farthest in distance from the zones of adherence descend the most following MWL, which in most patients includes the lateral truncal tissues.[71] The estimated skin resections may be simulated by performing "pinch tests", which may also help determine the translation of pull (distance from the pinched area that tissues are affected).[72]

Scars from prior surgeries are important to document, as a reduction in blood supply may require technical modifications during surgery. Commonly, rectus diastasis may be discovered. Ventral hernias are reducible or nonreducible, and the edges of the hernia may be palpated. A breast examination should be performed, noting masses, position of the nipple areola complex, and skin envelope quality. Asymmetries are pointed out to the patient. Lateral thoracic skin rolls are noted. Standardized photographs are taken.

Investigations

A proper medical work-up is essential. Preoperative clearances from internists, psychiatrists, and other physicians that care for the patient are the rule. Investigations include a chest X-ray, electrocardiogram, CBC, coagulation profile, pre-albumin, albumin, pregnancy screen in females of child-bearing age, and a mammogram if breast surgery is considered.[73] Abdominal CT in cases of suspected hernias will aid surgical planning.

Patient preoperative counseling and education

Preoperative counseling exploring the patient's goals, expectations, and areas of greatest concern aids in patient selection. Patients are questioned on areas of the body of greatest priority requiring correction, especially when multiple procedures are performed. Education regarding the areas of the body that may be contoured concurrently and discussion as to the appropriate staging of procedures is undertaken.

Patients must be made aware of the lengthy scars that occur with large skin resections, and must be willing to trade a better contour with the resultant scar. Although gentle tissue handling, meticulous wound closure and postoperative scar therapies attempt to create inconspicuous scars, some incisions tend to heal with raised, reddened, or even hypertrophic scars.

Education must focus on pre- and postoperative expectations, the length of the surgical procedures, as well as the nature and length of recovery following multiple procedures. As the majority of surgeons use drains in the initial postoperative period, information regarding drain care should be given. Patients must have appropriate social support at home in order for a smooth recovery to occur. No lifting of items heavier than 10 pounds is a good rule of thumb for patients undergoing abdominal procedures.

Abstinence from medications that predispose to bleeding, including herbal medications is important. Tobacco use is a relative or absolute contraindication for body contouring by most surgeons. Smoking cessation helps to minimize flap loss and wound complications such as dehiscence and infection.[74,75] Although there is no consensus, a commonly used guideline is abstinence from tobacco or nicotine replacement therapies for at least 4 weeks prior to and 4 weeks post-elective cosmetic or reconstructive procedures.[76]

Informed consent is a key element of preoperative counseling. Patients must understand that body contouring after MWL may require multiple stages, and possible revisionary surgeries. The surgeon's revision policy must be emphasized to patients and the difference between secondary procedures (further skin tightening) and revisions understood. In general, MWL patients experience mild to moderate amounts of skin relaxation postoperatively, resulting in the need for further skin resections. There is also the possibility of contour irregularities and postoperative "dog-ears" at the extents of resection. A comprehensive guide to informed consent in body contouring patients following MWL is available from the American Society of Plastic Surgeons.[77]

Patient selection

Patients presenting following MWL should be at or around their goal weight, and be weight-stable for at least 3 months prior to body contouring surgery. This usually corresponds to a period of 12–18 months following bariatric surgery. A BMI <35 kg/m^2 is acceptable; a BMI >35 kg/m^2 portends increased risk of surgical complications.[78–80] Ideally, patients undergoing body contouring after MWL should be within 10–15% of their goal weight and have had no large fluctuations in their weight (weight-stable) over the past 3–6 months.[48]

Aesthetic outcomes are improved with a lower BMI. In general, a BMI of 25–30 kg/m^2 is ideal, and patients with a BMI >32 kg/m^2 may have more limited aesthetic outcomes.[81,82] Also, a high BMI increases the rate of complications, especially thrombotic complications such as deep venous thrombosis.[83,84] Patients with high BMIs are counseled to further lose weight and return again at a more ideal BMI. A notable exception to this guideline is the patient with the disabling giant pannus, or panniculus morbidus. These patients will generally benefit from the removal of abdominal excess in order to improve ambulation, quality of life, hygiene, and further their weight loss.[85]

Patients with severe medical co-morbidities, psychiatric co-morbidities, unrealistic expectations, and patients currently using tobacco are preoperatively optimized. These issues are reassessed at the second preoperative visit and surgical management is offered only once improved or resolved.

The authors consider systemic medical disease that precludes general anesthesia an absolute contraindication for body contouring surgery. Relative contraindications include active smoking, BMI >35 kg/m^2, uncorrected coagulopathies, severe disorders that affect wound healing, and systemic medical disease that place the patient at high risk for surgery.

Psychological considerations

Post-bariatric body contouring

MWL is considered by many to be a "life-altering event". Such is the same with body contouring procedures. Patients should be congratulated on their weight loss. Pre- and postoperative

counseling as to the usual postoperative course is essential. Family and social supports aid in the recovery period.

Prior to bariatric surgery, up to one-third of patients have at least one psychiatric diagnosis; approximately 40% of patients undergoing bariatric surgery are undergoing some form of psychiatric treatment.[86,87] Mood disorders, personality disorders, and poor body image are most common. Patients with a history of bipolar disorder and schizophrenia must be offered surgery with caution. A high index of suspicion must be maintained with liberal preoperative psychiatric clearances. Following MWL, many psychiatric conditions reportedly improve, albeit transiently.[88] Quality of life, however, has been found to improve following body contouring surgery, independent of mood.[89]

Patient safety and intraoperative considerations

Any body contouring surgery should be performed in a fully accredited ambulatory care facility or hospital. An operating room staff familiar with body contouring is essential for efficiency and timeliness of the surgery. Anesthesiologists should be familiar with the post-bariatric patient and sensitive to the physiological and structural changes that are associated (*Table 30.3*).[90]

Prevention of hypothermia is crucial. With lengthy procedures involving the creation of large wounds, exposing the majority of the patient's body, all patients must be monitored carefully. A temperature of at least 35°C should be maintained. The authors perform pre-warming for all body contouring patients in the pre-anesthesia holding area with forced-air warming blankets. Warming continues in the operating room with elevated basal room temperatures, forced-air blankets, warmed fluids if needed, and operating table warming pads.

Venous thrombosis prevention is integral. Surgeries are lengthy and abdominal wall tightening or reconstruction is common, elevating intra-abdominal pressures and predisposing to deep vein thrombosis (DVT) and pulmonary embolism. A preoperative history for risk factors for DVT and careful prophylaxis reduces these rates. Factors such as increased age, malignancy, history of spontaneous miscarriages, inherited or acquired thrombophilia, use of exogenous estrogens, pregnancy, and previous venous thromboembolism should alert the plastic surgeon of increased risk.[91–93]

Guidelines from the American College of Chest Physicians in prevention of DVT are available.[94] Early ambulation, mechanical lower extremity compression devices applied pre-induction, and prophylactic doses of blood thinners may be used.[91] Improved efficacy does not occur when chemoprophylaxis is given preoperatively compared to within 6–12 h of the surgery. However, a higher risk of bleeding occurs

Table 30.3 Safety and intraoperative considerations in body contouring

Procedures should be performed in a fully accredited ambulatory facility or hospital
Prevention of hypothermia is crucial
Venous thrombosis prevention is essential
Be aware of patient positioning
Length of surgery is important

when given within 2 h of surgery.[95] Currently, no clear evidence based guidelines for chemoprophylaxis in the plastic surgery population exist.

Patient positioning may improve the ease of surgery and prevent untoward complications secondary to pressure. Prone positioning is often required and pressure must be minimized to points such as the breasts, genitals, and face. Endotracheal tube positioning must be maintained. Compression on the eyes must be avoided, as blindness has been reported following prone positioning.[96] When prone, patients should be placed in 15° of Trendelenburg to prevent excessive pressures on the globes.[97,98] Neural and vascular compression may occur.[99]

Length of surgery is an important consideration. Combining multiple body contouring procedures is frequent and can significantly increase operative time. Time is increased when turning the patient is required. There is no consensus on the time limits for body contouring surgery. However, fewer procedures performed and less operative time generally result in a lower complication rate.

Surgical techniques by anatomic region

Abdominal contouring

Abdominoplasty procedures are explored in Chapter 25. Abdominoplasty is reviewed here with specific reference to the MWL patient (see *Box 30.1*).

Deformity/patient evaluation

The abdominal area is the most common reason patients seek plastic surgical consultation after MWL. Along with aesthetic concerns, a hanging abdominal pannus may be symptomatic, causing recurrent intertrigo and infections in skin folds, hindering ambulation, and making intimacy difficult. Following abdominoplasty or panniculectomy after MWL, patients indicate a consistent improvement in body image and subjective quality of life.[100]

Evaluation of the patient presenting for abdominal contouring, in addition to a complete history, includes:

> **Box 30.1 Abdominal contouring in the MWL patient**
>
> - A panniculectomy is primarily a reconstructive procedure aiming to remove skin and fat from the anterior abdominal area in patients that are not at their optimal weight. The term abdominoplasty is primarily an aesthetic procedure involving the removal of abdominal skin and fat, along with tightening of the abdominal wall musculature, and repositioning of the umbilicus.
> - Ventral and umbilical hernias are common in the MWL population. A high index of suspicion must be maintained and structural anomalies sought preoperatively.
> - Vertical resection of trunk skin and fat (fleur-de-lis abdominoplasty) may be required to tighten the abdomen transversely. Care must be taken to minimize flap undermining.
> - In patients with skin and soft tissue excess circumferentially, a procedure such as a lower bodylift or belt lipectomy may result in a more aesthetic result than a panniculectomy or abdominoplasty alone.
> - The genital area or mons may require thinning and resuspension.
> - In the patient with the giant pannus (panniculus morbidus), special equipment including supportive lifts aid in resection.

- Quality, elasticity of abdominal skin
- Presence of multiple skin rolls
- Degree of adiposity, deflation of skin rolls
- Evaluation of intra-abdominal versus extra-abdominal adiposity
- Presence or absence of rectus diastasis
- Presence or absence of ventral hernias, umbilical hernias
- Surgical scars
- Extent of excess tissues laterally and circumferentially
- Co-existing genital deformities, including mons ptosis.

Operative planning and techniques

A panniculectomy is a functional operation designed to relieve symptoms related to an overhanging abdominal pannus. It is performed for patients with higher BMIs or more severe medical co-morbidities. It is considered a functional, reconstructive procedure removing only skin and fat. Skin flap undermining is limited, and no plication is performed. The risks of a traditional abdominoplasty are minimized. In patients who have lost a considerable amount of weight, the umbilical stalk may be quite long and preclude its use, resulting in excision and possibly the creation of a neo-umbilicus.

The term panniculectomy is in contrast to abdominoplasty, which is traditionally performed for aesthetic purposes and includes not only the removal of skin and fat, but includes abdominal wall and umbilical repositioning. The patient is usually at or around their goal weight.

The assessment of tissue excesses, not only anteriorly, but also laterally and circumferentially, is important. A panniculectomy or abdominoplasty will resect skin and fat anteriorly; however if excess in skin and fat extends laterally and posteriorly, these areas are not addressed. Large dog-ears laterally may occur in this case. Conversion to alternative procedures such as a lower bodylift, liposuction, or belt lipectomy will correct larger lateral deformities. This should be documented and discussed with the patient preoperatively. In the case of panniculectomy/abdominoplasty, the extent of the resection laterally should be discussed. Dog-ears may be minimized or avoided in many cases by marking the lateral extents of the pannus in the standing position.

Old surgical scars must be considered. The elevation of flaps surrounding prior healed incisions is always concerning in regards to blood supply. Limitation of undermining (up to the scar) reduces the risk of skin flap necrosis. Risk factors for skin necrosis should also be sought preoperatively and if present, dissection should be minimized.

With the introduction of minimally-invasive bariatric surgical procedures, abdominal wall incisional hernias are becoming less common. Care must be taken to ensure that the abdominal cavity will accommodate the reduction of intra-abdominal contents without causing excessive tension on the abdominal wall reconstruction. If not, the patient is first treated with supportive care with an abdominal binder and counseled to lose further weight prior to reconstruction.

Abdominal wall reconstruction for ventral or umbilical hernias may be accessed through the low transverse abdominal incision. Small to moderate ventral hernia repairs may easily be combined with other body contouring procedures. However, more extensive hernias require wider dissection and lysis of adhesions. In these cases, the amount of concomitant procedures is decreased for safety reasons.[73] It is the author's preference to avoid using prosthetic materials for abdominal wall reconstruction if avoidable due to the higher risk in this population of wound dehiscence and infection. Components separation of the abdominal wall is an excellent technique for repair of ventral hernias and may avoid the use of mesh prosthetics.[101]

Final scar placement must be taken into consideration. The inferior margin for the transverse resection is planned 6 cm superior to the vulvar commissure in females and from the base of the penis in males. This position allows the final scar to be hidden in the patient's underwear.

Variations in abdominal contouring and reconstruction

In patients with significant epigastric laxity, a vertical trunk excision may be combined with the low transverse excision, creating a fleur-de-lis type abdominoplasty *(Fig. 30.1)*.[102,103] It is wise to limit undermining at the edges of the vertical excision, to preserve as many local perforators as possible, and to avoid excessive triple-point tension to preserve flap viability.[104] Umbilical inset is made within the vertical incision; creating a cut-out for the inset will create an unaesthetic widened umbilicus over time. Defatting superior to the cephalad limit of the vertical excision will reduce the resultant dog-ear. Advantages to the fleur-de-lis abdominoplasty include the ability to contour the epigastrium and enhance waist definition *(Fig. 30.2)*. Disadvantages include the additional vertical abdominal scar and potential for overtightening at the waist in males, creating a feminine appearing torso.

Ptosis of the pubic/mons area is frequently encountered in the MWL patient. Resuspension with nonabsorbable sutures from the anterior abdominal fascia to the superficial fascial system of the pubic area at three to five points helps reposition this area *(Figs 30.3, 30.4)*. Sub-scarpal defatting of the pubic area may be required to match abdominal flap thickness. If mons resuspension is performed, the patient is advised preoperatively that there may be a temporary change in the angle of urine stream.

Extreme cases of pubic ptosis accompanied by excess pubic fat in males results in a buried penis, in which the shaft and glans of the penis are concealed from view *(Fig. 30.5)*.[105] Increases in abdominal fat may contribute to this condition, as the penis is tethered by the suspensory ligament, while the abdominal fat is not.[106] With recurrent episodes of infection, persistent moisture, and superficial skin breakdown, cicatricial changes occur, trapping the penis. Buried penis is a debilitating condition, interfering with normal urinary function, proper hygiene, and making sexual intercourse difficult.[107] Correction of such deformities is complex, and multiple techniques have been developed.[108–110]

Special consideration is made for the giant pannus. Associated with a high BMI, a giant pannus causes significant morbidity. Interference with ambulation, hygiene issues including recurrent intertrigo and rashes, and chronic pannus lymphedema may be alleviated with resection.[111,112] Since a large mass of tissue may be present, special lifts provide access to incision sites.[78,113] Steinman pins may be placed superficially into the edge of the pannus, bearing in mind that an incisional or umbilical hernia may be present. These pins may be connected to a Hoyer hydrolic lift. Elevation allows

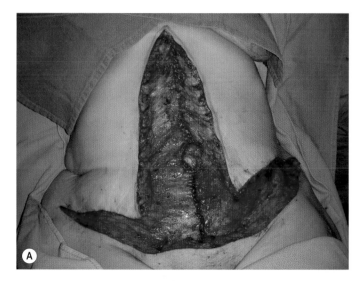

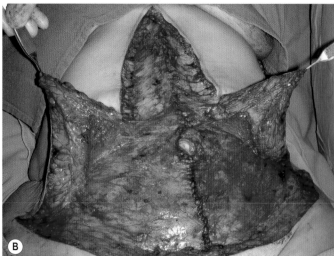

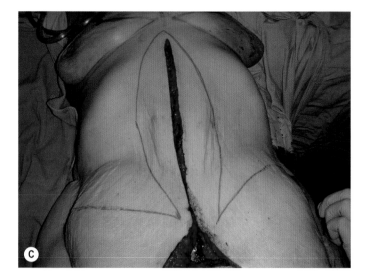

Fig. 30.1 Surgical technique for fleur-de-lis (FDL) abdominoplasty. **(A)** Estimated resection marked. Undermining of skin flaps is minimized. **(B)** Transverse resection of tissues performed first, followed by resection in the vertical axis. **(C)** Preservation of abdominal wall perforating vessels minimizes risk of flap necrosis and wound healing complications. Minimal undermining is key.

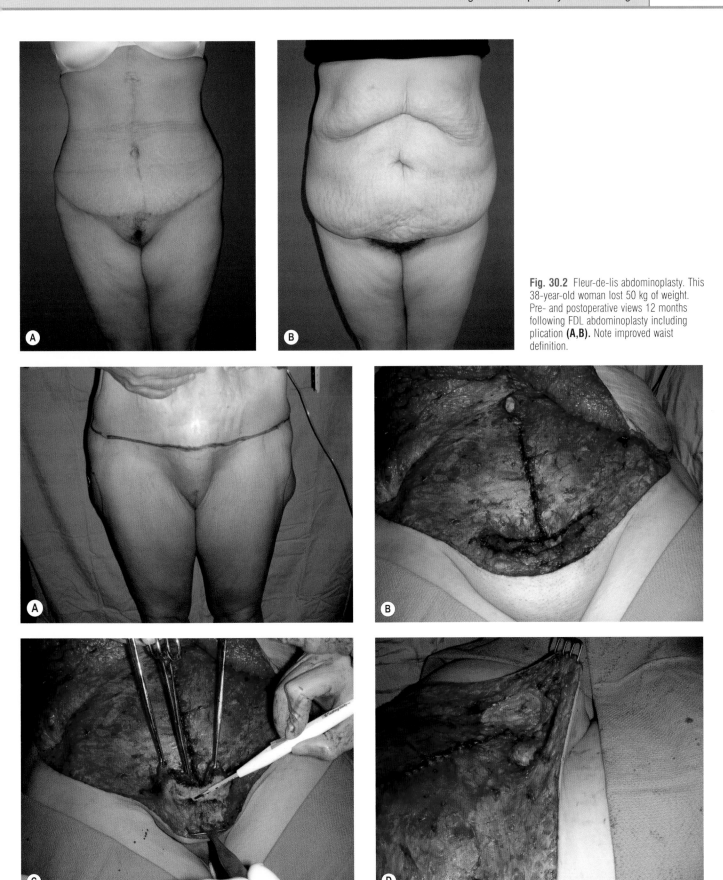

Fig. 30.2 Fleur-de-lis abdominoplasty. This 38-year-old woman lost 50 kg of weight. Pre- and postoperative views 12 months following FDL abdominoplasty including plication **(A,B)**. Note improved waist definition.

Fig. 30.3 Mons correction and resuspension. The patient is marked for abdominoplasty with caudal resection line shown, 6 cm superior to the anterior vulvar commissure **(A)**. Following abdominal wall plication, resection of deep adipose tissue beneath the mons is performed. The thickness of the mons should match that of the abdominal flap. The wedge-shaped resection extends to the symphysis pubis, while avoiding the vaginal vault **(B–D)**.

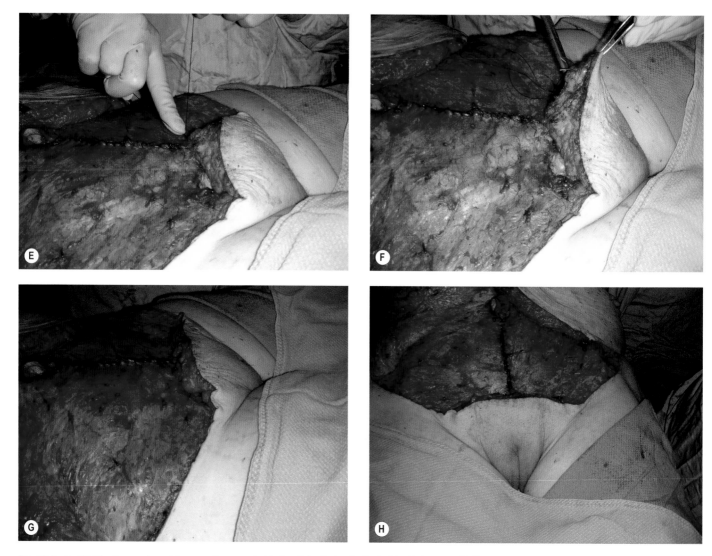

Fig. 30.3, cont'd The deep surface of the mons is suspended to the abdominal wall with 3–5 braided sutures **(E,F)**. A reduction of the fullness and ptosis of the mons is seen **(G,H)**.

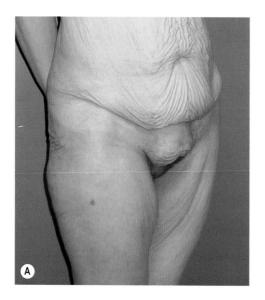

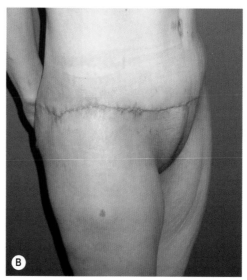

Fig. 30.4 Mons ptosis correction. A 49-year-old woman with significant mons ptosis. Pre- and postoperative views following correction and suspension with abdominoplasty **(A,B)**. Note improved genital contour with reduction in mons volume and improvement in position.

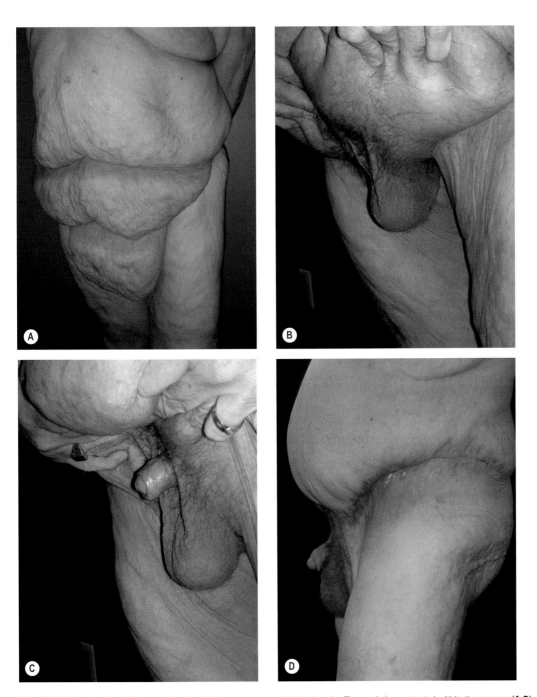

Fig. 30.5 Buried penis. A 53-year-old male with large pannus and buried penis. The penis has retracted within the pannus **(A,B)**. Manual extraction is possible in this case **(C)**. Improved appearance and exposure of the genitals are seen following panniculectomy **(D)**.

venous drainage from the pannus and better control of large blood vessels. Hemostasis with surgical clips or ties is essential. In most cases, umbilical excision is necessary *(Fig. 30.6)*.

Complications

Local complications including hematoma, seroma, wound infection, and wound dehiscence may be seen in the early postoperative period. Asymmetries involving scar position and contour are possible. Lateral dog-ears are common, but avoidable if care is taken in surgical planning or choice of procedure (e.g., conversion to circumferential truncal surgery). Resuspension of the genital area may cause a temporary alteration in the stream of urine.

Other complications include deep vein thrombosis, pulmonary embolism, over- or under-resection. Relapse, with recurrence of tissue laxity is common and may require further skin tightening procedures.

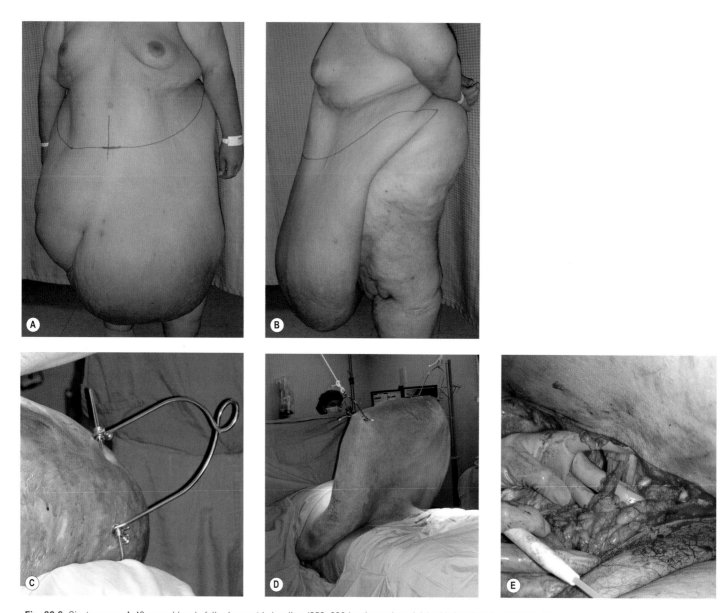

Fig. 30.6 Giant pannus. A 42-year-old male following gastric banding (352–236 kg change in weight) with functionally disabling giant pannus preoperatively **(A,B)**. Orthopedic pins are inserted through the edge of the pannus, held with traction bows and used to suspend the pannus above the patient **(C,D)**. Commonly, large blood vessels are encountered and ligated **(E)**. Total resected pannus weight was 61 kg.

Lower bodylift (LBL)/buttock contouring

Lower bodylift (belt lipectomy) is covered in Chapter 27. It is reviewed here with specific reference to the MWL patient (see *Box 30.2*).

Box 30.2 **Lower bodylift**

- In patients with excess skin and fat circumferentially, an isolated abdominal procedure is not the ideal choice. A lower bodylift or belt lipectomy will provide a more aesthetic result.
- Discontinuous undermining of the soft tissues of the lateral thigh will aid in optimal tissue resection and tension.
- Meticulous repair of the SFS will support the tension across the wound in a LBL and help prevent poor scarring.
- In many cases, flattening of the buttocks may occur without the preservation of autologous fat.

Deformity/patient evaluation

In many MWL patients, abdominal contouring alone is insufficient. Deflation of soft tissues in the lateral thighs and buttocks may need surgical correction. Often deflated, ptotic buttocks with loose skin and adiposity in the lateral thigh accompany a hanging pannus. A number of procedures address these deformities, including the belt lipectomy, lower bodylift, circumferential torsoplasty, all achieve circumferential trunk contouring.[81,114–116] The buttocks, abdomen and thighs must be treated as a single unit. Advancements using the superficial fascial system (SFS) by Lockwood, as well as autologous buttocks auto-augmentation with local de-epithelialized gluteal flaps to restore buttock projection and shape, have improved results.[117–119]

In addition to the patient evaluation described in the abdominal section, assessment of the lateral thigh and buttocks region is essential. The quality, elasticity, and quantity of skin in these areas are assessed and the translation of pull determined with a pinch test. The volume and location of fat deposits is documented. Buttocks projection and volume in the buttocks area is determined to aid in operative planning and the need for auto-augmentation of the buttocks with local flaps.

Patient selection

The ideal patient for a circumferential lower body contouring procedure is a patient with an optimal BMI, a deflated skin-fat envelope with descent of the buttocks and lateral thigh tissues, who is in good health and has realistic expectations. The patient must be counseled on the extent of scarring and post-operative expectations.

Staging of procedures in the MWL patient is important. In patients undergoing both lower body circumferential contouring procedures and medial thigh-lifting procedures, it is advisable to stage the procedures. It is the preference of the authors to perform the lower bodylifting procedure in a first stage, followed by the medial thigh-lifting procedure in a second stage. Further details are discussed below.

Markings

Markings for circumferential lower body procedures vary depending on individual morphology. Placing the resection more superiorly allows more control over the excision of flank rolls, provides moderate elevation force on the lateral thighs, and accentuates the waist. This may be ideal in the female patient wishing further waist definition, but may be less than ideal for the male patient who does not wish for a feminized silhouette.[71] Buttock reshaping with autologous gluteal flaps is more difficult with this higher positioning. Resections placed more inferiorly allow greater elevation on the lateral thigh tissues as compared with higher resections. Buttocks reshaping is also easier. Waist definition may be enhanced in this case by rectus plication and the addition of a vertical abdominal skin resection. Choice of resection depends on individual body type and surgical goals. The authors prefer to keep the resection low (inferior) to prevent gluteal flattening, add control to lateral thigh contour, and to keep the final scar position reliably covered by most undergarments.

In the supine position, with the abdominal skin on stretch, a distance of 6 cm is marked from the superior aspect of the vulvar commissure in females, or the base of the penis in males. Posterior markings are made with the patient facing away from the surgeon. The superior anchor line posteriorly is determined in the midline and extended bilaterally to the mid-axillary line. Vertical reference marks are spaced 6 cm apart. Laterally, the amount of tissues to be resected is estimated with a pinch test with the legs slightly abducted, and marked accordingly. This creates the lateral margins of the inferior resection line. The inferior resection line is then drawn. A transition zone between the posterior and anterior resections is marked, usually in the mid-axillary line. The areas within the resection lines that are to be preserved for autologous buttocks augmentation are marked.

With the patient facing the surgeon, and the patient holding the abdominal skin on vertical stretch, the points marking the lower lateral margin of resection bilaterally are gently connected to the point 6 cm superior to the vulvar commissure in the midline. This is the inferior margin of resection of the abdominal contouring portion of the procedure. Areas of adjunct liposuction are marked *(Fig. 30.7)*.

Operative technique

Video 1

Although initially described as a three-position procedure by Lockwood, the authors believe a two-position procedure (prone, then supine) to be adequate.[119–121] Routine Foley catheter, warming blankets and sequential compression devices are used. Circumferential sterile prepping of the lower body is performed. Beginning in the prone position, the gluteal flaps to be preserved for buttock augmentation are de-epithelialized. Next, the superior anchor line is incised and an inferiorly based flap is created, avoiding the de-epithelialized gluteal flaps. The inferior line is checked during the procedure and adjusted to ensure reasonable closure and the resection is completed.

Laterally, the buttock flaps are undermined and absorbable sutures are used to shape the flaps for increased projection and gluteal augmentation. Inferior to the flaps, moderate undermining is performed in order to accommodate the buttocks flap volume *(Fig. 30.8)*. The lateral thigh region is mobilized with the Lockwood discontinuous undermining device (Byron Medical, Tucson AZ) passed into the subcutaneous tissue *(Fig. 30.9)*. The legs are abducted to decrease lateral tension and towel clips are used to hold the wound together. Closure is performed over drains. The lateral dog-ears are temporarily stapled closed.

In the supine position, the procedure continues as a traditional abdominoplasty. Attention must be paid to flexion at the waist as a high resection in the posterior body will lead to greater tension on the back wound, allowing a less aggressive anterior resection. Absorbable sutures placed in the lateral aspect of the wound to coapt the SFS is essential. Drains are placed in the abdominal wound and closure in the usual fashion is performed. Representative cases are shown in *Figures 30.10 and 30.11*.

Postoperative care

The patient is kept in the beach-chair position, with the waist flexed. Perioperative antibiotics are administered. Mobilization with assistance is encouraged on postoperative day 1 and the Foley catheter is removed at this time. Chemoprophylaxis for venous thromboembolism and maintenance of pneumatic compression devices continues. The expected duration of hospitalization is 2 nights, however this may vary depending on the patient's condition and the number of concomitant procedures performed. Drains are removed when output is <30 cc in a 24-hour period.

Vertical thigh-lift

Deformity/patient evaluation

The thighs are a difficult area to treat in the MWL patient. No single procedure can address changes in both the medial and lateral thighs (see *Box 30.3*). A lower bodylift (LBL) may contour the lateral thighs, but leave the medial thighs

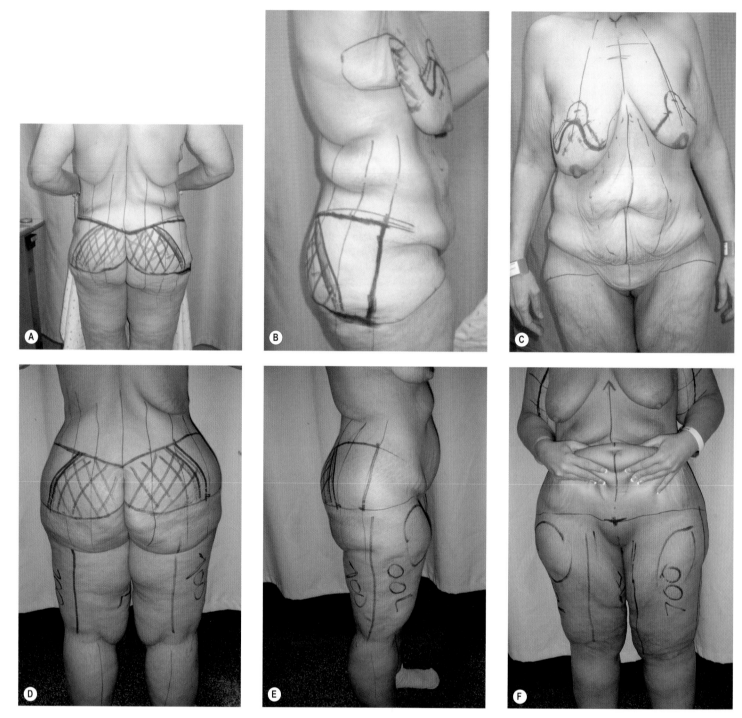

Fig. 30.7 Lower bodylift markings. Examples of two patients marked for circumferential lower bodylift. On the posterior views **(A,D),** the red hashed areas indicate gluteal fat tissue that will be preserved for buttock reshaping. Note the difference in body types of these patients, but both will benefit from preserving gluteal fat. On lateral views **(B,E),** the extent of lateral skin resection is noted. Anterior views **(C,F)** demonstrate the low position of the transverse scar. With the abdominal tissues on upward stretch, the final transverse scar position is demonstrated **(F).** The second patient **(D–F)** is marked for additional extensive debulking liposuction, thus facilitating improved results for the second stage vertical medial thigh-lift.

minimally affected, while a vertical medial thigh-lift may tighten the inner thigh, leaving the lateral thigh untouched.

MWL produces characteristic changes in the medial thighs. Inferior descent of the soft tissues, as well as significant deflation may occur. The skin-fat envelope of the thigh is less tightly adherent medially than laterally, resulting in significant soft tissue descent in this area with MWL.[122] Although

this gives the impression of vertical excess, it in fact is primarily horizontal excess that needs to be addressed.

Earlier methods of correcting the medial thigh region were crescentic and aimed at placing the scar in the groin and perineal crease. A vertical vector of pull towards the groin is achieved and can treat minor medial thigh laxity, only treating the upper-third of the thigh.[123,124] Due to frequent

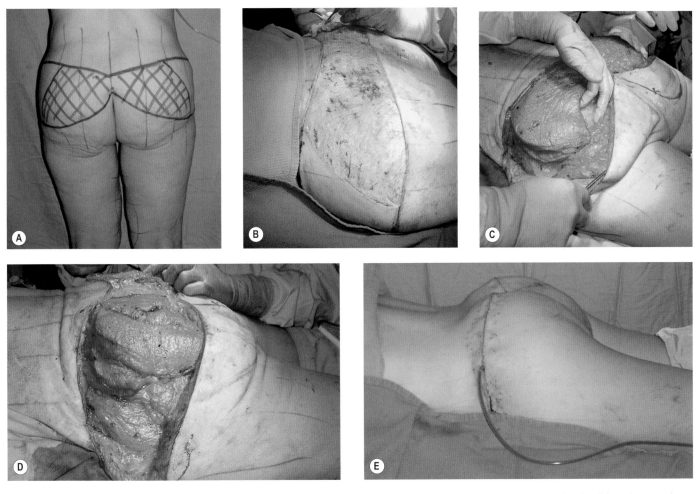

Fig. 30.8 Lower bodylift gluteal reshaping technique. Preoperative markings for lower bodylift are shown. Hashed marks demonstrate areas for gluteal fat pad preservation **(A)**. De-epithelialization of the area of gluteal fat preservation is performed, preserving full thickness flaps, while laterally excision is deeper. The fat pad is undermined laterally for rotation. Inferiorly, subcutaneous pocket is created to accommodate volume **(B,C)**. Rotation of the lateral portion of the flap inferiorly into the subcutaneous pocket with suture to the deep fascia is shown **(D)**. Enhanced buttock projection is achieved with dermal surface plication. Final operative result is shown **(E)**.

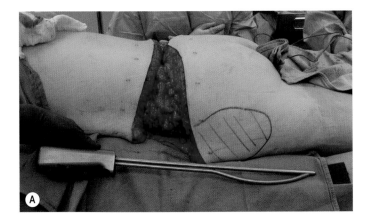
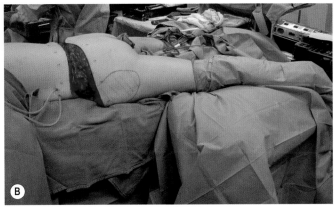

Fig. 30.9 Lower bodylift. Intraoperative use of Lockwood undermining device of the lateral thighs **(A)**. Leg abduction over a sterile side table or additional arm boards decreases tension off of lateral closure **(B)**.

complications including scar widening, vulvar deformity, and recurrence of ptosis, a modification of the upper medial thigh-lift involved anchoring the inner thigh to Colles' fascia.[125] Advantages to this procedure include avoiding a medial longitudinal scar, the ability to perform this in conjunction with a lower bodylift, decreased recovery and operative time as compared with a vertical thigh-lift. However, laxity of the distal third of the medial thigh is minimally improved with this procedure. Many MWL patients with severe skin envelope deflation require more powerful procedures.

The aim of a vertical medial thigh-lift is to primarily correct horizontal laxity with the resection of a vertical component,

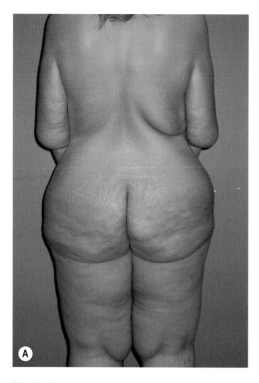 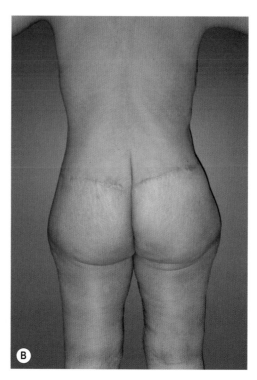

Fig. 30.10 Lower bodylift with debulking liposuction. A 39-year-old woman s/p 45 kg weight loss **(A)**. A first stage lower bodylift with 9 L debulking liposuction of the thighs was followed by a second stage vertical medial thigh-lift six months following initial procedure **(B)**. Mid-back rolls were corrected with a lateral chest excision concurrent with a mastopexy at the second stage.

Box 30.3 Thigh-lift

- The thigh must be conceptually divided into lateral and medial areas. Procedures such as the lower bodylift, and lateral thigh-lift may affect the lateral thigh, but minimally tighten the medial thigh tissues. Conversely, a medial thigh-lift will only affect medial tissues, leaving the lateral tissues primarily unaffected.
- In a vertical thigh-lift procedure, the extent of resection distally may be altered depending on the skin redundancy at the knee, as well as patient preference and acceptance of the length of scar.
- In patients with minimally deflated thighs requesting thigh-lift, further weight reduction may be necessary. Alternatively, staged debulking procedures are required prior to excisional procedures.
- The lymphatic structures of the leg are primarily concentrated medially and deep to the plane of the saphenous vein until the vessels begin to converge in the femoral triangle. Inadvertent injury to the lymphatics during thigh-lift procedures may result in lymphedema of the lower extremity.

focusing tension on the medial thigh as a cylinder. The thigh may be thought of as two components, the firm and unyielding inner core composed of bone and muscle, and the outer skin and soft tissue envelope.[122] The widest aspect of the thigh is located 2–3 cm below the perineal crease. The only transverse component of excision in a vertical thigh-lift is at the superior aspect of the incision, used to remove the resultant dog-ear in the proximal thigh. Depending on the distal extent of skin laxity, the scar may be shortened, or lengthened towards the medial knee.

A history of lymphedema or significant varicosities is important to document. Physical examination should include the degree and distal extent of skin laxity and quality. A pinch test of the medial and lateral thighs will demonstrate the amount of possible skin resection and translation of pull. The amount of lipodystrophy and whether or not the thighs are deflated should be documented. Any signs of lymphedema should raise concern.

Discussion with the patient regarding his or her preferences in the areas to be contoured is imperative. This will impact the order and staging of procedures. For example, if a patient is to undergo a lower bodylift (to correct outer thighs) and medial thigh-lift (to correct medial thighs), the lower bodylift procedure is generally performed in the first stage, followed by a second stage medial thigh-lift.

Patient selection

Selection of surgical procedure is based on quality, quantity, and extent of skin excess, the amount and position of adiposity, surgeon and patient preference, and patient willingness to accept scar in exchange for improved contour.

In patients with mild to moderate skin laxity localized to the upper thigh with minimal adiposity, a crescentic transversely based excision in the groin and perineal creases with suspension to Colles' fascia may provide vertical pull, while keeping the scar hidden.

In patients with greater degrees of skin laxity in the medial thigh, and mild to moderate adiposity, a vertically-based excision of the medial thigh (vertical medial thigh-lift) with a transverse component in the groin and perineal creases may

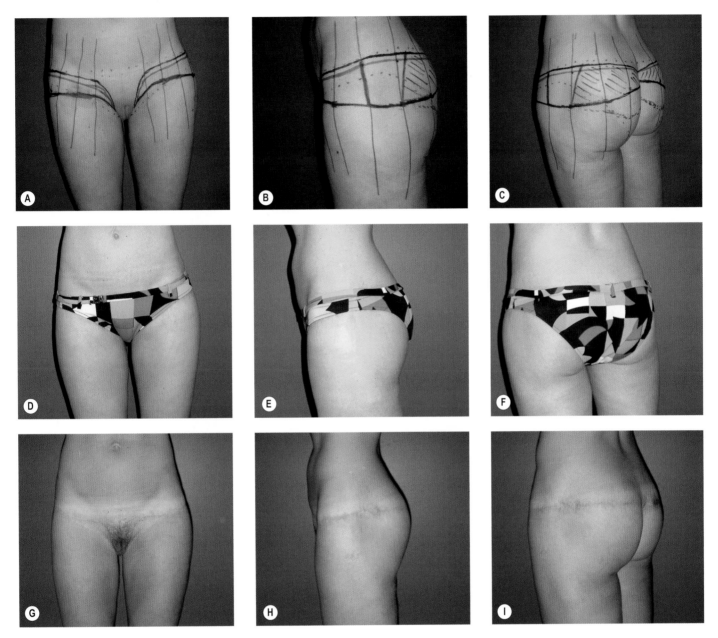

Fig. 30.11 Lower bodylift without abdominoplasty. A 49-year-old woman s/p 36 kg weight loss. Patient had good skin tone and minimal skin excess of the abdomen and the patient was marked fro a lower bodylift without abdominoplasty. The red line is the proposed scar position, based on the distance the superior incision will move on stretch. Anteriorly, the scars extend parallel to the groin crease **(A–C)**. Postoperative views at 8 months show scar position well hidden in undergarment **(D–F)**. Note the anterior scars come very close to the mons to prevent them from descending onto the anterior thigh **(G–I)**.

suffice. Adjunct liposuction may be used. The distal extent of vertical resection may be altered and lengthened to the level of the knee in more extreme cases of skin excess.

In the MWL patient with residual thigh adiposity (non-deflated) and skin excess, either further weight reduction is recommended, or an initial debulking liposuction procedure of the medial thigh area is performed, followed by a second stage vertical medial thigh-lift.

Skin excess and adiposity in the lateral thighs does not respond well to medial thigh-lifting alone. Procedures such as a lower bodylift or lateral thigh-lift are required to address these deformities, usually in a separate stage to the medial thigh procedure.

Markings

With the patient in the supine position with legs abducted, the line of incision in the groin crease is made beginning 4 cm lateral to the midline of the mons. A pinch test estimates the crescentic resection in the groin crease. Next, the vertical resection marks are made. The proposed scar position is marked. The thigh tissues are pulled posteriorly to simulate the result of the thigh-lift of the anterior tissues. The anterior anchor line is marked with this maneuver. The posterior mark is made with a similar traction anteriorly. Reference lines are placed every 6 cm perpendicular to the resection. Bilateral thigh markings are compared for symmetry *(Fig. 30.12)*.

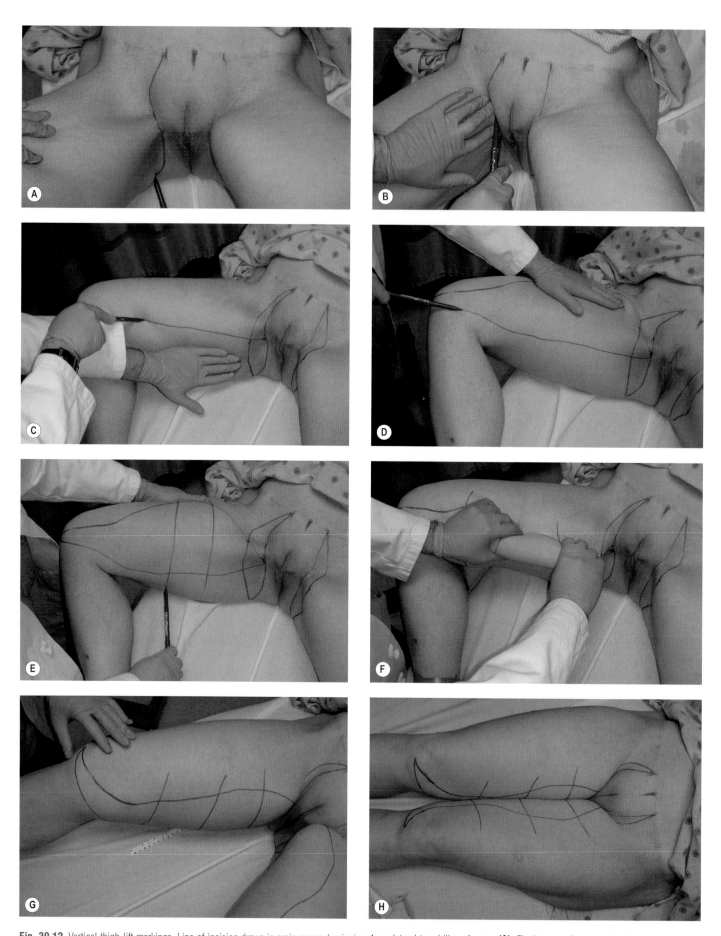

Fig. 30.12 Vertical thigh-lift markings. Line of incision drawn in groin crease beginning 4 cm lateral to midline of mons **(A).** Pinch test estimates vertical component of skin resection **(B).** Anterior line of resection drawn by placing posterior traction with left hand and marking along mid-thigh, demonstrating estimated scar position **(C).** Posterior line of resection drawn by applying anterior traction with nondominant hand and marking along mid-thigh **(D).** Transverse reference lines drawn for tissue alignment during closure **(E).** Estimated margins of resection are checked **(F).** Distally, the resection crosses the knee in the mid-axial position and curves under the patella **(G).** Symmetry is checked **(H).**

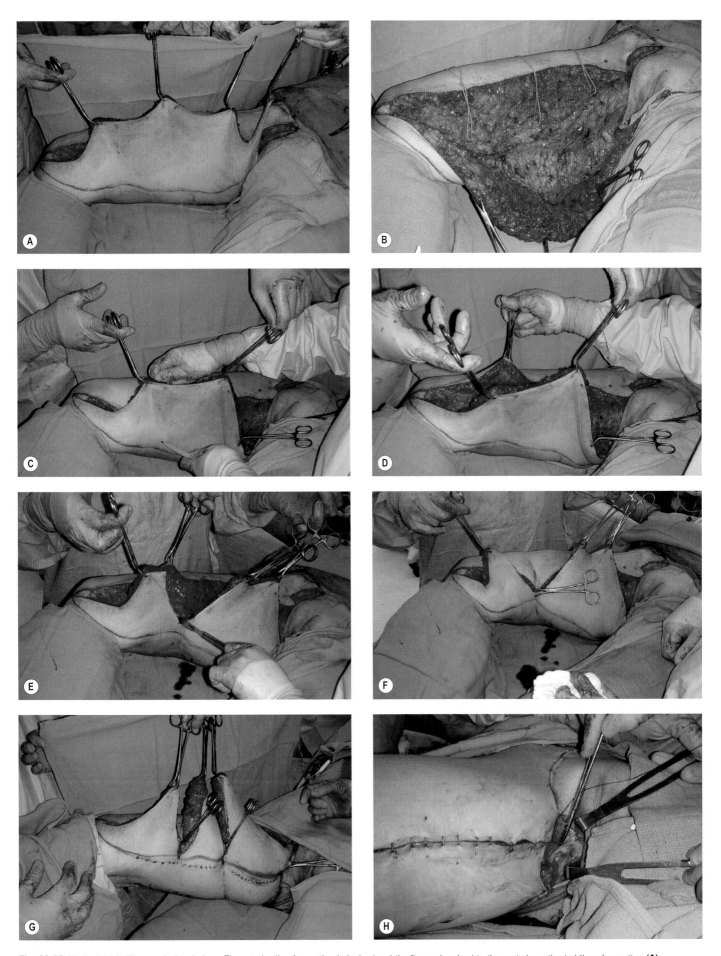

Fig. 30.13 Vertical thigh-lift – surgical technique. The anterior lie of resection is incised and the flap undermined to the posterior estimated line of resection **(A)**. Identification and preservation of the saphenous vein (marked with vessel loops). The pane of dissection is superficial to the vein **(B)**. Towel clips hold the flap while an everted towel clip placed at the edge of the anterior incision line is used as a flap marker **(C,D)**. The flap is incised at intervals and secured with towel clips **(E,F)**. The posterior line of resection is remarked between the towel clips and incised **(G)**. Braided nylon sutures approximate the SFS of the thigh to Colles' fascia **(H)**.

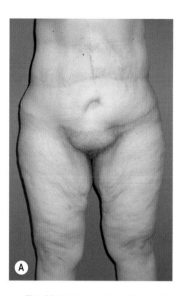
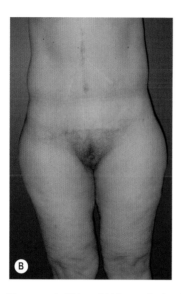
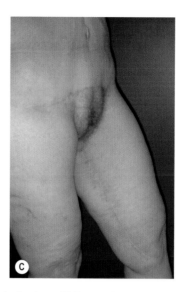
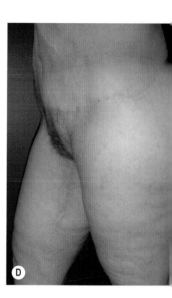

Fig. 30.14 Vertical thigh-lift. A 52-year-old woman s/p 60 kg weight loss and prior abdominoplasty. **(A)** Preoperatively. Postoperative views 1 year after revision abdominoplasty and vertical medial thigh-lift without having had a lower bodylift **(B–D)**.

If including any degree of horizontal skin resection adjacent to the groin area, the degree to which any downward traction is transmitted to the genital area in females is assessed. Labial spreading with exposure of the labia minora postoperatively may occur and care must be taken to minimize this risk.

Operative technique (Fig. 30.13)

The legs are prepped and draped circumferentially. Additional arm boards are placed laterally to support the legs in abduction. Incision of the anterior line, followed by flap elevation towards the posterior line is performed. The saphenous vein is identified and preserved. The posterior incision line is checked for the ability to close, and dissection carried out. Resection of the horizontal component occurs in a superficial plane to preserve lymphatics. The lymphatic drainage of the leg is concentrated medially. Multi-layered closure over drains, followed by circumferential compressive wraps is performed. A representative case is shown in *Figure 30.14*.

An alternative approach to correcting the medial thigh area has been described by Cram and Aly.[122] Vertical resection is also used in this technique, with the option of a transverse perineal resection if necessary to correct the resultant dog-ear. A similar resection is marked, however, the "double ellipse" technique is used to avoid over-resection. The procedure begins with aggressive suction lipectomy in the proposed area of excision in order to completely defat the area. The ellipse is tailor-tacked to simulate closure. Adjustments are made. The resection is performed segmentally from distal to proximal and each section closed with staples temporarily prior to advancing. This prevents excessive intraoperative edema from forming and helps avoid the inability to close. Dog-ears at the superior aspect of resection may be corrected with a transverse excision in the perineal crease. Small to moderate amounts of residual fullness distally may be ameliorated with localized liposuction.

Postoperative care

Ambulation is encouraged the evening of surgery; the legs remain elevated; 4 weeks in compressive stockings including the feet aids in edema prevention. Drains are removed when the output is <30 cc in a 24-hour period.

Complications

Virtually all patients undergoing medial thigh-lifting procedures develop varying degrees of temporary lower extremity edema. Compression garments and leg elevation may aid in minimizing edema in the early period. In the majority of cases, edema resolves within months. Disabling lymphedema of the lower extremity is one of the most feared complications that may occur following any thigh-lifting procedure. Careful and superficial dissection in the femoral triangle may help avoid lymphedema.

If including any horizontal resection of skin adjacent to the groin, labial spreading is possible and is a leading cause of medicolegal action in thigh-reduction procedures.[122] More common complications such as hematoma, seroma, poor scarring and asymmetries are also possible.

Contouring of the arms, breast, upper trunk, and male chest in the massive weight loss patient

Brachioplasty and axillary contouring; mastopexy and breast reshaping; upper bodylift after weight loss and gynecomastia in the massive weight loss patient are covered in Volume V, Chapter 24.

Staging and combination procedures

Unlike many patients presenting for correction of specific areas, the post-bariatric patient often presents requesting a number of areas be treated. Careful preoperative considerations need to be evaluated. Factors including medical status, length of procedure, vectors of tension, surgeon experience, operative assistance, and cost to the patient play a role.

There is a paucity of information regarding the safety and complication rates in patients undergoing multiple concomitant procedures. The MWL population differs significantly from the nonweight loss population. A recent study by Coon et al., demonstrated that multiple procedures may be combined safely in the body contouring patient.[126] Aggregate minor complication rates were higher than with single-procedures and there was no significant increase on a per-procedure basis.

Although no consensus exists, many surgeons believe that stages should be separated by a minimum of 3 months. A patient should be back to their preoperative health status prior to a second stage. There is no strong data to suggest a defined limit for operative time during each stage.[127,128]

When faced with a patient requesting multiple procedures, the order in which they are carried out may vary from patient to patient. Assessing an individual's desires regarding the areas of the body of priority is a must. Patient desires combined with surgeon preference and the patient's overall medical condition will help decide the order of procedures.[128] In general, if a lower bodylift and medial thigh-lift are considered, the circumferential truncal procedure should be done in a first stage. This will set the foundation for following procedures and may safely be combined with upper body procedures such as breast surgery or brachioplasty. This is our preference for the following reasons:

1. The LBL will have a more immediate impact on the patient's overall body shape and therefore, body image.

2. The LBL will relax over time allowing medial and inferior rotation of the medial thigh tissues.

3. If LBL and medial thigh-lift procedures were performed at the same time, patient recovery would be more difficult, and may also be taxing on the surgical team.

If an upper bodylift procedure to treat back rolls and a circumferential lower body procedure is to be undertaken, the upper bodylift should be performed in a second stage following the truncal procedure. If upper body and lower body posterior contouring procedures are performed concomitantly, competing, opposing tensions may lead to banding with less aesthetic contouring compared with when the procedures were staged. There is a description of a single-staged total bodylift for complete torso correction. A combination of lower bodylifts, upper bodylifts, and circumferential abdominoplasty are performed concomitantly. Brachioplasty, breast surgery, and liposuction are commonly done at this single stage. While a complication rate of 76% was noted and mostly related to wound healing issues,[129] the authors considered single-stage total bodylift to be a safe and effective technique in selected patients if performed by a plastic surgeon and team experienced in body contouring surgery.[129,130]

Complications/secondary procedures

The majority of complications from post-bariatric body contouring are wound related. Small areas of wound breakdown or dehiscence, along with suture extrusion are common occurrences.

Seromas occur not infrequently.[131] Serial aspiration is performed with a large-gauge needle, usually on a weekly basis until resolution occurs. In some instances, ultrasound-guided drainage may be required. Techniques to avoid seromas in the body contouring patient include sutures to secure the undersurface of the flap to the deep tissues, the use of tissue sealants (off-label use), and the use of multiple drains.[132,133]

Although variable between surgeons, removal of drains generally occurs when drainage is <30 cc over a 24-hour period. However, some routinely remove drains at 2 weeks and rely less on the amount of drainage. If the amount of drainage continues to be substantial at 2–3 weeks postoperatively, the injection of dilute doxycycline (100 mg in 5 cc of saline) into the drain tubing may be used. Following injection, the drain is left off-suction for 4 hours. Suction is reapplied. Although anecdotal, some report improvement in seroma formation following this technique.[134]

BMI at the time of surgery may impact complication rates.[80] Three or more procedures in a single stage may increase the risk of blood transfusion and increase the length of postoperative hospital stay.[135] The risk of complications is not significantly different following bariatric surgery as compared with massive dietetic weight reduction.[136] Recurrence of varying amounts of skin laxity may also occur, sometimes requiring secondary procedures (mostly involving further skin tightening). In many cases, relapse or skin loosening is expected,[77] and patients advised of the possible need for secondary procedures to address this finding.

Body contouring centers of excellence

Like their bariatric surgery counterparts, plastic surgeons are realizing that an organized center of excellence, dedicated to body contouring can have multiple benefits.[137] Even following MWL, specialized resources are necessary for some in order to further, or maintain their goals. Dedicated, multidisciplinary centers may improve the safety and efficacy of weight loss surgery and post-bariatric reconstruction.[61] Patients benefit from on-site nutritional assessments at the initial consultation. Standardized screening is facile, and evaluation by all team members occurs. The idea of a team approach allows the plastic surgeon to perform more procedures in a single stage, as operative time is significantly decreased. Research and innovation may flourish associated with a center of excellence, as databases and quality assurance measures can be used.[64]

Access the complete references list online at **http://www.expertconsult.com**

17. Pories WJ, Swanson MS, MacDonald KG, et al. Who would have thought it? An operation proves to be the most effective therapy for adult-onset diabetes mellitus. *Ann Surg*. 1995;222(3):339–352.

51. Anon. A review of bariatric surgery procedures. *Plast Reconstr Surg*. 2006;117(1 Suppl):8S–13S.

72. Aly AS, ed. Belt lipectomy. In: *Body contouring after massive weight loss*. St Louis: Quality Medical; 2006:71–145.

   The authors describe their experience with circumferential belt lipectomy. Technical aspects and review of results is discussed. This procedure should be considered for any patients with circumferential truncal excess who are well informed about the possible risks of the procedure.

73. Rubin JP, Nguyen V, Schwentker A. Perioperative management of the post-gastric-bypass patient presenting for body contour surgery. *Clin Plast Surg*. 2004;31(4):601–610, vi.

76. Krueger JK, Rohrich RJ. Clearing the smoke: the scientific rationale for tobacco abstention with plastic surgery. *Plast Reconstr Surg*. 2001;108(4):1063–1077.

80. Coon D, Gusenoff JA, Kannan N, et al. Body mass and surgical complications in the postbariatric reconstructive patient: analysis of 511 cases. *Ann Surg*. 2009;249(3):397–401.

92. Davison SP, Venturi ML, Attinger CE, et al. Prevention of venous thromboembolism in the plastic surgery patient. *Plast Reconstr Surg*. 2004;114(3):43E–51E.

   Review of current guidelines and procedures used to decrease the risk of venous thromboembolism specifically regarding the plastic surgery patient.

114. Lockwood T. Lower bodylift with superficial fascial system suspension. *Plast Reconstr Surg*. 1993;92(6):1112–1125.

   The author presents his experience with patients undergoing lower bodylift alone or in conjunction with other body contouring procedures. Key technical elements regarding lower bodylift are highlighted and results are reviewed.

122. Cram A, Aly A. Thigh reduction in the massive weight loss patient. *Clin Plast Surg*. 2008;35(1):165–172.

   A review of the authors' technique and experience with vertical medial thigh-lifts in the massive weight loss patient.

126. Coon D, Michaels 5th J, Gusenoff JA, et al. Multiple procedures and staging in the massive weight loss population. *Plast Reconstr Surg*. 2010;125(2):691–698.

   Principles in staging of multiple procedures and evaluation of outcomes are discussed.

31

Aesthetic genital surgery

Gary J. Alter

SYNOPSIS

- Male and female aesthetic genital surgery can greatly enhance confidence if a real or perceived deformity exists.
- Many new genital surgeries have been developed.
- In the male, penile enlargement surgery can result in severe deformities, which can often be reconstructed.
- Hidden penis, penoscrotal web, and scrotum reduction surgeries are very successful with a low complication rate.
- Labia minora and clitoral hood reduction performed by the "extended central wedge" excision gives a natural appearance with very high patient satisfaction.
- Mons pubic lifting and labia majora reduction, with or without fat excision, increase self-esteem.
- As with all aesthetic surgeries, genital surgery requires the same meticulous attention to detail.

Introduction

Identity and self-esteem are intimately related to a person's image of his or her genitalia. Self-esteem can be impaired if a person feels inadequate compared with a perceived ideal. A normal man may consider his penis to be too small or a woman may judge her genital appearance as unsightly. These feelings develop from self-comparisons with pornographic photos or videos, media attention, or comments from a sexual partner or friend.

Patient awareness has led to significant demand for aesthetic genital surgery. Recently, new techniques to enhance the appearance of male and female genitalia have been developed, based partially on improved reconstructive pediatric and adult surgical procedures. Considerable aesthetic improvement in the genital appearance is now possible. The surgery is challenging and requires strict attention to detail and meticulous technique.

Male genital aesthetic surgery

Introduction

Several procedures are now available to enhance or improve the aesthetic appearance of the penis or scrotum. Penile lengthening is performed by releasing the suspensory ligament of the penis followed by the use of penile weights or stretching devices. Penile girth is increased by either injecting fat or by inserting dermal fat grafts or allografts such as AlloDerm into the dartos fascia. Penoscrotal webbing may be corrected with one or several Z-plasties, often combined with excision of the web skin. An enlarged, low-hanging scrotum can be reduced and lifted. The hidden or buried penis is corrected with a suprapubic lipectomy, possible upper pubic skin resection, and stabilization of pubic and penoscrotal skin.

Men are very resistant to psychiatric evaluation prior to penile enlargement surgery. Many of the men presenting for penile enlargement have significant generalized self-esteem issues, so refusal to perform the surgery may be justified. The psychological motivations of a man with a hidden penis, penoscrotal webbing, scrotal enlargement, or true congenital deformities are different from those of a man with a normal sized penis who desires only enlargement, so his care is usually more rewarding for both the patient and the surgeon.

Measurements

Schonfeld and Beebe[1] determined that the length of the fully stretched flaccid penis correlated closely with the erect penis. The dorsal length from the junction of the penopubic skin to the tip of the glans in the fully stretched flaccid penis correlated closely to the erect penis. Erect girth or circumference correlated with girth measurements of the flaccid penis according to a more complicated ratio.

Da Ros and Teloken et al.[2] performed artificial erections on 150 Caucasian men, measuring penis length from the center of the pubic bone to the tip of the glans and penis circumference at the corona and base. Average penis length was 5.7 inches; 18 were shorter than 4.7 inches and 18 longer than 6.3 inches. Circumference at the base of the penis ranged from 3.5 to 5.9 inches (average 4.7) and at the coronal groove from 3.2–5.5 inches (average 4.4).

Wessells *et al.*[3] compared the relationship between penile length in the flaccid stretched and in erect states and also concluded that there was a positive relationship. The average flaccid stretched penile length was 11 cm, while the average erect penile length was 12.5 cm. The correlation between stretched length and erect length was $r^2=0.769$. Average flaccid circumference was 10 cm with an average erect circumference of 12.5 cm, and, therefore, correlation was not favorable for circumference. They also state that a thick pubic fat pad decreases visible flaccid penile length but not functional penile length during intercourse.

Patient selection/examination

The patient is evaluated both standing and supine to determine variations that change with gravity. While standing, the penis is checked for concealment owing to descent of the pubic fat pad and escutcheon from gravity, since supine positioning often eliminates this abnormality. A protuberant abdomen with excess skin and fat may overhang the penis and functionally interfere with sexual intercourse, so he may need an abdominoplasty in addition to a suprapubic lipectomy and skin excision. The amount of suprapubic fat between the pubic symphysis and the skin should be evaluated to determine potential length improvement from suprapubic lipectomy or liposuction. Penis position must be checked to see if it is partially encircled by the scrotum. The underside of the penis should be examined for penoscrotal webbing that causes an aesthetically or functionally shorter penis. Supine measurements are taken from the pubic bone and from the skin over the pubis to the tip of the glans on full stretch while the penis is at 90° to the abdomen. Circumference is measured at the base and corona with the penis on full stretch. The penis should be palpated for Peyronie's plaques, which are firm scars on the tunica albuginea.

It is important to question and evaluate function prior to penile surgery. Urinary and orgasmic function should be normal but are not affected by these procedures.

The patient is asked if he has any erectile difficulties or penile curvature. Most men have some minor curvatures, but these are not bothersome and are not an issue. However, if girth surgery is considered, any known or suspected curvature should be documented. The patient is asked to present photographs showing his erect penis from various angles. If the patient is unwilling to present photographs, an erection can be obtained, and then photographed, by patient self-stimulation or by intracavernosal injection of prostaglandin E1. This pharmacologic agent is injected with a 30-gauge needle transversely into the cavernosal bodies at the base of the penis. The injected dosage usually is 10 μg in the normal male. The patient should be cautioned about the possibility of priapism and the necessity for mandatory reversal of the erection if it persists longer than 4 hours. The erection can be immediately reversed with a low-dose intracavernosal injection of phenylephrine, which is routinely performed to reverse a pharmacologic erection at the end of surgery.

Once the diagnosis is made, the possible procedures are discussed with the patient, as well as risks and benefits. Penoscrotal webbing and extensive suprapubic fat and pubic descent may not be presenting complaints, but the physician must describe these abnormalities and possible corrective surgery. Each individual is evaluated to determine the best method to achieve his goals, since several procedures are available depending on the patient's anatomy. He must have a realistic understanding of the design and limitations of the surgery in order to prevent misconceptions and dissatisfaction. Exaggerated promises lead to patient disappointment, depression, and hostility; therefore, honesty, clear communication, and compassion are mandatory for both patient and physician. Because not all malpractice carriers will cover physicians for penile enlargement procedures, verification of coverage is recommended.

Anatomy

The suspensory ligament of the penis is a thick, triangular band extending from the linea alba and the upper portion of the symphysis pubis and arcuate ligament to the dorsal midline of the penis.[4] It derives from the outer investing fascia of the abdomen and divides into a sling at the junction of the fixed and mobile portions of the penis. In addition, thickened bands of Scarpa's fascia, called the fundiform ligaments, firmly attach to the rectus fascia above the pubic symphysis and extend onto the dorsal and lateral penis, possibly restricting penile excursion.[5]

The skin of the penis is thin, hairless (more distal), and has loose connections with the deeper structures of the penis. No adipose tissue is present under the skin. The superficial or subcutaneous fascia of the penis (dartos fascia) is continuous with the Scarpa's and Camper's fascias of the lower abdomen and extends to the corona of the penis. The dartos fascia contains scattered smooth muscle cells. Branches of the superficial external pudendal vessels provide the blood supply to the dartos fascia and skin. The internal pudendal system, which includes the deep dorsal arteries and veins and the cavernosal and urethral vessels, usually communicates with the external pudendal system only at the glans and corona.[6] Because the dartos fascia is highly vascular, it provides an excellent tissue bed for grafts. Buck's fascia invests the shaft of the penis deep to the dartos fascia. The dorsal nerves of the penis supply erogenous sensation to the glans penis. The deep dorsal vessels and the dorsal nerve travel in the pudendal canal along the ischial ramus and then pass ventrally along the margin of the inferior ramus of the pubis in the deep perineal pouch. The neurovascular bundles pierce the perineal membrane ½ inch from the symphysis pubis and continue within Buck's fascia of the penis. Each of the two deep dorsal arteries lies between the deep dorsal vein in the midline and the dorsal nerves of the penis laterally.

Penile enlargement

Penile lengthening

Penile lengthening is achieved by releasing the suspensory ligament of the penis and the postoperative use of penile weights or stretching devices *(Fig. 31.1A)*.[7–10] The ligament is patient has a shortage of penile skin. Penile length gain is disputed in most cases, and the VY flap can actually cause the penis to appear either longer or shorter in the flaccid state. The VY flap is based distally at the penopubic junction varying from a small (2–3 cm) to a large base. The larger flap encompasses the entire dorsal base of the penis and part of the scrotum, which causes interruption of a significant portion of the proximal penile dartos fascia and skin. The blood supply and lymphatic drainage of the penis is thus partially interrupted which can cause healing complications such as flap tip loss, poor wound healing with wound dehiscence, and postoperative swelling. Healing problems predispose to hypertrophic or wide scars, which create hairless pubic scars and depressions *(Figs 31.2A, 31.3A)*. The large VY flap also advances thick, hair-bearing tissue onto the penis, which frequently creates an unnatural hump at the penile base and the appearance of a low-hanging penis.[13–16] The penis can appear surrounded by the scrotum (scrotalization) with an overhanging large pubic fat pad, which makes the penis look shorter and hidden. A VY flap can also create 'dog-ears' at the distal scrotal flap incision. Smaller VY advancement flaps cause less frequent problems, but wound and aesthetic complications also occur.

Outcomes

It is difficult to interpret the results of penile lengthening, because no standardized measurement technique exists, and no mainstream studies have been published.

Suspensory ligament release alone may rarely increase flaccid penile length 1–2 cm, but often no gain is achieved. Real flaccid and erect length gain may be obtained by using penile weights or penile stretching devices. Patients can use these devices without undergoing ligament release, but the ligament release frees more of the penis to be expanded, thereby possibly increasing the amount of eventual length gain. A patient should not undergo release of the suspensory ligament unless he is willing to use the stretching devices. Approximately one week after surgery, the patient suspends the weights or devices from the end of the penis several times daily over a period of months to years, stretching the corporal bodies. The amount of weight required as well as the duration and frequency of use are still evolving. Other devices are available to produce constant penile stretching and traction.

The amount of length gain achieved is controversial, and most patients probably do not achieve any significant increase even with stretching devices. Actual length gains of several inches are rare, but may occur if a suprapubic lipectomy is also performed on thick subcutaneous tissue. However, anecdotal flaccid as well as erect increases of several inches have been reported by some compulsive weight-users. In fact, a one-half to one-inch gain is considered very successful, albeit very uncommon.

An occasional patient may complain of penile shortening after release of the suspensory ligament. Since there is a dead space between the pubic symphysis and the corpora, it is possible for the corpora to reattach in a shortened position. This dead space can be filled by a proximal or distal based fat flap transposed from the medial spermatic cord *(Fig. 31.4)*. However, most doctors tell the patients to stretch the penis after the release without filling the space.

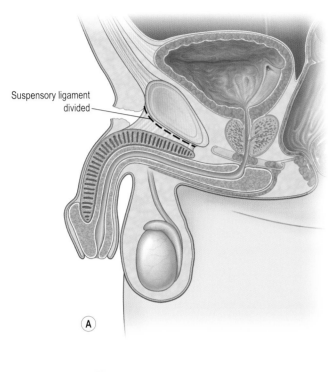

Suspensory ligament divided

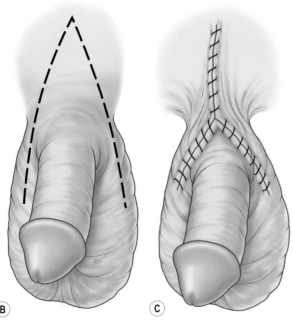

Fig. 31.1 Method commonly used for penile lengthening that often causes penile deformities. **(A)** The suspensory ligament is released. **(B)** A large VY advancement flap is designed. **(C)** The flap is advanced, resulting in hair on the proximal penile shaft, bilateral dog-ears, and a lower-hanging penis.

released only one fingerbreadth by cutting directly on the periosteum throughout the length of the midline pubic symphysis. The release is usually performed through a 3–4 cm lower transverse incision just above the penopubic junction, but many surgeons advance infrapubic skin onto the penis using a VY advancement flap *(Fig. 31.1B,C)*.[11,12] This VY flap theoretically increases penile length or gives the penis the appearance of increased flaccid length, which may occur if the

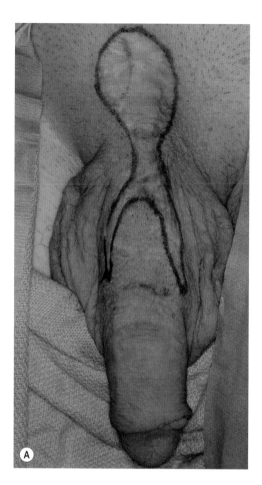

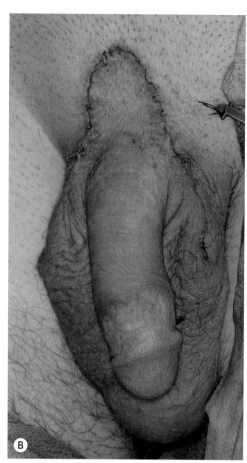

Fig. 31.2 Complete reversal of VY advancement flap. **(A)** The scar is marked for excision. The marking at the base of the VY flap on the left is the estimated location for the reapproximation of the flap to the pubic hairline. **(B)** Complete reversal of the VY flap resulting in a semicircular incision line. Hair on the VY flap is aligned with the pubic hair.

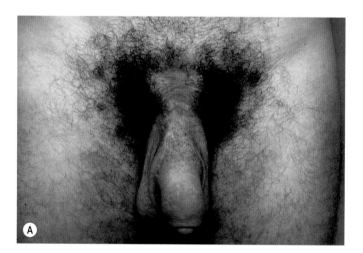

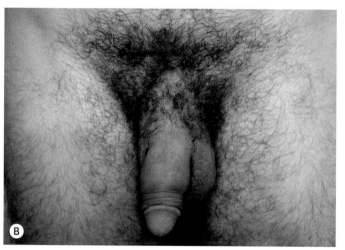

Fig. 31.3 Patient who had release of the suspensory ligament, a large VY advancement flap, and fat injections. **(A)** The deformity shows a low-lying penis, hair on the proximal shaft, bilateral dog-ears at the penoscrotal junction, a short-appearing penis, wide pubic scars, and fat in the shaft. **(B)** Reconstruction after partial reversal of the VY advancement flap, correction of the VY dog-ears, scar revisions, and selective removal of fat. Complete reversal of the VY flap was not possible due to previous partial loss of a portion of the VY flap.

Penile instability is very rare after suspensory ligament release and usually results from an overly aggressive release of the corporal bodies from the ischiopubic rami. If the release is limited to one fingerbreadth on the midline of the pubic symphysis, this will not occur. Dorsal nerve or vessel injuries are prevented by staying directly on the pubic periosteum of the midline of the symphysis with the penis on full stretch and by not releasing the corpora laterally. A mild decrease in the elevation of the erection can occur with release but is not problematic.

Girth increase treatment

Techniques to increase penile girth are in a constant state of evolvement and are associated with the largest incidence of complications. The difficulty of achieving girth enhancement is the necessity to create a symmetrical relatively cylindrical phallus. Any graft that may resorb can cause visual or functional deformities. Thus, many techniques have been used with varying success.

Simultaneous lengthening and girth enhancement procedures are not performed by some physicians, because weight use needs to be delayed several weeks owing to penile swelling and discomfort, which risks premature ligament reattachment. Moreover, the complication rate increases if both operations are performed simultaneously, resulting in wound problems and decreased graft survival. A girth procedure is sometimes performed once length is achieved.

Fat injections

Autologous fat injections into the dartos fascia are still used by some physicians to increase penile thickness. The fat is moveable and gives a somewhat spongy texture to the penis. Less than 50% of injected fat normally survives in other parts of the body. Ideally, small amounts of fat (10–20 cc) are injected in multiple tunnels. Small amounts of total injected fat produce only minimal girth gain but do not have much risk of complications. Complications include asymmetry of the sides of the penis, nodules with bulging and concavities, and loss of penile rigidity due to an overabundance of fat (*Figs 31.3, 31.5A*).

Dermal and dermal fat grafts

Girth enlargement is also performed by inserting either dermal or dermal fat strips into the dartos fascia or by wrapping dermal fat sheets circumferentially between the dartos and Buck's fascias.[7–10] The strips can be placed through either a partial circumcision incision or a transverse pubic incision. The sheet graft, which is not commonly performed, is usually placed through a hemi-circumcision incision and wrapped about 80% of the circumference of the penis with the urethra left uncovered. The grafts are sutured proximally and distally to prevent migration. Usually, the dermal fat grafts 'take' well and provide circumference girth increase from 2–4 cm. However, difficulties with penile immobilization and the thickness of the grafts increase the risk of poor 'take' and subsequent severe complications such as restriction of erection with penile shortening or penile curvature. The procedure is far more invasive than fat injections and requires several hours of surgery. Donor site scars from the buttock crease, suprapubic region, or flanks can be very unsightly. Nodules and fat reabsorption are less common with dermal fat grafts than fat injections. Significant penile edema and induration exist for 6 weeks postoperation, and relatively

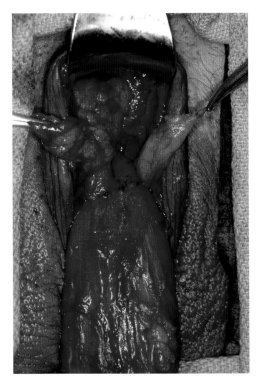

Fig. 31.4 Bilateral fat flaps from the medial spermatic cords are transposed to the midline to fill the dead space at the penile base.

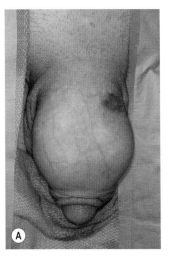
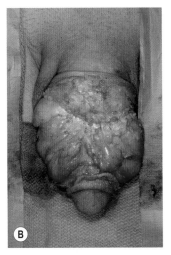
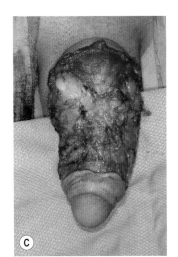
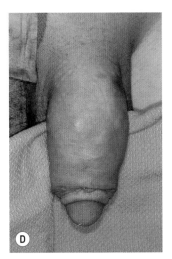

Fig. 31.5 (A) Patient with large volume of injected penile fat that is causing obvious convexities. **(B)** Circumcision incision reveals diffuse fat deposits **(C)**. Residual fat after contouring **(D)**. Penis appearance after closure. It is very difficult to achieve ideal symmetrical contouring.

normal texture returns in 4–6 months. Wrapping a sheet of dermal-fat grafts, rather than inserting strips, provides smooth texture with less risk of ridges and displacement. Penile skin loss has been seen with dermal fat grafts.

Allograft dermal matrix grafts

Alloderm use for girth expansion was motivated by the unpredictability of dermal fat graft 'take' with its cosmetically unappealing donor site scars. Layers of Alloderm are inserted in a plane above the Buck's fascia and stabilized proximally and distally. Theoretically, the Alloderm is a matrix for the ingrowth of tissue and becomes integrated into the area. However, this does not always occur, so the Alloderm can be isolated within a capsule. Since Alloderm does not stretch, the patient may complain of loss of length or curvature. Patients may also complain of an unnatural feel of the penis, displacement of the Alloderm, asymmetry, and visual and palpable deformities. Many cases of infected Alloderm have occurred resulting in chronic infections and chronic skin sinuses with or without skin loss.

True corporal girth increase can be obtained by making lengthwise incisions through the tunica albuginea at the 3 and 9 o'clock locations and then patching these defects with Alloderm or long saphenous vein grafts.[17] This procedure was derived from penile straightening operations for Peyronie's disease. However, most of the results are anecdotal with no large series. The risk of erectile dysfunction is theoretically possible if infection or poor healing occurs, since the erectile chamber is violated.

Other techniques are being tried to increase girth by using tissue engineering with biodegradable scaffolds.[18]

Reconstruction of penile enlargements

Patients present with a diverse array of deformities and reconstructive issues.[15,16] They may have a combination of penile lengthening with VY flaps and/or fat injections, or penile lengthening with Alloderm, etc. The patient must prioritize his reconstructive goals, because complete correction of all the deformities may not be possible at one operation, if at all. He may want only limited fat or Alloderm removal, partial or no VY flap reversal, or minimal scar revisions. Realistic expectations must be emphasized.

Reversal of VY advancement flap

The most common repair is partial or complete reversal of the VY advancement flap with excision of the wide scars (*Figs 31.2, 31.3*).[14–16] Reversal and scar revision eradicates the unsightly dorsal penile hump and proximal penile hair-bearing tissue by re-draping the penis with the normal shaft skin. The penile skin is elevated to its normal position by aligning the hair on the 'V' flap with the pubic hair. The suprapubic concavity and unsightly scars are usually also corrected by partially or completely reversing the VY flap, excising scar tissue, mobilizing Scarpa's fascia and skin from both sides of the vertical scar, and approximating the wound. Complete VY reversal resulting in a semicircular incision is ideal, but it is often impossible or undesirable. Part of the flap tip may have necrosed after the first procedure or

must be excised on this revision to prevent tip flap loss. The patient may have had multiple circumcisions after fat injections stretched the penile skin. Therefore, the adequacy of shaft skin needs to be determined intraoperatively to insure that complete reversal of the flap does not shorten the penis (either real or illusory) and restrict an erection. A pharmacologic erection achieved by intracavernosal injection of Prostaglandin E1 helps to determine skin adequacy. No restriction of erection should occur by pulling on the erect penis. If there is inadequate penile skin for complete reversal, partial reversal is performed which results in an inverted Y-shaped scar with a shorter vertical limb (*Figs 31.3B, 31.6*). The resulting 'Y' scar is more noticeable than the scar from complete reversal.

Reversing the VY flap can cause scrotal 'dog-ears', which are usually followed along the lateral scrotum. The method of closure and 'dog-ear' excision is determined by judging the tightness of the penile skin, taking care not to restrict an erection. Do not eliminate skin discrepancy or 'dog-ears' by making a circular incision through the skin and dartos fascia at the penile base, since prolonged lymphedema or skin loss can occur. Alternatively, the 'dog-ear' is excised from the mid-portion on the lateral side of the incision, creating a lateral dart instead of following the 'dog-ear' medially around the penile base (*Fig. 31.6*).

Excision and scar revision require meticulous skin closure without tension, thus reducing the potential for re-developing a hypertrophic scar. A suction drain is used. Despite careful wound closure, minor healing problems often occur at the common junction of the flaps of the 'Y' with the partial reversal. In addition, some spreading of the scar is common.

Re-release of the suspensory ligament is performed only if the patient complains of penile shortening, since the risk of injury to the dorsal neurovascular structures is increased. In order to prevent reattachment of the corpora bodies to the symphysis in a shortened position, a fat flap or flaps transposed from spermatic cord lipomatous tissue should be placed between the corpora and the pubic symphysis (*Fig. 31.4*).

Fat removal

Most patients with fat injections do not want complete removal of the fat. They usually complain of nodules or penile asymmetry with various concavities or convexities. Removal of fat nodules and/or penile contouring is performed through a limited or complete circumcision incision, a medial raphe incision, or part of a previous VY incision (*Fig. 31.5*). Shaft incisions are cosmetically unacceptable and unnecessary. Deforming or firm fat deposits are removed first followed by contouring of the residual fat. Over-resection of fat creates unsightly concavities, so perform contouring by removing small increments of the deforming fat.

Complete removal of most of the fat can lead to significant complications, so attempts to dissuade the patient from this should be made. If performed, complete fat removal or excision of large diffuse areas of injected fat is usually performed through a circumcision or hemi-circumcision incision. The fat deposits are removed, preserving as much dartos fascia as possible, even if some fat remains. Despite all attempts to leave dartos fascia, a high complication rate occurs;

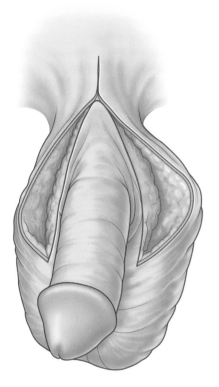
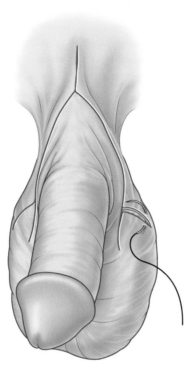

Fig. 31.6 Partial reversal of VY advancement flap. **(A)** The VY flap is reversed as much as possible while preserving penile length. **(B)** Dog-ears are removed by making lateral darts. The can also be removed by extending the incision along the lateral scrotum.

lymphedema may persist for up to 6 months, skin attachment to the Buck's fascia may occur, and fibrous attachments from the dorsal corpora to the pubic subcutaneous tissue and skin can shorten the penis. These skin and fibrous attachments may necessitate Kenalog injections. However, another difficult operation may be required to release this scar tissue and transpose unilateral or bilateral fat flaps to fill the dead space or the area of the skin attachment.

If VY flap reversal is performed, simultaneous removal of fat nodules or deforming fat deposits is limited. Fat is removed through a several centimeter tunnel on one or both sides of the most distal aspect of the VY incisions without undermining the V flap, and/or through a limited circumcision incision. One side of the penis must be kept relatively inviolate to assure adequate lymphatic and blood drainage. However, a proximal medial raphe incision in a patient with a large VY flap reversal may injure the remaining nontraumatized proximal dartos fascia. Removal of large diffuse fat deposits should rarely be done at the same time as the VY reversal, since further flap disruption and dartos fascia injury decrease vascularity of the flap and possibly prolong edema. This large fat removal should not be done earlier than 6 months after VY flap reversal, allowing time for revascularization of the scarred areas.

Dermal fat graft and Alloderm removal

Dermis, dermal fat grafts, and Alloderm present with a variety of different problems, including penile shortening, curvature, and areas of induration.[3] Removal of the grafts are performed though one or a combination of circumcision, median raphe, or low pubic incisions. An indurated, scarred graft that is not adhered to the Buck's fascia can be removed without much difficulty, thereby correcting the deformity *(Fig. 31.7)*.

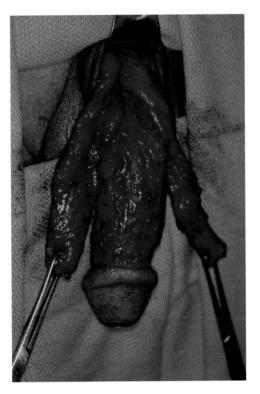

Fig. 31.7 Alloderm was elevated off the Buck's fascia without much difficulty. Fat flaps will be placed at the penile base to prevent scar formation with penile restriction (see Fig. 31.4).

However, the graft may be extensively adhered to the Buck's fascia, so extreme care must be used to prevent injury to the dorsal neurovascular structures. Loupe magnification is usually necessary. Removal of the scarred dermal graft or Alloderm may eliminate the deformity, curvature, or penile restriction, but full return of penile length or straightening may not occur due to permanent scarring of the skin, dartos, or Buck's fascia. Leave as much dartos fascia as possible to prevent skin adhesions to Buck's fascia. Unilateral or bilateral spermatic cord fat flaps are usually used to fill dead space at the penopubic junction to prevent penile shortening *(Fig. 31.4)*. Closed suction drains are used.

Postoperative care

Any significant fat removal or degloving of the penis usually requires a small closed suction drain placed through a pubic stab incision. The dressing used around the penis after any of these surgeries is crucial to recovery, since it will help prevent hematomas and swelling that can lead to secondary deformities. A thin Duoderm dressing is loosely wrapped around the penis followed by a loose Coban wrap. This dressing is not removed for a minimum of 2 days but frequently longer. It is then replaced with a circumferential loose Tegaderm wrap. Drains are kept until they cease draining.

Outcomes

Reconstruction of the complications of these procedures is challenging. These patients are often psychologically devastated, since they started with self-esteem issues that led to their initial penile enlargement operation. Thus, the reconstructions must be done with extreme care in order to regain the patient's penile form, function, and psychological health. The outcome for most patients with reconstruction is usually satisfactory to achieve their goals. There is a low complication rate if meticulous technique is used. However, more than one operation is often necessary. The vast majority of these patients are able to resume normal sex lives without being self-conscious after correction of their deformities.

Penoscrotal web

Scrotal skin extending onto the ventral penile shaft causes an obtuse angle to the penoscrotal junction, thereby obscuring the normal definition to the junction of the scrotum and penis *(Fig. 31.8A)*. The penis appears longer with more functional length if the penoscrotal junction is well defined. The cause of this webbing maybe congenital but is more often caused by over-resection of the ventral penile skin during circumcision. Webbing can cause discomfort during intercourse or when wearing a condom.

A mild web is eliminated using a single or double Z-plasty with the vertical limb centered along the median raphe at the penoscrotal junction.[19,20] Transposition of the flaps lengthens the shortened web and sharpens the penoscrotal junction, which gives the appearance of more ventral length. If the patient has a more severe penoscrotal web with significant excess skin, then the web is excised along the median raphe *(Fig. 31.8B,C)*. The amount of skin that can be excised without causing circumferential penile constriction is determined by giving the patient a pharmacologic erection with an intracavernosal injection of Prostaglandin E1. The excess is then removed and a Z-plasty at the penoscrotal web is made, which prevents a recurrent web re-forming from a scar contracture *(Fig. 31.8D,E)*.

A VY advancement flap can also be used to eliminate a penoscrotal web but care must be taken to prevent scrotal 'dog-ears'.[21,22]

Scrotal enlargement

The scrotum can be enlarged and low-hanging secondary to increased laxity from aging, congenital enlargement, or stretching secondary to a scrotal hydrocele or varicocele *(Fig. 31.9A)*. Enlargement from lymphedema is beyond the extent of this chapter. An enlarged scrotum can cause discomfort or a loss of self-esteem. Reduction of the scrotum can be performed in many ways, but the preferred technique maintains the normal sack-like appearance. If a varicocele or hydrocele is present, it should be corrected first or at the same time to prevent recurrent scrotal stretching.

The posterior scrotum should usually be saved due to its superior lymphatic drainage. Preliminary markings are made with the patient in the standing position in front of a mirror and are checked intraoperatively with the patient in the lithotomy position. Usually, the scrotum is reduced by a horizontal excision of the mid to upper scrotum. However, a lower horizontal excision can be performed if a unilateral scrotal enlargement is present with one testicle significantly lower than the other.

The markings depend on whether the patient has a significant penoscrotal web. If so, the patient is given a pharmacologic erection with Prostaglandin E1 intraoperatively prior to making final markings. The web is bunched in the midline without causing tightness around the penile circumference *(Fig. 31.9B–D)*. Markings are then made for a transverse crescent excision of upper and mid-scrotum angling up towards each pubic region. If the skin is bunched at the penoscrotal junction, lateral 'dog-ears' usually do not occur. If they do, then an inverted 'V' on the right and left lateral scrotum is marked, creating a downward incision. The skin and underlying dartos fascia are excised. The closure may be adjusted to maintain normal scrotal shape *(Fig. 31.9E)*. The dartos is reapproximated with 4-0 reabsorbable sutures, and the skin is closed with a subcuticular reabsorbable suture. A Penrose or closed suction drain is placed.

Meticulous hemostasis is important, since a hematoma is the most common complication. There is sometimes a color and tissue mismatch between the two sides of the incision line, which can make the eventual scar more noticeable. Therefore the patient must be shown this preoperatively, so that he will not be surprised after surgery. Most patients are extremely pleased with the result, both for aesthetic and comfort reasons *(Fig. 31.9F,G)*.

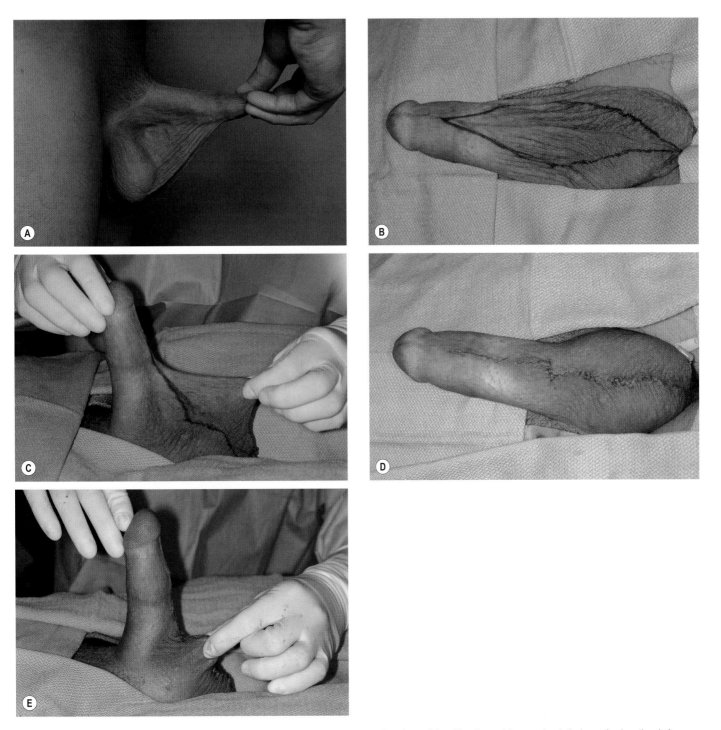

Fig. 31.8 Patient with severe penoscrotal web almost certainly caused by an overly aggressive circumcision. The circumcision scar is relatively proximal on the shaft.
(A) Side view showing severe penoscrotal web and relative deficiency of normal penile skin. **(B,C)** Skin to be excised. Markings are made with a pharmacologically induced erection. **(D,E)** Penis after skin excision with obvious elimination of the web. Notice the Z-plasty at the penoscrotal junction and the drain.

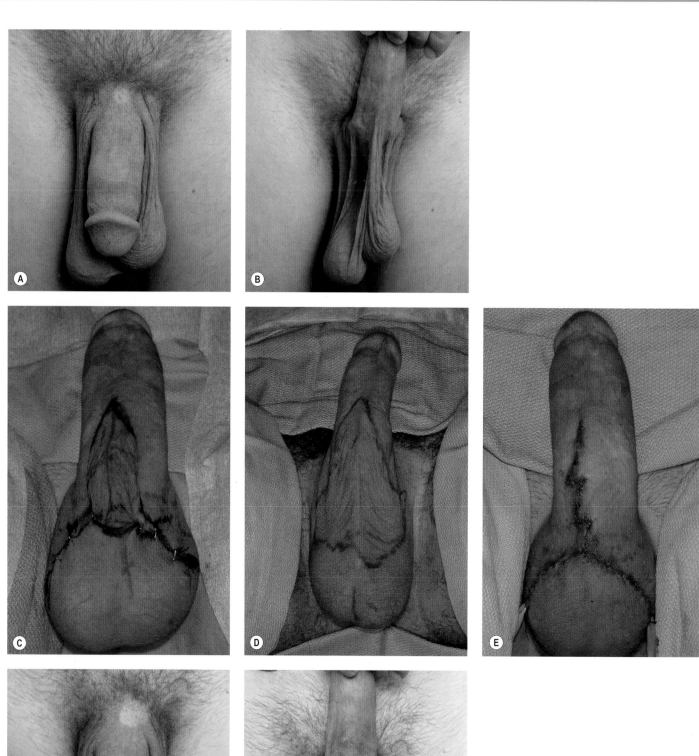

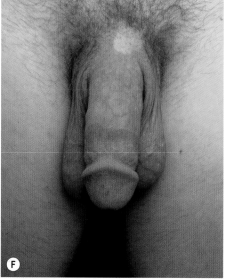

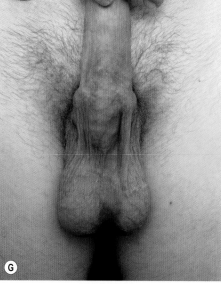

Fig. 31.9 A 27-year-old man for scrotum reduction due to excess skin and laxity. **(A,B)** Notice that the scrotum hangs lower than the penis and that he has a large penoscrotal web. **(C)** The area to be excised is verified with a pharmacologically induced erection. The penoscrotal web is bunched first with tacking sutures. The horizontal excision is then stapled closed and adjusted for an asymmetrical scrotum. **(D)** Skin to be excised (different patient but similar situation). **(E)** The scrotum at the termination of the procedure. There are Z-plasties at the penoscrotal junction. There are no lateral dog-ears because the penoscrotal web was bunched in the midline. **(F,G)** The result at 3 ½ months. The scars are difficult to see. The scrotum does not hang lower than the penis, and the web is eliminated.

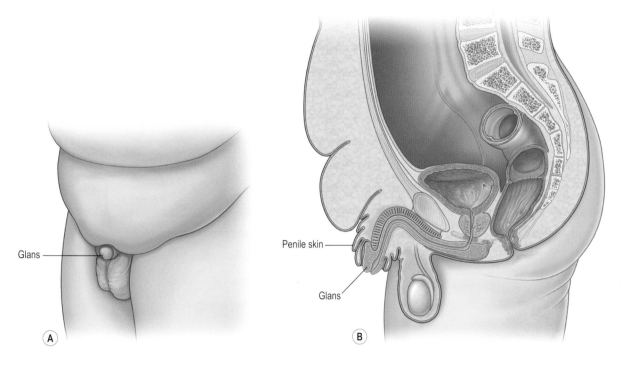

Fig. 31.10 The typical hidden or buried penis. **(A)** The penis is buried in the pubic fat and scrotum. **(B)** The penile shaft skin is not firmly attached to the corporal bodies, so the corporal bodies telescope proximally inside the pubis and scrotum.

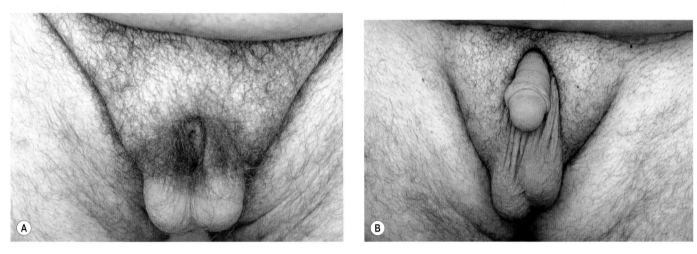

Fig. 31.11 (A) A 32-year-old obese, uncircumcised man with a severe buried penis. **(B)** View at 3 months postoperatively revealing a normal-sized penis. Notice that the pubic skin and fat were excised, which elevates the penopubic skin.

Hidden penis

The terms hidden, concealed, and buried all refer to a penis in which the functional and visual penile length is obscured (*Figs 31.10, 31.11A, 31.12A,B, 31.13A*).[22–41] Penile corporal length may be normal but not visible. Congenital buried penis is uncommon. More often, the penis shaft may be buried below the surface of the pubic skin by a large suprapubic fat pad, obesity, or pubic skin and fat descent from aging or weight loss.[39] Other causes of a hidden penis are an

overly aggressive circumcision, an abdominoplasty with aggressive release of dartos fascia attachments to Scarpa's fascia, or penile lengthening using an ill-advised large pubic VY advancement flap. Buried or hidden penis has severe effects on self-esteem, causing the patient to avoid locker rooms, sport participation, and sexual intimacy. Chronic dampness from a buried penis can cause penile inflammation and destruction of penile skin such as balanitis xerotica obliterans. This section describes the surgical technique to correct the buried adult and pediatric penis on the patient with

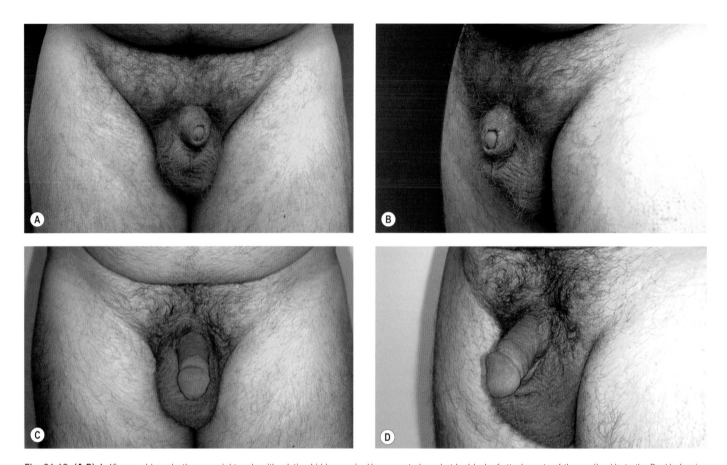

Fig. 31.12 (A,B) A 45-year-old modestly overweight male with relative hidden penis. He was not obese but had lack of attachments of the penile skin to the Buck's fascia. **(C,D)** Two months after a suprapubic dermatolipectomy with liposuction and tacking of the pubic and penoscrotal skin. Notice the mild pubic concavity.

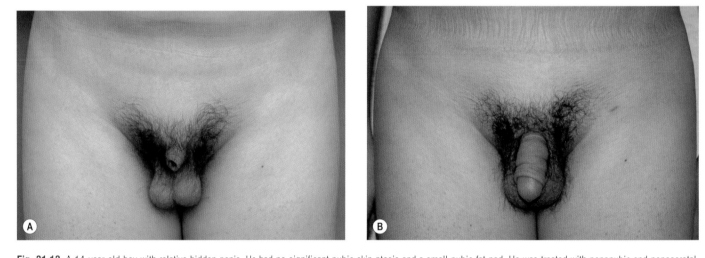

Fig. 31.13 A 14-year-old boy with relative hidden penis. He had no significant pubic skin ptosis and a small pubic fat pad. He was treated with penopubic and penoscrotal tacking and pubic liposuction. **(A)** Preoperation. **(B)** Postoperation at 3 months. He still has residual edema of his penile shaft, which should resolve in another several months.

adequate penile shaft skin. Treatment of inadequate shaft skin with skin grafts or local flaps is beyond the scope of this chapter.[42,43]

Surgery is partially derived from the principles and techniques used to correct the pediatric buried penis. These patients usually have inadequate attachments of the Buck's fascia to the skin and dartos fascia, so the corporal bodies telescope proximally without the skin and dartos covering. Since the corporal bodies may bury into the pubic fat or into the scrotum, it is necessary to reattach and stabilize the dartos and skin to the corporal bodies dorsally and ventrally to assure success.[39]

Surgical technique

Examining the patient in the standing position is required for an accurate diagnosis.

If the patient has excess pubic fat, it should be removed and restricting bands of Scarpa's fascia released to increase penile visual and functional length. Moreover, aging and weight gain and loss causes suprapubic skin and fat to descend, concealing the penis when the patient is standing. Combining fat and skin excision in the aging male with pubic flap stabilization provides a more attractive and youthful appearance to the escutcheon while increasing visual, and often, functional penile length. On occasion, the patient may not have significant pubic fat or skin descent *(Fig. 31.13)*. In these cases, the patient undergoes an incision at the penopubic junction with stabilization of the dorsal penile skin to the tunica albuginea of the penis (see below). Evaluate the penoscrotal junction, since the ventral penis must be stabilized to this skin, oftentimes with correction of a penoscrotal web.

Preoperative markings are made with the patient standing to determine the amount of excess skin. If excess skin is excised to raise the escutcheon, a transverse crescent incision is made well above the level of the pubic hair. If the patient is obese, the incision is made just inferior to the panniculus fold *(Fig. 31.14)*.[39,44] It is uncommon to remove more than a few centimeters of transverse skin, because the pubic skin retracts somewhat with fat removal. On rare occasions of massive obesity, part of the panniculus fat and skin needs to be excised.

Fat is incised to the rectus fascia and the flap of skin and fat is elevated off the rectus fascia to the pubic symphysis between the external rings. The pubic, inguinal, and upper scrotal areas are infiltrated with the usual tumescent fluid.

The pubic area is uniformly liposuctioned to eliminate the fat pad with fat tapering in the inguinal areas and upper scrotum to prevent a pubic concavity. A 1–2 cm layer of subcutaneous fat with its fibrous tissue is kept on the dermal side. Frequently, limited sharp dissection of fat is also performed to remove excess fat resistant to liposuction. Suprapubic fat removal is contoured to match the abdominal side of the incision. Some medial spermatic cord fat is removed, but overly aggressive fat removal in the inguinal regions can cause genital lymphedema and injury to the superficial sensory nerves of the genitalia. The buried corporal bodies are seen and freed from the deep subcutaneous tissue. The suspensory ligament is occasionally partially released. In order to prevent adhesion of the released penis to the pubic symphysis after suspensory ligament release, a fat flap from the lipomatous tissue adjacent to a spermatic cord can be transposed to fill the space (see above).

Tacking this fibrofatty tissue of the suprapubic skin to the rectus fascia maintains the upward position of the escutcheon and stabilizes dorsal penile skin to the penis *(Fig. 31.14B)*. In order to prevent the corporal bodies from retracting under the penile skin into the scrotum and pubis, tacking sutures of No.1 polydioxanone (PDS) sutures on a CTX needle are placed from the fibrous fatty tissue of the flap to the rectus fascia. A No.0 or 2-0 polydioxanone (PDS) on a CT needle may be used on a child. A pharmacologic erection is created by an intracavernosal injection of Prostaglandin E1. Care is then taken not to restrict the erection during placement of the sutures. The first row of three sutures is placed between the external inguinal rings near the pubic symphysis to the subdermal tissue 1–2 cm. cephalad to the penopubic junction. Usually three or four rows of three sutures are placed. Try to prevent excessive dimpling or a deep suprapubic concavity. A closed

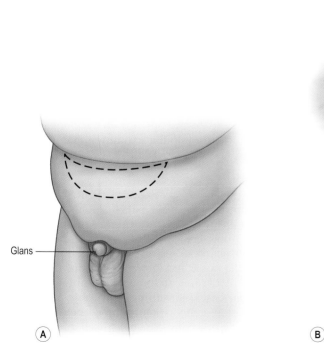

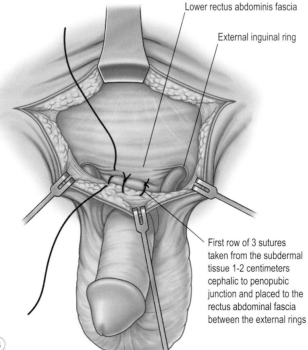

Lower rectus abdominis fascia

External inguinal ring

First row of 3 sutures taken from the subdermal tissue 1-2 centimeters cephalic to penopubic junction and placed to the rectus abdominal fascia between the external rings

Glans

Fig. 31.14 (A) A low transverse incision is made below the panniculus line. Skin excision depends on whether skin excess is present. Pubic fat is removed with liposuction and excision. **(B)** The pubic flap is stabilized to the rectus fascia with rows of tacking sutures.

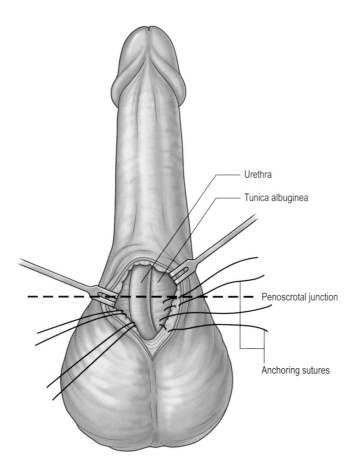

Fig. 31.15 An incision is made at the penoscrotal junction. If a web is present, correction is done with a Z-plasty and/or skin excision. Tacking sutures are taken bilaterally from the tunica albuginea proximal to the penoscrotal junction to the subdermal skin.

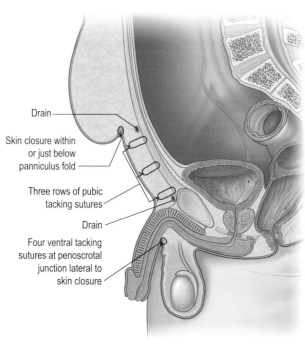

Fig. 31.16 The patient at the end of surgery with stabilization of the pubic skin to the rectus fascia and of the ventral penile skin to the tunica albuginea. The penile skin and corporal bodies are now stabilized as one synchronous unit.

suction drain is placed from the pubic symphysis, around the right side, and under the deep closure of the wound.

Despite suprapubic tacking, the corpora still tend to retract into the scrotum if the ventral skin is not stabilized *(Fig. 31.15)*. Many of these patients also have penoscrotal webbing, which is corrected at the same time (see above). A midline or Z-plasty incision is made at or just inferior to the penoscrotal junction and dissection is performed through the dartos fascia to the corpus spongiosum and tunica albuginea. A pharmacologic erection is induced. Two 2-0 tacking polydioxanone (PDS) sutures on an SH needle are placed at the penoscrotal junction on each side of the urethra horizontally from tunica albuginea to ventral subdermal dartos fascia just inferior to the lateral penoscrotal junction.[39,44] These sutures stabilize the ventral penile skin to the corpora and prevent retraction into fat or scrotum. Care must be taken not to cause excessive skin dimpling from the tacking sutures, but some dimpling is necessary. The dartos fascia and skin are closed *(Fig. 31.16)*.

The patient with no pubic skin excess and mild pubic fat does not need a transverse upper pubic incision *(Fig. 31.13)*. Instead, tacking is performed from the dorsal penopubic subdermal tissue to the proximal dorsal tunica albuginea.[45,46] A 3–4 cm incision is made just cephalad to the penopubic junction. Dissection proceeds to the dorsal corporal bodies. A pharmacologic erection is induced. Longitudinal blunt dissection is performed at the 10 and 2 o'clock location of the Buck's fascia of the penis lateral to the dorsal arteries, and

preferably, lateral to the dorsal nerves. No cutting is performed which could transect the dorsal nerves. Once the tunica albuginea is visible in each of the two locations, two 2-0 Ethibond sutures on an SH needle are placed next to each other *(Fig. 31.17A,B)*. Each of the two sutures on each side is then placed through the subdermal tissue of the penopubic junction to stabilize the skin to the tunica. All four sutures are then tied. A No. 10F round closed suction drain is placed and brought out through a separate stab incision. If mild fat is present, then pubic liposuction is performed with care not to disturb the tacking sutures. The wound is then closed. These patients usually also need penoscrotal tacking.

At the conclusion of any hidden penis procedure, the penis should be prominent and inward pressure on the glans should not allow the penis to bury into the scrotum or abdomen.

Outcomes

Hidden penis surgery is very successful. Patient self-esteem is dramatically improved as most patients have been tormented throughout life by this malady. Complications include an overly concave pubic area, which is much less common with the use of liposuction to remove most of the pubic fat. Tacking sutures in the pubic and scrotal region may not hold over time in a minority of cases, so some skin dimpling during initial placement of the tacking sutures is probably necessary to assure adequate skin stabilization to the corporal bodies. The penopubic tacking procedure is usually used if secondary surgery is needed on patients in whom the pubic tacking sutures did not successfully hold. Repeat penoscrotal tacking may occasionally be necessary, but this is a relatively minor procedure.

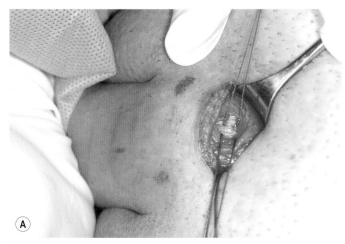

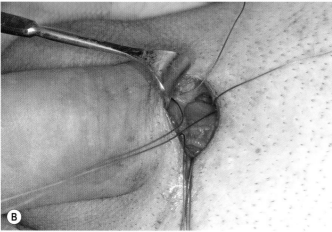

Fig. 31.17 Penopubic tacking on a patient with relative hidden penis and no significant pubic ptosis or fat pad. **(A)** Tacking sutures are placed in the tunica albuginea at the penopubic junction. Two sutures are placed each at the 10 and 2 o'clock positions. The dorsal arteries and dorsal nerves are bluntly dissected away for suture placement. The marks are the locations at the penopubic junction where the sutures will be placed. **(B)** The tacking sutures are placed from the tunica albuginea to the subdermis at the penopubic junction.

Female genital aesthetic surgery

Introduction

Female aesthetic genital ideal is a function of cultural influences or each woman's personal concept of beauty. In recent years, women are more aware of their genital appearance due to the popularity of genital hair removal and the proliferation of pornographic photographic material. Therefore, women compare themselves to others and create an aesthetic ideal. If a woman feels deformed or abnormal, she will have resulting embarrassment or loss of self-esteem.[47–50] These women frequently refrain from social and sexual situations that may require visualization of their genitals, including wearing tight swimsuits, group showers, or sexual intimacy. They often avoid gynecological exams and are too self-conscious to mention their concerns to the doctor, who frequently dismisses them. There is no standard of genital aesthetic ideal. However, most consider ideals as (1) symmetrical labia minora that do not protrude past the labia majora, especially when

standing; (2) a clitoral hood that is reasonably short and non-protuberant with no extra folds; (3) full labia majora without redundant skin but not overly fatty which can cause an unsightly bulge in clothes, and (4) a mons pubis that has mild fullness but does not protrude in clothes.[51] Due to surgical innovations, these results can be achieved in most cases. Reassurance concerning normal variations of the labia may be adequate to allay some women's insecurities, but others seek surgical correction, which achieves improved confidence.

In addition, many women with enlarged labia minora or majora or clitoral hood complain of discomfort during sexual intercourse, with exercise, or when wearing tight clothing. Massively enlarged labia cause difficulty with hygiene, interfere with sexual intercourse, hamper urinary self-catheterization, and cause chronic inflammation.

Anatomy

Knowledge of the vulvar anatomy is necessary to prevent clitoral injury and loss of sensation *(Fig. 31.18)*. The glans clitoris is visible under the prepuce, which is an extension of the clitoral hood. The clitoral body is attached to the pubic symphysis by the suspensory ligament and then each corporal body diverges inferior and lateral to attach bilaterally to the ischiopubic ramus. The frenula are folds of skin extending from the glans clitoris to merge with an extension of the clitoral hood to form the labia minora.

The external genitalia have extensive blood supply.[52] It consists of branches from the external superficial pudendal artery, the internal pudendal artery, and frequent contributions from the internal circumflex artery. The external superficial pudendal artery anastomoses with the posterior labial artery, a branch of the internal pudendal artery, in the labium majora. Multiple arterial arches in the labium minora arise from this initial anastomosis, which provide a rich blood supply.

Labia minora reduction

Labia minora enlargement is congenital in most cases, but some women claim enlargement with age, after childbirth, chronic irritation, or hormones.[53–57] Labia minora reduction is indicated in women as young as 12 years old, when the enlargement severely affects self-esteem or causes discomfort. Fear of embarrassment of one's genitals is a powerful anti-social force. Most women want straight, thin, light-colored, symmetrical labia minora.

Most physicians correct protuberant or asymmetrical labia minora by excising or trimming the abnormal areas using a scissor, knife, clamp or laser and oversewing them.[47,53–58] The advantages of this technique are the short operative time and the creation of light colored labial edges. Disadvantages include elimination of the normal labial edge with the replacement of a longitudinal scar line that is often irregular and scalloped, the higher incidence of chronic discomfort, and a relatively high incidence of asymmetry and over-resection. In addition it is often difficult with the trimming technique to maintain the normal transition between the frenulum of the clitoris, the clitoral hood, and the labium. Other surgeons have reported W-plasties to reduce the protruding labia or S-shaped labial incisions, but these also eliminate the normal labial edge.[59,60] The ideal for any cosmetic procedure is to

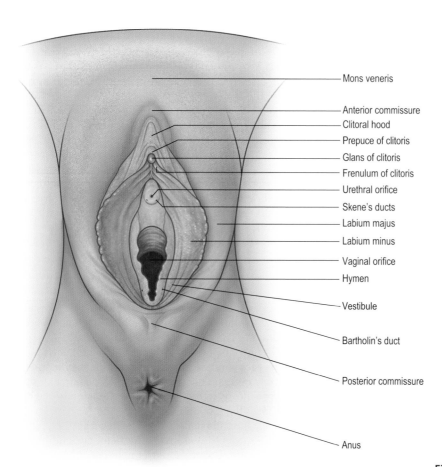

Mons veneris

Anterior commissure
Clitoral hood
Prepuce of clitoris
Glans of clitoris
Frenulum of clitoris
Urethral orifice
Skene's ducts
Labium majus
Labium minus
Vaginal orifice
Hymen

Vestibule

Bartholin's duct

Posterior commissure

Anus

Fig. 31.18 Female external genitalia.

preserve normal anatomy including the normal labial edge. The removal of medial and lateral de-epithelialized labial ellipses eliminates the protrusion but the total length of the labium remains elongated.[48] The extended central wedge technique, which excises a wedge or 'V' of the most protuberant labium and reapproximates the edges, preserves the normal anatomy of the labial edge.[61] Its only disadvantages are a longer operative time, more surgical expertise, and occasional persistence of darker labial pigment.[62,63] Other physicians have reported the use of an inferior wedge, but this maintains the thickness of the labium and has a higher complication rate.[64–66] Another variation of a central wedge using a Z-plasty has also been reported.[67,68]

Surgical technique

Preoperatively, the woman is examined in the lithotomy position with her head elevated. While using a mirror to visualize her genitalia, she indicates her concerns. The proposed surgical plan for central wedge excision is explained and illustrated.[61]

Labia minora vary greatly in length, thickness, and form. Therefore, the surgical markings vary depending on the anatomy. The clitoral hood is evaluated to determine protrusion, symmetry, location of hyperkeratotic darkened skin, the presence of extra folds, and the amount of clitoral glans size and exposure. Evaluate the posterior introitus for a high posterior lip or for gaping due to a previous episiotomy. A large 'V' or central wedge is excised from the most protuberant

portion of each labium *(Fig. 31.19A,B)*. The wedge is adjusted when asymmetry is present. Excellent symmetry can usually be achieved even in very asymmetrical patients. Usually, the most darkly pigmented skin is removed.

The operation is usually performed under general or regional anesthesia in the lithotomy position. The upper labial incision of the wedge is usually placed at or just posterior to the convergence of the glans frenulum with the clitoral hood. The amount of labium excised is determined to achieve a straight, nonredundant labium that can be closed without tension and without causing an overly tight introitus, which is usually insured by placing two fingerbreadths in the vagina. The medial 'V' extends internally to terminate distal to the hymeneal ring. The lateral 'V' is curved anterior in a hockey-stick design to eliminate a 'dog-ear' and to excise a redundant lateral clitoral hood or lateral hood folds *(Fig. 31.19C)*. Thus, the medial and lateral Vs are asymmetrical. On rare occasions, another unilateral or bilateral posterior 'V' is necessary to achieve symmetry or adequate reduction.

Conservative infiltration of the labia is performed with lidocaine with epinephrine and Marcaine after marking. The skin and vaginal mucosa are de-epithelialized with care to leave as much subcutaneous tissue as possible, because a good subcutaneous tissue closure is mandatory to prevent dehiscence of the closure or fistulae. The subcutaneous tissue of the anterior and posterior labium is reapproximated, usually in two layers, with 5-0 Monocryl on an atraumatic TF needle *(Fig. 31.19D)*. Loupe magnification is usually necessary to achieve accurate approximation. The internal and external

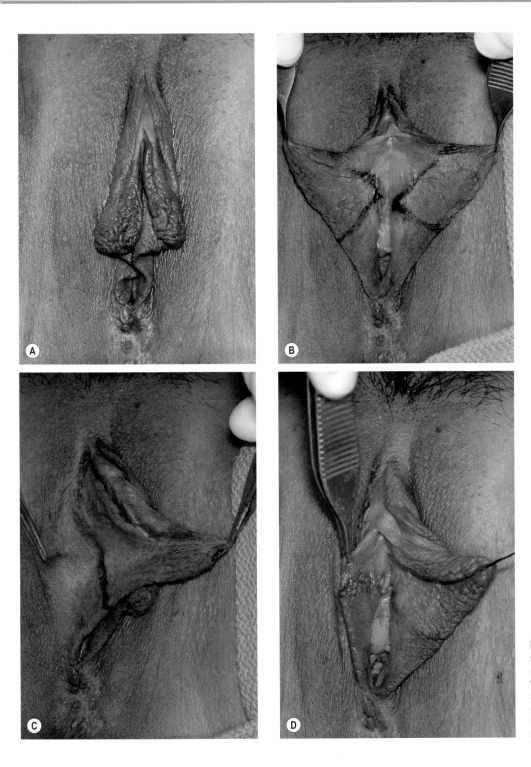

Fig. 31.19 A 47-year-old underwent labia reduction and lateral clitoral hood reduction. **(A)** Preoperation. **(B)** Internal 'V' markings with the labia open. **(C)** External hockey stick 'V' marking extending along the lateral clitoral hood to the anterior hood. **(D)** The completed right side compared to the left side.

subcutaneous 'dog-ears' are excised. The labial edges and medial and lateral closures are re-approximated with interrupted, horizontal mattress 5-0 Monocryl on a TF needle. Running sutures can be used on the deepest portion of the medial incision line or occasionally on the most lateral labium. The lateral clitoral hood is closed with running 5-0 Monocryl in the subcutaneous tissue and a running subcuticular 5-0 Monocryl on the skin. The only suture line on the leading edge of the labium is a small transverse line *(Fig. 31.19E)*. If possible, the labia should protrude only slightly past the introitus, but this may not be possible if the labia are massively enlarged.

If the clitoral hood has extra vertical medial folds or medial hypertrophic skin, these can be excised with vertical ellipses. In this case, the lateral 'V' labial excision can stop at the lateral labium. Occasionally, the patient may have redundant horizontal folds, which can be excised with a conservative transverse ellipse. However, this can result in overexposure of the glans clitoris that can cause hypersensitivity or an unacceptable aesthetic appearance. More aggressive clitoral hood reduction with clitoral repositioning (clitoropexy) can be performed but is beyond the scope of this chapter as is clitoral glans and shaft reduction.

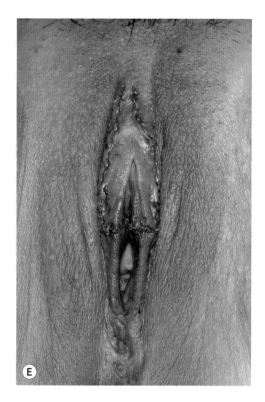

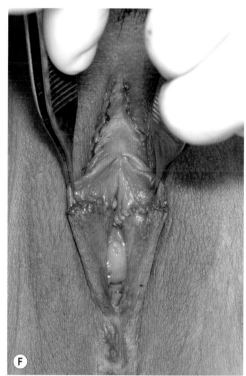

Fig. 31.19, cont'd (E) Postoperation.
(F) Postoperation with the labia open.

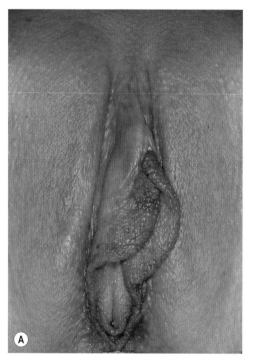

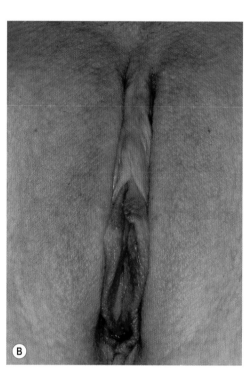

Fig. 31.20 A 50-year-old woman underwent labia minora and lateral clitoral hood reduction. **(A)** Preoperation. **(B)** Postoperation at 3 months

If the introitus is too tight or if the posterior lip is too high, a midline incision can be made at the 6 o'clock position with a careful aesthetic closure of the resulting 'dog-ears'. If a perineoplasty or posterior vaginal repair or tightening is performed at the same time as a large labia minora reduction, care needs to be taken to insure that the introitus is not overly tight. This can be prevented by delaying the perineal and vaginal repair distal to the hymeneal ring until the labia reduction is completed, which allows for introital adjustments during this closure.

Outcomes

Patients heal well with normal appearing labia minora *(Figs 31.19F, 31.20, 31.21)*. The most common complications are a slight separation of the labial edge closure or a small fistula, but these occur in less than 2% of cases if the above guidelines are followed. Major dehiscence is rare if performed as stated. A minor separation or fistula can be easily repaired in 4–6 months under local anesthesia. Chronic scar discomfort or interference with intercourse are very rare and can be

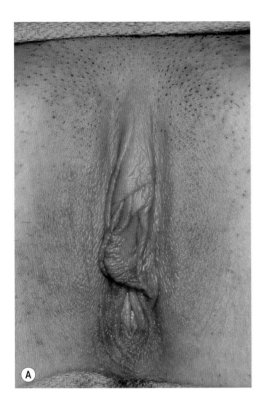 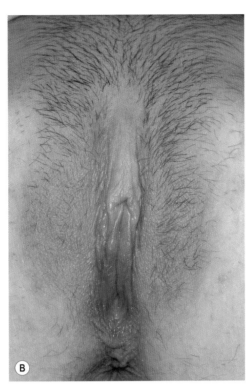

Fig. 31.21 A 44-year-old woman underwent labia minora and medial-lateral clitoral hood reduction. **(A)** Preoperation. **(B)** Postoperation at 3 months.

corrected. On occasion, the labia can stretch or the scars may spread, which can easily be reduced. If the labia still protrude too far after maximal 'V' excision, then medial and lateral elliptical excisions can be performed later, but this is rarely necessary.

The central wedge technique is a major advance over trimming or techniques requiring long suture lines along the labial edges. Patient satisfaction with the central wedge and most other carefully performed techniques easily exceeds 90%.

Labia majora reduction

The youthful labia majora have fullness with no significant excess skin. Protuberance can either result from an overly fatty, full majora or a majora with excess skin or a combination of both *(Fig. 31.22)*. Excess hanging skin can be congenital, postpartum or caused by weight loss or aging. Excess protuberant fat can be congenital or due to weight gain. The women should also be evaluated for significant mons pubis lipodystrophy or descent. If the woman has a deficiency of fullness, fat can be injected into the majora. The majora are over-filled with fat with the knowledge that some of the fat will eventually resorb.

The patient for labia majora reduction is marked preoperatively under her supervision with a hand mirror while standing and lying in the lithotomy position.[7] Depending on the patient, she may need skin and/or fat excision. The skin excess is removed bilaterally from the medial portion of each labium as a crescent excision extending from the anterior to the posterior labial commissures *(Fig. 31.23A)*.[51] The medial incision line is usually placed just lateral to the medial hairline of each labium, but it can be placed slightly more medial if a reasonable skin match is present. Skin excision depends on each woman but it is usually mandatory to leave at least 2 cm of pigmented labium lateral to the lateral excision line,

which usually insures preservation of enough skin to prevent introital gaping while fully abducting the legs. If in doubt, be conservative. The amount of crescent excision varies depending on symmetry and whether skin excess extends posteriorly. The anterior and posterior incision lines should not meet in the midline but should extend laterally in a fusiform manner. Fat removal from the majora is usually not performed. If fat is to be removed, the location and amount is determined preoperatively. Over-resection can result in an aged appearance.

Surgery is performed in the lithotomy position. Local anesthetic with lidocaine and Marcaine with epinephrine are injected. After symmetry is checked, the skin excisions are made and checked again for symmetry. If fat is to be excised, superficial Colles fascia is opened, and fat is conservatively removed with electrocautery using meticulous hemostasis to prevent a hematoma. The superficial Colles is then closed with 4-0 or 5-0 Monocryl *(Fig. 31.23B)*. Drains are used only if a very large volume fat excision is performed. The subdermal tissue is closed with 5-0 Monocryl catching some superficial Colles fascia to eliminate dead space. The skin is closed with a running subcuticular closure of 5-0 Monocryl.

Complications are unusual. Hematomas are rare and asymmetry can occur. Contrast of the color and tissue texture between the medial and lateral skin is common, so the location of the incision lines are placed to minimize this contrast. Patients generally do not object if they are counseled preoperatively.

Care must be taken not to overly resect labia majora skin, which can cause a gaping introitus with resulting vaginal dryness, discomfort in clothes, and an aesthetic deformity. Extreme care must be taken in patients who have had or anticipate a medial thigh lift. Loosening of the thigh lift Colles fascia tacking sutures can cause posterior migration of the thigh skin, which can pull the majora laterally and open the introitus.

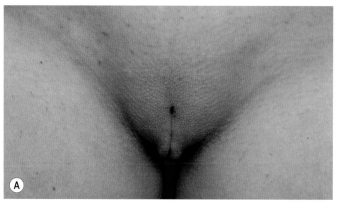

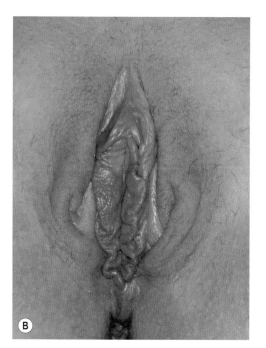

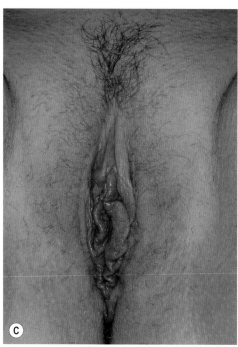

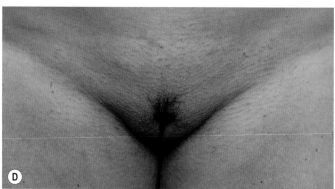

Fig. 31.22 A 40-year-old woman underwent labia majora reduction with skin removal only. **(A,B)** Preoperation. **(C,D)** Postoperation at 5 months.

Labia minora and majora reduction can be performed at the same time with the minora performed first.

Mons pubis descent and lipodystrophy

A protuberant mons pubis fat pad without skin excess can be reduced with liposuction through bilateral groin incisions. The patient with massive weight gain or large volume weight loss may have a very protuberant mons pubis fat pad with excess skin and ptosis *(Figs 31.24A,B 31.25A,B)*. Physicians have tried to correct this deformity through mons elevation in association with an abdominoplasty or by just lifting the pubic area, but these attempts often fail. The use of a midline incision to eliminate the excess pubic skin and fat results in an unsightly vertical or 'T' scar. A natural pubic lift with mons reduction can be achieved with a combination of horizontal skin excision; undermining of the mons fat pad; liposuction of the mons pubis, upper labia majora, and inguinal regions; and fat excision of the residual deforming fat pad. Stabilization of the fibrofatty tissue of the pubic skin

flap to the rectus fascia by tacking sutures prevents recurrent pubic descent.[51]

The patient should be evaluated in the standing position. The location of the anterior labial commissure should be at the pubic symphysis, so manual elevation of ptotic skin and panniculus helps determine the amount of skin excision required to achieve this lift. No more than several centimeters of skin excision are usually necessary, since the pubic skin will modesty contract after fat removal. Over-resection of skin can give an abnormally elevated appearance to the anterior commissure. The horizontal incision is placed just inferior to the panniculus fold or at a previous abdominoplasty scar. The incision line extends just long enough to remove the redundant skin without causing a 'dog-ear'. On rare occasions, the incision may extend to both anterior superior spines.

The surgery is performed supine if only a mons pubis lift is performed. If a simultaneous labia majora reduction is to be done, then the patient is placed in the lithotomy position with both areas prepped. The upper incision is made and carried down to the rectus fascia. The flap is dissected to the pubic symphysis and fat elevated off the rectus between the

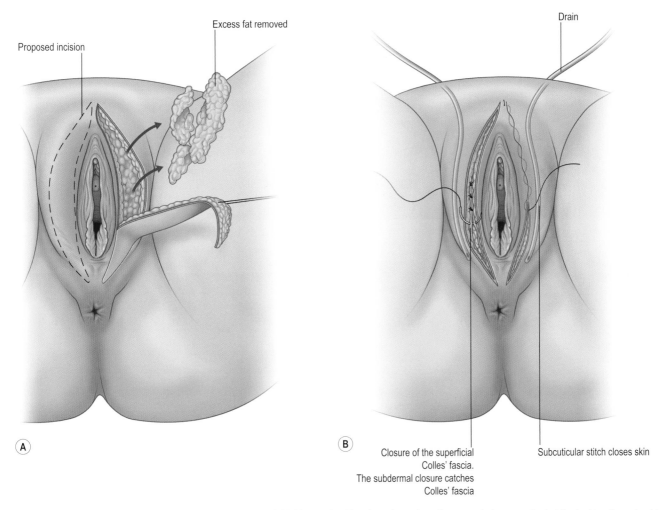

Fig. 31.23 (A) Illustration of the skin crescent removed from the medial labium majus. The shape depends on the amount of excess skin, but the incision lines should not meet in the midline. Fat is excised. **(B)** The closure is performed in layers. Colles fascia is closed if fat is removed. A drain is placed if a large amount of fat is removed. The subdermal layer is closed while also catching Colles fascia to reduce dead space. The skin is closed with a subcuticular suture.

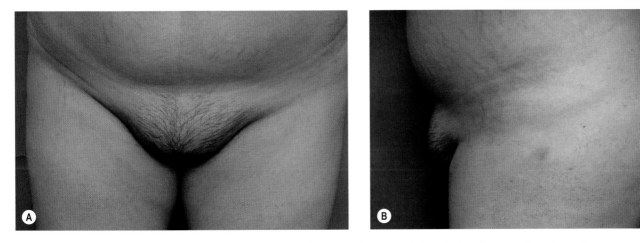

Fig. 31.24 A 19-year-old woman with a large pubic fat pad and excess skin. She underwent a pubic lift and pubic fat removal. **(A,B)** Preoperation.

external rings. The inferior incision of the crescent is made and removed along with some pubic fat *(Fig. 31.26A)*. The pubic flap, upper labia majora, and inguinal areas are infiltrated with the usual tumescence fluid. The pubic flap is liposuctioned and residual fat is sharply excised, leaving a flap thickness of 1–2 cm. The surrounding areas are suctioned to prevent a pubic concavity. The majora can be liposuctioned at this time or an open fat resection can be done from above followed by bilateral insertion of closed suction drains. Tacking sutures of No.1 polydioxanone (PDS) on a CTX needle are placed from the pubic flap to the rectus fascia and closure is done similarly to that of hidden penis (see above) *(Figs 31.14, 31.26B)*.

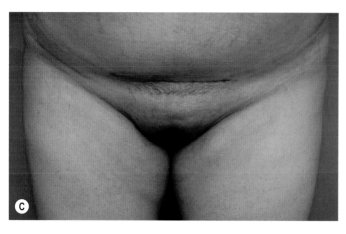

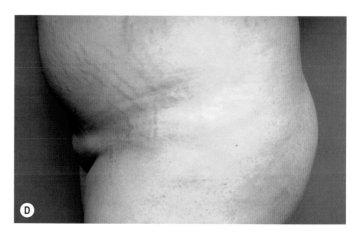

Fig. 31.24, cont'd   (C,D) Postoperation at 2 months.

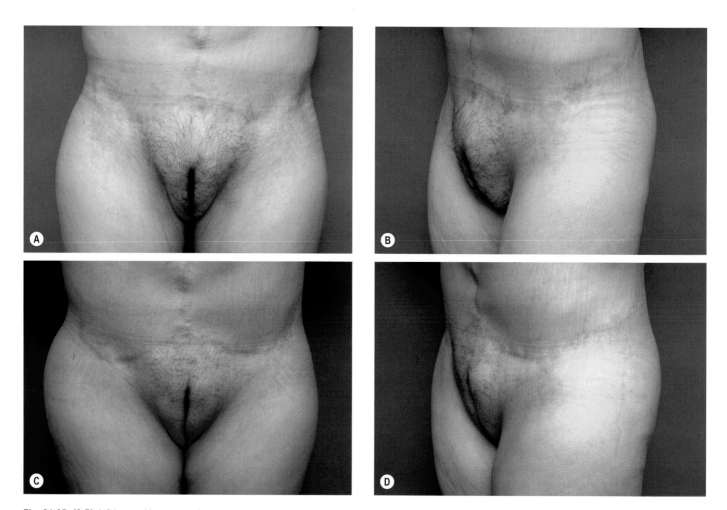

Fig. 31.25 (A,B) A 34-year-old woman underwent pubic lift and labia majora reduction. The patient has a protuberant mons fat pad and enlarged labia majora. **(C,D)** Ten months after pubic lift. She could benefit from more pubic liposuction but declined.

Labia majora skin and fat excision can be performed simultaneously with a pubic lift. However, this should probably not be done if the patient has had a previous medial thigh lift. The previous thigh lift incision added to the medial labia majora and pubic lift incisions can theoretically cause vascular insufficiency to the remaining majora and lateral perineal skin. In these cases, the patient can return later for the labia majora reduction.

The woman should be told that a pubic concavity or incomplete correction might result. Over-elevation of the pubis can cause an abnormally high location of the anterior labial commissure and a short escutcheon. The patients are generally very happy with the outcome as long as good judgment is used and the limitations and expected outcome are explained preoperatively *(Figs 31.24, 31.25).*

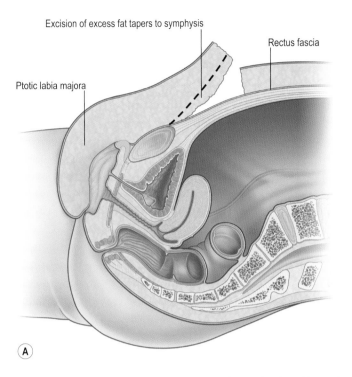

Excision of excess fat tapers to symphysis

Rectus fascia

Ptotic labia majora

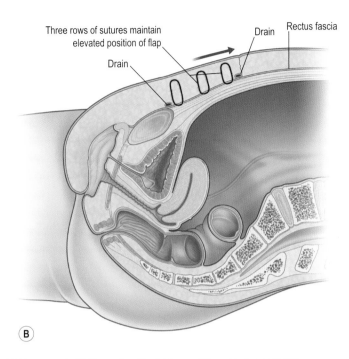

Three rows of sutures maintain elevated position of flap

Drain

Rectus fascia

Drain

Fig. 31.26 (A) A small amount of fat is excised and tapered to the pubic symphysis. Most fat is removed with liposuction. The thickness of the pubic flap cephalad matches the abdominal side. **(B)** Three rows of tacking sutures are usually placed with care to minimize dimpling. The pubic region along with the labia majora and anterior labial commissure are pulled up. A closed suction drain is placed from the pubic symphysis along the right side, then under the deep closure.

Conclusion

Over the past decades, innovative techniques have been developed to successfully treat a variety of genital aesthetic deformities. Often, these procedures enable men and women to overcome psychologically crippling feelings of low self-esteem. Unfortunately, misinformation is widespread. Male and female aesthetic genital techniques will continue to evolve, with more data and experience. Most patients achieve substantially improved self-esteem, justifying the continued exploration of new and better methods.

Access the complete references list online at **http://www.expertconsult.com**

9. Alter GJ. Penile enhancement surgery. *Tech in Urol.* 1998;4:70.

15. Alter GJ. Reconstruction of deformities resulting from penile enlargement surgery. *J Urol.* 1997;158:2153.
    This paper is the most comprehensive article describing reconstruction of deformities of penile enlargement surgeries.

16. Alter GJ. Reconstruction of the penis for complications of penile enlargement surgery. In: Graham Jr SD, Keane TE, eds. *Glenn's Urologic Surgery.* Philadelphia: Wolters Kluwer/Lippincott Williams &Wilkins; 2010:537–543.

39. Alter GJ, Ehrlich RM. A new technique for correction of the hidden penis in adults and children. *J Urol.* 1999;161:455.
    This article is the first paper to outline ventral tacking sutures but also discusses pubic tacking techniques. The discussion explains indications and pitfalls.

42. Pestana IA, Greenfield JM, Walsh M, et al. Management of the 'buried' penis in adulthood; an overview. *Plast Reconstr Surg.* 2009;124:1186–1195.

44. Alter GJ. Surgery to correct hidden penis: Surgical techniques. *J Sex Med.* 2006;3:939–942.

This graphic article updates and illustrates the technique for correction of hidden or buried penis in the usual pediatric and adult patient.

47. Hodgkinson DJ, Hait G. Aesthetic vaginal labioplasty. *Plast Reconstr Surg.* 1984;74:414.

48. Choi HY, Kim KT. A new method for aesthetic reduction to the labia minora (the deepithelialized reduction labiaplasty). *Plast Reconstr Surg.* 2000;105:419.

51. Alter GJ. Management of the mons pubis and labia majora in the massive weight loss patient. *Aesthet Surg J.* 2009;29:432–442.

This is the only article that explicitly explains and illustrates the techniques for correction of the protuberant or ptotic mons pubis and also the method for labia majora reduction.

61. Alter GJ. Aesthetic labia minora and clitoral hood reduction using extended central wedge resection. *Plast Reconstr Surg.* 2008;122:1780–1789.

This is the seminal article on the central wedge or 'V' excision labiaplasty with methods and results in 407 patients. It also discusses the advantages and disadvantages of alternative techniques.

Index

Note: **Boldface** roman numerals indicate volume. Page numbers followed by f refer to figures; page numbers followed by t refer to tables; page numbers followed by b refer to boxes.

*Note: **Boldface** roman numerals indicate volume. Page numbers followed by f refer to figures; page numbers followed by t refer to tables; page numbers followed by b refer to boxes.*

Note: **Boldface** *roman numerals indicate volume. Page numbers followed by f refer to figures; page numbers followed by t refer to tables; page numbers followed by b refer to boxes.*

Note: **Boldface** *roman numerals indicate volume. Page numbers followed by f refer to figures; page numbers followed by t refer to tables; page numbers followed by b refer to boxes.*

*Note: **Boldface** roman numerals indicate volume. Page numbers followed by f refer to figures; page numbers followed by t refer to tables; page numbers followed by b refer to boxes.*

Note: **Boldface** *roman numerals indicate volume. Page numbers followed by f refer to figures; page numbers followed by t refer to tables; page numbers followed by b refer to boxes.*

Note: **Boldface** roman numerals indicate volume. Page numbers followed by f refer to figures; page numbers followed by t refer to tables; page numbers followed by b refer to boxes.

Note: **Boldface** roman numerals indicate volume. Page numbers followed by f refer to figures; page numbers followed by t refer to tables; page numbers followed by b refer to boxes.

*Note: **Boldface** roman numerals indicate volume. Page numbers followed by f refer to figures; page numbers followed by t refer to tables; page numbers followed by b refer to boxes.*

Note: **Boldface** roman numerals indicate volume. Page numbers followed by f refer to figures; page numbers followed by t refer to tables; page numbers followed by b refer to boxes.

Note: **Boldface** *roman numerals indicate volume. Page numbers followed by f refer to figures; page numbers followed by t refer to tables; page numbers followed by b refer to boxes.*

Note: **Boldface** *roman numerals indicate volume. Page numbers followed by f refer to figures; page numbers followed by t refer to tables; page numbers followed by b refer to boxes.*

*Note: **Boldface** roman numerals indicate volume. Page numbers followed by f refer to figures; page numbers followed by t refer to tables; page numbers followed by b refer to boxes.*

Note: **Boldface** roman numerals indicate volume. Page numbers followed by f refer to figures; page numbers followed by t refer to tables; page numbers followed by b refer to boxes.

*Note: **Boldface** roman numerals indicate volume. Page numbers followed by f refer to figures; page numbers followed by t refer to tables; page numbers followed by b refer to boxes.*

*Note: **Boldface** roman numerals indicate volume. Page numbers followed by f refer to figures; page numbers followed by t refer to tables; page numbers followed by b refer to boxes.*

Note: **Boldface** roman numerals indicate volume. Page numbers followed by f refer to figures; page numbers followed by t refer to tables; page numbers followed by b refer to boxes.

*Note: **Boldface** roman numerals indicate volume. Page numbers followed by f refer to figures; page numbers followed by t refer to tables; page numbers followed by b refer to boxes.*

*Note: **Boldface** roman numerals indicate volume. Page numbers followed by f refer to figures; page numbers followed by t refer to tables; page numbers followed by b refer to boxes.*

Note: **Boldface** roman numerals indicate volume. Page numbers followed by f refer to figures; page numbers followed by t refer to tables; page numbers followed by b refer to boxes.

Note: **Boldface** roman numerals indicate volume. Page numbers followed by f refer to figures; page numbers followed by t refer to tables; page numbers followed by b refer to boxes.

Note: **Boldface** roman numerals indicate volume. Page numbers followed by f refer to figures; page numbers followed by t refer to tables; page numbers followed by b refer to boxes.

Note: **Boldface** *roman numerals indicate volume. Page numbers followed by f refer to figures; page numbers followed by t refer to tables; page numbers followed by b refer to boxes.*

*Note: **Boldface** roman numerals indicate volume. Page numbers followed by f refer to figures; page numbers followed by t refer to tables; page numbers followed by b refer to boxes.*

Note: **Boldface** roman numerals indicate volume. Page numbers followed by f refer to figures; page numbers followed by t refer to tables; page numbers followed by b refer to boxes.

Note: **Boldface** roman numerals indicate volume. Page numbers followed by f refer to figures; page numbers followed by t refer to tables; page numbers followed by b refer to boxes.

Note: **Boldface** *roman numerals indicate volume. Page numbers followed by f refer to figures; page numbers followed by t refer to tables; page numbers followed by b refer to boxes.*

Note: **Boldface** *roman numerals indicate volume. Page numbers followed by f refer to figures; page numbers followed by t refer to tables; page numbers followed by b refer to boxes.*

*Note: **Boldface** roman numerals indicate volume. Page numbers followed by f refer to figures; page numbers followed by t refer to tables; page numbers followed by b refer to boxes.*

*Note: **Boldface** roman numerals indicate volume. Page numbers followed by f refer to figures; page numbers followed by t refer to tables; page numbers followed by b refer to boxes.*

Note: **Boldface** *roman numerals indicate volume. Page numbers followed by f refer to figures; page numbers followed by t refer to tables; page numbers followed by b refer to boxes.*

Note: **Boldface** *roman numerals indicate volume. Page numbers followed by f refer to figures; page numbers followed by t refer to tables; page numbers followed by b refer to boxes.*

Note: **Boldface** roman numerals indicate volume. Page numbers followed by f refer to figures; page numbers followed by t refer to tables; page numbers followed by b refer to boxes.

Note: **Boldface** *roman numerals indicate volume. Page numbers followed by f refer to figures; page numbers followed by t refer to tables; page numbers followed by b refer to boxes.*

Note: **Boldface** roman numerals indicate volume. Page numbers followed by f refer to figures; page numbers followed by t refer to tables; page numbers followed by b refer to boxes.

*Note: **Boldface** roman numerals indicate volume. Page numbers followed by f refer to figures; page numbers followed by t refer to tables; page numbers followed by b refer to boxes.*

Note: **Boldface** roman numerals indicate volume. Page numbers followed by f refer to figures; page numbers followed by t refer to tables; page numbers followed by b refer to boxes.

Note: **Boldface** *roman numerals indicate volume. Page numbers followed by f refer to figures; page numbers followed by t refer to tables; page numbers followed by b refer to boxes.*

*Note: **Boldface** roman numerals indicate volume. Page numbers followed by f refer to figures; page numbers followed by t refer to tables; page numbers followed by b refer to boxes.*

*Note: **Boldface** roman numerals indicate volume. Page numbers followed by f refer to figures; page numbers followed by t refer to tables; page numbers followed by b refer to boxes.*

Note: **Boldface** roman numerals indicate volume. Page numbers followed by f refer to figures; page numbers followed by t refer to tables; page numbers followed by b refer to boxes.

Note: **Boldface** *roman numerals indicate volume. Page numbers followed by f refer to figures; page numbers followed by t refer to tables; page numbers followed by b refer to boxes.*

Note: **Boldface** roman numerals indicate volume. Page numbers followed by f refer to figures; page numbers followed by t refer to tables; page numbers followed by b refer to boxes.

Note: **Boldface** roman numerals indicate volume. Page numbers followed by f refer to figures; page numbers followed by t refer to tables; page numbers followed by b refer to boxes.

*Note: **Boldface** roman numerals indicate volume. Page numbers followed by f refer to figures; page numbers followed by t refer to tables; page numbers followed by b refer to boxes.*

*Note: **Boldface** roman numerals indicate volume. Page numbers followed by f refer to figures; page numbers followed by t refer to tables; page numbers followed by b refer to boxes.*

*Note: **Boldface** roman numerals indicate volume. Page numbers followed by f refer to figures; page numbers followed by t refer to tables; page numbers followed by b refer to boxes.*

Note: **Boldface** roman numerals indicate volume. Page numbers followed by f refer to figures; page numbers followed by t refer to tables; page numbers followed by b refer to boxes.

*Note: **Boldface** roman numerals indicate volume. Page numbers followed by f refer to figures; page numbers followed by t refer to tables; page numbers followed by b refer to boxes.*

Note: **Boldface** roman numerals indicate volume. Page numbers followed by f refer to figures; page numbers followed by t refer to tables; page numbers followed by b refer to boxes.

Note: **Boldface** roman numerals indicate volume. Page numbers followed by f refer to figures; page numbers followed by t refer to tables; page numbers followed by b refer to boxes.

Note: **Boldface** *roman numerals indicate volume. Page numbers followed by f refer to figures; page numbers followed by t refer to tables; page numbers followed by b refer to boxes.*

*Note: **Boldface** roman numerals indicate volume. Page numbers followed by f refer to figures; page numbers followed by t refer to tables; page numbers followed by b refer to boxes.*

Note: **Boldface** roman numerals indicate volume. Page numbers followed by f refer to figures; page numbers followed by t refer to tables; page numbers followed by b refer to boxes.

Note: **Boldface** *roman numerals indicate volume. Page numbers followed by f refer to figures; page numbers followed by t refer to tables; page numbers followed by b refer to boxes.*

*Note: **Boldface** roman numerals indicate volume. Page numbers followed by f refer to figures; page numbers followed by t refer to tables; page numbers followed by b refer to boxes.*

Note: **Boldface** roman numerals indicate volume. Page numbers followed by f refer to figures; page numbers followed by t refer to tables; page numbers followed by b refer to boxes.